PCF

MW00744869

PALLIATIVE CARE FORMULARY

Canadian edition

Published by palliativedrugs.com Ltd.

Palliativedrugs.com Ltd
Hayward House Study Centre
Nottingham University Hospitals NHS Trust, City Campus
Nottingham NG5 1PB
United Kingdom

www.palliativedrugs.com

A catalogue record for this book is available from the British Library.

ISBN 978 0-9552547-4-1

Typeset by Alden Prepress Services Private Limited, Chennai, India
Printed by Friesens Corporation, Canada

DISCLAIMER

Every effort has been made to ensure the accuracy of this text, and that the best information available has been used. However, palliativedrugs.com Ltd neither represents nor guarantees that the practices described herein will, if followed, ensure safe and effective patient care. The recommendations contained in this book reflect the editors' judgement regarding the state of general knowledge and practice in the field as of the date of publication. Recommendations such as those contained in this book can never be all-inclusive, and thus will not be appropriate in all and every circumstance. Those who use this book should make their own determinations regarding specific safe and appropriate patient-care practices, taking into account the personnel, equipment, and practices available at the hospital or other facility at which they are located. Neither palliativedrugs.com Ltd nor the editors can be held responsible for any liability incurred as a consequence of the use or application of any of the contents of this book. Mention of specific product brands does not imply endorsement. As always, clinicians are advised to make themselves familiar with manufacturer's recommendations and precautions before prescribing what is, for them, a new drug.

EDITORIAL STAFF

Editors-in-Chief
Robert Twycross DM Oxon, FRCP London
Emeritus Clinical Reader in Palliative Medicine, Oxford University

Andrew Wilcock DM Nottm, FRCP London
Macmillan Clinical Reader in Palliative Medicine and Medical Oncology,
Nottingham University
Consultant Physician, Hayward House, Nottingham University Hospitals NHS Trust,
City Campus

Canadian Editors
Mervyn Dean MB ChB, CCFP
Consultant Physician in Palliative Care, Western Memorial Regional Hospital,
Corner Brook, NL

Bruce Kennedy BSc(Pharm), MBA
Clinical Pharmacy Specialist Palliative Care, Palliative Care Program,
Fraser Health, Surrey BC

UK Senior Editor
Julie Mortimer BPharm, MRPharmS
Malcolm Mortimer Media, Nottingham

UK Editors
Sarah Charlesworth BPharm, MRPharmS
Specialist Pharmacist, Palliative Care Information and Website Management,
Hayward House, Nottingham University Hospitals NHS Trust, City Campus

Shelagh French BPharm, MRPharmS, MBA
Independent Pharmacist, Nottingham

Paul Howard BMedSci BM BS Nottm, MRCP London
Consultant in Palliative Medicine, Duchess of Kent House,
Berkshire West Primary Care Trust

CONTENTS

PREFACE

We are pleased to introduce the Canadian edition of the *Palliative Care Formulary* (*PCF*) to our readers. Although written primarily with cancer patients in mind, the contents of *PCF* are more widely applicable to any form of end-stage progressive disease. Thus, sections relating to general medical topics, e.g. COPD, diabetes mellitus, are important parts of the book.

PCF includes a number of clinical guidelines. To enhance their usefulness in practice, each set of guidelines is limited to no more than two pages, and references are not included. We welcome feedback on these. We also encourage donation of other people's guidelines for posting on our website (e-mail copies to hq@palliativedrugs.com).

The Canadian edition of *PCF* is one of a growing family of country-specific editions. The parent *PCF* is produced in the UK, and is mirrored in the United States of America by the *Hospice and Palliative Care Formulary* (*HPCF*USA). There are also German, Italian, and Polish editions. In each country, the target audience remains the same, namely doctors, pharmacists, and other health professionals caring for patients receiving palliative care.

As always, readers should satisfy themselves as to the appropriateness of any information in *PCF* before applying it in practice. *PCF* often refers to uses of drugs which are outside the scope of their marketing licence. The use of drugs in this way has implications for the prescriber, and is discussed on p.xvii.

Editors-in-chief
March 2010

ACKNOWLEDGEMENTS

The production of a book of this nature depends partly on the help and advice of numerous colleagues. In relation to this edition, we acknowledge with gratitude the support of close colleagues, particularly Patrick Costello, Vincent Crosby, Claudia Bausewein, Karen Power, Constanze Remi, and Claire Stark Toller, and those members of palliativedrugs.com who have provided feedback on one or more of the monographs or contributed to the Syringe Driver Survey Database. With this Canadian edition, we are particularly grateful to the following for their advice in relation to part or all of a chapter:
Off-label use of drugs, Judith Bedford-Jones, Alison Gardner, Special Access Programme Enquiries Department;
Chapter 1, Pippa Hawley (laxatives);
Chapter 2, Yahya Ismail (heart failure); Simon Noble (LMWH);
Chapter 3, David Baldwin, Ian Johnston, Alan Kaplan, Anne Tattersfield (asthma and COPD);
Chapter 4, Ken Gillman (serotonin toxicity);
Chapter 5, Jo Chambers, Felicity Murtagh (renal effects of opioids);
Chapter 6, Andrew Davies (candidosis); Vaughan Keeley (AIEs); Tony Tavenor (*Helicobacter pylori* gastritis);
Chapter 12, Joe Coffey, Russell Kilpatrick;
Chapter 14, Lynda Brook, Susie Lapwood (prescribing for children); Richard Burden, Judith Palmer (prescribing in renal impairment), Rachel Howard (drug concentration interpretation);
Chapter 16, Roger Knaggs, John MacKenzie, Jim Mason;
Chapter 17, Judith Bedford-Jones, Alison Gardner;
Chapter 22, Andrew Staniforth;
Chapter 23, Martin Lennard;
Appendix 2, Sue North, Cameron Zaremba;
Appendix 3, Avril Jackson, Willem Scholten, Gisela Wieser-Herbeck.
We are most grateful to Karen Isaac for her secretarial assistance, Pat Trozzo for assistance with Canadian drug names, spellings and medical terminology, and Cheryl Gnanapragasam for additional pharmaceutical support.

ABOUT www.palliativedrugs.com

We encourage readers of *PCF* to register with the website, and to participate fully in this online community. The website provides additional on-line information for thousands of members world-wide:

- **Bulletin Board** enables members to seek help and offer advice
- **Latest additions** informs members about the latest changes to the Formulary and website
- **News** informs members about drug-related news including changes in drug availability and/or formulation
- **Document library** (previously **Research, Audit and Guidelines (RAG) Panel**) acts as a repository for guidelines, policies and other documents donated by members
- **Syringe Driver Survey Database** has >1,000 observational compatibility reports of drug combinations given by continuous subcutaneous infusion (CSCI)
- **Online bookshop** enables members to purchase copies of *PCF* online.

We are constantly striving to improve the site and its resources, and welcome feedback via hq@palliativedrugs.com. We would also encourage readers to participate in the website satisfaction surveys.

We are committed to keeping www.palliativedrugs.com a free-access resource. Please help us do this by completing market research surveys when invited to do so from time to time.

MONOGRAPHS AVAILABLE ELSEWHERE

The contents of this edition of the *Palliative Care Formulary* are mostly restricted to drugs currently available and used in palliative care in Canada. Monographs of other drugs used in palliative care in the UK and/or the USA are listed below.

www.palliativedrugs.com and *Palliative Care Formulary* 3rd edition (PCF)
Chapter 1 GI: propantheline
Chapter 2 Cardiovascular: etamsylate
Chapter 3 Respiratory: chemical mucolytics (carbocisteine, mecysteine)
Chapter 4 CNS: duloxetine
        orphenadrine
Chapter 5 Analgesics: nefopam
        flurbiprofen
        dihydrocodeine
        diamorphine
        buprenorphine (with guidelines for TD patches)
Chapter 7 Endocrine: ibandronic acid
        demeclocycline
Chapter 9 Nutrition and blood: epoetin
Chapter 26 Oral nutritional supplements (products are UK-specific).

Hospice and Palliative Care Formulary 2nd edition (HPCFUSA)
Pharmaco-economics in the USA
Chapter 1 GI: propantheline
Chapter 4 CNS: chloral hydrate
        chlorpromazine
        quetiapine
        duloxetine
        orphenadrine
Chapter 5 Analgesics: choline magnesium salicylate
        hydrocodone
        buprenorphine
        nalbuphine
Chapter 7 Endocrine: demeclocycline
Chapter 9 Nutrition and blood: epoetin
Appendix: Medicare/Medicaid conditions of hospice participation.

GETTING THE MOST OUT OF PCF

The literature on the pharmacology of pain and other symptom management in end-stage disease is growing continually, and it is impossible for anyone to be totally familiar with it. This is where *PCF* comes into its own as a major accessible resource for prescribing clinicians involved in palliative care.

PCF is not an easy read, indeed it was never intended that it would be read from cover to cover. It is essentially a reference book – to study the monograph of an individual drug, or class of drugs, with fairly specific questions in mind.

Drugs marked with an asterisk (*) should generally be used only by, or after consultation with, a specialist palliative care service.

PCF is *not* a comprehensive manual of pain and symptom management. For more comprehensive advice, the reader should consult one or more of the numerous books about palliative care or symptom management which are currently available. In Canada, *Symptom Relief in Palliative Care* (Dean et al 2006, Radcliffe Publishing, Oxford; ISBN 1 85775 6290) should be seen as the companion book to *PCF*.

Readers should also be aware of *Opioids in Cancer Pain* 2nd edition (Davis *et al.* 2009, OUP). This provides a wealth of additional data, and will be particularly useful for clinical teachers and Palliative Medicine Fellows.

Drugs costs

The prices listed in *PCF* for both prescription drugs and OTC products are derived from current wholesale prices from a national wholesaler, and are given in Canadian dollars unless stated otherwise. A common mark-up percentage was applied to the wholesale pricing for OTC products to provide an anticipated market price. Variation will occur, dependent upon local retail market conditions. Further, drugs bought on contract are generally much cheaper.

Prices under $5 have been rounded up to a half dollar; prices over $5 are rounded up to a full dollar. Prices change over time, and the prices given in this edition of *PCF* should be regarded as a rough guide rather than currently exact.

Drugs included in provincial and territorial government prescription drug programmes vary across the country. It may be necessary to prescribe an alternative if a drug recommended in *PCF* is not available through the local programme. However, both third party insurers and government programmes may cover the cost of a particular drug if the prescribing physician requests a special authorization for a named patient.

Indications, cautions, and contra-indications

Indications, cautions, and contra-indications listed in Product Monographs sometimes vary between different manufacturers of the same drug, and between the same manufacturer in different countries. In an international work of this kind, there inevitably is a degree of 'syncretism' and selection. Thus, when using a drug for the first time, the prescriber should familiarize themselves with the indications, cautions, and contra-indications as listed in their national Product Monograph. Be aware that a caution in some countries becomes a contra-indication in another, and *vice versa*.

In this edition of *PCF*, we have *not* included universal contra-indications (e.g. history of hypersensitivity to the drug), and have generally *not* included a contra-indication from the Product Monograph if the use of the drug in the stated circumstance is accepted prescribing practice in palliative care.

As always, a cautious approach is generally necessary when prescribing for the frail elderly, patients with hepatic impairment, renal impairment, and respiratory insufficiency (see p.486).

The use of drugs for unlicensed (off-label) indications is common in palliative care (and indeed in all areas of medical practice) and is discussed on p.xvii.

Undesirable effects of drugs

In *PCF*, the term 'undesirable effect' is used rather than side effect or adverse effect. Wherever possible, undesirable effects are categorized as:

- very common (>10%)
- common (<10%, >1%)
- uncommon (<1%, >0.1%)
- rare (<0.1%, >0.01%)
- very rare (<0.01%).

PCF includes information on the very common and common undesirable effects. Selected other undesirable effects are also included, e.g. uncommon or rare ones which may have serious consequences. The manufacturer's Product Monograph should be consulted for a full list of undesirable effects.

Reliable knowledge and levels of evidence

Research is the pursuit of reliable knowledge. The gold standard for drug treatment is the randomized controlled trial (RCT) or, better, a systematic review of homogeneous RCTs.

Over the last 25 years, numerous systems have been published for categorizing levels of evidence and the strength of the derived recommendations. Box A reproduces the system used by the *British Medical Journal*. This checklist is based on material published by three main sources, namely the US Agency for Health Care Policy and Research, the NHS Management Executive, and the North of England Guidelines Group.[1,2,3]

Box A	A scheme for categorizing evidence and grading recommendations[4]		
Category	**Level of evidence**	**Grade**	**Strength of recommendations**
Ia	Evidence obtained from a meta-analysis of RCTs	A	Directly based on Category I evidence without extrapolation
Ib	Evidence from at least one RCT		
IIa	Evidence obtained from at least one well-designed controlled study without randomization	B	Directly based on Category II evidence or by extrapolation from Category I evidence
IIb	Evidence obtained from at least one other well-designed quasi-experimental study		
III	Evidence obtained from well-designed non-experimental descriptive studies, such as comparative studies, correlation studies and case studies	C	Directly based on Category III evidence or by extrapolation from Category I or II evidence
IV	Evidence obtained from expert committee reports or opinions and/or clinical experiences of respected authorities	D	Directly based on Category IV evidence or by extrapolation from Category I, II, or III evidence. This grading indicates that directly applicable clinical studies of good quality are absent or not readily available

However, it is important to recognize that the RCT is *not* the only source of reliable knowledge. Broadly speaking, sources of knowledge can be conveniently grouped under three headings:

- *instrumental*, includes RCT data and data from other high-quality studies
- *interactive*, refers to anecdotal data (shared clinical experience), including retrospective and prospective surveys
- *critical*, data unique to the individual in question (e.g. personal choice) and societal/cultural factors (e.g. financial and logistic considerations).[5]

Relying on one type of knowledge alone is *not* good practice. All three sources must be exploited in the process of therapeutic decision-making.

Pharmaceutical company information

Although the manufacturer's Product Monograph is an important source of information about a drug, it is important to remember that many published studies are sponsored by the drug company in question. This can lead to a conflict of interest between the desire for objective data and the need to make one's own drug as attractive as possible.[6] It is thus best to treat information from company representatives as inevitably biased. The information provided by *PCF* is commercially independent, and should serve as a counterbalance to manufacturer bias.

We should also remember that it is often safer to stick with the 'old favorite', and not seek to be among the first to prescribe a newly released product – which may simply be a 'me-too' drug rather than a true innovation.[6]

Generic drugs

It is the policy of *PCF* to use generic drug names, and to encourage generic prescribing. With occasional exceptions, e.g. SR diltiazem, nifedipine and theophylline, there is little reliable evidence that different preparations of the same drug are significantly different in terms of bio-availability and efficacy.[7] However, including the proprietary (brand) name of a strong opioid analgesic on the prescription and dispensing label, particularly in the case of oral morphine, is good practice because it helps to reduce the scope for confusion over the various available formulations.

Literature references

In choosing references, articles in hospice and palliative care journals have frequently been selected preferentially. Such journals are likely to be more readily available to our readers, and often contain detailed discussion.

It is not feasible to reference every statement in *PCF*. However, readers are invited to enter into constructive dialogue with the Editorial Team via the *Bulletin Board* on www.palliativedrugs.com.

Electronic sources of information

As far as possible, Canadian sources have been given prominence in *PCF*. However, some UK sources have inevitably been included. To facilitate access to the relevant documents, website details are given below.

Canadian free access resources

Canadian Agency for Drugs and Technology in Health (CADTH, formerly CCOHTA) Database: available from www.cadth.ca/index.php/en/hta/reports-publications/search
Gives access to free, full-text systematic reviews, health technology assessments (HTAs) and economic assessments from a Canadian perspective. A free email alert service is available.

Drug Product Database, Health Canada: available from
www.hc-sc.gc.ca/dhp-mps/prodpharma/databasdon/index-eng.php
Contains product-specific information on human pharmaceutical and biological drugs, veterinary drugs and disinfectant products approved for use in Canada. Also allows access to some product monographs.

Canadian resources, subscription required
Electronic Compendium of Pharmaceuticals and Specialties (e-CPS): available from http://www.pharmacists.ca/content/products/ecps_english.cfm

UK free access resources
Bandolier (evidence-based articles for health professionals): available from www.medicine.ox.ac.uk/bandolier

Current Problems in Pharmacovigilance: available via MHRA website at www.mhra.gov.uk/home/idcplg?IdcService=SS_GET_PAGE&nodeId=368

Drug Safety Update: available via MHRA website at www.mhra.gov.uk/Publications/Safetyguidance/DrugSafetyUpdate/index.htm

MeReC Bulletin: available via National Prescribing Centre website at www.npc.co.uk/ebt/merec.htm

National Institute for Health and Clinical Excellence (NICE) guidelines: available from www.nice.org.uk/
Evidence-based cost-effectiveness guidelines for health professionals, with simplified versions for the general public.

UK manufacturers' Summary of Product Characteristics (SPCs), broadly equivalent to the Canadian Product Monographs, available from www.medicines.org.uk

UK and international resources, subscription required
British National Formulary: two editions/year, March and September. Latest edition available from www.bnf.org

The Cochrane Library: available at http://www3.interscience.wiley.com/cgi-bin/mrwhome/106568753/AccessCochraneLibrary.html #canada. Collection of evidence-based systematic reviews. Access temporarily free in Canada

Pharmaceutical Journal (official weekly journal of the Royal Pharmaceutical Society of Great Britain): available from www.pjonline.com

---

1 Agency for Health Care Policy and Research (1992) Acute pain management, operative or medical procedures and trauma 92-0032. In: *Clin Pract Guidel Quick Ref Guide Clin.* AHCPR Publications, Rockville, Maryland, USA, pp. 1–22.
2 DoH (1996) *Clinical Guidelines: Using Clinical Guidelines to Improve Patient Care Within the NHS.* Department of Health: NHS Executive, Leeds.
3 Eccles M et al. (1996) North of England evidence based guidelines development project: methods of guideline development. *British Medical Journal.* 312: 760–762.
4 BMJ Publishing Group (2009) Resources for authors. Checklists and forms: clinical management guidelines. Available from: http://resources.bmj.com/bmj/authors/checklists-forms/clinical-management-guidelines
5 Aoun SM and Kristjanson LJ (2005) Challenging the framework for evidence in palliative care research. *Palliative Medicine.* 19: 461–465.
6 Angell M (2004) *The Truth About the Drug Companies: how they deceive us and what to do about it.* Random House, New York.
7 National Prescribing Centre (2000) Modified-release preparations. *MeReC Bulletin.* 11: 13–16.

USING LICENSED DRUGS FOR OFF-LABEL PURPOSES

In palliative care, up to 1/4 of all prescriptions are for licensed drugs given for an off-label indication or in doses, formulations or a route not covered by the licence,[1,2] and this is reflected in the recommendations contained in *PCF*. The symbol † is used to draw attention to such use. However, it is impossible to highlight every example of off-label use. Often it is simply a matter of the route or dose being different from those in the manufacturer's Product Monograph. Thus, it is important to recognize that the approval and licensing process for drugs regulates the marketing activities of pharmaceutical companies and not a practitioner's prescribing practice. Off-label use of drugs is often appropriate and may represent standard practice.[3]

The approval and licensing process

All new therapeutic products intended for sale in Canada must undergo an extensive clinical trial, approval and licensing process.[4] New drugs are evaluated by the Health Products and Food Branch (HPFB) of Health Canada. After receiving satisfactory evidence of quality, safety and efficacy via the pharmaceutical company's New Drug Submission, the HPFB issues a marketing authorization (licence), known as a Notice of Compliance (NOC), and a Drug Identification Number (DIN). This allows the pharmaceutical company to market and supply the product in Canada for specific indications and at specified doses in a defined patient population. These are all listed in its Product Monograph and other labelling information. Restrictions are imposed by the HPFB if evidence of safety and efficacy is unavailable in particular patient groups, e.g. children. Once a NOC is received, the manufacturer can apply for listing on provincial and territorial drug formularies, which means that the drug will be covered for reimbursement, either in full or in part, by the healthcare plan which manages that formulary.[4,5] Once a product is marketed, further clinical trials and experience may reveal other indications. For these to become licensed, additional evidence needs to be submitted via a Supplemental New Drug Submission.[4,5] The considerable expense of this, perhaps coupled with a small market for the new indication, often means that a revised application is not made.

Prescribing outside the licence

In Canada, there is no law or formal advice from professional bodies governing the off-label prescribing of licensed drugs. However, it is accepted that a physician may legally prescribe and use, or advise using:
- unlicensed medicines which are:
  - ▷ specially prepared (compounded) products *or*
  - ▷ imported or supplied for a named patient through Health Canada's Special Access Programme (SAP)
- licensed drugs for indications or in doses, formulations or routes outside the licensed recommendations, i.e. off-label
- drugs for conditions for which there are no other treatments (even in the absence of strong evidence)
- for individuals not covered by the licence, e.g. children
- unlicensed drugs in clinical trials, providing the trial has been approved by the HPFB.[6]

In addition, a physician may override the warnings and precautions given in the licence. The responsibility for the consequences of these actions lies with the prescriber.[3,6] Further, although drugs prescribed outside the licence can be dispensed by pharmacists and administered by nurses or midwives, it is good professional practice for them to inform themselves about the use of the drug in the proposed off-label indication, and of any potential safety issues, before doing so.[7]

In some provinces and territories, some nurses, midwives and pharmacists have limited prescribing powers. Depending on the province/territory, they may either act as independent prescribers or prescribe under the direction of a physician. Providing they meet the SAP's required criteria for practitioner status, they are eligible to request unlicensed drugs under the SAP (see p.xx).

Prescription of a drug (whether licensed use/route or not) requires the prescriber, in the light of published evidence, to balance both the potential good and the potential harm which might ensue. Prescribers and other health professionals have a duty to act with reasonable care and skill in a manner consistent with the practice of professional colleagues of similar standing. Thus, when prescribing, administering or dispensing drugs outside the terms of the licence, they must:
• inform themselves fully about the published evidence supporting the intended off-label use[7–9]
• assure themselves of the quality of the particular product.

It is possible to draw a hierarchy of degrees of reasonableness relating to the use of unlicensed drugs (Figure 1).[10] The more dangerous the medicine and the more flimsy the evidence the more difficult it is to justify its prescription. Further, it is good practice to report any undesirable effects of off-label drugs to the Canadian MedEffect programme (www.hc-sc.gc.ca/dhp-mps/medeff/index-eng.php).[3]

It has also been recommended that when prescribing a drug outside its licence, a prescriber should:
• record in the patient's records the reasons for the decision to prescribe outside the licensed indications
• ensure that the patient (and family as appropriate) is as fully informed as possible about the expected benefits and potential risks (undesirable effects, drug interactions, etc.) of the treatment, ideally in sufficient detail to allow them to give informed consent; the Patient Package Insert obviously does not contain information about unlicensed indications
• inform other professionals, e.g. pharmacist, nurses, family practitioner, involved in the care of the patient to avoid misunderstandings and to ensure appropriate monitoring.[3,6,7,10,11]

However, in palliative care, the use of drugs for off-label indications or by unapproved routes is so widespread that such an approach is impractical. Indeed, a survey in the UK showed that <5% of palliative medicine specialists *always* obtain verbal or written consent, document in the notes or inform other professionals when using licensed drugs for unlicensed purposes/routes.[12] Concern was expressed that not only would it be impractical to do so, but it would be burdensome for the patient, increase anxiety and might result in refusal of beneficial treatment. Some 1/2 to 2/3 indicated that they would *sometimes* obtain verbal consent (53%), document in the notes (41%) and inform other professionals (68%) when using treatments which are not widely used within the specialty, e.g. ketamine, octreotide, ketorolac.

This is a grey area and each clinician must decide how explicit to be; an appropriate level of counselling and a sensitive approach is essential. Some institutions have policies in place and have produced information cards or leaflets for patients and caregivers (Box B). In the UK, a position statement has also been produced by the Association for Palliative Medicine and the Pain Society (Box C).

Status	*The drug*	*Published data*	*The illness*
Licensed for the intended indication	Well known; generally safe	Recommended in standard textbooks	Life-threatening
Licensed for another indication; other related products licensed for the intended indication	Well known; some clear undesirable effects	Well-documented studies in peer-reviewed journals	Severe
	Well known; has serious undesirable effects *or* Little studied; no clear undesirable effects	Only poor quality studies reported	
A licensed product; not licensed for the intended indication, nor are similar medicines	Little studied; has serious undesirable effects	Only anecdotal evidence published	Mild
Drug/product not licensed at all	Not studied	No published data available	Trivial

Most reasonable → Least reasonable

Figure 1 Factors influencing the reasonableness of prescribing decisions.[10]

Box B Example of a patient information leaflet about the use of medicines outside their licence

Use of Medicines in Unapproved Ways

This leaflet contains important information about your medicines, please read it carefully.

Before a medicine can be marketed, approval must be obtained from Health Canada by the manufacturer. Health Canada approves the ways in which the medicine can be marketed: for which conditions, in what doses, and which age groups. Manufacturers are obliged to include with all their medicines a Patient Package Insert which, by law, must be limited to the details of the Health Canada approval.

In practice, medicines are often prescribed in ways which are not approved by Health Canada. However, this will only be done when there is research and experience to support such 'off-label' use.

You will know if one of your medicines is being used in an unapproved way when you read the Patient Package Insert supplied by the manufacturer. You will notice that the information in it is not fully relevant to how you are taking the medicine.

Medicines used commonly 'off-label' include some antidepressants and anti-epileptics (anti-seizure drugs) which are used to relieve some types of pain. Also, because it is generally more comfortable and convenient, some medicines are often injected subcutaneously (under the skin) instead of being injected into a vein or muscle.

If you have any questions or concerns about your medicines, particularly in relation to 'off-label' use, your doctor or pharmacist will be happy to address them.

The Special Access Programme (SAP)

Practitioners who are authorized to treat patients with drugs listed in Schedule F of the Food and Drug Regulations can gain access to limited supplies of drugs which are not licensed for sale in Canada through the SAP. In some provinces and territories, health professionals other than physicians, e.g. nurses, midwives and pharmacists, are allowed to prescribe and may thus qualify as practitioners for purposes of requesting SAP drugs. Individuals should consult their provincial or territorial professional regulatory body to ascertain their Schedule F prescriber status, and submit any relevant documentation to the SAP with their request for consideration as a practitioner.[13] Lists of professional bodies are available from: www.cna-aiic.ca/CNA/nursing/regulation/ regbodies/default_e.aspx (nurses), http://cmrc-ccosf.ca/node/2 (midwives) and www.napra.org/ pages/Licensing_Registration/Authorities.aspx?id=1971 (pharmacists).

SAP drugs can be requested for patients with serious or life-threatening conditions when conventional treatments have failed, are unavailable or are unsuitable. Access is considered on a case-by-case basis, taking into account the nature of the emergency and/or any compassionate grounds.[4,14]

Full guidance on applying for the SAP and an application form can be downloaded from: www.hc-sc.gc.ca/dhp-mps/acces/index-eng.php

1 Atkinson C and Kirkham S (1999) Unlicensed uses for medication in a palliative care unit. *Palliative Medicine.* **13**: 145–152.
2 Todd J and Davies A (1999) Use of unlicensed medication in palliative medicine. *Palliative Medicine.* **13**: 466.
3 de Paulsen N (2005) The regulatory gap: off-label drug use in Canada. *University of Toronto Faculty of Law Review.* **63**: 183–211.
4 Health Products and Food Branch (2006) Access to Therapeutic Products. The Regulatory Process in Canada. Health Canada, Ottawa. Available from: www.hc-sc.gc.ca/ahc-asc/alt_formats/hpfb-dgpsa/pdf/pubs/access-therapeutic_acces-therapeutique-eng.pdf
5 Health Canada (2007) Drug licensing process. Introduction to the current system. Available from: www.hc-sc.gc.ca/dhp-mps/ homologation-licensing/system/intro-eng.php
6 Canadian Medical Association legal department (2009) Personal communication.
7 Friesen M (2008) Off-label prescribing. Veering off the beaten path. *Pharmacy Practice.* **February**: 26–29.
8 Palacioz K (2003) Off-label uses of Neurontin (gabapentin). Detail document 190812. *Pharmacist'sLetter/Prescriber's Letter.* **19 (August)**: 1–4.
9 Gazarian M et al. (2006) Off-label use of medicines: consensus recommendations for evaluating appropriateness. *Medical Journal of Australia.* **185**: 544–548.

Box C The recommendations of the Association for Palliative Medicine and the Pain Society (UK)

The use of drugs beyond licence in palliative care and pain management

1 This statement should be seen as reflecting the views of a responsible body of opinion within the clinical specialties of palliative medicine and pain management.

2 The use of drugs beyond licence should be seen as a legitimate aspect of clinical practice.

3 The use of drugs beyond licence in palliative care and pain management practice is currently both necessary and common.

4 Choice of treatment requires partnership between patients and health professionals, and informed consent should be obtained, whenever possible, before prescribing any drug. Patients should be informed of any identifiable risks and details of any information given should be recorded. It is often unnecessary to take additional steps when recommending drugs beyond licence.

5 Patients, carers, and health professionals need accurate, clear and specific information that meets their needs. The Association for Palliative Medicine and the Pain Society should work with pharmaceutical companies to design accurate information for patients and their carers about the use of drugs beyond licence.

6 Health professionals involved in prescribing, dispensing, and administering drugs beyond licence should select those drugs that offer the best balance of benefit against harm for any given patient.

7 Health professionals should inform, change, and monitor their practice with regard to drugs beyond licence in the light of evidence from audit and published research.

8 The Department of Health should work with health professionals and the pharmaceutical industry to enable and encourage the extension of product licences where there is evidence of benefit in circumstances of defined clinical need.

9 Organizations providing palliative care and pain management services should support therapeutic practices that are underpinned by evidence and advocated by a responsible body of professional opinion.

10 There is urgent need for the Department of Health to assist healthcare professionals to formulate national frameworks, guidelines and standards for the use of drugs beyond licence. The Pain Society and the Association for Palliative Medicine should work with the Department of Health, NHS Trusts, voluntary organizations and the pharmaceutical industry to design accurate information for staff, patients and their carers in clinical areas where drugs are used beyond their licence (off-label). Practical support is necessary to facilitate and expedite surveillance and audit which are essential to develop this initiative.

10 Ferner R (1996) Prescribing licensed medicines for unlicensed indications. *Prescribers' Journal.* **36**: 73–79.

11 Cohen P (1997) Off-label use of prescription drugs: legal, clinical and policy considerations. *European Journal of Anaesthesiology.* **14**: 231–235.

12 Pavis H and Wilcock A (2001) Prescribing of drugs for use outside their licence in palliative care: survey of specialists in the United Kingdom. *British Medical Journal.* **323**: 484–485.

13 Health Canada (2009) Personal communication SAP drugs department.

14 Health Canada (2008) Release of final Special Access Programme (SAP) for drugs guidance document. Available from: www.hc-sc.gc.ca/dhp-mps/alt_formats/hpfb-dgpsa/pdf/acces/sapg3_pasg3-eng.pdf

DRUG NAMES

Canadian approved names are used throughout *PCF*. These are generally the same as United States Adopted Names (USANs). Proprietary (brand) names are generally not included. In contrast, all drugs marketed within the European Union are known by their recommended International Non-proprietary Names (rINNs). Differences between Canadian approved names, USANs and rINNs are listed in Table 1.

Formerly, drugs in the UK were known by their British Approved Names (BANs). Where a BAN differs from the rINN, the BAN has also been included in Table 1 to aid understanding of the older UK literature. As a further aid to understanding UK literature, the UK conventional names for combination products, such as codeine and acetaminophen (paracetamol) or diphenoxylate and atropine, are shown in Table 2, e.g. co-codamol or co-phenotrope.

Table 1 Drug names relevant to palliative care for which the Canadian approved name, USAN, rINN and/or BAN differ

Canadian approved name	USAN	rINN	Former BAN
Acetaminophen	Acetaminophen	Paracetamol	–
Aluminum	Aluminum	Aluminium	–
Amphetamine	Amphetamine	Amfetamine	Amphetamine
Beclomethasone	Beclomethasone	Beclometasone	Beclomethasone
Benzathine penicillin	Benzathine penicillin	Benzathine benzylpenicillin	Benzathine penicillin
Benztropine	Benztropine	Benzatropine	Benztropine
Calcitonin	Calcitonin	Calcitonin (salmon)	Salcatonin
Carboxymethylcellulose	Carboxymethylcellulose	Carmellose	–
Cephalexin (etc.)	Cephalexin (etc.)	Cefalexin (etc.)	Cephalexin (etc.)
Chlorpheniramine	Chlorpheniramine	Chlorphenamine	Chlorpheniramine
Cholestyramine	Cholestyramine	Colestyramine	Cholestyramine
Cyclosporine	Cyclosporine	Ciclosporin	Cyclosporin
Dextroamphetamine	Dextroamphetamine	Dexamfetamine	Dexamphetamine
Dicyclomine	Dicyclomine	Dicycloverine	Dicyclomine
Diethylstilbestrol	Diethylstilbestrol	Diethylstilbestrol	Stilboestrol
Dimethicone	Dimethicone	Dimeticone	Dimethicone
Epinephrine	Epinephrine	Epinephrine	Adrenaline
Estradiol	Estradiol	Estradiol	Oestradiol
Furosemide	Furosemide	Furosemide	Frusemide
Glyburide	Glyburide	Glibenclamide	–
Glycerin	Glycerin	Glycerol	Glycerine
Glycopyrrolate	Glycopyrrolate	Glycopyrronium	–
Guaifenesin	Guaifenesin	Guaifenesin	Guaiphenesin
Hyoscine (used in relation to the *butylbromide* salt; scopolamine is used for the *hydrobromide* salt)	Scopolamine	Hyoscine	–
Indomethacin	Indomethacin	Indometacin	Indomethacin
Isoproterenol	Isoproterenol	Isoprenaline	–
Levothyroxine	Levothyroxine	Levothyroxine	Thyroxine
Lidocaine	Lidocaine	Lidocaine	Lignocaine
Meclizine	Meclizine	Meclozine	–

continued

Table I Continued

Canadian approved name	USAN	rINN	Former BAN
Meperidine	Meperidine	Pethidine	–
Methenamine	Methenamine	Methenamine	Hexamine
Methotrimeprazine	Methotrimeprazine	Levomepromazine	Methotrimeprazine
Mineral oil	Mineral oil	Liquid paraffin	–
Mitoxantrone	Mitoxantrone	Mitoxantrone	Mitozantrone
Nitroglycerin	Nitroglycerin	Glyceryl trinitrate	–
Oxethazine	Oxethazine	Oxetacaine	Oxethazine
Penicillin G	Penicillin G	Benzylpenicillin	–
Penicillin V	Penicillin V	Phenoxymethylpenicillin	–
Phenobarbital	Phenobarbital	Phenobarbital	Phenobarbitone
Phytonadione	Phytonadione	Phytomenadione	–
Procaine penicillin	Procaine penicillin	Procaine benzylpenicillin	Procaine penicillin
Propoxyphene	Propoxyphene	Dextropropoxyphene	–
Psyllium	Psyllium	–	Ispaghula
Rifampin	Rifampin	Rifampicin	–
Salbutamol	Albuterol	Salbutamol	–
Scopolamine (used in relation to the *hydrobromide* salt; hyoscine is used for the *butylbromide* salt)	Scopolamine	Hyoscine	–
Simethicone[a]	Simethicone	Simeticone	Simethicone
Sodium cromoglycate	Cromolyn sodium	Sodium cromoglicate	Sodium cromoglycate
Sulfasalazine	Sulfasalazine	Sulfasalazine	Sulphasalazine
Sulfonamides	Sulfonamides	Sulfonamides	Sulphonamides
Tetracaine	Tetracaine	Tetracaine	Amethocaine
Trihexyphenidyl	Trihexyphenidyl	Trihexyphenidyl	Benzhexol
Trimeprazine	Trimeprazine	Alimemazine	Trimeprazine
Vitamin A	Vitamin A	Retinol	Vitamin A

a. silica-activated dimethicone; known in some countries as (di)methylpolysiloxane.

Table 2 UK names for combination products

Contents	UK name
Acetaminophen-codeine phosphate	Co-codamol
Acetaminophen-dihydrocodeine[a]	Co-dydramol
Acetaminophen-propoxyphene[a]	Co-proxamol
Aluminum hydroxide-magnesium hydroxide	Co-magaldrox
Amoxicillin-clavulanate	Co-amoxiclav
Atropine-diphenoxylate	Co-phenotrope
Sulfamethoxazole-trimethoprim[b]	Co-trimoxazole

a. not available in Canada
b. also known as cotrimoxazole in Canada.

LIST OF ABBREVIATIONS

Drug administration

In 2005, the US Joint Commission on Accreditation of Healthcare Organizations (JCAHO) published National Patient Safety Goals. These include a series of recommendations about ways in which confusion (and thus errors) can be reduced by avoiding the use of certain abbreviations on prescriptions. The full set of recommendations is available at www.jointcommission.org/PatientSafety/DoNotUseList/. These recommendations have been adopted by the Institute for Safe Medication Practices Canada (ISMP Canada).[1] Although some traditional abbreviations remain acceptable (e.g. Table 3), other commonly used abbreviations are not. Thus, ISMP now recommends that the following are written in full:

- at bedtime
- once daily
- each morning
- every other day.

These four recommendations have also been adopted in *PCF*. However, several other abbreviations which are now unacceptable on prescriptions are still used in *PCF*.

Although the following conventions have *not* been adopted in *PCF*, readers should be aware of the following recommendations for handwritten and printed prescriptions, and other printed medical matter, e.g. packaging, patient records:
- include a space between the drug dose and the unit of measure, e.g. 25 mg, not 25mg
- write 'per' instead of an oblique (mistaken for a figure 1), e.g. 200 mg per day, not 200mg/day
- use 'subcut' or 'subcutaneous' instead of SC (mistaken for SL)
- write 'less than' or 'greater than' instead of < and > (mistaken for a letter L or figure 7; or written the wrong way round and thus signifying the opposite of the intended meaning).

Table 3 Abbreviations used in *PCF* for the times of drug administration

Times	Canada and USA	Latin	UK	Latin
Twice daily	b.i.d.	*bis in die*	b.d.	*bis die*
Three times daily	t.i.d.	*ter in die*	t.d.s.	*ter die sumendus*
Four times daily	q.i.d.	*quarta in die*	q.d.s.	*quarta die sumendus*
Every 4 hours etc.	q4h	*quaque quarta hora*	q4h	*quaque quarta hora*
Rescue medication (as needed/required)	p.r.n.	*pro re nata*	p.r.n.	*pro re nata*
Give immediately	stat		stat	

a.c.	ante cibum (before food)
amp	ampoule containing a single dose (compare with vial)
CIVI	continuous intravenous infusion
CR	controlled-release (used for proprietary SR products only when it is part of the brand name); see SR
CSCI	continuous subcutaneous infusion
EC	enteric-coated
ED	epidural
ER	extended-release (used for proprietary SR products only when it is part of the brand name); see SR

IM	intramuscular
IT	intrathecal
IV	intravenous
IVI	intravenous infusion
OTC	over the counter (i.e. can be obtained without a prescription)
p.c.	post cibum (after food)
PO	per os, by mouth
POM	prescription only medicine
PR	per rectum
PV	per vaginum
SC	subcutaneous
SL	sublingual
SR	sustained-release (preferred generic term for all slow-release products)
TD	transdermal
vial	sterile container with a rubber bung containing either a single or multiple doses (compare with amp)
WFI	water for injections

General

*	specialist use only
†	off-label use
BNF	British National Formulary
BP	British Pharmacopoeia
CADTH	Canadian Agency for Drugs and Technologies in Health
CDSA	Controlled Drugs and Substances Act
CHM	Commission on Human Medicines (UK)
CPS	Compendium of Pharmaceuticals and Specialities
CSM	Committee on Safety of Medicines (UK; now part of CHM)
EMEA	European Medicines Agency
EORTC	European Organisation for Research and Treatment of Cancer
FDA	Food and Drug Administration (USA)
HPFB	Health Products and Food Branch (of Health Canada)
IASP	International Association for the Study of Pain
MCA	Medicines Control Agency (UK; now MHRA)
MHRA	Medicines and Healthcare products Regulatory Agency (UK; formerly MCA)
NYHA	New York Heart Association
NICE	National Institute for Health and Clinical Excellence (UK)
NOC	Notice of Compliance
PCS	Palliative care service
PEG	percutaneous endoscopic gastrostomy
rINN	recommended International Non-proprietary Name
SAP	Special Access Programme
SPC	Summary of Product Characteristics (UK; broadly equivalent to the Canadian Product Monograph)
UK	United Kingdom
USA	United States of America
USP	United States Pharmacopoeia
VAS	visual analogue scale, 0–100mm
WHO	World Health Organization

Medical

ACD	anemia of chronic disease
ACE	angiotensin-converting enzyme
ADH	antidiuretic hormone (vasopressin)
AUC	area under the plasma concentration–time curve
β_2	beta 2 adrenergic (receptor)
BUN	blood urea nitrogen

CHF	congestive heart failure
CNS	central nervous system
COX	cyclo-oxygenase; alternative, prostaglandin synthase
COPD	chronic obstructive pulmonary disease
CRP	C-reactive protein
CSF	cerebrospinal fluid
CT	computed tomography
δ	delta-opioid (receptor)
D_2	dopamine type 2 (receptor)
DIC	disseminated intravascular coagulation
DVT	deep vein thrombosis
ECG	electrocardiogram (also known as EKG)
ECT	electroconvulsive therapy
FEV_1	forced expiratory volume in 1 second
FRC	functional residual capacity
FSH	follicle-stimulating hormone
FVC	forced vital capacity of lungs
GABA	gamma-aminobutyric acid
GI	gastro-intestinal
Hgb	hemoglobin
HIV	human immunodeficiency virus
H_1, H_2	histamine type 1, type 2 (receptor)
Ig	immunoglobulin
INR	international normalized ratio
κ	kappa-opioid (receptor)
LABA	long-acting β_2-adrenergic receptor agonist
LFTs	liver function tests
LH	luteinizing hormone
LMWH	low molecular weight heparin
MAOI	mono-amine oxidase inhibitor
MARI	mono-amine re-uptake inhibitor
MRI	magnetic resonance imaging
MSU	mid-stream specimen of urine
μ	mu-opioid (receptor)
NaSSA	noradrenergic and specific serotoninergic antidepressant
NDRI	norepinephrine (noradrenaline) and dopamine re-uptake inhibitor
NG	nasogastric
NJ	nasojejunal
NMDA	N-methyl D-aspartate
NNH	number needed to harm, i.e. the number of patients needed to be treated in order to harm one patient sufficiently to cause withdrawal from a drug trial
NNT	number needed to treat, i.e. the number of patients needed to be treated in order to achieve 50% improvement in one patient compared with placebo
NRI	norepinephrine (noradrenaline) re-uptake inhibitor
NSAID	non-steroidal anti-inflammatory drug
$PaCO_2$	arterial partial pressure of carbon dioxide
PaO_2	arterial partial pressure of oxygen
PCA	patient-controlled analgesia
PE	pulmonary embolus/embolism
PEF	peak expiratory flow
PG	prostaglandin
PPI	proton pump inhibitor
PUB	gastro-intestinal perforation, ulceration or bleeding (in relation to serious GI events caused by NSAIDs)
RCT	randomized controlled trial
RIMA	reversible inhibitor of mono-amine oxidase type A
RTI	respiratory tract infection
SNRI	serotonin and norepinephrine (noradrenaline) re-uptake inhibitor
SSRI	selective serotonin re-uptake inhibitor

TCA	tricyclic antidepressant
TIBC	total iron-binding capacity; alternative, plasma transferrin concentration
Tl_{CO}	transfer factor of the lung for carbon monoxide
UTI	urinary tract infection
VEGF	vascular endothelial growth factor
VIP	vaso-active intestinal polypeptide
WBC	white blood cell

Units

cm	centimetre(s)
cps	cycles per sec
dL	decilitre(s)
g	gram(s)
Gy	Gray(s), a measure of radiation
h	hour(s)
Hg	mercury
kg	kilogram(s)
L	litre(s)
mg	milligram(s)
microL	microlitre(s)
micromol	micromole(s)
mL	millilitre(s)
mm	millimetre(s)
mmol	millimole(s)
min	minute(s)
mosmol	milli-osmole(s)
msec	millisecond(s)
nm	nanometre(s)
nmol	nanomole(s); alternative, nM
sec	second(s)

1 Institute for Safe Medication Practices Canada (2006) Eliminate use of dangerous abbreviations, symbols, and dose designations. *ISMP Canada Safety Bulletin.* **6(4)**: 1–2.

1: GASTRO-INTESTINAL SYSTEM

ANTACIDS

Antacids taken by mouth to neutralize gastric acid include:
* magnesium salts
* aluminum hydroxide
* calcium carbonate
* sodium bicarbonate.

*Magnesium salts are laxative and can cause diarrhea; **aluminum salts** constipate.* Most proprietary antacids contain a mixture of **magnesium salts** and **aluminum salts** so as to have a neutral impact on intestinal transit. With doses of >100–200mL/24h, the effect of **magnesium salts** tends increasingly to override the constipating effect of **aluminum**.[1]

The sodium content of some antacids may be detrimental in patients on salt-restricted diets, e.g. those with hypertension or heart failure; Gaviscon® Liquid (available OTC) contains Na⁺ 53mg/5mL (equivalent to 4.6mmol/10mL dose) compared with 0.1nmol/10mL in **aluminum hydroxide-magnesium hydroxide** suspension (e.g. Almagel®). Regular use of **sodium bicarbonate** may cause sodium loading and metabolic alkalosis. **Calcium carbonate** may cause rebound acid secretion about 2h after each dose, and regular use may cause hypercalcemia, particularly if taken with **sodium bicarbonate**.

Aluminum hydroxide binds dietary phosphate. It is of benefit in patients with hyperphosphatemia in renal failure. Long-term complications of phosphate depletion and osteomalacia are not an issue in advanced cancer.

In post-radiation esophagitis and candidosis which is causing painful swallowing, an **aluminum hydroxide-magnesium hydroxide** suspension containing **oxethazine**, a local anesthetic, can be helpful. Give 5–10mL (without fluid) 15min a.c. & at bedtime, and p.r.n. before drinks. This should be regarded as short-term symptomatic treatment while time and specific treatment of the underlying condition permits healing of the damaged mucosa. Alternatively, **lidocaine** viscous oral suspension 2% (or a compounded **lidocaine** suspension) can be used (see p.449).

The following should be borne in mind:
* *the administration of antacids should be separated from the administration of EC tablets;* direct contact between EC tablets and antacids may result in damage to the enteric coating with consequential exposure of the drug to gastric acid, and of the stomach mucosa to the drug
* except for **sodium bicarbonate**, antacids delay gastric emptying and may thereby modify drug absorption.

- most antacid tablets feel gritty when sucked; some patients dislike this
- some proprietary products are fruit-flavoured, e.g. Tums® (chewable tablet)
- the cheapest single-ingredient product is **aluminum hydroxide** chewable tablets (Amphojel®)
- the cheapest single-ingredient **magnesium** product is **milk of magnesia liquid** (generic), containing **magnesium hydroxide** 80mg/mL
- the cheapest **aluminum-magnesium** combination product is a generic store brand liquid product
- some antacids contain additional substances for use in specific situations, e.g. alginates (see below), **simethicone** (see p.3)
- magnesium-containing antacids should be used with caution in patients with renal impairment (see p.491); **calcium carbonate** is preferable.

Antacids are now generally only used p.r.n. for occasional dyspepsia; H_2-receptor antagonists (see p.15) and PPIs (see p.19) are used when continuous gastric acid reduction is indicated.[2]

Supply
See also **Simethicone**, p.3.

Aluminum hydroxide
Amphojel® (Aurium Pharma)
Tablets chewable 600mg, 28 days @ 1 t.i.d. & at bedtime = $27; *mint flavour.*
Oral suspension (sugar-free) 320mg/5mL, 28 days @ 10mL t.i.d. & at bedtime = $38; *mint flavour.*

Aluminum hydroxide-magnesium hydroxide
Almagel 200® (Laboratoire Atlas)
Oral suspension (sugar-free) aluminum hydroxide 200mg, **magnesium hydroxide** 200mg/5mL, 28 days @ 10mL t.i.d. & at bedtime = $13; *low Na^+.*

Calcium carbonate
Tums® (GlaxoSmithKline)
Tablets chewable regular strength, 500mg; extra strength, 750mg; ultra strength, 1,000mg; 28 days @ 2 t.i.d. & at bedtime = $7, $13 and $19 respectively; *low Na^+, fruit flavour.*

With **oxethazine**
Mucaine® suspension (Aurium Pharma)
Oral suspension aluminum hydroxide 300mg, **magnesium hydroxide** 100mg, **oxethazine** 10mg/5mL, 28 days @ 10mL t.i.d. a.c. & at bedtime = $77.

---

1 Morrissey J and Barreras R (1974) Antacid therapy. *New England Journal of Medicine.* **290**: 550–554.
2 NICE (2004) Dyspepsia. Management of dyspepsia in adults in primary care. In: *Clinical Guideline 17.* National Institute for Clinical Excellence. Available from: www.nice.org.uk/page.aspx?o=CG017

ALGINATE PRODUCTS

Included for general information. Alginate products are generally *not recommended* as antacids for palliative care patients.

Class: Alginate.

Indications: Acid reflux ('heartburn').

Pharmacology
Antacid products containing alginic acid or sodium alginate prevent esophageal reflux pain by forming an inert low-density raft on the top of the acidic stomach contents. Both acid and air bubbles are necessary to produce the raft. Compound alginate products may thus be less effective if used with drugs which reduce acid (e.g. an H_2-receptor antagonist or a PPI) or products which reduce air bubbles (i.e. an antifoaming agent/antiflatulent).

Gaviscon® Liquid, a sodium alginate product, is a weak antacid; most of the antacid content adheres to the alginate raft. This neutralizes acid which seeps into the esophagus around the raft but does nothing to correct the underlying causes, e.g. lax lower esophageal sphincter, hyperacidity, delayed gastric emptying, obesity. Indeed, alginate-containing products are no better than **simethicone**-containing antacids in the treatment of acid reflux.[1] Compound alginate products have been largely superseded by acid suppression with PPIs and H_2-receptor antagonists.

Onset of action <5min.
Duration of action 1–2h.

Cautions
Gaviscon® Liquid contains Na^+ 53mg/5mL (equivalent to 4.6mmol/10mL dose). It should not be used in patients requiring a salt-restricted diet, e.g. those with fluid retention, heart failure or renal impairment.

Dose and use
Several products are available but none is recommended. For patients already taking an alginate product and who are reluctant to change to **aluminum hydroxide–magnesium hydroxide** (or similar option), and if there are grounds for limiting sodium intake, choose one with a low sodium content, e.g. Gaviscon Heartburn Relief Tablets® (22mg Na^+/tablet).

Supply
Gaviscon® Liquid and tablets are available OTC.

Gaviscon Liquid® (GlaxoSmithKline)
Oral suspension (sugar-free) **sodium alginate** 250mg, **aluminum hydroxide** 100mg/5mL, 340mL bottle = $13 and 600mL bottle = $20; *53mg Na^+/5mL.*

Gaviscon Heartburn Relief Tablets® (GlaxoSmithKline)
Tablets chewable **alginic acid** 200mg, **magnesium carbonate** 40mg, 100 tablets = $20; *22mg Na^+/tablet.*

Gaviscon Heartburn Relief Extra Strength Tablets® (GlaxoSmithKline)
Tablets chewable **alginic acid** 313mg, **magnesium carbonate** 63mg, 60 tablets = $20; *35mg Na^+/tablet.*

Maalox Nighttime® (Novartis)
Oral suspension **sodium alginate** 275mg, calcium carbonate 300mg, **magnesium carbonate** 125mg/5mL, 350mL bottle = $12; *45mg Na/5mL, mint flavour.*

---

1 Pokorny C et al. (1985) Comparison of an antacid/dimethicone mixture and an alginate/antacid mixture in the treatment of oesophagitis. *Gut.* **26**: A574.

SIMETHICONE

Class: Antifoaming agent (antiflatulent).

Indications: Acid dyspepsia (including acid reflux), gassy dyspepsia, †hiccup (if associated with gastric distension).

Pharmacology
Simethicone (silica-activated dimethicone or dimethylpolysiloxane) is a mixture of liquid dimethicones with silicon dioxide. It is an antifoaming agent present in several single-agent products (e.g. Ovol®) and some combination antacids (e.g. Diovol Plus® and Maalox antacid with anti-gas®). By facilitating belching, simethicone eases flatulence, distension and postprandial gastric discomfort. Simethicone-containing antacids are as effective as alginate-containing

products in the treatment of acid reflux.[1] Simethicone-containing antacids should be used in preference to **alginate** products because they are more effective antacids, are cheaper, and contain less sodium.

Onset of action <5min.

Duration of action 1–2h.

Cautions

With high doses of mixed **aluminum–magnesium** antacids (>100–200mL/day), the laxative effect of **magnesium** tends to override the constipating effect of **aluminum**.[2]

Dose and use

Practice varies. Some centres initially prescribe simethicone alone; others use a combination antacid as a 'general purpose' antacid (and thus minimize the number of products kept in stock). Typical regimens include:

- simethicone alone:
  ▷ 40–125mg t.i.d. p.c. and bedtime (plus p.r.n.)
  ▷ maximum 500mg/day
- combination antacid:
  ▷ Diovol Plus® or Maalox antacid with anti-gas® suspension 5mL t.i.d. p.c. and bedtime (plus p.r.n.)
  ▷ if necessary, increase to 10–30mL/dose.

Supply

A selection of products only.

Simethicone

Ovol® (Church and Dwight)

Tablets chewable 80mg, 180mg, 28 days @ 80mg q.i.d. = $26.

Gas X® (Novartis)

Tablets chewable 80mg, 125mg, 28 days @ 80mg q.i.d. = $31.

Phazyme® (GlaxoSmithKline)

Capsule softgel 95mg, 180mg, 28 days @ 95mg q.i.d. = $35.

With antacids

Diovol Plus® (Church & Dwight)

Tablets simethicone 25mg, **aluminum hydroxide–magnesium carbonate** co-dried gel 300mg, **magnesium hydroxide** 100mg, 28 days @ 2 q.i.d. = $34.

Oral suspension simethicone 25mg, **aluminum hydroxide** 165mg, **magnesium hydroxide** 200mg/5mL, 28 days @ 20mL q.i.d. = $68.

Diovol Plus AF Tablets® (Church & Dwight)

Tablets chewable simethicone 25mg, **calcium carbonate** 200mg, **magnesium hydroxide** 200mg, 28 days @ 2 q.i.d. = $47.

Gelusil® (Wellspring)

Tablets chewable simethicone 25mg, **aluminum hydroxide** 200mg, **magnesium hydroxide** 200mg, 28 days @ 2 t.i.d. & at bedtime = $53.

Maalox Antacid Quick Dissolve with anti-gas® (Novartis)

Tablets chewable simethicone 60mg, **calcium carbonate** 1g, 28 days @ 2 q.i.d. = $40.

Oral suspension simethicone 20mg, **aluminum hydroxide** 200mg, **magnesium hydroxide** 200mg/5mL, 28 days @ 20mL q.i.d. = $74.

---

1 Pokorny C et al. (1985) Comparison of an antacid/dimethicone mixture and an alginate/antacid mixture in the treatment of oesophagitis. *Gut.* **26**: A574.

2 Morrissey J and Barreras R (1974) Antacid therapy. *New England Journal of Medicine.* **290**: 550–554.

ANTIMUSCARINICS

Indications: Smooth muscle spasm (e.g. bladder, intestine), motion sickness (**scopolamine (hyoscine)** *hydrobromide* TD), drying secretions (including surgical premedication, †sialorrhea, †drooling, †death rattle (noisy respiratory secretions) and †inoperable intestinal obstruction), †paraneoplastic pyrexia and sweating.

Contra-indications: See individual monographs.

Pharmacology

Antimuscarinics are classified chemically as tertiary amines or quaternary ammonium compounds. The naturally-occurring belladonna alkaloids, **atropine** and **scopolamine (hyoscine)** *hydrobromide*, are tertiary amines, whereas the numerous semisynthetic and synthetic derivatives fall into both categories. Thus, **dicyclomine, oxybutynin** and **tolterodine** are tertiary amines, and **glycopyrrolate, propantheline** (not Canada) and **hyoscine (scopolamine)** *butylbromide* are quaternary ammonium compounds.

Except for **scopolamine hydrobromide**, which causes CNS depression at therapeutic doses, the tertiary amines stimulate the brain stem and higher centres, producing mild central vagal excitation and respiratory stimulation. At toxic doses, all the tertiary amines, including **scopolamine hydrobromide** cause CNS stimulation resulting in agitation and delirium. Synthetic tertiary amines generally cause less central stimulation than the naturally-occurring alkaloids. Quaternary ammonium compounds do not cross the blood-brain barrier in any significant amount, and accordingly do not have any central effects.[1] They are also less well absorbed from the GI tract.

Peripheral antimuscarinic effects are a class characteristic (Box 1.A), and have been summarized as:

'*Dry as a bone, blind as a bat, red as a beet, hot as a hare, mad as a hatter.*'

However, at least five different types of muscarinic receptors have been identified,[2] and newer drugs tend to be more selective in their actions. Thus, **oxybutynin** and **tolterodine** are relatively selective for muscarinic receptors in the urinary tract (see p.411).

Box 1.A Peripheral antimuscarinic effects

Visual
Mydriasis
Loss of accommodation } blurred vision (and thus may impair driving ability)

Cardiovascular
Tachycardia, palpitations
Extrasystoles
Arrhythmias } also related to norepinephrine potentiation and a quinidine-like action

Gastro-intestinal
Dry mouth
Heartburn (relaxation of lower esophageal sphincter)
Constipation

Urinary tract
Hesitancy of micturition
Retention of urine

Skin
Reduced sweating
Flushing

Except when a reduction of oropharyngeal secretions is intended, dry mouth is an almost universal *undesirable* effect with this class of drugs. The secretion of saliva is mainly under the control of the autonomic nervous system. Food in the mouth causes reflex secretion of saliva, and so does stimulation by acid of afferent vagal fibres in the lower esophagus. Stimulation of the parasympathetic nerves causes profuse secretion of watery saliva, whereas stimulation of the sympathetic nerve supply causes the secretion from only the submaxillary glands of small quantities of saliva rich in organic constituents.[3] If the parasympathetic supply is interrupted, the salivary glands atrophy, whereas interruption of the sympathetic supply has no such effect. The muscarinic receptors in salivary glands are very responsive to antimuscarinics and inhibition of salivation occurs at lower doses than required for other antimuscarinic effects.[4] This reduces the likelihood of undesirable effects when antimuscarinics are given to reduce salivation. In some patients, a reduction in excess saliva results in improved speech.[5]

To reduce the risk of undesirable effects, e.g. the development of an agitated delirium (central antimuscarinic syndrome), the concurrent use of two antimuscarinic drugs should generally be avoided (Box 1.B). Likewise, the concurrent use of an antimuscarinic and an opioid should be avoided as far as possible. Both cause constipation (by different mechanisms) and, if used together, will result in an increased need for laxatives, and may even result in a paralytic ileus. On the other hand, **morphine** and **hyoscine butylbromide** or **glycopyrrolate** are sometimes purposely combined in terminally ill patients with inoperable intestinal obstruction in order to prevent colic and to reduce vomiting.[6]

Box 1.B   Drugs with antimuscarinic effects used in palliative care (Canada)[a]

Antidepressants	Antipsychotics (typical)
TCAs, e.g. amitriptyline, imipramine	phenothiazines, e.g.
paroxetine (SSRI)	chlorpromazine
Antihistamines, e.g.	methotrimeprazine
chlorpheniramine	prochlorperazine
dimenhydrinate	Antisecretory drugs
promethazine	belladonna alkaloids
Antiparkinsonians, e.g.	atropine
orphenadrine	scopolamine (hyoscine)
procyclidine	glycopyrrolate
Antipsychotics (atypical)	Antispasmodics, e.g.
olanzapine	dicyclomine
	oxybutynin
	tolterodine

a. meperidine/pethidine, an opioid (not recommended), also has antimuscarinic effects.

Antimuscarinics used as antispasmodics and/or antisecretory drugs differ in their pharmacokinetic characteristics (Table 1.1). Availability and fashion are probably the main influences in choice of drug.

Table 1.1   Pharmacokinetic details of antimuscarinic drugs used for death rattle

	Bio-availability	Plasma halflife	Duration of action (antisecretory)
Atropine	'readily absorbed' PO, SL	4h	no data
Glycopyrrolate	<5% PO	1.7h	7h
Hyoscine (scopolamine) butylbromide	8–10% PO	5–6h	<2h[a]
Scopolamine (hyoscine) hydrobromide	60–80% SL	5–6h	1–9h

a. in volunteers; possibly longer in moribund patients.

Cautions

Concurrent treatment with two antimuscarinic drugs will increase the likelihood of undesirable effects, and of central toxicity, i.e. restlessness, agitation, delirium. Children, the elderly, and patients with renal or hepatic impairment are more susceptible to the central effects of antimuscarinics.

Various drugs not generally considered antimuscarinic have been shown to have detectable antimuscarinic activity by means of a radioreceptor assay, including **codeine, digoxin, dipyridamole, isosorbide, nifedipine, prednisone, ranitidine, theophylline, warfarin.**[7] Theoretically, these drugs could exacerbate toxicity, particularly in debilitated elderly patients.

The increased GI transit time produced by antimuscarinics may allow increased drug absorption from some formulations, e.g. **digoxin** and **nitrofurantoin** from tablets and **potassium** from SR tablets, but reduced absorption from others, e.g. **acetaminophen** tablets. Dissolution and absorption of SL tablets (e.g. **nitroglycerin**) may be reduced because of decreased saliva production.

Because antimuscarinics competitively block the final common (cholinergic) pathway through which prokinetics act,[8] concurrent prescription with **metoclopramide** and **domperidone** should be avoided if possible.

Use with caution in myasthenia gravis, conditions predisposing to tachycardia (e.g. thyrotoxicosis, heart failure, β-adrenergic receptor agonists), and bladder outflow obstruction (prostatism). Use in hot weather or pyrexia may lead to heatstroke. Likely to exacerbate acid reflux. Narrow-angle glaucoma may be precipitated in those at risk, particularly the elderly.

Dose and use
Antispasmodic

Antimuscarinics are used to relieve smooth muscle spasm in the bladder (see **oxybutynin**, p.411) and rectum.

Antispasmodic and antisecretory

Antimuscarinics are used to reduce intestinal colic and intestinal secretions, particularly gastric, associated with inoperable organic intestinal obstruction in terminally ill patients (Table 1.2).

Table 1.2 Antisecretory and antispasmodic drugs: typical SC doses

Drug	Stat and p.r.n. doses	CSCI dose/24 h
Atropine	400microgram	1,000–2,000microgram
Glycopyrrolate	200microgram	600–1,200microgram
Hyoscine (scopolamine) butylbromide	20mg	20–300mg[a]
Scopolamine (hyoscine) hydrobromide	400microgram	1,200–2,000microgram

a. death rattle 20–60mg, some centres use up to 120mg; intestinal obstruction 60–300mg.

Antisecretory
Sialorrhea and drooling

Indicated particularly in patients with ALS/MND, advanced Parkinson's disease or with various disorders of the head and neck. Several regimens have been recommended, including:
- **atropine** 1% ophthalmic solution, 4 drops SL q4h p.r.n. (Note: drop size varies with applicator and technique, dose per drop may vary from 200–500microgram, i.e. 800microgram–2mg/dose)
- compounded **glycopyrrolate** PO (see p.465)
- **scopolamine hydrobromide** 1mg/3 days TD.[9]

A regimen of **atropine** 1% 500microgram (1 drop) SL b.i.d. has been reported[10] but a controlled trial found 500microgram (2 drops) SL q.i.d. no better than placebo.[11]

When antimuscarinics are contra-indicated, not tolerated or ineffective, **botulinum toxin** injections (with ultrasound guidance) into the parotid and submandibular glands offer an alternative approach. Generally effective in ≤1–2 weeks, with benefit lasting 3–4 months.[12–16]

Death rattle (noisy respiratory secretions)

In Canada, antimuscarinic drugs for death rattle are generally given SC.[17] See Table 1.2 and Guidelines, p.10. In some countries the SL route is preferred, particularly in home care because it circumvents the need for injections. Treatment regimens, all off-label, are based mainly on local clinical experience, e.g.:

- **atropine** 1% ophthalmic solution, 4 drops SL q4h p.r.n. (Note: drop size varies with applicator and technique, dose per drop may vary from 200–500microgram, i.e. 800microgram–2mg/dose)
- **glycopyrrolate** 100microgram SL q6h p.r.n. (see p.465)

Paraneoplastic pyrexia and sweating

Antimuscarinic drugs are used in the treatment of paraneoplastic pyrexia (Box 1.C).

Box 1.C   Symptomatic drug treatment of paraneoplastic pyrexia and sweating

Prescribe an antipyretic:
- acetaminophen 500–1,000mg q.i.d. or p.r.n. (generally less toxic than an NSAID)
- NSAID, e.g. ibuprofen 200–400mg t.i.d. or p.r.n. (or the locally preferred alternative).

If the sweating does not respond to an NSAID, prescribe an antimuscarinic drug:
- amitriptyline 25–50mg at bedtime (may cause sedation, dry mouth, and other antimuscarinic effects)
- scopolamine hydrobromide 1mg/3 days TD[18]
- glycopyrrolate up to 2mg PO t.i.d.[19]

If an antimuscarinic fails, other options include:
- propranolol 10–20mg b.i.d.–t.i.d.
- cimetidine 400–800mg b.i.d.[20]
- olanzapine 5mg b.i.d.[21]
- thalidomide 100mg at bedtime.[22,23]

Thalidomide is generally seen as the last resort even though the response rate appears to be high.[22] This is because it can cause an irreversible painful peripheral neuropathy, and may also cause drowsiness (see p.405).

Overdose

In the past, **physostigmine**, a cholinesterase inhibitor, was sometimes administered to correct antimuscarinic toxicity/poisoning. This is no longer recommended because **physostigmine** itself can cause serious toxic effects, including cardiac arrhythmias and seizures.[24–26] A benzodiazepine can be given to control marked agitation and seizures. Phenothiazines should not be given because they will exacerbate the antimuscarinic effects, and could precipitate an acute dystonia (see Drug-induced movement disorders, p.561). Anti-arrhythmics are not advisable if arrhythmias develop; but hypoxia and acidosis should be corrected.

Supply

See individual monographs: **glycopyrrolate** (p.465), **hyoscine (scopolamine) butylbromide** (p.11), **scopolamine (hyoscine) hydrobromide** (p.195), **oxybutynin** (p.411).

Atropine sulfate (generic)
Injection 400microgram/mL, 1mL ampoule = $1.50; 600microgram/mL, 1mL ampoule = $1.50.
Ophthalmic solution 1%, 5mL bottle = $3.50.

Minims® atropine sulfate (Chauvin)
Ophthalmic solution (single-dose units) 1%, 0.5mL single-dose unit = $2.

---

1 Sweetman SC (ed) (2005) *Martindale: The Complete Drug Reference* (34e). Pharmaceutical Press, London, p. 475.
2 Caulfield M and Birdsall N (1998) International Union of Pharmacology. XVII. Classification of muscarinic acetylcholine receptors. *Pharmacological Review.* **50**: 279–290.

3 Ganong WF (1979) *Review of Medical Physiology* (9e). Lange Medical Publications, pp. 177–181.
4 Ali-Melkkila T *et al.* (1993) Pharmacokinetics and related pharmacodynamics of anticholinergic drugs. *Acta Anaesthesiologica Scandinavica.* **37**: 633–642.
5 Rashid H *et al.* (1997) Management of secretions in esophageal cancer patients with glycopyrrolate. *Annals of Oncology.* **8**: 198–199.
6 Twycross RG and Wilcock A (2001) *Symptom Management in Advanced Cancer* (3e). Radcliffe Medical Press, Oxford, pp. 113–114.
7 Tune I *et al.* (1992) Anticholinergic effects of drugs commonly prescribed for the elderly; potential means of assessing risk of delirium. *American Journal of Psychiatry.* **149**: 1393–1394.
8 Schuurkes JAJ *et al.* (1986) Stimulation of gastroduodenal motor activity: dopaminergic and cholinergic modulation. *Drug Development Research.* **8**: 233–241.
9 Talmi YP *et al.* (1990) Reduction of salivary flow with transdermal scopolamine: a four-year experience. *Otolaryngology and Head and Neck Surgery.* **103**: 615–618.
10 Hyson HC *et al.* (2002) Sublingual atropine for sialorrhea secondary to parkinsonism: a pilot study. *Movement Disorders.* **17**: 1318–1320.
11 De Simone GG *et al.* (2006) Atropine drops for drooling: a randomized controlled trial. *Palliative Medicine.* **20**: 665–671.
12 Lipp A *et al.* (2003) A randomized trial of botulinum toxin A for treatment of drooling. *Neurology.* **61**: 1279–1281.
13 Mancini F *et al.* (2003) Double-blind, placebo-controlled study to evaluate the efficacy and safety of botulinum toxin type A in the treatment of drooling in parkinsonism. *Movement Disorders.* **18**: 685–688.
14 Ellies M *et al.* (2004) Reduction of salivary flow with botulinum toxin: extended report on 33 patients with drooling, salivary fistulas, and sialadenitis. *Laryngoscope.* **114**: 1856–1860.
15 Jongerius P *et al.* (2004) Effect of botulinum toxin in the treatment of drooling: a controlled clinical trial. *Pediatrics.* **114**: 620–627.
16 Ondo WG *et al.* (2004) A double-blind placebo-controlled trial of botulinum toxin B for sialorrhea in Parkinson's disease. *Neurology.* **62**: 37–40.
17 Bennett M *et al.* (2002) Using anti-muscarinic drugs in the management of death rattle: evidence based guidelines for palliative care. *Palliative Medicine.* **16**: 369–374.
18 Mercadante S (1998) Hyoscine in opioid-induced sweating. *Journal of Pain and Symptom Management.* **15**: 214–215.
19 Klaber M and Catterall M (2000) Treating hyperhidrosis. Anticholinergic drugs were not mentioned. *British Medical Journal.* **321**: 703.
20 Pittelkow M and Loprinzi C (2003) Pruritus and sweating in palliative medicine. In: D Doyle *et al.* (eds) *Oxford Textbook of Palliative Medicine* (3e). Oxford University Press, Oxford, pp. 573–587.
21 Zylicz Z and Krajnik M (2003) Flushing and sweating in an advanced breast cancer patient relieved by olanzapine. *Journal of Pain and Symptom Management.* **25**: 494–495.
22 Deaner P (2000) The use of thalidomide in the management of severe sweating in patients with advanced malignancy: trial report. *Palliative Medicine.* **14**: 429–431.
23 Calder K and Bruera E (2000) Thalidomide for night sweats in patients with advanced cancer. *Palliative Medicine.* **14**: 77–78.
24 Aquilonius SM and Hedstrand U (1978) The use of physostigmine as an antidote in tricyclic anti-depressant intoxication. *Acta Anaesthesiologica Scandinavica.* **22**: 40–45.
25 Caine ED (1979) Anticholinergic toxicity. *New England Journal of Medicine.* **300**: 1278.
26 Newton RW (1975) Physostigmine salicylate in the treatment of tricyclic antidepressant overdosage. *Journal of the American Medical Association.* **231**: 941–943.

Guidelines: Management of death rattle (noisy respiratory secretions)

Death rattle is a term used to describe noisy rattling breathing which occurs in about 50% of patients near the end of life. It is caused by fluid pooling in the hypopharynx, and arises from one or more sources:

- saliva (most common)
- respiratory tract infection
- pulmonary edema
- gastric reflux.

Rattling breathing can also occur in patients with a tracheostomy and infection. Because the patient is generally semiconscious or unconscious, drug treatment for death rattle is mainly for the benefit of relatives, other patients and staff.

Non-drug treatment

- ease the family's distress by explaining that the semiconscious/unconscious patient is not distressed by the rattle
- position the patient semiprone to encourage postural drainage; but upright or semirecumbent if the cause is pulmonary edema or gastric reflux
- oropharyngeal suction but, because it is distressing to many moribund patients, generally reserve for unconscious patients.

Drug treatment
Saliva
Because they do not affect existing secretions, an antisecretory drug should be given SC (see Table) or SL (see Box A), as soon as the onset of the rattle is detected. SL use is off-label and less well supported by the literature.

Table Antimuscarinic antisecretory drugs for death rattle: typical SC doses

Drug	Stat SC and p.r.n. doses	CSCI dose/24h
Atropine	400microgram	1,200–2,000microgram
Glycopyrrolate	200microgram	600–1,200microgram
Hyoscine (scopolamine) *butylbromide*	20mg	20–120mg
Scopolamine (hyoscine) *hydrobromide*	400microgram	1,200–2,000microgram

---

Box A Antimuscarinic antisecretory drugs for death rattle: typical SL doses

Atropine 1% ophthalmic solution, 4 drops SL q4h p.r.n. (Note: drop size varies with applicator and technique, dose per drop may vary from *200–500*microgram, i.e. 800microgram–2mg/dose).

Glycopyrrolate 0.01% oral solution, 1mL (100microgram) SL q6h p.r.n.; A 0.05% solution (500microgram/mL) can be compounded from glycopyrrolate powder (see Box B).

Note:

- by injection, the efficacy of the different drugs is broadly similar; the rattle is reduced in 1/2–2/3 of patients
- the onset of action of glycopyrrolate is slower compared with scopolamine (hyoscine) *hydrobromide*
- scopolamine (hyoscine) *hydrobromide* crosses the blood-brain barrier and possesses anti-emetic and sedative properties, but there is also a risk of developing or exacerbating delirium
- atropine also crosses the blood-brain barrier but tends to stimulate rather than sedate; concurrent use with midazolam or haloperidol is more likely to be necessary.

continued

Box B Examples of compounded oral solutions of glycopyrrolate

Based on glycopyrrolate injection
Glycopyrrolate 100microgram/mL (1mg/10mL)
Combine 25mL of Ora-Plus® and 25mL of Ora-Sweet®; add to 50mL preservative-free glycopyrrolate injection USP 200microgram/mL to make up to 100mL, and mix well. Stable for 35 days at room temperature or in a refrigerator (refrigeration minimizes risk of microbial contamination).

Based on glycopyrrolate powder
Glycopyrrolate 500microgram/mL (5mg/10mL)
Add 5mL of glycerin to 50mg of glycopyrrolate powder and mix to form a smooth paste. Add 50mL of Ora-Plus® in portions and mix well. Add sufficient Ora-Sweet® or Ora-Sweet SF® to make a total volume of 100mL.
This solution is stable for 90 days at room temperature or in a refrigerator.

Respiratory tract infection
Occasionally, it is appropriate to prescribe an antibiotic in an imminently dying patient if death rattle is caused by profuse purulent sputum associated with an underlying chest infection:
- e.g. ceftriaxone, mix 1g ampoule with 2.1mL lidocaine 1% (total volume 2.6–2.8mL), and give 250mg–1g SC/IM once daily
- some centres use larger volumes of lidocaine 1% (up to 4mL) and administer a divided dose at separate SC/IM sites once daily or b.i.d.

Pulmonary edema
Consider furosemide 20–40mg SC/IM/IV q2h p.r.n.
Note: beware precipitating urinary retention.

Gastric reflux

Consider metoclopramide 20mg SC/IV q3h p.r.n., but do not use concurrently with an antimuscarinic because the latter blocks the prokinetic effect of the former.

Rattling breathing causing distress to a patient
In a semiconscious patient, if rattling breathing is associated with breathlessness, supplement the above with an opioid (e.g. morphine) ± an anxiolytic sedative (e.g. midazolam).

HYOSCINE (SCOPOLAMINE) BUTYLBROMIDE

Class: Antimuscarinic.

Indications: Smooth muscle spasm (e.g. bladder, GI tract), †drying secretions (including sialorrhea, drooling, death rattle/noisy respiratory secretions and inoperable bowel obstruction), †paraneoplastic pyrexia and sweating.

Contra-indications: Narrow-angle glaucoma (unless moribund), myasthenia gravis (unless moribund).

Pharmacology

Hyoscine (scopolamine) butylbromide is an antimuscarinic (see p.5) and has both smooth muscle relaxant (antispasmodic) and antisecretory properties. It is a quaternary compound and, unlike **scopolamine (hyoscine) hydrobromide**, it does not cross the blood-brain barrier. In consequence, it does not have a central anti-emetic effect or cause drowsiness.

Oral bio-availability, based on urinary excretion, is <1%.[1] Thus, any antispasmodic effect reported after PO administration probably relates to a local contact effect on the GI mucosa.[2] In an RCT, hyoscine butylbromide 10mg t.i.d. PO and **acetaminophen (paracetamol)** 500mg t.i.d. both significantly reduced the severity of intestinal colic by >50%.[3] However, the difference between the benefit from these two drugs (both given in suboptimal doses) and placebo was only 0.5cm on a 10cm scale of pain intensity. This is of dubious clinical importance.[4] Thus the therapeutic value of PO hyoscine butylbromide for intestinal colic remains debatable.

The main uses for hyoscine butylbromide in palliative care are as an antispasmodic and antisecretory drug in inoperable GI obstruction, and as an antisecretory drug for death rattle. In an open non-randomized trial of hyoscine butylbromide 60mg/24h CSCI vs. **octreotide** 300microgram/24h CSCI, **octreotide** resulted in a more rapid reduction in the volume of gastric aspirate (by 75% vs. 50%) and improvement in nausea, although it was possible to remove nasogastric tubes in both groups after about 5 days.[5,6] However, higher doses of hyoscine butylbromide, e.g. 120–200mg/24h, have not been compared with **octreotide**.

In healthy volunteers, a bolus injection of 20mg has a maximum antisecretory duration of action of 2h.[7] However, the same dose by CSCI is often effective for 1 day in death rattle. Hyoscine butylbromide and **scopolamine hydrobromide** act faster than **glycopyrrolate** for this indication,[8,9] but the overall efficacy is generally the same[10] with death rattle reduced in 1/2–2/3 of patients.

Bio-availability <1% PO.[1]
Onset of action <10min SC/IM/IV; 1–2h PO.[11]
Time to peak plasma concentration 15min–2h PO.[1]
Plasma halflife 1–5h.[1]
Duration of action <2h in volunteers; probably longer in moribund patients.[7]

Cautions

Competitively blocks the prokinetic effect of **metoclopramide** and **domperidone**.[1,12] Increases the peripheral antimuscarinic effects of antihistamines, phenothiazines and TCAs (see Antimuscarinics, p.5).

Use with caution in conditions predisposing to tachycardia (e.g. thyrotoxicosis, heart failure, β-adrenergic receptor agonists), and bladder outflow obstruction (prostatism). Likely to exacerbate acid reflux. Narrow-angle glaucoma may be precipitated in those at risk, particularly the elderly. Use in hot weather or pyrexia may lead to heatstroke.

Undesirable effects

For full list, see manufacturer's Product Monograph.
Peripheral antimuscarinic effects (see p.5).

Dose and use

Inoperable intestinal obstruction with colic[13,14]
• start with 20mg SC stat and 60mg/24h CSCI
• if necessary, increase to 120mg/24h
• maximum reported dose 300mg/24h.

Some centres add **octreotide** 300–500microgram/24h if hyoscine butylbromide 120mg/24h fails to relieve symptoms adequately.

For patients with obstructive symptoms without colic, **metoclopramide** (see p.185) should be tried before an antimuscarinic because the obstruction is often more functional than organic.

Death rattle (noisy respiratory symptoms)
- start with 20mg SC stat, 20–60mg/24h CSCI, and/or 20mg SC q1h p.r.n.
- some centres use higher doses, namely 60–120mg/24h CSCI[9]

For use of alternative antimuscarinics, see Guidelines, p.10.

Supply
Buscopan® (Boehringer Ingelheim)
Tablets 10mg, 28 days @ 20mg q.i.d. = $79.
Injection 20mg/ml, 1ml amp = $5.

1　Boehringer Ingelheim GmbH *Data on file*.
2　Tytgat GN (2007) Hyoscine butylbromide: a review of its use in the treatment of abdominal cramping and pain. *Drugs*. **67**: 1343–1357.
3　Mueller–Lissner S *et al.* (2006) Placebo- and paracetamol-controlled study on the efficacy and tolerability of hyoscine butylbromide in the treatment of patients with recurrent crampy abdominal pain. *Alimentary Pharmacology & Therapeutics*. **23**: 1741–1748.
4　Farrar JT *et al.* (2000) Defining the clinically important difference in pain outcome measures. *Pain*. **88**: 287–294.
5　Mercadante S *et al.* (2000) Comparison of octreotide and hyoscine butylbromide in controlling gastrointestinal symptoms due to malignant inoperable bowel obstruction. *Supportive Care in Cancer*. **8**: 188–191.
6　Ripamonti C *et al.* (2000) Role of octreotide, scopolamine butylbromide, and hydration in symptom control of patients with inoperable bowel obstruction and nasogastric tubes: a prospective randomized trial. *Journal of Pain and Symptom Management*. **19**: 23–34.
7　Herxheimer A and Haefeli L (1966) Human pharmacology of hyoscine butylbromide. *Lancet*. **ii**: 418–421.
8　Back I *et al.* (2001) A study comparing hyoscine hydrobromide and glycopyrrolate in the treatment of death rattle. *Palliative Medicine*. **15**: 329–336.
9　Bennett M *et al.* (2002) Using anti-muscarinic drugs in the management of death rattle: evidence based guidelines for palliative care. *Palliative Medicine*. **16**: 369–374.
10　Hughes A *et al.* (2000) Audit of three antimuscarinic drugs for managing retained secretions. *Palliative Medicine*. **14**: 221–222.
11　Sanches Martinez J *et al.* (1988) Clinical assessment of the tolerability and the effect of IK-19 in tablet form on pain of spastic origin. *Investigacion Medica International*. **15**: 63–65.
12　Schuurkes JAJ *et al.* (1986) Stimulation of gastroduodenal motor activity: dopaminergic and cholinergic modulation. *Drug Development Research*. **8**: 233–241.
13　De-Conno F *et al.* (1991) Continuous subcutaneous infusion of hyoscine butylbromide reduces secretions in patients with gastrointestinal obstruction. *Journal of Pain and Symptom Management*. **6**: 484–486.
14　Ripamonti C *et al.* (2001) Clinical-practice recommendations for the management of bowel obstruction in patients with end-stage cancer. *Supportive Care in Cancer*. **9**: 223–233.

PROKINETICS

Prokinetics accelerate gastro-intestinal transit by a neurohumoral mechanism. The term is restricted to drugs which co-ordinate antroduodenal contractions and accelerate gastroduodenal transit (Table 1.3). This excludes other drugs which enhance intestinal transit such as bulk-forming agents and other laxatives, and drugs which cause diarrhea by increasing GI secretions, e.g. **misoprostol**. Some drugs increase contractile motor activity but not in a co-ordinated fashion, and so do not reduce transit time, e.g. **bethanechol**. Such drugs are promotility but not prokinetic.

Table 1.3 Gastric prokinetics[1]

Class	Examples	Site of action
D$_2$-receptor antagonist	Domperidone	Stomach
	Metoclopramide	Stomach
5HT$_4$-receptor agonist	Metoclopramide	Stomach → jejunum
Motilin agonist	Erythromycin	Stomach

Except for **erythromycin**, prokinetics act by triggering a cholinergic system in the wall of the GI tract (Table 1.4, Figure 1.1).[2] This action is impeded by opioids. Further, antimuscarinic drugs competitively block cholinergic receptors on the intestinal muscle fibres (and elsewhere).[3] Thus, all drugs with antimuscarinic properties reduce the impact of prokinetic drugs; the extent of this depends on several factors, including the respective doses of the interacting drugs and times of administration. Thus, generally, the concurrent administration of prokinetics and antimuscarinic drugs is best avoided. On the other hand, even if the peripheral prokinetic effect is completely blocked, **domperidone** and **metoclopramide** will still exert an anti-emetic effect at the dopamine receptors in the area postrema (see p.187).

Table 1.4 Comparison of prokinetic drugs[2]

Drug	Erythromycin	Domperidone	Metoclopramide
Mechanism of action			
Motilin agonist	+	−	−
D_2-receptor antagonist	−	+	+
$5HT_4$-receptor agonist	−	−	+
Response to treatment[a]			
Gastric emptying (mean % acceleration)	45	30	20
Symptom relief (mean % improvement)	50	50	40

a. all percentages rounded to nearest 5%.

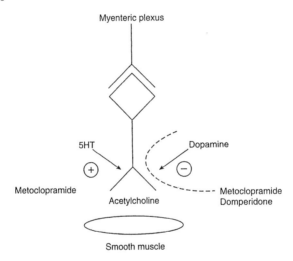

Myenteric plexus

5HT   Dopamine

Metoclopramide

Acetylcholine   Metoclopramide Domperidone

Smooth muscle

Figure 1.1 Schematic representation of drug effects on antroduodenal co-ordination via a postganglionic effect on the cholinergic nerves from the myenteric plexus.
⊕ stimulatory effect of 5HT triggered by metoclopramide; ⊖ inhibitory effect of dopamine; - - - blockade of dopamine inhibition by metoclopramide and domperidone.

Erythromycin, an antibiotic, is the only available motilin agonist.[4] It has been used mainly in diabetic gastroparesis when other prokinetics have proved inadequate.[5,6] A systematic review suggests that, overall, its prokinetic effect is greater than that of **metoclopramide** (Table 1.4). However, it may cause intestinal colic and, in healthy people, it often causes diarrhea. There is also concern about bacterial resistance developing. In some patients, tolerance to its prokinetic effects develops over time.[7] However, some patients have taken **erythromycin** 250mg b.i.d. for more than a year without apparent loss of its prokinetic effect.[8]

Prokinetics are used in various conditions in palliative care (Box 1.D). D_2-receptor antagonists block the dopaminergic 'brake' on gastric emptying induced by stress, anxiety and nausea from any cause. In contrast, $5HT_4$-receptor agonists have a direct excitatory effect which in theory gives them an advantage over the D_2-receptor antagonists particularly for patients with gastric stasis or functional intestinal obstruction. However, when used for dysmotility dyspepsia, **metoclopramide** is no more potent than **domperidone** in standard doses.[9,10]

> **Box 1.D** Indications for prokinetics in palliative care
>
> Gastro-esophageal reflux
>
> Gastroparesis
>   dysmotility dyspepsia
>   paraneoplastic autonomic neuropathy
>   spinal cord compression
>   diabetic autonomic neuropathy
>
> Functional gastro-intestinal obstruction
>   drug-induced, e.g. opioids
>   cancer of head of pancreas
>   neoplastic mural infiltration (linitis plastica)

1 Debinski H and Kamm M (1994) New treatments for neuromuscular disorders of the gastrointestinal tract. *Gastrointestinal Journal Club.* **2**: 2–11.
2 Sturm A *et al.* (1999) Prokinetics in patients with gastroparesis: a systematic analysis. *Digestion.* **60**: 422–427.
3 Schuurkes JAJ *et al.* (1986) Stimulation of gastroduodenal motor activity: dopaminergic and cholinergic modulation. *Drug Development Research.* **8**: 233–241.
4 Janssens J *et al.* (1990) Improvement of gastric emptying in diabetic gastroparesis by erythromycin. Preliminary studies. *New England Journal of Medicine.* **322**: 1028–1031.
5 Erbas T *et al.* (1993) Comparison of metoclopramide and erythromycin in the treatment of diabetic gastroparesis. *Diabetes Care.* **16**: 1511–1514.
6 Smith DS and Ferris CD (2003) Current concepts in diabetic gastroparesis. *Drugs.* **63**: 1339–1358.
7 Dhir R and Richter JE (2004) Erythromycin in the short- and long-term control of dyspepsia symptoms in patients with gastroparesis. *Journal of Clinical Gastroenterology.* **38**: 237–242.
8 Hunter A *et al.* (2005) The use of long-term, low-dose erythromycin in treating persistent gastric stasis. *Journal of Pain and Symptom Management.* **29**: 430–433.
9 Loose FD (1979) Domperidone in chronic dyspepsia: a pilot open study and a multicentre general practice crossover comparison with metoclopramide and placebo. *Pharmatheripeutica.* **2**: 140–146.
10 Moriga M (1981) A multicentre double blind study of domperidone and metoclopramide in the symptomatic control of dyspepsia. In: G Towse (ed) *International congress and symposium series: Progress with Domperidone, a gastrokinetic and anti-emetic agent* (No. 36). Royal Society of Medicine, London, pp. 77–79.

H$_2$-RECEPTOR ANTAGONISTS

Class: Gastroprotective drugs.

Indications: Chronic episodic dyspepsia, acid reflux, prevention and treatment of peptic ulceration (including NSAID-induced ulceration), †reduction of malabsorption and fluid loss in short bowel syndrome (**cimetidine**), †prevention of degradation of pancreatin supplements (**cimetidine**).

Pharmacology

H$_2$-receptor antagonists reduce both gastric acid output and the volume of gastric secretions.[1] **Ranitidine** is a good choice in terms of convenience and safety. **Cimetidine**, alone among H$_2$-receptor antagonists, can cause serious cytochrome P450-related drug interactions (see Cautions below and Cytochrome P450, p.551). None of the H$_2$-receptor antagonists, including **cimetidine**, alters the metabolism of **morphine**.[2]

Prophylactic treatment with a standard dose of an H$_2$-receptor antagonist reduces the incidence of NSAID-induced *duodenal* ulcers.[3] Prevention of *gastric* erosions and ulcers is seen only with a double dose.[4] In patients taking NSAIDs, **ranitidine** (compared with **omeprazole**) is less effective and slower in *healing* gastroduodenal ulcers (63% vs. 80% at 8 weeks) and in *preventing* relapse (59% vs. 72% over 6 months) (Table 1.5).[3,5]

Bio-availability cimetidine 60–70% PO; **ranitidine** 50% PO.

Onset of action <1h.

Time to peak plasma concentration cimetidine 1–3h PO, 15min IM; **ranitidine** 2–3h PO.

Plasma halflife cimetidine 2h; **ranitidine** 2–3h.

Duration of action cimetidine 7h; ranitidine 8–12h.

Table 1.5 Comparison of gastroprotective agents[3–7]

	Prevent NSAID-GU	Prevent NSAID-DU	Heal NSAID-GU	Heal NSAID-DU
Misoprostol	+	+	+	+
H$_2$-receptor antagonists	+[a]	+	+[b]	+[b]
Proton pump inhibitors	+	+	+[c]	+[c]

a. double dose necessary to protect against gastric ulcers
b. rate of healing decreased if NSAID continued
c. rate of healing unchanged if NSAID continued.

Cautions

Serious drug interactions: the increase in gastric pH caused by all H$_2$-receptor antagonists decreases the absorption of **itraconazole** and **ketoconazole**; an increased dose may be needed to avoid antifungal treatment failure. **Cimetidine** binds to microsomal cytochrome P450 and inhibits the metabolism of **warfarin**, IV **lidocaine** (but not ED **lidocaine** or **bupivacaine**), some calcium antagonists (**diltiazem, nifedipine**), **pentoxifylline, theophylline, chlormethiazole** (not Canada), **diazepam**, TCAs, **moclobemide, phenytoin, methadone** and **fluorouracil**. **Cimetidine** inhibits the renal clearance of **procainamide** and **quinidine**.[8]

Hepatic impairment, renal impairment (see Table 1.7). **Cimetidine** causes a transient rise in the plasma concentrations of **carbamazepine**. It also increases plasma concentrations of some benzodiazepines (including **alprazolam** and **diazepam**), some SSRIs (including **citalopram, paroxetine** and **sertraline**), **mirtazapine, alfentanil, fentanyl, methadone, mefloquine, tacrine** (not Canada) and **zolmitriptan**.[8,9] There are inconsistent reports of **cimetidine** and **ranitidine** increasing the plasma concentration of **midazolam**.[8]

Undesirable effects

See manufacturer's Product Monograph.
Cimetidine occasionally causes gynecomastia.

Dose and use

Cochrane review: H$_2$-receptor antagonists (double-dose), **misoprostol** and PPIs are effective at preventing chronic NSAID-related endoscopic peptic ulcers. **Misoprostol** 400microgram daily is less effective than 800microgram and is still associated with diarrhea. Of all these treatments, only **misoprostol** 800microgram daily has been definitely shown to reduce the overall incidence of ulcer complications (perforation, hemorrhage or obstruction).[4] PPIs definitely reduce the incidence of re-bleeding from endoscopically confirmed peptic ulcers,[10] and may reduce the incidence of ulcer complications.[7]

Because **cimetidine** is responsible for several serious drug interactions, **ranitidine** is preferable in palliative care. However, H$_2$-receptor antagonists have been largely superseded by PPIs as the gastroprotective drugs of choice (see p.19).[11] H$_2$-receptor antagonists are second-line treatment for gastro-esophageal reflux disease, non-ulcer dyspepsia and uninvestigated dyspepsia.

The dose and duration of treatment is least with duodenal ulceration and most with reflux esophagitis and prophylaxis for NSAID-induced peptic ulcer, although the dose for ulcer healing can be doubled if the initial response is poor (Table 1.6). **Ranitidine** is more effective if taken at bedtime rather than with the evening meal.[12] Parenteral formulations are available for IM and IV use if treatment is considered necessary in a patient with severe nausea and vomiting. Some centres use 50mg SC b.i.d.–q.i.d. (off-label route) without evidence of local inflammation.

In renal impairment, the dose of **cimetidine** should be adjusted according to creatinine clearance (Table 1.7). **Cimetidine** is removed by hemodialysis, but not by peritoneal dialysis. For **ranitidine**, reduce the dose to 150mg at bedtime in severe renal impairment, (creatinine clearance < 30mL/min) but increase to 150mg b.i.d. if an ulcer fails to respond at the lower dose.

Table 1.6 Recommended treatment regimens for H$_2$-receptor antagonists

Indication	Cimetidine	Ranitidine
Duodenal ulcer[a,b]	400mg b.i.d. or 800mg at bedtime for 4+ weeks	150mg b.i.d. or 300mg at bedtime for 4–8 weeks
Gastric ulcer[a,b]	400mg b.i.d. or 800mg at bedtime for 6+ weeks	150mg b.i.d. or 300mg at bedtime for 4–8 weeks
Prophylaxis for NSAID-associated peptic ulcer	800mg b.i.d. indefinitely	300mg b.i.d. indefinitely
Reflux esophagitis	400mg q.i.d. for 4–8 weeks	150mg b.i.d. or 300mg at bedtime for 8–12 weeks
†Short bowel syndrome	400mg b.i.d. or 800mg at bedtime indefinitely	
†To reduce degradation of pancreatin supplements	200–400mg 1h a.c.	150mg 1h a.c.

a. 8 weeks for NSAID-induced ulcer
b. dose can be doubled if initial response is poor.

Table 1.7 Dose adjustment for cimetidine in renal impairment

Creatinine clearance (mL/min)	Dose of cimetidine
>50	No change in dose
30–50	200mg q.i.d.
15–30	200mg t.i.d.
0–15	200mg b.i.d.

Supply
Cimetidine (generic)
Tablets 200mg, 300mg, 400mg, 600mg, 800mg, 28 days @ 400mg b.i.d. or 800mg at bedtime = $8 and $7 respectively.

Ranitidine (generic)
Tablets 150mg, 300mg, 28 days @ 150mg b.i.d. or 300mg at bedtime = $23 and $22 respectively.
Oral solution 75mg/5mL, 28 days @ 150mg b.i.d. = $66.
Injection 25mg/mL, 2mL amp = $2.50.

Zantac$^®$ (GSK)
Tablets 150mg, 300mg, 28 days @ 150mg b.i.d. or 300mg at bedtime = $11; *a 75mg Zantac$^®$ tablet is available OTC.*
Oral solution (sugar-free) 75mg/5mL, 28 days @ 150mg b.i.d. = $125; contains 7.5% alcohol, mint flavour.
Injection 25mg/mL, 2mL amp = $3.

1 Williams JG and Strunin L (1985) Pre-operative intramuscular ranitidine and cimetidine. Double blind comparative trial, effect on gastric pH and volume. *Anaesthesia.* **40**: 242–245.
2 Mojaverian P et al. (1982) Cimetidine does not alter morphine disposition in man. *British Journal of Clinical Pharmacology.* **14**: 809–813.
3 Hollander D (1994) Gastrointestinal complications of nonsteroidal anti-inflammatory drugs: prophylactic and therapeutic strategies. *American Journal of Medicine.* **96**: 274–281.
4 Rostom A et al. (2002) Prevention of NSAID-induced gastroduodenal ulcers. *Cochrane Database Systematic Review.* **10**: CD002296.
5 Yeomans N et al. (1998) A comparison of omeprazole with ranitidine for ulcers associated with nonsteroidal anti-inflammatory drugs. Acid suppression trial. *New England Journal of Medicine.* **338**: 719–726.
6 Hawkins C and Hanks G (2000) The gastroduodenal toxicity of nonsteroidal anti-inflammatory drugs. A review of the literature. *Journal of Pain and Symptom Management.* **20**: 140–151.
7 Hooper L et al. (2004) The effectiveness of five strategies for the prevention of gastrointestinal toxicity induced by non-steroidal anti-inflammatory drugs: systematic review. *British Medical Journal.* **329**: 948.

8 Baxter K (ed) (2006) *Stockley's Drug Interactions* (7e). Pharmaceutical Press, London.
9 Sorkin E and Ogawa C (1983) Cimetidine potentiation of narcotic action. *Drug Intelligence and Clinical Pharmacy.* **17**: 60–61.
10 Leontiadis GI et al. (2005) Systematic review and meta-analysis of proton pump inhibitor therapy in peptic ulcer bleeding. *British Medical Journal.* **330**: 568.
11 NICE (2004) Dyspepsia. Management of dyspepsia in adults in primary care. In: *Clinical Guideline 17.* National Institute for Clinical Excellence. Available from: www.nice.org.uk/page.aspx?o=CG017
12 Johnston DA and Wormsley KG (1988) The effect of food on ranitidine-induced inhibition of nocturnal gastric secretion. *Alimentary Pharmacology and Therapeutics.* **2**: 507–511.

MISOPROSTOL

Class: Prostaglandin analogue, gastroprotective drug.

Indications: Healing of duodenal ulcers, prevention and healing of NSAID-induced gastric and duodenal ulcers.

Contra-indications: Women of childbearing potential should not be started on misoprostol until pregnancy is excluded (misoprostol increases uterine tone).

Pharmacology

Misoprostol is a synthetic PG analogue with gastric antisecretory and protective properties. After oral administration, it is rapidly converted to an active free acid. Misoprostol helps *prevent* NSAID-related gastroduodenal erosions and ulcers.[1–3] In relation to *healing* NSAID-related gastroduodenal injury, misoprostol and PPIs are equally effective.[4] In one RCT, PPIs were more effective at preventing relapse (relapse rate: PPI 39%, misoprostol 52%, placebo 73%).[4] However, a systematic review indicates that the evidence for prophylactic benefit is much stronger for misoprostol than for PPIs.[3] The use of misoprostol is limited by its tendency to cause diarrhea and intestinal colic.

Bio-availability 90% PO.
Onset of action <30min.
Time to peak plasma concentration 30min.
Plasma halflife 1–2h for free acid.
Duration of action 2–4h.

Cautions

Women of childbearing age should use effective contraception.
Conditions where hypotension might precipitate severe complications, e.g. cerebrovascular disease, cardiovascular disease.

Undesirable effects

For full list, see manufacturer's Product Monograph.
Diarrhea (may necessitate stopping treatment), colic, dyspepsia, flatulence, nausea and vomiting, abnormal vaginal bleeding (intermenstrual, menorrhagia, postmenopausal), rashes, dizziness.

Dose and use

Cochrane review: Misoprostol, PPIs, and double-dose H$_2$-receptor antagonists are effective at *preventing* chronic NSAID-related endoscopic peptic ulcers. Misoprostol 400microgram daily is less effective than 800microgram and is still associated with diarrhea. Of all these treatments, only misoprostol 800microgram daily has been definitely shown to reduce the overall incidence of ulcer complications (perforation, hemorrhage or obstruction).[5] PPIs definitely reduce the incidence of re-bleeding from endoscopically confirmed peptic ulcers,[6] and may reduce the incidence of ulcer complications.[3]

NSAID-associated ulcers may be treated with an H$_2$-receptor antagonist, a PPI or misoprostol. In most cases, the causal NSAID need not be discontinued during treatment.[4,7] Consideration should be given to switching to a less toxic NSAID (see p.248).

Prophylaxis against NSAID-induced ulcers
200microgram b.i.d.–q.i.d. taken with the NSAID.

NSAID-associated ulceration
- 200microgram t.i.d. with meals & at bedtime *or*
- 400microgram b.i.d. (breakfast and bedtime) for 4–8 weeks.[1]

If causes diarrhea, give 200microgram t.i.d. & at bedtime; avoid **magnesium salts**.

Supply
Misoprostol (generic)
Tablets 200microgram, 28 days @ 200microgram b.i.d. = $25.

1 Bardhan KD et al. (1993) The prevention and healing of acute NSAID-associated gastroduodenal mucosal damage by misoprostol. British Journal of Rheumatology. **32**: 990–995.
2 Silverstein FE et al. (1995) Misoprostol reduces serious gastrointestinal complications in patients with rheumatoid arthritis receiving nonsteroidal anti-inflammatory drugs. Annals of internal medicine. **123**: 241–249.
3 Hooper L et al. (2004) The effectiveness of five strategies for the prevention of gastrointestinal toxicity induced by non-steroidal anti-inflammatory drugs: systematic review. British Medical Journal. **329**: 948.
4 Hawkey C et al. (1998) Omeprazole compared with misoprostol for ulcers associated with nonsteroidal anti-inflammatory drugs. New England Journal of Medicine. **338**: 727–734.
5 Rostom A et al. (2002) Prevention of NSAID-induced gastroduodenal ulcers. Cochrane Database Systematic Reviews. **10**: CD002296.
6 Leontiadis GI et al. (2005) Systematic review and meta-analysis of proton pump inhibitor therapy in peptic ulcer bleeding. British Medical Journal. **330**: 568.
7 Hawkins C and Hanks G (2000) The gastroduodenal toxicity of nonsteroidal anti-inflammatory drugs. A review of the literature. Journal of Pain and Symptom Management. **20**: 140–151.

PROTON PUMP INHIBITORS

Class: Gastroprotective drugs.

Indications: Licensed indications vary between products; consult the manufacturers' product monographs for details; they include acid dyspepsia, acid reflux, peptic ulceration, prevention and treatment of NSAID-induced ulceration, eradication of *Helicobacter pylori* (with antibiotics).

Pharmacology
Proton pump inhibitors (PPIs) reduce gastric acid output but, in contrast to H_2-receptor antagonists, do not reduce the volume of gastric secretions. Because they are all rapidly degraded by acid, they are formulated as EC granules or tablets. These dissolve in the duodenum where the drug is rapidly absorbed to be selectively taken up by gastric parietal cells and converted into active metabolites. These irreversibly inhibit the proton pump (H^+/K^+-ATPase) and thereby block gastric acid secretion. Elimination is predominantly by metabolism in the liver to inactive derivatives excreted mainly in the urine. The plasma halflives of PPIs are mostly < 2h but, because they irreversibly inhibit the proton pump, the antisecretory activity continues for several days until new proton pumps are synthesized.

When treating peptic ulceration **lansoprazole** 30mg daily is as effective as **omeprazole** 40mg daily, and **pantoprazole** 40mg daily is as effective as **omeprazole** 20mg daily.[1] However, **omeprazole** shows a dose-response curve above the standard dose of 20mg daily, whereas no further benefit is seen by increasing the dose of **lansoprazole** and **pantoprazole** above 30mg and 40mg daily respectively.[2,3] Thus, **omeprazole** 40mg daily is superior to **lansoprazole** 60mg daily and **pantoprazole** 80mg daily in the management of severe gastro-esophageal reflux disease (esophagitis and stricture).[4]

The bio-availability of **lansoprazole** is reduced by food and the manufacturer recommends that it should be given each morning 1h before breakfast. However, the reduced bio-availability appears not to reduce efficacy.[5–7] In one study comparing **lansoprazole** given either before or after food, acid suppression was comparable with both regimens after 1 week (although on day 1 it was significantly less when taken after food).[8] Pharmacokinetic data are shown in Table 1.8.

Onset of action <2h.

Duration of action >1 day.

Table 1.8 Pharmacokinetic details of PPIs given PO[9]

	Bio-availability (%)	Time to peak plasma concentration (h)	Plasma halflife (h)
Esomeprazole	64 (40mg single dose) 89 (40mg once daily for 5 days)	1–2	1.2 for 20mg 1.5 for 40mg
Lansoprazole	80–90	1.5–2	1–2
Omeprazole	60	3–6	0.5–3
Pantoprazole	77	2–2.5	1[a]
Rabeprazole	52	1.6–5	1

a. increases to 3–6h in cirrhosis.

Cautions

Serious undesirable drug reactions: ocular damage,[10] impaired hearing, angina, hypertension. Most cases of ocular damage have been reported with IV **omeprazole**.[11] PPIs possibly cause vasoconstriction by blocking H^+/K^+-ATPase. Because the retinal artery is an end-artery, anterior ischemic optic neuropathy may result. If the PPI is stopped, visual acuity may improve. Some patients have become permanently blind, in some instances after 3 days. Impaired hearing and deafness have also been reported, again mostly with IV **omeprazole**. A similar mechanism may be responsible for the angina and hypertension included in the US manufacturer's list of undesirable effects for **omeprazole**.

Severe hepatic impairment. Note: concern about serious cardiac events (infarction, death) with esomeprazole and omeprazole is now considered to be groundless.[12]

All PPIs increase gastric pH, and this can affect the absorption of other drugs. The European Medicines Agency (EMEA) recommends that PPIs should not be used concurrently with **atazanavir**, because of a study in which **omeprazole** reduced the trough plasma concentrations and AUC of **atazanavir** by 75%. Increasing the **atazanavir** dose by 33% did not compensate for this decrease.[13] **Omeprazole** also reduces **indinavir** levels, and should not be used concurrently.[14] Further, **omeprazole** and **rabeprazole** decrease the absorption of **ketoconazole**; **omeprazole** also reduces the absorption of **itraconazole** from capsules but not oral solution. Increased azole doses may be necessary to avoid treatment failure; alternatively, giving the azole with an acidic drink, e.g. Cola, minimizes the interaction.[14] Conversely, increased gastric pH with **omeprazole** increases the bio-availability of **digoxin** by 10%.[14]

PPIs are metabolized by the CYP450 family of liver enzymes (see Cytochrome P450, p.551). However, clinically important interactions are rare with PPIs.[15,16] Sedation and gait disturbances have been reported when **omeprazole** was given with **diazepam**, **flurazepam**, or **lorazepam**. **Omeprazole** levels are increased by some macrolides (**clarithromycin**, **erythromycin**) and azole antifungals (**fluconazole**, **ketoconazole**, **voriconazole**).[14]

The antithrombotic effect of **clopidogrel** (a pro-drug activated by CYP2C19) is reduced by concurrent administration with a PPI, including **rabeprazole**.[17–19] The evidence in relation to **pantoprazole** is equivocal.[17,18] Although **pantoprazole** is said not to inhibit CYP2C19,[18] and thus could be safe in this respect, the safest option would be to prescribe an H_2-receptor antagonist instead. e.g. **ranitidine**. No other significant CYP450 drug–drug interactions have been identified with **pantoprazole** or **rabeprazole**.[14,20]

Undesirable effects

For full list, see manufacturer's Product Monograph.

Common (<10%, >1%): headache, abdominal pain, nausea, vomiting, diarrhea or constipation, flatulence.

Dose and use

Cochrane review: PPIs, **misoprostol**, and double-dose H_2-receptor antagonists are effective at *preventing* chronic NSAID-related endoscopic peptic ulcers. **Misoprostol** 400microgram daily is less effective than 800microgram and is still associated with diarrhea. Of all these treatments, only **misoprostol** 800microgram daily has been definitely shown to reduce the overall incidence of ulcer complications (perforation, hemorrhage or obstruction).[21] PPIs definitely reduce the incidence of re-bleeding from endoscopically confirmed peptic ulcers,[22] and may reduce the incidence of ulcer complications.[23]

PPIs are preferable to H_2-receptor antagonists for the treatment of dyspepsia, gastro-esophageal reflux disease and peptic ulcers, including NSAID-induced peptic ulcers (for comparison with H_2-receptor antagonists, see Table 1.5, p.16).[24] PPIs are used together with antibiotics for the eradication of *Helicobacter pylori* (see p.367).

The choice of PPI is often determined by the local Drug and Therapeutics Committee, with cost being the overriding consideration. However, **pantoprazole** (available in PO and parenteral formulations) and **rabeprazole** (available only in PO formulations) cause fewer drug-drug interactions, and are preferable from a purely clinical perspective. For recommended dose regimens, see the manufacturers' Product Monographs.

Omeprazole has been used in the management of acute bleeding from an endoscopically proven peptic ulcer, either PO or IV.[22] **Omeprazole** has been used parenterally in palliative care to treat painful reflux esophagitis in patients too ill or unable to take PO medication. Although not approved for SC administration, it has been used successfully by this route for ≤4 days.[25]

Supply

Pantoprazole (generic)
Tablets EC 20mg, 40mg, 28 days @ 40mg each morning = $39.
Injection (powder for reconstitution with 0.9% saline and use as an IV injection/infusion) 40mg vial = $11.

Pantoloc® (Altana)
Tablets EC 20mg, 40mg, 28 days @ 40mg each morning = $61.
Injection (powder for reconstitution with 0.9% saline and use as an IV injection/infusion) 40mg vial = $15.

Rabeprazole (generic)
Tablets EC 10mg, 20mg, 28 days @ 20mg each morning = $28.

Pariet® (Janssen-Ortho)
Tablets EC 10mg, 20mg, @ 20mg each morning = $39.

Esomeprazole magnesium trihydrate
Nexium® (AstraZeneca)
Delayed release tablet 20mg, 40mg, 28 days @ 40mg each morning = $63.
Sachet of EC delayed release granules (for dispersal in water) 10mg/sachet, 28 days @ 20mg each morning = $126.

Lansoprazole (generic)
Delayed release capsules 15mg, 30mg, 28 days @ 30mg each morning = $42.

Prevacid® (Tap Pharmaceuticals)
Delayed release capsules enclosing EC granules 15mg, 30mg, 28 days @ 30mg each morning = $60.
Delayed release tablets orodispersible (FasTab®) strawberry flavour 15mg, 30mg, 28 days @ 30mg each morning = $60.

Omeprazole (generic)
Capsules enclosing EC granules 10mg, 20mg, 28 days @ 20mg each morning = $31.

Losec® (AstraZeneca)
Delayed release capsules 10mg, 20mg, 28 days @ 20mg each morning = $33.
Delayed release tablets 10mg, 20mg, 28 days @ 20mg each morning = $66.

1 DTB (1997) Pantoprazole – a third proton pump inhibitor. *Drug and Therapeutics Bulletin.* **35**: 93–94.
2 Dammann H *et al.* (1993) The effects of lansoprazole, 30 or 60mg daily, on intragastric pH and on endocrine function in healthy volunteers. *Alimentary Pharmacology and Therapeutics.* **7**: 191–196.
3 Koop H *et al.* (1996) Intragastric pH and serum gastrin during administration of different doses of pantoprazole in healthy subjects. *European Journal of Gastroenterology and Hepatology.* **8**: 915–918.
4 Jaspersen D *et al.* (1998) A comparison of omeprazole, lansoprazole and pantoprazole in the maintenance treatment of severe reflux oesophagitis. *Alimentary Pharmacology and Therapeutics.* **12**: 49–52.
5 Andersson T (1990) Bioavailability of omeprazole as enteric coated (EC) granules in conjunction with food on the first and seventh days of treatment. *Drug Investigations.* **2**: 184–188.
6 Delhotal-Landes B *et al.* (1991) The effect of food and antacids on lansoprazole absorption and disposition. *European Journal of Drug Metabolism and Pharmacokinetics.* **3**: 315–320.
7 Moules I *et al.* (1993) Gastric acid inhibition by the proton pump inhibitor lansoprazole is unaffected by food. *British Journal of Clinical Research.* **4**: 153–161.
8 Brummer RJM and Geerling BJ (1995) Acute and chronic effect of lansoprazole and omeprazole in relation to food intake. *Gut.* **37**: 127.
9 Anonymous (2007) Compendium of Pharmaceuticals and Specialities: The Canadian Drug Reference for Health Professionals. *Canadian Pharmacists Association, Ottawa.*
10 Schonhofer P *et al.* (1997) Ocular damage associated with proton pump inhibitors. *British Medical Journal.* **314**: 1805.
11 Schonhofer P (1994) Intravenous omeprazole and blindness. *Lancet.* **343**: 665.
12 Health Canada (2008). Available from: www.hc-sc.gc.ca/ahc-asc/media/advisories-avis/_2008/2008_34-eng.php
13 European Agency for the Evaluation of Medicinal Products (2004) Important new pharmacokinetic data demostrating that REYATAZ (atazanavir sulphate) combined with NORVIR (ritonavir) and omeprazole should not be co-administered. In: *EMEA public statement.* Available from: www.emea.europa.eu/pdfs/human/press/pus/20264904en.pdf
14 Baxter K (ed) (2006) *Stockley's Drug Interactions* (7e). Pharmaceutical Press, London.
15 Andersson T (1996) Pharmacokinetics, metabolism and interactions of acid pump inhibitors. Focus on omeprazole, lansoprazole and pantoprazole. *Clinical Pharmacokinetics.* **31**: 9–28.
16 Tucker G (1994) The interaction of proton pump inhibitors with cytochrome P450. *Alimentary Pharmacology and Therapeutics.* **8**: 33–38.
17 Ho M *et al.* (2009) Risk of adverse outcomes associated with concomitant use of clopidogrel and proton pump inhibitors following acute coronary syndrome. *Journal of the American Medical Association.* **301**: 937–944.
18 Juurlink DN *et al.* (2009) A population-based study of the drug interaction between proton pump inhibitors and clopidogrel. *Canadian Medical Association Journal.* **180**: 713–718.
19 Society for Cardiovascular Angiography and Interventions (2009) A national study of the effect of individual proton pump inhibitors on cardiovascular outcomes in patients treated with clopidogrel following coronary stenting: The Clopidogrel Medco Outcomes Study. Available from: www.scai.org/drlt1.aspx?PAGE_ID=5870
20 Steinijans W (1996) Lack of pantoprazole drug interactions in man: an updated review. *International Journal of Clinical Pharmacology and Therapeutics.* **34**: S31–S50.
21 Rostom A *et al.* (2002) Prevention of NSAID-induced gastroduodenal ulcers. *Cochrane Database Systematic Review.* **10**: CD002296.
22 Leontiadis GI *et al.* (2005) Systematic review and meta-analysis of proton pump inhibitor therapy in peptic ulcer bleeding. *British Medical Journal.* **330**: 568.
23 Hooper L *et al.* (2004) The effectiveness of five strategies for the prevention of gastrointestinal toxicity induced by non-steroidal anti-inflammatory drugs: systematic review. *British Medical Journal.* **329**: 948.
24 NICE (2004) Dyspepsia. Management of dyspepsia in adults in primary care. In: *Clinical Guideline 17.* National Institute for Clinical Excellence. Available from: www.nice.org.uk/page.aspx?o=CG017
25 Agar M *et al.* (2004) The use of subcutaneous omeprazole in the treatment of dyspepsia in palliative care patients. *Journal of Pain and Symptom Management.* **28**: 529–531.

LOPERAMIDE

Class: Antidiarrheal.

Indications: Acute non-specific diarrhea; chronic diarrhea associated with inflammatory bowel disease; reducing volume of discharge for ileostomies, colostomies and other intestinal resections.

Contra-indications: Colitis (ulcerative, infective, or antibiotic-associated).

Pharmacology

Loperamide is a potent μ-opioid receptor agonist.[1] Although well absorbed from the GI tract, it is almost completely metabolized by the liver where it is conjugated and excreted via the bile. Further, although highly lipophilic,[2] loperamide is a substrate for the efflux membrane transporter, P-glycoprotein, in the blood-brain barrier and it is actively excluded from the CNS.[3,4] Consequently, loperamide acts almost exclusively via a local effect in the GI tract[1] and the maximum therapeutic impact may not manifest for 16–24h, which has implications for dosing.[4]

Loperamide also has an effect on other peripheral μ-opioid receptors, including those which are activated in the presence of inflammation.[5] Accordingly, it is currently under investigation as a possible topical analgesic for painful skin ulcers.

Like **morphine** and other μ-receptor agonists, loperamide decreases propulsive intestinal activity and increases non-propulsive activity.[2,6] It also has an intestinal antisecretory effect mediated by calmodulin antagonism, which is a property not shared by other opioids.[7–9] Paradoxically, loperamide also reduces sodium-dependent uptake of glucose and other nutrients from the small GI tract.[10] Tolerance does not occur. Unlike **diphenoxylate**, loperamide has no analgesic effect in therapeutic and supratherapeutic doses (but see Cautions). CNS effects have been observed rarely in children under 2 years of age who received excessive doses.[11,12] Loperamide is about 3 times more potent than **diphenoxylate** and 50 times more potent than **codeine**.[13] as an antidiarrheal agent. It is longer acting and, if used regularly, generally needs to be given only b.i.d. The following regimens are approximately equivalent:
- loperamide 2mg b.i.d.
- **diphenoxylate** 2.5mg q.i.d. (in **diphenoxylate/atropine**, e.g. Lomotil®)
- **codeine phosphate** 60mg q.i.d.

Bio-availability 10% PO.
Onset of action about 1h; maximum effect 16–24h.[14]
Time to peak plasma concentration 2.5h (oral solution); 4–6h (caplets, capsules, tablets).[15,16]
Plasma halflife 11h.[15]
Duration of action up to 3 days.[17]

Cautions

Inhibitors of P-glycoprotein (e.g. **cyclosporine, clarithromycin, erythromycin, intraconazole, ketoconazole, quinidine, ritonavir, verapamil**) may allow loperamide to cross the blood-brain barrier and thus potentially manifest central opioid effects.[3] Although available evidence is inconclusive for individual drugs, caution should be exercised when using loperamide with any medication known to inhibit P-gycoprotein. Severe hepatic impairment leads to increased plasma concentrations with a risk of CNS effects.

Undesirable effects

For full list, see manufacturer's Product Monograph.
Excessive use of loperamide may cause symptomatic constipation or fecal impaction associated with overflow diarrhea and/or urinary retention.

A patient on **clozapine** (an atypical antipsychotic) died of toxic megacolon after taking loperamide during an episode of food poisoning. Additive inhibition of intestinal motility was considered the precipitating cause.[18]

Dose and use

Ensure that the diarrhea is not secondary to fecal impaction.

Acute diarrhea
- start with 4mg PO stat
- continue with 2mg after each loose bowel action for up to 5 days
- maximum recommended dose 16mg/24h.

Chronic diarrhea
If symptomatic treatment is appropriate, the same initial approach is used for 2–3 days, after which a prophylactic b.i.d. regimen is instituted based on the needs of the patient during the previous 24h, plus 2mg after each loose bowel action. The effective dose varies widely. In palliative care, it is occasionally necessary to increase the dose to as much as 32mg/24h; *this is twice the recommended maximum daily dose.*

Supply

Loperamide (generic)
Tablets 2mg, 28 days @ 2mg q.i.d. = $43; also available OTC.
Oral solution 1mg/5mL, 28 days @ 2mg q.i.d. = $188; also available OTC.

Imodium® (McNeil)
Caplets 2mg, 28 days @ 2mg q.i.d. = $101; also available OTC.
Quick dissolve tablets 2mg, 28 days @ 2mg q.i.d. = $121; also available OTC.
Oral solution 2mg/15mL, 28 days @ 2mg q.i.d. = $102 OTC.

1 Shannon H and Lutz E (2002) Comparison of the peripheral and central effects of the opioid agonists loperamide and morphine in the formalin test in rats. *Neuropharmacology.* **42**: 253–261.
2 Ooms L *et al.* (1984) Mechanisms of action of loperamide. *Scandinavian Journal of Gastroenterology.* **19 (suppl 96)**: 145–155.
3 Heykants J *et al.* (1974) Loperamide (R 18553), a novel type of antidiarrheal agent. Part 5: The pharmacokinetics of loperamide in rats and man. *Arzneimittel-Forschung.* **24**: 1649–1653.
4 Sadeque A *et al.* (2000) Increased drug delivery to the brain by P-glycoprotein inhibition. *Clinical Pharmacology and Therapeutics.* **68**: 231–237.
5 Nozaki-Taguchi N and Yaksh TL (1999) Characterization of the antihyperalgesic action of a novel peripheral mu-opioid receptor agonist–loperamide. *Anesthesiology.* **90**: 225–234.
6 Van Nueten JM *et al.* (1974) Loperamide (R 18553), a novel type of antidiarrheal agent. Part 3: *In vitro* studies on the peristaltic reflex and other experiments on isolated tissues. *Arzneimittel-Forschung.* **24**: 1641–1645.
7 Merritt J *et al.* (1982) Loperamide and calmodulin. *Lancet.* **1**: 283.
8 Zavecz J *et al.* (1982) Relationship between anti-diarrheal activity and binding to calmodulin. *European Journal of Pharmacology.* **78**: 375–377.
9 Daly J and Harper J (2000) Loperamide: novel effects on capacitative calcium influx. *Cellular and Molecular Life Sciences.* **57**: 149–157.
10 Klaren P *et al.* (2000) Effect of loperamide on Na+/D-glucose cotransporter activity in mouse small intestine. *Journal of Pharmacy and Pharmacology.* **52**: 679–686.
11 Friedli G and Haenggeli CA (1980) Loperamide overdose managed by naloxone. *Lancet.* **ii**: 1413.
12 Minton N and Smith P (1987) Loperamide toxicity in a child after a single dose. *British Medical Journal.* **294**: 1383.
13 Schuermans V *et al.* (1974) Loperamide (R18553), a novel type of antidiarrhoeal agent. Part 6: clinical pharmacology. Placebo-controlled comparison of the constipating activity and safety of loperamide, diphenoxylate and codeine in normal volunteers. *Arzneimittel-Forschung Drug Research.* **24**: 1653–1657.
14 Dreverman JWM and van der Poel AJ (1995) Loperamide oxide in acute diarrhoea: a double-blind placebo-controlled trial. *Alimentary Pharmacology and Therapeutics.* **9**: 441–446.
15 Killinger J *et al.* (1979) Human pharmacokinetics and comparative bioavailability of loperamide hydrochloride. *Journal of Clinical Pharmacology.* **19**: 211–218.
16 McNeil Consumer and Specialty Pharmaceuticals (2006). *Data on file.*
17 Heel R *et al.* (1978) Loperamide: A review of its pharmacological properties and therapeutic efficacy in diarrhoea. *Drugs.* **15**: 33–52.
18 Eronen M *et al.* (2003) Lethal gastroenteritis associated with clozapine and loperamide. *American Journal of Psychiatry.* **160**: 2242–2243.

LAXATIVES

Constipation is common in advanced cancer,[1] particularly in immobile patients with small appetites and those receiving constipating drugs such as opioids.[2,3] Exercise and increased dietary fibre are rarely feasible options.[4] Although some strong opioids are less constipating than **morphine** (e.g. **fentanyl**),[5] most patients receiving any opioid regularly will need a laxative concurrently.[1] Thus, as a general rule, all patients prescribed **morphine** (or other opioid) should also be prescribed a laxative (see Guidelines, p.26).

About 1/3 of patients also need rectal measures[6,7] either because of failed oral treatment or electively, e.g. in bedbound debilitated elderly patients, or patients with paralysis (see Guidelines, p.27).

There are several classes of laxatives (Box 1.E).[8,9] At doses commonly used, **docusate sodium** acts mainly by lowering surface tension, thus enabling water to percolate into the substance of the feces; at higher doses it will also act as a contact (stimulant) laxative (see p.29).

Opioids cause constipation by decreasing propulsive intestinal activity and increasing non-propulsive activity, and also by enhancing the absorption of fluid and electrolytes.[2,10] Contact (stimulant) laxatives reduce intestinal ring contractions and thus facilitate propulsive activity. In this way, they provide a logical approach to the correction of opioid-induced constipation. However, in practice, a combination of a peristaltic stimulant and a fecal softener is often prescribed,[11,12] although a recent study found no additional benefit when docusate was added to sennosides.[13]

> **Box 1.E**   Classification of commonly used laxatives
>
> **Bulk-forming agents (fibre)**
> Methylcellulose
> Psyllium husk, (e.g. Metamucil®)
> Sterculia (e.g. Normacol®)
>
> **Lubricants**
> Mineral oil
>
> **Surface-wetting agents**
> Docusate sodium
> Docusate calcium
>
> **Osmotic laxatives**
> Lactulose syrup
> Magnesium hydroxide suspension (Milk of Magnesia®)
> Magnesium sulfate (Epsom Salts)
> Magnesium citrate (Citro-Mag)
>
> **Contact (stimulant) laxatives**
> Bisacodyl
> Sennosides

Few RCTs of laxatives have been completed in palliative care patients:
- **sennosides** vs. **lactulose**[14]
- **sennosides** vs. **misrakasneham** (an Ayurvedic herbal remedy)[15]
- **sennosides–lactulose** vs. **magnesium hydroxide–mineral oil**.[16]

There were no significant differences between these treatments.

1 Miles C *et al.* (2005) Laxatives for the management of constipation in palliative care patients
2 Kurz A and Sessler DI (2003) Opioid-induced bowel dysfunction: pathophysiology and potential new therapies. *Drugs.* **63**: 649–671.
3 Pappagallo M (2001) Incidence, prevalence, and management of opioid bowel dysfunction. *American Journal of Surgery.* **182 (suppl 5A)**: 11s–18s.
4 Mancini IL *et al.* (2000) Opioid type and other clinical predictors of laxative dose in advanced cancer patients: a retrospective study. *Journal of Palliative Medicine.* **3**: 49–56.
5 Radbruch L *et al.* (2000) Constipation and the use of laxatives: a comparison between transdermal fentanyl and oral morphine. *Palliative Medicine.* **14**: 111–119.
6 Twycross RG and Lack SA (1986) *Control of Alimentary Symptoms in Far Advanced Cancer.* Churchill Livingstone, Edinburgh, pp. 173–174.
7 Twycross RG and Harcourt JMV (1991) The use of laxatives at a palliative care centre. *Palliative Medicine.* **5**: 27–33.
8 Tramonte S *et al.* (1997) The treatment of chronic constipation in adults. A systematic review. *Journal of General Internal Medicine.* **12**: 15–24.
9 Kamm MA (2003) Constipation and its management. *British Medical Journal.* **327**: 459–460.
10 Beubler E (1983) Opiates and intestinal transport: *in vivo* studies. In: LA Turnberg (ed) *Intestinal secretion.* Smith Kline and French, Herefordshire, pp. 53–55.
11 Avila JG (2004) Pharmacologic treatment of constipation in cancer patients. *Cancer Control.* **11**: 10–18.
12 McMillan SC (2004) Assessing and managing opiate-induced constipation in adults with cancer. *Cancer Control.* **11**: 3–9.
13 Hawley PH and Byeon JJ (2008) A comparison of sennosides-based bowel protocols with and without docusate in hospitalized patients with cancer. *Journal of Palliative Medicine.* **11**: 575–581.
14 Agra Y *et al.* (1998) Efficacy of senna versus lactulose in terminal cancer patients treatment with opioids. *Journal of Pain and Symptom Management.* **15**: 1–7.
15 Ramesh P *et al.* (1998) Managing morphine-induced constipation: a controlled comparison of an Ayurvedic formulation and senna. *Journal of Pain and Symptom Management.* **16**: 240–244.
16 Sykes N (1991) A clinical comparison of lactulose and senna with magnesium hydroxide and liquid paraffin emulsion in a palliative care population. [Cited in Miles CL *et al.* (2006) Laxatives for the management of constipation in palliative care patients. The Cochrane Database of Systematic Reviews. CD003448]

Guidelines: Opioid-induced constipation

Most patients taking an opioid need a laxative. Thus, as a general rule, all patients prescribed an opioid should also be prescribed a laxative, with the aim of achieving a regular bowel movement without straining every 1–3 days.

A standardized protocol is likely to enhance management. However, occasionally, rather than automatically changing to sennosides (see below), it may be more appropriate to optimize a patient's existing regimen.

1 Ask about the patient's past and present bowel habit and use of laxatives; record the date of last bowel movement.

2 Palpate for fecal masses in the line of the colon; examine the rectum digitally if the bowels have not been open for >3 days or if the patient reports rectal discomfort or has diarrhea suggestive of fecal impaction with overflow.

3 For inpatients, keep a daily record of bowel movements.

4 Encourage fluids generally, and fruit juice and fruit specifically.

5 When an opioid is prescribed, unless contra-indicated (e.g. bowel obstruction), also prescribe sennosides:
   • generally start with 17.2mg at bedtime and each morning
   • if no response after 24 hours, increase to 25.8mg at bedtime and each morning
   • if no response after a further 24 hours, consider adding a third daytime dose
   • if necessary, consider increasing to a maximum of 34.4mg t.i.d.

6 During dose titration and subsequently, if ⩾3 days since last bowel movement, give laxative suppositories, e.g. glycerin 2.6g and bisacodyl 10mg, or a micro-enema. If these are ineffective, administer a phosphate enema and possibly repeat the next day.

7 If the maximum dose of sennosides is ineffective:
   • halve the dose and add an osmotic laxative, e.g. lactulose 20mL b.i.d. or magnesium hydroxide (Milk of Magnesia®) 15–30mL b.i.d., and titrate as necessary *or*
   • prescribe SC methylnaltrexone.

Methylnaltrexone

Because constipation in advanced disease is generally multifactorial in origin, methylnaltrexone ($41 per 12mg vial) is likely to augment rather than replace laxatives.
• marketed as a SC injection for use in patients with 'advanced illness' and opioid-induced constipation despite treatment with laxatives
• 50% of patients given methylnaltrexone have a bowel movement within 4 hours, without loss of analgesia or the development of opioid withdrawal symptoms
• dose recommendations:
   ▷ for patients weighing 38–61kg, start with 8mg on alternate days
   ▷ for patients weighing 62–114kg, start with 12mg on alternate days
   ▷ outside this range, give 150*microgram*/kg on alternate days
   ▷ the interval between administrations can be varied, either extended or reduced, but not more than once daily
• in severe renal impairment (creatinine clearance < 30mL/minute) reduce the dose:
   ▷ for patients weighing 38–61kg, reduce to 4mg
   ▷ for patients weighing 62–114kg, reduce to 6mg
   ▷ outside this range, reduce to 75*microgram*/kg, rounding up the dose volume to the nearest 0.1mL
• methylnaltrexone is contra-indicated in cases of known or suspected GI obstruction
• common undesirable effects include abdominal pain, diarrhoea, flatulence, and nausea; these generally resolve after a bowel movement.

---

8 Alternatively, switch completely to an osmotic laxative, e.g. lactulose 20–40mL b.i.d.–t.i.d. or magnesium hydroxide (Milk of Magnesia®) 15–60mL b.i.d.

9 An osmotic laxative (lactulose, magnesium hydroxide) may be preferable in patients with a history of colic with stimulant laxatives (senna, bisacodyl).

Guidelines: Bowel management in paraplegia and tetraplegia

Theoretically, management is determined by the level of the spinal cord lesion:
- above T12–L1 = cauda equina intact → spastic GI tract with preserved sacral reflex; generally responds to digital stimulation of the rectum; the presence of an anal reflex suggests an intact sacral reflex
- below T12–L1 = cauda equina involved → flaccid GI tract; generally requires digital evacuation of the rectum
- a lesion at the level of the conus medullaris (the cone shaped distal end of the spinal cord, surrounded by the sacral nerves) may manifest a mixture of clinical features.

However, in practice, management tends to follow a common pathway.

Aims

1 Primary: to achieve the controlled regular evacuation of normal formed feces:
- every day in long-term paraplegia/tetraplegia, e.g. post-traumatic
- every 1–3 days in advanced cancer.

2 Secondary: to prevent both incontinence (feces too soft, over-treatment with laxatives) and an anal fissure (feces too hard, under-treatment with laxatives).

Oral measures

3 In debilitated patients with a poor appetite, a bulking agent is unlikely to be helpful, and may result in a soft impaction.

4 Particularly if taking morphine or another constipating drug, an oral contact (stimulant) laxative should be prescribed, e.g. sennosides 17.2mg b.i.d., bisacodyl tablets 5–10mg b.d. The dose should be carefully titrated to a level which results in normal feces *in the rectum* but without causing an uncontrolled evacuation.

5 In relatively well patients with a good appetite (probably the minority):
- maintain a high fluid intake
- encourage a high roughage diet, e.g. wholegrain cereals, wholemeal foods, greens, bran or a bulk-forming laxative, e.g. psyllium (ispaghula) husk.

6 Beware:
- the prescription of docusate sodium, a fecal softener, may result in a soft fecal impaction of the rectum, and fecal leakage through a patulous anus
- oral bisacodyl in someone not on opioids may cause multiple uncontrolled evacuations, at the wrong time and in the wrong place.

continued

Rectal measures

7 Initially, if impacted with feces, empty the rectum digitally. Then, develop a daily routine:
- as soon as convenient after waking up in the morning, insert 2 glycerin suppositories, or 1–2 bisacodyl suppositories (10–20mg), or a micro-enema deep into the rectum, and wait for 1.5–2 hours
- because the bisacodyl acts only after absorption and biotransformation, bisacodyl suppositories must be placed against the rectal wall, and not into feces
- the patient should be encouraged to have a hot drink after about 1 hour in the hope that it will stimulate a gastro-colonic reflex
- if there is a strong sacral reflex, some feces will be expelled as a result of the above two measures
- to ensure complete evacuation of the rectum and sigmoid colon, digitally stimulate the rectum
- insert gloved and lubricated finger (either soap or gel)
  - ▷ rotate finger 3–4 times
  - ▷ withdraw and wait 5 minutes
  - ▷ if necessary, repeat 3–4 times
  - ▷ check digitally that rectum is fully empty.

8 Patients who are unable to transfer to the toilet or a commode will need nursing assistance. Sometimes it is easiest for a patient to defecate onto a pad while in bed in a lateral position.

9 If the above measures do not achieve complete evacuation of the rectum and sigmoid colon, proceed to digital evacuation (more likely with a flaccid bowel). A pattern will emerge for each patient, allowing the rectal measures to be adjusted to the individual patient's needs and response.

PSYLLIUM HUSK

Included for general information. Psyllium husk is *not recommended* as a laxative in palliative care patients. It may sometimes be helpful in regulating the consistency of feces (making them more formed) in a patient with a colostomy/distal ileostomy.

Class: Bulk-forming laxative.

Indications: Colostomy/ileostomy regulation, anal fissure, hemorrhoids, diverticular disease, irritable bowel syndrome, ulcerative colitis.

Contra-indications: Dysphagia, bowel obstruction, colonic atony, fecal impaction.

Pharmacology

Psyllium is derived from the husks of an Asian plant, *Plantago ovata*. It has very high water-binding capacity, is partly fermented in the colon, and increases bacterial cell mass, thereby further increasing fecal bulk. Like other bulk-forming laxatives, psyllium stimulates peristalsis by increasing fecal mass. Its water-binding capacity also helps to make loose feces more formed in some patients with a colostomy/distal ileostomy.

Onset of action full effect obtained only after several days.

Duration of action best taken regularly to obtain a consistent ongoing effect; may continue to act for 2–3 days after the last dose.

Cautions
Adequate fluid intake should be maintained to avoid bowel obstruction.

Undesirable effects
For full list, see manufacturer's Product Monograph.
Flatulence, abdominal distension, fecal impaction, bowel obstruction.

Dose and use
Psyllium swells in contact with fluid and needs to be swallowed quickly before it absorbs water. Stir the powder briskly in 240mL of water and swallow immediately; carbonated water can be used if preferred. Alternatively, the powder can be mixed with a vehicle such as jam, and followed by 100–200mL of water. Give 3.3–3.4g each morning–t.i.d., preferably after meals; not immediately before bedtime.

Supply
Metamucil Fibre® (Proctor & Gamble)
Wafers 3.4g per 2 wafers, 24 per box = $8; *apple or cinnamon flavour.*
Capsules 525mg, 100 capsules = $20.
Powder Smooth Texture 3.3g per 5.95g of powder, 72 doses = $20; *sugar-free; orange, pink lemonade or berry burst flavour.*

CONTACT (STIMULANT) LAXATIVES

Indications: Prevention and treatment of constipation.

Contra-indications: Large intestinal obstruction.

Pharmacology
Sennosides is a mixture of two naturally occurring plant glycosides (sennosides A and B). It is inactive and passes unabsorbed and unchanged through the small intestine; it is then hydrolyzed by *bacterial* glycosidases in the large intestine to yield an active metabolite.[1] Systemic absorption of sennosides or the active metabolite is small. The laxative effect is through direct contact with the submucosal (Meissner's) plexus and the deeper myenteric (Auerbach's) plexus, resulting in both a secretory and a motor effect in the large intestine. The motor effect precedes the secretory effect, and is the more important laxative action. There is a decrease in segmenting muscular activity and an increase in propulsive waves. Differences in bacterial flora may explain differences in individual response to **sennosides**.

    Bisacodyl has a similar laxative effect to **sennosides**.[1] However, it is hydrolyzed by intestinal enzymes and thus acts on both the small and large intestines. When applied directly to the intestinal mucosa in normal subjects, **bisacodyl** induces powerful propulsive motor activity within minutes.[2]

    Few RCTs of laxatives have been completed in palliative care patients:
- **sennosides** vs. **lactulose**[3]
- **sennosides** vs. **misrakasneham** (an Ayurvedic herbal remedy)[4]
- **sennosides** and **lactulose** vs. **magnesium hydroxide** and **mineral oil**.[5]

There were no significant differences between these treatments. However, because they relax the intestinal ring contractions induced by opioids, contact laxatives should be considered the laxatives of choice for patients taking opioids. Compared to **lactulose**, **sennosides**:
- are faster acting
- come in liquid and tablet formulations (the latter may be crushed)
- cause no drug–drug interactions
- are easier to use in fluid-restricted cardiac patients
- may be taken by patients on a galactose-free diet.

Onset of action
Bisacodyl tablets 10–12h; suppositories 20–60min.
Sennosides 6–12h.

Undesirable effects

For full list, see manufacturer's Product Monograph.
Intestinal colic, diarrhea. **Bisacodyl** suppositories may cause local rectal inflammation, and/or fecal discharge.

Dose and use

Because of the constipating effect of opioids (and other drugs), the doses recommended here for contact (stimulant) laxatives sometimes exceed those recommended in the manufacturers' Product Monographs.

Sennosides are widely used as the PO contact laxative of first choice. However, the mode of action of **bisacodyl** (it acts on both small and large intestines) suggests that it may be preferable in some patients. At some centres, the laxative of choice is **sennosides** combined with **docusate sodium**. However, published data suggest that patients generally respond as well to **sennosides** alone.[6]

All palliative care services should have a protocol for the management of opioid-induced constipation (see Guidelines, p.26).[7–10] Likewise, there is need for a protocol for patients with paraplegia and tetraplegia (see Guidelines, p.27).

For many people, the optimum time for taking sennosides is at bedtime, backed up by a second dose in the morning. The onset of action, 6–12h after administration, is then likely to coincide with the natural postprandial increase in intestinal propulsive activity (gastrocolic reflex) which peaks in many people during the hour after a meal, particularly breakfast.[11] However, if a patient experiences laxative-induced colic, a smaller dose should be given more frequently, e.g. t.i.d–q.i.d.

Sennosides

When an opioid is prescribed, unless contra-indicated (e.g. bowel obstruction):
- start with **sennosides** 17.2mg at bedtime and each morning
- if no response after 24h, increase to 25.8mg at bedtime and each morning
- if no response after a further 24h, consider adding a third daytime dose
- if necessary, consider increasing to a maximum of 34.4mg t.i.d.
- if the maximum dose of **sennosides** is ineffective, halve the dose and add an osmotic laxative (see Guidelines, p.26).

During dose titration and subsequently, if ⩾3 days elapse since last bowel movement, rectal measures should be considered. Note: at some centres, 12mg tablets are used in order to reduce the number of tablets to be taken.

Bisacodyl

- start with 10–20mg PO at bedtime
- if necessary, increase by stages to 20mg PO t.i.d.
- by suppository: 10–20mg PR once daily.

Supply

Sennosides (generic)
Tablets total **sennosides**/tablet 8.6mg, 12mg, 28 days @ 2 tablets b.i.d. = $12 and $16 respectively.

Senokot® (Purdue Frederick)
Tablets standardized **sennosides**/tablet 8.6mg, 28 days @ 2 tablets b.i.d. = $17.

Oral syrup standardized **sennosides** 1.7mg/mL, 28 days @ 10mL b.i.d. = $33.

Combination products
Docusate sodium and sennosides (generic)
Tablets docusate sodium 50mg, **sennosides** 8.6mg, 28 days @ 2 tablets b.i.d. = $20.

Senokot-S® (Purdue)
Tablets docusate sodium 50mg, **sennosides** 8.6mg, 28 days @ 2 tablets b.i.d. = $30.

Bisacodyl (generic)
Tablets EC 5mg, 28 days @ 10mg at bedtime = $5.
Suppositories 10mg, 28 days @ 10mg once daily = $37.

Dulco-lax® (Boehringer Ingelheim)
Tablets EC 5mg, 28 days @ 10mg at bedtime = $15.
Suppositories 5mg, 10mg, 28 days @ 10mg once daily = $48.

1 Jauch R et al. (1975) Bis-(p-hydroxyphenyl)-pyridyl-2-methane: the common laxative principle of bisacodyl and sodium picosulfate. Arzneimittel-Forschung Drug Research. **25**: 1796–1800.
2 De Schryver AM et al. (2003) Effects of a meal and bisacodyl on colonic motility in healthy volunteers and patients with slow-transit constipation. Digestive Diseases Sciences. **48**: 1206–1212.
3 Agra Y et al. (1998) Efficacy of senna versus lactulose in terminal cancer patients treatment with opioids. Journal of Pain and Symptom Management. **15**: 1–7.
4 Ramesh P et al. (1998) Managing morphine-induced constipation: a controlled comparison of an Ayurvedic formulation and senna. Journal of Pain and Symptom Management. **16**: 240–244.
5 Sykes N (1991) A clinical comparison of lactulose and senna with magnesium hydroxide and liquid paraffin emulsion in a palliative care population. [Cited in Miles CL et al. (2006) Laxatives for the management of constipation in palliative care patients. The Cochrane Database of Systematic Reviews. CD003448]
6 Hawley PH and Byeon JJ (2008) A comparison of sennosides-based bowel protocols with and without docusate in hospitalized patients with cancer. Journal of Palliative Medicine. **11**: 575–581.
7 Levy MH (1996) Pharmacologic treatment of cancer pain. New England Journal of Medicine. **335**: 1124–1132.
8 Pappagallo M (2001) Incidence, prevalence, and management of opioid bowel dysfunction. American Journal of Surgery. **182 (suppl 5A)**: 11s–18s.
9 Bouvy ML et al. (2002) Laxative prescribing in relation to opioid use and the influence of pharmacy-based intervention. Journal of Clinical Pharmacy and Therapeutics. **27**: 107–110.
10 Herndon CM et al. (2002) Management of opioid-induced gastrointestinal effects in patients receiving palliative care. Pharmacotherapy. **22**: 240–250.
11 Guyton A and Hall J (eds) (2006) Textbook of Medical Physiology (11e). Elsevier Saunders, Philadelphia.

DOCUSATE SODIUM

Class: Surface-wetting agent (fecal softener).

Indications: Constipation, hemorrhoids, anal fissure, bowel preparation before abdominal radiography, †partial bowel obstruction.

Pharmacology

Although sometimes classified as a stimulant laxative, docusate sodium (docusate) is principally an emulsifying and wetting agent and has a relatively weak effect on GI transit. Docusate lowers surface tension, thereby allowing water and fats to penetrate hard, dry feces. It also stimulates fluid secretion by the small and large intestines.[1,2] Docusate does not interfere with protein or fat absorption.[3] Docusate has been evaluated in several groups of elderly patients; frequency of defecation increased and the need for enemas decreased almost to zero.[4–6] Given these clinical results, it is surprising that, in a study in normal subjects, docusate did not increase fecal weight.[7]

In palliative care, docusate is not recommended as the sole laxative except in patients with partial bowel obstruction.[8] Although sometimes used together with a contact (stimulant) laxative for the management of opioid-induced constipation, published data indicate that patients generally respond equally well to **sennosides** alone.[9]
Onset of action 12–72h.

Cautions

Docusate enhances the absorption of **mineral oil**, and this combination should be avoided.[10]

Undesirable effects
For full list, see manufacturer's Product Monograph.
Diarrhea, nausea, colic, rashes. Docusate syrup can cause an unpleasant after-taste or burning sensation; this is minimized by drinking plenty of water after taking the syrup.

Dose and use
Docusate is often used alone in patients with persistent partial bowel obstruction. Dose varies according to individual need:
- generally start with 100mg b.i.d.
- if necessary, increase to 200mg b.i.d.–t.i.d.

Supply
Docusate (generic)
Capsules 100mg, 240mg, 28 days @ 100mg b.i.d. or 240mg b.i.d. = $4 and $6 respectively.
Syrup 4mg/1mL, 28 days @100mg b.i.d. = $61.
Oral drops 50mg/5mL, 28 days @ 100mg b.i.d. = $181.

Colace® (Wellspring)
Capsules 100mg, 28 days @ 100mg b.i.d. = $17.
Syrup 4mg/mL, 28 days @100mg b.i.d. = $61.
Oral drops 10mg/mL, 28 days @100mg b.i.d. = $186.

Combination products
With **sennosides** (generic)
Tablets docusate sodium 50mg, **sennosides** 8.6mg, 28 days @ 1 tablet b.i.d. = $10.

Senokot S® (Purdue)
Tablets docusate sodium 50mg, **sennosides** 8.6mg, 28 days @ 1 tablet b.i.d. = $15.

1 Donowitz M and Binder H (1975) Effect of dioctyl sodium sulfosuccinate on colonic fluid and electrolyte movement. *Gastroenterology.* **69**: 941–950.
2 Moriarty K et al. (1985) Studies on the mechanism of action of dioctyl sodium sulphosuccinate in the human jejunum. *Gut.* **26**: 1008–1013.
3 Wilson J and Dickinson D (1955) Use of dioctyl sodium sulfosuccinate (aerosol O.T.) for severe constipation. *Journal of the American Medical Association.* **158**: 261–263.
4 Cass L and Frederik W (1956) Doxinate in the treatment of constipation. *American Journal of Gastroenterology.* **26**: 691–698.
5 Harris R (1957) Constipation in geriatrics. *American Journal of Digestive Diseases.* **2**: 487–492.
6 Hyland C and Foran J (1968) Dicotyl sodium sulphosuccinate as a laxative in the elderly. *Practitioner.* **200**: 698–699.
7 Chapman R et al. (1985) Effect of oral dioctyl sodium sulfosuccinate on intake-output studies of human small and large intestine. *Gastroenterology.* **89**: 489–493.
8 Twycross R et al. (2009) *Symptom Management in Advanced Cancer* (4e). palliativedrugs.com, Nottingham, pp. 108–111.
9 Hawley PH and Byeon JJ (2008) A comparison of sennosides-based bowel protocols with and without docusate in hospitalized patients with cancer. *Journal of Palliative Medicine.* **11**: 575–581.
10 Godfrey H (1971) Dangers of dioctyl sodium sulfosuccinate in mixtures. *Journal of the American Medical Association.* **215**: 643.

LACTULOSE

Class: Osmotic laxative.

Indications: Constipation, †hepatic encephalopathy.

Contra-indications: Intestinal obstruction, galactosemia.

Pharmacology
Lactulose is a synthetic disaccharide, a combination of galactose and fructose, which is not absorbed by the small intestine.[1] It is a 'small bowel flusher', i.e. through an osmotic effect, lactulose deposits a large volume of fluid into the large intestine. Lactulose is fermented in the large intestine to acetic, formic and lactic acids, hydrogen and carbon dioxide, with an increase in

fecal acidity, which also stimulates peristalsis. The low pH discourages the proliferation of ammonia-producing organisms and thereby reduces the absorption of ammonium ions and other nitrogenous compounds; hence its use in hepatic encephalopathy.[2] Lactulose does not affect the management of diabetes mellitus; 15mL contains 19 calories, but because bio-availability is negligible (about 3%), the number of calories absorbed is much lower.

Few RCTs of lactulose have been completed in palliative care patients:
- **senna** vs. **lactulose**[3]
- **senna** and **lactulose** vs. **magnesium hydroxide** and **mineral oil**.[4]

There were no significant differences between these treatments.

Onset of action up to 48h.

Undesirable effects

For full list, see manufacturer's Product monograph.
Abdominal bloating, discomfort and flatulence, diarrhea, colic.

Dose and use

Lactulose is used particularly in patients who experience colic with contact (stimulant) laxatives, or who fail to respond to contact (stimulant) laxatives alone.
- starting dose 15mL b.i.d. and adjust according to need
- in hepatic encephalopathy, 30–50mL t.i.d.; adjust dose to produce 2–3 soft fecal evacuations per day.

Supply

Lactulose (generic)
Oral solution 10g/15mL, 28 days @ 15mL b.i.d. = $23.

1 Schumann C (2002) Medical, nutritional and technological properties of lactulose. An update. *European Journal of Nutrition.* **41** (suppl 1): 117–25.
2 Zeng Z *et al.* (2006) Influence of lactulose on the cognitive level and quality of life in patients with minimal hepatic encephalopathy. *Chinese Journal of Clinical Rehabilitation.* **10**: 165–167.
3 Agra Y *et al.* (1998) Efficacy of senna versus lactulose in terminal cancer patients treatment with opioids. *Journal of Pain and Symptom Management.* **15**: 1–7.
4 Sykes N (1991) A clinical comparison of lactulose and senna with magnesium hydroxide and liquid paraffin emulsion in a palliative care population. [Cited in Miles CL et al. (2006) Laxatives for the management of constipation in palliative care patients. The Cochrane Database of Systematic Reviews. CD003448]

POLYETHYLENE GLYCOL (MACROGOL)

Class: Osmotic laxative.

Indications: Constipation, †fecal impaction.

Contra-indications: Severe inflammatory conditions of the intestines, intestinal obstruction.

Pharmacology

Polyethylene glycol acts by virtue of an osmotic action in the intestines, thereby producing an increase in fecal volume which induces a laxative effect. Polyethylene glycol is unchanged in the GI tract, virtually unabsorbed and has no known pharmacological activity. Any absorbed polyethylene glycol is excreted via the urine.

At some centres in Germany, it is the first-line laxative for opioid-induced constipation (often supplemented with a contact/stimulant laxative).[1] In an open study in 27 adults of its use in fecal impaction without concurrent rectal measures, polyethylene glycol 3,350 cleared the impaction in 44% in ≤1 day, 85% in ≤2 days, and 89% in ≤3 days.[2,3]

Onset of action 1–2 days for constipation; 1–3 days for fecal impaction.

Undesirable effects

For full list, see manufacturer's Product Monograph.

Uncommon (<1%, >0.1%): abdominal bloating, discomfort, borborygmi, nausea.

Very rare (<0.01%): electrolyte shift (edema, shortness of breath, dehydration and heart failure).

Dose and use

Each 17g dose is taken in 250mL of water.

Constipation

• start with 17g once daily
• if necessary, increase progressively to 17g t.i.d. (this is three times the manufacturer's dose recommendation).

Although it is more expensive than **lactulose** (another osmotic laxative), it is more effective and better tolerated.[4]

Fecal impaction

• 8 doses (8 x 17g) on day 1, to be taken in <6h
• patients with cardiovascular impairment should restrict intake to not more than 2 doses/h
• repeat on days 2 and 3 p.r.n.

Most patients do not need the full dose on the second day.

Supply

Lax-A-Day® (Pharmascience)
Oral powder polyethylene glycol 3,350 510g bottle, (30 doses) = $37.

RestoraLAX® (Schering-Plough)
Oral powder polyethylene glycol 3,350 17g/sachet, 28 days @ 1sachet once daily = $50; 510g bottle (30 doses) = $32.

1 Wirz S and Klaschik E (2005) Management of constipation in palliative care patients undergoing opioid therapy: is polyethylene glycol an option? *American Journal of Hospice and Palliative Care.* **22**: 375–381.
2 Culbert P et al. (1998) Highly effective oral therapy (polyethylene glycol/electrolyte solution) for faecal impaction and severe constipation. *Clinical Drug Investigation.* **16**: 355–360.
3 Culbert P et al. (1998) Highly effective new oral therapy for faecal impaction. *British Journal of General Practice.* **48**: 1599–1600.
4 Attar A et al. (1999) Comparison of a low dose polyethylene glycol electrolyte solution with lactulose for treatment of chronic constipation. *Gut.* **44**: 226–230.

MAGNESIUM SALTS

Class: Osmotic laxative.

Indications: Constipation, particularly in patients who experience colic with contact (stimulant) laxatives, or who fail to respond to the latter.

Pharmacology

Magnesium ions are poorly absorbed from the gut. Their action is mainly osmotic but other factors may be important, e.g. the release of cholecystokinin.[1,2] Magnesium ions also decrease absorption or increase secretion in the small bowel. Total fecal PGE_2 increases progressively as the dose of magnesium hydroxide is raised from 1.2 to 3.2g daily.[3] Also see **Magnesium**, p.429.

Magnesium hydroxide mixture BP contains about 8% of hydrated magnesium oxide. Magnesium sulfate is more potent and tends to produce a large volume of liquid feces. It often leads to a sense of distension and the sudden passage of offensive liquid feces which is socially inconvenient; it is very difficult to adjust the dose to produce a normal soft result.

An RCT of magnesium hydroxide and **mineral oil** vs. **senna** and **lactulose** failed to differentiate between the two combination treatments.[4]

Cautions
Risk of hypermagnesemia in patients with renal impairment.

Dose and use
Magnesium hydroxide mixture USP
For opioid-induced constipation (see p.26), as an alternative to **lactulose** when an osmotic laxative is indicated:
- if the maximum dose of **sennosides** is ineffective, halve the dose and add magnesium hydroxide 15–30mL b.i.d., and titrate as necessary
- alternatively, switch completely to magnesium hydroxide 15–60mL b.i.d.

Magnesium hydroxide (or **lactulose**) may be preferable in patients with a history of colic with contact (stimulant) laxatives (see p.32).

Magnesium sulfate
A typical dose is 4–10g of crystals once daily *before breakfast*; dissolve in warm water and take with extra fluid.

Supply
Selected products only; all are available OTC.
Magnesium hydroxide
Magnesium Hydroxide Mixture USP
Oral suspension hydrated magnesium oxide 415mg (7.1mmol elemental magnesium)/5mL, 500mL bottle = $8, *do not store in a cold place.*

Phillips Milk of Magnesia® (Bayer)
Tablets 311mg, Bottle of 100 = $9.
Oral suspension 400mg/5mL, 769mL bottle = $13; cherry, mint, original flavours.

Magnesium sulfate
Oral solution magnesium sulfate (Epsom Salts) 4–5g/10mL can be compounded.

---

1 Donowitz M (1991) Magnesium-induced diarrhea and new insights into the pathobiology of diarrhea. *New England Journal of Medicine.* **324**: 1059–1060.
2 Harvey R and Read A (1975) Mode of action of the saline purgatives. *American Heart Journal.* **89**: 810–813.
3 Donowitz M and Rood R (1992) Magnesium hydroxide: new insights into the mechanism of its laxative effect and the potential involvement of prostaglandin E2. *Journal of Clinical Gastroenterology.* **14**: 20–26.
4 Sykes N (1991) A clinical comparison of lactulose and senna with magnesium hydroxide and liquid paraffin emulsion in a palliative care population. [Cited in Miles CL et al. (2006) Laxatives for the management of constipation in palliative care patients. The Cochrane Database of Systematic Reviews. CD003448]

RECTAL PRODUCTS

Indications: Constipation and fecal impaction if oral laxatives are ineffective.

Treatment strategy
One third of patients receiving **morphine** continue to need rectal measures (laxative suppositories, enemas and/or digital evacuation) either regularly or intermittently despite oral laxatives.[1,2] Sometimes these measures are elective, e.g. in paraplegics and in the very old and debilitated (Box 1.F; also see Guidelines, p.27).

In the UK, most patients needing laxative suppositories receive both **glycerin** and **bisacodyl**. **Glycerin** is hygroscopic, and draws fluid into the rectum, thereby softening and lubricating any feces in the rectum. The laxative effect of **bisacodyl** is the result of local direct contact with the rectal mucosa after dissolution of the suppository and after metabolism by intestinal bacteria to an active metabolite (see p.29). The minimum time for response is thus generally >20min, and may be up to 3h.[3] (Defecation a few minutes after the insertion of a **bisacodyl** suppository is the result of ano-rectal stimulation.) **Bisacodyl** suppositories occasionally cause fecal leakage, even after a successful evacuation.

Osmotic micro-enemas contain mainly **sodium citrate** and **sodium lauryl sulfoacetate** with several excipients, including **glycerin** and sorbitol. **Sodium lauryl sulfoacetate** is a wetting agent (similar to **docusate sodium**), whereas **sodium citrate** draws fluid into the intestine by osmosis, an action enhanced by sorbitol, and displaces bound water from the feces. Osmotic standard enemas contain phosphates, which draw fluid into the rectum by osmosis. Digital evacuation is the ultimate approach to fecal impaction; the need for this can be reduced by using oral **polyethylene glycols** (see p.33).[4,5]

Box 1.F   Rectal measures for the relief of constipation or fecal impaction

Suppositories (must be placed in contact with rectal mucosa)
Glycerin 2.6g, has a hygroscopic and lubricant action; also said to be a rectal stimulant but this is unsubstantiated.

Bisacodyl 10mg, after hydrolysis by enteric enzymes, stimulates propulsive activity.[6]

Enemas
Lubricant enema (130mL) contains mineral oil; this is generally instilled and left overnight before giving a stimulant laxative suppository or an osmotic enema.

Osmotic micro-enemas (5mL) contain sodium citrate, sodium lauryl sulfoacetate, glycerin, and sorbitol.

Osmotic standard enemas (65–130mL), contain phosphates.

Supply
Suppositories
Glycerin
Suppositories glycerin 2.34g, in adult suppository of 2.6g, 28 days @ 2.6g once daily = $7.

Bisacodyl (generic)
Suppositories 10mg, 28 days @ 10mg once daily = $37.

Dulco-lax® (Boehringer Ingelheim)
Suppositories 5mg, 10mg, 28 days @ 10mg once daily = $48.

Enemas
Fecal softener enema
Fleet® Ready-to-use Mineral Oil enema (Johnson & Johnson-Merck), **mineral oil** 100%, 130mL, 1 enema = $11.

Osmotic micro-enemas
These all contain **sodium citrate**, **sodium lauryl sulfoacetate**, **glycerin** and sorbitol and are supplied in 5ml single-dose disposable packs with nozzle:

Microlax Micro Enema® (McNeil Consumer Healthcare), **sodium citrate** 90mg, **sodium lauryl sulfoacetate** 9mg, sorbitol 625mg/mL single dose with nozzle, 5mL = $2.

Osmotic standard enema
Fleet® Ready-to-use enema (Johnson & Johnson-Merck), **monobasic sodium phosphate** 20.8g, **dibasic sodium phosphate** 7.8g in 130mL, 1 enema = $8.

Fleet® Ready-to-use Pediatric enema (Johnson & Johnson-Merck), **monobasic sodium phosphate** 10.4g, **dibasic sodium phosphate** 3.9g in 65 ml, 1 enema = $8.

Enemol® (Pendopharm), **monobasic sodium phosphate** 20.8g, **dibasic sodium phosphate** 7.8g in 130mL, 1 enema = $5.

---

1 Twycross RG and Lack SA (1986) *Control of Alimentary Symptoms in Far Advanced Cancer.* Churchill Livingstone, Edinburgh, pp. 173–174.
2 Twycross RG and Harcourt JMV (1991) The use of laxatives at a palliative care centre. *Palliative Medicine.* **5**: 27–33.

3 Flig E et al. (2000) Is bisacodyl absorbed at all from suppositories in man? International Journal of Pharmaceutics. 196: 11–20.
4 Goldman M (1993) Hazards of phosphate enemas. Gastroenterology Today. 3: 16–17.
5 Culbert P et al. (1998) Highly effective oral therapy (polyethylene glycol/electrolyte solution) for faecal impaction and severe constipation. Clinical Drug Investigation. 16: 355–360.
6 von Roth W and von Beschke K (1988) Pharmakokinetik und laxierende wirkung von bisacodyl nach gabe verschiedener zubereitungsformen. Arzneimittel Forschung Drug Research. 38: 570–574.

PRODUCTS FOR HEMORRHOIDS

Because hemorrhoids can be more troublesome if associated with the evacuation of hard feces, constipation must be corrected (see Laxatives, p.24).

Peri-anal pruritus, soreness and excoriation are best treated by the application of a bland ointment or cream. Suppositories are often not effective because they are inserted into the rectum, bypassing the anal canal where the medication is needed.

Soothing products containing mild astringents (e.g. **bismuth subgallate**, **zinc sulfate**, **hamamelis/witch hazel**) often provide symptomatic relief in hemorrhoids. Some products also contain vasoconstrictors and/or antiseptics.

Lidocaine ointment is used mainly to relieve pain associated with an anal fissure but will also relieve pruritus ani. Local anesthetic ointments are absorbed through the anal mucosa and, if applied excessively, could theoretically produce a systemic effect. They should be used for only a few days because all 'caines' can cause contact dermatitis.

Corticosteroids may be helpful if local inflammation is exacerbating discomfort. Infection (e.g. Herpes simplex) must first be excluded; and treatment limited to 7–10 days. Pain associated with spasm of the internal anal sphincter may be helped by topical **nitroglycerin** ointment (see p.53).

Dose and use
Topical products should be applied:
- t.i.d.–q.i.d. for the first 24h
- then b.i.d. and after defecation for 5–7 days or longer if necessary
- then daily for 3–5 days after symptoms have cleared.

Local anesthetic-containing products to ease painful defecation can also be applied b.i.d., p.r.n. (including before defecation if possible).

Supply
Various OTC products are available, and are not included here. The following list is highly selective.

Astringent
Anusol® (McNeil Consumer Healthcare)
Ointment zinc sulphate 0.5%, 30g = $8.

Local anesthetic
Lidocaine (generic)
Ointment 5%, 35g = $9

Xylocaine® (Astra Zeneca)
Ointment lidocaine 5%, 35g = $10.

Local anesthetic plus astringent
Anusol Plus® (McNeil Consumer Healthcare)
Ointment pramoxine 1%, **zinc sulfate** 0.5%, 30g = $10.

Corticosteroid plus astringent
Generic
Ointment hydrocortisone 0.5%, **zinc sulfate** 0.5%, 30g = $13.
Anusol HC ® (McNeil Consumer Healthcare)
Ointment hydrocortisone 0.5%, **zinc sulfate** 0.5%, 30g = $24.

Corticosteroid plus local anesthetic and astringent
Anugesic®HC (McNeil Consumer Health)
Ointment hydrocortisone 0.5%, **pramoxine** 1%, **zinc sulfate** 0.5%, 30g = $28.

PANCREATIN

Class: Enzyme supplement.

Indications: †Symptomatic steatorrhea caused by biliary and/or pancreatic obstruction, e.g. cancer of the pancreas.

Pharmacology

Steatorrhea (the presence of undigested fecal fat) typically results in pale, bulky, offensive, frothy and greasy feces which flush away only with difficulty; associated with abdominal distension, increased flatus, loss of weight, and mineral and vitamin deficiency (A, D, E and K).

Pancreatin is a standardized preparation of porcine lipase, protease and amylase. Pancreatin hydrolyzes fats to glycerol and fatty acids, degrades protein into amino acids, and converts starch into dextrin and sugars. Because it is inactivated by gastric acid, pancreatin is best taken with food (or immediately before or after food). Gastric acid secretion may be reduced by giving a H_2-receptor antagonist, e.g. **ranitidine**, an hour before meals or a PPI once daily. Concurrent use of antacids further reduces gastric acidity. EC products, such as Creon®, deliver a higher enzyme concentration in the duodenum provided the granules are swallowed whole without chewing.

Cautions

Fibrotic strictures of the colon have developed in children with cystic fibrosis who have used high-strength preparations of pancreatin. This has not been reported in adults or in patients without cystic fibrosis. Creon® has not been implicated.

If mixing with food or drinks:
- avoid very hot food or drinks because heat inactivates pancreatin
- do not mix the capsule contents with alkaline foods or drinks, e.g. dairy products, because this degrades the EC coating
- take immediately after mixing because the EC coating starts to dissolve if left to stand.

Undesirable effects

For full list, see manufacturer's Product Monograph.
Very common (>10%): abdominal pain.
Common (<10%, >1%): nausea and vomiting, constipation or diarrhea, allergic skin reactions.

Dose and use

There are several different pancreatin products, of which Creon® is a good choice. Capsule strength denotes lipase unit content. Thus, Creon 10® contains 10,000 units and Creon 25® contains 25,000 units.

In adults, start with Creon® 10. The granules in the capsules are EC and, if preferred, may be added to fluid or soft food and *swallowed without chewing*:
- Creon® 10, initially give 1–2 capsules with each meal
- Creon® 25, initially give 1 capsule with each meal.

The dose is adjusted upwards according to fecal size, consistency, and number. Extra capsules may be needed if snacks are taken between meals. If the pancreatin continues to seem ineffective, prescribe a PPI or H_2-receptor antagonist concurrently, and review.

Supply

Creon® (Solvay)
A standardized preparation obtained from pigs; *there is no non-porcine alternative.*
Capsules enclosing EC granules Creon 5®, lipase 5,000 units, amylase 16,600 units, protease 18,750 units, 28 days @ 2 t.i.d. = $31.
Capsules enclosing EC granules Creon 10®, lipase 10,000 units, amylase 33,200 units, protease 37,500 units, 28 days @ 2 t.i.d. = $49.
Capsules enclosing EC granules Creon 25®, lipase 25,000 units, amylase 74,000 units, protease 62,500 units, 28 days @ 2 t.i.d. = $153.

2: CARDIOVASCULAR SYSTEM

FUROSEMIDE

Class: Loop diuretic.

Indications: Edema, †malignant ascites associated with portal hypertension and hyper-aldosteronism (with **spironolactone**), †bronchorrhea.

Contra-indications: Hepatic encephalopathy, anuric renal failure.

Pharmacology

Furosemide inhibits sodium (and hence water) resorption from the ascending limb of the loop of Henlé in the renal tubule. It also increases urinary excretion of K^+, H^+, Cl^- and Mg^{2+}. Diuretics such as furosemide are the standard first-line therapy for the treatment of symptomatic fluid overload in congestive heart failure (CHF) (Figure 2.1).[1-3]

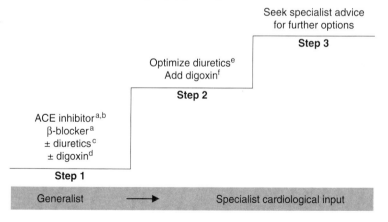

Figure 2.1 Drug treatment for CHF caused by left ventricular systolic dysfunction. For more detail, see published guidelines.[1,4]

a. in all patients who are stable, i.e. minimal or no signs of fluid overload or depletion, even if asymptomatic
b. if an ACE inhibitor is not tolerated, substitute an angiotensin-II antagonist, e.g. losartan; if an angiotensin-II antagonist is not tolerated, substitute hydralazine and isosorbide dinitrate
c. in patients with signs of fluid overload
d. in patients with atrial fibrillation
e. combine a loop diuretic with spironolactone (see p.42)
f. if not already taking it, i.e. patients in sinus rhythm.

Furosemide alone has little effect on ascites associated with cirrhosis, massive liver metastases and portal hypertension, even when used in daily doses of 100–200mg PO.[5,6] The use of furosemide in malignant ascites is generally best limited to when treatment alone with **spironolactone** 300–400mg daily is insufficient (see p.42).

A diuretic-induced reduction in plasma volume can activate several neurohumoral systems, e.g. renin–aldosterone–angiotensin, resulting in impaired renal perfusion and increased Na^+ and water resorption. These changes reduce the effect of the diuretic and contribute to renal impairment. **Octreotide** 300microgram SC b.i.d. (see p.395) can suppress this diuretic-induced activation of the renin-aldosterone-angiotensin system and its addition has improved renal function and Na^+ and water excretion in patients with cirrhosis and ascites receiving furosemide and **spironolactone**.[7,8]

Nebulized furosemide 20–40mg attenuates experimentally-induced cough and dyspnea,[9–11] and also allergen-induced asthma,[12] possibly via an effect on vagal sensory nerve endings. The reduction in breathlessness may result from increasing sensory traffic to the brain stem from sensitized slowly adapting pulmonary stretch receptors, but shows wide individual variability, is of short duration (generally <2h) and systemic absorption can be sufficient to induce a diuresis.[11] In moderate–severe COPD, compared with placebo, nebulized furosemide reduced breathlessness during endurance testing, but *not* incremental exercise testing.[13] Although significant bronchodilation was also seen, it may have been due to the exercise[14] rather than the nebulized furosemide.

Nebulized furosemide has also been used to relieve severe breathlessness in palliative care patients.[15,16] However, controlled trials have failed to demonstrate benefit.[17,18] Further, in one study,[17] 5/7 patients reported a deterioration in their breathing after furosemide; it is thus recommended that the use of nebulized furosemide is restricted to closely controlled circumstances. Anecdotally, nebulized furosemide is of benefit in bronchorrhea.[19]

In heart failure, compared with bolus IV doses, furosemide by CIVI appears to provide a greater diuresis and a better safety profile.[20] Furosemide is effective when given by SC injection. Diuresis persists for about 4h, reaching a maximum at 2–3h, and urine output is significantly increased. This provides a useful alternative route of administration when IV or IM injections are problematic.[21,22]

Bio-availability 60–70% PO, but reduced by gastro-intestinal edema in CHF.
Onset of action 30–60min PO; 2–5min IV; 30min SC.[22]
Time to peak plasma concentration no data; peak *effect* at 1–2h PO.
Plasma halflife 30–120min in healthy subjects, 50min–6h in heart failure, 10h in end-stage renal disease.
Duration of action 4–6h PO; 2h IV; 4h SC.[22]

Cautions

Increased risk of hypokalemia with corticosteroids, β_2-agonists, **theophylline**, **amphotericin** and **carbenoxolone** (not Canada); increased risk of hyponatremia with **carbamazepine**; increased risk of hypotension with ACE inhibitors and TCAs; increased risk of nephrotoxicity with NSAIDs; increased risk of **lithium** toxicity. Furosemide-induced hypokalemia increases the risk of **digoxin** toxicity and may also increase the toxicity of other drugs which prolong the QT interval; maintain adequate plasma K^+ concentrations during concurrent use.[23]

Reduced diuretic effect of furosemide with **phenytoin** (up to 50% reduction), **indomethacin** and possibly other NSAIDs; may need to increase the furosemide dose. **Cholestyramine** and **colestipol** decrease absorption of furosemide; give furosemide 2–3h before the resin.[23]

Withdrawal: Some patients receive long-term diuretic therapy for hypertension, or non-heart failure ankle edema. This often become inappropriate as physical deterioration progresses, and may lead to postural hypotension and prerenal failure. In such circumstances the dose of furosemide should be reduced and possibly discontinued altogether. However, the withdrawal of diuretics requires careful monitoring to prevent the subsequent insidious onset of CHF.[24]

Undesirable effects

For full list, see manufacturer's Product Monograph.
Transient pain at the site of SC injection.[22]
Frequency not stated: headache, dizziness, fever, fatigue, weakness, restlessness, blurred vision, tinnitus, deafness (generally after rapid injection, may be permanent), hypotension, bone marrow depression, hypokalemia, hyponatremia, hypocalcemia, hyperglycemia, hyperuricemia,

dehydration, thirst, nausea, anorexia, acute pancreatitis, interstitial nephritis, urinary retention (in patients with prostatic hypertrophy), may precipitate gout, muscle cramps, pruritus, rash, photosensitivity.

Dose and use
CHF
- start with 40mg each morning
- usual maintenance dose 40–80mg each morning
- usual maximum dose 160mg each morning.

Ascites
Use only as a supplement to **spironolactone** (see p.42):
- start with 40mg each morning
- usual maintenance dose 20–40mg each morning
- usual maximum dose 160mg each morning.

Incompatibility: Furosemide injection is alkaline. It should not be mixed or diluted with glucose solutions or other acidic fluids.[25,26] When given by CSCI, furosemide injection should be diluted with 0.9% saline. It should not be mixed in the same syringe with any other drugs.

Supply
Furosemide (generic)
Tablets 20mg, 40mg, 80mg, 28 days @ 40mg each morning = $2.00.
Injection 10mg/mL, 2mL amp = $1.50, 4mL amp = $3, 25mL amp = $20.

Lasix® (Sanofi-Aventis)
Tablets 20mg, 40mg, 500mg, 28 days @ 40mg or 500mg each morning = $4, or $87 respectively.
Oral solution (sugar-free) 50mg/5mL, 28 days @ 40mg each morning = $32.

1 NICE (2003) Management of chronic heart failure in adults in primary and secondary care. In: *Clinical Guideline 5*. National Institute for Clinical Excellence. Available from: www.nice.org.uk/guidance/CG5/niceguidance/pdf/English
2 McMurray JJ and Pfeffer MA (2005) Heart failure. *Lancet*. **365**: 1877–1889.
3 Faris R et al. (2006) Diuretics for heart failure. *Cochrane Database of Systematic Reviews*. CD003838.
4 Arnold JM et al. (2006) Canadian Cardiovascular Society consensus conference recommendations on heart failure 2006: diagnosis and management. *Canadian Journal of Cardiology*. **22**: 23–45. [Erratum appears in Canadian Journal of Cardiology. 2006 Mar 1;22(3):271.]
5 Fogel M et al. (1981) Diuresis in the ascitic patient: a randomized controlled trial of three regimens. *Journal of Clinical Gastroenterology*. **3**: 73–80.
6 Amiel S et al. (1984) Intravenous infusion of frusemide as treatment for ascites in malignant disease. *British Medical Journal*. **288**: 1041.
7 Kalambokis G et al. (2005) Renal effects of treatment with diuretics, octreotide or both, in non-azotemic cirrhotic patients with ascites. *Nephrology, Dialysis, Transplantation*. **20**: 1623–1629.
8 Kalambokis G et al. (2006) The effects of treatment with octreotide, diuretics, or both on portal hemodynamics in nonazotemic cirrhotic patients with ascites. *Journal of Clinical Gastroenterology*. **40**: 342–346.
9 Bianco S et al. (1989) Protective effect of inhaled furosemide on allergen-induced early and late asthmatic reactions. *New England Journal of Medicine*. **321**: 1069–1073.
10 Ventresca P et al. (1990) Inhaled furosemide inhibits cough induced by low-chloride solutions but not by capsaicin. *American Review of Respiratory Disease*. **142**: 143–146.
11 Moosavi SH et al. (2006) Effect of inhaled furosemide on air hunger induced in healthy humans. *Respiratory Physiology and Neurobiology*. **156**: 1–8.
12 Nishino T et al. (2000) Inhaled furosemide greatly alleviates the sensation of experimentally induced dyspnea. *American Journal of Respiratory and Critical Care Medicine*. **161**: 1963–1967.
13 Ong KC et al. (2004) Effects of inhaled furosemide on exertional dyspnea in chronic obstructive pulmonary disease. *American Journal of Respiratory and Critical Care Medicine*. **169**: 1028–1033.
14 Natif N et al. (1998) Improved breathing capacity during exercise in severe obstructive airway disease. *Respiration and Physiology*. **112**: 145–154.
15 Shimoyama N and Shimoyama M (2002) Nebulized furosemide as a novel treatment for dyspnea in terminal cancer patients. *Journal of Pain and Symptom Management*. **23**: 73–76.
16 Kohara H et al. (2003) Effect of nebulized furosemide in terminally ill cancer patients with dyspnea. *Journal of Pain and Symptom Management*. **26**: 962–967.
17 Stone P et al. (2002) Re: nebulized furosemide for dyspnea in terminal cancer patients. *Journal of Pain and Symptom Management*. **24**: 274–275; author reply 275–276.
18 Wilcock A et al. (2008) Randomised, placebo-controlled trial of nebulised furosemide for breathlessness in patients with cancer. *Thorax*. **63**: 872–875.
19 Twycross R et al. (2009) *Symptom Management in Advanced Cancer* (4e). palliativedrugs.com, Nottingham, pp. 160–166.

20 Salvador DR et al. (2005) Continuous infusion versus bolus injection of loop diuretics in congestive heart failure. *Cochrane Database of Systematic Reviews.* CD003178.
21 Goenaga MA et al. (2004) Subcutaneous furosemide. *Annals of Pharmacotherpy.* **38**: 1751.
22 Verma AK et al. (2004) Diuretic effects of subcutaneous furosemide in human volunteers: a randomized pilot study. *Annals of Pharmacotherapy.* **38**: 544–549.
23 Baxter K (ed) (2006) *Stockley's Drug Interactions* (7e). Pharmaceutical Press, London.
24 Walma E et al. (1997) Withdrawal of long term diuretic medication in elderly patients: a double blind randomised trial. *British Medical Journal.* **315**: 464–468.
25 Chiu MF and Schwartz ML (1997) Visual compatibility of injectable drugs used in the intensive care unit. *American Journal of Health System Pharmacy.* **54**: 64–65.
26 Trissel LA et al. (1997) Compatibility of parenteral nutrient solutions with selected drugs during simulated Y-site administration. *American Journal of Health System Pharmacy.* **54**: 1295–1300.

SPIRONOLACTONE

Class: Potassium-sparing diuretic; aldosterone antagonist.

Indications: Ascites and peripheral edema associated with portal hypertension and hyperaldosteronism (i.e. cirrhosis, hepatocellular cancer, massive hepatic metastases), CHF, nephrotic syndrome, primary hyperaldosteronism, hypokalemia.

Contra-indications: Hyperkalemia, Addison's disease, anuria, severe renal impairment.

Pharmacology

Spironolactone and two metabolites (7α-thiomethyl-spironolactone and canrenone) bind to cytoplasmic mineralocorticoid receptors and function as aldosterone antagonists. In the distal tubules of the kidney, this results in a potassium-sparing diuretic effect. Hyperaldosteronism is a concomitant of ascites associated with portal hypertension (a *transudate* with a relatively low albumin concentration, best indicated by a serum-ascites albumin difference or gradient of $\geqslant 11$g/L), i.e. cirrhosis, hepatocellular cancer, massive hepatic metastases.[1,2] Most evidence comes from cirrhosis, but spironolactone in a median daily dose of 200–300mg is successful in the majority of patients with these conditions (90% in cirrhosis).[1-6] Spironolactone alone is the initial drug of choice, it is as safe and effective as spironolactone + **furosemide** and requires less frequent dose adjustments.[4,5] In contrast, treatment with even large PO doses of a loop diuretic alone, e.g. **furosemide** 200mg, generally fails to reduce ascites.[7] Even if paracentesis becomes necessary, diuretics should be continued as they reduce the rate of recurrence.[4] Note: paracentesis is generally preferable for patients with predominantly peritoneal (an *exudate* with relatively high albumin concentration, best indicated by a serum-ascites albumin gradient of $\leqslant 11$g/L) or chylous ascites as these are unlikely to respond to diuretics,[3,6] and also for patients with a tense distended abdomen in need of rapid relief, and those unable to tolerate spironolactone.

A diuretic-induced reduction in plasma volume can increase the activity of various closely related neurohumoral systems, e.g. the renin-aldosterone-angiotensin system, sympathetic nervous system, ADH secretion, which results in impaired renal perfusion and increased Na^+ and water resorption. These changes reduce the effect of the diuretic and contribute to renal impairment. In patients with cirrhosis receiving spironolactone $\pm$ **furosemide**, improved renal function and diuresis is seen with co-administration of **octreotide** 300microgram SC b.i.d. (see p.395) or **clonidine** 75microgram PO b.i.d. (see p.50) due to inhibition of the renin-aldosterone-angiotensin (**octreotide** and **clonidine**) and sympathetic nervous (**clonidine**) systems.[8-10] Patients in the **clonidine** study were considered to have an overactive sympathetic nervous system based on a higher than normal serum norepinephrine level.[10]

Spironolactone is also added in a low dose (12.5–50mg daily) to standard treatment for patients with severe symptomatic CHF (see Figure 2.1, p.39).[11-14] Its aldosterone antagonist action helps reduce vascular and myocardial fibrosis, sympathetic nervous system activation, baroreceptor dysfunction and K^+ and Mg^{2+} depletion.[15]

Spironolactone (but not its metabolites) has several actions independent of the mineralocorticoid receptor, including an anti-inflammatory effect. This involves the inhibition of the nuclear factor-κB pathway involved in the production of pro-inflammatory cytokines.[16] Longer-acting analogues of spironolactone may thus be developed as anti-inflammatory drugs.

Bio-availability about 90%.
Onset of action 2–4h; maximum effect 7h (single dose), 2–3 days (multiple doses).
Time to peak plasma concentration 2–3h; active metabolites 3–4.5h PO.
Plasma halflife 1–1.5h; active metabolites 14–16.5h (multiple doses).
Duration of action >24h (single dose), 2–3 days (multiple doses).

Cautions

Serious drug interactions: risk of hyperkalemia with potassium supplements (avoid concurrent use), table salt substitutes (contain both potassium and sodium chlorides), potassium-sparing diuretics, ACE inhibitors and angiotensin II receptor antagonists, particularly if other risk factors also present, e.g. elderly, renal impairment, diabetes.[17]

Elderly; hepatic impairment, renal impairment. Initial drowsiness and dizziness (may impair driving). May induce hyponatremia, particularly if used with other diuretics. May induce reversible hyperchloremic metabolic acidosis in patients with decompensated hepatic cirrhosis. Natriuretic effect reduced by **aspirin**, **indomethacin** and possibly other NSAIDs. Spironolactone increases the plasma concentration of **digoxin** by up to 25% and can interfere with **digoxin** plasma concentration assays; measure free **digoxin** levels using a chemiluminescent assay.[17]

Undesirable effects

For full list, see manufacturer's Product Monograph
Very common (>10%): CNS disturbances (drowsiness, lethargy, confusion, headache, fever, ataxia, fatigue), gastro-intestinal disturbances (anorexia, dyspepsia, nausea, vomiting, peptic ulceration, colic).
Common (<10%, >1%): gastritis, hyperkalemia, gynecomastia.[18]

Dose and use
Cirrhotic or malignant ascites
Elimination of ascites may take 10–28 days:
- monitor body weight and renal function
- start with 100–200mg each morning with food; give in divided doses if it causes nausea and vomiting
- if necessary, increase by 100mg every 3–7 days to achieve a weight loss of 0.5–1kg/24h (<0.5kg/24h when peripheral edema absent)
- a typical maintenance dose is 200–300mg/24h; maximum dose 400–600mg/24h[1,2,5,7]
- if not achieving the desired weight loss with spironolactone 300–400mg/24h, consider adding **furosemide** 40–80mg each morning
- in cirrhosis, **furosemide** is generally increased in 40mg steps every 3 days to a maximum of 160mg/24h[4,5,19,20]
- if Na^+ falls to <120mmol/L, temporarily stop diuretics
- if K^+ falls to <3.5mmol/L, temporarily stop or decrease the dose of **furosemide**; if it rises to >5.5mmol/L, halve the dose of spironolactone; if >6mmol/L, temporarily stop spironolactone
- if creatinine rises to >150micromol/L, temporarily stop diuretics.[4]

Severe CHF (NYHA class III or IV disease)
The following is based on several sets of published guidelines:
- do *not* prescribe spironolactone unless serum K^+ <5mmol/L and creatinine <200micromol/L
- start with 12.5–25mg once daily; check serum K^+ and creatinine after 4–7 days
- if necessary, *after 1 month*, increase to 50mg once daily; check serum K^+ and creatinine after 1 week
- if K^+ rises to >5mmol/L, halve the dose; if >5.5mmol/L, stop spironolactone completely
- it is particularly important to monitor potassium levels when spironlactone and an ACE inhibitor are prescribed concurrently.[11,14,15]

Supply

Spironolactone (generic)
Tablets 25mg, 100mg, 28 days @ 200mg each morning = $12.

Aldactone® (Pfizer)
Tablets 25mg, 100mg, 28 days @ 200mg each morning = $19.

Spironolactone suspension can also be compounded for individual patients.[21]

1 Greenway B et al. (1982) Control of malignant ascites with spironolactone. British Journal of Surgery. **69**: 441–442.

2 Fernandez-Esparrach G et al. (1997) Diuretic requirements after therapeutic paracentesis in non-azotemic patients with cirrhosis. A randomized double-blind trial of spironolactone versus placebo. Journal of Hepatology. **26**: 614–620; erratum 1430.

3 Pockros P et al. (1992) Mobilization of malignant ascites with diuretics is dependent on ascitic fluid characteristics. Gastroenterology. **103**: 1302–1306.

4 Moore KP et al. (2003) The management of ascites in cirrhosis: report on the consensus conference of the International Ascites Club. Hepatology. **38**: 258–266.

5 Santos J et al. (2003) Spironolactone alone or in combination with furosemide in the treatment of moderate ascites in nonazotemic cirrhosis. A randomized comparative study of efficacy and safety. Journal of Hepatology. **39**: 187–192.

6 Becker G et al. (2006) Malignant ascites: systematic review and guideline for treatment. European Journal of Cancer. **42**: 589–597.

7 Fogel M et al. (1981) Diuresis in the ascitic patient: a randomized controlled trial of three regimens. Journal of Clinical Gastroenterology. **3**: 73–80.

8 Kalambokis G et al. (2005) Renal effects of treatment with diuretics, octreotide or both, in non-azotemic cirrhotic patients with ascites. Nephrology, Dialysis, Transplantation. **20**: 1623–1629.

9 Kalambokis G et al. (2006) The effects of treatment with octreotide, diuretics, or both on portal hemodynamics in nonazotemic cirrhotic patients with ascites. Journal of Clinical Gastroenterology. **40**: 342–346.

10 Lenaerts A et al. (2006) Effects of clonidine on diuretic response in ascitic patients with cirrhosis and activation of sympathetic nervous system. Hepatology. **44**: 844–849.

11 NICE (2003) Management of chronic heart failure in adults in primary and secondary care. In: Clinical Guideline 5. National Institute for Clinical Excellence. Available from: www.nice.org.uk/guidance/CG5/niceguidance/pdf/English

12 Veterans Health Administration (2003) The Pharmacologic Management of Chronic Heart Failure. Department of Veterans Affairs, Washington DC. Available from: www.guideline.gov/summary/summary.aspx?doc_id=5184

13 McMurray JJ and Pfeffer MA (2005) Heart failure. Lancet. **365**: 1877–1889.

14 Arnold JM et al. (2006) Canadian Cardiovascular Society consensus conference recommendations on heart failure 2006: diagnosis and management. Canadian Journal of Cardiology. **22**: 23–45. [Erratum appears in Can J Cardiol. 2006 Mar 1;22(3):271.]

15 Swedberg K et al. (2005) Guidelines for the diagnosis and treatment of chronic heart failure: full text (update 2005). European Heart Journal. Available from: 10.1093/eurheartj/ehi205

16 Sonder SU et al. (2006) Effects of spironolactone on human blood mononuclear cells: mineralocorticoid receptor independent effects on gene expression and late apoptosis induction. British Journal of Pharmacology. **148**: 46–53.

17 Baxter K (ed) (2006) Stockley's Drug Interactions (7e). Pharmaceutical Press, London.

18 Williams EM et al. (2006) Use and side-effect profile of spironolactone in a private cardiologist's practice. Clinical Cardiology. **29**: 149–153.

19 Gines P et al. (1987) Comparison of paracentesis and diuretics in the treatment of cirrhotics with tense ascites. Gastroenterology. **93**: 234–241.

20 Sharma S and Walsh D (1995) Management of symptomatic malignant ascites with diuretics: two case reports and a review of the literature. Journal of Pain and Symptom Management. **10**: 237–242.

21 Allen LV Jr and Erickson MA 3rd (1996) Stability of ketoconazole, metolazone, metronidazole, procainamide hydrochloride, and spironolactone in extemporaneously compounded oral liquids. American Journal of Health System Pharmacy. **53**: 2073–2078.

SYSTEMIC LOCAL ANESTHETICS

Local anesthetics and their orally administered congeners are sometimes useful as third- or fourth-line drugs in the treatment of neuropathic pain. An analgesic effect has been reported when such drugs have been administered systemically:[1]

- **lidocaine** TD, CSCI, IVI[2,3]
- **flecainide** PO (see p.47)
- **mexiletine** PO (see p.48)
- **tocainide** PO.

The mechanism by which they provide relief is not fully understood, but probably includes blockade of sodium channels. This stabilizes the nerve membrane and thus suppresses injury-induced hyperexcitability in the peripheral and central nervous systems. Antidepressants and anti-epileptics which benefit neuropathic pain also have membrane stabilizing properties, e.g. **carbamazepine, amitriptyline.**[4]

A systematic review of 32 RCTs, mostly of IV **lidocaine** and PO **mexiletine**, for neuropathic pain of various causes concluded that systemic local anesthetics are better than placebo and as effective as **amantadine, carbamazepine, gabapentin, morphine** (Box 2.A).[1] Even so, despite the occasional impressive anecdotal account, RCT evidence of benefit is not overwhelming. Thus, the overall degree of improvement is small, and some studies suggest that not all components of neuropathic pain are relieved, e.g. constant pain and allodynia to touch improve but cold-induced allodynia does not.[5,6] Benefit is inconsistent in some types of pain, e.g. diabetic neuropathy, and absent in others, e.g. cancer-related neuropathic pain.[1,7,8] Further, in elderly patients (mean age 77 years), **lidocaine** 5mg/kg IVI over 2h provides no greater analgesic benefit than 1mg/kg, despite producing higher serum levels which were potentially toxic in some patients.[9]

Box 2.A Systemic local anesthetics and neuropathic pain[1]

Of overall benefit in:
- trigeminal neuralgia
- post-herpetic neuralgia
- diabetic neuropathy
- lumbosacral radiculopathy
- post-stroke pain
- chronic post-surgery pain
- chronic post-trauma pain
- spinal cord injury pain
- complex regional pain syndrome.

Not of benefit in:
- cancer-related neuropathy (but see main text)
- HIV-related neuropathy.

Lidocaine dose used ranged from 1mg/kg IV over 2–3min to 1–5mg/kg IVI over 30min–2h. Mexiletine median dose 600mg/24h (range 300–1,200mg/24h). Improvement equivalent to a reduction of 10mm on a 100mm VAS, but about 50% of patients achieve an improvement of ≥30%.

Although improvement lasting 8–20 weeks following a single dose of IV **lidocaine** has been reported in patients with central pain syndrome, generally benefit is limited to a few hours.[10] Thus, the need for ongoing relief will necessitate CIVI or CSCI **lidocaine** or the use of an oral analogue, e.g. **mexiletine**. However, the response to IV **lidocaine** does not reliably predict subsequent benefit from **mexiletine** and undesirable effects can limit its chronic use.[5,11]

There are case reports of patients with cancer-related neuropathic pain benefiting from **lidocaine**:
- IV, e.g. 1–2mg/kg over 15–20min[12]
- CIVI, e.g. 0.5–1mg/kg/h[12,13]
- CSCI, e.g. 4 or 10% **lidocaine** hydrochloride solution, generally 10–80mg/h; 100–160mg/h reported in younger patients (age ~60years).[13,14]

Continuous infusions have been given for up to 6 months.[14] As a minimum, some suggest monitoring serum levels 1–3 days after commencement or dose escalation and when toxicity is suspected.[13]

Analgesia is generally seen with serum levels of 1.5–5microgram/mL and severe neurotoxicity with levels ≥10microgram/mL.[3,15] However, there is large interindividual variation and the beneficial/toxic effect relates more to the amount of free local anesthetic (unbound to protein), rather than the total serum level (bound plus unbound).[16]

With a continuous infusion, accumulation of **lidocaine** and its active metabolites, e.g. monoethylglycinexylidide and glycinexylidide can occur and lead to toxicity. Particular caution is required in the elderly in whom clearance is already reduced.[16–18] For example, two elderly patients (≥70 years) despite normal renal/liver function and receiving a relatively small dose of **lidocaine** (200–300mg/day), developed severe drowsiness after 10 days.[19]

Generally, developing toxicity should be clinically obvious because as serum levels rise, there is a progressive worsening of neurotoxicity:
- lightheadedness, dizziness
- circumoral numbness
- tinnitus
- visual changes
- dysarthria
- muscle spasm
- seizures
- coma
- respiratory arrest.

However, the monitoring of serum levels is the most effective way of maintaining a consistent and safe **lidocaine** dose.[3,17,19]

Prolonged toxicity has also been reported when 10mL of 2% viscous **lidocaine** was used hourly for a painful mouth ulcer (twice the recommended daily dose), and was probably partly caused by accumulation of metabolites.[18]

More recently the TD route has been used to treat localized non-cancer peripheral neuropathic pain. Modest benefit, i.e. a reduction of 10–20mm on a 100mm VAS, is seen with 1–4 **lidocaine** 5% patches covering the maximally painful area.[2]

In conclusion, certainly in cancer-related neuropathic pains, systemic local anesthetics should be considered for use only when the combination of a strong opioid + NSAID + TCA + anti-epileptic are ineffective or poorly tolerated. Even then, **ketamine** (see p.468) may be preferable because:
- the serum level does not need to be monitored
- it can be given PO
- it is more effective than **lidocaine** in spinal cord injury pain.[20]

1 Challapalli V et al. (2005) Systemic administration of local anesthetic agents to relieve neuropathic pain. *Cochrane Database of Systematic Reviews*. CD003345.
2 Meier T et al. (2003) Efficacy of lidocaine patch 5% in the treatment of focal peripheral neuropathic pain syndromes: a randomized, double-blind, placebo-controlled study. *Pain*. **106**: 151–158.
3 Devulder J et al. (1993) Neuropathic pain in a cancer patient responding to subcutaneously administered lignocaine. *The Clinical Journal of Pain*. **9**: 220–223.
4 Devor M (2006) Sodium channels and mechanisms of neuropathic pain. *Journal of Pain*. **7**: S3–S12.
5 Attal N et al. (2000) Intravenous lidocaine in central pain: a double-blind, placebo-controlled, psychophysical study. *Neurology*. **54**: 564–574.
6 Attal N et al. (2004) Systemic lidocaine in pain due to peripheral nerve injury and predictors of response. *Neurology*. **62**: 218–225.
7 Ellemann K et al. (1989) Trial of intravenous lidocaine on painful neuropathy in cancer patients. *Clinical Journal of Pain*. **5**: 291–294.
8 Bruera E et al. (1992) A randomized double-blind crossover trial of intravenous lidocaine in the treatment of neuropathic cancer pain. *Journal of Pain and Symptom Management*. **7**: 138–140.
9 Baranowski AP et al. (1999) A trial of intravenous lidocaine on the pain and allodynia of postherpetic neuralgia. *Journal of Pain and Symptom Management*. **17**: 429–433.
10 Backonja M and Gombar KA (1992) Response of central pain syndromes to intravenous lidocaine. *Journal of Pain and Symptom Management*. **7**: 172–178.
11 Chong S et al. (1997) Pilot study evaluating local anesthetics administered systemically for treatment of pain in patients with advanced cancer. *Journal of Pain and Symptom Management*. **13**: 112–117.
12 Thomas J et al. (2004) Intravenous lidocaine relieves severe pain: results of an inpatient hospice chart review. *Journal of Palliative Medicine*. **7**: 660–667.
13 Ferrini R (2000) Parenteral lidocaine for severe intractable pain in six hospice patients continued at home. *Journal of Palliative Medicine*. **3**: 193–200.
14 Massey GV et al. (2002) Continuous lidocaine infusion for the relief of refractory malignant pain in a terminally ill pediatric cancer patient. *Journal of Pediatric Hematology/Oncology*. **24**: 566–568.
15 Ferrante FM et al. (1996) The analgesic response to intravenous lidocaine in the treatment of neuropathic pain. *Anesthesia and Analgesia*. **82**: 91–97.
16 Rosenberg PH et al. (2004) Maximum recommended doses of local anesthetics: a multifactorial concept. *Regional Anesthesia and Pain Medicine* **29**: 564–575; discussion 524.
17 Brose W and Cousins M (1991) Subcutaneous lidocaine for treatment of neuropathic pain. *Pain*. **45**: 145–148.
18 Yamashita S et al. (2002) Lidocaine toxicity during frequent viscous lidocaine use for painful tongue ulcer. *Journal of Pain and Symptom Management*. **24**: 543–545.
19 Tei Y et al. (2005) Lidocaine intoxication at very small doses in terminally ill cancer patients. *Journal of Pain and Symptom Management*. **30**: 6–7.
20 Kvarnstrom A et al. (2004) The analgesic effect of intravenous ketamine and lidocaine on pain after spinal cord injury. *Acta Anaesthesiologica Scandinavica*. **48**: 498–506.

*FLECAINIDE

Class: 1C anti-arrhythmic.

Indications: Cardiac arrhythmias, †neuropathic pain.

Contra-indications: Cardiogenic shock, bradycardia, 2nd or 3rd degree AV block or bundle branch block in the absence of rescue pacing or an indwelling pacemaker (see manufacturer's Product Monograph for more details). Do not give concurrently with **ritonavir** or **fosamprenavir**.

Pharmacology

Flecainide is a chemical congener of **lidocaine**. It is a membrane stabilizer, i.e. it inhibits sodium ion channels in nerve membranes, thereby suppressing injury-induced hyperexcitability in the peripheral and central nervous systems.[1] Flecainide is approved for use in the prevention and treatment of ventricular and supraventricular arrhythmias but, like **mexiletine** (see p.48), it is sometimes used to treat nerve injury pain, generally after treatment failure with a combination of strong opioid + NSAID + TCA + anti-epileptic (see Systemic local anesthetics, p.44). Benefit is reported in about 2/3 of patients with cancer, but there have been no RCTs.[2–4] Flecainide has a narrow therapeutic index, and some patients experience psychoneurological and cardiac toxicity within the recommended therapeutic range.[5,6]

When used as prophylaxis against arrhythmias after recent myocardial infarction (<2 years), flecainide was associated with an increased incidence of sudden death.[7] Thus, when used as an anti-arrhythmic, the manufacturer recommends that treatment is started in hospital. However, at some centres, flecainide for neuropathic pain is started on an outpatient basis without an ECG provided the patient is in normal rhythm, is not in heart failure and has no history of myocardial infarction. Alternative treatments include **ketamine** (see p.468), **methadone** (see p.327) and spinal analgesia (see p.521).

Bio-availability 90–95% PO.

Onset of action 0.5–2h as an anti-arrhythmic.

Time to peak plasma concentration 1.5–6h PO.

Plasma halflife 12–27h.

Duration of action 15–23h as an anti-arrhythmic.

Cautions

Correct electrolyte disturbances, e.g. of K^+, Ca^{2+}, Mg^{2+}, before starting treatment. Hepatic and renal impairment. Risk of myocardial depression increased by β-adrenergic receptor antagonists (β-blockers), calcium-channel blockers and hypokalemia; risk of arrhythmia if used with a pro-arrhythmic drug, e.g. TCAs.

Flecainide is metabolized by, and inhibits, CYP2D6 (see Cytochrome P450, p.551). Plasma concentration increased by **amiodarone** (reduce flecainide dose by 1/3 to 1/2 and monitor plasma concentrations), **cimetidine**, **propranolol** and **quinine**, and decreased by smoking.[8] In contrast, flecainide elimination may be increased by about 1/3 by **phenytoin**, **phenobarbital** and **carbamazepine**.

Undesirable effects

For full list, see manufacturer's Product Monograph

Very common (>10%): dizziness, dyspnea.

Common (<10%, >1%): headache, fatigue, malaise, drowsiness or insomnia, vertigo, anxiety, depression, fever, hypesthesia, paresis, ataxia, tremor, weakness, paresthesia, double/blurred vision, tinnitus, palpitations, tachycardia, sinus node dysfunction, chest pain, nausea, vomiting, anorexia, abdominal pain, constipation or diarrhea, rash, abnormal LFTs.

Dose and use

Flecainide is not a first-line adjuvant analgesic (see Systemic local anesthetics, p.44). *Generally, antidepressants should be stopped at least 48h before starting flecainide.* Initial doses are comparable

to those used in cardiology:
- start with 50mg b.i.d.
- usual dose 100mg b.i.d.
- maximum dose 200mg b.i.d.

The use of a test dose of **lidocaine** 2–5mg/kg IVI has been suggested as a means of predicting whether flecainide or **mexiletine** will be of benefit.[9] However, this is not a reliable guide.[10] Further, in cancer patients, **lidocaine** 5mg/kg IV over 30min is no more effective than placebo.[11–13]

Overdose

A single dose of 800mg, i.e. twice the maximum recommended daily dose, is potentially life-threatening.[5] Symptoms of overdose include sedation, delirium, coma, seizures, respiratory arrest, hypotension, sinus arrest, AV block, and asystole. Treatment is supportive and may necessitate the use of anti-epileptic and anti-arrhythmic drugs. **Sodium bicarbonate** may reverse QRS prolongation, bradycardia and hypotension. Hemodialysis is not of benefit.

Supply

Flecainide (generic)
Tablets 50mg, 100mg, 28 days @ 100mg b.i.d. = $45.

Tambocor® (3M)
Tablets 50mg, 100mg, 28 days @ 100mg b.i.d. = $64.

1 Devor M (2006) Sodium channels and mechanisms of neuropathic pain. *Journal of Pain.* **7**: S3–S12.
2 Dunlop R et al. (1988) Analgesic effects of oral flecainide. *Lancet.* **1**: 420–421.
3 Sinnott C et al. (1991) Flecainide in cancer nerve pain. *Lancet.* **337**: 1347.
4 Chong S et al. (1997) Pilot study evaluating local anesthetics administered systemically for treatment of pain in patients with advanced cancer. *Journal of Pain and Symptom Management.* **13**: 112–117.
5 Nestico PF et al. (1988) New antiarrhythmic drugs. *Drugs.* **35**: 286–319.
6 Bennett M (1997) Paranoid psychosis due to flecainide toxicity in malignant neuropathic pain. *Pain.* **70**: 93–94.
7 Cardiac arrhythmia suppression trial (CAST) (1989) Investigators' preliminary report: effect of encainide and flecainide on mortality in a randomized trial of arrhythmia suppression after myocardial infarction. *New England Journal of Medicine.* **321**: 406–412.
8 Baxter K (ed) (2006) *Stockley's Drug Interactions* (7e). Pharmaceutical Press, London.
9 Galer B et al. (1996) Response to intravenous lidocaine infusion predicts subsequent response to oral mexiletine: a prospective study. *Journal of Pain and Symptom Management.* **12**: 161–167.
10 Jarvis B and Coukell AJ (1998) Mexiletine. A review of its therapeutic use in painful diabetic neuropathy. *Drugs.* **56**: 691–707.
11 Ellemann K et al. (1989) Trial of intravenous lidocaine on painful neuropathy in cancer patients. *Clinical Journal of Pain.* **5**: 291–294.
12 Challapalli V et al. (2005) Systemic administration of local anesthetic agents to relieve neuropathic pain. *Cochrane Database of Systematic Reviews.* CD003345.
13 Bruera E et al. (1992) A randomized double-blind crossover trial of intravenous lidocaine in the treatment of neuropathic cancer pain. *Journal of Pain and Symptom Management.* **7**: 138–140.

*MEXILETINE

Class: 1B anti-arrhythmic.

Indications: Ventricular arrhythmias, neuropathic pain.

Contra-indications: Cardiogenic shock, bradycardia, 2nd or 3rd degree AV block or bundle branch block in the absence of rescue pacing or an indwelling pacemaker (see manufacturer's Product Monograph for more details).

Pharmacology

Mexiletine is a chemical congener of **lidocaine**. It is a membrane stabilizer, i.e. it inhibits sodium ion channels in nerve membranes, thereby suppressing injury-induced hyperexcitability in the peripheral and central nervous systems.[1] Oral mexiletine is well absorbed. About 40% is bound to albumin and α_1-acid glycoprotein. It is metabolized in the liver by CYP2D6 and CYP1A2 to inactive metabolites and smaller doses/dose reduction should be considered for patients with moderate–severe hepatic impairment or severe renal impairment (creatinine clearance <10mL/min).

Mexiletine is approved for the treatment of ventricular arrhythmias but, like **flecainide** (see p.47), it is sometimes used to treat painful peripheral neuropathies, generally after treatment failure with a combination of strong opioid + NSAID + TCA + anti-epileptic (see Systemic local anesthetics, p.44). RCTs have shown benefit in painful diabetic neuropathy,[2–6] and in peripheral nerve injury pain from several other causes,[7–11] but not in that associated with HIV.[12,13] However, in painful diabetic neuropathy, it has an NNT of 10 compared with 2.4 for TCAs.[14] In open-label studies, benefit has been reported in 2/3 of patients with cancer-related neuropathic pain.[15,16] Although it has been used in central post-stroke and spinal cord injury pain,[9,17] a systematic review states that mexiletine is *inactive* in central pain.[14]

Undesirable effects can limit the long-term use of mexiletine;[15] it has a narrow therapeutic index and some patients experience psychoneurological and cardiac toxicity even within the recommended therapeutic range.[18] Alternative treatments include **ketamine** (see p.468), **methadone** (see p.327) and spinal analgesia (see p.521).

Bio-availability 80–90% PO.
Onset of action 1–3h.
Time to peak plasma concentration 2–3h.
Plasma halflife 5–17h.
Duration of action 6–8h.

Cautions

Moderate–severe hepatic impairment, severe renal impairment (creatinine clearance <10mL/min). Risk of esophageal ulceration. Opioids reduce the rate and extent of absorption. Risk of myocardial depression with other anti-arrhythmics (→ hypotension); risk of arrhythmia if used with a pro-arrhythmic drug, e.g. a TCA. Effect reduced by drugs causing hypokalemia (e.g. loop and thiazide diuretics). Plasma concentration of mexiletine increased by inhibitors of CYP2D6 and CYP1A2, e.g. **fluvoxamine, propafenone quinidine** and decreased by inducers of CYP2D6 and CYP1A2, e.g. **phenytoin** and **rifampin**. Mexiletine increases the plasma concentration of caffeine and **theophylline** (see Cytochrome P450, p.551).[19]

Undesirable effects

For full list, see manufacturer's Product Monograph
Very common (>10%): dizziness, lightheadedness, nervousness, inco-ordination, tremor, ataxia, gastro-intestinal distress, nausea, vomiting.
Common (<10%, >1%): confusion, headache, drowsiness or insomnia, depression, weakness, numbness of extremities, paresthesia, nystagmus, blurred vision, tinnitus, dizziness, chest pain, cardiac arrhythmias, palpitations, angina, dyspnea, xerostomia, nausea, constipation or diarrhea, arthralgia, rash.

Dose and use

Mexiletine is not a first-line adjuvant analgesic (see Systemic local anesthetics, p.44). *Generally, antidepressants should be stopped at least 48h before starting mexiletine.* Compared with use in cardiology, the initial dose of mexiletine is low:
• start with 50mg t.i.d. if necessary, increase by 50mg t.i.d. every week
• median dose 600mg/24h (range 300–1,200mg/24h)[20]
• maximum dose 10mg/kg/24h.
To reduce the risk of esophageal irritation and ulceration, mexiletine should be taken sitting upright with a glass of water and preferably with food; the latter may also help to minimize undesirable effects by delaying absorption and thereby reducing the maximum plasma concentration. Alternatively, give a smaller dose more frequently.

The use of a test dose of **lidocaine** 2–5mg/kg IVI has been suggested as a means of predicting whether mexiletine or **flecainide** will be of benefit.[21] However, this is not a reliable guide.[22,23] Further, in cancer patients, **lidocaine** 5mg/kg IV over 30min is no more effective than placebo.[20,24,25]

Overdose

The ingestion of a single dose of >2.4g, i.e. twice the maximum recommended daily dose, is potentially life-threatening.[18] Symptoms of overdose include sedation, delirium, coma, seizures, respiratory arrest, hypotension, sinus arrest, AV block, asystole and nausea and vomiting. Treatment is supportive and may necessitate the use of anti-epileptic and anti-arrhythmic drugs. **Sodium bicarbonate** may reverse QRS prolongation, bradycardia and hypotension. Hemodialysis is not of benefit.

Supply

Mexiletine (generic)
Capsules 100mg, 200mg, 28 days @ 200mg t.i.d. = $92.

1 Devor M (2006) Sodium channels and mechanisms of neuropathic pain. *Journal of Pain.* **7**: S3–S12.
2 Dejgard A et al. (1988) Mexiletine for treatment of chronic painful diabetic neuropathy. *Lancet.* **1**: 9–11.
3 Stracke H et al. (1994) Mexiletine in treatment of painful diabetic neuropathy. *Medica Klinische. (Munich).* **89**: 124–131.
4 Matsuoka K et al. (1997) Double blind trial of mexiletine on painful diabetic polyneuropathy. *Diabetologia.* **40**: A559.
5 Oskarsson P et al. (1997) Efficacy and safety of mexiletine in the treatment of painful diabetic neuropathy. The Mexiletine Study Group. *Diabetes Care.* **20**: 1594–1597.
6 Wright JM et al. (1997) Mexiletine in the symptomatic treatment of diabetic peripheral neuropathy. *Annals of Pharmacotherapy.* **31**: 29–34.
7 Chabal C et al. (1992) The use of oral mexiletine for the treatment of pain after peripheral nerve injury. *Anaesthesiology.* **76**: 513–517.
8 Galer BS et al. (1996) Response to intravenous lidocaine infusion predicts subsequent response to oral mexiletine: a prospective study. *Journal of Pain and Symptom Management.* **12**: 161–167.
9 Kalso E et al. (1998) Systemic local-anaesthetic-type drugs in chronic pain: a systematic review. *European Journal of Pain.* **2**: 3–14.
10 Wallace MS et al. (2000) Efficacy of oral mexiletine for neuropathic pain with allodynia: a double-blind, placebo-controlled, crossover study. *Regional Anesthesia and Pain Medicine.* **25**: 459–467.
11 Fassoulaki A et al. (2002) The analgesic effect of gabapentin and mexiletine after breast surgery for cancer. *Anesthesia and Analgesia.* **95**: 985–991.
12 Kemper C et al. (1998) Mexiletine for HIV-infected patients with painful peripheral neuropathy: a double-blind, placebo-controlled, crossover treatment trial. *Journal of Acquired Immuno-Deficiency Syndromes.* **19**: 367–372.
13 Kieburtz K et al. (1998) A randomized trial of amitriptyline and mexiletine for painful neuropathy in HIV infection. AIDS Clinical Trial Group 242 Protocol Team. *Neurology.* **51**: 1682–1688.
14 Sindrup S and Jensen T (1999) Efficacy of pharmacological treatments of neuropathic pain: an update and effect related to mechanism of drug action. *Pain.* **83**: 389–400.
15 Chong S et al. (1997) Pilot study evaluating local anesthetics administered systemically for treatment of pain in patients with advanced cancer. *Journal of Pain and Symptom Management.* **13**: 112–117.
16 Sloan P et al. (1999) Mexiletine as an adjuvant analgesic for the management of neuropathic cancer pain. *Anesthesia and Analgesia.* **89**: 760–761.
17 Chiou-Tan F et al. (1996) Effect of mexiletine on spinal cord injury dysaesthetic pain. *American Journal of Physical Medicine and Rehabilitation.* **75**: 84–87.
18 Nestico PF et al. (1988) New antiarrhythmic drugs. *Drugs.* **35**: 286–319.
19 Baxter K (ed) (2006) *Stockley's Drug Interactions* (7e). Pharmaceutical Press, London.
20 Challapalli V et al. (2005) Systemic administration of local anesthetic agents to relieve neuropathic pain. *Cochrane Database of Systematic Reviews.* CD003345.
21 Galer B et al. (1996) Response to intravenous lidocaine infusion predicts subsequent response to oral mexiletine: a prospective study. *Journal of Pain and Symptom Management.* **12**: 161–167.
22 Jarvis B and Coukell AJ (1998) Mexiletine. A review of its therapeutic use in painful diabetic neuropathy. *Drugs.* **56**: 691–707.
23 Attal N et al. (2000) Intravenous lidocaine in central pain: a double-blind, placebo-controlled, psychophysical study. *Neurology.* **54**: 564–574.
24 Ellemann K et al. (1989) Trial of intravenous lidocaine on painful neuropathy in cancer patients. *Clinical Journal of Pain.* **5**: 291–294.
25 Bruera E et al. (1992) A randomized double-blind crossover trial of intravenous lidocaine in the treatment of neuropathic cancer pain. *Journal of Pain and Symptom Management.* **7**: 138–140.

*CLONIDINE

Class: α-adrenergic receptor agonist.

Indications: Hypertension, menopausal hot flashes, †migraine prophylaxis, †pain poorly responsive to epidural or intrathecal **morphine** and **bupivacaine**, †spasticity, †diarrhea or †gastroparesis related to autonomic dysfunction in diabetes mellitus, †sweating.

Contra-indications: Cardiac conduction defects.

Pharmacology

Clonidine is a mixed α_1- and α_2-adrenergic receptor agonist (mainly α_2). It reduces the responsiveness of peripheral blood vessels to vasoconstrictor and vasodilator substances, and to sympathetic nerve stimulation.[1] Clonidine can cause a reduction in venous return and mild bradycardia, resulting in a reduced cardiac output.

Clonidine also attenuates the opioid withdrawal syndrome, indicating an interaction with the opioid system. It appears to have synergistic analgesic effects with opioids.[2] Reproducible pain relief in some patients with neuropathic pain has been observed, particularly when given via the ED or IT routes.[3–6] ED clonidine is effective in cancer-related neuropathic pain, generally as an 'add-on' drug (see Spinal analgesia, p.521). It is particularly useful for patients who do not respond to high-dose systemic opioids or who tolerate them poorly, and for those who fail to respond to spinal **morphine** plus **bupivacaine**.[7,8] Although a typical dose is 150–300microgram/24h ED, benefit has been reported in some patients with IT doses of ≤1mg/24h.[6] Further, solo treatment with high-dose ED clonidine, i.e. a bolus of 10microgram/kg followed by an infusion of 6microgram/kg/h, provides effective postoperative analgesia.[9] Benefit has also been reported in patients receiving clonidine by CSCI, with increasing benefit in a few patients with doses of up to 1.5mg/24h.[10]

ED clonidine is absorbed into the systemic circulation producing significant plasma concentrations (reflected clinically by drowsiness and cardiovascular effects), reaching a peak after 20min. IT clonidine produces similar effects; sedation occurs within 15–30min and lasts 1–2h.[6,11,12] The analgesic effect of clonidine can be reversed by α-adrenergic receptor antagonists but not by **naloxone**.[5] Clonidine can thus be used in the management of unexpected acute pain in addicts receiving **naltrexone** (see p.345). It is probable that clonidine analgesia is mediated by an agonist effect at α_2-adrenergic receptors or imidazoline receptors resulting in:

- peripheral and/or central suppression of sympathetic transmitter release[5,13]
- presynaptic inhibition of nociceptive afferents[14]
- post-synaptic inhibition of spinal cord neurones[15,16]
- facilitation of brain stem pain modulating systems.[17]

In patients with spinal cord injury, the addition of clonidine reduces muscle spasticity which has failed to respond to maximal doses of **baclofen**.[18,19] In healthy volunteers, clonidine induces muscular relaxation and reduces pain caused by distension in the stomach, colon and rectum.[20,21] In patients with diabetic-related intestinal autonomic neuropathy, clonidine improves symptoms of gastroparesis and chronic diarrhea.[22–24] The improvement in diarrhea is due partly to the stimulation of α_2-adrenergic receptors on enterocytes, which promotes intestinal fluid and electrolyte absorption, inhibits anion secretion and may also modify intestinal motility.[23,24]

There is RCT evidence that clonidine relieves sweating in menopausal women (with or without hot flashes), and sweating in both men and women resulting from hormonal manipulation by drugs (e.g. **tamoxifen**) or surgery (e.g. castration).[25,26] However, some trials have found no difference from placebo.[27,28]

In patients with cirrhosis receiving **spironolactone** ± **furosemide**, improved renal function and diuresis is seen with co-administration of clonidine 75microgram PO b.i.d. (see p.42) due to inhibition of the renin-aldosterone-angiotensin and sympathetic nervous systems.[29,30] Patients were considered to have an overactive sympathetic nervous system based on a higher than normal serum norepinephrine level.[30]

About 1/2 of a dose of clonidine is excreted unchanged by the kidneys, and most of the remainder is metabolized by the liver to inactive metabolites. Accumulation occurs in renal impairment, extending its halflife up to 40h.

Bio-availability 75–100% PO; 60% TD.[31]
Onset of action 30–60min IV, PO; 2–3 days TD.
Time to peak plasma concentration 1.5–5h PO; 20min ED; 2 days TD.
Plasma halflife 12–16h.
Duration of action 8–24h PO; 24h TD.

Cautions

Severe coronary insufficiency, recent myocardial infarction, stroke, peripheral vascular disease. May precipitate depression in susceptible patients. Abrupt curtailment of long-term treatment likely to cause agitation, sympathetic overactivity, rebound hypertension; therefore withdraw treatment progressively over 2–4 days (ED) or 1 week (PO).

Effects reduced or abolished by drugs with α-adrenergic receptor antagonist activity, e.g. **mirtazapine**, TCAs (e.g. **amitriptyline, clomipramine, desipramine, imipramine**), and antipsychotic drugs.[32]

TD patches (not Canada) contain metal in the backing and must be removed before MRI to avoid burns.[33]

Undesirable effects

For full list, see manufacturer's Product Monograph.

Very common (>10%): sedation and dry mouth (initially), dizziness, transient pruritus and erythema (TD route).

Common (<10%, >1%): headache, fatigue, lethargy, depression (long-term use), nervousness, nocturnal restlessness, hypotension (after bolus injection), peripheral vasoconstriction, nausea, vomiting, anorexia, constipation, sodium and water retention, nocturia, sexual dysfunction, local reactions (e.g. rash, hyperpigmentation, excoriation) with TD route.

Dose and use

Clonidine is available as a tablet, but can also be administered as a TD patch (not Canada),[4,34] by CSCI, and spinally. TD is generally better tolerated than PO.

Spinal analgesia

ED clonidine is generally given with **morphine** and **bupivacaine** (see p.521). A typical ED regimen would be:
- a test bolus dose of 50–150microgram in 5mL saline injection over 5min
- if relief obtained, 150–300microgram/24h by infusion.

Clonidine is also used IT. A typical IT regimen would be:
- a test bolus dose of 50microgram in 5mL saline injection over 5min
- if relief obtained, 50–150microgram/24h by infusion.

Spasticity

Generally used as an adjunct to maximum dose of **baclofen**:
- start with 50microgram PO b.i.d.
- if necessary, increase by 50microgram every 3–7 days
- usual maximum dose 200microgram b.i.d.

Gastroparesis or diarrhea related to autonomic dysfunction in diabetes mellitus
- start with 50microgram PO b.i.d.
- if necessary, increase by 50microgram every 24h
- usual maintenance dose 150microgram b.i.d.
- usual maximum dose for diabetic gastroparesis 300microgram b.i.d.
- usual maximum dose for diabetic diarrhea 600microgram b.i.d.

Hormonal/menopausal sweating
- start with 50microgram PO b.i.d.
- if necessary, increase by 50microgram every 3–7 days
- usual maintenance dose 50–100microgram b.i.d.

Supply

Clonidine (generic)
Tablets 100microgram, 200microgram, 28 days @ 100microgram b.i.d. = $10.

Dixarit® (Boehringer Ingelheim)
Tablets 25microgram, 28 days @ 50microgram b.i.d. = $33.

Catapres® (Boehringer Ingelheim)
Tablets 100microgram, 200microgram, 28 days @ 100microgram b.i.d. = $12.

Clonidine injection is not commercially available in Canada, but can be imported through the Special Access Programme (see p.xx).

1　Hieble JP and Ruffolo RR (1991) Therapeutic applications of agents interacting with alpha-adrenoceptors. In: RR Ruffolo (ed) *Alpha-adrenoceptors: molecular biology, biochemistry and pharmacology* Vol 8. Karger, Basel, pp. 180–220.

2　Siddall PJ et al. (2000) The efficacy of intrathecal morphine and clonidine in the treatment of pain after spinal cord injury. *Anesthesia and Analgesia.* **91**: 1493–1498.

3　Glynn C et al. (1988) A double-blind comparison between epidural morphine and epidural clonidine in patients with chronic noncancer pain. *Pain.* **34**: 123–128.

4　Zeigler D et al. (1992) Transdermal clonidine versus placebo in painful diabetic neuropathy. *Pain.* **48**: 403–408.

5　Quan D et al. (1993) Clonidine in pain management. *Annals of Pharmacotherapy.* **27**: 313–315.

6　Ackerman LL et al. (2003) Long-term outcomes during treatment of chronic pain with intrathecal clonidine or clonidine/opioid combinations. *Journal of Pain and Symptom Management.* **26**: 668–677.

7　Eisenach JC et al. (1995) Epidural clonidine analgesia for intractable cancer pain. The Epidural Clonidine Study Group. *Pain.* **61**: 391–399.

8　Chen H et al. (2004) Contemporary management of neuropathic pain for the primary care physician. *Mayo Clinic Proceedings.* **79**: 1533–1545.

9　deKock M et al. (1999) Epidural clonidine or bupivacaine as the sole analgesic agent during and after abdominal surgery. *Anesthesiology.* **90**: 1354–1362. [Erratum appears in *Anesthesiology* (1999) **91**: 602.]

10　Glynn C (1997) Personal communication.

11　Malinovsky JM et al. (2003) Sedation caused by clonidine in patients with spinal cord injury. *British Journal of Anaesthesia.* **90**: 742–745.

12　Wells J and Hardy P (1987) Epidural clonidine. *Lancet.* **i**: 108.

13　Langer SZ et al. (1980) Recent developments in noradrenergic neurotransmission and its relevance to the mechanism of action of certain antihypertensive agents. *Hypertension.* **2**: 372–382.

14　Calvillo O and Ghignone M (1986) Presynaptic effect of clonidine on unmyelinated afferent fibers in the spinal cord of the cat. *Neuroscience Letters.* **64**: 335–339.

15　Yaksh T (1985) Pharmacology of spinal adrenergic systems which modulate spinal nociceptive processing. *Pharmacology, Biochemistry and Behaviour.* **22**: 845–858.

16　Michel MC and Insel PA (1989) Are there multiple imidazoline binding sites? *TIPS.* **10**: 342–344.

17　Sagen J and Proudfit H (1985) Evidence for pain modulation by pre- and postsynaptic noradrenergic receptors in the medulla oblongata. *Brain Research.* **331**: 285–293.

18　Weingarden S and Belen J (1992) Clonidine transdermal system for treatment of spasticity in spinal cord injury. *Archives of Physical Medicine and Rehabilitation.* **73**: 876–877.

19　Yablon S and Sipski M (1993) Effect of transdermal clonidine on spinal spasticity: a case series. *American Journal of Physical Medicine and Rehabilitation.* **72**: 154–156.

20　Thumshirn M et al. (1999) Modulation of gastric sensory and motor functions by nitrergic and alpha2-adrenergic agents in humans. *Gastroenterology.* **116**: 573–585.

21　Viramontes BE et al. (2001) Effects of an alpha(2)-adrenergic agonist on gastrointestinal transit, colonic motility, and sensation in humans. *American Journal of Physiology Gastrointestinal and Liver Physiology.* **281**: G1468–1476.

22　Rosa-Silva L et al. (1995) Treatment of diabetic gastroparesis with oral clonidine. *Alimentary Pharmacology and Therapeutics.* **9**: 179–183.

23　Fedorak R et al. (1985) Treatment of diabetic diarrhea with clonidine. *Annals of Internal Medicine.* **102**: 197–199.

24　Fedorak R and Field M (1987) Antidiarrheal therapy prospects for new agents. *Digestive Diseases and Science.* **32**: 195–205.

25　Goldberg R et al. (1994) Transdermal clonidine for ameliorating tamoxifen-induced hot flashes. *Journal of Clinical Oncology.* **12**: 155–158.

26　Pandya K et al. (2000) Oral clonidine in postmenopausal patients with breast cancer experiencing tamoxifen-induced hot flashes: a university of Rochester Cancer Centre community clinical oncology program study. *Annals of Internal Medicine.* **132**: 788–793.

27　Salmi T and Punnonen R (1979) Clonidine in the treatment of menopausal symptoms. *International Journal of Gynaecology and Obstetrics.* **16**: 422–461.

28　Loprinzi C et al. (1994) Transdermal clonidine for ameliorating post-orchidectomy hot flashes. *Journal of Urology.* **151**: 634–636.

29　Kalambokis G et al. (2005) Renal effects of treatment with diuretics, octreotide or both, in non-azotemic cirrhotic patients with ascites. *Nephrology, Dialysis, Transplantation.* **20**: 1623–1629.

30　Lenaerts A et al. (2006) Effects of clonidine on diuretic response in ascitic patients with cirrhosis and activation of sympathetic nervous system. *Hepatology.* **44**: 844–849.

31　Toon S et al. (1989) Rate and extent of absorption of clonidine from a transdermal therapeutic system. *Journal of Pharmacy and Pharmacology.* **41**: 17–21.

32　Baxter K (ed) (2006) *Stockley's Drug Interactions* (7e). Pharmaceutical Press, London, p. 667.

33　Institute for Safe Medication Practices (2004) Medication Safety Alert. Burns in MRI patients wearing transdermal patches. Available from: www.ismp.org/Newsletters/acutecare/articles/20040408.asp?ptr=y

34　Davis K et al. (1991) Topical application of clonidine relieves hyperalgesia in patients with sympathetically maintained pain. *Pain.* **47**: 309–317.

NITROGLYCERIN

Class: Nitrate.

Indications: Angina, left ventricular failure, anal fissure, †smooth muscle spasm pain (particularly of the esophagus, rectum and anus or cutaneous leiomyomas),[1] †biliary and †renal colic.

Contra-indications: Severe hypotension (systolic < 90mmHg), aortic or mitral stenosis, cardiac tamponade, constrictive pericarditis, hypertrophic obstructive cardiomyopathy, marked anemia, severe hypovolemia, raised intracranial pressure, narrow-angle glaucoma. Concurrent use of **sildenafil, tadalafil and vardenafil** (may precipitate hypotension and myocardial infarction).[2]

Pharmacology

Nitroglycerin relaxes smooth muscle in blood vessels and the GI tract, and may thus improve dysphagia and odynophagia associated with esophagitis and esophageal spasm.[3,4]

In patients with anal fissure, nitroglycerin relieves pain, improves quality of life and aids healing. It is more effective than botulinum toxin but less effective than surgery.[5–9] In chronic anal fissure, nitroglycerin ointment 0.2–0.4% applied b.i.d. to the anal canal is as effective and as well tolerated as SR **nifedipine** 20mg PO b.i.d.[10] It also relieves painful rectal spasm. Thus, if nitroglycerin is ineffective or poorly tolerated, consider the use of **nifedipine** (see p.56) or other smooth muscle relaxants, e.g. **hyoscine (scopolamine) butylbromide** (see p.11).

Nitroglycerin produces its smooth muscle relaxant effects via its metabolism to nitric oxide (NO), which stimulates guanylate cyclase. This results in an increase in cyclic guanosine monophosphate which reduces the amount of intracellular calcium available for muscle contraction.[11] NO appears to have an important role in the regulation of distal esophageal peristalsis and relaxation of the lower esophageal sphincter. A wider role of NO in pain is evident but is yet to be clarified. NO is produced when the NMDA-receptor is stimulated by excitatory amino acids (see **ketamine**, p.468) and may be important in the development of opioid tolerance as NO synthase inhibitors attenuate the development of analgesic tolerance.[12] TD nitroglycerin enhances pain relief in cancer patients and, as a topical gel, reduces local pain and inflammation.[13–18] In patients with lung cancer, a TD patch for 5 days with each cycle of chemotherapy increases the frequency and duration of response. This may reflect improved perfusion of the tumour, thereby increasing drug delivery or decreasing hypoxia (a factor associated with drug resistance).[19]

It is rapidly absorbed through the buccal mucosa but orally it is inactivated by extensive first-pass metabolism in the gastro-intestinal mucosa and liver. Many patients on long-acting or TD nitrates develop tolerance, i.e. experience a reduced therapeutic effect. Tolerance is generally prevented if nitrate levels are allowed to fall for 4–8h in every 24h (a 'nitrate holiday'). This may not be possible for patients with persistent pain. If tolerance develops, it will be necessary to increase the dose to restore efficacy.

Bio-availability 40% SL.
Onset of action 1–3min SL; 30–60min ointment or TD patch.
Time to peak plasma concentration 3–6min SL; 2h TD.
Plasma halflife 1–3min SL; 2–4min TD.
Duration of action 30–60min SL; 8h ointment; 24h TD patch.

Cautions

Severe hepatic or renal impairment, hypothyroidism, malnutrition, hypovolemia, hypoxemia, hypothermia, recent myocardial infarction.

Exacerbates the hypotensive effect of other drugs. Drugs causing dry mouth may reduce the effect of sublingual nitrates. Topically applied nitroglycerin can be absorbed in sufficient quantities to cause undesirable systemic effects.

TD patches which contain metal in the backing, e.g. Transderm-Nitro® (but not Nitro-Dur®) must be removed before MRI to avoid burns.[20]

Undesirable effects

For full list, see manufacturer's Product Monograph.
Very common (>10%): headache.
Common (<10%, >1%): flushing, dizziness, postural hypotension, tachycardia (paradoxical bradycardia also reported), nausea, local stinging, itching or burning sensation after SL spray or rectal administration.
These effects generally settle with continued use.

Dose and use

For intermittent dysphagia and/or odynophagia, administer 5–15min a.c.
- start with 400–500microgram SL
- if necessary, increase to a maximum single dose of 1mg
- instruct the patient to swallow or spit out tablet once pain relief is obtained
- repeat p.r.n.

For persistent spasm consider:
- nitroglycerin TD patches
- orally active nitrates, e.g. **isosorbide mononitrate**.

For pain due to anal fissure, use 0.2–0.4% rectal ointment (see Supply), apply a pea-sized quantity or 2.5cm length of ointment to the anal rim b.i.d. for 6–8 weeks.[5]

Supply

Nitroglycerin (generic)
Aerosol spray 400microgram/metered dose, 200-dose unit = $9.

Nitrostat® (Pfizer)
Tablets SL 300microgram, 600microgram, 100 = $13; *store in the original glass container; because of degradation, unused tablets should be discarded after 8 weeks.*

Nitrolingual® (Sanofi-Aventis)
Aerosol spray 400microgram/metered dose, 200-dose unit = $15.

TD products
Nitro-Dur® (Schering-Plough)
TD patch 200microgram/h (approx 5mg/24h), 400microgram/h (approx 10mg/24h), 600microgram/h, (approx 15mg/24h), 800microgram/h (approx 20mg/24h), 28 days @ 1 patch daily = $17, $20, $20 and $34 respectively.

Transderm-Nitro® (Novartis)
TD patch 200microgram/h (approx 5mg/24h), 400microgram/h (approx 10mg/24h), 600microgram/h, (approx 15mg/24h), 28 days @ 1 patch daily = $19, $22 and $22, respectively.

Topical
Nitrol® (Paladin)
Ointment 2%, 60g = $39.

Rectal ointments
Rectal ointment 0.2%, can be compounded by diluting 2% nitroglycerin ointment (Nitrol®, Paladin, 60g = $39) 1:10 with petrolatum.[21]

This is not a complete list.

1 George S et al. (1997) Pain in multiple leiomyomas alleviated by nifedipine. *Pain.* **73**: 101–102.
2 Baxter K (ed) (2009) Stockley's Drug Interactions (online edition). Pharmaceutical Press, London. Available from: www.medicinescomplete.com/mc/stockley/current/ (subscription required)
3 McDonnell F and Walsh D (1999) Treatment of odynophagia and dysphagia in advanced cancer with sublingual glyceryl trinitrate. *Palliative Medicine.* **13**: 251–252.
4 Tutuian R and Castell DO (2006) Review article: oesophageal spasm – diagnosis and management. *Alimentary Pharmacology and Therapeutics.* **23**: 1393–1402.
5 Lund J and Scholefield J (1997) A randomised, prospective, double-blind, placebo-controlled trial of glyceryl trinitrate ointment in treatment of anal fissure. *Lancet.* **349**: 11–14.
6 Griffin N et al. (2004) Quality of life in patients with chronic anal fissure. *Colorectal Disease.* **6**: 39–44.
7 Solomon M and Smith S (2004) Review: medical therapies are less effective than surgery for anal fissure. Available from: http://ebm.bmjjournals.com/cgi/reprint/9/4/112
8 Thornton MJ et al. (2005) Manometric effect of topical glyceryl trinitrate and its impact on chronic anal fissure healing. *Diseases of the Colon and Rectum.* **48**: 1207–1212.
9 Fruehauf H et al. (2006) Efficacy and safety of botulinum toxin a injection compared with topical nitroglycerin ointment for the treatment of chronic anal fissure: a prospective randomized study. *American Journal of Gastroenterology.* **101**: 2107–2112.
10 Mustafa NA et al. (2006) Comparison of topical glyceryl trinitrate ointment and oral nifedipine in the treatment of chronic anal fissure. *Acta Chirurgica Belgica.* **106**: 55–58.
11 Hashimoto S and Kobayashi A (2003) Clinical pharmacokinetics and pharmacodynamics of glyceryl trinitrate and its metabolites. *Clinical Pharmacokinetics.* **42**: 205–221.
12 Elliott K et al. (1994) The NMDA receptor antagonists, LY274614 and MK-801, and the nitric oxide synthase inhibitor, NG-nitro-L-arginine, attenuate analgesic tolerance to the mu-opioid morphine but not to kappa opioids. *Pain.* **56**: 69–75.

13 Ferreira S *et al.* (1992) Blockade of hyperalgesia and neurogenic oedema by topical application of nitroglycerin. *European Journal of Pharmacology.* **217**: 207–209.

14 Berrazueta J *et al.* (1994) Local transdermal glyceryl trinitrate has an antiinflammatory action on thrombophlebitis induced by sclerosis of leg varicose veins. *Angiology.* **5**: 347–351.

15 Lauretti G *et al.* (1999) Oral ketamine and transdermal nitroglycerin as analgesic adjuvants to oral morphine therapy and amitriptyline for cancer pain management. *Anesthesiology.* **90**: 1528–1533.

16 Lauretti GR *et al.* (2002) Double-blind evaluation of transdermal nitroglycerine as adjuvant to oral morphine for cancer pain management. *Journal of Clinical Anesthesia.* **14**: 83–86.

17 El-Sheikh SM and El-Kest E (2004) Transdermal nitroglycerine enhanced fentanyl patch analgesia in cancer pain management. *Egyptian Journal of Anaesthesia.* **20**: 291–294.

18 Paoloni JA *et al.* (2004) Topical glyceryl trinitrate treatment of chronic noninsertional achilles tendinopathy. A randomized, double-blind, placebo-controlled trial. *Journal of Bone and Joint Surgery American Volume.* **86-A**: 916–922.

19 Yasuda H *et al.* (2006) Randomized phase II trial comparing nitroglycerin plus vinorelbine and cisplatin with vinorelbine and cisplatin alone in previously untreated stage IIIB/IV non-small-cell lung cancer. *Journal of Clinical Oncology.* **24**: 688–694.

20 Institute for Safe Medication Practices (2004) Medication Safety Alert. Burns in MRI patients wearing transdermal patches. Available from: www.ismp.org/Newsletters/acutecare/articles/20040408.asp?ptr=y

21 DTB (1998) Glyceryl trinitrate for anal fissure? *Drug and Therapeutics Bulletin.* **36**: 55–56.

NIFEDIPINE

Class: Calcium-channel blocker.

Indications: Prophylaxis of stable angina, hypertension, †Raynaud's phenomenon (use immediate release formulation) †severe smooth muscle spasm pain (particularly of the esophagus, rectum and anus, cutaneous leiomyomas),[1–5] †intractable hiccup.[6,7]

Contra-indications: Cardiogenic shock, severe aortic stenosis, acute or unstable angina (normal-release capsules PO or SL may cause hypotension and reflex tachycardia precipitating myocardial or cerebrovascular ischemia). *Do not use within 1 month of myocardial infarction.*

Pharmacology

Calcium-channel blockers inhibit the influx of calcium into cells, thereby modifying cell function, e.g. smooth muscle contraction and neural transmission.[8] They have an antinociceptive effect and augment opioid analgesia. Nifedipine may help hiccup by relieving esophageal spasm or by interference with neural pathways involved in hiccup.[6,7,9] In chronic anal fissure, SR nifedipine 20mg PO b.i.d. provides similar outcomes to **nitroglycerin** ointment 0.2–0.4% (see p.53) applied b.i.d. to the anal canal.[10]

Nifedipine exhibits most of its effects on blood vessels, less on the myocardium and has no anti-arrhythmic activity. It rarely precipitates heart failure because any negative inotropic effect is offset by a reduction in left ventricular work. Nifedipine undergoes extensive first-pass metabolism in the liver to inactive metabolites that are excreted in the urine. Higher plasma concentrations are seen in slow metabolizers, which are more prevalent in South American, South Asian and Black African populations.[11,12] Hepatic impairment increases bio-availability and halflife.

Bio-availability 90% PO (normal-release capsules); 50–70% (SR tablets Apotex®) 77% (Adalat® XL).

Onset of action 15min (normal-release capsules).

Time to peak plasma concentration 1–2h PO (normal-release capsules); 4h (SR tablets Apotex®); 6h (Adalat® XL).

Plasma halflife 5h (normal-release capsules); 10h (SR tablets Apotex®).

Duration of action 8h (normal-release capsules); 12 or 24h (SR tablets, depending on brand).

Cautions

Serious drug interactions: augments the hypotensive and negative inotropic effects of other drugs, e.g. α- and β-adrenergic receptor antagonists, **chlorpromazine**, **vardenafil**.[13]

May exacerbate angina; discontinue nifedipine if angina occurs 30–60min after the first dose. May precipitate or worsen heart failure; avoid in patients with significantly impaired cardiac function or heart failure. Hepatic impairment, may impair glucose tolerance and worsen diabetes mellitus.

Nifedipine is metabolized by and inhibits CYP3A4 and CYP2D6; it also inhibits CYP1A2 and CYP2C8/9. Plasma concentration increased by grapefruit juice, **cimetidine** (reduce nifedipine dose by 50%), **fluoxetine**, **fluconazole** and **itraconazole**; reduced by **phenobarbital**, **phenytoin** and **rifampin**. Nifedipine increases plasma concentrations of **tacrolimus** and **theophylline**; may increase or reduce plasma concentrations of **quinidine** (see Cytochrome P450, p.551).[13]

Undesirable effects

For full list, see manufacturer's Product Monograph.

Common (<10%, >1%): headache, dizziness, vasodilation, peripheral edema, nausea.

Uncommon (<1%, >0.1%): asthenia, lethargy, malaise, agitation, nervousness, sleep disorder, tremor, vertigo, abnormal vision, chest pain, tachycardia, palpitations, postural hypotension, edema, dyspnea, dry mouth, dyspepsia, abdominal pain, diarrhea or constipation, rash, pruritus, sweating.

Dose and use

Patients with angina should not bite into or use a normal-release capsule SL because of the risk of rapid-onset hypotension and reflex tachycardia, which could lead to myocardial or cerebrovascular ischemia.

- start with 10mg PO/SL stat, and 10–20mg t.i.d. with food, or SR 20mg b.i.d. or 30–60mg once daily
- in achalasia use 10–20mg SL 30min a.c.
- usual maximum dose 60–80mg/24h.

Up to 160mg/24h has been used for intractable hiccup with concurrent **fludrocortisone** 0.5–1mg to overcome associated orthostatic hypotension.[7]

Supply

Nifedipine (generic)
Capsules 5mg, 10mg, 28 days @ 10mg t.i.d. = $41.
Tablets SR 10mg, 20mg 28 days @ 10mg b.i.d. = $25.

Adalat® XL (Bayer)
Tablets SR 20mg, 30mg, 60mg, 28 days @ 30mg once daily = $36.

1 Cargill G et al. (1982) Nifedipine for relief of esophageal chest pain. New England Journal of Medicine. **307**: 187–188.
2 Al-Waili N (1990) Nifedipine for intestinal colic. Journal of the American Medical Association. **263**: 3258.
3 Celik A et al. (1995) Hereditary proctalgia fugax and constipation: report of a second family. Gut. **36**: 581–584.
4 George S et al. (1997) Pain in multiple leiomyomas alleviated by nifedipine. Pain. **73**: 101–102.
5 McLoughlin R and McQuillan R (1997) Using nifedipine to treat tenesmus. Palliative Medicine. **11**: 419–420.
6 Lipps DC et al. (1990) Nifedipine for intractable hiccups. Neurology. **40**: 531–532.
7 Brigham B and Bolin T (1992) High dose nifedipine and fludrocortisone for intractable hiccups. Medical Journal of Australia. **157**: 70.
8 Castell DO (1985) Calcium-channel blocking agents for gastrointestinal disorders. American Journal of Cardiology. **55**: 210B–213B.
9 Williams M (2004) The management of hiccups in advanced cancer. CME Cancer Medicine. **2**: 68–70.
10 Mustafa NA et al. (2006) Comparison of topical glyceryl trinitrate ointment and oral nifedipine in the treatment of chronic anal fissure. Acta Chirurgica Belgica. **106**: 55–58.
11 Sowunmi A et al. (1995) Ethnic differences in nifedipine kinetics: comparisons between Nigerians, Caucasians and South Asians. British Journal of Clinical Pharmacology. **40**: 489–493.
12 Castaneda-Hernandez G et al. (1996) Interethnic variability in nifedipine disposition: reduced systemic plasma clearance in Mexican subjects. British Journal of Clinical Pharmacology. **41**: 433–434.
13 Baxter K (ed) (2006) Stockley's Drug Interactions (7e). Pharmaceutical Press, London.

LOW MOLECULAR WEIGHT HEPARIN (LMWH)

Indications: Surgical thromboprophylaxis (**dalteparin, enoxaparin, tinzaparin**), medical thromboprophylaxis (**dalteparin, enoxaparin**), treatment of thrombo-embolism (**dalteparin, enoxaparin, nadroparin, tinzaparin**), prevention of clotting in extracorporeal circuits during hemodialysis (**dalteparin, nadroparin, tinzaparin**), unstable angina and non-Q wave myocardial infarction (**dalteparin, enoxaparin, nadroparin**), †thrombophlebitis migrans, †disseminated intravascular coagulation (DIC).

Contra-indications: Active major bleeding, suspected or confirmed immune-mediated heparin-induced thrombocytopenia (HIT) with a LMWH, known bleeding diathesis, severe uncontrolled hypertension, hemorrhagic stroke, diabetic or hemorrhagic retinopathy, bacterial endocarditis, injury or surgery involving the brain, spinal cord, eyes or ears, spinal analgesia (if *treatment* dose of LMWH, increased risk of spinal hematoma), IM use (risk of hematoma at the injection site).
Note: variation exists in what manufacturers consider to be a contra-indication or a caution; see individual Product Monographs.

Pharmacology

Several varieties of low molecular weight heparin (LMWH) are now available, e.g. **dalteparin, enoxaparin, nadroparin**, and **tinzaparin**. All LMWH is derived from porcine heparin and some patients may need to avoid it because of hypersensitivity, or for religious or cultural reasons. The most appropriate non-porcine alternative is **fondaparinux**.[1–3]

LMWH acts by potentiating the inhibitory effect of antithrombin III on factor Xa and thrombin. It has a relatively higher ability to potentiate factor Xa inhibition than to prolong plasma clotting time (APTT), which cannot be used to guide dosing.[1] Anti-factor Xa activity levels can be measured if necessary, e.g. if a patient is at increased risk of bleeding, but routine monitoring is not generally required because the dose is determined by the patient's weight.

LMWH is as effective as unfractionated heparin for the treatment of DVT and pulmonary embolism (PE) and is now considered the initial treatment of choice.[1,4] Other advantages include a longer duration of action which allows administration once daily, and possibly a better safety profile, e.g. fewer major hemorrhages.[5,6]

Compared with non-cancer patients, those with cancer are about three times more likely to experience recurrent thrombo-embolism, *despite* optimal oral anticoagulant treatment (e.g. 21% vs. 7% of patients).[7] The increased risk results from the cancer-related pro-inflammatory state, activation of the coagulation cascade by procoagulant proteins expressed by the cancer, damage to blood vessel walls and venous stasis in addition to other general risk factors (Box 2.B). Major bleeding is also more likely in patients with cancer, irrespective of the INR.[8] In patients with cancer,

---

Box 2.B Risk factors for thrombo-embolism in medical patients[2,15–21]

Age ⩾40 years, particularly >60 years
Immobility
Obesity
Cancer, particularly metastatic and of the pancreas, stomach, bladder, ovary, uterus, kidney, or lung; also hematological
Chronic respiratory or cardiac disease
Other serious medical conditions, e.g. sepsis, lower limb weakness (including spinal cord compression), inflammatory bowel disease, collagen disorder
Varicose veins/chronic venous insufficiency
Previous thrombo-embolism
Cancer chemotherapy, e.g. platinum compounds, 5-FU, mitomycin-C, thalidomide
Growth factors, e.g. granulocyte colony stimulating factor, erythropoietin
Radiation therapy, e.g. to the pelvis
Hormone therapy, e.g. oral contraceptives, hormone replacement, tamoxifen, anastrozole, and possibly progestins
Thrombophilia

LMWH is more effective than **warfarin**, with a similar (or reduced) risk of bleeding.[9-12] Thus, LMWH is considered superior to **warfarin** for the treatment of thrombo-embolism in patients with cancer (UK specialist guidelines)[13] and is recommended for at least the first 3–6 months of indefinite anticoagulation for thrombo-embolism in patients with cancer (USA specialist guidelines).[4,14]

LMWH is the preferred choice for indefinite anticoagulation in patients for whom maintaining a stable INR is likely to be, or turns out to be, difficult (risking either therapeutic failure or hemorrhagic complications) or those who have recurrent thrombo-embolism despite a therapeutic INR.

LMWH is also the treatment of choice for *chronic* DIC; this commonly presents as recurrent thromboses in both superficial and deep veins which do not respond to **warfarin**. The antifibrinolytic drug **tranexamic acid** should not be used in DIC because it increases the risk of end-organ damage from microvascular thromboses. For recurrent thrombo-embolism despite LMWH, exclude heparin-induced thrombocytopenia (HIT), check patient adherence and seek the advice of a hematologist.

LMWH interacts with growth factors, other blood components and vascular cells. An anticancer effect has been seen, possibly via inhibiting cancer-cell growth, angiogenesis and metastasis.[22-25] Survival is improved in cancer patients receiving LMWH compared with unfractionated heparin, or when LMWH is given in addition to chemotherapy compared with chemotherapy alone. This effect cannot be attributed to differences in thrombosis or complications of bleeding and the improvement was greatest in those whose life expectancy was >6 months at the outset of treatment. However, such use of LMWH is not currently recommended outside of a clinical trial.[1]

For pharmacokinetic details, see Table 2.1. LMWH is likely to be superseded by specific factor Xa inhibitors, e.g. **fondaparinux**.[1-3] Some of these need be administered only once weekly, e.g. **idraparinux** (not Canada).[26]

Table 2.1 Selected pharmacokinetic details for dalteparin, enoxaparin and tinzaparin[27-30]

	Dalteparin	Enoxaparin	Tinzaparin
Bio-availability SC[a]	87%	100%	87%
Onset of action	3min IV 2–4h SC	5min IV 3h SC	5min IV 2–3h SC
Time to peak plasma activity[a]	4h SC	2–6h SC	4–5h SC
Plasma activity halflife[a]	2h IV 3–5h SC	2–4.5h IV 4.5–7h SC	1.5h IV 3–4h SC
Duration of action	10–24h SC	>24h SC	24h

a. based on anti-factor Xa activity.

Cautions

Note: variation exists in what manufacturers consider to be a contra-indication or a caution; see individual Product Monographs.

Serious drug interactions: enhanced anticoagulant effect with anticoagulant/antiplatelet drugs, e.g. NSAIDs (particularly **ketorolac**).

Increased risk of hemorrhage if underlying bleeding diathesis (e.g. thrombocytopenia), recent cerebral hemorrhage, recent neurological or ophthalmic surgery, uncontrolled hypertension, diabetic or hypertensive retinopathy, current or past peptic ulcer.

Risk of spinal (intrathecal or epidural) hematoma in patients undergoing spinal puncture or with an indwelling spinal catheter, particularly if concurrently receiving a drug which affects hemostasis. Spinal analgesia may be used in patients on *thromboprophylactic* doses of LMWH but monitor for neurological impairment.

Severe hepatic impairment: reduced synthesis of clotting factors increases the risk of bleeding. Caution (e.g. consider dose reduction) is recommended for **dalteparin**, **enoxaparin** (also possible risk of accumulation) and **tinzaparin**.

Severe renal impairment: dose reduction is recommended for **enoxaparin** and **nadroparin** and may be necessary for **dalteparin** and **tinzaparin** (see below).

Inhibition of aldosterone secretion by heparin/LMWH may cause hyperkalemia. The risk appears to increase with duration of therapy and is higher in patients with diabetes mellitus, chronic renal failure, acidosis and those taking potassium supplements or potassium-sparing drugs. The UK CSM recommends measuring plasma potassium in such patients before starting heparin and regularly thereafter, particularly if heparin is to be continued for >1 week, although a specific frequency is not stated.

Undesirable effects
For full list, see manufacturers' Product Monographs
Common (<10%, >1%): headache, dizziness, pain at the injection site, minor bleeding (generally hematoma at the injection site), major bleeding in surgical patients receiving thromboprophylaxis and patients being treated for DVT or PE, tachycardia, chest pain, peripheral edema, hypotension, hypertension, anemia, nausea, constipation, reversible increases in liver transaminase enzymes, back pain, hematuria.
Uncommon (<1%, >0.1%): major bleeding in patients receiving thromboprophylaxis, thrombocytopenia (see below), abdominal pain, diarrhea.

Heparin-induced thrombocytopenia (HIT)
Both standard heparin and LMWH can cause thrombocytopenia (platelet count $<100 \times 10^9$/L). An early (<4 days) mild fall in platelet count is often seen after starting heparin therapy, particularly after surgery. This corrects spontaneously despite the continued use of heparin and is asymptomatic.[31] However, in <1% of patients, immune HIT develops, associated with heparin-dependent IgG antibodies (Box 2.C).[31–33] The antibodies form a complex with platelet factor 4

Box 2.C Diagnosis and management of heparin-induced thrombocytopenia (HIT)[32,33,35,36]

High clinical suspicion for HIT
- platelet count fall below the normal range or by >50%, generally after 5–10 days of heparin use, sometimes sooner and occasionally several days after heparin has been stopped
- new thrombotic or thrombo-embolic event
- necrosis or erythematous plaques at injection sites.
If any of the above occur, evaluate probability of HIT and obtain advice from a hematologist.

Diagnosis
Based on both the clinical probability (see Table 2.2) and laboratory tests, e.g.:
- platelet activation assay using washed platelets
- antigen-based high-sensitivity assay of platelet factor 4/heparin IgG antibodies.

Therapeutic approach
If high probability of HIT, while awaiting results of laboratory test:
- stop heparin or LMWH
- start treatment with a non-heparin anticoagulant, e.g. danaparoid, lepirudin, argatroban whether or not there is clinical evidence of a DVT.
Do not:
- use warfarin alone because this may increase the risk of venous limb gangrene
- prescribe warfarin until the platelet count has recovered
- give prophylactic platelet transfusions.

The non-heparin anticoagulant should be continued until the INR has been at a therapeutic level for two consecutive days.

Preventing recurrence
- record the diagnosis in the patient's notes as a serious allergy
- warn the patient to avoid the future use of heparin and LMWH
- issue an antibody card.

Note: for full Canadian guidelines see www.tigc.org/eguidelines/hit05.htm

---

Table 2.2 Estimating the pre-laboratory-test probability of HIT: the 'four Ts' (adapted from Warkentin and Heddle 2003)[34]

	Score		
	2	1	0
Feature present			
Thrombocytopenia	>50% fall or platelet nadir 20–100×10⁹/L	30–50% fall or platelet nadir 10–19×10⁹/L	<30% fall or platelet nadir <10×10⁹/L
Timing of platelet count fall or other sequela	Clear onset after 5–10 days; or <1 day if heparin exposure within past 100 days	Onset of thrombocytopenia after 10 days, or unclear due to missing counts	Platelet count fall too early (without recent heparin exposure)
Thrombosis or other sequela	New thrombosis, skin necrosis or post-heparin bolus acute systemic reaction	Progressive or recurrent thrombosis, erythematous skin lesions or suspected thrombosis not yet proven	None
Other cause of thrombocytopenia present	None	Possible	Definite
Combine the scores for the four individual features to obtain a total score			
Probability of HIT	6–8 high	4–5 intermediate	0–3 low

and bind to the platelet surface, causing disruption of the platelets and a release of procoagulant material. HIT manifests as venous or arterial thrombo-embolism which may be fatal.

HIT is less common with prophylactic regimens (low doses) than with therapeutic ones (higher doses) and with LMWH rather than unfractionated heparin. Cross-reactivity between unfractionated heparin and LMWH is rare. HIT typically develops 5–10 days after starting heparin, but rarely >15 days. Routine monitoring of the platelet count is recommended (see p.62). *LMWH should be stopped immediately if there is a fall in the platelet count below the normal range or by >50% and the advice of a hematologist obtained.*

Because the procoagulant material released by the disintegrating platelets increases the risk of thrombosis, anticoagulation should be continued with a non-heparin anticoagulant, such as **danaparoid** (a heparinoid), **lepirudin** (a hirudin derivative) or **argatroban** (a direct thrombin inhibitor) even if there is no clinically evident thrombosis.[32,34]

The risk of HIT with **fondaparinux** (a synthetic factor Xa inhibitor) is also likely to be low.[32] If possible, surgery should be avoided in patients with HIT for at least 3 months, after which they generally become antibody negative. Even so, for patients with a history of HIT, if subsequent thromboprophylaxis or anticoagulation for a thrombo-embolism is required, a non-heparin anticoagulant should be used.[32] For patients requiring dialysis with HIT or a history of HIT, seek specialist advice.

Dose and use

The Thrombosis Interest Group of Canada have published recommendations on prophylaxis and treatment of thromboembolism in cancer patients.[4] More specific guidelines are available in the USA.[14] Anticoagulation should be considered for those who:
- develop a DVT (indefinite anticoagulation, using LMWH for at least 3–6 months)[14]
- sustain a PE (indefinite anticoagulation, using LMWH for at least 3–6 months)[14]
- are hospitalized and bedbound as a result of an acute medical illness for ⩾3 days (short-term thromboprophylactic anticoagulation).[16]

Generally, indefinite anticoagulation is discontinued only if contra-indications develop, or when the patient reaches the stage when symptom relief alone is appropriate, e.g. in the last few weeks of life.

If patients undergoing curative treatment for cancer experience thrombo-embolism and are deemed to have only a transient risk factor, duration of treatment is generally 3 months (DVT) or 6 months (PE). Long-term anticoagulation should be considered following a second episode of thrombo-embolism, or for those with a first episode considered to have a significant ongoing risk factor. Thrombo-embolism in a 'cured' cancer patient may be related to disease recurrence. If truly idiopathic, a minimum of 6–12 months of anticoagulation is recommended but long-term anticoagulation should be considered.

In patients at high risk of recurrent thrombo-embolism for whom anticoagulation is contra-indicated, an inferior vena caval filter may be an option, but requires careful patient selection.

SC injection

May cause transient stinging and local bruising.[37] Rotate injection sites daily, e.g. between left and right anterolateral and left and right posterolateral abdominal wall; introduce the total length of the needle vertically into the thickest part of a skin fold produced by squeezing the skin between the thumb and forefinger. Do not rub the injection site.

For the manufacturers' recommended sites for injection, see respective Manufacturers' Product Monographs and **dalteparin** and **enoxaparin** monographs (p.66 and p.70). The long-term use of SC injections is not acceptable to some patients with cancer (about 15% in one survey).[38]

Severe renal impairment (creatinine clearance <30mL/min)

Clearance of **enoxaparin** is reduced by up to 65% and **tinzaparin** clearance is decreased by up to 25%. The manufacturers recommend dose reduction for **enoxaparin** (see p.70) and **nadroparin**. The anti-factor Xa activity halflives of **dalteparin** and **tinzaparin** are prolonged, and specialist guidelines suggest monitoring anti-factor Xa activity to guide dosing in severe renal impairment.[1] For example, the dose of **tinzaparin** should be reduced if anti-factor Xa activity exceeds 1.5 units/mL (usual range 1–1.2 units/mL).[39]

During hemodialysis, the IV or extracorporeal circuit dose of **dalteparin** and **tinzaparin** should be reduced in patients with acute renal failure, or with chronic renal failure and an increased risk of bleeding. Specialist guidelines suggest using unfractionated heparin IV instead of LMWH in severe renal impairment but the evidence is grade 2C; i.e. not based on RCT.[1,14]

Routine platelet count monitoring

All patients should have a baseline platelet count before starting LMWH. Those who have received unfractionated heparin in the last 3 months should have a repeat platelet count after 24h to exclude rapid-onset HIT due to pre-existing antibodies. Subsequently, and for all patients, a platelet count should be monitored every 2–4 days from days 4–14.[32]

Thromboprophylaxis

For **dalteparin** and **enoxaparin** monographs, see p.66 and p.70 respectively.

Patients with cancer undergoing surgery

Patients with cancer undergoing major surgery are at high risk of thrombo-embolism; they have twice the risk of developing a DVT and three times the risk of a fatal PE.[40] Abdominal and pelvic surgery is particularly high-risk.[41,42]

The dose of **tinzaparin** in high-risk surgical patients is:
- 50 units/kg 2h before surgery, then 50 units/kg every 24h for 7–10 days or
- 4,500 units 12h before surgery, then 4,500 units every 24h for 7–10 days

However, 4 weeks of thromboprophylaxis is more effective than 1 week and thromboprophylaxis should be continued for 2–4 weeks after hospital discharge in patients with cancer (and in non-cancer patients >60 years old or with a history of thrombo-embolism).[4,16,43,44]

Patients with cancer with indwelling venous catheters

The presence of a central (subclavian) or peripheral indwelling venous catheter can lead to catheter-related thrombosis. It occurs in up to 2/3 of patients and is symptomatic in 10–30%, although more recent figures suggest the incidence is falling (5–15%), possibly as a result of improved catheter materials and placement. Routine thromboprophylaxis with LMWH is not recommended because RCTs have shown no benefit from their use (e.g. **enoxaparin** 40mg daily), or from low-dose **warfarin** (1mg daily).[45–48]

Patients with cancer who are immobile or confined to bed because of a concurrent acute medical illness

Compared with surgical patients, thromboprophylaxis is underused in medical patients, even though mortality and morbidity from thrombo-embolism (major/fatal PE) and its treatment (major/fatal hemorrhage) are higher in medical patients.[49]

Hospitalized cancer patients will be at high risk of venous thrombo-embolism and specialist guidelines recommend that they should be considered for thromboprophylaxis when an acute medical illness is likely to render them bedbound for ≥3 days, particularly in the presence of one or more additional risk factors (Box 2.B).[1,41] Duration of treatment is generally ≤2 weeks.[19] If anticoagulation is contra-indicated, use graduated compression stockings instead.[16]

Thromboprophylaxis appears acceptable to palliative care inpatients,[50] and should be considered in patients meeting the above criteria. However, thromboprophylaxis is less relevant for cancer patients with a poor performance status in their last few weeks of life, i.e. when symptom relief alone would be the most appropriate treatment for any fresh thrombo-embolic episode.

Patients with cancer undertaking long-distance air travel

The evidence for an association between prolonged travel and venous thrombo-embolism is controversial.[16] The risk appears greatest in journeys of >6h and in those travellers with one or more pre-existing risk factors (see Box 2.B, p.58). Although there is insufficient evidence to support routine thromboprophylaxis in any group, all travellers should follow some general recommendations (Box 2.D). The need for additional measures in those deemed to be at an increased risk (e.g. patients with cancer) should be made on an individual basis (Box 2.D).

Box 2.D Recommendations for preventing thrombo-embolism in long-distance travel (>6h)[16]

General recommendations for all travellers
Avoid constrictive clothing around the waist and legs.
Avoid dehydration.
Frequently stretch the calf muscles by moving the feet up and down.

Additional recommendations for travellers with one or more risk factors for thrombo-embolism (see Box 2.B, p.58)
Properly fitted, below-knee graduated compression stockings, providing 15–30mmHg of pressure at the ankle *or*
A single prophylactic dose of LMWH (e.g. enoxaparin 40mg) 2–4h before departure.

Treatment

For **dalteparin** and **enoxaparin** monographs, see p.66 and p.70 respectively.

DVT and PE

- uncomplicated DVT or PE are increasingly treated on an outpatient basis.[51] Some centres use a fixed-dose regimen (see Box 2.B, p.58):[52]
- general guidance is to give **tinzaparin**, 175 units/kg SC once daily for at least 5 days or until the INR has been in the therapeutic range for two successive days
- US guidelines (more specific to patients with cancer) advise giving **tinzaparin** 175 units/kg SC once daily for the first 3–6 months of indefinite anticoagulation[14]
- **dalteparin** or **enoxaparin**, see p.66 or p.70.

If **warfarin** is used, the LMWH should be continued until the INR is ≥2 on two consecutive days.

In palliative care, LMWH is preferable because hemorrhagic complications with **warfarin** occur in nearly 50% (possibly related to a poor performance status, drug interactions and hepatic impairment). Most patients agreeing to the indefinite use of LMWH have found it acceptable.[37,53,54] Compared with **warfarin**, treatment with LMWH is easier to monitor with less need for blood tests and frequent dose adjustments.

Disseminated intravascular coagulation (DIC)
- confirm the diagnosis:
  ▷ thrombocytopenia (platelet count $<150 \times 10^9$/L in 95% of cases)
  ▷ decreased plasma fibrinogen concentration
  ▷ elevated plasma D-dimer concentration, a fibrin degradation product (85% of cases)
  ▷ prolonged prothrombin time and/or partial thromboplastin time.[55]

A normal plasma fibrinogen concentration (200–250mg/100mL) is also suspicious because fibrinogen levels are generally raised in cancer (e.g. 450–500mg/100mL) unless there is extensive liver disease. Infection and cancer both may be associated with an increased platelet count which likewise may mask an evolving thrombocytopenia.
- *do not use* **warfarin** *because it is ineffective*
- for chronic DIC presenting with recurrent thromboses, give LMWH as for treatment of DVT
- for chronic or acute DIC presenting with hemorrhagic manifestations (e.g. ecchymoses, hematomas), seek specialist advice.

Thrombophlebitis migrans
- *do not use* **warfarin** because it is ineffective
- generally responds rapidly to small doses of LMWH
- continue treatment indefinitely
- if necessary, titrate the LMWH dose to maximum allowed according to weight.[56]

Overdose
In emergencies, **protamine sulfate** can be used to reverse the effects of **tinzaparin**:
- for each 100 units of **tinzaparin**, give 1mg of **protamine sulfate**
- give a maximum of 50mg by IV injection over 10min.
- Give a further 0.5mg of **protamine sulfate** per 100 units of **tinzaparin** after 2–4h if APTT still prolonged.

Note: the anti-factor Xa activity of **tinzaparin** or **nadroparin** cannot be completely neutralized even by high doses of **protamine sulfate** (maximum reversal ~60%).

In three patients who bled after surgery or an invasive procedure, a single dose of recombinant activated **factor VIIa** concentrate 20–30microgram/kg IV successfully reversed anticoagulation from LMWH. It did not precipitate thrombosis, despite all patients having risk factors for hypercoagulation, e.g. protein S deficiency, antiphospholipid antibody syndrome, cancer-related surgery.[57]

Supply
Dalteparin and **enoxaparin**: see respective monographs, p.66 and p.70.

Nadroparin Calcium
Fraxiparine® (GlaxoSmithKline)
Injection 9,500 units/mL, 0.2mL (1,900 units) syringe = $10, 0.3mL (2,850 units) syringe = $10, 0.4mL (3,800 units) syringe = $10, 0.6mL (5,700 units) syringe = $10, 0.8mL (7,600 units) syringe = $10, 1mL (9,500 units) syringe = $10.

Fraxiparine Forte® (GlaxoSmithKline)
Injection 19,000 units/mL, 0.6mL (114,000 units) syringe = $20, 0.8mL (15,200 units) syringe = $20, 1mL (19,000 units) syringe = $20.

Tinzaparin
Innohep® (Leo)
Injection 10,000 units/mL, 0.35mL (3,500 units) syringe = $6, 0.45mL (4,500 units) syringe = $8, 2mL (20,000 units) vial = $35.
Injection 20,000 units/mL, 0.5mL (10,000 units) syringe = $18, 0.7mL (14,000 units) syringe = $25, 0.9mL (18,000 units) syringe = $32, 2mL (40,000 units) vial = $70.

1 Baglin T et al. (2006) Guidelines on the use and monitoring of heparin. *British Journal of Haematology.* **133**: 19–34.

2 Blann AD and Lip GY (2006) Venous thromboembolism. *British Medical Journal.* **332**: 215–219.

3 Cohen AT et al. (2006) Efficacy and safety of fondaparinux for the prevention of venous thromboembolism in older acute medical patients: randomised placebo controlled trial. *British Medical Journal.* **332**: 325–329.

4 The Thrombosis Interest Group of Canada (2007) Cancer and venous thrombo-embolic disease. A significant issue (only online). Available from: *www.tigc.org/eguidelines/cancer06.htm*

5 Van Dongen CJ et al. (2004) Fixed dose subcutaneous low molecular weight heparins versus adjusted dose unfractionated heparin for venous thromboembolism. *Cochrane Database of Systematic Reviews.* **4**: CD001100.

6 Quinlan D et al. (2004) Low-molecular weight heparin compared with intravenous unfractionated heparin for treatment of pulmonary embolism. *Annals of Internal Medicine.* **140**: 175–183.

7 Prandoni P et al. (2002) Recurrent venous thromboembolism and bleeding complications during anticoagulant treatment in patients with cancer and venous thrombosis. *Blood.* **100**: 3484–3488.

8 Streiff MB (2006) Long-term therapy of venous thromboembolism in cancer patients. *Journal of the National Comprehensive Cancer Network.* **4**: 903–910.

9 Meyer G et al. (2002) Comparison of low-molecular-weight heparin and warfarin for the secondary prevention of venous thromboembolism in patients with cancer: a randomized controlled study. *Archives of Internal Medicine.* **162**: 1729–1735.

10 Lee A et al. (2003) Low molecular weight heparin versus a coumarin for the prevention of recurrent venous thromboembolism in patients with cancer. *New England Journal of Medicine.* **349**: 146–153.

11 Iorio A et al. (2003) Low-molecular-weight heparin for the long-term treatment of symptomatic venous thromboembolism: meta-analysis of the randomized comparisons with oral anticoagulants. *Journal of Thrombosis and Haemostasis.* **1**: 1906–1913.

12 Hull RD et al. (2006) Long-term low-molecular-weight heparin versus usual care in proximal-vein thrombosis patients with cancer. *American Journal of Medicine.* **119**: 1062–1072.

13 Baglin TP et al. (2005) Guidelines on oral anticoagulation (warfarin): third edition-2005 update. *British Journal of Haematology.* **132**: 277–285.

14 Buller HR et al. (2004) Antithrombotic therapy for venous thromboembolic disease: the Seventh ACCP Conference on Antithrombotic and Thrombolytic Therapy. *Chest.* **126 (suppl 3)**: 401S–428S.

15 Samama MM et al. (1999) A comparison of enoxaparin with placebo for the prevention of venous thromboembolism in acutely ill medical patients. Prophylaxis in Medical Patients with Enoxaparin Study Group. *New England Journal of Medicine.* **341**: 793–800.

16 Geerts WH et al. (2004) Prevention of venous thromboembolism: the seventh ACCP Conference on Antithrombotic and Thrombolytic Therapy. *Chest.* **126 (suppl)**: 338s–400s.

17 De Cicco M (2004) The prothrombotic state in cancer: pathogenic mechanisms. *Critical Reviews in Oncology Hematology.* **50**: 187–196.

18 Deitcher SR and Gomes MP (2004) The risk of venous thromboembolic disease associated with adjuvant hormone therapy for breast carcinoma: a systematic review. *Cancer.* **101**: 439–449.

19 Leizorovicz A and Mismetti P (2004) Preventing venous thromboembolism in medical patients. *Circulation.* **110**: IV13–19.

20 Leizorovicz A et al. (2004) Randomized, placebo-controlled trial of dalteparin for the prevention of venous thromboembolism in acutely ill medical patients. *Circulation.* **110**: 874–879.

21 Chew HK et al. (2006) Incidence of venous thromboembolism and its effect on survival among patients with common cancers. *Archives of Internal Medicine.* **166**: 458–464.

22 Cunningham RS (2006) The role of low-molecular-weight heparins as supportive care therapy in cancer-associated thrombosis. *Seminars in Oncology.* **33**: S17–26; quiz S41–12.

23 Klerk CP et al. (2005) The effect of low molecular weight heparin on survival in patients with advanced malignancy. *Journal of Clinical Oncology.* **23**: 2130–2135.

24 Khorana AA and Fine RL (2004) Pancreatic cancer and thromboembolic disease. *Lancet Oncology.* **5**: 655–663.

25 Hettiarachchi RJ et al. (1999) Do heparins do more than just treat thrombosis? The influence of heparins on cancer spread. *Journal of Thrombosis and Haemostasis.* **82**: 947–952.

26 Prandoni P (2004) Toward the simplification of antithrombotic treatment of venous thromboembolism. *Annals of Internal Medicine.* **140**: 925–926.

27 Bara L and Samama M (1990) Pharmacokinetics of low molecular weight heparins. *Acta Chirurgica Scandinavica Supplementum.* **556 (suppl)**: 57–61.

28 Dawes J (1990) Comparison of the pharmacokinetics of enoxaparin (Clexane) and unfractionated heparin. *Acta Chirurgica Scandinavica Supplementum.* **556 (suppl)**: 68–74.

29 Fareed J et al. (1990) Pharmacologic profile of a low molecular weight heparin (enoxaparin): experimental and clinical validation of the prophylactic antithrombotic effects. *Acta Chirurgica Scandinavica Suppl.* **556 (suppl)**: 75–90.

30 Fossler MJ et al. (2001) Pharmacodynamics of intravenous and subcutaneous tinzaparin and heparin in healthy volunteers. *American Journal of Health System Pharmacy.* **58**: 1614–1621.

31 Warkentin T et al. (1995) Heparin-induced thrombocytopenia in patients treated with low molecular weight heparin or unfractionated heparin. *New England Journal of Medicine.* **332**: 1330–1335.

32 Keeling D et al. (2006) The management of heparin-induced thrombocytopenia. (Guidelines of the Haemostasis and Thrombosis Task Force of the British Committee for Standards in Haematology). *British Journal of Haematology.* **133**: 259–269.

33 Hirsh J et al. (2001) Heparin and low-molecular-weight heparin: mechanisms of action, pharmacokinetics, dosing, monitoring, efficacy, and safety. *Chest.* **119 (suppl)**: 64s–94s.

34 Warkentin TE and Heddle NM (2003) Laboratory diagnosis of immune heparin-induced thrombocytopenia. *Current Hematology Reports.* **2**: 148–157.

35 Warkentin TE and Greinacher A (2004) Heparin-induced thrombocytopenia: recognition, treatment, and prevention: the seventh ACCP Conference on Antithrombotic and Thrombolytic Therapy. *Chest.* **126 (suppl)**: 311s–337s.

36 The Thrombosis Interest Group of Canada (2006) Heparin induced thrombocytopenia (only online). Available from: www.tigc.org/eguidelines/hit05.htm

37 Noble SI and Finlay IG (2005) Is long-term low-molecular-weight heparin acceptable to palliative care patients in the treatment of cancer related venous thromboembolism? A qualitative study. *Palliative Medicine.* **19**: 197–201.

38 Wittkowsky AK (2006) Barriers to the long-term use of low-molecular weight heparins for treatment of cancer-associated thrombosis. *Journal of Thrombosis and Haemostasis.* **4**: 2090–2091.

39 Leo Laboratories *Personal communication.*

40 Kakkar AK and Williamson RC (1999) Prevention of venous thromboembolism in cancer patients. *Seminars in Thrombosis and Hemostasis.* **25**: 239–243.

41 Cunningham MS *et al.* (2006) Prevention and management of venous thromboembolism in people with cancer: a review of the evidence. *Clinical Oncology (Royal College of Radiologists).* **18**: 145–151.

42 Negus JJ *et al.* (2006) Thromboprophylaxis in major abdominal surgery for cancer. *European Journal of Surgical Oncology.* **32**: 911–916.

43 Bergqvist D *et al.* (2002) Duration of prophylaxis against venous thromboembolism with enoxaparin after surgery for cancer. *New England Journal of Medicine.* **346**: 975–980.

44 Kher A and Samama MM (2005) Primary and secondary prophylaxis of venous thromboembolism with low-molecular-weight heparins: prolonged thromboprophylaxis, an alternative to vitamin K antagonists. *Journal of Thrombosis and Haemostasis.* **3**: 473–481.

45 Geerts WH *et al.* (2001) Prevention of venous thromboembolism. *Chest.* **119 (suppl)**: 132s–175s.

46 Tesselaar ME *et al.* (2004) Risk factors for catheter-related thrombosis in cancer patients. *European Journal of Cancer.* **40**: 2253–2259.

47 Couban S *et al.* (2005) Randomized Placebo-Controlled Study of Low-Dose Warfarin for the Prevention of Central Venous Catheter-Associated Thrombosis in Patients With Cancer. *Journal of Clinical Oncology.* **23**: 4063–4069.

48 Verso M *et al.* (2005) Enoxaparin for the Prevention of Venous Thromboembolism Associated With Central Vein Catheter: A Double-Blind, Placebo-Controlled, Randomized Study in Cancer Patients. *Journal of Clinical Oncology.* **23**: 4057–4062.

49 Monreal M *et al.* (2004) The outcome after treatment of venous thromboembolism is different in surgical and acutely ill medical patients. Findings from the RIETE registry. *Journal of Thrombosis and Haemostasis.* **2**: 1892–1898.

50 Noble SI *et al.* (2006) Acceptability of low molecular weight heparin thromboprophylaxis for inpatients receiving palliative care: qualitative study. *British Medical Journal.* **332**: 577–580.

51 Wells PS *et al.* (2005) A randomized trial comparing 2 low-molecular-weight heparins for the outpatient treatment of deep vein thrombosis and pulmonary embolism. *Archives of Internal Medicine.* **165**: 733–738.

52 Monreal M *et al.* (2004) Fixed-dose low-molecular-weight heparin for secondary prevention of venous thromboembolism in patients with disseminated cancer: a prospective cohort study. *Journal of Thrombosis and Haemostasis.* **2**: 1311–1315.

53 Johnson M (1997) Problems of anticoagulation within a palliative care setting: an audit of hospice patients taking warfarin. *Palliative Medicine.* **11**: 306–312.

54 Johnson M and Sherry K (1997) How do palliative physicians manage venous thromboembolism? *Palliative Medicine.* **11**: 462–468.

55 Spero J *et al.* (1980) Disseminated intravascular coagulation: findings in 346 patients. *Journal of Thrombosis and Haemostasis.* **43**: 28–33.

56 Walsh-McMonagle D and Green D (1997) Low-molecular weight heparin in the management of Trousseau's syndrome. *Cancer.* **80**: 649–655.

57 Firozvi K *et al.* (2006) Reversal of low-molecular-weight heparin-induced bleeding in patients with pre-existing hypercoagulable states with human recombinant activated factor VII concentrate. *American Journal of Hematology.* **81**: 582–589.

DALTEPARIN

Class: Low molecular weight heparin (LMWH).

Indications: Surgical and medical thromboprophylaxis, treatment of thromboembolism, prevention of clotting in extracorporeal circuits during hemodialysis or hemofiltration, unstable angina, non-Q wave myocardial infarction, †thrombophlebitis migrans, †disseminated intravascular coagulation (DIC).

Contra-indications: Active major bleeding, known bleeding diathesis, confirmed or suspected immune-mediated heparin-induced thrombocytopenia (HIT), bacterial endocarditis, injury or surgery to the CNS, eyes or ears, spinal analgesia (if *treatment* dose of LMWH, increased risk of spinal hematoma), IM use (risk of hematoma at the injection site), active peptic ulcer, cerebral hemorrhage, severe uncontrolled hypertension, diabetic or hemorrhagic retinopathy, other conditions or diseases with an increased risk of hemorrhage.

Pharmacology

Dalteparin acts by potentiating the inhibitory effect of antithrombin III on factor Xa and thrombin. It has a relatively higher ability to potentiate factor Xa inhibition than to prolong plasma clotting time (APTT) which cannot be used to guide dosing. Anti-factor Xa levels can be measured if necessary, e.g. if a patient is at increased risk of bleeding, but routine monitoring is not generally required because the dose is determined by the patient's weight. LMWH is as effective as unfractionated heparin for the treatment of DVT and PE and is now the initial treatment of choice.[1,2] Other advantages include a longer duration of action which allows administration once daily and possibly a better safety profile, e.g. fewer major hemorrhages.[1–5] LMWH is the treatment of choice for *chronic* DIC; this commonly presents as recurrent thromboses in both superficial and deep veins which do not respond to **warfarin**. The antifibrinolytic drug **tranexamic acid** should not be used in DIC because it increases the risk of end-organ damage from microvascular thromboses. All LMWH is derived from porcine heparin and some patients may need to avoid it because of hypersensitivity, or for religious or cultural reasons. The most appropriate non-porcine alternative is **fondaparinux**.[6,7]

Bio-availability 87% SC (based on plasma anti-factor Xa activity).
Onset of action 3min IV; 2–4h SC.
Time to peak plasma anti-factor Xa activity 4h SC.
Plasma anti-factor Xa activity halflife 2h IV; 6h IV in hemodialysis patients; 3–5h SC.
Duration of action 10–24h SC.

Cautions

Serious drug interactions: enhanced anticoagulant effect with anticoagulant/antiplatelet drugs, e.g. NSAIDs.

Risk of spinal (intrathecal or epidural) hematoma in patients undergoing spinal puncture or with indwelling spinal catheter, particularly if concurrently receiving a drug which affects hemostasis; spinal analgesia may be used cautiously in patients on *thromboprophylactic* doses of dalteparin but monitor for neurological impairment.

Other risk factors for bleeding include serious concurrent illness, chronic heavy consumption of alcohol, use of platelet inhibiting drugs, renal failure, age, and possibly female gender. In severe liver disease, the manufacturer recommends dose reduction but gives no definite guidance. In severe renal impairment (creatinine clearance <30mL/min) and those on hemodialysis the anti-factor Xa activity halflife of dalteparin is prolonged, and dose reduction may be required.

Inhibition of aldosterone secretion by heparin/LMWH may cause hyperkalemia. The risk appears to increase with duration of therapy; patients with diabetes mellitus, chronic renal failure, acidosis and those taking potassium supplements or potassium-sparing drugs are more susceptible. The UK CSM recommends that plasma potassium should be measured in such patients before starting heparin and monitored regularly thereafter, particularly if heparin is to be continued for >7 days.

Undesirable effects

For full list, see manufacturer's Product Monograph
Common (<10%, >1%): hematoma at the injection site, mild thrombocytopenia which reverses with continued treatment.
Uncommon (<1%, >0.1%): major bleeding (e.g. GI, retroperitoneal, intracranial, surgical sites), thrombocytopenia during prophylaxis.

Both standard heparin and LMWH can cause thrombocytopenia (platelet count $<100 \times 10^9$/L). An early (<4 days) mild fall in platelet count is often seen after starting heparin therapy, particularly after surgery. This corrects spontaneously despite the continued use of heparin and is asymptomatic.[8] However, occasionally, an immune heparin-induced thrombocytopenia (HIT) develops, associated with heparin-dependent IgG antibodies (see LMWH, p.60).[3,8] Dalteparin should be stopped immediately if there is a fall in the platelet count of >50% and the advice of a hematologist obtained. Anticoagulation should be continued with either a hirudin derivative, e.g. **lepirudin**, a heparinoid, e.g. **danaparoid**, or a direct thrombin inhibitor, e.g. **argatroban**, even if there is no clinically evident thrombosis (see p.61).[9]

Dose and use

All patients should have a baseline platelet count before starting LMWH. Those who have received unfractionated heparin in the last 3 months should have a repeat platelet count after 24h to exclude rapid-onset HIT due to pre-existing antibodies. Subsequently, for all patients, the platelet count should be monitored every 2–4 days from days 4–14.[10]

May cause transient stinging and local bruising. Inject SC, rotate sites daily between the left and right anterolateral abdominal wall, posterolateral abdominal wall and lateral thigh; introduce the total length of the needle vertically into the thickest part of a skin fold produced by squeezing the skin between the thumb and forefinger. Do not rub the injection site.

The anti-factor Xa activity halflife of dalteparin is prolonged in patients with severe renal impairment and those requiring hemodialysis. The manufacturer recommends a dose reduction may be required. Specialist guidelines suggest using IV unfractionated heparin instead of LMWH in severe renal impairment but the evidence is not strong (grade 2C, i.e. not based on RCT).[11]

Thromboprophylaxis
Patients with cancer undergoing surgery
- give 5,000 units SC once daily, starting the evening before surgery
- continue for 2–4 weeks;[12] 4 weeks is more effective than I week[13,14]
- consider additional mechanical measures such as graduated compression stockings or intermittent pneumatic compression.

Patients with cancer who are immobile or confined to bed because of a concurrent acute medical illness
- give 5,000 units SC once daily (see LMWH, p.63)
- duration of therapy is generally ⩽2 weeks[15,16]
- if anticoagulation is contra-indicated, use graduated compression stockings instead.[12]

Thromboprophylaxis appears acceptable to palliative care inpatients,[17] and should be considered in patients meeting the recommended criteria (see p.62). However, thromboprophylaxis is increasingly irrelevant for cancer patients with a poor performance status in the last few weeks of life, i.e. at a time when symptom relief alone would be the most appropriate treatment for any fresh thrombo-embolic episode.

Patients with cancer undertaking long-distance air travel (>6h)
- if a LMWH is deemed necessary (see p.63), prescribe three injections (one each for the outward and return journeys, and one spare)
- provide training in the correct administration of the injection (see the information on self-administration included in the patient information leaflet)
- self-administer 5,000 units SC 2–4h before departure[12]
- if there is a stop over, followed by another long flight, another injection is not necessary unless the second flight is more than 24h after the first.

Treatment
DVT and PE in patients with cancer: initial treatment
- confirm diagnosis radiologically (e.g. ultrasound, CT pulmonary angiography)
- manufacturer's recommendation:
  ▷ 200 units/kg (up to a maximum total dose of 18,000 units) SC once daily for I month, followed by
  ▷ 150 units/kg (up to a maximum total dose of 18,000 units) SC once daily for 1–5 months
- USA guidelines for patients with cancer:
  ▷ 150 units/kg SC once daily indefinitely.[11]

DVT and PE in patients with cancer: ongoing treatment
Indefinite anticoagulation should be considered for patients who have a DVT, a sudden and severe PE or a persistent major risk factor for thrombo-embolism such as cancer[11] (see Box 2.B, p.58). In patients with cancer, long-term LMWH appears more effective than **warfarin**, with a similar (or reduced) risk of bleeding.[18–20] **Warfarin** should be reserved for those patients whose cancer is relatively stable. When switching to **warfarin**, LMWH should be continued for 2 days after achieving a therapeutic INR. Patients undergoing anticancer treatments should receive LMWH.

In palliative care, because hemorrhagic complications with **warfarin** occur in nearly 50% (possibly related to drug interactions and hepatic impairment), LMWH (e.g. dalteparin 150 units/kg SC once daily) is preferable. It has been used indefinitely and is acceptable to patients.[21–23] Generally, indefinite anticoagulation is discontinued only if contra-indications develop, or when the patient reaches the stage when symptom relief alone is appropriate, e.g. in the last few weeks of life.

Some centres use a fixed low-dose regimen, independent of body weight (Box 2.E). With this regimen, 15% of patients did not complete the first week (6% experienced a major bleed,

5% required a smaller dose of dalteparin due to abnormal coagulation and 2% had massive recurrent PE. Subsequently, almost 80% of patients received chemotherapy, 27% experienced transient thrombocytopenia (generally related to the chemotherapy) and 23% required surgery or an invasive procedure. Major bleeding occurred in 5% (fatal in 3%) and minor bleeding in 8%. Recurrent thrombo-embolism occurred in 9%. Complications were no higher in patients with liver or brain metastases, thrombocytopenia, or those undergoing surgical or invasive procedures.[24]

Box 2.E Modified dalteparin regimen in patients with metastatic cancer and venous thrombo-embolism[24]

First week
Give dalteparin in a dose according to body weight (see DVT and PE, p.68).

Subsequent weeks (continue indefinitely)
Dalteparin in a fixed-dose of 10,000 units SC once daily.
If DVT recurs
Increase the fixed-dose of dalteparin to 12,500 units SC once daily.
If PE occurs/recurs
Consider an inferior vena caval filter.

Dose modifications
Thrombocytopenia
If the platelet count falls below 50×10^9/L reduce the dose of dalteparin to 5,000 units SC once daily.
If the platelet count falls below 10×10^9/L reduce the dose of dalteparin to 2,500 units SC once daily.

Surgical procedures
Give dalteparin 5,000 units SC once daily for the first 4 days postoperatively and then return to the patient's usual dose.
Other invasive procedures (e.g. biopsy)
Give dalteparin 5,000 units SC on the day of the procedure and then return to the patient's usual dose.

Disseminated intravascular coagulation (DIC)
- confirm the diagnosis (see p.64)
- *do not use **warfarin** because it is ineffective*
- *for chronic* DIC presenting with recurrent thromboses, give dalteparin as for treatment of DVT
- *for chronic or acute* DIC presenting with hemorrhagic manifestations (e.g. ecchymoses and hematomas), seek specialist advice.

Thrombophlebitis migrans
- *do not use **warfarin** because it is ineffective*
- generally responds rapidly to small doses, e.g. 2,500–5,000 units SC once daily
- continue treatment indefinitely[2,25]
- if necessary, titrate dose to maximum allowed according to weight, i.e. 200 units/kg.

Overdose
In emergencies, **protamine sulfate** can be used to reverse the effects of dalteparin:
- for each 100 units of dalteparin, give 1mg of **protamine sulfate**
- give a maximum of 50mg by IV injection over 10min
- give a further 0.5mg of **protamine sulfate** per 100 units of dalteparin after 2–4h if APTT still prolonged.
Note: the anti-factor Xa activity of dalteparin is not completely neutralized by **protamine sulfate** (maximum reversal about 60%).

Supply
Fragmin® (Pfizer)

Injection (prefilled single dose syringe for SC injection) 12,500 units/mL, 0.2mL (2,500 units) = $6; 25,000 units/mL, 0.2mL (5,000 units) = $11, 0.3mL (7,500 units) = $16, 0.4mL (10,000 units) = $22, 0.5mL (12,500 units) = $27, 0.6mL (15,000 units) = $32, 0.72mL (18,000 units) = $38.

Injection (for SC or IV use) 10,000 units/mL, 1mL amp (10,000 units) = $17.

Injection (multiple dose vial for SC injection) 25,000 units/mL, 3.8mL (95,000 units) = $159.

1 Quinlan D et al. (2004) Low-molecular weight heparin compared with intravenous unfractionated heparin for treatment of pulmonary embolism. *Annals of Internal Medicine*. **140**: 175–183.

2 Van Dongen CJ et al. (2004) Fixed dose subcutaneous low molecular weight heparins versus adjusted dose unfractionated heparin for venous thromboembolism. *Cochrane Database of Systematic Reviews*. **4**: CD001100.

3 Hirsh J et al. (2001) Heparin and low-molecular-weight heparin: mechanisms of action, pharmacokinetics, dosing, monitoring, efficacy, and safety. *Chest*. **119 (suppl)**: 64s–94s.

4 Prandoni P (2001) Heparins and venous thromboembolism: current practice and future directions. *Journal of Thrombosis and Haemostasis*. **86**: 488–498.

5 Fareed J et al. (2003) Pharmacodynamic and pharmacokinetic properties of enoxaparin: implications for clinical practice. *Clinical Pharmacokinetics*. **42**: 1043–1057.

6 Blann AD and Lip GY (2006) Venous thromboembolism. *British Medical Journal*. **332**: 215–219.

7 Cohen AT et al. (2006) Efficacy and safety of fondaparinux for the prevention of venous thromboembolism in older acute medical patients: randomised placebo controlled trial. *British Medical Journal*. **332**: 325–329.

8 Warkentin T et al. (1995) Heparin-induced thrombocytopenia in patients treated with low molecular weight heparin or unfractionated heparin. *New England Journal of Medicine*. **332**: 1330–1335.

9 Warkentin TE and Greinacher A (2004) Heparin-induced thrombocytopenia: recognition, treatment, and prevention: the seventh ACCP Conference on Antithrombotic and Thrombolytic Therapy. *Chest*. **126 (suppl)**: 311s–337s.

10 Keeling D et al. (2006) The management of heparin-induced thrombocytopenia. *British Journal of Haematology*. **133**: 259–269.

11 Buller HR et al. (2004) Antithrombotic therapy for venous thromboembolic disease: the Seventh ACCP Conference on Antithrombotic and Thrombolytic Therapy. *Chest*. **126 (suppl 3)**: 401S–428S.

12 Geerts WH et al. (2004) Prevention of venous thromboembolism: the seventh ACCP Conference on Antithrombotic and Thrombolytic Therapy. *Chest*. **126 (suppl)**: 338s–400s.

13 Bergqvist D et al. (2002) Duration of prophylaxis against venous thromboembolism with enoxaparin after surgery for cancer. *New England Journal of Medicine*. **346**: 975–980.

14 Kher A and Samama MM (2005) Primary and secondary prophylaxis of venous thromboembolism with low-molecular-weight heparins: prolonged thromboprophylaxis, an alternative to vitamin K antagonists. *Journal of Thrombosis and Haemostasis*. **3**: 473–481.

15 Leizorovicz A and Mismetti P (2004) Preventing venous thromboembolism in medical patients. *Circulation*. **110**: IV13–19.

16 Leizorovicz A et al. (2004) Randomized, placebo-controlled trial of dalteparin for the prevention of venous thromboembolism in acutely ill medical patients. *Circulation*. **110**: 874–879.

17 Noble SI et al. (2006) Acceptability of low molecular weight heparin thromboprophylaxis for inpatients receiving palliative care: qualitative study. *British Medical Journal*. **332**: 577–580.

18 Meyer G et al. (2002) Comparison of low-molecular-weight heparin and warfarin for the secondary prevention of venous thromboembolism in patients with cancer: a randomized controlled study. *Archives of Internal Medicine*. **162**: 1729–1735.

19 Lee A et al. (2003) Low molecular weight heparin versus a coumarin for the prevention of recurrent venous thromboembolism in patients with cancer. *New England Journal of Medicine*. **349**: 146–153.

20 Hull RD et al. (2006) Long-term low-molecular-weight heparin versus usual care in proximal-vein thrombosis patients with cancer. *American Journal of Medicine*. **119**: 1062–1072.

21 Johnson M (1997) Problems of anticoagulation within a palliative care setting: an audit of hospice patients taking warfarin. *Palliative Medicine*. **11**: 306–312.

22 Johnson M and Sherry K (1997) How do palliative physicians manage venous thromboembolism? *Palliative Medicine*. **11**: 462–468.

23 Noble SI and Finlay IG (2005) Is long-term low-molecular-weight heparin acceptable to palliative care patients in the treatment of cancer related venous thromboembolism? A qualitative study. *Palliative Medicine*. **19**: 197–201.

24 Monreal M et al. (2004) Fixed-dose low-molecular-weight heparin for secondary prevention of venous thromboembolism in patients with disseminated cancer: a prospective cohort study. *Journal of Thrombosis and Haemostasis*. **2**: 1311–1315.

25 Walsh-McMonagle D and Green D (1997) Low-molecular weight heparin in the management of Trousseau's syndrome. *Cancer*. **80**: 649–655.

ENOXAPARIN

Class: Low molecular weight heparin (LMWH).

Indications: Prevention of thrombo-embolism in surgical patients and hospitalized, bedbound medical patients (acute respiratory failure, NYHA class III or IV cardiac insufficiency); treatment of thrombo-embolism; treatment of unstable angina or non-Q-wave myocardial infarction concurrently with ASA, †thrombophlebitis migrans, †disseminated intravascular coagulation (DIC).

Contra-indications: Active major bleeding, thrombocytopenia with positive aggregation test in the presence of enoxaparin, known bleeding diathesis, bacterial endocarditis, spinal analgesia if on *treatment* dose of enoxaparin (increased risk of spinal hematoma), IM use (risk of hematoma at the injection site), active gastric or duodenal ulcer, severe uncontrolled hypertension, diabetic or hemorrhagic retinopathy, injury or surgery to the brain, spinal cord, eyes or ears, cerebral hemorrhage, spinal/epidural analgesia if on *treatment* dose of enoxaparin, or conditions or diseases with an increased risk of hemorrhage.

Pharmacology

Enoxaparin acts by potentiating the inhibitory effect of antithrombin III on factor Xa and thrombin. It has a relatively higher ability to potentiate factor Xa inhibition than to prolong plasma clotting time (APTT) which cannot be used to guide dosing. Anti-factor Xa levels can be measured if necessary, e.g. if a patient is at increased risk of bleeding, but routine monitoring is not generally required because the dose is determined by the patient's weight. In renal impairment excretion of enoxaparin is reduced and increased bleeding can occur. LMWH is as effective as unfractionated heparin for the treatment of DVT and PE and is now the initial treatment of choice.[1,2] Other advantages include a longer duration of action which allows administration once daily and possibly a better safety profile, e.g. fewer major hemorrhages.[1–5] LMWH is the treatment of choice for *chronic* DIC; this commonly presents as recurrent thromboses in both superficial and deep veins which do not respond to **warfarin**. The antifibrinolytic drug **tranexamic acid** should not be used in DIC because it increases the risk of end-organ damage from microvascular thromboses. All LMWH is derived from porcine heparin and some patients may need to avoid it because of hypersensitivity, or for religious or cultural reasons. The most appropriate non-porcine alternative is **fondaparinux.**[6,7]

Bio-availability 100% SC (based on plasma anti-factor Xa activity).
Onset of action 5min IV; 3h SC.[8]
Time to peak plasma anti-factor Xa activity 2–6h SC.
Plasma anti-factor Xa activity halflife 2–4.5h IV;[9,10] 4.5–7h SC.
Duration of action >24h SC.[5]

Cautions

Serious drug interactions: enhanced anticoagulant effect with anticoagulant/antiplatelet drugs, e.g. NSAIDs.

Risk of spinal (intrathecal or epidural) hematoma in patients undergoing spinal puncture or with indwelling spinal catheter, particularly if concurrently receiving a drug which affects hemostasis; spinal analgesia may be used cautiously in patients on *thromboprophylactic* doses of enoxaparin but monitor for neurological impairment.

In severe liver disease consider reducing the dose. In severe renal impairment (creatinine clearance <30mL/min) the clearance of enoxaparin is decreased by 65%, and the dose should be reduced.

Inhibition of aldosterone secretion by heparin/LMWH may cause hyperkalemia. The risk appears to increase with duration of therapy; patients with diabetes mellitus, chronic renal failure, acidosis and those taking potassium supplements or potassium-sparing drugs are more susceptible. The UK CSM recommends that plasma potassium should be measured in such patients before starting heparin and monitored regularly thereafter, particularly if heparin is to be continued for >1 week.

Undesirable effects

For full list, see manufacturer's Product Monograph.
Common (<10%, >1%): pain at the injection site, minor bleeding (generally hematoma or ecchymosis at the injection site), major bleeding in surgical patients and patients being treated for DVT or PE (e.g. retroperitoneal or intracranial), thrombocytopenia, anemia, ecchymosis, reversible increases in transaminases (rarely associated with increased bilirubin levels).
Uncommon (<1%, >0.1%): major bleeding associated with prophylactic treatment, hematuria.

Both standard heparin and LMWH can cause thrombocytopenia (platelet count $<100 \times 10^9$/L). An early (<4 days) mild fall in platelet count is often seen after starting heparin therapy, particularly after surgery. This corrects spontaneously despite the continued use of heparin and is asymptomatic.[11] However, occasionally, an immune heparin-induced thrombocytopenia (HIT) develops associated with heparin-dependent IgG antibodies (see LMWH, p.60).[3,11] Enoxaparin should be stopped immediately if there is a fall in the platelet count $>50\%$ and the advice of a hematologist obtained. Anticoagulation should be continued with either a hirudin derivative, e.g. **lepirudin**, a heparinoid, e.g. **danaparoid**, or a direct thrombin inhibitor, e.g. **argatroban**, even if there is no clinically evident thrombosis (see LMWH, p.61).

Dose and use

All patients should have a baseline platelet count before starting LMWH. Those who have received unfractionated heparin in the last 3 months should have a repeat platelet count after 24h to exclude rapid-onset HIT due to pre-existing antibodies. Subsequently, for all patients, the platelet count should be monitored every 2–4 days from days 4–14.[12]

May cause transient stinging and local bruising. Inject SC; rotate injection sites between left and right anterolateral and left and right posterolateral abdominal wall; introduce the total length of the needle vertically into the thickest part of a skin fold produced by squeezing the skin between the thumb and forefinger. Do not rub the injection site.

In severe renal impairment (creatinine clearance <30mL/min), the dose of enoxaparin should be reduced to a maximum of 30mg SC daily (thromboprophylaxis) or 1mg/kg SC daily (treatment). The manufacturer also advises measuring anti-factor Xa activity to monitor the anticoagulant effect. Specialist guidelines suggest using IV unfractionated heparin instead of LMWH but the evidence is not strong (grade 2C, i.e. not based on RCT).[13]

Thromboprophylaxis
Patients with cancer undergoing surgery
- give 40mg SC once daily, starting 12h before surgery
- twice-daily dosing: 30mg b.i.d., with initial dose within 12–24h after surgery, and every 12h until risk of DVT has diminished or the patient is adequately anticoagulated on warfarin
- continue for 2–4 weeks;[14] 4 weeks is more effective than 1 week[15,16]
- consider additional mechanical measures such as graduated compression stockings or intermittent pneumatic compression.[14]

Patients with cancer who are immobile or confined to bed because of a concurrent acute medical illness
- give 40mg SC once daily (see p.63)
- duration of therapy is generally $\leqslant 2$ weeks[17,18]
- if anticoagulation is contra-indicated, use graduated compression stockings instead.[14]

Thromboprophylaxis appears acceptable to palliative care inpatients,[19] and should be considered in patients meeting the recommended criteria (see p.62). However, thromboprophylaxis is increasingly irrelevant for cancer patients with a poor performance status in the last few weeks of life, i.e. at a time when symptom relief alone would be the most appropriate treatment for any fresh thrombo-embolic episode.

Patients with cancer undertaking long-distance air travel ($>6h$)
- if a LMWH is deemed necessary (see p.63), prescribe three injections (one each for the outward and return journeys, and one spare)
- provide training in the correct administration of the injection (see the information on self-administration included in the patient information leaflet)
- self-administer 40mg SC 2–4h before departure[14]
- if there is a stop over, followed by another long flight, another injection is not necessary unless the second flight is >24h after the first.

Treatment

DVT and PE in patients with cancer: initial treatment

- confirm diagnosis radiologically (e.g. ultrasound, CT pulmonary angiography)
- general guidance is to give 1.5mg/kg SC once daily for at least 5 days or until the INR has been in the therapeutic range for two successive days
- US guidelines more specific to patients with cancer advise giving 1mg/kg SC b.i.d. for at least the first 3–6 months of indefinite anticoagulation.[13]

DVT and PE in patients with cancer: ongoing treatment

Indefinite anticoagulation should be considered for patients who have a DVT, a sudden and severe PE or a persistent major risk factor such as cancer[13] (see Box 2.E, p.69). In patients with cancer, long-term LMWH appears more effective than **warfarin**, with a similar (or reduced) risk of bleeding.[20–22] **Warfarin** should be reserved for those patients whose cancer is relatively stable. When switching to **warfarin**, LMWH should be continued for 2 days after achieving a therapeutic INR. Patients undergoing anticancer treatments should receive LMWH.

In palliative care, because hemorrhagic complications with **warfarin** occur in nearly 50% (possibly related to drug interactions and hepatic impairment), LMWH is preferable. It has been used indefinitely and is acceptable to patients.[23–25] Generally, indefinite anticoagulation is discontinued only if contra-indications develop, or when the patient reaches the stage when symptom relief alone is appropriate, e.g. in the last few weeks of life.

Some centres use a fixed low-dose regimen, independent of body weight (see Box 2.E, p.69).

Disseminated intravascular coagulation (DIC)

- confirm the diagnosis (see LMWH, p.64)
- *do not use* **warfarin** *because it is ineffective*
- *for chronic* DIC presenting with recurrent thromboses, give enoxaparin as for treatment of DVT
- *for chronic or acute* DIC presenting with hemorrhagic manifestations (e.g. ecchymoses and hematomas), seek specialist advice.

Thrombophlebitis migrans

- *do not use* **warfarin** *because it is ineffective*
- generally responds rapidly to small doses, e.g. ≤60mg/day
- continue treatment indefinitely[26]
- if necessary, titrate dose to maximum allowed according to weight, i.e. 1.5mg/kg SC once daily.

Overdose

In emergencies, **protamine sulfate** can be used to reverse the effects of enoxaparin:

- for each 1mg (100 units) of enoxaparin, give 1mg of **protamine sulfate** if <8h since the overdose, or 0.5mg if >8h
- give a maximum of 50mg by slow IV injection over 10min
- give a further 0.5mg of **protamine sulfate** per 100 units of enoxaparin after 2–4h if APTT still prolonged.

Note: even with high doses of protamine sulfate, the anti-factor Xa activity of enoxaparin is not completely neutralized (maximum reversal ~60%).

Supply

Lovenox® (Sanofi-Aventis)
Injection (single dose syringe for SC injection) 100mg/mL, 0.3mL (30mg, 3,000 units) = $7, 0.4mL (40mg, 4,000 units) = $9, 0.6mL (60mg, 6,000 units) = $14, 0.8mL (80mg, 8,000 units) = $18, 1mL (100mg, 10,000 units) = $22.
Injection (multidose vial) 100mg/mL, 3mL (300mg, 30,000 units) = $66.

Lovenox HP® (Sanofi-Aventis)
Injection (single dose syringe for SC injection) 150mg/mL, 0.8mL (120mg, 12,000 units) = $27, 1mL (150mg, 15,000 units) = $33.

1 Quinlan D *et al.* (2004) Low-molecular weight heparin compared with intravenous unfractionated heparin for treatment of pulmonary embolism. *Annals of Internal Medicine.* **140**: 175–183.
2 Van Dongen CJ *et al.* (2004) Fixed dose subcutaneous low molecular weight heparins versus adjusted dose unfractionated heparin for venous thromboembolism. *Cochrane Database of Systematic Reviews.* **4**: CD001100.
3 Hirsh J *et al.* (2001) Heparin and low-molecular-weight heparin: mechanisms of action, pharmacokinetics, dosing, monitoring, efficacy, and safety. *Chest.* **119 (suppl)**: 64s–94s.
4 Prandoni P (2001) Heparins and venous thromboembolism: current practice and future directions. *Journal of Thrombosis and Haemostasis.* **86**: 488–498.
5 Fareed J *et al.* (2003) Pharmacodynamic and pharmacokinetic properties of enoxaparin: implications for clinical practice. *Clinical Pharmacokinetics.* **42**: 1043–1057.
6 Blann AD and Lip GY (2006) Venous thromboembolism. *British Medical Journal.* **332**: 215–219.
7 Cohen AT *et al.* (2006) Efficacy and safety of fondaparinux for the prevention of venous thromboembolism in older acute medical patients: randomised placebo controlled trial. *British Medical Journal.* **332**: 325–329.
8 Fareed J *et al.* (1990) Pharmacologic profile of a low molecular weight heparin (enoxaparin): experimental and clinical validation of the prophylactic antithrombotic effects. *Acta Chirurgica Scandinavica Supplementum.* **556 (suppl)**: 75–90.
9 Bara L and Samama M (1990) Pharmacokinetics of low molecular weight heparins. *Acta Chirurgica Scandinavica Supplementum.* **556 (suppl)**: 57–61.
10 Dawes J (1990) Comparison of the pharmacokinetics of enoxaparin (Clexane) and unfractionated heparin. *Acta Chirurgica Scandinavica Supplementum.* **556 (suppl)**: 68–74.
11 Warkentin T *et al.* (1995) Heparin-induced thrombocytopenia in patients treated with low molecular weight heparin or unfractionated heparin. *New England Journal of Medicine.* **332**: 1330–1335.
12 Keeling D *et al.* (2006) The management of heparin-induced thrombocytopenia. *British Journal of Haematology.* **133**: 259–269.
13 Buller HR *et al.* (2004) Antithrombotic therapy for venous thromboembolic disease: the Seventh ACCP Conference on Antithrombotic and Thrombolytic Therapy. *Chest.* **126 (suppl 3)**: 401S–428S.
14 Geerts WH *et al.* (2004) Prevention of venous thromboembolism: the seventh ACCP Conference on Antithrombotic and Thrombolytic Therapy. *Chest.* **126 (suppl)**: 338s–400s.
15 Bergqvist D *et al.* (2002) Duration of prophylaxis against venous thromboembolism with enoxaparin after surgery for cancer. *New England Journal of Medicine.* **346**: 975–980.
16 Kher A and Samama MM (2005) Primary and secondary prophylaxis of venous thromboembolism with low-molecular-weight heparins: prolonged thromboprophylaxis, an alternative to vitamin K antagonists. *Journal of Thrombosis and Haemostasis.* **3**: 473–481.
17 Leizorovicz A and Mismetti P (2004) Preventing venous thromboembolism in medical patients. *Circulation.* **110**: IV13–19.
18 Samama MM *et al.* (1999) A comparison of enoxaparin with placebo for the prevention of venous thromboembolism in acutely ill medical patients. Prophylaxis in Medical Patients with Enoxaparin Study Group. *New England Journal of Medicine.* **341**: 793–800.
19 Noble SI *et al.* (2006) Acceptability of low molecular weight heparin thromboprophylaxis for inpatients receiving palliative care: qualitative study. *British Medical Journal.* **332**: 577–580.
20 Meyer G *et al.* (2002) Comparison of low-molecular-weight heparin and warfarin for the secondary prevention of venous thromboembolism in patients with cancer: a randomized controlled study. *Archives of Internal Medicine.* **162**: 1729–1735.
21 Lee A *et al.* (2003) Low molecular weight heparin versus a coumarin for the prevention of recurrent venous thromboembolism in patients with cancer. *New England Journal of Medicine.* **349**: 146–153.
22 Hull RD *et al.* (2006) Long-term low-molecular-weight heparin versus usual care in proximal-vein thrombosis patients with cancer. *American Journal of Medicine.* **119**: 1062–1072.
23 Johnson M (1997) Problems of anticoagulation within a palliative care setting: an audit of hospice patients taking warfarin. *Palliative Medicine.* **11**: 306–312.
24 Johnson M and Sherry K (1997) How do palliative physicians manage venous thromboembolism? *Palliative Medicine.* **11**: 462–468.
25 Noble SI and Finlay IG (2005) Is long-term low-molecular-weight heparin acceptable to palliative care patients in the treatment of cancer related venous thromboembolism? A qualitative study. *Palliative Medicine.* **19**: 197–201.
26 Walsh-McMonagle D and Green D (1997) Low-molecular weight heparin in the management of Trousseau's syndrome. *Cancer.* **80**: 649–655.

TRANEXAMIC ACID

Class: Antifibrinolytic.

Indications: Prevention of bleeding after dental extraction in hemophilia or postoperatively, hemorrhagic complications after thrombolytic treatment, menorrhagia, epistaxis, hereditary angioedema, †subarachnoid hemorrhage, †surface bleeding from ulcerating tumours on the skin, in the nose, mouth, pharynx and other hollow organs (lungs, stomach, rectum, bladder, uterus).

Contra-indications: Active thrombo-embolic disease, e.g. recent thrombo-embolism, disseminated intravascular coagulation (DIC); severe renal impairment (creatinine clearance <30mL/min).

Pharmacology

Tranexamic acid is a synthetic antifibrinolytic drug which blocks the binding of plasminogen and plasmin to fibrin, thereby preventing dissolution of hemostatic plugs.[1] It is also a weak direct inhibitor of plasmin. Tranexamic acid is excreted in the urine mainly unchanged.

Tranexamic acid is a potential option in cancer patients for the management of surface bleeding both externally and internally.[2] It should *not* be used in DIC even when hemorrhagic manifestations (ecchymoses and hematomas) are predominant because clot formation is the trigger for further intravascular coagulation and platelet consumption, and an increased risk of end-organ damage from microvascular thromboses. Although the Product Monograph gives severe renal impairment as a contra-indication, there are reports of its use in this circumstance in reduced doses (see Table 2.3 below).[3,4]

Bio-availability 30–50% PO; minimal with an oral rinse.

Onset of action (route-dependent) 1–3h.

Time to peak plasma concentration 3h PO.

Plasma halflife 2h.

Duration of action 24h.

Table 2.3 Doses in renal impairment[4]

Creatinine clearance (mL/min)	PO dose	IV dose
50–80	15mg/kg b.i.d.	10mg/kg b.i.d.
10–50	15mg/kg once daily	10mg/kg once daily
<10	15mg/kg every 2 days	10mg/kg every 2 days

Cautions

Serious drug interactions: increased risk of thrombosis with other thrombogenic drugs.

History of thrombo-embolism, renal impairment. In both microscopic and macroscopic hematuria there is a risk of clot formation causing ureteric obstruction or urinary retention.[5]

Undesirable effects

For full list, see manufacturer's Product Monograph.

Nausea, vomiting, abdominal pain, diarrhea (generally settle if the dose is reduced), disturbances in colour vision (discontinue drug).

Dose and use

For general approach to the management of surface bleeding, see Box 2.F.

The following recommendations are taken mainly from anecdotal reports.

As an oral rinse for local bleeding

As a mouthwash, tranexamic acid can be used as a 4–5% aqueous solution, 10mL q.i.d.[2]

Surface bleeding from any site[11,13]

- 1.5g PO stat and 1g t.i.d.
- if bleeding not subsiding after 3 days, increase dose to 1.5–2g t.i.d.
- usual maximum dose 2g q.i.d.
- discontinue 1 week after cessation of bleeding or reduce to 500mg t.i.d.
- restart if bleeding occurs, and possibly continue indefinitely.

Parenteral use may occasionally be indicated, e.g. in patients with bleeding and complete dysphagia due to esophageal cancer:

- 10mg/kg IV over 5–10min t.i.d.–q.i.d.

Note: in renal impairment the dose should be reduced (Table 2.3).

Box 2.F   Management of surface bleeding

Physical
Gauze applied with pressure for 10min soaked in:
* epinephrine (1 in 1,000) 1mg in 1mL *or*
* tranexamic acid 500mg in 5mL   } use standard ampules.

Silver nitrate sticks applied to bleeding points in the nose and mouth, and on skin nodules and fungating tumours.
Hemostatic dressings, i.e. alginate (e.g. Kaltostat®).

Diathermy.
Specialist therapy:
   LASER
   embolization.[6,7]

Drugs
Review existing medication
Discontinue aspirin and/or other platelet-impairing NSAID.
Prescribe an NSAID which does not impair platelet function (see Table 5.4, p.248), or acetaminophen instead.

Topical
Sucralfate paste 2g (two 1g tablets crushed in 5mL KY jelly).[8]
Sucralfate suspension 2g in 10mL b.i.d. for the mouth and rectum.[9]
Tranexamic acid 5g in 50mL warm water b.i.d. for rectal bleeding[10] (e.g. 10 ampules of undiluted injection).
1% alum solution.

Systemic
Antifibrinolytic drug, e.g. tranexamic acid.[11]
Desmopressin (augments platelet function).[12]

Radiation therapy
Teletherapy and brachytherapy are both used to control hemorrhage from:
   skin   bladder
   lungs   uterus
   esophagus   vagina
   rectum

Topical application for bleeding from fungating cancer in the skin[14]

* solution (10%): use injection, 500mg in 5mL, soak into gauze and apply with pressure for 10min, then leave *in situ* with a dressing *or*
* paste (3.3%): use tablets, 2g crushed in 60g base (e.g. hydrophilic petrolatum) and apply b.i.d.; cover with a dressing[15]
* Topical solution for bleeding from cancer in rectum, bladder or pleura.[10,16]

Generally used only if PO tranexamic acid has failed:
* 5g in 50mL of water, instilled at body temperature once daily–b.i.d. (e.g. 10 ampules of undiluted injection).

Supply
Tranexamic acid (generic)
Injection 100mg/mL, 5mL, 10mL, 50mL ampule = $19, $36 and $189 respectively.

Cyklokapron® (Pfizer)
Tablets 500mg, 28 days @ 500mg t.i.d. = $104.
Injection 100mg/mL, 5mL, 10mL ampule = $23 and $43 respectively.

---

1   Verstraete M (1985) Clinical application of inhibitors of fibrinolysis. *Drugs*. **29**: 236–261.
2   Dunn CJ and Goa KL (1999) Tranexamic acid: a review of its use in surgery and other indications. *Drugs*. **57**: 1005–1032.
3   Andersson L et al. (1978) Special considerations with regard to the dosage of tranexamic acid in patients with chronic renal diseases. *Urological Research*. **6 (2)**: 83–88.
4   Lacy C et al. (eds) (2003) *Lexi-Comp's Drug Information Handbook* (11e). Lexi-Comp and the American Pharmaceutical Association, Hudson, Ohio.
5   Schultz M and van der Lelie H (1995) Microscopic haematuria as a relative contraindication for tranexamic acid. *British Journal of Haematology*. **89**: 663–664.
6   Broadley K et al. (1995) The role of embolization in palliative care. *Palliative Medicine*. **9**: 331–335.
7   Rankin E et al. (1988) Transcatheter embolisation to control severe bleeding in fungating breast cancer. *European Journal of Surgical Oncology*. **14**: 27–32.
8   Regnard C and Makin W (1992) Management of bleeding in advanced cancer: a flow diagram. *Palliative Medicine*. **6**: 74–78.
9   Kochhar R et al. (1988) Rectal sucralfate in radiation proctitis. *Lancet*. **332**: 400.
10 McElligott E et al. (1991) Tranexamic acid and rectal bleeding. *Lancet*. **337**: 431.
11 Dean A and Tuffin P (1997) Fibrinolytic inhibitors for cancer-associated bleeding problems. *Journal of Pain and Symptom Management*. **13**: 20–24.
12 Mannucci P (1997) Desmopressin (DDAVP) in the treatment of bleeding disorders: the first 20 years. *Blood*. **90**: 2515–2521.
13 Seto AH and Dunlap DS (1996) Tranexamic acid in oncology. *Annals of Pharmacology*. **30**: 868–870.
14 Twycross R et al. (2009) *Symptom Management in Advanced Cancer* (4e). palliativedrugs.com, Nottingham, p. 236.
15 Kennedy B, Personal communication.
16 deBoer W et al. (1991) Tranexamic acid treatment of haemothorax in two patients with malignant mesothelioma. *Chest*. **100**: 847–848.

3: RESPIRATORY SYSTEM

BRONCHODILATORS

Palliative care clinicians caring for patients with end-stage COPD need to be aware of the latest management guidelines. Further, some patients with cancer also suffer from COPD or asthma and occasionally both. Concurrent COPD can be a major cause of breathlessness, notably in lung cancer, but may be unrecognized, and so go untreated.

The guidelines provided here (Box 3.A–Box 3.C) for the use of bronchodilators in patients with asthma and COPD are based on the recommendations of the Canadian Network for Asthma Care and the Canadian Thoracic Society.[1,2] These have much in common with international guidelines produced by the Global Initiative for Asthma (GINA), and the Global Initiative for Chronic Obstructive Lung Disease (GOLD), although there are some differences in emphasis.[3,4]

Generally, the guidelines should be followed. However, for patients whose prognosis is only weeks or 2–3 months (particularly those having difficulty with metered-dose inhalers (MDIs)), regularly scheduled short-acting nebulized bronchodilators are often preferable. If a patient is receiving long-term PO corticosteroids for another indication (see p.381), it is often possible to discontinue inhaled corticosteroids.

Inhalation delivers the drug directly to the bronchi and enables a smaller dose to work more quickly and with fewer undesirable systemic effects. β₂-Adrenergic receptor agonists (β₂-agonists), e.g. **salbutamol** (see p.86), **formoterol** and **salmeterol** (see p.89), act directly on bronchial smooth muscle to cause bronchodilation whereas antimuscarinics, e.g. **ipratropium** (see p.84) and **tiotropium** (see p.85), act by reducing the vagal tone to the airways. Both classes of drug improve breathlessness by airway bronchodilation and/or reducing air-trapping at rest (static hyperinflation) and on exertion (dynamic hyperinflation). A reduction in hyperinflation probably explains why clinical benefit may be seen in patients with COPD with little or no change in the FEV_1.

β₂-Agonists are used in both asthma and COPD; antimuscarinic drugs in COPD and *acute* asthma. Their use is often combined in COPD and *acute* asthma (Box 3.B, p.81; Box 3.C, p.82). In asthma, bronchodilators are generally combined with inhaled corticosteroids (Box 3.A, p.80; Box 3.B, p.81; also see p.94).

In asthma and COPD, when the above do not bring about adequate relief, a third class of bronchodilators, the methylxanthines, are sometimes used systemically, i.e. PO SR **theophylline**. Because they have a narrow therapeutic window, their use requires careful monitoring to avoid toxicity.

β-Adrenergic receptor blocking drugs (β-blockers), both cardioselective and non-selective, are contra-indicated in patients with asthma. They should also be avoided in patients with COPD, unless there are compelling reasons for their use, e.g. severe glaucoma. In such circumstances, a cardioselective β-blocker should be used with extreme caution under specialist guidance.

Box 3.A Management of chronic asthma in adults, based on references[1,5]

Start at the appropriate point on the continuum. The aim is to achieve and maintain prolonged control:
- daytime symptoms ≤twice/week
- need for rapid-acting reliever inhaler ≤twice/week
- no nocturnal symptoms, limitation of activity or exacerbations
- no missed work or school
- normal lung function, i.e. >90% of predicted or personal best.

In addition to drug treatment, discuss ways of minimizing exposure to environmental allergens, and provide a written action plan for use in the event of deterioration. Before starting an add-on therapy, check compliance, inhaler technique, treat any co-morbidities and, as far as possible, eliminate trigger factors.

Very mild (intermittent) asthma: as-needed reliever medication
Inhaled rapid-acting β_2-agonist p.r.n., e.g. salbutamol, terbutaline.

Mild (persistent) asthma: reliever medication + single controller
Start or move to here if reliever medication is needed >three times/week (aside from pre-exercise dose).
Regular low dose of inhaled corticosteroid (beclomethasone 400microgram/24h or equivalent)[a]
+ inhaled rapid-acting β_2-agonist p.r.n., e.g. salbutamol, terbutaline.
Alternatively, if unable or unwilling to use an inhaled corticosteroid, and/or concurrent allergic rhinitis:
- regular oral leukotriene modifier, e.g. montelukast.
Less preferable alternatives include:
- regular oral SR theophylline
- regular inhaled sodium cromoglycate.

Moderate asthma: reliever medication + one or two controllers
Start or move to here if symptoms occur:
- *daily*
- *at night more than once/week and*
- *are uncontrolled or only partly controlled by the regimen above.*
Regular low dose of inhaled corticosteroid[a]
+ regular inhaled LABA (e.g. salmeterol aerosol inhalation 50microgram b.i.d. or formoterol dry powder inhalation 12microgram b.i.d.)[b]
+ inhaled rapid-acting β_2-agonist p.r.n.
Increase the dose of inhaled corticosteroid if control not achieved within 3–4 months.
Alternatives to adding an inhaled LABA include the following, given regularly:
- increase to a medium (e.g. budesonide 400–800microgram/24h)[a] or high (e.g. budesonide 800–1,600microgram/24h) dose of inhaled corticosteroid alone; administer via a large-volume spacer
- add an oral leukotriene modifier
- add oral SR theophylline.

Severe asthma: reliever medication + two or more controllers
Start or move to here if symptoms occur:
- *daily and are continual*
- *frequently at night, and*
- *are uncontrolled or only partly controlled by the regimen above.*
Regular medium or high dose of inhaled corticosteroid[a]
+ regular inhaled LABA b.i.d.[b]
+ inhaled rapid-acting β_2-agonist p.r.n.
If above inadequate, add one of the following:
- oral leukotriene modifier
- oral SR theophylline.
Refer to asthma clinic for consideration of further options, e.g. oral corticosteroids.

continued

Box 3.A Continued

Very severe asthma: reliever medication + two or more controllers and oral glucocorticoid
Move to here if symptoms occur:
• *daily and are continual*
• *frequently at night, and*
• *are uncontrolled or only partly controlled by regimen above.*
Regular high dose of inhaled corticosteroid[a]
+ regular inhaled LABA b.i.d.[b]
+ inhaled rapid-acting β_2-agonist p.r.n.
If above inadequate, add one of the following:
• oral leukotriene modifier
• oral SR theophylline
If above inadequate add oral corticosteroids.

Stepping down
If good control for ⩾3 months, consider moving to the next regimen below on the continuum. If treatment includes medium- or high-dose inhaled corticosteroids, 50% reduction should be attempted every 3 months until a low dose is reached.

a. see Table 3.4, p.96 for comparative daily doses of inhaled corticosteroids
b. inhaled LABA should not be used alone because of concern over an increase in severe asthma exacerbations and asthma-related deaths.

Box 3.B Severe acute asthma, based on summary of recommendations from the Canadian Asthma Consensus Report 1999[6,7]

Characterized by persistent breathlessness despite usual bronchodilators, respiratory rate often > 30breaths/min, speaking in words rather than sentences, hunched position, chest retraction, agitation, tachycardia (>120beats/min) and a low peak expiratory flow rate (<60% of best). It requires urgent treatment with:
• oxygen, to keep SaO_2 ⩾92%
• inhaled rapid-acting β_2-agonist, e.g. salbutamol, delivered by (according to the need for expedient treatment and availability):
  ▷ MDI with spacer or dry powder inhaler, 4–6 puffs (inhaled one at a time), repeated every 15–30min, *or*
  ▷ oxygen-driven nebulizer, 5mg, repeated every 10–20min
• systemic corticosteroids, e.g. prednisone 40–60mg PO stat & once daily or hydrocortisone 100mg IV stat & q.d.s.; PO is as effective as IV.

If little response (or with β-blocker-induced bronchospasm), continue above and:
• add nebulized ipratropium bromide (e.g. 500microgram)
• magnesium IV.

If continued poor response (life-threatening asthma), ideally admit to intensive care, continue treatment as above and also consider:
• epinephrine IM or IV
• salbutamol IV
• theophylline (not in first 4h)
• assisted ventilation, e.g. intubation and mechanical ventilation.

Box 3.C   Palliative bronchodilator therapy in COPD[2]

Smoking and medication (e.g. β-blockers) may cause bronchoconstriction and should be avoided.

Treatment depends on the severity of symptoms and their effect on lifestyle; most patients need only a single drug but a few require combined treatment.

Assess benefit in terms of improvement in symptoms, activities of daily living, exercise capacity, and rapidity of symptom relief; discontinue if ineffective.

The choice of drug(s) should take into account the benefit obtained from a trial of the drug, undesirable effects, patient preference and cost.

For breathlessness and exercise limitation, consider the following:
- inhaled short-acting β₂-agonist or short-acting antimuscarinic bronchodilator p.r.n.; if symptoms persist, either use both together or go to next bullet
- if symptoms persist or frequent exacerbations[a], add regular inhaled LABA or long-acting antimuscarinic bronchodilator; if symptoms persist, either use both together or go to next bullet
- if symptoms persist, add theophylline[b]
- in severe COPD, if symptoms persist ± frequent exacerbations[a] use a regular inhaled LABA and an inhaled high-dose corticosteroid in one preparation (maintenance oral corticosteroid is not recommended[c]).

a. >2 episodes requiring antibiotics or oral corticosteroid per annum
b. requires caution, particularly in the elderly, monitoring of blood levels and for risk of drug–drug interaction; can be used earlier in patients unable to use inhaled therapy
c. if unavoidable in patients with advanced COPD, keep dose to a minimum and prescribe appropriate prophylactic treatment for osteoporosis.

Diagnosing asthma and COPD

The diagnosis of asthma or COPD is mainly based on the history and examination, supported by objective tests and, ultimately, the response to treatment.

Objective tests are recommended to try to confirm a diagnosis of asthma before long-term therapy is started, e.g. examining peak expiratory flow variability over a period of 2 weeks or evaluating the effect on lung function of a bronchodilator or course of oral corticosteroid (Box 3.D). Spirometry is the preferred method of measuring airflow limitation and its reversibility (asthma), but peak expiratory flow (PEF) can be an important aid in diagnosis.[6] For COPD, a post-bronchodilator ratio of $FEV_1/FVC < 0.7$ is widely accepted as the diagnostic criteria for

---

Box 3.D   Bronchodilator reversibility test[6,8,9]

These tests are done to detect patients whose FEV_1 or PEF increases substantially, i.e. are asthmatic.

Response
Measure FEV_1 or PEF:
- before and 15min after an inhaled short-acting β₂-agonist either by MDI + spacer *or* nebulizer
- before and after 10–14 days of an inhaled corticosteroid or oral prednisone.

Interpretation
Reversibility is suggested by:
- an increase in FEV_1 that is both greater than 180mL and ⩾12% (preferably 15%)
- an increase in PEF that is ⩾12% (preferably 20%).

However, because some patients with untreated asthma may not improve to this degree and because of the poor repeatability of the test, the results are best considered a guide only, to be used with the clinical assessment and response to regular therapy.

COPD. In the elderly, the results should be adjusted for height and age to reduce the risk of a false positive diagnosis.[2]

In palliative care, unless asthma is suspected, reversibility testing is likely to have a minor role. When airflow obstruction is suspected, evaluating the impact on symptoms of a 1–2 weeks trial of a bronchodilator is a more pragmatic and probably more relevant approach than a reversibility test.

Delivery devices

Pressurized metered dose inhalers (MDIs) are the most commonly prescribed delivery device. However, they are difficult to master, and the correct inhaler technique should be carefully explained to the patient and subsequently checked.[1] The patient should be instructed to inhale slowly and, if possible, then hold their breath for 10sec. With an MDI, even with a good technique, 80% of a dose is deposited in the mouth and oropharynx.

If inhaler technique does not improve with training, or in patients with poor inspiratory effort, consider using an MDI plus a large-volume (650–850mL) spacer device to deliver single-dose actuations. There should be minimal delay between actuation and inhalation, but normal (tidal) breathing is as effective as taking a single breath. Build up of static on plastic and polycarbonate spacers attracts drug particles and reduces drug delivery. To reduce static, spacers should be washed according to the manufacturer's information. Spacers should be replaced every 6–12 months.[10]

Dry powder inhalers, e.g. Turbuhalers® and breath-actuated MDIs are other options. Patients generally prefer Turbuhalers® over an MDI ± a spacer, but they are not suited to patients with poor inspiratory effort. Breath-actuated MDIs are triggered at low inspiratory flow rates, are popular with patients and are the easiest to use correctly.[8]

Nebulizers are more expensive and not as convenient as an MDI but may be preferable in patients with a poor inhaler technique, e.g. children, the frail, and patients with end-stage disease. Because of improved drug delivery, there may be better symptom relief.[11] However, the higher doses administered can increase the risk of undesirable effects and their use should be carefully monitored (also see Nebulized drugs, p.537).

There is no evidence to suggest that a nebulizer is superior to any inhaler device for the delivery of a β_2-agonist or corticosteroid for the treatment of stable asthma, or to an MDI + spacer in treating moderate–severe acute exacerbations.[6] In patients with COPD and a good inhaler technique, nebulized bronchodilator therapy is only indicated in severe acute exacerbations[3] or when there is distressing or disabling breathlessness despite maximal therapy using inhalers.

Breathlessness can be improved in most patients with lung cancer and concurrent COPD by a combination of a β_2-agonist and an antimuscarinic bronchodilator; this is equally effective when given by an MDI + a spacer or by nebulizer (see Nebulized drugs, p.537).[12]

Propellants

In Canada, hydrofluoroalkane-134a (HFA) has now replaced chlorofluorocarbons (CFC) as the propellant in all MDIs containing bronchodilators. Compared with CFC, 'clogging' is more likely with HFA because of a reduced exit velocity, and cleaning of the nozzle after use is recommended, particularly with drugs suspended rather than dissolved in the propellant, e.g. **salbutamol**.

Supply

Inhaler aids and spacer devices
Optichamber® Advantage (Respironics) large-volume spacer, latex-free
Chamber with mask = $17 (medium or small); $21 (large).

Aerochamber Max® (Trudell Medical)
Chamber with mouthpiece = $44, with infant or pediatric mask = $70, with adult mask = $75.
Aerochamber Pediatric ACBoyz/ACGirlz® (Trudell Medical)
Chamber with mouthpiece = $40.

Spacechamber® (CareStream Medical)
Chamber with mask = $25 (pediatric); $23 (adult).

1 Becker A et al. (2005) Summary of recommendations from the Canadian Asthma Consensus guidelines, 2003 and Canadian Pediatric Asthma Consensus Guidelines, 2003 (updated to December 2004). *Canadian Medical Association Journal.* **173 (6 suppl)**: S1–S56.

2 O'Donnell DE et al. (2007) Canadian Thoracic Society recommendations for management of chronic obstructive pulmonary disease – 2007 update. *Canadian Respiratory Journal.* **14 (suppl B)**: 5B–32B.

3 NHLBI/WHO (2008) Global Initiative for Chronic Obstructive Lung Disease. Strategy for the diagnosis management and prevention of chronic obstructive pulmonary disease. Available from: www.goldcopd.com

4 NHLBI/WHO (2008) Global Initiative for Asthma (GINA). Pocket guide for asthma management and prevention. Available from: www.ginasthma.com

5 Balter MS et al. (2009) Management of asthma in adults. *Canadian Medical Association Journal.* DOI:10.1503/cmaj.080007.

6 Boulet LP et al. (1999) Canadian asthma consensus report, 1999. *Canadian Medical Association Journal.* **161 (11 suppl)**: S1–62.

7 Hodder R et al. (2009) Management of acute asthma in adults in the emergency department: nonventilatory management. *Canadian Medical Association Journal.* DOI:10.1503/cmaj.080072.

8 Lenney J et al. (2000) Inappropriate inhaler use: assessment of use and patient preference of seven inhalation devices. *Respiratory Medicine.* **94**: 496–500.

9 BTS/SIGN (2009) British Guideline on the Management of Asthma. A National Clinical Guideline. Revised edition June 2009. British Thoracic Society and Scottish Intercollegiate Guidelines Network. Available from: http://www.sign.ac.uk/pdf/sign101.pdf

10 DTB (2000) Inhaler devices for asthma. *Drug and Therapeutics Bulletin.* **38**: 9–14.

11 Tashkin DP et al. (2007) Comparing COPD treatment: nebulizer, metered dose inhaler, and concomitant therapy. *American Journal of Medicine.* **120**: 435–441.

12 Congelton J and Muers M (1995) The incidence of airflow obstruction in bronchial carcinoma, its relation to breathlessness and response to bronchodilator therapy. *Respiratory Medicine.* **89**: 291–296.

IPRATROPIUM BROMIDE

Class: Quaternary ammonium antimuscarinic bronchodilator.

Indications: Reversible airways obstruction, particularly in COPD.

Pharmacology

In patients with COPD, cholinergic vagal efferent nerves to the airways activate muscarinic receptors resulting in increased resting bronchial tone and mucus secretion.[1] Antimuscarinics block these effects and cause bronchodilation. Short-acting antimuscarinics improve pulmonary function, breathlessness and exercise performance, but have less consistent benefit on quality of life.[2] For patients with mild COPD (MRC grade 2) causing breathlessness and exercise limitation, an inhaled short-acting antimuscarinic bronchodilator or a short-acting β_2-adrenergic receptor agonist (β_2-agonist) are recommended as initial treatment on a p.r.n. basis; if symptoms persist, their use can be combined. If patients remain symptomatic, either a regular inhaled long-acting antimuscarinic bronchodilator (**tiotropium**, see p.85) or an inhaled long-acting β_2-agonist (LABA) can be added (see Inhaled LABAs, p.89). Ipratropium is not recommended for moderate–severe COPD (see Box 3.C, p.82). An inhaled short-acting antimuscarinic bronchodilator plus a short-acting β_2-agonist is recommended to relieve breathlessness in acute exacerbations of COPD.[2]

Antimuscarinic bronchodilators have no role in the management of chronic asthma, but nebulized ipratropium bromide is used in severe acute exacerbations (see Box 3.B, p.81).[3,4]

Bio-availability 10–20% of the dose reaches the lower airways.

Onset of action 3–30min asthma; 15min COPD.

Peak response 1.5–3h asthma; 1–2h COPD.

Plasma halflife 2.3–3.8h.

Duration of action 4–8h.

Cautions

Bladder neck obstruction, prostatic hypertrophy. Nebulized solution reaching the eye may precipitate narrow-angle glaucoma in susceptible patients.

Undesirable effects

For full list, see manufacturer's Product Monograph.

Headache, nausea and dry mouth. Rarely visual accommodation changes, tachycardia, paradoxical bronchoconstriction, gastro-intestinal motility changes and urinary retention. Nebulized drug droplets may reach the eye and there have been isolated reports of eye pain, mydriasis, increased intra-ocular pressure and narrow-angle glaucoma.

Dose and use

In most patients, administration t.i.d. is sufficient.

Aerosol inhalation

- generally 20–40microgram (1–2 puffs) p.r.n. up to t.i.d.–q.i.d.; however, in mild COPD (MRC grade 2), guidelines include doses of 40–60microgram (2–3 puffs) p.r.n. up to q4h[2]
- 20–40microgram (1–2 puffs) before exercise in exercise-induced bronchoconstriction in COPD.

Nebulizer solution

- use with a mouthpiece to minimize any nebulized drug entering the eye
- 250–500microgram p.r.n. up to t.i.d.–q.i.d. in COPD; generally given q.i.d. in an exacerbation of COPD
- 500microgram q6h–q4h in acute exacerbation of asthma.

Supply

Ipratropium bromide (generic)
Nebulizer solution (single-dose units) 125microgram/mL, 20×2mL (250microgram) = $15; 250microgram/mL, 20×1mL (250microgram), 20×2mL (500microgram) = $15; *may be diluted with sterile 0.9% saline.*
Nebulizer solution (multiple-dose bottle) 250microgram/mL, 20mL = $12; *may be diluted with sterile 0.9% saline.*

Atrovent® (Boehringer Ingelheim)
Aerosol inhalation (CFC-free) Atrovent HFA®, 20microgram/metered inhalation, 28 days @ 40microgram (2 puffs) t.i.d. = $17.

1 Gross NJ et al. (1989) Cholinergic bronchomotor tone in COPD. Estimates of its amount in comparison with that in normal subjects. *Chest.* **96**: 984–987.
2 O'Donnell DE et al. (2007) Canadian Thoracic Society recommendations for management of chronic obstructive pulmonary disease – 2007 update. *Canadian Respiratory Journal.* **14 (suppl B)**: 5B–32B.
3 Becker A et al. (2005) Summary of recommendations from the Canadian Asthma Consensus guidelines, 2003 and Canadian Pediatric Asthma Consensus Guidelines, 2003 (updated to December 2004). *Canadian Medical Association Journal.* **173 (6 suppl)**: S1–S56.
4 Rodrigo GJ (2003) Inhaled therapy for acute adult asthma. *Current Opinion in Allergy and Clinical Immunology.* **3**: 169–175.

TIOTROPIUM

Class: Quaternary ammonium antimuscarinic bronchodilator.

Indications: Maintenance treatment of airways obstruction in COPD.

Contra-indications: Hypersensitivity to **atropine** or its derivatives, including **ipratropium**, lactose intolerance.

Pharmacology

Tiotropium bromide is structurally related to **ipratropium bromide** but is longer acting and thus has the convenience of once daily administration.[1-3] Its main effect is to inhibit muscarinic M_3-receptors in airway smooth muscle and mucous glands, and M_1-receptors in parasympathetic ganglia. Because it is a quaternary compound, relatively little tiotropium is absorbed into the systemic circulation. However, a small amount of tiotropium is excreted renally unchanged and, theoretically at least, accumulation could occur in patients with moderate–severe renal impairment.

A recent systematic review has shown that in patients with COPD, tiotropium is more effective than **ipratropium** in improving lung function, relieving breathlessness, reducing exacerbations, exacerbation-related hospitalizations, and improving quality of life.[4] It improves lung function significantly more than **salmeterol**, but the difference is unlikely to be clinically significant.[5] It is cost-effective, although not cost-saving.[4] Tiotropium should be considered when symptoms are unrelieved by the use of an inhaled short-acting antimuscarinic bronchodilator (**ipratropium**, see p.84) or a short-acting β_2-adrenergic receptor agonist (β_2-agonist, e.g. **salbutamol**, see below) given alone or in combination on a p.r.n. basis (see Box 3.C, p.82). If symptoms persist despite the use of tiotropium, an inhaled long-acting β_2-agonist (LABA) should be added.[6]

Tiotropium has a relatively slow onset of bronchodilation and it should not be used as rescue therapy for acute bronchospasm.[7] Patients receiving tiotropium should use a short-acting β_2-agonist, e.g. **salbutamol**, as a rescue bronchodilator;[6] **ipratropium** should not be used as it has a slower onset of action and the muscarinic receptors will already be occupied by tiotropium.[8]

Bio-availability 20% reaches the lower airways.
Onset of action ≤30min.
Peak response 1–3h.
Plasma halflife 5–6 days.
Duration of action >24h.

Cautions

Bladder neck obstruction, prostatic hypertrophy, moderate–severe renal impairment (creatinine clearance ≤50mL/min). Powder accidentally sprayed into the eye may precipitate narrow-angle glaucoma in susceptible patients.

Undesirable effects

For full list, see manufacturer's Product Monograph.
Very common (>10%): dry mouth (generally mild and transient; settles after 3–5 weeks of use).
Common (<10%, >1%): constipation, candidosis, sinusitis, epistaxis, pharyngitis, cough.
Uncommon (<1%, >0.1%): tachycardia, palpitations, urinary retention.

Dose and use

Regular administration of 1 capsule once daily via the HandiHaler® inhalation device.

Supply

Spiriva® (Boehringer Ingelheim)
Dry powder inhalation capsules for use with the HandiHaler® device, 18microgram/capsule, 28 days @ 1 capsule once daily = $63; *contain lactose.*

1 Barnes PJ (2000) The pharmacological properties of tiotropium. *Chest.* **117 (suppl)**: 63s–66s.
2 Hvizdos KM and Goa KL (2002) Tiotropium bromide. *Drugs.* **62**: 1195–1203; discussion 1204–1195.
3 Gross NJ (2004) Tiotropium bromide. *Chest.* **126**: 1946–1953.
4 Barr RG et al. (2006) Tiotropium for stable chronic obstructive pulmonary disease: A meta-analysis. *Thorax.* **61**: 854–862.
5 Brusasco V et al. (2003) Health outcomes following treatment for 6 months with once daily tiotropium compared with twice daily salmeterol in patients with COPD. *Thorax.* **58**: 399–404.
6 O'Donnell DE et al. (2007) Canadian Thoracic Society recommendations for management of chronic obstructive pulmonary disease – 2007 update. *Canadian Respiratory Journal.* **14 (suppl B)**: 5B–32B.
7 Calverley PMA (2000) The timing and dose pattern of bronchodilation with tiotropium in stable COPD [abstract P523]. *European Respiratory Journal.* **16 (suppl 31)**: 56s.
8 Sutherland ER and Cherniack RM (2004) Management of chronic obstructive pulmonary disease. *New England Journal of Medicine.* **350**: 2689–2697.

SALBUTAMOL

Class: β_2-Adrenergic receptor agonist (sympathomimetic).

Indications: Asthma and other conditions associated with reversible airways obstruction.

Pharmacology

Short-acting β_2-adrenergic receptor agonists (β_2-agonists, e.g. salbutamol, **terbutaline**) have an important role in the management of chronic asthma and COPD and acute exacerbations of both (see Bronchodilators, p.79).[1,2] They have a predominantly β_2-adrenergic agonist bronchodilator effect and, at low doses, do not have a major impact on the heart. With increasing dose, tachycardia can occur and rarely prolongation of the QT interval which may predispose to *torsade de pointes*, a ventricular tachyarrhythmia (see Prolongation of the QT interval in palliative care, p.543).

In chronic asthma, short-acting β_2-agonists should be used only p.r.n. at the minimum dose and frequency required.[2] They are not recommended for regular use because this appears to be of little benefit in controlled studies. Further, regular use has also been associated with poorer asthma control in one study.[3] Thus, the need to use a short-acting β_2-agonist $\geqslant$3 times a week is one indication for the introduction of an inhaled corticosteroid (see Box 3.A, p.80).[2]

In mild (MRC grade 2) COPD, for breathlessness and exercise limitation, either a short-acting β_2-agonist or a short-acting antimuscarinic bronchodilator can be used p.r.n. If symptoms persist, the alternative can be tried or their use combined (see Box 3.C, p.82).[1]

Plasma potassium concentration should be monitored in severe asthma because β_2-agonists, particularly when used with **theophylline** and inhaled corticosteroids, can cause *hypokalemia* which further increases the QT interval and risk of arrhythmia.

On the other hand, salbutamol via a metered dose inhaler (MDI) or nebulizer is more convenient and equally as effective as **insulin** and **dextrose** for the treatment of *hyperkalemia* in uremic patients.[4] The use of an MDI and a spacer device is more accessible and quicker acting compared with the nebulized route.[5] A β_2-agonist with both **insulin** and **dextrose** may be more effective than the alternative treatments used alone. Thus, the combined treatment is probably better in severe hyperkalemia (i.e. $\geqslant$6mmol/L), and in patients who fail to respond to one or other treatment.[4,6]

Bio-availability 10–20% of the dose reaches the lower airways.
Onset of action 5min inhaled; 3–5min nebulized.
Peak response 0.5–2h inhaled; 1.2h nebulized.
Plasma halflife 4–6h inhaled and nebulized.
Duration of action 4–6h inhaled and nebulized.

Cautions

Serious drug interaction: increased risk of hypokalemia with corticosteroids, diuretics, **theophylline**.

Hyperthyroidism, myocardial insufficiency, hypertension, diabetes mellitus (risk of keto-acidosis if given by CIVI).

Undesirable effects
For full list, see manufacturer's Product Monograph.
Common (<10%, >1%): tremor, headaches, tachycardia.
Uncommon (<1%, >0.1%): mouth and throat irritation from dry powder inhalation.

Dose and use
Asthma
In acute exacerbations of asthma, β_2-agonists can be given repeatedly by MDI + spacer or a nebulizer until symptoms improve. In severe episodes which do not respond to a rapid-acting β_2-agonist plus a systemic corticosteroid, nebulized β_2-agonists should be combined with nebulized **ipratropium** (see Box 3.B, p.81).[7]

Aerosol inhalation
Chronic asthma
- 100–200microgram (1–2 puffs) p.r.n. up to q.i.d.
- 200microgram (2 puffs) before exercise in exercise-induced bronchoconstriction.
Acute asthma
- 100microgram (1 puff) via a spacer, repeated p.r.n. up to every 30–60sec until symptoms and lung function improve; there is no definite maximum dose, although some have suggested 20–40 puffs.[7]

Nebulizer solution
Chronic asthma
- 2.5–5mg p.r.n. up to q.i.d. in patients for whom inhalers are unsuitable.

Acute asthma
- 5mg every 15–20min via an oxygen-driven nebulizer (see Box 3.B, p.81).

COPD
In acute exacerbations of COPD, bronchodilator use should be optimized (see Box 3.C, p.82);[1] both nebulizers and inhalers can be used to administer inhaled therapy during severe exacerbations.[8]

In stable COPD, some guidelines suggest that patients with distressing or disabling breathlessness despite maximal bronchodilator therapy using inhalers can be considered for nebulizer therapy. However, there is no good evidence that nebulizer therapy is more helpful than inhalers in stable disease, and the equipment is expensive and requires maintenance.[8,9]

Aerosol inhalation
- 100–200microgram (1–2 puffs) p.r.n. up to q.i.d.

Nebulizer solution
- 2.5–5mg p.r.n. up to q.i.d. via an oxygen-driven nebulizer unless the patient is hypercapnic or acidotic when compressed air should be used. If oxygen therapy is required by such patients, administer simultaneously by nasal cannula.

Emergency treatment of hyperkalemia
Stop and think! Are you justified in correcting a potentially fatal complication in a moribund patient?
The use of β_2-agonists for this indication is included here to allow practitioners to institute therapy without undue delay. However, this is only part of the management of hyperkalemia and specialist advice should be obtained as necessary:
- when ECG abnormalities are present, first give **calcium gluconate** 10mL of 10% solution IV to protect against arrhythmia; this is important because initially β_2-agonists may transiently increase the plasma potassium concentration[5,6]
- 1,200microgram (12 puffs) inhaled over 2min via a spacer device *or*
- 10–20mg nebulized (use 5mg/mL formulation) over 10–30min
- effective within 5–30min; duration of effect 1–2h or more
- if necessary, repeat dose[4]
- others use smaller doses, 2.5mg nebulized every 20min as tolerated
- if above ineffective or hyperkalemia severe (i.e. ⩾6mmol/L), combine above with **insulin** and **dextrose**.[6]

Supply
Salbutamol (generic)
Aerosol inhalation (CFC-free) 100microgram/metered inhalation, 28 days @ 200microgram (2 puffs) *p.r.n.* up to q.i.d. = $9.
Nebulizer solution (single-dose units) 0.5mg/mL, 20×2.5mL (1.25mg) = $8; 1mg/mL, 20×2.5mL (2.5mg) = $13; 2mg/mL, 20×2.5mL (5mg) = $24; *may be diluted with sterile 0.9% saline.*

Airomir® (Graceway)
Aerosol inhalation (CFC-free) 100microgram/metered inhalation, 28 days @ 200microgram (2 puffs) *p.r.n.* up to q.i.d. = $10.

Ventolin® (GlaxoSmithKline)
Aerosol inhalation (CFC-free) Ventolin HFA®, 100microgram/metered inhalation, 28 days @ 200microgram (2 puffs) *p.r.n.* up to q.i.d. = $17.
Dry powder inhalation blisters for use with Ventolin Diskus® device, 200microgram/blister, 28 days @ 200microgram (1 blister) *p.r.n.* up to q.i.d. = $27.
Nebulizer solution (multiple-dose bottle for use with a nebulizer or ventilator) 5mg/mL, 10mL = $11; *may be diluted with sterile 0.9% saline.*

Nebulizer solution (single-dose units for use with nebulizer) Nebules®, 1mg/mL, 20×2.5mL (2.5mg) = $23; 2mg/mL, 20×2.5mL (5mg) = $43; *may be diluted with sterile 0.9% saline if administration time >10min is required.*

1 O'Donnell DE et al. (2007) Canadian Thoracic Society recommendations for management of chronic obstructive pulmonary disease – 2007 update. *Canadian Respiratory Journal.* **14 (suppl B)**: 5B–32B.
2 Becker A et al. (2005) Summary of recommendations from the Canadian Asthma Consensus guidelines, 2003 and Canadian Pediatric Asthma Consensus Guidelines, 2003 (updated to December 2004). *Canadian Medical Association Journal.* **173 (6 suppl)**: S1–S56.
3 Sears M (2000) Short-acting inhaled B-agonists: to be taken regularly or as needed? *Lancet.* **355**: 1658–1659.
4 Mahoney BA et al. (2005) Emergency interventions for hyperkalaemia. *Cochrane Database of Systematic Reviews.* **2**: CD003235.
5 Mandelberg A et al. (1999) Salbutamol metered-dose inhaler with spacer for hyperkalemia: how fast? How safe? *Chest.* **115**: 617–622.
6 Evans KJ and Greenberg A (2005) Hyperkalemia: a review. *Journal of Intensive Care Medicine* **20**: 272–290.
7 Boulet LP et al. (1999) Canadian asthma consensus report, 1999. *Canadian Medical Association Journal.* **161 (11 suppl)**: S1–62.
8 NHLBI/WHO (2008) Global Initiative for Chronic Obstructive Lung Disease. Strategy for the diagnosis management and prevention of chronic obstructive pulmonary disease. Available from: www.goldcopd.com
9 O'Donnell DE et al. (2003) Canadian Thoracic Society recommendations for management of chronic obstructive pulmonary disease – 2003. *Canadian Respiratory Journal.* **10 (suppl A)**: 5A–33A.

INHALED LONG-ACTING β₂-ADRENERGIC RECEPTOR AGONISTS (LABAs)

Class: β₂-Adrenergic receptor agonist (sympathomimetic).

Indications: Reversible airways obstruction in patients requiring long-term regular bronchodilator therapy. **Formoterol** can be used to relieve asthma symptoms, or to prevent exercise-induced bronchospasm (approved for Oxeze® Turbuhaler only).

Contra-indications: **Salmeterol** should not be used for the relief of acute asthma because of its slow onset of action.

Pharmacology

The selective, long-acting β₂-adrenergic receptor agonists (LABAs) **salmeterol** and **formoterol** have a bronchodilating effect which lasts for 12h.[1] **Salmeterol** has a relatively slow onset of action. **Formoterol** has an onset of action similar to **salbutamol** and can thus also be used as a reliever inhaler,[2] or to prevent exercise-induced bronchospasm.

In patients with asthma, inhaled LABAs are added when symptoms are inadequately relieved by a regular low-dose inhaled corticosteroid (see Box 3.A, p.80).[3] The addition of inhaled LABAs to inhaled corticosteroids improves lung function, symptoms, and decreases exacerbations more effectively than increasing the dose of inhaled steroids alone.[4,5] However, the findings of post-marketing studies generally have been less impressive and safety concerns have been identified. When used *without* an inhaled corticosteroid, **salmeterol** has been associated with increased exacerbations of life-threatening and fatal asthma.[6,7] High doses of **formoterol** (e.g. ≥24microgram b.i.d.) may also be associated with an increased incidence of severe asthma exacerbations.[8] Thus inhaled LABAs should *not* be used in asthma without inhaled cortico-steroids (see Cautions).[3,9] Inhalers are available which combine inhaled LABAs and inhaled corticosteroids. There is no difference in efficacy compared with the use of separate inhalers. However, reducing the number of inhalations and inhalers required may aid patient adherence and also guarantees that inhaled LABAs are not used alone without corticosteroids.[1]

In patients with COPD, **salmeterol** or **formoterol** ± a long-acting antimuscarinic (**tiotropium**, p.85) should be considered when symptoms are unrelieved by the use of an inhaled short-acting β₂-adrenergic receptor agonist (β₂-agonist, e.g. **salbutamol**, p.86) or a short-acting antimuscarinic bronchodilator (**ipratropium**, p.84) given alone or in combination on a p.r.n. basis (see Box 3.C, p.82).[10] Inhaled LABAs and long-acting antimuscarinic bronchodilators are equally effective in terms of improving lung function, relieving breathlessness, reducing exacerbations and hospitalizations, and improving quality of life.[11] For pharmacokinetic details see Table 3.1.

Table 3.1 Pharmacokinetics of inhaled LABAs

	Formoterol	Salmeterol
Bio-availability	30–50% of the delivered dose reaches the lungs (Turbuhaler®)	Approximately 10% of the delivered dose reaches the lungs (aerosol)[12]
Onset of action	1–3min	10–20min
Peak response	5–10min	≤30min[12]
Plasma halflife	≤8h	≤8h (plasma concentration low or undetectable after therapeutic doses)[12]
Duration of action	About 12h	12–16h[12]

Cautions

Serious drug interactions: increased risk of hypokalemia with corticosteroids, diuretics, theophylline.

Inhaled LABAs should *not* be used without inhaled corticosteroids in asthma because of concern over an increase in severe asthma exacerbations and asthma-related deaths. To ensure safe use, Health Canada has advised that in chronic asthma:[7]
- **salmeterol** and **formoterol** can only be used with an appropriate dose of inhaled corticosteroid as determined by a physician
- LABAs are not a substitute for inhaled or oral corticosteroids
- Serevent®, Foradil®, Symbicort® or Advair® should never be used to treat acute or sudden onset of asthma symptoms and attacks
- Oxeze® may be used to treat acute or sudden onset of asthma symptoms in patients ≥6 years
- medical attention should be sought if a patient's use of asthma medications becomes less effective, or if more inhalations than usual are required
- patients must not stop or reduce their asthma therapy without first consulting their prescribing physician. Abruptly stopping medications may result in deteriorating asthma control, which can be life-threatening
- patients with asthma who have any questions about their current prescription or treatment should contact their physician or pharmacist directly.

Hyperthyroidism, cardiovascular disease, arrhythmias, susceptibility to QT prolongation or concurrent use of drugs that prolong the QT interval (see p.543), hypertension, paradoxical bronchoconstriction (discontinue and use alternative treatment), severe liver cirrhosis (**formoterol**), diabetes mellitus (may cause hyperglycemia; monitor blood glucose).

Undesirable effects

For full list, see manufacturer's Product Monograph.
Common (<10%, >1%): headache, tremor, palpitations, muscle cramps.
Uncommon (<1%, >0.1%): tachycardia.
Rare (<0.1%) or very rare (<0.01%): arrhythmias, e.g. atrial fibrillation, supraventricular tachycardia, QT interval prolongation, paradoxical bronchoconstriction.

Dose and use
Asthma
An inhaled LABA should be added *only* if p.r.n. treatment with a short-acting β_2-agonist *and* regular prophylactic therapy with an inhaled corticosteroid is insufficient to control symptoms (see Box 3.A, Moderate asthma, p.80).[9]
COPD
An inhaled LABA may be used either alone or together with **tiotropium** for maintenance treatment in COPD, where symptoms persist with p.r.n. use of a short-acting β_2-agonist or short-acting antimuscarinic bronchodilator (see Box 3.C, p.82).[10]

Formoterol

The dose varies with formulation and indication (Table 3.2).

Table 3.2 Adult doses of formoterol

Formulation	Foradil® (dry powder)	Oxeze® (turbuhaler)
Asthma		
Starting dose	12microgram b.i.d.	6–12microgram daily–b.i.d.
Maximum dose	24microgram b.i.d.	24microgram b.i.d.
Relief of bronchospasm or use before exercise		
	n/a	6–12microgram p.r.n.
COPD		
Starting dose	12microgram b.i.d.	n/a
Maximum dose	24microgram b.i.d.	n/a

Salmeterol

Asthma and COPD:
• 50microgram b.i.d.

Supply

Formoterol fumarate
Foradil® (Novartis)
Dry powder inhalation capsules for use with the inhaler device supplied, 12microgram/capsule, 28 days @ 1 capsule b.i.d. = $47.

Formoterol fumarate dihydrate
Oxeze®Turbuhaler (AstraZeneca)
Dry powder inhalation Oxeze® 6 Turbuhaler®, 6microgram/metered inhalation, 28 days @ 2 puffs b.i.d. = $66.
Dry powder inhalation Oxeze® 12 Turbuhaler®, 12microgram/metered inhalation, 28 days @ 1 puff b.i.d. = $44.

Salmeterol
Serevent® (GlaxoSmithKline)
Dry powder inhalation blisters for use with Diskus® device, salmeterol (as xinafoate) 50microgram/blister, 28 days @ 50microgram (1 blister) b.i.d. = $57.

With corticosteroids
Formoterol
Symbicort® (AstraZeneca)
Dry powder inhalation Symbicort® 100 Turbuhaler®, formoterol (as fumarate dihydrate) 6microgram, budesonide 100microgram/metered inhalation, 28 days @ 2 puffs b.i.d. = $60.
Dry powder inhalation Symbicort® 200 Turbuhaler®, formoterol (as fumarate dihydrate) 6microgram, budesonide 200microgram/metered inhalation, 28 days @ 1 puff b.i.d. = $39.

Salmeterol
Advair® (GlaxoSmithKline)
Dry powder inhalation Advair 125®, salmeterol (as xinafoate) 25microgram, fluticasone propionate 125microgram/metered inhalation, 28 days @ 2 puffs b.i.d. = $96.
Dry powder inhalation Advair 250®, salmeterol (as xinafoate) 25microgram, fluticasone propionate 250microgram/metered inhalation, 28 days @ 1 puff b.i.d. = $68.

Advair Diskus® (GlaxoSmithKline)
Dry powder inhalation Advair 100 Diskus®, blisters for use with Diskus® device, salmeterol (as xinafoate) 50microgram, fluticasone propionate 100microgram/blister, 28 days @ 1 blister b.i.d. = $81.

Dry powder inhalation Advair 250 Diskus® blisters for use with Diskus® device, salmeterol (as xinafoate) 50microgram, fluticasone propionate 250microgram/blister, 28 days @ I blister b.i.d. = $96.

Dry powder inhalation Advair 500 Diskus® blisters for use with Diskus® device, salmeterol (as xinafoate) 50microgram, fluticasone propionate 500microgram/blister, 28 days @ I blister b.i.d. = $137.

I   Kips JC and Pauwels RA (2001) Long-acting inhaled beta(2)-agonist therapy in asthma. *American Journal of Respiratory and Critical Care Medicine.* **164**: 923–932.
2   Becker A et al. (2005) Summary of recommendations from the Canadian Asthma Consensus guidelines, 2003. *Canadian Medical Association Journal.* **173 (6 suppl):** S3–11.
3   Lemiere C et al. (2004) Adult Asthma Consensus Guidelines update 2003. *Canadian Respiratory Journal.* **11 Suppl A**: 9A–18A.
4   Pauwels RA et al. (1997) Effect of inhaled formoterol and budesonide on exacerbations of asthma. Formoterol and Corticosteroids Establishing Therapy (FACET) International Study Group. *New England Journal of Medicine.* **337**: 1405–1411.
5   Shrewsbury S et al. (2000) Meta-analysis of increased dose of inhaled steroid or addition of salmeterol in symptomatic asthma (MIASMA). *British Medical Journal.* **320**: 1368–1373.
6   Nelson HS et al. (2006) The Salmeterol Multicenter Asthma Research Trial: a comparison of usual pharmacotherapy for asthma or usual pharmacotherapy plus salmeterol. *Chest.* **129**: 15–26.
7   Health Canada (2005) Safety information about a class of asthma drugs known as long-acting beta-2 agonists. Available from: http://www.hc-sc.gc.ca/ahc-asc/media/advisories-avis/_2005/2005_107_e.html
8   Palliativedrugs.com (2005) October Newsletter. Available from: www.palliativedrugs.com
9   Becker A et al. (2005) Summary of recommendations from the Canadian Asthma Consensus guidelines, 2003 and Canadian Pediatric Asthma Consensus Guidelines, 2003 (updated to December 2004). *Canadian Medical Association Journal.* **173 (6 suppl)**: S1–S56.
10 O'Donnell DE et al. (2007) Canadian Thoracic Society recommendations for management of chronic obstructive pulmonary disease – 2007 update. *Canadian Respiratory Journal.* **14 (suppl B)**: 5B–32B.
11 Barr RG et al. (2006) Tiotropium for stable chronic obstructive pulmonary disease: A meta-analysis. *Thorax.* **61**: 854–862.
12 Cazzola M et al. (2002) Clinical pharmacokinetics of salmeterol. *Clinical Pharmacokinetics.* **41**: 19–30.

THEOPHYLLINE

Class: Methylxanthine.

Indications: Reversible airways obstruction.

Contra-indications: Uncontrolled cardiac arrhythmias, seizure disorders.

Pharmacology

Because of its inferior safety and efficacy, theophylline should only be considered in patients with asthma and COPD after the use of an inhaled corticosteroid and an inhaled LABA (see Box 3.A, p.80 and Box 3.C, p.82).[1–3]

Theophylline shares the actions of the other xanthine alkaloids (e.g. caffeine) on the CNS, myocardium, kidney and smooth muscle. It has a relatively weak CNS effect but a more powerful relaxant effect on bronchial smooth muscle. It probably acts by inhibiting cyclic nucleotide phosphodiesterase. This leads to an accumulation of cyclic AMP which prevents the use of intracellular calcium for muscle contraction. In addition, an immunomodulator effect on cells important in airway inflammation has been shown at plasma concentrations as low as 5mg/L.[4,5] Other effects include an improvement in respiratory muscle strength, the release of catecholamines from the adrenal medulla, inhibition of catechol-O-methyl transferase and blockade of adenosine receptors, all of which may play a part in the beneficial effect of theophylline.

Theophylline is metabolized by the liver. Its therapeutic index is narrow and some patients experience toxic effects even in the therapeutic range. Plasma concentrations of theophylline are influenced by infection, hypoxia, smoking, various drugs, hepatic impairment, thyroid disorders, and heart failure; all these can make the use of theophylline difficult. Steady-state theophylline levels are attained within 3–4 days of adjusting the dose of a SR preparation. Blood for theophylline levels should be taken 6–8h after the last dose or immediately before the next dose.

Because it is not possible to ensure bio-equivalence between different SR theophylline products, they should be prescribed by brand name and should not be interchanged.
Bio-availability ⩾90%; 80% SR.
Onset of action 40–60min PO; immunomodulation ⩽3 weeks.
Plasma halflife 6–12h.
Duration of action 12h SR theophylline PO; immunomodulation several days.

Cautions

Elderly, cardiac disease, hypertension, hyperthyroidism and hypothyroidism, peptic ulcer, hepatic failure, pyrexia. May potentiate hypokalemia associated with β_2-adrenergic receptor agonists (β_2-agonists), corticosteroids, diuretics and hypoxia.[6,7] High-dose **loperamide** (32mg/24h) reduces the absorption of PO theophylline.

Theophylline is metabolized mainly by CYP1A2, and to some extent by CYP3A4 and CYP2E1 and there are numerous interactions (Box 3.E; see also Cytochrome P450, p.551).

Box 3.E Interactions between theophylline and other drugs involving CYP450[7]

Plasma concentrations of theophylline

Increased by	Decreased by
Acyclovir	Smoking
Allopurinol	Heavy drinking
β-Blockers	Carbamazepine
Barbiturates	Isoproterenol HCl
Cimetidine	Phenytoin
Clarithromycin	Rifampin
Diltiazem	Ritonavir
Erythromycin	St John's wort
Fluconazole	Sulfinpyrazone
Fluvoxamine	
Leukotriene inhibitors/antagonists	
Mexiletine	
Oral contraceptives	
Quinolone antibacterials	
Troleandomycin (not Canada)	
Verapamil	

Undesirable effects

For full list, see manufacturer's Product Monograph.
Common (<10%, >1%): headache, dyspepsia, nausea, vomiting; risk of seizures and arrhythmias increases as serum levels increase; hyperpnea (fast breathing) when given IV.

Dose and use

An SR formulation should be used:[3]
- usual starting dose 200mg b.i.d. (or 400mg once daily if a 24h-release tablet is used); increase after 1 week
- in the elderly or patients weighing <70kg, the usual maintenance dose is 300mg b.i.d. (or 600mg once daily if a 24h-release tablet is used)
- in younger heavier patients, the usual maintenance dose is 400mg b.i.d. (or 800mg once daily if a 24h-release tablet is used)
- in patients whose symptoms manifest diurnal fluctuation, a larger evening or morning dose is appropriate to ensure maximum therapeutic benefit when symptoms are most severe
- samples for drug plasma concentration monitoring should be taken 4–6h after a PO dose of theophylline SR
- the recommended therapeutic range is 55–110micromol/L (10–20mg/L).

However, some patients may experience unacceptable undesirable effects even within the recommended therapeutic range and for them a lower range may suffice, e.g. 28–83micromol/L (5–15mg/L). Ultimately, the clinical response, rather than the serum level, will determine the need for dose adjustment.

Normal-release oral liquids are available if patients are unable to swallow SR formulations, e.g. those being fed by enteral feeding tubes (see Administering drugs via enteral feeding tubes, p.531).

Generally, because it has a narrow therapeutic index, and dehydration, hepatic and renal impairment increase the risk of toxicity, theophylline should be withdrawn in the terminal phase.

Supply

Sustained-release
Theophylline (Generic.)
Tablets SR (12h-release) 100mg, 200mg, 300mg, 28 days @ 300mg b.i.d. = $8.

Uniphyl SRT® (Purdue)
Tablets SR (24h-release) 400mg, 600mg, 28 days @ 400mg, 600mg daily = $15 and $19 respectively.

Normal-release
Theophylline elixir (generic)
Oral liquid (elixir) 80mg/15mL, 28 days @ 100mg t.i.d. = $7.

Theolaire® liquid (Graceway)
Oral liquid (elixir) 80mg/15mL, 28 days @ 100mg t.i.d. = $43.

1 Boulet LP et al. (1999) Canadian asthma consensus report, 1999. Canadian Medical Association Journal. **161 (11 suppl)**: S1–62.
2 Lemiere C et al. (2004) Adult Asthma Consensus Guidelines update 2003. Canadian Respiratory Journal. **11 Suppl A**: 9A–18A.
3 O'Donnell DE et al. (2007) Canadian Thoracic Society recommendations for management of chronic obstructive pulmonary disease – 2007 update. Canadian Respiratory Journal. **14 (suppl B)**: 5B–32B.
4 Sullivan P et al. (1994) Anti-inflammatory effects of low-dose oral theophylline in atopic asthma. Lancet. **343**: 1006–1008.
5 Kidney J et al. (1995) Immunomodulation by theophylline in asthma. Demonstration by withdrawal of therapy. American Journal of Respiratory and Critical Care Medicine. **151**: 1907–1914.
6 Sweetman SC (ed) (2005) Martindale: The Complete Drug Reference (34e). Pharmaceutical Press, London, pp. 798–806.
7 Baxter K (ed) (2006) Stockley's Drug Interactions (7e). Pharmaceutical Press, London.

INHALED CORTICOSTEROIDS

Indications: Reversible and irreversible airways obstruction, †stridor, †lymphangitic carcimomatosis, †radiation pneumonitis, †cough after insertion of a bronchial stent (see Nebulized drugs, p.537).

Pharmacology:

Inhaled corticosteroids reduce airway inflammation. **Fluticasone** and the hydrofluoroalkane-134a (HFA) formulation of **beclomethasone** (Qvar®) are given in a smaller dose than **budesonide**. For **fluticasone**, this is because the drug itself is twice as potent as **budesonide**, whereas for Qvar®, it is because the formulation delivers a greater fraction of smaller particles to the lung, approximately doubling its potency compared with the **budesonide** dry powder formulation (see Dose and use, Table 3.4). **Ciclesonide** and **mometasone** (not Canada) are relatively new inhaled corticosteroids.

Inhaled corticosteroids reach the systemic circulation via both the pulmonary circulation and the gastro-intestinal tract. Long-term high-dose inhaled corticosteroids have been associated with adrenal suppression, and deaths from Addisonian crisis (acute adrenal failure) have rarely occurred (see Cautions).[1,2] Total daily doses of **budesonide** ≤1,500microgram or equivalent do not generally lead to adrenal suppression. However, there is significant variation amongst individuals, and formulation and duration of treatment are also important. Canadian guidelines do not consider routine supplementation with systemic corticosteroids to cover stressful periods (e.g. infection, surgery) in patients on long-term high-dose *inhaled* corticosteroids necessary.[2] However, UK guidelines recommend that systemic corticosteroids should be considered in these circumstances in patients receiving **budesonide** >800microgram/24h or equivalent.

Inhaled corticosteroids are the most effective preventer drug in asthma and there is a low threshold for their use (see Box 3.A, p.80).[2–4] Improvement in symptoms generally takes 3–7 days, but maximal improvement in airway inflammation may take weeks. If low doses fail to improve symptoms, the preferred approach is to add an inhaled long-acting β_2-adrenergic receptor agonist (LABA), e.g. **salmeterol** (p.89), before increasing the dose of inhaled corticosteroid (see Box 3.A, Moderate asthma, p.80).[3,4]

Alternatives to inhaled LABAs include increasing the inhaled corticosteroid to a medium or high dose, or adding a leukotriene-receptor antagonist given PO (**montelukast, zafirlukast**). The latter complement the anti-inflammatory effect of inhaled corticosteroids, but are less effective than LABAs. They have also been used in patients unwilling or unable to take inhaled corticosteroids, but provide less effective control.[2–4] If medium or high-dose inhaled corticosteroids are used, they should be continued only if they have clear benefit over the lower doses. Once sustained improvement has been achieved, attempts should generally be made to reduce to the minimum effective dose. Specialist review by a pulmonologist is recommended for patients who need long-term high-dose inhaled corticosteroid; and the risk of osteoporosis considered.[2]

Inhaled corticosteroids have a less well-defined role in COPD. They are recommended, together with an inhaled LABA, for patients with severe disease ($FEV_1 < 50\%$ predicted) who are symptomatic despite an inhaled LABA + **tiotropium**, or have frequent exacerbations ($\geqslant 2$ per annum) (see Box 3.C, p.82).[5] Studies in COPD have generally used high-dose inhaled corticosteroids, e.g. **fluticasone** 1,000microgram/24h; despite this, the overall clinical benefit of inhaled corticosteroids is relatively small.[6–8] For example, although the annual exacerbation rate is reduced by about 20% compared with placebo, in absolute terms this represents a reduction from 1.1 to 0.9 per patient with NNTs of 4 and 32 to prevent one exacerbation and one exacerbation requiring hospitalization per annum respectively.[6] This relatively small benefit must be balanced on an individual patient basis against the undesirable effects of using inhaled corticosteroids.

The only evidence to support the other indications for inhaled or nebulized corticosteroids listed above is clinical experience.

For pharmacokinetic details, see Table 3.3.

Table 3.3 Pharmacokinetics of inhaled corticosteroids in asthma

	Beclomethasone dipropionate[9–11]	Budesonide[a 12]	Fluticasone propionate[a 12]
Bio-availability	62%[b] CFC-containing and CFC-free aerosol inhalers	39% Turbuhaler® 6% Nebuamps®	30% aerosol inhaler 14% powder inhaler
Onset of action	Days to weeks	Days to weeks	Days to weeks
Time to peak plasma concentration	30–60min[b] CFC-containing and CFC-free aerosol inhalers	5–10min Turbuhaler® 10–30min Nebuamps®	1–2h powder inhaler
Plasma halflife	3h[b] CFC-containing and CFC-free aerosol inhalers	2–3h	8h

a. data from Micromedex

b. values for beclomethasone 17-*monopropionate*, the form in which most of the dipropionate reaches the circulation.

Cautions

Active or quiescent tuberculosis, mycetoma, immunosuppression. Patients receiving long-term high-dose inhaled corticosteroids should be warned not to abruptly stop treatment and should be given the advice contained in steroid treatment cards which are issued by some centres (see Box 7.G, p.385), particularly if they are also taking oral corticosteroids or drugs which may inhibit corticosteroid metabolism by cytochrome P450, e.g. protease inhibitors.

Undesirable effects

For full list, see manufacturer's Product Monograph.

Oropharyngeal candidosis, sore throat, hoarse voice, paradoxical bronchospasm, hypersensitivity reactions (e.g. rash), thinning and bruising of the skin. There is good evidence for adrenal suppression whereas that on osteoporosis is mixed, but for both of these effects, the risk is greatest in patients receiving long-term high-dose corticosteroids, which exceed the recommended maximum, e.g. **budesonide** 1,600microgram/24h or equivalent.[2,5]

Prolonged use of inhaled corticosteroids is associated with an increased risk of glaucoma and cataract, particularly in those aged over 40 years.[13–15] Worsening diabetes has been reported in a patient receiving **fluticasone** ≥1,000microgram/24h.[16] In COPD, an increased frequency of pneumonia has been observed.[6,7]

Dose and use

Aerosol or dry powder inhalation

Although breath-actuated dry powder inhalers are available, MDIs are generally used first-line:
- check the patient's inhaler technique
- use a large-volume spacer device if the patient is on an MDI, particularly when they:
  ▷ have a poor inhaler technique
  ▷ are using a high dose (Table 3.4)
  ▷ develop a hoarse voice, sore throat or oral candidosis
- instruct patient to rinse mouth after use to reduce systemic availability and oral candidosis
- in asthma, start with a dose appropriate to severity, e.g. for mild persistent asthma **beclomethasone** 200microgram b.i.d. or equivalent (Table 3.4), and titrate to the lowest dose effective against symptoms (see Box 3.A, p.80); b.i.d. dosing is generally preferred but, if subsequently the asthma is controlled on a low dose, e.g. 100–200microgram/24h, once daily administration could be considered.[17]
- in COPD, consider adding inhaled corticosteroids to a combination of an inhaled LABA + **tiotropium** for patients with severe disease ($FEV_1 < 50\%$ predicted) who remain symptomatic ± experience frequent exacerbations, e.g. **fluticasone** 500microgram b.i.d.[5]

Inhalers which combine a corticosteroid and a LABA are available.

Nebulizer solution

- **budesonide** 1–2mg b.i.d.; occasionally more.

Table 3.4 Approximate equivalent doses (microgram/24h) for inhaled corticosteroids in adults with asthma[2,3]

	Low-dose	Medium-dose	High-dose
Beclomethasone HFA aerosol inhaler + spacer (Qvar®)	≤250	>250–500	>500
Budesonide Turbuhaler Nebulizer solution	≤400 ≤1,000	>400–800 >1,000–2,000	>800 >2,000
Fluticasone HFA aerosol inhaler + spacer *or* dry powder inhaler	≤250	>250–500	>500

Supply

Beclomethasone
Qvar® (Graceway)
Hand-actuated aerosol inhalation (CFC-free) 50microgram, 100microgram/metered inhalation, 28 days @ 100microgram (1 puff) b.i.d. = $18.

Budesonide
Pulmicort® (AstraZeneca)

Dry powder inhalation Turbuhaler®, 100microgram, 200microgram, 400microgram/metered inhalation, 28 days @ 200microgram (1 puff) b.i.d. = $19.
Nebulizer solution (single-dose units) Nebuamps®, 125microgram/mL, 20 × 2mL (250microgram) = $9; 250microgram/mL, 20 × 2mL (500microgram) = $18; 500microgram/mL, 20 × 2mL (1mg) = $36.

Fluticasone

Flovent® (GlaxoSmithKline)
Aerosol inhalation (CFC-free) Flovent HFA®, 50microgram, 125microgram, 250microgram/ metered inhalation, 28 days @ 125microgram (1 puff) b.i.d. = $21.
Dry powder inhalation Flovent Diskus®, blisters for use with Diskus® device, 50microgram, 100microgram, 250microgram, 500microgram/blister, 28 days @ 100microgram (1 blister) b.i.d. = $24.

For combined products containing inhaled corticosteroids and LABAs, see Inhaled long-acting β₂-adrenergic receptor agonists (LABAs), p.91.

1 Tattersfield AE et al. (2004) Safety of inhaled corticosteroids. *Proceedings of the American Thoracic Society.* **1**: 171–175.
2 Boulet LP et al. (1999) Canadian asthma consensus report, 1999. *Canadian Medical Association Journal.* **161 (11 suppl)**: S1–62.
3 Lemiere C et al. (2004) Adult Asthma Consensus Guidelines update 2003. *Canadian Respiratory Journal.* **11 (suppl A)**: 9A–18A.
4 Becker A et al. (2005) Summary of recommendations from the Canadian Asthma Consensus guidelines, 2003 and Canadian Pediatric Asthma Consensus Guidelines, 2003 (updated to December 2004). *Canadian Medical Association Journal.* **173 (6 suppl)**: S1–S56.
5 O'Donnell DE et al. (2007) Canadian Thoracic Society recommendations for management of chronic obstructive pulmonary disease – 2007 update. *Canadian Respiratory Journal.* **14 (suppl B)**: 5B–32B.
6 Calverley PM et al. (2007) Salmeterol and fluticasone propionate and survival in chronic obstructive pulmonary disease. *New England Journal of Medicine.* **356**: 775–789.
7 Kardos P et al. (2007) Impact of salmeterol/fluticasone propionate versus salmeterol on exacerbations in severe chronic obstructive pulmonary disease. *American Journal of Respiratory and Critical Care Medicine.* **175**: 144–149.
8 Niewoehner DE and Wilt TJ (2007) Inhaled corticosteroids for chronic obstructive pulmonary disease: a status report. *American Journal of Respiratory and Critical Care Medicine.* **175**: 103–104.
9 Daley-Yates PT et al. (2001) Beclomethasone dipropionate: absolute bioavailability, pharmacokinetics and metabolism following intravenous, oral, intranasal and inhaled administration in man. *British Journal of Clinical Pharmacology.* **51**: 400–409.
10 Harrison LI et al. (2002) Pharmacokinetics of beclomethasone 17-monopropionate from a beclomethasone dipropionate extrafine aerosol in adults with asthma. *European Journal of Clinical Pharmacology.* **58**: 197–201.
11 Woodcock A et al. (2002) Modulite technology: pharmacodynamic and pharmacokinetic implications. *Respiratory Medicine* **96 (suppl D)**: S9–15.
12 Harrison TW and Tattersfield AE (2003) Plasma concentrations of fluticasone propionate and budesonide following inhalation from dry powder inhalers by healthy and asthmatic subjects. *Thorax.* **58**: 258–260.
13 Cumming R and Mitchell P (1999) Inhaled corticosteroids and cataract. Prevalence, prevention and management. *Drug Safety.* **20**: 77–84.
14 Carnahan M and Goldstein D (2000) Ocular complications of topical, peri-ocular, and systemic corticosteroids. *Current Opinion in Ophthalmology.* **11**: 478–483.
15 Jick S et al. (2001) The risk of cataract among users of inhaled steroids. *Epidemiology.* **12**: 229–234.
16 Faul JL et al. (1998) High dose inhaled corticosteroids and dose dependent loss of diabetic control. *British Medical Journal.* **317**: 1491.
17 Chisholm S et al. (1998) Once-daily budesonide in mild asthma. *Respiratory Medicine.* **92**: 421–425.

OXYGEN

Indications: Breathlessness on exertion (intermittent use); breathlessness at rest (continuous use).

Pharmacology

Oxygen is prescribed for breathless patients to increase alveolar oxygen tension and decrease the work of breathing necessary to maintain a given arterial oxygen tension. The concentration given varies with the underlying condition. The prescription of oxygen in patients with cancer must be carefully considered: used inappropriately, oxygen can have serious or fatal effects (see Cautions and Box 3.F). Home oxygen should be prescribed only after careful evaluation.[1,2]

Breathlessness is a complex sensation which does not simply relate to oxygen tension. Thus, there is great variation in the response to oxygen which cannot be reliably predicted by the level of oxygen saturation at rest, the degree of desaturation on exercise or by the degree of improvement in oxygen saturation.[3–5]

One short-term study in cancer-related breathlessness suggests that oxygen is generally better than air in severely hypoxic patients (oxygen saturation $SaO_2 < 90\%$).[6] Short- and long-term (7 days) studies which have included mainly patients with lesser degrees of hypoxia/normoxia have found no significant difference in the benefit achieved with oxygen or piped air delivered by nasal prongs.[3-5,7]

This suggests that a sensation of airflow is an important determinant of benefit.[8-12] Thus, these patients should be encouraged to test the benefit of a cool draft (open window or fan) before being offered oxygen.

Ideally, patients should undergo a formal evaluation, e.g. shuttle walk test, symptom scores/diaries to examine the benefit of oxygen, e.g. in breathlessness, exercise capacity and quality of life.[2] These need to be tailored to the circumstances of each patient. As a minimum, a trial of oxygen therapy can be given via nasal prongs for 10–15min and levels of breathlessness evaluated.

Initial oxygen saturation is a poor predictor of who will benefit subjectively, and the degree of symptom relief should be used to help guide the dose of oxygen ultimately given. However, a pulse oximeter will help identify those patients who are severely hypoxic for whom it appears reasonable to give sufficient oxygen to achieve an $SaO_2 > 90\%$. If benefit is obtained, review again after a longer period of use, e.g. 3–4 days.[7] If the patient has persisted in using the oxygen and has found it useful, it can be continued but, if the patient has any doubts about its benefit, it should be discontinued.

Helium 79%–oxygen 21% mixture is less dense and viscous than air.[13] Its use helps to reduce the respiratory work required to overcome upper airway obstruction.[14-16] It can be used as a temporary measure in patients breathless at rest while more definitive therapy is arranged. A high concentration/non-rebreathing mask must be used for optimal benefit, and the patient's voice will be squeaky. Mixtures containing higher concentrations of oxygen are also available, e.g. **helium** 72%–oxygen 28%. This improves exercise capacity, oxygen saturation and breathlessness in patients with lung cancer.[17] However, this approach is expensive (each cylinder lasts only 2–3h), and limited by the practical difficulties of transporting a large gas cylinder. Nonetheless, there appears to be increasing interest in the use of **helium**–oxygen mixtures, e.g. to improve exercise capacity in patients with COPD or in acute exacerbations of asthma or COPD.[18]

Cautions

Patients with hypercapnic ventilatory failure who are dependent on hypoxia for their respiratory drive. Patients should be advised of the fire risks of oxygen therapy:
- no smoking in the vicinity of the cylinder
- no open flames, including candles, matches and gas stoves
- keep away from sources of heat, e.g. radiators and direct sunlight.

Undesirable effects (Box 3.F)

Box 3.F Undesirable effects of oxygen therapy[2]

Psychological dependence:
- increased anxiety
- increased likelihood of excessive use
- excessive restriction of normal activities
- withdrawal difficult.

Apparatus restricts activities.

Oxygen mask may cause claustrophobia.

Nasal prongs may cause dryness and soreness of the nasal mucosa.

If necessary, humidification is noisy and not always effective.

Impaired communication.

Social stigmatization.

Cost.

Masks and nasal cannulae

Masks are either constant or variable performance masks. Constant supply masks provide an almost constant supply of 28% oxygen over a wide range of oxygen supply (generally 4L/min) irrespective of the patients breathing pattern. The flow rate should be adjusted for optimal patient comfort and symptom relief. *Constant supply masks should be used when an accurate delivery of oxygen is necessary, i.e. in patients at risk of hypercapnic respiratory failure.* With variable performance masks, the concentration of oxygen supplied to the patient varies with the rate of flow of the oxygen (2L/min is recommended and provides 24% oxygen) and with the patients breathing pattern.

Nasal cannulae are best suited to chronic use but they are the least accurate. The concentration of oxygen delivered is dependent on factors other than flow rate and, at 2L/min, oxygen concentrations can vary 24–35%.[19]

Prescribing oxygen

Oxygen is generally poorly prescribed. Ideally, an inpatient oxygen prescription should include the flow rate, the concentration, the delivery device, the duration, and the method of monitoring treatment of oxygen, on a specific oxygen prescription chart.[20,21] Palliative care services should develop their own standards and guidelines for the use of oxygen, incorporating information for prescribing oxygen at home based on the programme available in their province/territory.

Short-term/intermittent

High concentration oxygen (60%) is given for pneumonia, pulmonary embolism and fibrosing alveolitis. In these situations, a low arterial oxygen (PaO_2) is generally associated with normal or low levels of carbon dioxide ($PaCO_2$). High concentrations of oxygen are also given in acute asthma; $PaCO_2$ levels are generally subnormal, so raised levels in the presence of hypoxia are indicative of near fatal asthma and ventilation needs to be considered urgently (see Box 3.B, p.81).
Low concentration oxygen ($\leqslant$28%) is reserved for patients with ventilatory failure related to COPD and other causes. The aim is to improve breathlessness caused by hypoxemia without worsening pre-existing CO_2 retention. Intermittent (short-burst) oxygen can be considered for episodic breathlessness not relieved by other treatments in patients with advanced cancer, COPD, interstitial lung disease and heart failure.[1,2] For exercise-induced breathlessness, some patients use oxygen before the exercise and others afterwards to aid recovery. However, studies have shown inconsistent benefit from this strategy in patients with COPD.[22–26] Ideally, oxygen should only be prescribed after a formal evaluation has shown benefit in breathlessness and/or exercise tolerance.[1,2]

Long-term/continuous

Long-term oxygen ($\geqslant$15h/day) can be considered for use in patients with severe disabling breathlessness because of cancer and other progressive life-threatening diseases.[1] More specifically in patients with:
- COPD or cystic fibrosis with PaO_2 <55mmHg (7.3kPa)
- COPD or cystic fibrosis with PaO_2 $\leqslant$60mmHg (8kPa) when there is secondary polycythemia or nocturnal hypoxemia (SaO_2 below 90% for at least 30% of the night) or peripheral edema or evidence of pulmonary hypertension
- interstitial lung disease and PaO_2 $\leqslant$60mmHg (8kPa)
- pulmonary hypertension, without parenchymal lung involvement and $\leqslant$60mmHg (8kPa)
- obstructive sleep apnea who remain hypoxic during sleep despite nasal continuous positive airway pressure (CPAP)
- heart failure and PaO_2 <55mmHg (7.3kPa) or nocturnal hypoxemia
- neuromuscular or skeletal disorders causing inspiratory muscle weakness, either alone or together with ventilatory support.[1]

Long-term oxygen therapy prolongs survival only in patients with severe COPD.[27] Correction of hypoxia reduces pulmonary vascular resistance and the load on the right side of the heart. Ideally, the evaluation for long-term oxygen therapy should be done by a specialist, i.e. respiratory physician. For example, in patients with COPD, blood gas tensions should be measured before treatment when the patient's condition is stable (e.g. not less than 4 weeks after an exacerbation) on two occasions at least 3 weeks apart to ensure the criteria are met (see first bullet above). When treatment is commenced, blood gas tensions should be measured to ensure that the set flow is achieving a PaO_2 of >8kPa without an unacceptable rise in $PaCO_2$. It is more economical to use a concentrator if oxygen is given >8h/day (equivalent to 21 cylinders per month). If necessary, two concentrators can be linked by tubing and a Y-connector to deliver higher flow rates (6–8L/min).

Ambulatory oxygen therapy can be prescribed in patients who fulfil the criteria for long-term oxygen therapy who are mobile and wish to leave the home. It can also be considered for patients who are not hypoxic at rest but desaturate on exertion, by at least 4% to a level below 90%, whose walking distance and/or breathlessness improves when using oxygen, to keep SaO_2 > 90%, in a formal evaluation, e.g. shuttle walk test.[1,2,28] In patients with cancer and SaO_2 > 90% at rest, ambulatory oxygen was no better than air; although desaturation with exercise was not evaluated.[4]

Travel by air

Patients with lung conditions who wish to travel by air should be given specific advice (Box 3.G).

Box 3.G Air travel and oxygen[29]

Air travel exacerbates hypoxemia in patients with lung disease and may cause compensatory hyperventilation and tachycardia.

Aircraft cabins are pressurized, generally to reflect an altitude of about 8,000ft. This is equivalent to breathing a PO_2 of 15% instead of 21% at sea level. Even in the healthy, blood oxygen levels (PaO_2) will fall to about 55–65mmHg (7–8.5kPa).

Low risk

Patients who can walk 50m on the level at a steady pace without oxygen, breathlessness or needing to stop are unlikely to experience problems with reduced cabin pressure.

High risk

- severe COPD or asthma
- cystic fibrosis
- severe restrictive disease (including chest wall and respiratory muscle disease), particularly with blood gas abnormalities
- previous air travel intolerance with respiratory symptoms (breathlessness, chest pain, confusion or syncope)
- co-morbidity worsened by hypoxemia (cerebrovascular disease, coronary artery disease, heart failure)
- <6 weeks since hospital discharge for acute respiratory illness.

Evaluation

If in doubt, or a hypoxic challenge required, refer to a respiratory specialist.
Generally, the following is recommended:

- clinical, history and examination (previous flying experience, breathlessness, cardio-respiratory disease)
- spirometry, FEV_1% predicted
- pulse oximetry (place the probe on a warm ear or finger long enough to obtain a stable reading)
- blood gases are preferable if hypercapnia is known or suspected:

SaO_2 when breathing air	Recommendation
> 95%	Oxygen *not* required
92–95% with no risk factor[a]	Oxygen *not* required
92–95% with risk factor[a]	Hypoxic challenge test with arterial or capillary measurements[b]
< 92%	In-flight oxygen required (2–4L/min)
On long-term oxygen therapy	Increase flow rate, e.g. by 2–4L/min

a. see list above; also if hypercapnia, FEV_1 <50% predicted, lung cancer, ventilator support, <6 weeks since hospital discharge for an exacerbation of chronic lung or cardiac disease
b. patient breathes 15% oxygen at sea level to mimic air cabin conditions; interpretation: PaO_2 >55mmHg (>7.4kPa), oxygen not required; PaO_2 <50mmHg (<6.6kPa), in-flight oxygen 2L/min required; PaO_2 50–55mmHg (6.6–7.4kPa) borderline result, consider a walk test.

In-flight oxygen provision

- generally airlines charge for providing in-flight oxygen (fees and services vary considerably)
- passengers may carry their own small, full oxygen cylinders with them as hand luggage for medical use, provided they have airline approval; a charge may be made for this service, in addition to a charge for in-flight oxygen
- the airline must be informed at the time of the booking, and at least 1 month before the flight
- the airline will issue a form to be completed by the patient and GP/hospital specialist; the airline's Medical Officer then evaluates the patient's needs
- in-flight oxygen is usually prescribed at a rate of 2–4L/min and given by nasal cannulae to be used when the plane is at cruising altitude; can be switched off at the start of descent.

For guidance on specific diseases, patients oxygen-dependent at sea level, and those requiring ventilation, see the full guidance.[29]

General advice

- *medical insurance*, ensure fully covered for medical costs that may arise related to the lung disease, including the cost of an air ambulance
- *documentation,* have a medical letter on their person detailing condition and medication
- *medication*, take a full supply of all medication as hand luggage, e.g. well-filled reliever and preventer inhalers
- *equipment*, e.g. portable battery-operated nebulizers may be used at the discretion of the cabin crew, but the airline must be notified in advance (an inhaler + spacer is an alternative)
- *ground transportation,* airports can usually provide transport assistance
- *DVT prophylaxis,* see Box 2.D, p.63.

Supply
Home oxygen

Contact the home oxygen programme in the relevant province or territory for further details.

1 Royal College of Physicians of London (1999) *Domiciliary oxygen therapy services: clinical guidelines and advice for prescribers.* Royal College of Physicians, London.

2 Booth S et al. (2004) The use of oxygen in the palliation of breathlessness. A report of the expert working group of the scientific committee of the association of palliative medicine. *Respiratory Medicine.* **98**: 66–77.

3 Booth S et al. (1996) Does oxygen help dyspnea in patients with cancer? *American Journal of Respiratory and Critical Care Medicine.* **153**: 1515–1518.

4 Bruera E et al. (2003) A randomized controlled trial of supplemental oxygen versus air in cancer patients with dyspnea. *Palliative Medicine.* **17**: 659–663.

5 Philip J et al. (2006) A randomized, double-blind, crossover trial of the effect of oxygen on dyspnea in patients with advanced cancer. *Journal of Pain and Symptom Management.* **32**: 541–550.

6 Bruera E et al. (1993) Effects of oxygen on dyspnoea in hypoxaemic terminal cancer patients. *Lancet.* **342**: 13–14.

7 Abernathy A et al. (2009) Palliation of refractory dyspnea: A randomised, controlled, double-blind study of oxygen vs. medical air (NCT00327873). *Journal of the American Medical Association.* In Press.

8 Schwartzstein R et al. (1987) Cold facial stimulation reduces breathlessness induced in normal subjects. *American Review of Respiratory Disease.* **136**: 58–61.

9 Burgess K and Whitelaw W (1988) Effects of nasal cold receptors on pattern of breathing. *Journal of Applied Physiology.* **64**: 371–376.

10 Freedman S (1988) Cold facial stimulation reduces breathlessness induced in normal subjects. *American Review of Respiratory Diseases.* **137**: 492–493.

11 Kerr D (1989) A bedside fan for terminal dyspnea. *American Journal of Hospice Care.* **89**: 22.

12 Liss H and Grant B (1988) The effect of nasal flow on breathlessness in patients with chronic obstructive pulmonary disease. *American Review of Respiratory Disease.* **137**: 1285–1288.

13 Boorstein J et al. (1989) Using helium–oxygen mixtures in the emergency management of acute upper airway obstruction. *Annals of Emergency Medicine.* **18**: 688–690.

14 Lu T-S et al. (1976) Helium–oxygen in treatment of upper airway obstruction. *Anesthesiology.* **45**: 678–680.

15 Rudow M et al. (1986) Helium–oxygen mixtures in airway obstruction due to thyroid carcinoma. *Canadian Anaesthesiology Society Journal.* **33**: 498–501.

16 Khanlou H and Eiger G (2001) Safety and efficacy of heliox as a treatment for upper airway obstruction due to radiation-induced laryngeal dysfunction. *Heart and Lung.* **30**: 146–147.

17 Ahmedzai SH et al. (2004) A double-blind, randomised, controlled Phase II trial of Heliox28 gas mixture in lung cancer patients with dyspnoea on exertion. *British Journal of Cancer.* **90**: 366–371.

18 Laude EA and Ahmedzai SH (2007) Oxygen and helium gas mixtures for dyspnoea. *Current Opinion in Supportive & Palliative Care.* **1**: 91–95.

19 Bazuaye E et al. (1992) Variability of inspired oxygen concentration with nasal cannulas. *Thorax.* **47**: 609–611.

20 Bateman NT and Leach RM (1998) ABC of oxygen. Acute oxygen therapy. *British Medical Journal.* **317**: 798–801.

21 Dodd ME et al. (2000) Audit of oxygen prescribing before and after the introduction of a prescription chart. *BMJ.* **321**: 864–865.

22 Killen J and Corris P (2000) A pragmatic assessment of the placement of oxygen when given for exercise induced dyspnoea. *Thorax.* **55**: 544–546.

23 McKeon JL et al. (1988) Effects of breathing supplemental oxygen before progressive exercise in patients with chronic obstructive lung disease. *Thorax.* **43**: 53–56.

24 Nandi K et al. (2003) Oxygen supplementation before or after submaximal exercise in patients with chronic obstructive pulmonary disease. *Thorax.* **58**: 670–673.

25 Stevenson NJ and Calverley PM (2004) Effect of oxygen on recovery from maximal exercise in patients with chronic obstructive pulmonary disease. *Thorax.* **59**: 668–672.

26 Roberts CM (2004) Short burst oxygen therapy for relief of breathlessness in COPD. *Thorax.* **59**: 638–640.

27 Crockett A et al. (2001) A review of long-term oxygen therapy for chronic obstructive pulmonary disease. *Respiratory Medicine.* **95**: 437–443.

28 Bradley J et al. (2005) Short-term ambulatory oxygen for chronic obstructive pulmonary disease. *Cochrane Database of Systematic Reviews.* **4**: CD004356.

29 BTS Standards of Care Committee (2004) Managing passengers with respiratory disease planning air travel. British Thoracic Society. Available from: http://www.brit-thoracic.org.uk/Portals/0/Clinical%20Information/Air%20Travel/Guidelines/FlightRevision04.pdf

DRUGS FOR COUGH

General strategy

Coughing helps clear the central airways of foreign matter, secretions or pus and should generally be encouraged.[1] It is pathological when:

- ineffective
- it adversely affects sleep, rest, eating, or social activities
- it causes other symptoms such as muscle strain, rib fracture, vomiting, syncope, headache, or urinary incontinence.

The primary aim is to identify and treat the cause of the distressing cough but, when this is not possible or is inappropriate, an antitussive is generally indicated (Box 3.H and Figure 3.1).[2] However, protussives (expectorants) can be used to make sputum less tenacious, and thus easier to expectorate (Box 3.H and Figure 3.1). Generally, nebulized 0.9% saline is the protussive of choice but sometimes an irritant mucolytic (e.g. **guaifenesin**) or a chemical mucolytic (e.g. **acetylcysteine**) may be preferable.

Box 3.H Drugs for cough

Protussives (expectorants)
Topical mucolytics
Nebulized 0.9% saline
Chemical inhalations
   e.g. menthol and eucalyptus

Irritant mucolytics
Ammonium chloride
Guaifenesin

Chemical mucolytics
Acetylcysteine

Antitussives
Peripheral
Simple syrup USP
Benzonatate (not Canada)
Leukotriene antagonist
   zafirlukast
   montelukast
Local anesthetics (nebulized)
NSAIDs
   indomethacin
   sulindac
Thromboxane synthase/thromboxane
   receptor antagonists (not Canada)

Central
GABA agonists
   baclofen
Opioids
   codeine
   hydrocodone
   hydromorphone
   morphine
   methadone
Opioid derivatives
   dextromethorphan

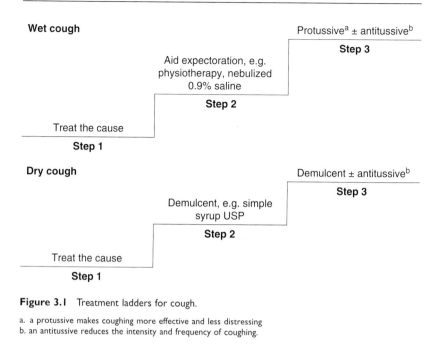

Figure 3.1 Treatment ladders for cough.

a. a protussive makes coughing more effective and less distressing
b. an antitussive reduces the intensity and frequency of coughing.

1 Twycross R *et al.* (2009) *Symptom Management in Advanced Cancer* (4e). palliativedrugs.com, Nottingham, pp. 160–166.
2 Homsi J *et al.* (2001) Important drugs for cough in advanced cancer. *Supportive Care in Cancer.* **9**: 565–574.

GUAIFENESIN

Class: Protussive (irritant mucolytic expectorant).

Indications: Symptomatic management of cough associated with upper respiratory tract infection and bronchitis; †non-infective cough associated with thick tenacious sputum.

Contra-indications: Guaifenesin combined with **dextromethorphan** should not be taken concurrently with an MAOI (but see p.140).

Pharmacology
Mechanism of action unknown.[1] As with other mucolytic expectorants, guaifenesin is said to stimulate the production of more profuse and therefore less viscid bronchial secretions.[2] Expectorants are also gastric irritants and may cause nausea and vomiting at higher doses. Guaifenesin is well absorbed from the GI tract. Its metabolites are excreted in the urine.
Bio-availability probably high.
Onset of action 30–60min.
Plasma halflife 1h.
Duration of action 2–3h.

Cautions
Continuing use of >600mg/day may result in urolithiasis.

Undesirable effects

For full list, see manufacturer's Product Monograph.
Drowsiness, headache, dyspepsia, nausea, vomiting, urolithiasis, rash.

Dose and use

- 200mg q2h p.r.n. and/or 200–400mg q4h
- maximum recommended total daily dose 2.4g.

Supply

Guaifenesin (generic)
Oral solution 100mg/5mL, 28 days @ 10mL q6h = $64.

Robitussin® Liquid (Wyeth)
Oral solution 100mg/5mL, 100mL, 250mL, 28 days @ 10mL q6h = $74.

Robitussin Extra Strength® Liquid (Wyeth)
Oral solution 200mg/5mL, 100mL, 250mL, 28 days @ 5mL q6h = $37.

---

1 Thomas J (1990) Guaiphenesin – an old drug now found to be effective. *Australian Journal of Pharmacy.* **71**: 101–103.
2 Irwin RS *et al.* (1998) Managing cough as a defense mechanism and as a symptom. A consensus panel report of the American College of Chest Physicians. *Chest.* **114 (suppl)**: 133s–181s.

ACETYLCYSTEINE

Class: Chemical mucolytic.

Indications: Reduction of sputum viscosity.

Contra-indications: Active peptic ulceration.

Pharmacology

Acetylcysteine reduces the viscosity of bronchial secretions and facilitates expectoration. It alters the physical and chemical characteristics of the mucin components of sputum to a more 'normal' pattern (by reducing fructose and sulfate content and increasing the proportion of sialomucins). In patients with COPD, mucolytics reduce the number of exacerbations and days of illness but the benefit appears small and their routine use remains debatable.[1–3] However, some individual patients benefit from their use and a therapeutic trial may be justified if all other approaches have failed, particularly in patients with more severe COPD and frequent or prolonged exacerbations.

Undesirable effects

For full list, see manufacturer's Product Monograph.
Occasional dyspepsia, diarrhea, rash.

Dose and use

- start with 200mg q6h–q2h via nebulizer
- maximum dose 2g q2h via nebulizer.

Supply

Acetylcysteine (generic)
Nebulizer solution 200mg/mL, 10mL, 30mL vial = $10 and $21 respectively.

Mucomyst® (Wellspring)
Nebulizer solution 200mg/mL, 10mL, 30mL vial = $9 and $20 respectively.

---

1 Stey C *et al.* (2000) The effect of oral N-acetylcysteine in chronic bronchitis: quantitative systematic review. *European Respiratory Journal.* **16**: 253–262.
2 Poole P and Black P (2001) Oral mucolytic drugs for exacerbations of chronic obstructive pulmonary disease: systematic review. *British Medical Journal.* **322**: 1271–1274.
3 NHLBI/WHO (2008) Global Initiative for Chronic Obstructive Lung Disease. Strategy for the diagnosis management and prevention of chronic obstructive pulmonary disease. Available from: www.goldcopd.com

ANTITUSSIVES

Antitussives can be divided into peripherally-acting and centrally-acting agents. The former include local pharyngeal soothing agents (demulcents) and local anesthetics and their derivatives.[1] The centrally-acting antitussives are almost exclusively opioids or opioid derivatives. Because in palliative care the opioid antitussives are generally used in preference to local anesthetics and their derivatives, they are given precedence in this section.

Demulcents

These contain soothing substances such as syrup or glycerin. The high sugar content stimulates the production of saliva and soothes the oropharynx. The associated swallowing may also interfere with the cough reflex. The sweet taste itself may be antitussive by stimulating the release of endogenous opioids in the brain stem, and this may contribute to the large placebo effect seen in controlled trials of demulcents.[2] However, the antitussive effect of demulcents is generally short-lived and there is no evidence that combination products are better than **simple syrup USP** (5mL t.i.d.–q.i.d.). Thus, if **simple syrup USP** is ineffective, there is little point in trying combination products.

Opioids

Opioids act primarily by suppressing the cough reflex centre in the brain stem. Opioids appear less effective for cough caused by upper airway disorders, e.g. upper respiratory tract infection, possibly because laryngeal cough involves opioid insensitive central mechanisms and/or reflects a different reflex (i.e. an expiration reflex).[3] **Codeine** and **dextromethorphan** are common ingredients in combination products for cough but often in small and probably ineffective doses. Although **dextromethorphan** is a synthetic opioid derivative, its antitussive action is not mediated via opioid receptors. The effective dose of **codeine** or **dextromethorphan** is often greater than the dose recommended by manufacturers of combination products.[4] Thus, the benefit of combination products may reside mainly in the sugar content (see demulcents).[2]

Many centres use **hydrocodone** in preference to **codeine**, on the grounds that it causes fewer undesirable GI and CNS effects.[5] If **hydrocodone** is ineffective, **morphine** should be prescribed.[6]

For patients already receiving strong opioids, if a p.r.n. dose relieves the cough, continue to use it in this way or increase the regular dose of the opioid. However, if no benefit is obtained from a p.r.n. dose, there is little point in further regular dose increments. Some patients with cough but no pain benefit from a bedtime dose of **morphine** to prevent cough disturbing sleep. *If a patient is already receiving a strong opioid for pain relief it is nonsense to prescribe* **codeine** *or* **hydrocodone** *as well.*

Local anesthetics

Nebulized local anesthetics have been used as antitussives in patients with cough caused by cancer. They probably act locally by inhibiting the sensory nerves in the airways involved in the cough reflex but there could be a central effect as well. However, their use has not been formally evaluated; thus they should be considered only when other avenues have failed, including nebulized 0.9% saline.

Suggested doses are 5mL of either 2% **lidocaine** or 0.25% **bupivacaine** t.i.d.–q.i.d. Use is limited by:
• unpleasant taste
• oropharyngeal numbness
• risk of bronchoconstriction
• a short duration of action (10–30min).[4]

Even so, there are anecdotal reports of patients with chronic lung disease, sarcoidosis or cancer, in whom a single treatment with nebulized **lidocaine** 400mg relieved cough for 1–8 weeks.[7–9]

Management strategy
Correct the correctable

If possible, the cause of the cough should be treated specifically, e.g. antibacterials for infection. However, when the cause of the cough is not amenable to specific treatment or is unknown, measures should be taken to suppress the cough (see Figure 3.1, p.103).

Drug treatment

If a locally soothing demulcent (e.g. **simple syrup USP** 5mL t.i.d.–q.i.d.) is inadequate, consider a centrally-acting opioid antitussive, for example:

- **codeine** oral solution 12.5–25mg (2.5–5mL) t.i.d.–q.i.d.
- **hydrocodone:**
  ▷ start with 5mg **hydrocodone** (1 tablet or 5mL oral solution) b.i.d.
  ▷ if necessary, increase to 10–15mg **hydrocodone** (2–3 tablets or 10–15mL syrup) q4h[5]
  ▷ the manufacturer's recommended maximum dose is 6 tablets or 30mL syrup (= 30mg **hydrocodone**) per 24h.

If **codeine** or **hydrocodone** are not effective, switch to **morphine**:

- start with 5–10mg q.i.d.–q4h (but 2.5–5mg q.i.d.–q4h if not switching from **codeine** or **hydrocodone**)
- if necessary, increase the dose until the cough is relieved or until undesirable effects prevent further escalation (see p.302).

> If a patient is already receiving a strong opioid for pain relief it is nonsense to prescribe **codeine** or a second strong opioid for cough suppression.

If opioid antitussives are unsatisfactory, other possible treatments include:

- **sodium cromoglycate** 10mg inhaled q.i.d. improved cough in a single case report of a patient with lung cancer within 36–48h;[10]
- **baclofen** 10mg PO t.i.d. or 20mg PO once daily has an antitussive effect in healthy volunteers and in patients with ACE inhibitor cough; 2–4 weeks of therapy is required to attain maximum effect[1,11]
- **gabapentin** 100mg PO b.i.d. up to 800mg PO b.i.d. is reported to have an antitussive effect in idiopathic chronic cough.[12]

Supply

Simple syrup USP
Oral solution 28 days @ 5mL q.i.d. = $7.

Codeine phosphate (generic)
Oral solution 5mg/mL 28 days @ 15mg q.i.d. = $10.

Hydrocodone bitartrate
Hycodan® (BMS)
Tablets 5mg, 28 days @ 1 q.i.d. = $102.
Oral solution 5mg/5mL, 28 days @ 5mL q.i.d. = $66.

Morphine sulfate (generic)
Oral solution 5mg/5mL 28 days @ 5mg q.i.d. = $12.
Also see **morphine**, p.307 for other products.

1 Dicpinigaitis PV (2006) Current and future peripherally-acting antitussives. *Respiratory Physiology and Neurobiology.* **152**: 356–362.
2 Eccles R (2006) Mechanisms of the placebo effect of sweet cough syrups. *Respiratory Physiology and Neurobiology.* **152**: 340–348.
3 Bolser DC (2006) Current and future centrally acting antitussives. *Respiratory Physiology Neurobiology.* **152**: 349–355.
4 Fuller R and Jackson D (1990) Physiology and treatment of cough. *Thorax.* **45**: 425–430.
5 Homsi J et al. (2002) A phase II study of hydrocodone for cough in advanced cancer. *American Journal of Hospice and Palliative Care.* **19** (1): 49–56.
6 Homsi J et al. (2001) Important drugs for cough in advanced cancer. *Supportive Care in Cancer.* **9**: 565–574.
7 Howard P et al. (1977) Lignocaine aerosol and persistent cough. *British Journal of Diseases of the Chest.* **71**: 19–24.
8 Stewart C and Coady T (1977) Suppression of intractable cough. *British Medical Journal.* **1**: 1660–1661.
9 Saunders R and Kirkpatrick M (1984) Prolonged suppression of cough after inhalation of lidocaine in a patient with sarcoid. *Journal of the American Medical Association.* **252**: 2452–2457.
10 Moroni M et al. (1996) Inhaled sodium cromoglycate to treat cough in advanced lung cancer patients. *British Journal of Cancer.* **74**: 309–311.
11 Dicpinigaitis P et al. (1998) Inhibition of capsaicin-induced cough by the gamma-aminobutyric acid agonist baclofen. *Journal of Clinical Pharmacology.* **38**: 364–367.
12 Mintz S and Lee JK (2006) Gabapentin in the treatment of intractable idiopathic chronic cough: case reports. *American Journal of Medicine.* **119**: e13–15.

4: CENTRAL NERVOUS SYSTEM

PSYCHOTROPICS

Psychotropic drugs are primarily used to alter a patient's psychological state.[1] They are classified by the WHO as:
• anxiolytic sedatives
• antipsychotics (neuroleptics)
• antidepressants
• psychostimulants
• psychodysleptics.

Generally, smaller doses should be used in debilitated patients with advanced cancer than in physically fit patients, particularly if they are already receiving a strong opioid or another psychotropic.[2] Close supervision is essential, particularly during the first few days. Either a reduction in dose because of drug accumulation or a further increase because of a lack of response may be needed. A few patients respond paradoxically when prescribed psychotropics, e.g. **diazepam** (become more distressed) or **amitriptyline** (become wakeful and restless at night). Other patients derive little benefit from a benzodiazepine, e.g. **diazepam**, but are helped by an antipsychotic, e.g. **haloperidol**. Tricyclic antidepressants (TCAs) are widely used to relieve neuropathic pain; dose escalation is often limited by undesirable effects.

The drugs which are featured in this chapter are purposely restricted (Box 4.A). It is better to learn to use a small number of drugs well than to have limited experience with all possible alternatives.

Box 4.A   Psychotropics: preferred drugs

Benzodiazepines
Diazepam (universally available but cannot be given SC, cheap)
Midazolam (used SC, mainly in imminently dying patients)
Clonazepam (anti-epileptic, adjuvant analgesic)
Lorazepam (status epilepticus, quick-acting SL)
Oxazepam or temazepam (night sedative)

Typical antipsychotics
Haloperidol
Prochlorperazine
Methotrimeprazine (if drowsiness desirable; also used for intractable vomiting)

Atypical antipsychotics
Olanzapine (also used for intractable vomiting)
Risperidone

Antidepressants
Methylphenidate (if prognosis <2–3 months)
Sertraline or citalopram
Mirtazapine
Amitriptyline, nortriptyline, or desipramine

---

1 Stahl S (2000) *Essential Psychopharmacology: Neuroscientific Basis and Practical Applications (2e).* Cambridge University Press, Cambridge.
2 Wagner B and O'Hara D (1997) Pharmacokinetics and pharmacodynamics of sedatives and analgesics in the treatment of agitated critically ill patients. *Clinical Pharmacokinetics.* **33**: 426–453.

BENZODIAZEPINES

Class: Anxiolytic sedatives.

Contra-indications: Unless for end-of-life care: acute or severe pulmonary insufficiency, sleep apnea syndrome, severe liver disease, myasthenia gravis. Also see individual monographs.

Pharmacology
Benzodiazepines are a group of drugs which:
• reduce anxiety and aggression
• sedate and improve sleep
• relax muscles
• suppress seizures
• reduce nausea and vomiting in specific contexts.
Benzodiazepines bind to a specific site on the $GABA_A$-receptor and, as agonists, enhance the inhibitory effect of GABA. Subtypes of the $GABA_A$-receptor exist in different regions of the brain, and differ in their sensitivity to benzodiazepines. **Flumazenil** is a specific benzodiazepine antagonist, and can be used to reverse the sedative effects of benzodiazepines. Endogenous ligands for the benzodiazepine binding site include peptide and steroid molecules, but their physiological function is not yet understood.
Although the relationship is non-linear, the plasma halflife of a benzodiazepine and its pharmacologically active metabolites reflect its duration of action (Figure 4.1); those with long halflives can be taken once daily, preferably at bedtime. Intermediate-acting agents (e.g. **oxazepam** and **temazepam**) are used mainly for night sedation; they are metabolized in one step to inactive compounds. Some long-acting agents (e.g. **diazepam** and **chlordiazepoxide**) are

---

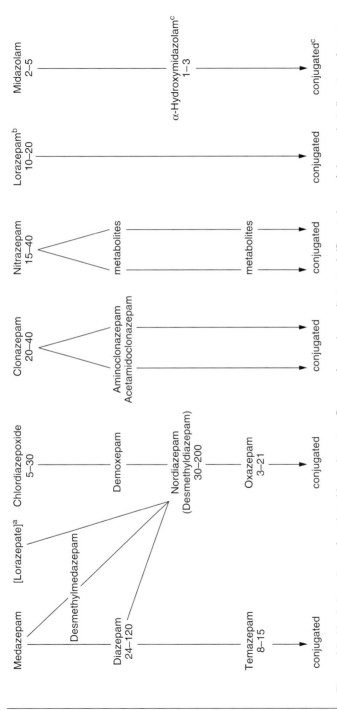

Figure 4.1 Metabolic pathways for selected benzodiazepines. Figures refer to plasma elimination halflives in hours of pharmacologically active substances.

a. lorazepate is a pro-drug
b. lorazepam does not use the P450 hepatic metabolic pathway and avoids interactions relating to competitive inhibition of metabolism
c. α-hydroxymidazolam glucuronide is an active substance, about 10 times less potent than both the unconjugated form and midazolam; accumulation in severe renal failure may lead to prolonged sedation.

converted to a long-lasting active metabolite (nordiazepam). Differences in the pharmacological profile of different benzodiazepines are relatively minor (Table 4.1) but potency varies considerably (Table 4.2). Compared with its other properties, **clonazepam** has relatively more antiseizure activity.

Table 4.1 Pharmacological properties of selected benzodiazepines[1]

Drug name	Anxiolytic	Night sedative	Muscle relaxant	Anti-epileptic
Diazepam	+++	++	+++	+++
Lorazepam	+++	++	+	+[a]
Clonazepam	+	+++	+	+++
Nitrazepam	++	+++	+	++
Oxazepam	+++	+	0	0
Temazepam	+	0[a]	0	0

Pharmacological activity: 0 = minimal effect; + = slight; ++ = moderate; +++ = marked.

a. the failure to show a major anti-epileptic effect with lorazepam or a significant night sedative effect with temazepam emphasizes a limitation of a single dose study in volunteers.

Table 4.2 Approximate equivalent anxiolytic-sedative doses[2]

Drug	Dose
Clonazepam	250microgram
Lorazepam	500microgram
Midazolam	1.5–2mg
Diazepam	5mg
Nitrazepam	5mg
Temazepam	10mg
Chlordiazepoxide	15mg
Oxazepam	15mg

Cautions

Benzodiazepines with long halflives accumulate when given repeatedly and undesirable effects may manifest only after several days or weeks. Caution is required in mild–moderate hepatic impairment and renal impairment. Because their central depressant effect can depress respiration, caution is required in chronic respiratory disease. However, they are relatively safe in overdose.

Because benzodiazepines can cause physical and psychological dependence, patients with a history of substance abuse should be monitored closely. Further, if treatment is discontinued, taper gradually to avoid withdrawal symptoms, e.g. by 1/8 of the daily dose every 2 weeks.

Undesirable effects

For full list, see manufacturer's Product Monograph.

The main undesirable effects of benzodiazepines are dose-dependent drowsiness, impaired psychomotor skills (e.g. impaired driving ability) and hypotonia (manifesting as unsteadiness/ataxia), with an increased risk (almost double) of femoral fracture in the elderly.[3] Their effects are exacerbated by alcohol.

Choice of benzodiazepine

Choice of benzodiazepine will depend on several factors, including:
- indication for use
- availability, either of the drug itself or of a suitable formulation for the intended route of administration, e.g. SL, SC
- efficacy
- cost
- fashion (Box 4.B).

Box 4.B   Benzodiazepines commonly used in palliative care

Diazepam (universally available but cannot be given SC, cheap)
Midazolam (used SC, mainly in imminently dying patients)
Clonazepam (anti-epileptic, adjuvant analgesic)
Lorazepam (status epilepticus, quick-acting SL)
Oxazepam or temazepam (night sedative)

Alprazolam is widely used in some countries for the short-term management of anxiety, particularly panic attacks.[4,5] Tolerance commonly occurs, necessitating dose escalation. Its relatively short duration of action means that tolerant patients may experience break-through (episodic) panic attacks during the night. These resolve if the patient is switched to a long-acting benzodiazepine such as **diazepam** or **clonazepam**, and possibly an SSRI such as **sertraline** (with a view to phasing out the benzodiazepine after 1–2 months).

However, there are no hard data that **alprazolam** has a greater abuse liability than other benzodiazepines.[6] Even so, despite claims of benefit in depression, **alprazolam** has no place in palliative care as an antidepressant.[7]

Dose and use

Benzodiazepines are essential drugs in palliative care (Box 4.C).

Apart from sedation at the very end of life, the most common uses of benzodiazepines are anxiety and/or insomnia. Thus, a benzodiazepine is indicated for short-term relief (2–4 weeks) of severe anxiety which is disabling to the individual, occurring alone or associated with insomnia. However, for prolonged treatment, an SSRI may be preferable (see p.155). There may also be a place for **gabapentin** and **pregabalin** in the management of anxiety (see p.220 and p.224). *The use of a benzodiazepine to treat mild anxiety is generally inappropriate; listening, explaining, and more specific psychological measures are preferable.*

Likewise, a benzodiazepine should be used to treat short-term insomnia only when it is severe and disabling, and after other (correctable) causes have been treated appropriately, e.g. analgesics for pain or an antidepressant for a depressive illness, and non-drug measures.[16–19] A recent meta-analysis confirmed that, in people >60 years of age, the NNT was 13 but the NNH was 6.[20] The undesirable effects were cognitive impairment, day-time drowsiness, ataxia and falls. Even low doses of short halflife benzodiazepines increase the risk of falls.[21]

However, patients dying of cancer may on average have higher levels of anxiety and fear compared with the general population, and thus a higher use of night sedatives (as adjuvant short-term treatment) is likely. The non-benzodiazepine sedative 'Z' drugs, e.g. **zopiclone**, have been recommended as night sedatives.[22,23] However, there is no strong evidence that this group of drugs have any advantages compared with the much cheaper benzodiazepines.[24] Nonetheless, at some centres, **zopiclone** is used as an alternative night sedative if a benzodiazepine is ineffective.

The role of benzodiazepines in the management of intractable pruritus is debatable.[25] There are contradictory reports in relation to **diazepam**[26,27] and **nitrazepam**.[27,28] In one patient with cancer of the pancreas and cholestatic pruritus, a CSCI of **midazolam** was effective 'within a few hours' (2mg bolus followed by 1mg/h, increasing by 1mg/h every 15min 'as needed for itching'), whereas **lorazepam** 1mg q6h or 2mg at bedtime (and several other psychotropic drugs) was ineffective.[29] The affinity of **midazolam** for the GABA-receptor is 5–6 times greater than that of **lorazepam**,[30] and it is possible that this is the explanation for the difference in the response to the two benzodiazepines.[31] (For alternative approaches to the management of cholestatic pruritus, see Box 5.O, p.339.)

Benzodiazepines are often of benefit in anticipatory nausea before chemotherapy, and in some cases of refractory nausea and vomiting, both after chemotherapy[32,33] and postoperatively.[11] (Alternative approaches to anticipatory nausea include relaxation, hypnosis and other psychological approaches.)[12,13]

Box 4.C   Benzodiazepines in palliative care

Short-term night sedation
Short-acting drugs
- midazolam (halflife 2–5h; not available in oral formulations in Canada)
- zopiclone (halflife 2–5h) is marketed as a night sedative but is relatively expensive; it is not a benzodiazepine but acts on the same receptors.

Intermediate-acting drugs
- temazepam 7.5–30mg PO at bedtime, occasionally more (halflife 8–15h)
- †oxazepam 15–30mg PO at bedtime, occasionally more (halflife 3–21h).

Some patients with insomnia respond better to an antipsychotic drug or a TCA.

Anxiety and panic disorder
Intermediate-acting drugs
- lorazepam 1–2mg PO or SL b.i.d.–t.i.d. (halflife 10–20h)
- oxazepam 10–15mg PO b.i.d.–t.i.d. (halflife 3–21h).

SL lorazepam tablets are used at some centres for episodes of acute severe distress, e.g. respiratory panic attacks. For regular use, give at bedtime or b.i.d.

Long-acting drugs
- diazepam 2–20mg PO at bedtime (halflife 24–120h)
- †clonazepam 500microgram–1mg at bedtime (halflife 20–40h).

Although manufacturers often recommend administration in divided doses for diazepam and clonazepam, their long plasma halflives mean that administration once daily at bedtime will generally be equally effective, and easier for the patient.

Acute psychotic agitation
- lorazepam 2mg PO/IM every 30min until settled. Surprisingly, this is as effective as haloperidol 5mg every 30min.[8]

Muscle relaxant
- diazepam 2–10mg PO at bedtime, occasionally more
- baclofen is a useful non-benzodiazepine alternative, particularly if diazepam is too sedative and anxiety is not an associated problem, or if long-term use is anticipated.

Anti-epileptic
Acute treatment[9]
- clonazepam 1mg IV over 30sec (injection not Canada)
- diazepam 10mg IV over 2–4min; can be given rectally in status epilepticus (see p.114 and p.205)
- lorazepam 4mg IV over 2min
- †midazolam 10mg IV over 2min; the injection can be given buccally in status epilepticus (see p.205).

If necessary, give two more doses at 10min intervals.[10]

Chronic treatment
- clonazepam 500microgram–1mg PO at bedtime
- increase by 500microgram every 3–5 days up to 2–4mg, occasionally more
- doses above 2mg can be divided, e.g. 2mg at bedtime and 1mg each morning.

Myoclonus
Same choice as for seizure control, but lower doses, e.g.:
- diazepam 5mg PO at bedtime
- †midazolam 5mg SC stat and 10mg/24h CSCI in moribund patients.

Neuropathic pain
Clonazepam is sometimes used as a second or third choice (see p.237 and p.118).

Nausea and vomiting
Anticipatory nausea and, if refractory, post-chemotherapy or postoperatively:[11–13]
- lorazepam 0.5mg SL p.r.n.
- †midazolam 10–20mg/24h CSCI.

Alcohol withdrawal
Same choice as for seizure (see above) with dose and route dependent on severity of withdrawal syndrome.[14,15]

---

1   Ansseau M et al. (1984) Methodology required to show clinical differences between benzodiazepines. *Current Medical Research and Opinion*. **8**: 108–113.
2   BNF (2008) Section 4.1. Hypnotics and anxiolytics. In: *British National Formulary* (No. 55). British Medical Association and Royal Pharmaceutical Society of Great Britain, London. Current BNF available from: www.bnf.org/bnf/bnf/current/
3   Grad R (1995) Benzodiazepines for insomnia in community-dwelling elderly: a review of benefit and risk. *Journal of Family Practice*. **41**: 473–481.
4   Pollack MH et al. (1993) Long-term outcome after acute treatment with alprazolam or clonazepam for panic disorder. *Journal of Clinical Psychopharmacology*. **13**: 257–263.
5   Woodman CL et al. (1994) Predictors of response to alprazolam and placebo in patients with panic disorder. *Journal of Affective Disorders*. **30**: 5–13.
6   Rush CR et al. (1993) Abuse liability of alprazolam relative to other commonly used benzodiazepines: a review. *Neuroscience and Biobehavioral Reviews*. **17**: 277–285.
7   Kravitz HM et al. (1993) Alprazolam and depression: a review of risks and benefits. *Journal of Clinical Psychiatry*. **54 (suppl)**: 78–84; discussion 85.
8   Foster S et al. (1997) Efficacy of lorazepam and haloperidol for rapid tranquilization in the psychiatric emergency room setting. *International Clinical Psychopharmacology*. **12**: 175–179.
9   Rey E et al. (1999) Pharmacokinetic optimization of benzodiazepines therapy for acute seizures. Focus on delivery routes. *Clinical Pharmacokinetics*. **36**: 409–424.
10 BNF (2008) Section 4.8.2 Drugs used in status epilepticus. In: *British National Formulary* (No. 55). British Medical Association and Royal Pharmaceutical Society of Great Britain, London. Current BNF available from: www.bnf.org/bnf/bnf/current/
11 Di Florio T and Goucke CR (1999) The effect of midazolam on persistent postoperative nausea and vomiting. *Anaesth Intensive Care*. **27**: 38–40.
12 Aapro MS et al. (2005) Anticipatory nausea and vomiting. *Support Care Cancer*. **13**: 117–121.
13 Mandala M et al. (2005) Midazolam for acute emesis refractory to dexamethasone and granisetron after highly emetogenic chemotherapy: a phase II study. *Support Care Cancer*. **13**: 375–380.
14 Peppers M (1996) Benzodiazepines for alcohol withdrawal in the elderly and in patients with liver disease. *Pharmacotherapy*. **16**: 49–57.
15 Chick J (1998) Review: benzodiazepines are more effective than neuroleptics in reducing delirium and seizures in alcohol withdrawal. *Evidence-Based Medicine*. **3**: 11.
16 Morin CM et al. (1994) Nonpharmacological interventions for insomnia: a meta-analysis of treatment efficacy. *American Journal of Psychiatry*. **151**: 1172–1180.
17 Murtagh DR and Greenwood KM (1995) Identifying effective psychological treatments for insomnia: a meta-analysis. *Journal of Consulting and Clinical Psychology*. **63**: 79–89.
18 Smith MT et al. (2002) Comparative meta-analysis of pharmacotherapy and behavior therapy for persistent insomnia. *American Journal of Psychiatry*. **159**: 5–11.
19 Hugel H et al. (2004) The prevalence, key causes and management of insomnia in palliative care patients. *Journal of Pain and Symptom Management*. **27**: 316–321.
20 Glass J et al. (2005) Sedative hypnotics in older people with insomnia: meta-analysis of risks and benefits. *British Medical Journal*. **331**: 1169.
21 Wang PS et al. (2001) Hazardous benzodiazepine regimens in the elderly: effects of half-life, dosage, and duration on risk of hip fracture. *American Journal of Psychiatry*. **158**: 892–898.
22 Lenhart SE and Buysse DJ (2001) Treatment of insomnia in hospitalized patients. *Annals of Pharmacotherapy*. **35**: 1449–1457.
23 Montplaisir J et al. (2003) Zopiclone and zaleplon vs benzodiazepines in the treatment of insomnia: Canadian consensus statement. *Human Psychopharmacology*. **18**: 29–38.
24 Anonymous (2005) Benzodiazepines and newer hypnotics. *MeReC Bulletin*. **15**: 17–20.
25 Twycross RG et al. (2003) Itch: scratching more than the surface. *Quarterly Journal of Medicine*. **96**: 7–26.
26 Hagermark O (1973) Influence of antihistamines, sedatives, and aspirin on experimental itch. *Acta Dermato-Venereologica*. **53**: 363–368.
27 Muston H et al. (1979) Differential effect of hypnotics and anxiolytics on itch and scratch. *Journal of Investigative Dermatology*. **72**: 283.
28 Ebata T et al. (1998) Effects of nitrazepam on nocturnal scratching in adults with atopic dermatitis: a double-blind placebo-controlled crossover study. *British Journal of Dermatology*. **138**: 631–634.
29 Prieto LN (2004) The use of midazolam to treat itching in a terminally ill patient with biliary obstruction. *Journal of Pain and Symptom Management*. **28**: 531–532.
30 Hanley DF and Kross JF (1998) Use of midazolam in the treatment of refractory status epilepticus. *Clinical Therapeutics*. **20**: 1093–1105.
31 Prommer E (2005) Re: Pruritus in patients with advanced cancer. *Journal of Pain and Symptom Management*. **30**: 201–202.
32 Maher J (1981) Intravenous lorazepam to prevent nausea and vomiting associated with cancer chemotherapy. *Lancet*. **1**: 91–92.
33 Bishop J et al. (1984) Lorazepam: a randomized, double-blind, crossover study of a new antiemetic in patients receiving cytotoxic chemotherapy and prochlorperazine. *Journal of Clinical Oncology*. **2**: 691–695.

DIAZEPAM

Class: Benzodiazepine.

Indications: Short-term treatment of anxiety, agitation (including delirium tremens during alcohol withdrawal), muscle spasm, myoclonus, epilepsy, status epilepticus, peri-operative sedation, †insomnia.

Contra-indications: Acute or severe pulmonary insufficiency, sleep apnea syndrome, severe liver disease, myasthenia gravis. Do not use alone for depression, mixed anxiety-depression or psychosis.

Pharmacology

Diazepam is a typical benzodiazepine with GABA-potentiating actions in the CNS, notably spinal cord, hippocampus, cerebellum and cerebrum. At all these sites, diazepam reduces neuronal activity. Diazepam is relatively devoid of autonomic effects and does not significantly reduce locomotor activity at low doses, or depress **amphetamine**-induced excitation. In high doses, it activates the drug metabolizing enzymes in the liver. Diazepam also possesses dependence liability and may produce withdrawal symptoms, but has a wide margin of safety against poisoning. Standard parenteral formulations are oil-based or an oil-in-water emulsion (the oil-based injection is no longer marketed in Canada), and absorption from muscle after IM injection is slower and more variable than after PO and PR administration. Diazepam has a long plasma halflife and several active metabolites, one of which has a plasma halflife of up to 120h in the elderly. Because of marked interindividual variation, the effects of a constant dose will vary greatly. Doses for individual patients are determined empirically.
Bio-availability almost 100% PO; 80–100% PR (rectal gel or oil-based injection); 67–84% PR (suppository).[1]
Onset of action 15min PO; 1–5min IV (oil-based injection).[1]
Time to peak plasma concentration 30–90min PO; 5–90min PR (rectal gel or oil-based injection);[1] ⩽15min IV (oil-based injection), ⩾15min IV (Diazemuls®); 1–1.5h IM (oil-based injection), 2h IM (Diazemuls®).
Plasma halflife 24–48h; active metabolite nordiazepam 48–120h.
Duration of action 3–30h, situation dependent; may be only 15min–1h after a single IV dose.[1]

Cautions

Concurrent administration with other sedative drugs, including strong opioids, old age, debilitation, chronic respiratory disease, mild–moderate hepatic impairment, renal impairment. If given IV can cause hypotension and transient apnea. Accumulation of active metabolites may necessitate a dose reduction after several days. History of alcohol or drug abuse.

Diazepam is metabolized via the cytochrome P450 group of liver enzymes which gives rise to several potentially important drug interactions (see Cytochrome P450, p.551); **amiodarone**, **cimetidine**, **fluconazole**, **metronidazole**, **omeprazole**, **valproic acid** all inhibit the clearance of diazepam, resulting in an enhanced and more prolonged effect.[2,3] Genetic polymorphism occurs and some people are slow metabolizers (whites 3–5%, Asians 20%); this also results in an enhanced and more prolonged effect (see Cytochrome P450, p.557).

Undesirable effects

For full list, see manufacturer's Product Monograph.
Drowsiness, muscle flaccidity, unsteadiness (ataxia). When given IV, the oil-based solution may cause painful thrombophlebitis. Paradoxical reactions have been reported: insomnia, anxiety, excitement, rage, hallucinations, increased muscle spasticity.

Dose and use

Typical doses for diazepam are shown in Table 4.3. The initial dose will depend on the patient's age, general condition, previous use of diazepam and other benzodiazepines, the intensity of distress, and the urgency of relief. Generally, elderly and debilitated patients should be started on low doses.

Table 4.3 Dose recommendations for diazepam

Indication	Stat & p.r.n. doses	Common range
Anxiety[a]	2–10mg PO	2–20mg PO at bedtime
Muscle spasm[b] Multifocal myoclonus	2–5mg PO	2–10mg PO at bedtime
Anti-epileptic[c,d]	10mg PR/IV	10–30mg at bedtime

a. given as an adjunct to non-drug approaches, e.g. relaxation therapy and massage
b. if localized, consider injection of a trigger point with local anesthetic or acupuncture
c. acute use but in the moribund can be used as a convenient substitute for long-term oral anti-epileptic therapy (also see Midazolam, p.115)
d. to reduce the risk of thrombophlebitis, inject IV diazepam slowly (rate not exceeding 5mg (1mL)/min) into a large vein, e.g. the antecubital vein.

Although the Product Monograph for diazepam recommends administration in divided doses, its long plasma halflife means that administration at bedtime will generally be equally effective, and easier for the patient. In an agitated moribund patient, b.i.d.–t.i.d. dosing is sometimes indicated so as to reduce the number of hours awake. Rectal diazepam is useful in a crisis or if the patient is moribund:
- suppositories 10mg (compounded)
- rectal gel 5–10mg in 1–2mL
- parenteral formulation administered with a blunt (needle-free) cannula.

If injections are necessary, preferably switch to **midazolam** (see below) or **lorazepam** (*not* CSCI; see p.119). Patients occasionally react paradoxically, i.e. become more distressed; if this happens, **haloperidol** (see p.128) or **olanzapine** (see p.134) should be given instead.

Supply

Diazepam (generic)
Tablets 2mg, 5mg, 10mg, 28 days @ 5mg at bedtime = $2.
Oral solution 1mg/mL, 28 days @ 5mg at bedtime = $12.

Diazemuls® (Actavis)
Injection (oil-in-water emulsion) 5mg/mL, 2mL amp = $2.50.

Diastat® (Valeant)
Rectal gel (prefilled unit-dose rectal delivery system) 5mg/mL, 5mg (1mL) single-dose unit = $76; 10mg (2mL) single-dose unit = $76; 15mg (3mL) single-dose unit = $76.

---

1 AHFS (2009) Benzodiazepines general statement (pharmacokinetics). AHFS Drug Information 2009 (online edition). Available from: www.ahfsdruginformation.com/ (subscription required).
2 Klotz U and Reimann I (1980) Delayed clearance of diazepam due to cimetidine. *New England Journal of Medicine.* **302**: 1012–1014.
3 Wagner B and O'Hara D (1997) Pharmacokinetics and pharmacodynamics of sedatives and analgesics in the treatment of agitated critically ill patients. *Clinical Pharmacokinetics.* **33**: 426–453.

MIDAZOLAM

Class: Benzodiazepine.

Indications: Anesthetic induction/maintenance agent, sedative for minor procedures, sedation for mechanically ventilated ICU patients, †myoclonus, †epilepsy, †status epilepticus, †terminal agitation,[1,2] †intractable hiccup,[3] †nausea and vomiting.[4,5]

Contra-indications: Unless for end-of-life care: acute or severe pulmonary insufficiency, sleep apnea syndrome, severe liver disease, myasthenia gravis.

Pharmacology

Midazolam is a short-acting, water-soluble benzodiazepine with GABA-potentiating actions in the CNS, notably spinal cord, hippocampus, cerebellum and cerebrum. At all these sites, midazolam reduces neuronal activity. In single doses for sedation, midazolam is 3 times more potent than **diazepam**; as an anti-epileptic, it is twice as potent. With multiple doses, **diazepam** will gain in potency because of its prolonged plasma halflife, i.e. 24–120h versus 2–5h for midazolam. In the elderly, the plasma halflife of midazolam is prolonged up to 3 times and in some intensive care patients having CIVI for sedation, the plasma halflife may be prolonged up to 6 times. It also may be prolonged in hepatic impairment and heart failure. An active metabolite, α-hydroxymidazolam glucuronide, has a receptor affinity about 1/10 that of midazolam. In severe renal impairment (creatinine clearance <10mL/min), accumulation can result in prolonged sedation.[6] The main advantage of midazolam in palliative care is that it is water-soluble and is compatible with most of the drugs commonly given by CSCI. It is better for IV injection because it does not cause thrombophlebitis; and can also be given by the buccal route as an alternative to SL **lorazepam**.[7]

When used in typical doses (see Table 4.4, p.116) in imminently dying patients, tolerance is not a practical problem. However, if much higher doses are used (e.g. >10–15mg/h CSCI), then a lack of response may be seen if the dose is further escalated. This relates in part to the fact that at these doses, maximum GABA-ergic inhibition has been reached.[8]

For severe terminal breathlessness, the combination of regular **morphine** and midazolam appears more effective than either drug alone (see p.307).[9]

In contrast to other benzodiazepines, midazolam may be of benefit in intractable (central) pruritus.[10,11] In one patient with cancer of the pancreas and cholestatic pruritus, a CSCI of midazolam was effective 'within a few hours' (2mg bolus followed by 1mg/h, increasing by 1mg/h every 15min 'as needed for itching'), whereas **lorazepam** 1mg q6h or 2mg at bedtime (and several other psychotropic drugs) was ineffective.[11] The affinity of midazolam for the GABA-receptor is 5–6 times greater than that of **lorazepam**,[12] and it is possible that this is the explanation for the difference in the response to the two benzodiazepines.[13] (For alternative approaches to the management of cholestatic pruritus, see Box 5.O, p.339.)

Bio-availability > 90% IM; 75% buccal; 35–44% PO.
Onset of action 5–10min SC; 2–3min IV; 15min buccal.
Time to peak plasma concentration 30min IM; 30min buccal; 60min PO.
Plasma halflife 2–5h; increased to about 10h by CSCI.
Duration of action 5mg <4h, interindividual variation.[14]

Cautions

Chronic respiratory disease, mild–moderate hepatic impairment, renal impairment, impaired cardiac function or low cardiac output. If given IV can cause hypotension, reduced myocardial contractility and transient apnea. History of alcohol or drug abuse.

Midazolam is a substrate of CYP3A4 (see Cytochrome P450, p.551). Plasma concentrations are increased by **cimetidine**, **clarithromycin**, **diltiazem**, **erythromycin** and **verapamil** (reduce midazolam dose by 50%), **aprepitant** and **cimetidine**. Midazolam concentrations are reduced by **carbamazepine**, **phenytoin** and **rifampin**.[15] When given PO, plasma concentrations of midazolam are increased by grapefruit juice, **fluconazole**, **itraconazole** and **ketoconazole**.

Undesirable effects

For full list, see manufacturer's Product Monograph.
Drowsiness.

Dose and use

Typical doses for midazolam are shown in Table 4.4. In practice, midazolam is mostly used in the terminal phase. If given IV rather than SC, smaller stat doses are generally used. The minimal interval between p.r.n. doses is typically 1h if SC, and 10–15min if IV.

Table 4.4 Dose recommendations for SC midazolam

Indication	Stat & p.r.n. doses	Common range
Muscle tension/spasm Multifocal myoclonus }	5mg SC	10–30mg/24h CSCI
Terminal agitation Terminal breathlessness Intractable hiccup }	5–10mg SC	30–60mg/24h CSCI[a]
Anti-epileptic	10mg SC	30–60mg/24h CSCI

a. reported upper dose range 120mg for hiccup; 240mg for agitation.

If an agitated patient does not settle on 30mg/24h, an antipsychotic (e.g. **haloperidol**) is best introduced before further increasing the dose of midazolam.

The use of midazolam for intractable hiccup is generally limited to a time when drowsiness is acceptable. For use in status epilepticus, see Anti-epileptics, p.205.

The use of midazolam for intractable hiccup is limited to patients in whom persistent distressing hiccup is contributing to terminal restlessness at a time when sedation is acceptable to aid symptom relief. For use in status epilepticus, see Figure 4.5, p.205.

Regimen for anticipatory nausea and vomiting, and refractory post-chemotherapeutic and postoperative nausea and vomiting:
- midazolam 10–20mg/24h CSCI.[4,5,16]

Some centres give midazolam buccally (off-label route). The contents of an ampoule of injection solution can be used.

Supply

Midazolam (generic)
Injection 1mg/mL, 2mL, 5mL, 10mL vial = $1.50, $4 and $5 respectively; 5mg/mL, 1mL, 2mL, 50mL amp = $4, $6 and $97 respectively.

---

1 Bottomley DM and Hanks GW (1990) Subcutaneous midazolam infusion in palliative care. *Journal of Pain and Symptom Management.* **5**: 259–261.
2 McNamara P et al. (1991) Use of midazolam in palliative care. *Palliative Medicine.* **5**: 244–249.
3 Wilcock A and Twycross R (1996) Case report: midazolam for intractable hiccup. *Journal of Pain and Symptom Management.* **12**: 59–61.
4 Di Florio T and Goucke CR (1999) The effect of midazolam on persistent postoperative nausea and vomiting. *Anaesthesia and Intensive Care.* **27**: 38–40.
5 Mandala M et al. (2005) Midazolam for acute emesis refractory to dexamethasone and granisetron after highly emetogenic chemotherapy: a phase II study. *Support Care Cancer.* **13**: 375–380.
6 Bauer T et al. (1995) Prolonged sedation due to accumulation of conjugated metabolites of midazolam. *Lancet.* **346**: 145–147.
7 McIntyre J et al. (2005) Safety and efficacy of buccal midazolam versus rectal diazepam for emergency treatment of seizures in children: a randomised controlled trial. *Lancet.* **366**: 205–210.
8 Cheng C et al. (2002) When Midazolam Fails. *Journal of Pain and Symptom Management.* **23**: 256–265.
9 Navigante AH et al. (2006) Midazolam as adjunct therapy to morphine in the alleviation of severe dyspnea perception in patients with advanced cancer. *Journal of Pain and Symptom Management.* **31**: 38–47.
10 Thomsen JS et al. (2002) Suppression of spontaneous scratching in hairless rats by sedatives but not by antipruritics. *Skin Pharmacology and Applied Skin Physiology.* **15**: 218–224.
11 Prieto LN (2004) The use of midazolam to treat itching in a terminally ill patient with biliary obstruction. *Journal of Pain and Symptom Management.* **28**: 531–532.
12 Hanley DF and Kross JF (1998) Use of midazolam in the treatment of refractory status epilepticus. *Clinical Therapeutics.* **20**: 1093–1105.
13 Prommer E (2005) Re: Pruritus in patients with advanced cancer. *Journal of Pain and Symptom Management.* **30**: 201–202.
14 Schwagmeier R et al. (1998) Midazolam pharmacokinetics following intravenous and buccal administration. *British Journal of Clinical Pharmacology.* **46**: 203–206.
15 Baxter K (ed) (2008) *Stockley's Drug Interactions* (8e). Pharmaceutical Press, London.
16 Aapro MS et al. (2005) Anticipatory nausea and vomiting. *Support Care Cancer.* **13**: 117–121.

CLONAZEPAM

Class: Benzodiazepine.

Indications: Epilepsy, †myoclonus, †anxiety,[1,2] †panic disorder, †restless legs syndrome,[3] †neuropathic pain.[4,5]

Contra-indications: Acute or severe pulmonary insufficiency, sleep apnea syndrome, severe liver disease, myasthenia gravis.

Pharmacology

Clonazepam is a typical benzodiazepine with GABA-potentiating actions in the CNS, notably spinal cord, hippocampus, cerebellum and cerebrum. At all these sites, clonazepam reduces neuronal activity. Clonazepam is extensively metabolized to inactive metabolites and the cytochrome CYP3A pathway may be important (see Cytochrome P450, p.551).
Bio-availability 100% PO.
Onset of action 20–60min PO; 5–10min SC.
Time to peak plasma concentration 1–4h.
Halflife 20–40h (mean 30h).
Duration of action 12h.

Cautions

Chronic respiratory disease, mild–moderate hepatic impairment, renal impairment, elderly or debilitated patients (may require dose reduction). Spinal or cerebellar ataxia. History of alcohol or drug abuse. Avoid abrupt withdrawal in epileptic patients (may precipitate status epilepticus).

Undesirable effects

For full list, see manufacturer's Product Monograph
Fatigue, drowsiness, muscular hypotonia and inco-ordination. These effects are generally transitory and can be minimized by starting with low doses at bedtime. In children, clonazepam has been associated with salivary hypersecretion and drooling.

Dose and use

See Table 4.5. Because of the development of tolerance to its anti-epileptic effect, clonazepam is generally reserved for the treatment of refractory tonic-clonic or partial seizures.[1–3]

Clonazepam has also been used successfully in some patients with neuropathic pain, including phantom limb,[6] post-herpetic,[7] diabetic,[8] and cancer-related[9] although there is no supporting RCT evidence.[5]

In countries where a parenteral formulation is available (not Canada), clonazepam can be administered by CSCI as an alternative to **midazolam** (see p.115). Although, because of its long halflife, it could be administered as a bolus injection once daily, preferably at bedtime.

Table 4.5 Dose recommendations for clonazepam

Indication	Stat & p.r.n. doses	Common range
Epilepsy	1mg PO	1mg at bedtime–8mg/24h PO in divided doses
Panic disorder	250microgram PO	500microgram–4mg PO at bedtime
Restless legs	250microgram PO	500microgram–2mg PO at bedtime
Neuropathic pain	500microgram PO	500microgram at bedtime–8mg/24h in divided doses PO

Supply

Clonazepam (generic)
Tablets 250microgram, 500microgram, 2mg, 28 days @ 2mg once daily = $6.

Rivotril® (Hoffman-La Roche)
Tablets 500microgram, 2mg, 28 days @ 2mg once daily = $11.

1 Davidson J and Moroz G (1998) Pivotal studies of clonazepam in panic disorder. *Psychopharmacology Bulletin.* **34**: 169–174.
2 Wulsin L et al. (1999) Clonazepam treatment of panic disorder in patients with recurrent chest pain and normal coronary arteries. *International Journal of Psychiatry and Medicine.* **29**: 97–105.
3 Joy M (1997) Clonazepam: benzodiazepine therapy for the restless legs syndrome. *ANNA Journal.* **24**: 686–689.
4 Reddy S and Patt R (1994) The benzodiazepines as adjuvant analgesics. *Journal of Pain and Symptom Management.* **9**: 510–514.
5 McQuay H et al. (1995) Anticonvulsant drugs for the management of pain: a systematic review. *British Medical Journal.* **311**: 1047–1052.
6 Bartusch S et al. (1996) Clonazepam for the treatment of lancinating phantom limb pain. *Clinical Journal of Pain.* **12**: 59–62.
7 Mamdani FS (1994) Pharmacologic management of herpes zoster and postherpetic neuralgia. *Canadian Family Physician.* **40**: 321–326, 329–332.
8 Young JP and Clarke BF (1985) Pain relief in diabetic neuropathy: the effectiveness of imipramine and related drugs. *Diabetic Medicine.* **2**: 363–366.
9 Hugel H et al. (2003) Clonazepam as an adjuvant analgesic in patients with cancer-related neuropathic pain. *Journal of Pain and Symptom Management.* **26**: 1073–1074.

LORAZEPAM

Class: Benzodiazepine.

Indications: Short-term treatment of anxiety or †insomnia, status epilepticus (injection), perioperative sedation, †nausea and vomiting (chemotherapy-related), †acute agitation or mania, †terminal agitation, †alcohol withdrawal (delirium tremens),[1] †serotonin toxicity.[2]

Contra-indications: Acute or severe pulmonary insufficiency, sleep apnea syndrome, severe liver disease, myasthenia gravis. Do not use alone for depression, anxiety-depression, psychosis, or delirium (unless alcohol withdrawal).[3]

Pharmacology

Lorazepam is a typical benzodiazepine with GABA-potentiating actions in the CNS, notably spinal cord, hippocampus, cerebellum and cerebrum. At all these sites, lorazepam reduces neuronal activity.[4] Like other benzodiazepines, lorazepam can cause amnesia. It is rapidly absorbed SL and PO. Despite being 85% protein-bound, it quickly reaches the CNS.[5] Lorazepam is glucuronidated in the liver to an inactive compound and is excreted both by the kidneys and in the bile (i.e. cytochrome P450 is not involved). The conjugated metabolite undergoes enterohepatic circulation. Duration of action does not correlate with plasma concentrations and can be up to 3 days.

Bio-availability 93% PO.

Onset of action 5min SL; 10–15min PO.

Time to peak plasma concentration 1h SL; 1–1.5h IM; 1–6h PO.

Plasma halflife 10–20h.

Duration of action 6–72h.

Cautions

History of alcohol or drug abuse. May lead to physical and psychological dependence. Concurrent administration with alcohol and/or other centrally acting drugs, e.g. TCAs, H_1-antihistamines, antipsychotics and opioids, may result in excessive sedation and/or delirium. The metabolism of lorazepam is retarded by **valproic acid**.[6] It has less interaction with **propoxyphene** than other benzodiazepines.[7] **Carbamazepine** and **rifampin** may decrease lorazepam levels.[8]

Although it has been used successfully as a sole agent in acute psychotic agitation (mania),[9,10] lorazepam should not be used alone in an agitated delirium because it is likely to exacerbate the condition.[3,11] May unmask or worsen pre-existing depression.

Undesirable effects

For full list, see manufacturer's Product Monograph.

Drowsiness, fatigue, impaired co-ordination, blurred vision, lightheadedness, memory impairment, insomnia, dysarthria, anxiety, decreased libido, depression, headaches, tachycardia, chest pain, dry mouth, constipation, diarrhea, nausea, vomiting, increased or decreased appetite, sweating, rash.

Dose and use

Lorazepam can be given SL, PO, PR, SC, IM, or IV. Specific SL tablets (Ativan® sublingual tablets) are available; these dissolve in about 20sec when placed under the tongue. The patient should avoid swallowing for about 2min to allow time for absorption.

SL tablets will not dissolve in the absence of saliva. In patients with a dry mouth, the SL tablet should be dissolved in a few drops of warm water, drawn up in a 1ml oral syringe and put between the patient's cheek and gum.[12]

If given by CSCI, there is a risk of precipitation.[13] Accidental intra-arterial administration, or extravasation close to an artery, has been associated with thrombosis and gangrene.

Status epilepticus

Lorazepam is now regarded as the benzodiazepine of choice in the control of status epilepticus (see p.205).[14]

Insomnia
- 2–4mg PO at bedtime

Anxiety[15]
- Img SL/PO stat and b.i.d.
- if necessary, increase to 2–6mg/24h.

Acute psychotic agitation
Use with **haloperidol** or **risperidone** to control psychotic agitation,[16] although some centres use it alone in this circumstance:[9,10]
- give 2mg PO every 30min until the patient is settled.[9]

Sedation in the imminently dying
Used at some centres instead of **midazolam**.[13,17] Generally use with an antipsychotic:
- 2–4mg IV stat
- 4–20mg/24h CIVI
- some centres use lorazepam 1–2mg SC q6–8h.

Supply
Lorazepam (generic)
Tablets 500microgram, Img, 2mg, 28 days @ 2mg b.i.d. = $4.
Injection 4mg/mL, ImL amp = $2.50. *For IV injection, dilute with an equal volume of WFI, 0.9% saline or 5% glucose (dextrose). For IM injection, administer deep into the muscle mass.*

Ativan® (Wyeth)
Tablets 500microgram, Img, 2mg, 28 days @ 2mg b.i.d. = $4.
Tablets SL 500microgram, Img, 2mg, 28 days @ 2mg b.i.d. = $12.

1 Peppers M (1996) Benzodiazepines for alcohol withdrawal in the elderly and in patients with liver disease. *Pharmacotherapy.* **16**: 49–57.
2 Brown T et al. (1996) Pathophysiology and management of the serotonin syndrome. *Annals of Pharmacotherapy.* **30**: 527–533.
3 Breitbart W et al. (1996) A double-blind trial of haloperidol, chlorpromazine, and lorazepam in the treatment of delirium in hospitalized AIDS patients. *American Journal of Psychiatry.* **153**: 231–237.
4 Ziemann U et al. (1996) The effect of lorazepam on the motor cortical excitability in man. *Experimental Brian Research.* **109**: 127–135.
5 Wagner B and O'Hara D (1997) Pharmacokinetics and pharmacodynamics of sedatives and analgesics in the treatment of agitated critically ill patients. *Clinical Pharmacokinetics.* **33**: 426–453.
6 Samara E et al. (1997) Effect of valproate on the pharmacokinetics and pharmacodynamics of lorazepam. *Journal of Clinical Pharmacology.* **37**: 442–450.
7 Abernethy D et al. (1985) Interaction of propoxyphene with diazepam, alprazolam and lorazepam. *British Journal of Clinical Pharmacology.* **19**: 51–57.
8 Bachmann KA and Jauregui L (1993) Use of single sample clearance estimates of cytochrome P450 substrates to characterize human hepatic CYP status in vivo. *Xenobiotica.* **23**: 307–315.
9 Foster S et al. (1997) Efficacy of lorazepam and haloperidol for rapid tranquilization in the psychiatric emergency room setting. *International Clinical Psychopharmacology.* **12**: 175–179.
10 Lenox R et al. (1992) Adjunctive treatment of manic agitation with lorazepam versus haloperidol: a double-blind study. *Journal of Clinical Psychiatry.* **53**: 47–52.
11 Salzman C et al. (1991) Parenteral lorazepam versus parenteral haloperidol for the control of psychotic disruptive behavior. *Journal of Clinical Psychiatry.* **52**: 177–180.
12 Nicholson A (2007) Lorazepam. In: *Bulletin board.* Palliativedrugs.com Ltd. Available from: www.palliativedrugs.org/forum/read.php?f=1&i=11203&t=11203
13 McCollam J et al. (1999) Continuous infusions of lorazepam, midazolam and propofol for sedation of the critically ill surgery trauma patient: a prospective, randomized comparison. *Critical Care Medicine.* **27**: 2454–2458.
14 Prasad K et al. (2005) Anticonvulsant therapy for status epilepticus. *Cochrane Database of Systematic Reviews.* **4**: CD003723.
15 MacLaren R et al. (2000) A prospective evaluation of empiric versus protocol-based sedation and analgesia. *Pharmacotherapy.* **20**: 662–672.
16 Currier G and Simpson G (2001) Risperidone liquid concentrate and oral lorazepam versus intramuscular haloperidol and intramuscular lorazepam for treatment of psychotic agitation. *Journal of Clinical Psychiatry.* **62**: 153–157.
17 Fainsinger R et al. (2000) Sedation for delirium and other symptoms in terminally ill patients in Edmonton. *Journal of Palliative Care.* **16 (2)**: 5–10.

ANTIPSYCHOTICS

Indications: Acute psychotic symptoms, mania and bipolar disorders, schizophrenia, †agitation, †delirium, †anti-emetic, intractable hiccup (**chlorpromazine** and †**haloperidol**), †treatment-resistant depression.[1]

Pharmacology

Antipsychotics are predominantly characterized by D_2-receptor antagonism. Dopamine has a central role in:

- the mesocorticolimbic system (midbrain reticular formation → hypothalamus, thalamus, frontal and limbic cortex). Implicated in reward, motivation, attention and arousal, dopamine is released in response to stimuli and thoughts perceived as relevant ('salience hypothesis'), particularly with regard to 'reward'. These effects are mediated by D_1 and D_2 receptors[2,3]
  the nigrostriatal system (substantia nigra → corpus striatum). Influences motor control. Dysregulation occurs in Parkinson's disease and many drug-induced movement disorders.

Psychosis is caused by dopaminergic dysfunction in the mesocorticolimbic system. Dopamine *excess* in the limbic cortex ('over attention' to stimuli and thoughts) is largely responsible for the 'positive' signs of psychoses (hallucinations, delusions).[2] Dopamine *deficiency* in the frontal cortex causes 'negative' signs (affective flattening, anhedonia, alogia, withdrawal).

The D_2-receptor antagonism of antipsychotics improves 'positive' signs but may worsen 'negative' signs because of the impact on the frontal cortex. The latter is due to excessive serotoninergic activity in the midbrain, acting on $5HT_2$ receptors, inhibiting dopaminergic neurons projecting to the frontal cortex. Many newer 'atypical' antipsychotics are dual $D_2/5HT_2$ receptor antagonists and their correction of serotoninergic overactivity may thus explain their effect on 'negative' symptoms (see below).[4]

The potency of antipsychotics is proportional to their D_2-receptor affinity and an antipsychotic effect is seen with ⩾60% D_2-receptor occupancy.[5] Dopamine modulation is also responsible for many of the undesirable effects of this class of drugs (see p.561). Both beneficial and undesirable effects vary between antipsychotics. This is partly because of differing affinities for D_2 and other receptors (Table 4.6). By convention, antipsychotics are classified as either 'typical' or 'atypical', despite marked variation within these groups:

- typicals:
  - ▷ butyrophenones, e.g. **haloperidol**
  - ▷ phenothiazines, e.g. **chlorpromazine, prochlorperazine, perphenazine**
- atypicals, e.g. **clozapine, risperidone, olanzapine, quetiapine.**

The broad receptor profile of phenothiazines (Table 4.6) accounts for their undesirable effects at muscarinic (see Box 1.A, p.5), adrenergic (e.g. postural hypotension), and histaminic (e.g. drowsiness) receptors. The D_2-specific action of **haloperidol** avoids such problems but increases the risk of extrapyramidal effects.

Table 4.6 Receptor affinities for selected antipsychotics[4,6]

	D_2	$5HT_{2A}$	$5HT_{2C}$	$5HT_3$	H_1	α_1	α_2	ACh_M
Chlorpromazine	+++	+++	++	−	+++	+++	(+)	++
Clozapine	+	+++	++	+	+++	+	+	+++
Haloperidol	+++	+	−	−	−	++	−	−
Perphenazine	+++	+++	+		+++	++	(+)	−
Prochlorperazine	+++	++	+	−	++	++	−	+
Olanzapine	++	+++	+	+	+	++	+	++
Quetiapine	+	+	(+)	−	++	+	++	−
Risperidone	+++	+++	++	−	++	+	+++	−

Affinity: +++ high, ++ moderate, + low, (+) borderline, − negligible or none; blank = no data.

A lower risk of extrapyramidal effects, the defining feature of atypicals, may relate to balanced D_2 and $5HT_2$-receptor antagonism[7] and/or a faster dissociation from, or lower affinity for, D_2-receptors.[5] The relatively lower doses used in comparative studies with typicals may also contribute to some of the observed differences. 5HT-receptor antagonism may contribute to the efficacy of some atypicals for negative symptoms and schizophrenia refractory to typicals, particularly **clozapine**, the agent of choice for refractory schizophrenia. However, the risk of agranulocytosis, and need for monthly WBC monitoring initially, limits its usefulness in palliative care.

Direct comparisons suggest that acute extrapyramidal effects would be avoided in one patient for every 3–6 patients treated with an atypical rather than a typical antipsychotic drug.[8,9] However, the difference is greatest relative to **haloperidol**; *atypicals do not cause fewer extrapyramidal symptoms than **chlorpromazine** in doses of up to 600mg/24h*.[10] Further, in a large RCT, although extrapyramidal effects accounted for more discontinuations of **perphenazine** compared with several atypicals (8% vs. 2–4%), overall discontinuation rates for undesirable effects or lack of efficacy were comparable.[11] All treatment groups experienced some degree of involuntary movement (13–17%), akathisia (5–9%) or extrapyramidal signs (4–8%).

Most studies are too short to evaluate adequately the risk of tardive dyskinesia. Available data suggest a 5 times lower risk with atypicals compared with **haloperidol** in the first year of use, although **haloperidol** doses were perhaps relatively higher.[12] Among atypicals, **clozapine** and **quetiapine** carry the lowest risk of extrapyramidal effects, and **risperidone** the highest.[13]

Acquisition costs for atypicals are higher than for typicals. At doses ≤12mg/24h, the overall tolerability of **haloperidol** is comparable.[14] Suggested reductions in long-term healthcare costs from the use of atypicals[15] may be less relevant in palliative care if drugs are used at lower doses and for shorter periods of time.

Equivalent doses of typicals have been estimated, predominantly from surveys of clinical practice, and provide a starting point if switching from one to another (Table 4.7).[16] Effective doses of atypicals are less variable, but cannot be described meaningfully in terms of dose equivalence. For pharmacokinetic details, see Table 4.8.

Table 4.7 Equivalent doses of typical antipsychotics[16]

Chlorpromazine	100mg
Haloperidol	3mg
Trifluoperazine	5mg
Perphenazine	8mg
Promazine	100mg

Table 4.8 Pharmacokinetic details for selected antipsychotics[17,18]

	Oral bio-availability (%)	Time to peak plasma concentration	Halflife (h)	Metabolism (predominant P450 iso-enzyme)
Haloperidol	60–70	2–6h (PO) 10–20min (SC)	13–35	Multiple
Chlorpromazine	10–25	2–4h (PO)	30	CYP2D6
Prochlorperazine	6 (14 buccal)	4h PO; 8h buccal single dose, 4h multiple doses	15–20	Multiple
Clozapine	50–60	2h	12	CYP1A2, CYP3A4
Risperidone	99	1–2h	24[a,b]	CYP2D6[c]
Olanzapine	60	5–8h	34[d] (52[e])	CYP1A2, CYP2D6
Quetiapine	100	1.5h	7[f] (10–14[e]) (12[g])	CYP3A4

a. for risperidone + active 9-hydroxy metabolite
b. clearance reduced by renal impairment: see Product Monograph
c. activity of 9-hydroxyrisperidone, the predominant CYP2D6 metabolite, is comparable to risperidone; thus overall clinical effect is not altered by CYP2D6 polymorphisms or inhibitors
d. unaffected by hepatic or renal impairment
e. in the elderly
f. clearance reduced by both renal and hepatic impairment
g. of active metabolite.

Cautions
For full list, see manufacturer's Product Monograph.

Stroke risk
A meta-analysis of RCTs in elderly patients with dementia has shown that, compared with placebo, the risk of stroke with **risperidone** is about 3 times higher.[19–21] A pooled analysis of RCTs of **olanzapine** in similar patients showed a similar increased risk of stroke, and a 2-fold increase in all-cause mortality.[22] The mechanism of this association is not known, but it is regarded as a class effect. Subsequent findings indicate an increased risk in all older patients, with or without dementia, for both typicals and atypicals (the relative risk with individual drugs is unclear).[13,23,24] The risk is greatest when first prescribed, and with higher doses.

Epilepsy
Antipsychotics cause a dose-dependent reduction in seizure threshold. The risk for individual agents approximates to the degree of sedation: **chlorpromazine** and **clozapine** carry a higher risk, **haloperidol** a lower risk. Many other psychotropic medications also alter seizure threshold. To minimize the risk, use the lowest risk antipsychotic (e.g. **haloperidol**) at the lowest effective dose. In palliative care, depot formulations are best avoided because they cannot be withdrawn quickly if problems occur.

Parkinson's disease
All antipsychotics exacerbate Parkinson's disease through D_2-receptor antagonism. The risk is lowest with **clozapine** and **quetiapine**. Alternatives should be used where possible, e.g. **trazodone** or a benzodiazepine for agitation, or non-dopaminergic anti-emetics for nausea such as an antihistaminic anti-emetic (see p.189), a $5HT_3$-receptor antagonist (see p.192), or a corticosteroid. Where psychotic symptoms occur in the context of Parkinson's disease or Lewy Body dementia:
- look for possible causes of delirium, e.g. sepsis
- consider a trial reduction of antiparkinsonian medication:
  ▷ reduce dopamine receptor agonists and antimuscarinic agents initially
  ▷ dopamine precursors, e.g. **levodopa**, are less likely to cause psychosis.[25]

If the above measures are unhelpful, commence **quetiapine** 12.5–25mg/24h; or **clozapine** for patients unable to tolerate **quetiapine**.[25]

Drug interactions
For full list, see manufacturer's Product Monograph.
Several pharmacodynamic interactions (additive sedation, hypotension and QT prolongation; reduced effect of antiparkinsonian medication) can be predicted from the receptor profile of antipsychotics.

In addition, potentially serious interactions may result from induction or inhibition of hepatic metabolism. CYP 3A4 inhibitors (e.g. some antifungal azoles, **cimetidine**, macrolide antibiotics, **aprepitant**) can significantly increase plasma levels of **quetiapine**, **pimozide** and **aripiprazole**. **Carbamazepine** and protease inhibitors exhibit varied interactions (see respective Product Monographs).

Antipsychotics are one of several classes of drugs which can prolong the QT interval, and at least theoretically increase the risk of cardiac tachyarrthymias, including the potentially fatal *torsade de pointes* (see Prolongation of the QT interval in palliative care, p.543). Generally, concurrent prescribing of two drugs which can significantly prolong the QT interval should be avoided.

Neuroleptic (antipsychotic) malignant syndrome
Neuroleptic (antipsychotic) malignant syndrome (NMS) is a potentially life-threatening reaction which occurs in <1% of those prescribed an antipsychotic (Box 4.D).[26,27] This idiosyncratic syndrome is associated with both typicals and atypicals.[28]

Most cases of NMS occur within 2 weeks of starting treatment or a dose increase. It is more common in patients also receiving **lithium**. It is important to distinguish NMS from serotonin toxicity (Table 4.9).[29]

NMS is a hypodopaminergic state, where progressive bradykinesia results in a state of immobilization, akinesia and stupor, accompanied by lead-pipe rigidity, fever, and autonomic

---

Box 4.D Clinical features of neuroleptic (antipsychotic) malignant syndrome

Essential
Severe muscle rigidity
Pyrexia ± sweating

Additional
Muteness → drowsiness
Tachycardia and elevated/labile blood pressure
Leukocytosis
Raised plasma creatine phosphokinase (CPK) ± other evidence of muscle injury, e.g. myoglobinuria

---

Table 4.9 Neuroleptic (antipsychotic) malignant syndrome (NMS) vs. serotonin toxicity[30]

NMS	Serotonin toxicity
Antipsychotic drugs	Serotoninergic drugs
Idiosyncratic reaction to normal doses	Dose-related toxicity
Relatively rare	Relatively common
Slow onset, slow progression (several days)	Rapid onset, rapid progression (hours)
Extrapyramidal signs (bradykinesia and 'lead-pipe' rigidity)	Upper motor neurone signs (clonus, hyperreflexia, spasticity)
Hypertonia = early feature	Hypertonia = late feature
Muteness → stupor	Hyperkinesia (agitation)
Improved by dopamine agonists (e.g. bromocriptine[a]), resolves slowly	Improved by 5-HT$_{2A}$ antagonists, resolves rapidly

a. bromocriptine is serotoninergic and would exacerbate serotonin toxicity.

instability. In serotonin toxicity, the discriminating signs of clonus, hyperreflexia, tremor, shivering and agitation make it difficult to confuse with NMS (see p.140).[30,31]

Symptoms indistinguishable from NMS have been reported in patients with Parkinson's disease when long-term treatment with **levodopa** and **bromocriptine** has been abruptly discontinued.[32-34] This has led to the suggestion that the syndrome would be better called *acute dopamine depletion syndrome*.[32]

Death occurs in up to 20% of cases, mostly as a result of respiratory failure. The use of a dopamine agonist, e.g. **bromocriptine**, halves the mortality.[35] Subsequent prescription of an antipsychotic carries a 30–50% risk of recurrence.[36]

NMS is self-limiting if the causal antipsychotic drug is discontinued (and an alternative antipsychotic *not* prescribed). Generally it resolves in 1–2 weeks unless caused by a depot antipsychotic, when it takes 4–6 weeks. Antipsychotics are *not* removed by hemodialysis. Specific measures include:
• discontinuation of the causal drug
• prescription of a muscle relaxant, e.g. a benzodiazepine
• in severe cases, prescription of **bromocriptine**.[35]
General supportive measures may need to extend to artificial hydration and nutrition. Complications such as hypoxia, acidosis and renal failure require appropriate acute management.

Undesirable effects
For full list, see manufacturer's Product Monograph.
These are summarized in Box 4.E; see text and individual drug monographs for relative risk with different drugs.

Box 4.E   Undesirable effects of antipsychotics

Extrapyramidal syndromes
Parkinsonism, akathisia, dystonia, tardive dyskinesia (see Drug-induced movement disorders, p.561).

Metabolic effects[13]
More common with typicals, and risperidone
Hyperprolactinemia resulting in amenorrhea, galactorrhea, gynecomastia, sexual dysfunction, osteoporosis.

More common with atypicals, particularly olanzapine and clozapine
Weight gain.
Dyslipidemia, possibly associated with weight gain.
Type 2 diabetes mellitus, both new onset and worsening of pre-existing disease; risk independent of weight gain.

Cardiovascular effects
QT prolongation (see Prolongation of the QT interval in palliative care, p.543); dose-related, affected by presence of other risk factors, highest risk with thioridazine and ziprasidone.[13]

Venous thrombo-embolism; risk possibly highest with atypicals.[37]

Stroke and increased risk of death in elderly patients (see Cautions).

Postural hypotension (α-adrenergic antagonism), particularly phenothiazines and clozapine; also seen with quetiapine and risperidone.

Miscellaneous[13]

Reduced seizure threshold (see Cautions).

Antimuscarinic effects (see Box 1.A, p.5); more with phenothiazines and clozapine.

Neuroleptic (antipsychotic) malignant syndrome (see text).

Agranulocytosis is seen in about 1% of patients taking clozapine, generally after 3–6 months.

Use of antipsychotics in palliative care
Nausea and vomiting
The D_2-receptor antagonism of all antipsychotics is likely to provide anti-emetic activity in the area postrema (chemoreceptor trigger zone). Where specific action at this site is required (e.g. most chemical causes of nausea; see p.179), a selective dopaminergic agent such as **haloperidol** is used.[38] However, most antipsychotics have moderate or high affinity at several receptors, some of which are involved in the transduction of emetic signals (see p.180). Thus, most antipsychotics are, to a variable extent, broad-spectrum anti-emetics. Of those available in Canada, **methotrimeprazine** and **olanzapine** are perhaps the most attractive in this respect.[39,40]

Delirium
Treatment of underlying causes, non-drug management (e.g. orientation strategies, correction of sensory deprivation) and prevention of complications are central to delirium management. When medication is required, antipsychotics (e.g. **haloperidol**) are often used, though evidence is limited and comparative studies with other psychotropics are lacking.[41–43]

    Trazodone is an alternative, particularly where sedation is required. Benzodiazepines (e.g. **lorazepam**) can paradoxically worsen agitation, but are preferred for delirium related to alcohol withdrawal, neuroleptic (antipsychotic) malignant syndrome or Parkinson's disease. Hallucinations in delirium respond to antipsychotics in hours–days whereas seemingly identical phenomena in a psychosis may not resolve for 1–2 weeks.

Agitation and challenging behaviours in dementia

Patients with dementia may become agitated for many reasons, including an appropriate response to a distressing situation. Possible precipitants should be treated or modified:

- intercurrent infections
- pain and/or other distressing symptoms
- environmental factors.

When no reversible cause is found, and agitation is mild, assurance that such behaviours are often self-limiting may suffice. Training in non-drug management of behavioural disturbances reduces the need for psychotropic medication.[44]

The first-line use of antipsychotics for behavioural disturbance in dementia is inappropriate and actively discouraged.[45–47] In addition to safety concerns (increased risk of stroke and overall mortality, see above), evidence of benefit compared with non-drug measures is limited. A recent large RCT for agitation or psychosis in patients with dementia found atypicals and typicals to be no better than placebo in all but a few secondary outcomes.[48] Taken together with other studies, the efficacy of antipsychotics in dementia is at best modest, and should be used only where other measures have failed.[49,50]

The use of alternative psychotropics including antidepressants, benzodiazepines, anti-epileptic drugs and cholinesterase inhibitors, has been proposed. However, evidence is even more limited than for antipsychotics, and certainly insufficient to allow clear evidence-based recommendations of one class over another.[50,51] Larger studies have not replicated the promising earlier results found with **trazodone**.[50] Despite this, the serious consequences of not treating severe agitation or psychosis in dementia are also recognized.[50] Where drug treatment is required, clinicians should be guided by the individual patient's symptoms and co-morbidities, and the clinician's familiarity with the agents available. Options include:

- **haloperidol**
- atypicals, e.g. **olanzapine, quetiapine, risperidone**
- cholinesterase inhibitors (benefit is marginal, but may be better tolerated).[51]

Whichever drug is selected, use the lowest effective dose, and attempt dose reduction every 2–3 months; many patients do not deteriorate when medication is withdrawn.[49,51,52]

Intractable hiccup

Chlorpromazine or **haloperidol** is used when more specific treatment, e.g. an antifoaming agent (antiflatulent) ± **metoclopramide** for gastric distension (see Prokinetics, p.13), and **baclofen** (see p.438) are ineffective.

Pain

In the past, antipsychotics were often used as part of an analgesic cocktail. However, in chronic pain, the combination of an antipsychotic with an antidepressant is no more effective than treatment with an antidepressant alone,[53] and when used with **morphine**, antipsychotics cause more sedation without more pain relief.[54] Even so, antipsychotics may be of benefit in selected highly anxious patients overwhelmed by persisting pain and insomnia.[55] Benefit may also be seen in patients whose pain escalates with the onset of delirium (acute confusion) and who derive no benefit from increased doses of opioids.[56]

1 Mahmoud RA et al. (2007) Risperidone for treatment-refractory major depressive disorder: a randomized trial. Annals of Internal Medicine. 147: 593–602.
2 Kapur S et al. (2005) From dopamine to salience to psychosis–linking biology, pharmacology and phenomenology of psychosis. Schizophrenia Research. 79: 59–68.
3 Boutrel B and Koob GF (2004) What keeps us awake: the neuropharmacology of stimulants and wakefulness-promoting medications. Sleep. 27: 1181–1194.
4 Shiloh R et al. (2006) Chapter 4. Antipsychotic drugs. In: Atlas of psychiatric pharmacotherapy (2e). Taylor & Francis, London.
5 Kapur S and Mamo D (2003) Half a century of antipsychotics and still a central role for dopamine D2 receptors. Prog Neuropsychopharmacol Biol Psychiatry. 27: 1081–1090.
6 NIMH (National Institute of Mental Health) (2006) National Institute of Mental Health's Psychoactive Drug Screening Program. University of North Carolina. Available from: http://pdsp.med.unc.edu/indexR.html
7 Meltzer HY (2004) What's atypical about atypical antipsychotic drugs? Current Opinion in Pharmacology. 4: 53–57.
8 Hunter RH et al. (2003) Risperidone versus typical antipsychotic medication for schizophrenia. Cochrane Database of Systematic Reviews. CD000440.
9 Wahlbeck K et al. (2000) Clozapine versus typical neuroleptic medication for schizophrenia. Cochrane Database of Systematic Reviews. CD000059.
10 Leucht S et al. (2003) New generation antipsychotics versus low-potency conventional antipsychotics: a systematic review and meta-analysis. Lancet. 361: 1581–1589.

11 Lieberman JA et al. (2005) Effectiveness of antipsychotic drugs in patients with chronic schizophrenia. New England Journal of Medicine. **353**: 1209–1223.

12 Correll CU et al. (2004) Lower risk for tardive dyskinesia associated with second-generation antipsychotics: a systematic review of 1-year studies. American Journal of Psychiatry. **161**: 414–425.

13 Haddad PM and Sharma SG (2007) Adverse effects of atypical antipsychotics: differential risk and clinical implications. CNS Drugs. **21**: 911–936.

14 Geddes J et al. (2000) Atypical antipsychotics in the treatment of schizophrenia: systematic overview and meta-regression analysis. British Medical Journal. **321**: 1371–1376.

15 Davies A et al. (1998) Risperidone versus haloperidol: II. cost-effectiveness. Clinical Therapeutics. **20**: 196–213.

16 Foster P (1989) Neuroleptic equivalence. Pharmaceutical Journal. **September 30**: 431–432.

17 Eiermann B et al. (1997) The involvement of CYP1A2 and CYP3A4 in the metabolism of clozapine. British Journal of Clinical Pharmacology. **44**: 439–446.

18 Finn E et al. (2005) Bioavailability and metabolism of prochlorperazine administered via the buccal and oral delivery route. Journal of Clinical Pharmacology. **45**: 1383–1390.

19 Wooltorton E (2002) Risperidone (Risperdal): increased rate of cerebrovascular events in dementia trials. Canadian Medical Association Journal. **167**: 1269–1270.

20 Bullock R (2005) Treatment of behavioural and psychiatric symptoms in dementia: implications of recent safety warnings. Current Medical Research and Opinion. **21**: 1–10.

21 Schneider LS et al. (2005) Risk of death with atypical antipsychotic drug treatment for dementia: meta-analysis of randomized placebo-controlled trials. Journal of the American Medical Association. **294**: 1934–1943.

22 Wooltorton E (2004) Olanzapine (Zyprexa): increased incidence of cerebrovascular events in dementia trials. Canadian Medical Association Journal. **170**: 1395.

23 Wang PS et al. (2005) Risk of death in elderly users of conventional vs. atypical antipsychotic medications. New England Journal of Medicine. **353**: 2335–2341.

24 Gill SS et al. (2007) Antipsychotic drug use and mortality in older adults with dementia. Annals of internal medicine. **146**: 775–786.

25 Weintraub D and Hurtig HI (2007) Presentation and management of psychosis in Parkinson's disease and dementia with Lewy bodies. American Journal of Psychiatry. **164**: 1491–1498.

26 Caroff S and Mann S (1993) Neuroleptic malignant syndrome. Medical Clinics of North America. **77**: 185–202.

27 Adnet P et al. (2000) Neuroleptic malignant syndrome. British Journal of Anaesthesia. **85**: 129–135.

28 Isbister GK et al. (2002) Comment: neuroleptic malignant syndrome associated with risperidone and fluvoxamine. Annals of Pharmacotherapy. **36**: 1293; author reply 1294.

29 Gillman PK (1999) The serotonin syndrome and its treatment. Journal of Psychopharmacology. **13**: 100–109.

30 Gillman P (2005) NMS and ST: chalk and cheese. In: British Medical Journal. Available from: http://bmj.bmjjournals.com/cgi/eletters/329/7478/1333

31 Gillman P (2004) Defining toxidromes: serotonin toxicity and neuroleptic malignant syndrome: A comment on Kontaxakis et al. In: Archives of General Hospital Psychiatry. Available from: www.annals-general-psychiatry.com/content/2/1/10/comments#41454

32 Keyser DL and Rodnitzky RL (1991) Neuroleptic malignant syndrome in Parkinson's disease after withdrawal or alteration of dopaminergic therapy. Archives of Internal Medicine. **151**: 794–796.

33 Mann S et al. (1991) Pathogenesis of neuroleptic malignant syndrome. Psychiatry Annals. **21**: 175–180.

34 Ong K et al. (2001) Neuroleptic malignant syndrome without neuroleptics. Singapore Medical Journal. **42**: 85–88.

35 Sakkas P et al. (1991) Pharmacotherapy of neuroleptic malignant syndrome. Psychiatry Annals. **21**: 157–164.

36 Wells A et al. (1988) Neuroleptic rechallenges after neuroleptic malignant syndrome: case report and literature review. Drug Intelligence and Clinical Pharmacy. **22**: 475–479.

37 Liperoti R et al. (2005) Venous thromboembolism among elderly patients treated with atypical and conventional antipsychotic agents. Archives of Internal Medicine. **165**: 2677–2682.

38 Buttner M et al. (2004) Is low-dose haloperidol a useful antiemetic? A meta-analysis of published and unpublished randomized trials. Anesthesiology. **101**: 1454–1463.

39 Passik SD et al. (2004) A phase I trial of olanzapine (Zyprexa) for the prevention of delayed emesis in cancer patients: a Hoosier Oncology Group study. Cancer Invest. **22**: 383–388.

40 Navari RM et al. (2005) A phase II trial of olanzapine for the prevention of chemotherapy-induced nausea and vomiting: a Hoosier Oncology Group study. Support Care Cancer. **13**: 529–534.

41 Centeno C et al. (2004) Delirium in advanced cancer patients. Palliative Medicine. **18**: 184–194.

42 Marcantonio ER (2005) Clinical management and prevention of delirium. Psychiatry. **4**: 68–72.

43 Grace JB and Holmes J (2006) The management of behavioural and psychiatric symptoms in delirium. Expert Opinion on Pharmacotherapy. **7**: 555–561.

44 Fossey J et al. (2006) Effect of enhanced psychosocial care on antipsychotic use in nursing home residents with severe dementia: cluster randomised trial. British Medical Journal. **332**: 756–761.

45 CSM (Committee on Safety of Medicines) (2004) Antipsychotic drugs and stroke. Available from: www.mhra.gov.uk/Safetyinformation/Safetywarningsalertsandrecalls/Safetywarningsandmessagesformedicines/CON1004298

46 Mowat D et al. (2004) CSM warning on atypical psychotics and stroke may be detrimental for dementia. British Medical Journal. **328**: 1262.

47 Health Canada (2005) Increased mortality associated with the use of atypical antipsychotic drugs in elderly patients with dementia. Notice to healthcare professionals. Available from: www.hc-sc.gc.ca/dhp-mps/medeff/advisories-avis/prof/_2005/atyp-antipsycho_hpc-cps-eng.php

48 Schneider LS et al. (2006) Effectiveness of atypical antipsychotic drugs in patients with Alzheimer's disease. New England Journal of Medicine. **355**: 1525–1538.

49 Howard R et al. (2001) Guidelines for the management of agitation in dementia. International Journal of Geriatric Psychiatry. **16**: 714–717.

50 Jeste DV et al. (2007) ACNP White Paper: Update on Use of Antipsychotic Drugs in Elderly Persons with Dementia. Neuropsychopharmacology.

51 Sink KM et al. (2005) Pharmacological treatment of neuropsychiatric symptoms of dementia: a review of the evidence. Journal of the American Medical Association. **293**: 596–608.

52 Lee PE *et al.* (2004) Atypical antipsychotic drugs in the treatment of behavioural and psychological symptoms of dementia: systematic review. *British Medical Journal.* **329**: 75.
53 Getto C et al. (1987) Antidepressants and chronic nonmalignant pain: a review. *Journal of Pain and Symptom Management.* **2**: 9–18.
54 Houde RW (1966) On assaying analgesics in man. In: RS Knighton and PR Dumke (eds) *Pain.* Little Brown, Boston, pp. 183–196.
55 Maltebie A and Cavenar J (1977) Haloperidol and analgesia: case reports. *Military Medicine.* **142**: 946–948.
56 Coyle N et al. (1994) Delirium as a contributing factor to 'crescendo' pain: three case reports. *Journal of Pain and Symptom Management.* **9**: 44–47.

HALOPERIDOL

Class: Butyrophenone.

Indications: Psychotic symptoms, Gilles de la Tourette's syndrome, agitation and delirium (including †disturbed nights in the elderly), †nausea and vomiting, †intractable hiccup.

Pharmacology

Haloperidol is a typical antipsychotic D_2-receptor antagonist. Steady-state plasma concentrations do not vary greatly between patients after injection but they vary considerably after PO administration. The metabolism of haloperidol is not as complex as that of the phenothiazines but, even so, there are many metabolites and some may contribute to its extrapyramidal effects.[1] It is not possible to relate clinical response to plasma haloperidol concentrations. Haloperidol in solution is odourless, colourless and tasteless and can be administered clandestinely in extreme situations.

Compared with **chlorpromazine**, haloperidol has less effect on the cardiovascular system and causes less drowsiness. It has no antimuscarinic properties,[2] but causes *more* extrapyramidal reactions (see Drug-induced movement disorders, p.561). In one study, haloperidol caused akathisia in $>50\%$ of schizophrenics.[3] The incidence in palliative care appears to be low, possibly because generally lower doses are used and the duration of treatment is relatively short.

Haloperidol is widely used in palliative care as an anti-emetic and for delirium. By virtue of its D_2-receptor antagonism, it has a profound inhibitory effect on the area postrema (chemoreceptor trigger zone). It is an effective anti-emetic postoperatively and in patients referred to specialist gastro-enterological clinics with multifactorial nausea.[4] Long-standing clinical experience in palliative care indicates that haloperidol is a good anti-emetic for many chemical causes of vomiting, e.g. **morphine**, **digoxin**, renal failure, hypercalcemia;[5,6] and also after radiation therapy.[7] However, no RCTs have been conducted in palliative care patients.[8] Haloperidol has also been used for obstructive vomiting in relatively small doses, e.g. 2–5mg SC.[9,10] Its benefit in this circumstance is difficult to understand. However, the affinity of haloperidol for D_2-receptors is 10 times that of **domperidone** (see p.187), marketed in many countries as a prokinetic drug.[11] Haloperidol might therefore correct gastric stasis induced by stress, anxiety or nausea from any cause.

Bio-availability 45–75% PO.[1]
Onset of action 10–15min SC; >1h PO.
Time to peak plasma concentration 2–6h PO; 10–20min SC.
Plasma halflife 13–35h.
Duration of action up to 24h, sometimes longer.

Cautions

Haloperidol can cause potentially fatal prolongation of the QT interval and *torsade de pointes*, particularly if given IV (off-label route) or at higher-than-recommended doses. Caution is required if any formulation of haloperidol is given to patients with an underlying predisposition, e.g. those with cardiac abnormalities, hypothyroidism, familial long QT syndrome, electrolyte imbalance (particularly hypokalemia or hypomagnesemia), or taking drugs which prolong the QT interval (see Prolongation of the QT interval in palliative care, p.543). If IV haloperidol is essential, ECG monitoring during administration is recommended.[12,13]

Parkinson's disease. Potentiation of CNS depression caused by other CNS depressants, e.g. anxiolytics, alcohol. Increased risk of extrapyramidal effects and possible neurotoxicity with **lithium**. Plasma concentration of haloperidol is approximately halved by concurrent use of **carbamazepine**.

Note: in the management of behavioural disturbances in elderly patients with dementia (agitation, restlessness, wandering, physical aggression, inappropriate sexual activity, culturally inappropriate behaviours, hoarding, cursing, shadowing, screaming, sleep disorders) there is often limited benefit with haloperidol compared with non-drug measures.[14–19] Given the excess mortality seen in these patients with all antipsychotics, their off-label use to control such behaviours must be actively discouraged.[20]

Undesirable effects

For full list, see manufacturer's Product Monograph.

Extrapyramidal effects (including tardive dyskinesia), hypothermia, sedation, hypotension, endocrine effects, blood disorders, alteration in liver function, neuroleptic (antipsychotic) malignant syndrome (see p.123).

Dose and use

Haloperidol exacerbates Parkinson's disease: use alternatives where possible (see p.187).

As a general rule, the dose of haloperidol is halved when switching from PO to SC.

Anti-emetic (for chemical/toxic causes of vomiting)
- start with 1mg PO stat & at bedtime (standard anti-emetic for **morphine**-induced vomiting at many centres)
- typical maintenance dose 1–2mg at bedtime (or 500microgram–1mg b.i.d.)
- if necessary, increase the total daily dose progressively to 5–10mg
- if 10mg at bedtime (or 5mg b.i.d.) is ineffective, review the cause of the vomiting; consider switching to **methotrimeprazine** (see p.130).

Delirium

If possible, correct underlying causes, and use non-drug measures (e.g. orientation strategies, correction of sensory deprivation).[21] When symptomatic drug treatment is required:
- patient distress mild–moderate and not an immediate danger to self or others:
  ▷ start with 500microgram stat
  ▷ repeat q2h p.r.n.
  ▷ if necessary, increase the dose progressively (e.g. → 1mg → 2mg etc.)[22]
  ▷ patient distress moderate–severe and/or an immediate danger to self or others
  ▷ start with 1–2mg stat, possibly combined with a benzodiazepine
  ▷ repeat q2h p.r.n.
  ▷ if necessary, increase the dose progressively (e.g. → 3mg → 5mg).
The maintenance dose is based on the initial cumulative dose needed to settle the patient; usual maximum ≤5mg/24h. Review daily, particularly if the underlying cause can be resolved. Other strategies include:
- prescribing a more sedating antipsychotic (e.g. **olanzapine** (see p.134), **quetiapine**) *or*
- the concurrent use of **trazodone** (see p.162) or a benzodiazepine (see p.108).
If necessary, seek advice from a psychogeriatrician. Note: for the management of terminal agitation, see p.228.

Behavioural problems in dementia

The management of delirium or psychosis should be distinguished from the long-term treatment of behavioural disturbance in dementia. Antipsychotics are generally not indicated in the latter (see p.126). Training in the non-drug management of behavioural disturbances reduces the need for psychotropic medication; medication is a last resort.[23] When used, dose reduction should be attempted every 2–3 months; many patients do not deteriorate when medication is withdrawn.[20,24,25]

Intractable hiccup

Haloperidol is generally used only when sequential therapeutic trials of **metoclopramide** (see p.185) ± an anti-foaming agent (see p.3) and **baclofen** (see p.438) have both failed:
- give haloperidol 1mg PO t.i.d.
- if no response, consider giving 5mg IV
- maintenance dose 1–3mg at bedtime.[26,27]
Another option is **gabapentin** (see p.220).[28]

Supply

Haloperidol (generic)
Tablets 500microgram, 5mg, 10mg, 20mg, 28 days @ 5mg at bedtime = $5.
Oral solution 2mg/mL, 28 days @ 5mg at bedtime = $8.
Injection 5mg/mL, 1mL ampoule = $5.

1 Vella-Brincat J and Macleod AD (2004) Haloperidol in palliative care. *Palliative Medicine.* **18**: 195–201.
2 de Leon J (2005) Benztropine equivalents for antimuscarinic medication. *American Journal of Psychiatry.* **162**: 627.
3 Wirshing D et al. (1999) Novel antipsychotics: comparison of weight gain liabilities. *Journal of Clinical Psychiatry.* **60**: 358–363.
4 Buttner M et al. (2004) Is low-dose haloperidol a useful antiemetic? A meta-analysis of published and unpublished randomized trials. *Anesthesiology.* **101**: 1454–1463.
5 Bentley A and Boyd K (2001) Use of clinical pictures in the management of nausea and vomiting: a prospective audit. *Palliative Medicine.* **15**: 247–253.
6 Stephenson J and Davies A (2006) An assessment of aetiology-based guidelines for the management of nausea and vomiting in patients with advanced cancer. *Supportive Care in Cancer.* **14**: 348–353.
7 Stoll BA (1962) Radiation sickness. *British Medical Journal.* **2**: 507–510.
8 Perkins P and Dorman S (2009) Haloperidol for the treatment of nausea and vomiting in palliative care patients. *Cochrane Database of Systematic Reviews.* **2**: CD006271. DOI: 006210.001002/14651858.CD1400627 1.pub1465 1852.
9 Ventafridda V et al. (1990) The management of inoperable gastrointestinal obstruction in terminal cancer patients. *Tumori.* **76**: 389–393.
10 Mercadante S (1995) Bowel obstruction in home-care cancer patients: 4 years experience. *Support Care Cancer.* **3**: 190–193.
11 Sanger G (1993) The pharmacology of anti-emetic agents. In: P Andrews and G Sanger (eds) *Emesis in Anti-Cancer Therapy: Mechanisms and Treatment.* Chapman and Hall, London, pp. 179–210.
12 FDA (2007) Information for healthcare professionals. Haloperidol (marketed as Haldol, Haldol decanoate and Haldol lactate). Food and Drugs Administration. Available from: www.fda.gov/Drugs/DrugSafety/PostmarketDrugSafetyInformationforPatientsandProviders/DrugSafetyInformationforHeathcareProfessionals/ucm085203.htm
13 Canadian Pharmacists Association (2009) Haloperidol. Compendium of pharmaceuticals and specialities (eCPS). Available from: www.pharmacists.ca/content/products/ecps_english.cfm
14 Schneider LS et al. (1990) A metaanalysis of controlled trials of neuroleptic treatment in dementia. *Journal of the American Geriatrics Society.* **38**: 553–563.
15 Devanand DP (1996) Antipsychotic treatment in outpatients with dementia. *International Psychogeriatrics.* **8 (suppl 3)**: 355–361; discussion 381–352.
16 Lanctot KL et al. (1998) Efficacy and safety of neuroleptics in behavioral disorders associated with dementia. *Journal of Clinical Psychiatry.* **59**: 550–561; quiz 562–553.
17 Ballard C and O'Brien J (1999) Treating behavioural and psychological signs in Alzheimer's disease. *British Medical Journal.* **319**: 138–139.
18 Schneider LS (1999) Pharmacologic management of psychosis in dementia. *Journal of Clinical Psychiatry.* **60 (suppl 8)**: 54–60.
19 Mowat D et al. (2004) CSM warning on atypical psychotics and stroke may be detrimental for dementia. *British Medical Journal.* **328**: 1262.
20 Howard R et al. (2001) Guidelines for the management of agitation in dementia. *International Journal of Geriatric Psychiatry.* **16**: 714–717.
21 Twycross R et al. (2009) *Symptom Management in Advanced Cancer* (4e). palliativedrugs.com, Nottingham, pp. 207–211.
22 British Geriatrics Society and Royal College of Physicians (2006) The prevention, diagnosis and management of delirium in older people. National Guidelines. Available from: www.rcplondon.ac.uk/pubs/books/pdmd/deliriumconciseguide.pdf
23 Fossey J et al. (2006) Effect of enhanced psychosocial care on antipsychotic use in nursing home residents with severe dementia: cluster randomised trial. *British Medical Journal.* **332**: 756–761.
24 Lee PE et al. (2004) Atypical antipsychotic drugs in the treatment of behavioural and psychological symptoms of dementia: systematic review. *British Medical Journal.* **329**: 75.
25 Sink KM et al. (2005) Pharmacological treatment of neuropsychiatric symptoms of dementia: a review of the evidence. *Journal of the American Medical Association.* **293**: 596–608.
26 Ives TJ et al. (1985) Treatment of intractable hiccups with intramuscular haloperidol. *American Journal of Psychiatry.* **142**: 1368–1369.
27 Scarnati RA (1979) Intractable hiccup (singultus): report of case. *Journal of the American Osteopathic Association.* **79**: 127–129.
28 Twycross R et al. (2009) *Symptom Management in Advanced Cancer* (4e). palliativedrugs.com, Notitngham, pp. 174–177.

METHOTRIMEPRAZINE

Class: Phenothiazine antipsychotic, anti-emetic.

Indications: Psychosis, terminal agitation, intractable pain (with strong opioids), nausea and vomiting.[1]

Pharmacology

Methotrimeprazine (rINN levomepromazine) is a typical antipsychotic drug, first introduced in the 1950s.[2,3] Like **chlorpromazine**, it is a potent antagonist at D_2, H_1, α_1-adrenergic and muscarinic receptors. However, methotrimeprazine is also a potent $5HT_2$-receptor antagonist.[4] Early clinical studies suggest that it possesses antidepressant properties.[5]

Many studies confirm that 25mg by injection has definite analgesic properties.[6-11] It is also a potent anti-emetic,[4,12,13] and is widely used as a second- or third-line agent in patients who fail to respond to less 'broad-spectrum' anti-emetics (see Anti-emetics, p.178).[13,14] Some centres also use methotrimeprazine in low doses (e.g. 2–5mg) as a first-line anti-emetic, provided a prokinetic anti-emetic (e.g. **metoclopramide**) is not indicated.

Doses ⩾25mg/24h tend to cause drowsiness, and also postural hypotension. **Olanzapine** (see p.000) and possibly **risperidone** (see p.136) are alternative broad-spectrum anti-emetics for those unable to tolerate methotrimeprazine.

Bio-availability 20–40% PO.[15]
Onset of action 30min.
Time to peak plasma concentration 2–3h PO; 30–90min SC.
Plasma halflife 15–30h, sometimes longer.[16]
Duration of action 12–24h.

Cautions

Parkinsonism, postural hypotension, antihypertensive medication, epilepsy, hypothyroidism, myasthenia gravis.

Undesirable effects

For full list, see manufacturer's Product Monograph.
Drowsiness, postural hypotension, antimuscarinic effects (see Box 1.A, p.5).

Dose and use
Anti-emetic
Generally used as a second- or third-line anti-emetic:
- start with 5–12.5mg PO/SC stat, at bedtime & p.r.n.
- if necessary, increase to 25–50mg/24h.

If used as a first-line anti-emetic:
- start with 2mg PO stat, at bedtime & p.r.n.
- if necessary, increase to 5mg PO at bedtime & p.r.n.

Terminal agitation ± delirium
Generally given only when a reduced level of consciousness is acceptable:
- 25mg SC stat, and q1h–q2h p.r.n.
- if necessary, increase to 50mg b.i.d., and q1h–q2h p.r.n.
- uncommon to need > 300mg/24h.[17,18]

Given its plasma halflife, most patients can be maintained satisfactorily on intermittent injections, 1–3 times/24h. However, at some centres, methotrimeprazine is given by CSCI. To reduce the likelihood of inflammatory reactions at the skin infusion site, dilute to the largest practical volume (see CSCI, Diluent section, p.515).

Analgesic
May be of benefit in a very distressed patient with severe pain unresponsive to other measures:
- stat dose 25mg PO/SC and at bedtime
- titrate dose according to response; usual maximum daily dose 100mg SC/200mg PO.

There are 2-drug compatibility data for methotrimeprazine in 0.9% saline with **oxycodone**. Incompatibility may occur with **dexamethasone, ketorolac, or octreotide**. For more details and 3-drug compatibility data, see Charts A4.1–A4.4 (p.591).
Compatibility data in WFI can be found on www.palliativedrugs.com Syringe Driver Survey Database.

Supply
Methotrimeprazine (generic)
Tablets 2mg, 5mg, 25mg, 50mg, 28 days @ 12.5mg at bedtime = $2.

Nozinan® (Sanofi-Aventis)
Injection 25mg/mL, 1mL amp = $4.

1 Prommer E (2005) The use of levomepromazine in palliative care. *European Journal of Palliative Care.* **12 (1)**: 8–10.
2 Courvoisier S *et al.* (1958) General pharmacodynamic properties of levomepromazine. *Comptes rendus des seances de la Societe de biologie et de ses filiales.* **7**: 1378–1382.
3 Ban T and Schwarz L (1963) Systematic studies with levomepromazine. *Journal of Neuropsychiatry.* **Nov/Dec**: 112–117.
4 Twycross RG *et al.* (1997) The use of low dose levomepromazine (methotrimeprazine) in the management of nausea and vomiting. *Progress in Palliative Care.* **5**: 49–53.
5 Antkiewicz-Michaluk L (1986) The influence of chronic treatment with antidepressant neuroleptics on the central serotonin system. *Polish Journal of Pharmacology and Pharmacy.* **38**: 359–370.
6 Montilla E *et al.* (1963) Analgesic effect of methotrimeprazine and morphine: a clinical comparison. *Archives of Internal Medicine.* **111**: 725–731.
7 Bloomfield S *et al.* (1964) Comparative analgesic activity of levomepromazine and morphine in patients with chronic pain. *Canadian Medical Association Journal.* **40**: 1156–1162.
8 Beaver W *et al.* (1966) A comparison of the analgesic effects of methotrimeprazine and morphine in patients with cancer. *Clinical Pharmacology and Therapeutics.* **5**: 436–446.
9 Minuck H (1972) Postoperative analgesia – comparison of methotrimeprazine and meperidine as postoperative analgesic agents. *Canadian Anesthetists Society Journal.* **19**: 87–96.
10 Davidsen O *et al.* (1979) Analgesic treatment with levomepromazine in acute myocardial infarction: A randomized clinical trial. *Acta Medica Scandinavica.* **205**: 191–195.
11 Bellens J *et al.* (1981) Analgesic treatment with levopromazine (Nozinan) and methadone in patients with acute myocardial infarction. *Ugeskrift nand Laeger.* **143**: 1313–1316.
12 Higi M *et al.* (1980) Pronounced anti-emetic activity of the antipsychotic drug levomepromazine (methotrimeprazine) in patients receiving cancer chemotherapy. *Journal of Cancer Research and Clinical Oncology.* **97**: 81–86.
13 Eisenchlas JH *et al.* (2005) Low-dose levomepromazine in refractory emesis in advanced cancer patients: an open-label study. *Palliative Medicine.* **19**: 71–75.
14 Kennett A *et al.* (2004) An open study of methotrimeprazine in the management of nausea and vomiting in patients with advanced cancer. *Support Care Cancer.* **13**: 715–721.
15 Bagli M *et al.* (1995) Bioequivalence and absolute bioavailability of oblong and coated levomepromazine tablets in CYP2D6 phenotyped subjects. *International Journal of Clinical Pharmacology and Therapeutics.* **33**: 646–652.
16 Dahl SG *et al.* (1977) Pharmacokinetics and relative bioavailability of levomepromazine after repeated administration of tablets and syrup. *European Journal of Clinical Pharmacology.* **11**: 305–310.
17 Johnson I and Patterson S (1992) Drugs used in combination in the syringe driver: a survey of hospice practice. *Palliative Medicine.* **6**: 125–130.
18 Regnard C and Tempest S (eds) (1998) *A Guide to Symptom Relief in Advanced Disease* (4e). Hochland and Hochland, Manchester.

PROCHLORPERAZINE

Class: Phenothiazine.

Indications: Nausea and vomiting, †vertigo in labyrinthine disorders.

Contra-indications: bone marrow depression.

Pharmacology

Prochlorperazine is a phenothiazine antipsychotic with general properties similar to those of **chlorpromazine** (see p.121). Prochlorperazine has been a popular anti-emetic for many years, particularly for nausea and vomiting caused by chemical stimulation of the chemoreceptor zone. Although it is not recommended for motion sickness, prochlorperazine is used for the short-term relief of vertigo in Meniere's disease.

Oral bio-availability is low because of high first-pass hepatic metabolism.[1] Buccal prochlorperazine (not available in Canada) is about 2.5 times more bio-available and the variance is much less. Prochlorperazine is rapidly metabolized via eight isoforms of cytochrome P450; most extensively by CYP 3A4, 2C19 and 2D6.[2,3] The multiple metabolic pathways suggest that clinically important drug interactions are unlikely.

Undesirable effects are generally less severe than those of **chlorpromazine** but, like all antipsychotics, prochlorperazine has a propensity to cause extrapyramidal effects.[4]

As with other antipsychotics, because prochlorperazine opposes the effects of dopamine agonists, e.g. **bromocriptine**, **levodopa** and other antiparkinsonian drugs, concurrent use should be avoided if possible.

Bio-availability 6% PO, 14% buccal.[3]

Onset of action 30–40min PO, 10–20min IM, 1h PR.[5]

Time to peak plasma concentration 4h PO, 8h buccal; 4h buccal when given regularly.[3]

Plasma halflife 15–20h.[3]

Duration of action 6–8h PO, PR (possibly longer when taken regularly); 12h buccal, IM.[3,5]

Cautions

Prochlorperazine is a potent irritant. Avoid direct contact of the oral solution or injection with the skin; do not give by CSCI (see Box 18.F, p.519). However, particularly in moribund patients, prochlorperazine has often been given successfully by bolus SC injection, i.e. without causing a significant local skin reaction.

Epilepsy, hepatic impairment, severe renal impairment. Drowsiness may affect the performance of skilled tasks, e.g. driving; the effect of alcohol is enhanced.

Drug interactions

Antimuscarinic effects will be more severe if given concurrently with other antimuscarinics; and sedation will be increased if combined with other sedative drugs. Extrapyramidal effects and neurotoxicity have occurred when given concurrently with **lithium**.[6]

Prochlorperazine increases the plasma concentration of **phenytoin** (mechanism unknown); if given concurrently, **phenytoin** levels must be monitored.

Compatibility

In solution, prochlorperazine is *incompatible* with **aminophylline, ampicillin**, barbiturates, calcium salts, **cephalothin, foscarnet, furosemide, hydrocortisone, hydromorphone, midazolam** and **penicillin G**.

Undesirable effects

For full list, see manufacturer's Product Monograph.
Very common (>10%): antimuscarinic effects (see p.5).
Frequency not stated: photosensitivity, slate-gray skin pigmentation, extrapyramidal reactions (see p.561), drug-induced parkinsonism, drowsiness, confusion, paradoxical psychotic behaviour and agitation, seizures, neuroleptic (antipsychotic) malignant syndrome (see p.123), postural hypotension, blood dyscrasias.

Dose and use

Canadian doses are expressed in terms of prochlorperazine *base*. In some countries, doses are expressed in terms of the relevant prochlorperazine *salt*. Thus: prochlorperazine base 5mg = prochlorperazine *mesylate* 7.6mg = prochlorperazine *maleate* 8.1mg = prochlorperazine *edisylate (edisilate)* 7.5mg.[7]

Because of the risk of photosensitivity, patients should be advised to use high-factor (25–30) sun screen cream and a wide–brimmed hat if going outdoors in fine weather.

Anti-emetic
Recommended maximum 40mg/24h (except for PR route):
• 5–10mg PO t.i.d.–q.i.d. *or*
• 5–10mg IM q3h–q4h *or*
• 2.5–10mg IV; may be repeated q3h–q4h p.r.n.
• 10mg PR t.i.d.–q.i.d.

Labyrinthine disorders
The following regimen is sometimes used:
• start with 5mg t.i.d.
• if necessary, increase to 10mg t.i.d.
• reduce gradually to 5mg once daily–b.i.d. after several weeks.

Supply
Prochlorperazine (generic)
Tablets *(as maleate)* 5mg, 10mg, 28 days @ 5mg q.i.d. = $13.
Injection *(as mesylate)* 10mg/2mL, 2mL amp = $2.
Suppositories 10mg, box of 10 = $9.

1 Taylor WB and Bateman DN (1987) Preliminary studies of the pharmacokinetics and pharmacodynamics of prochlorperazine in healthy volunteers. *British Journal of Clinical Pharmacology.* **23**: 137–142.
2 Collins JM et al. (2004) In-vitro characterization of the metabolism of prochlorperazine. *Clinical Pharmacology and Therapeutics.* **75**: 85.
3 Finn A et al. (2005) Bioavailability and metabolism of prochlorperazine administered via the buccal and oral delivery route. *Journal of Clinical Pharmacology.* **45**: 1383–1390.
4 Kawanishi C et al. (2007) Unexpectedly high prevalence of akathisia in cancer patients. *Palliative & Supportive Care.* **5**: 351–354.
5 Lacy C et al. (eds) (2003) *Lexi-Comp's Drug Information Handbook* (11e). Lexi-Comp and the American Pharmaceutical Association, Hudson, Ohio.
6 Baxter K (ed) (2006) *Stockley's Drug Interactions* (7e) Pharmaceutical Press, London.
7 Sweetman SC (ed) (2007) *Martindale: The Complete Drug Reference* (35e). Pharmaceutical Press, London, p. 917.

OLANZAPINE

Class: Atypical antipsychotic.

Indications: Acute psychosis, mania and bipolar disorders, schizophrenia, †agitation, †delirium; †anti-emetic, †paraneoplastic sweating.[1] †Poor response to or drug-induced movement disorders with **haloperidol**.

Pharmacology

Olanzapine is a potent D_1, D_2, D_3, D_4-receptor and $5HT_{2A}$, $5HT_{2C}$, $5HT_3$, $5HT_6$-receptor antagonist.[2–5] It also binds to other receptors, including α_1-adrenergic, H_1 and muscarinic receptors.[6] Olanzapine is used primarily in schizophrenia and other psychoses.[7] In a non-randomized comparison of olanzapine with **haloperidol** in the treatment of delirium, once daily doses (at bedtime) adjusted according to response were equally effective, with maximum benefit seen after 1 week.[8] Compared with **haloperidol**, olanzapine causes fewer drug-induced movement disorders, including tardive dyskinesia,[9] but dose-related weight gain is more common (40% vs. 12%).[10] Weight gain is greater than with **risperidone**.[11] It is metabolized in the liver by glucuronidation and, to a lesser extent, oxidation via the cytochrome P450 system (see p.551), primarily via CYP1A2 with a minor contribution via CYP2D6. The major metabolite is the 10-N-glucuronide which does not pass the blood-brain barrier. Elimination of metabolites is both renal (60%) and fecal (30%).[12] Clearance varies 4-fold among patients.[3,9]

Not surprisingly, given its receptor site affinities, olanzapine is a potent anti-emetic.[4,5,13] This has been confirmed in Phase 1 and Phase 2 trials in cancer patients receiving either moderately or highly emetogenic chemotherapy.[14,15]

Bio-availability 60%, sometimes > 80% PO.
Onset of action hours–days in delirium; days–weeks in psychoses.
Time to peak plasma concentration 5–8h, not affected by food.
Plasma halflife 34h; 52h in the elderly; shorter in smokers; unchanged in hepatic and renal impairment.
Duration of action 12–48h, situation dependent.

Cautions

Injections: fatalities from oversedation or cardiorespiratory depression have occurred after higher than approved doses or concurrent use with benzodiazepines. Monitor blood pressure, heart rate, respiratory rate and level of consciousness for at least 4h after IM olanzapine, and do not give parenteral benzodiazepines within 1h of IM olanzapine.
Dementia: because of an increase in mortality and cerebrovascular events,[16–18] olanzapine should not be used as first-line drug treatment for behavioural symptoms in elderly patients with dementia (see p.126).

Parkinson's disease (potentially can cause a deterioration). Epilepsy (*typical* antipsychotics and *atypical* **clozapine** lower seizure threshold; seizures reported uncommonly with **risperidone**). Elderly patients and those with renal or hepatic impairment. May cause or adversely affect diabetes mellitus; rare reports of keto-acidosis.

Omeprazole, carbamazepine, rifampin and tobacco exposure stimulate CYP1A2 and decrease olanzapine's plasma concentration; in contrast, **fluvoxamine**, an inhibitor of CYP1A2, increases the plasma concentration. Olanzapine potentiates the sedative effects of alcohol and other CNS depressants.

Undesirable effects
For full list, see manufacturer's Product Monograph.
Common (<10%, >1%): drowsiness, weight gain.
Uncommon (<1%, >0.1%): dry mouth, constipation, orthostatic hypotension,[19–21] agitation, nervousness, dizziness, peripheral edema.

The incidence and severity of drug-induced movement disorders are significantly less than with **haloperidol**.[9,22] Acute disorders are generally mild and are reversible if the dose is reduced and/or an antimuscarinic antiparkinsonian drug prescribed.

Dose and use
Schizophrenia
An atypical antipsychotic should be used preferentially:
- starting dose 5–10mg at bedtime
- increase if necessary to 20mg at bedtime.

Agitation and/or delirium
Used as an alternative to **haloperidol**:
- starting dose 2.5mg stat, p.r.n. & at bedtime
- increase if necessary to 5–10mg at bedtime.[23,24]

Anti-emetic
- start with 1.25–2.5mg stat, q2h p.r.n. & at bedtime
- if necessary, increase to 5mg at bedtime, occasionally to 5mg b.i.d.[4,5]

Orodispersible tablets are placed on the tongue and allowed to dissolve or dispersed in water, orange juice, apple juice, milk or coffee immediately before administration.

Supply
Olanzapine (generic)
Tablets 5mg, 28 days @ 5mg at bedtime = $71.

Zyprexa® (Lilly)
Tablets 2.5mg, 5mg, 7.5mg, 10mg, 15mg, 20mg, 28 days @ 5mg at bedtime = $108.
Tablets orodispersible (Zydis®) 5mg, 10mg, 15mg, 20mg, 28 days @ 5mg at bedtime = $108.
Injection (powder for reconstitution) 5mg/mL, 2mL vial = $31.

1   Zylicz Z and Krajnik M (2003) Flushing and sweating in an advanced breast cancer patient relieved by olanzapine. *Journal of Pain and Symptom Management.* **25**: 494–495.
2   Hale AS (1997) Olanzapine. *British Journal of Hospital Medicine.* **58**: 442–445.
3   Stephenson C and Pilowsky L (1999) Psychopharmacology of olanzapine. A review. *British Journal of Psychiatry Supplement.* **38**: 52–58.
4   Passik SD et al. (2002) A pilot exploration of the antiemetic activity of olanzapine for the relief of nausea in patients with advanced cancer and pain. *Journal of Pain and Symptom Management.* **23**: 526–532.
5   Srivastava M et al. (2003) Olanzapine as an antiemetic in refractory nausea and vomiting in advanced cancer. *Journal of Pain and Symptom Management.* **25**: 578–582.
6   Raedler T et al. (2000) In vivo olanzapine occupancy of muscarinic acetylcholine receptors in patients with schizophrenia. *Neuropsychopharmacology.* **23**: 56–68.
7   Fulton B and Goa K (1997) Olanzapine. A review of phamarcological properties and therapeutic efficacy in the management of schizophrenia and related psychoses. *Drugs.* **53**: 281–297.
8   Sipahimalani A and Masand P (1998) Olanzapine in the treatment of delirium. *Psychosomatics.* **39**: 422–430.
9   Beasley C et al. (1997) Efficacy of olanzapine: an overview of pivotal clinical trials. *Journal of Clinical Psychiatry.* **58 (suppl 10)**: 7–12.
10 Eli Lilly Company (2001) *Olanzapine. Clinical and Laboratory Experience. A Comprehensive Monograph.* Dextra Court, Basinstoke.
11 Wirshing DN et al. (1999) Novel antipsychotics: comparison of weight gain liabilities. *Journal of Clinical Psychiatry.* **60**: 358–363.
12 Callaghan J et al. (1999) Olanzapine. Pharmacokinetic and pharmacodynamic profile. *Clinical Pharmacokinetics.* **37**: 177–193.
13 Jackson WC and Tavernier L (2003) Olanzapine for intractable nausea in palliative care patients. *Journal of Palliative Medicine.* **6**: 251–255.

14 Passik SD *et al.* (2004) A phase I trial of olanzapine (Zyprexa) for the prevention of delayed emesis in cancer patients: a Hoosier Oncology Group study. *Cancer Invest.* **22**: 383–388.

15 Navari RM *et al.* (2005) A phase II trial of olanzapine for the prevention of chemotherapy-induced nausea and vomiting: a Hoosier Oncology Group study. *Support Care Cancer.* **13**: 529–534.

16 Wooltorton E (2004) Olanzapine (Zyprexa): increased incidence of cerebrovascular events in dementia trials. *Canadian Medical Association Journal.* **170**: 1395.

17 Bullock R (2005) Treatment of behavioural and psychiatric symptoms in dementia: implications of recent safety warnings. *Current Medical Research and Opinion.* **21**: 1–10.

18 Schneider LS *et al.* (2005) Risk of death with atypical antipsychotic drug treatment for dementia: meta-analysis of randomized placebo-controlled trials. *Journal of the American Medical Association.* **294**: 1934–1943.

19 Tollefson G *et al.* (1997) Olanzapine versus haloperidol in the treatment of schizophrenia and schizoaffective and schizophreniform disorders: results of an international collaborative trial. *American Journal of Psychiatry.* **154**: 457–465.

20 Conley R and Meltzer H (2000) Adverse events related to olanzapine. *Journal of Clinical Psychiatry.* **61**: 26–29.

21 Worrel J *et al.* (2000) Atypical antipsychotic agents: a critical review. *American Journal of Health-System Pharmacy.* **57**: 238–358.

22 Geddes J *et al.* (2000) Atypical antipsychotics in the treatment of schizophrenia: systematic overview and meta-regression analysis. *British Medical Journal.* **321**: 1371–1376.

23 Passik S and Cooper M (1999) Complicated delirium in a cancer patient successfully treated with olanzapine. *Journal of Pain and Symptom Management.* **17**: 191–223.

24 Meehan K *et al.* (2002) Comparison of rapidly acting intramuscular olanzapine, lorazepam, and placebo: A double-blind, randomized study in acutely agitated patients with dementia. *Neuropsychopharmacology.* **26**: 494–504.

RISPERIDONE

Class: Atypical antipsychotic.

Indications: Acute and chronic psychoses, manic phase of bipolar disorder †delirium, †poor response to or drug-induced movement disorders with **haloperidol**.

Pharmacology

Risperidone is a potent D_2-receptor and $5HT_{2A}$-receptor antagonist.[1] It also binds to α_1-adrenergic receptors and with lower affinity to H_1- and α_2-receptors. Unlike **olanzapine**, risperidone does *not* bind to muscarinic receptors. Compared with **haloperidol**, a high-potency typical antipsychotic, the incidence of drug-induced movement disorders is less.[2,3] This may be because of the balanced central antagonism of serotonin (5HT) and dopamine. Even so, a retrospective survey reported that >25% of patients developed akathisia or parkinsonism.[4]

Although in animal studies risperidone is 4–10 times less potent than **haloperidol** as a central D_2-receptor antagonist,[1] it is several times more potent as an antipsychotic, presumably because of the dual impact on both D_2- and $5HT_2$-receptors. In schizophrenia, risperidone has an earlier onset of action than **haloperidol**,[3,5,6] and is associated with fewer relapses.[7] In delirium, hallucinations respond to risperidone within hours but generally only after 1–2 weeks in a psychotic illness; this is true of all antipsychotics.

The major metabolite of risperidone is 9-hydroxyrisperidone. This hydroxylation is subject to debrisoquine-type genetic CYP2D6-related polymorphism but, because both risperidone and its major metabolite are equally active, the efficacy of risperidone is unaffected.[8] Risperidone is more slowly eliminated in the elderly and in patients with renal impairment. Doses of risperidone should be decreased in patients with hepatic impairment because the mean free fraction of risperidone is increased by up to 35% as a result of decreased levels of albumin and α_1-acid glycoprotein.[9]

Risperidone is as effective as **haloperidol** in treating delirium.[10] Its efficacy as an anti-emetic has not been fully evaluated but it could be better than **haloperidol** because of its antagonism of $5HT_2$-receptors (see **Methotrimeprazine**, p.130). A retrospective review of 20 cancer patients given risperidone 1mg at bedtime for refractory opioid-induced nausea and vomiting reported complete resolution of nausea in 1/2 and a partial response in the other 1/2, with cessation of vomiting in 2/3.[11]

Risperidone can cause a weight gain of several kg particularly over the first 2 months; this is generally less than with other atypical antipsychotics but may be more marked if it is given together with **valproic acid** or **lithium**.[3,4]

Bio-availability 99%.

Time to peak plasma concentration 1–2h, not affected by food.

Onset of action hours–days in delirium; days–weeks in psychoses.

Plasma halflife of active fraction (risperidone + 9-hydroxyrisperidone) 24h.

Duration of action 12–48h, situation dependent.

Cautions

Because of an increase in mortality and cerebrovascular events,[12-14] risperidone should not be used as first-line drug treatment for behavioural symptoms in elderly patients with dementia (see p.126).

Risperidone can cause orthostatic hypotension, particularly initially, because of α-adrenergic receptor antagonism. Parkinson's disease (potentially could cause deterioration). Epilepsy (no direct evidence of a deleterious effect but typical antipsychotics and **clozapine**, an atypical antipsychotic, lower seizure threshold). Elderly patients and those with renal or hepatic impairment.

Carbamazepine has been shown to decrease the combined plasma concentration of risperidone and 9-hydroxyrisperidone. A similar effect might be anticipated with other drugs which stimulate metabolizing enzymes in the liver. On initiation of **carbamazepine** or other hepatic enzyme-inducing drugs, the dose of risperidone should be re-evaluated and increased if necessary. Conversely, on discontinuation of such drugs, the dose of risperidone should be re-evaluated and decreased if necessary.

Phenothiazines, TCAs and some β-blockers may increase the plasma concentrations of risperidone but not the combined concentration of risperidone and its active metabolite. **Fluoxetine** may increase the plasma concentration of risperidone but the impact on the combined concentration is less. A dose reduction of risperidone should be considered when **fluoxetine** is added to risperidone therapy. Based on *in vitro* studies, the same interaction may occur with **haloperidol**.

Undesirable effects

For full list, see manufacturer's Product Monograph.

Common (<10%, >1%): insomnia, agitation, anxiety, headache, movement disorders (see below), drowsiness, weight gain.

Uncommon (<1%, >0.1%): drowsiness, fatigue, dizziness, impaired concentration, seizures, blurred vision, syncope, dyspepsia, nausea and vomiting, constipation, sexual dysfunction (including priapism and erectile dysfunction), urinary incontinence, rhinitis.

The incidence and severity of drug-induced movement disorders are significantly less than with **haloperidol**.[15-17] Acute disorders are generally mild and are reversible if the dose is reduced and/or an antimuscarinic antiparkinsonian drug prescribed (see Drug-induced movement disorders, p.561).

Dose and use

Despite being commonly given b.i.d. there is no advantage in dividing the total daily dose, which can conveniently be given at bedtime.[18] Doses above 10mg/24h generally do not provide added benefit and may increase the risk of drug-induced movement disorders.

Psychosis

An atypical antipsychotic should be used preferentially in chronic psychoses:
- start with 1mg b.i.d.
- if necessary, increase to 2mg b.i.d. and 3mg b.i.d. on successive days
- in elderly patients and those with severe hepatic or renal impairment, the starting dose should be halved to 500microgram b.i.d. (or 1mg once daily) and titration extended over 6 days.[19]

Delirium
- start with 500microgram b.i.d. & p.r.n.
- if necessary, increase by 500microgram b.i.d. every other day
- median maintenance dose is 1mg/24h
- uncommon to need >3mg/24h.[10]

Supply

Risperidone (generic)
Tablets 250microgram, 500microgram, 1mg, 2mg, 3mg, 4mg, 28 days @ 500microgram b.i.d. = $25.
Oral solution 1mg/1mL, 28 days @ 500microgram b.i.d. = $22.

Risperdal® (Janssen-Ortho)
Tablets 250microgram, 500microgram, 1mg, 2mg, 3mg, 4mg, 28 days @ 500microgram b.i.d. = $53.
Tablets orodispersible (M-tab®) 500microgram, 1mg, 2mg, 3mg, 4mg, 28 days @ 500microgram b.i.d. = $44.
Oral solution 1mg/1mL, 28 days @ 500microgram b.i.d. = $42; *may be diluted with mineral water, orange juice or black coffee, do not mix with cola or tea.*

1 Green B (2000) Focus on risperidone. *Current Medical Research and Opinion.* **16**: 57–65.
2 Tooley P and Zuiderwijk P (1997) Drug safety: experience with risperidone. *Advances in Therapy.* **14**: 262–266.
3 Wirshing D *et al.* (1999) Risperidone in treatment-refractory schizophrenia. *American Journal of Psychiatry.* **156**: 1374–1379.
4 Guille C *et al.* (2000) A naturalistic comparison of clozapine, risperidone and olanzapine in the treatment of bipolar disorder. *Journal of Clinical Psychiatry.* **61**: 638–642.
5 Couinard G (1993) A Canadian multicenter placebo-controlled study of fixed doses of risperidone and haloperidol in the treatment of chronic schizophrenic patients. *Journal of Clinical Psychopharmacology.* **13**: 25–40.
6 Rabinowitz J *et al.* (2001) Rapid onset of therapeutic effect of risperidone versus haloperidol in a double-blind randomized trial. *Journal of Clinical Psychiatry.* **62**: 343–346.
7 Csernansky J *et al.* (2002) A comparison of risperidone and haloperidol for the prevention of relapse in patients with schizophrenia. *New England Journal of Medicine.* **346**: 16–22.
8 Bork J *et al.* (1999) A pilot study on risperidone metabolism: the role of cytochromes P450 2D6 and 3A. *Journal of Clinical Psychiatry.* **60**: 469–476.
9 Snoecke E *et al.* (1995) Influence of age, renal and liver impairment on the pharmacokinetics of risperidone in man. *Psychopharmacology (Berl).* **122**: 223–229.
10 Sipahimalani A *et al.* (1997) Treatment of delirium with risperidone. *International Journal of Geriatric Psychopharmacology.* **1**: 24–26.
11 Okamoto Y *et al.* (2007) A retrospective chart review of the antiemetic effectiveness of risperidone in refractory opioid-induced nausea and vomiting in advanced cancer patients. *Journal of Pain and Symptom Management.* **34**: 217–222.
12 Wooltorton E (2002) Risperidone (Risperdal): increased rate of cerebrovascular events in dementia trials. *Canadian Medical Association Journal.* **167**: 1269–1270.
13 Bullock R (2005) Treatment of behavioural and psychiatric symptoms in dementia: implications of recent safety warnings. *Current Medical Research and Opinion.* **21**: 1–10.
14 Schneider LS *et al.* (2005) Risk of death with atypical antipsychotic drug treatment for dementia: meta-analysis of randomized placebo-controlled trials. *Journal of the American Medical Association.* **294**: 1934–1943.
15 Umbricht D and Kane J (1995) Risperidone: efficacy and safety. *Schizophrenia Bulletin.* **21**: 593–606.
16 Jeste D *et al.* (1999) Lower incidence of tardive dyskinesia with risperidone compared with haloperidol in older patients. *Journal of the American Geriatric Society.* **47**: 716–719.
17 Geddes J *et al.* (2000) Atypical antipsychotics in the treatment of schizophrenia: systematic overview and meta-regression analysis. *British Medical Journal.* **321**: 1371–1376.
18 Nair N (1998) Therapeutic equivalence of risperidone given once daily and twice daily in patients with schizophrenia. The Risperidone Study. *Journal of Clinical Psychopharmacology.* **18**: 10–110.
19 Luchins D *et al.* (1998) Alteration in the recommended dosing schedule for risperidone. *American Journal of Psychiatry.* **155**: 365–366.

ANTIDEPRESSANTS

The range of antidepressants has increased considerably in recent years (Box 4.F).[1,2] Factors dictating choice include availability, cost, fashion, and a desire to minimize undesirable effects. Thus, although **amitriptyline** is widely available, inexpensive and has equal or better efficacy than other antidepressants,[3,4] it causes more undesirable effects.[5]

Undesirable effects can also sometimes be a limiting factor with newer antidepressants. For example, nausea and anxiety are common reasons for discontinuing an SSRI.[6] For patients with epilepsy, an SSRI or **venlafaxine** are good choices because they are less likely to cause seizures.[7]

Most classifications of antidepressants do not include psychostimulants. However, they are used increasingly in palliative care, particularly in patients who have a concurrent depressive illness but have a prognosis of <2–3 months. There is no doubt that they have an antidepressant effect,[8] and it is necessary to consider them when discussing treatment options for depressed patients (Box 4.F). However, the fact that **dextroamphetamine** and **methylphenidate** can be effective within hours–days raises the question as to how conventional antidepressants actually work. A prolonged time course to clinical benefit is more consistent with an effect mediated through intracellular protein neo-synthesis rather than through presynaptic mono-amine re-uptake inhibition, which may partly be an epiphenomenon.

Box 4.F Classification of antidepressants according to principal actions[a]

Mono-amine re-uptake inhibitors (MARIs)
Serotonin and norepinephrine (SNRIs or dual inhibitors)
Amitriptyline,[b] imipramine,[b] venlafaxine, duloxetine
Serotonin (selective serotonin re-uptake inhibitors, SSRIs)
Sertraline, citalopram, paroxetine, fluoxetine
Norepinephrine (NRIs)
Nortriptyline,[b] desipramine,[b,c] maprotiline
Norepinephrine and dopamine (NDRIs)
Bupropion

Dopamine release
Dextroamphetamine, methylphenidate[d]

Receptor antagonists[e]
Trazodone (α_1, $5HT_2$)
Mirtazapine (central α_2, $5HT_2$, $5HT_3$); noradrenergic and specific serotoninergic anti-depressant, NaSSA

Mono-amine oxidase inhibitors (MAOIs)[f]
Phenelzine, tranylcypromine

a. abbreviated names broadly reflect those found elsewhere;[2] confusion is inevitable because S is used for *Selective*, *Specific*, and *Serotonin*
b. TCAs differ in their modes of action, and do not comprise a single discrete drug class
c. also has a clinically unimportant effect on serotonin re-uptake
d. to a lesser extent, also stimulate release of norepinephrine and/or serotonin
e. antagonism of pre-synaptic α_2 receptors increases norepinephrine and serotonin release. Antagonism of post-synaptic $5HT_2$- and/or $5HT_3$-receptors facilitates increased $5HT_{1A}$ binding; this enhances the antidepressant effect
f. MAOIs are included for completeness; their use is *not* recommended.

Choice of antidepressants

Each palliative care service needs to make its own limited list of preferred antidepressants, and become familiar with their use (Box 4.G). The Canadian Psychiatric Association and other organizations have produced guidelines for the treatment of depression.[9–13] However, most data regarding antidepressants relate to medically stable psychiatric outpatients, and not to physically debilitated patients with a short prognosis, or the very elderly with incipient or overt dementia.[14]

There are special situations in which a particular antidepressant class merits consideration as first-line treatment. For example:
- dual pre-synaptic re-uptake inhibitors (SNRIs, e.g. **amitriptyline**, **imipramine**, **duloxetine**) if neuropathic pain is a co-morbidity with depression
- SSRIs, and TCAs such as **amitriptyline** and **imipramine**, if depression is associated with marked anxiety
- **mirtazapine**, or TCAs such as **amitriptyline** and **imipramine**, if sedation or appetite stimulation are desirable.

Antidepressants take time to work, particularly when slow dose escalation is necessary (in psychiatry, the typical interval between dose increments is 4 weeks). With TCAs, the median response time for depression in older patients is said to be 2–3 months.[15] **Mirtazapine** and **venlafaxine** appear to be faster-acting.[16,17] However, recently published meta-analyses of a large number of RCTs suggest that generally much of the total effect of antidepressants comes within the first 2 weeks of treatment.[18–20]

Cerebral stimulants are being used increasingly in patients with a prognosis of <2–3 months. With **methylphenidate** it is possible to evaluate the response after 24h. If necessary and if not limited by undesirable effects, the dose can be increased every until a satisfactory result is achieved (see p.168).

Box 4.G PCF preferred antidepressants

First-line antidepressants
Psychostimulant, e.g. methylphenidate
Particularly if prognosis < 2–3 months.

SSRI, e.g. sertraline, citalopram
Particularly if prognosis > 2–3 months, and if associated anxiety.
If no response at all after 4 weeks, consider switching to a second-line antidepressant; if partial response, wait a further 2 weeks.

Second-line antidepressants
Mirtazapine (noradrenergic and specific serotoninergic antidepressant, NaSSA)
If no response after 4 weeks, consider switching to a TCA or seek advice from a psychiatrist.

Tricyclic antidepressant (TCA), e.g. amitriptyline or imipramine (SNRI)
If no response after 8 weeks, seek advice from a psychiatrist/psycho-oncologist.

Anxiety is often present in depressive illness and may be the presenting symptom, thereby masking the true diagnosis. Thus, although they are useful adjuncts in agitated depression the use of antipsychotics or anxiolytics (benzodiazepines) in anxious patients as the primary drug treatment for severe anxiety should be monitored carefully. Indefinite maintenance therapy is recommended for patients who have had > 3 depressive episodes in the preceding 5 years.[21]

Antidepressants and pain management

The use of antidepressants in pain management is now widespread. **Duloxetine** is the only one licensed for this purpose (see p.235). Most of the early RCTs related to **amitriptyline**, although other TCAs are also effective. SNRIs are generally better than selective re-uptake inhibitors (SSRIs and NRIs; see p.235). A CADTH Health Technology Assessment concluded that TCAs were a more cost-effective option for neuropathic pain than **gabapentin** and **pregabalin** (anti-epileptics) and **duloxetine** and **venlafaxine** (SNRIs). Although the differences in effectiveness between drug classes were not statistically significant, the number of patients needed to be treated to obtain a response in one patient (NNT) was always lowest with TCAs and highest with SNRIs, regardless of the design of the comparison and whether a response was classed as a 50% or a 30% reduction in pain. Further, switching all patients from TCAs to the recently-introduced SNRI **duloxetine** would increase government health costs by $171 million p.a.[22] However, some data suggest that certain newer antidepressants may have a niche position in the treatment of certain specific types of chronic pain states.[23]

Antidepressants and platelet function

SSRIs (e.g. **fluoxetine**, **paroxetine**, **sertraline**) and SNRIs (e.g. **amitriptyline**, **imipramine**, **venlafaxine**, **duloxetine**) decrease serotonin uptake from the blood by platelets. Because platelets do not synthesize serotonin, the amount of serotonin in platelets is reduced.[24] This adversely affects platelet aggregation.[25] After confounding factors have been controlled for, serotonin re-uptake inhibitors increase the risk of GI bleeding 3-fold.[26,27] This may be important in already high-risk patients. If an antidepressant is indicated in such patients, consider gastroprotection (although no direct evidence of benefit) or an alternative (e.g. **mirtazapine**).

Serotonin toxicity

Serotonin toxicity results from the ingestion of drug(s) which increase brain serotonin to levels sufficient to cause severe symptoms necessitating hospital admission and medical intervention.[28] Individuals vary in their susceptibility, but a continued increase in serotonin levels will inevitably lead to toxicity (cf. **digoxin** toxicity).

Serotonin toxicity has been characterized as a triad of neuro-excitatory features:

- *autonomic hyperactivity*; sweating, fever, mydriasis, tachycardia, hypertension, tachypnea, sialorrhea, diarrhea
- *neuromuscular hyperactivity*; tremor, clonus, myoclonus, hyperreflexia, and pyramidal rigidity (advanced stage)
- *altered mental status*; agitation, hypomania, and delirium (advanced stage).

Clonus (inducible, spontaneous or ocular), agitation, sweating, tremor and hyperreflexia are essential features. Spontaneous clonus, in the presence of a serotoninergic drug (Box 4.H), is the most reliable indicator of serotonin toxicity.[29]

Box 4.H Drugs with clinically relevant serotoninergic potency[28,30,31]

Antidepressants
Monoamine oxidase inhibitors (MAOIs)
All types (non-selective or selective type A/type B; reversible or irreversible)
e.g. moclobemide, phenelzine, tranylcypromine

Selective serotonin re-uptake inhibitors (SSRIs)
Citalopram, fluoxetine, fluvoxamine, paroxetine, sertraline

Serotonin and norepinephrine re-uptake inhibitors (SNRIs)
Clomipramine, duloxetine, imipramine, venlafaxine (but not other TCAs)

Psychostimulants (serotonin releasers)
Dextroamphetamine, methylenedioxymethamphetamine (MDMA, Ecstasy) (but not methylphenidate)

Other drugs
H$_1$-antihistamines (serotonin re-uptake inhibitors)
Chlorpheniramine, brompheniramine (but not other H$_1$-antihistamines)

Opioids (serotonin re-uptake inhibitors)
Dextromethorphan, propoxyphene, fentanils, methadone, pentazocine, meperidine, tramadol (but not other opioids)

Miscellaneous
MAOIs
Furazolidone, linezolid (antibiotics)
Methylene blue
Procarbazine (antineoplastic)
Selegiline (antiparkinsonian)

SNRI
Sibutramine (anorectic)

Because different drugs increase serotonin levels to differing degrees via different mechanisms, there is a characteristic degree of severity associated with each type of drug when taken by itself, either in normal therapeutic doses, or in overdose.

The older irreversible MAOIs have the greatest ability to increase serotonin levels. Thus an overdose of an MAOI like **tranylcypromine** alone will produce hyperpyrexia, and even death,[32] but not the RIMA **moclobemide**.[33]

Overdoses of SSRIs will cause serotoninergic effects but rarely (if ever) life-threatening serotonin toxicity.[34] Thus, death from serotonin toxicity is generally associated with the combination of two different types of drug which elevate serotonin levels via different mechanisms of action. Fatal combinations in overdose have been:

- MAOIs and SSRIs ($\geqslant$50% probability of life-threatening serotonin toxicity)[33,35]
- MAOIs with serotonin releasers, e.g. **dextroamphetamine** and **MDMA**, generally a result of illicit use
- SSRIs or SNRIs and triptans (antimigraine drugs).[36]

Opioids are relatively weak serotonin re-uptake inhibitors and may only cause symptoms in higher doses or susceptible individuals. Fatalities from serotonin toxicity involving opioids have been with **dextromethorphan, meperidine, tramadol**, and possibly **fentanyl**.[30]

The onset of toxicity is generally rapid and progressive, typically as the second drug reaches effective blood levels (one or two doses). Occasionally, recurrent mild symptoms may occur for weeks before the development of severe toxicity. The patient is often alert or agitated, with tremor (sometimes severe), myoclonus and hyperreflexia. Ankle clonus is generally demonstrable or, in severe toxicity, occurs spontaneously. Neuromuscular signs are initially greater in the lower limbs, then become more generalized as toxicity increases. Other symptoms include shaking, shivering (often including chattering of the teeth), and sometimes trismus.

Pyramidal rigidity is a late development in severe cases, and can impair respiration. Rigidity, a fever of $>38.5°C$ or deteriorating blood gases indicate life-threatening toxicity. Drugs which block $5\text{-}HT_{2A}$ post-synaptic receptors, e.g. **chlorpromazine**, prevent deaths from hyperpyrexia in animals and probably in humans too.

Generally give IM; the PO route is suitable only for patients with mild toxicity who, in the case of overdoses, have *not* received oral activated charcoal (Box 4.I).[37,38]

Box 4.I Treatment of serotonin toxicity[39]

Severe cases should be managed in an intensive care unit.
Discontinue causal medication (toxicity generally resolves within 24h).
Provide supportive care, e.g. IV fluids.
Symptomatic measures:
- benzodiazepines for agitation, myoclonus and seizures, e.g. midazolam 5–10mg SC p.r.n.
- $5HT_{2A}$ antagonists, e.g.:
  ▷ chlorpromazine 50–100mg IM
  ▷ olanzapine 10mg IM
  ▷ cyproheptadine 12mg PO stat followed by 8mg q6h and 2mg q2h p.r.n. until symptoms resolve; tablets can be crushed and given by enteral feeding tube
- stabilization of blood pressure:
  ▷ hypotension from MAOI interactions, give low doses of a sympathomimetic, e.g. epinephrine, norepinephrine, phenylephrine
  ▷ hypertension, give short-acting agents, e.g. nitroprusside (a vasodilator), esmolol (β-adrenergic receptor antagonist).
If severe hyperthermia ($>41°C$), consider immediate:
- sedation
- neuromuscular paralysis with a non-depolarizing agent, e.g. vecuronium
- ventilation.

Characteristics of selected classes of antidepressant
Tricyclic antidepressants (TCAs)
As noted in Box 4.F (see p.139), in terms of mechanisms of action, attempting to group TCAs under one heading is misleading. Collectively, TCAs have a range of actions, including:
- blockade of re-uptake by presynaptic terminals of:
  ▷ serotonin (5-hydroxytryptamine, 5HT) ⎱ responsible for antidepressant
  ▷ norepinephrine ⎰ and analgesic effects
- receptor blockade:
  ▷ muscarinic, responsible for benefit in urgency and bladder spasms
  ▷ H_1-histaminergic, responsible for sedation ⎱ tend to be correlated
  ▷ α_1-adrenergic, responsible for postural hypotension ⎰

The principal differences between TCAs relate to their monoamine re-uptake inhibiting properties. Thus, by virtue of an active metabolite with differing properties, **amitriptyline, clomipramine** and **imipramine** inhibit the presynaptic re-uptake of both serotonin and norepinephrine (SNRIs), whereas **desipramine** and **nortriptyline** are relatively selective norepinephrine re-uptake inhibitors (NRIs); they cause less postural hypotension, are less antimuscarinic, and are generally less sedative.

These differences are important, particularly for frail elderly patients, and may well determine which TCA is prescribed. All TCAs are Class 1A anti-arrhythmics, and can be pro-arrhythmic at higher doses, and in patients with pre-existing cardiac conduction disturbances.

Sedative effects are more common in physically ill patients, particularly if receiving other psycho-active drugs, including opioids. TCAs are widely used for chronic pain management (particularly neuropathic pain, see p.235) and for bladder spasms. The antimuscarinic effect of these drugs is responsible for their constipating effect (see p.5).

Before prescribing a TCA, practitioners should take into account:
- their poorer tolerability compared with other equally effective antidepressants
- the increased risk of cardiotoxicity
- their toxicity in overdose.

Selective serotonin re-uptake inhibitors (SSRIs)

SSRIs selectively block the presynaptic re-uptake of serotonin.[40,41] Compared with TCAs, SSRIs are unlikely to cause weight gain, sedation, delirium, cardiac arrhythmias or heart block. Apart from **paroxetine**, SSRIs do not have antimuscarinic effects but may cause extrapyramidal effects (see Drug-induced movement disorders, p.561). SSRIs can also cause serotonin toxicity, but generally only when given with a second drug which also increases synaptic serotonin concentrations (see p.140).

SSRIs often initially cause nausea as a consequence of increased serotonin activity in the GI tract and possibly via central $5HT_3$-receptors. $5HT_3$-receptor antagonists are effective anti-emetics in this situation.[42] Some SSRIs significantly inhibit the hepatic cytochrome P450 enzyme system, e.g. **fluvoxamine** (CYP1A2) and **paroxetine** (CYP2D6).[43] **Fluoxetine** is associated with a higher propensity for drug interactions.[12]

The efficacy of SSRIs in neuropathic pain relief is not completely clear.[23] In randomized controlled trials in diabetic neuropathy and post-herpetic neuralgia, **fluoxetine** and **zimelidine** (not Canada) were no better than placebo.[44–46] On the other hand, **paroxetine** and **sertraline** have been shown to relieve diabetic neuropathic pain.[47,48] Relief correlates with plasma drug concentrations; a **paroxetine** plasma concentration above 150 nmol/L provides relief similar to that obtained with **imipramine** and with fewer undesirable effects.[47] **Paroxetine** and **sertraline** are of value in some patients with pruritus (see Box 5.O p.339).[49]

St John's wort (Hypericum extract)

Although **St John's wort** is of benefit in mild–moderate depression, health professionals should *not* prescribe or advise its use by patients because of:
- uncertainty about appropriate doses
- variation in the nature of preparations
- potential serious interactions with other drugs (including oral contraceptives, anticoagulants and anti-epileptics).[12]

St John's wort is a popular OTC antidepressant. It is as effective as **imipramine** and **amitriptyline** in treating mild–moderate depression and causes fewer undesirable effects.[50–54] If OTC **St John's wort** is combined with prescription antidepressants, there is a risk of developing serotonin toxicity (see p.140).[55,56]

Mono-amine oxidase inhibitors (MAOIs)

Included for general information. MAOIs are *not recommended* as antidepressants in palliative care patients. MAOIs can cause serious adverse events when prescribed concurrently with various other drugs.

The use of an MAOI is potentially dangerous because of the risk of a hypertensive crisis precipitated by dietary factors and/or a drug interaction, and the risk of serotonin toxicity caused by a drug interaction (see p.140).

Hypertensive crises are mainly associated with the consumption of tyramine-containing foods, and the excessive production and accumulation of norepinephrine (Table 4.10). Hypertensive crises can also occur as a result of an interaction with a drug which has a direct or indirect sympathomimetic effect, e.g. **ephedrine**, **pseudephedrine**, **dextroamphetamine**, TCAs, and even SSRIs. They have also been reported when an MAOI and **meperidine** have been given concurrently, but not with other opioids (Box 4.J).[57–59] Typically, the patient experiences severe headache, and may suffer an intracranial hemorrhage.

Table 4.10 Tyramine-containing foods associated with MAOI-related syndrome

Alcohol	Meat (smoked or pickled)
red wine (white wine is safe)	Meat or yeast extracts
beer	Bovril
Broad bean pods	Oxo
Cheese (old)	Marmite
Fava beans	Pickled herring

Box 4.J A misleading report about morphine and MAOIs[57]

A patient who regularly took an MAOI and trifluoperazine 20mg/24h was given pre-operative promethazine 50mg IM and morphine 1mg IV followed by two doses of morphine 2.5mg IV. About 3min later she became unresponsive and hypotensive (systolic pressure 40mmHg); responding within 2min to IV naloxone. Although repeatedly referenced as such, this was not MAOI-related serotonin toxicity; it was a hypotensive response to IV morphine in someone chronically taking trifluoperazine, an α-adrenergic antagonist.

General cautions
- the possibility of a suicide attempt is inherent in major depression and persists until the antidepressant medication has induced a remission
- serotonin toxicity is a potential hazard with most antidepressants (see p.140)
- hyponatremia (usually in the elderly and possibly due to inappropriate secretion of ADH) has been associated with all types of antidepressants and should be considered in all patients who develop drowsiness, confusion or seizures when taking an antidepressant.

Undesirable effects
These vary from antidepressant to antidepressant (see individual drug monographs). A synopsis is contained in Table 4.11.

Switching antidepressants
When switching from one antidepressant to another, prescribers should be aware of the need for gradual and modest incremental increases of dose, of interactions between antidepressants and the risk of serotonin toxicity when combinations of serotoninergic antidepressants are prescribed.[12]

Alternative routes of administration
Generally, antidepressants are given PO, or not at all. However, in specific circumstances, the following routes have been utilized:
- buccal, e.g. **amitriptyline** by crushing and dissolving tablets and retaining the solution in the mouth[60]
- rectal, e.g. fluoxetine, imipramine or trazodone[61,62]
- IV, e.g. TCAs (**amitriptyline**, **clomipramine** and **imipramine**)[63–66] and SSRIs (**citalopram**); risk of a cardiac arrhythmia (*not* available as injections in Canada).

Table 4.11 Undesirable effects of antidepressant drugs[9]

Class and drug	Anti-muscarinic	Sedation	Insomnia/agitation	Postural hypotension	Nausea/GI	Sexual dysfunction	Weight gain	Specific effects	Inhibition of liver enzymes	Lethality in overdose
SNRIs								Serotonin toxicity[a] (see Box 4.H)		
Amitriptyline	++	++	–	++	–	++	++		++	High
Imipramine	++	++	++	++	–	++	++		++	High
Clomipramine	++	++	++	++	++	++	+		++	High
Venlafaxine	–	–	+	–	++	++	–	Dose-related hypertension	–	Low
NRIs										
Desipramine, nortriptyline	+	+	+	+	–	+	–		++	High
SSRIs								Serotonin toxicity[a] (see Box 4.H)		
Citalopram, sertraline	–	–	++	–	++	++	–		–	Low
Fluoxetine	–	–	++	–	++	++	–	Initial nausea and vomiting	++	Low
Paroxetine	+	–	++	–	++	++	–		++	Low
Receptor antagonists										
Trazodone	–	++	–	++	–	–	+	Priapism	?	Low
Mirtazapine	–	++	–	–	–	–	++		–	Low

Key: ++ = relatively common or strong; + = may occur or moderately strong; – = absent or rare/weak; ? = unknown/insufficient information.
Abbreviations: NRI = norepinephrine re-uptake inhibitor; SNRI = serotonin and norepinephrine re-uptake inhibitor; SSRI = selective serotonin re-uptake inhibitor.
a. antidepressants which inhibit serotonin re-uptake transport are all possible causes of serotonin toxicity, particularly if given in conjunction with a second drug which enhances serotonin release or also inhibits pre-synaptic re-uptake (see p.140).

Stopping antidepressants

Antidepressants are normally maintained for 6–12 months after resolution of the depression. In palliative care, this effectively means indefinitely. However, when a patient is close to death and swallowing has become burdensome, it is important to reduce the tablet burden. As with all psychotropic drugs, it is generally advisable to tail off the medication, and not stop it abruptly.

Abrupt cessation of antidepressant therapy (particularly an MAOI) after regular administration for >8 weeks may result in withdrawal phenomena.[67] Discontinuation reactions are different from recurrence of the primary psychiatric disorder. They generally start abruptly within a few days of stopping the antidepressant (or of reducing its dose) and may last up to 3 weeks. In contrast, a depressive relapse is uncommon in the first week after stopping an antidepressant, and symptoms tend to build up gradually and persist.

Discontinuation reactions vary, and depend on the class of antidepressant. Common symptoms include:
- GI disturbance (nausea, abdominal pain, diarrhea)
- sleep disturbance (insomnia, vivid dreams, nightmares)
- general somatic distress (sweating, lethargy, headaches)
- affective symptoms (low mood, anxiety, irritability).

With SSRIs the commonest symptoms are dizziness/lightheadedness and sensory abnormalities, e.g. numbness, paresthesia, and electric shock-like sensations (Box 4.K). **Citalopram** and **fluoxetine** are generally associated with fewer discontinuation symptoms.[12]

Discontinuation reactions generally resolve within 24h of re-instating antidepressant therapy, whereas the response is slower with a depressive relapse.

Box 4.K   SSRI withdrawal syndrome[68]

Somatic symptoms	Psychological symptoms
Disequilibrium	*Core*
Dizziness/lightheadness	Anxiety/agitation
Vertigo	Crying spells
Ataxia	Irritability
GI symptoms	*Other*
Nausea	Overactivity
Vomiting	Decreased concentration/slowed thinking
	Memory problems
Flu-like symptoms	Depersonalization
Fatigue	Lowered mood
Lethargy	Delirium
Myalgia	
Chills	
Sensory disturbance	
Paresthesia	
Sensations of electric shock	
Sleep disturbances	
Insomnia	
Vivid dreams	

Thus, ideally, to reduce the likelihood of discontinuation reactions, antidepressants which have been continuously prescribed for >8 weeks should be progressively reduced over 4 weeks. Tapering is unnecessary when switching between SSRIs. If a discontinuation reaction is suspected, the antidepressant should be restarted and reduced more gradually. However, if mild, re-assurance alone may be adequate ± a benzodiazepine to overcome insomnia.

---

1   Stahl S (1998) Basic psychopharmacology of antidepressants, part 1: antidepressants have seven distinct mechanisms of action. *Journal of Clinical Psychiatry.* **59**: 5–14.

2   Stahl S (2000) *Essential Psychopharmacology: Neuroscientific Basis and Practical Applications* (2e). Cambridge University Press, Cambridge, pp. 199–295.

3   Barbui C and Hotopf M (2001) Amitriptyline v. the rest: still the leading antidepressant after 40 years of randomised controlled trials. *British Journal of Psychiatry.* **178**: 129–144.

4   Thompson C (2001) Amitriptyline: still efficacious, but at what cost? *British Journal of Psychiatry.* **178**: 99–100.

5   Martin R et al. (1997) General practitioner's perception of the tolerability of antidepressant drugs: a comparison of selective serotonin reuptake inhibitors and tricyclic antidepressants. *British Medical Journal.* **314**: 646–651.

6   Trindade E et al. (1998) Adverse effects associated with selective reuptake inhibitors and tricyclic antidepressants: a meta-analysis. *Canadian Medical Association Journal.* **17**: 1245–1252.

7   Montgomery SA (2005) Antidepressants and seizures: emphasis on newer agents and clinical implications. *International Journal of Clinical Practice.* **59**: 1435–1440.

8   Homsi J et al. (2000) Psychostimulants in supportive care. *Supportive Care in Cancer.* **8**: 385–397.

9   APA (American Psychiatric Association) (2000) Practice guideline for the treatment of patients with major depressive disorder. Available from: www.guideline.gov/summary/summary.aspx?ss=15&doc_id=2605&nbr=1831

10 Canadian Psychiatric Association and Canadian Network for Mood and Anxiety Treatments (2001) Clinical guidelines for the treatment of depressive disorders. *Canadian Journal of Psychiatry.* **46 (suppl 1)**.

11 Lam RW and Kennedy SH (2004) Prescribing antidepressants for depression in 2005: recent concerns and recommendations. *Canadian Journal of Psychiatry.* **49**: 1–6.

12 NICE (2004) Depression: Management of depression in primary and secondary care. In: *National Clinical Practice Guideline Number 23.* National Institute for Clinical Excellence. Available from: www.nice.org.uk/page.aspx?o=236667

13 Fochtmann LJ and Gelenberg AJ (2005) Guideline watch: practice guideline for the treatment of patients with major depressive disorder. Available from: www.psychiatryonline.com/pracGuide/pracGuideTopic_7.aspx

14 Flint AJ (1998) Choosing appropriate antidepressant therapy in the elderly. A risk-benefit assessment of available agents. *Drugs Aging.* **13**: 269–280.

15 Reynolds C et al. (1998) Effects of age at onset of first lifetime episode of recurrent major depression on treatment response and illness course in elderly patients. *American Journal of Psychiatry.* **155**: 795–799.

16 Burrows G and Kremer C (1997) Mirtazapine: clinical advantages in the treatment of depression. *Journal of Clinical Psychopharmacology.* **1**: 34–39.

17 Thase M et al. (2001) Remission rates during treatment with venlafaxine or selective serotonin reuptake inhibitors. *British Journal of Psychiatry.* **178**: 234–241.

18 Posternak MA and Zimmerman M (2005) Is there a delay in the antidepressant effect? A meta-analysis. *Journal of Clinical Psychiatry.* **66**: 148–158.

19 Taylor MJ et al. (2006) Early onset of selective serotonin reuptake inhibitor antidepressant action: systematic review and meta-analysis. *Archives of General Psychiatry.* **63**: 1217–1223.

20 Tylee A and Walters P (2007) Onset of action of antidepressants. *British Medical Journal.* **334**: 911–912.

21 Edwards J (1998) Long term pharmacotherapy of depression. *British Medical Journal.* **316**: 1180–1181.

22 Iskedjian M et al. (2009) Anticonvulsants, serotonin-norepinephrine reuptake inhibitors, and tricyclic antidepressants in mangement of neuropathic pain: a meta-analysis and economic evaluation (Technology report number 116). Canadian Agency for Drugs and Technologies in Health, Ottawa. Available from: www.cadth.ca/index.php/en/hta/reports-publications/search/publication/870

23 Ansari A (2000) The efficacy of newer antidepressants in the treatment of chronic pain: a review of current literature. *Harvard Review of Psychiatry.* **7**: 257–277.

24 Ross S et al. (1980) Inhibition of 5-hydroxytryptamine uptake in human platelets by antidepressant agents in vivo. *Psychopharmacology.* **67**: 1–7.

25 Li N et al. (1997) Effects of serotonin on platelet activation in whole blood. *Blood Coagulation Fibrinolysis.* **8**: 517–523.

26 vanWalraven C et al. (2001) Inhibition of serotonin reuptake by antidepressants and upper gastrointestinal bleeding in elderly patients: retrospective cohort study. *British Medical Journal.* **323**: 655–657.

27 Paton C and Ferrier IN (2005) SSRIs and gastrointestinal bleeding. *British Medical Journal.* **331**: 529–530.

28 Gillman P (2006) Serotonin toxicity, serotonin syndrome: 2006 update, overview and analysis. Available from: www.psychotropical.com

29 Dunkley EJ et al. (2003) The Hunter Serotonin Toxicity Criteria: simple and accurate diagnostic decision rules for serotonin toxicity. *Quarterly Journal of Medicine.* **96**: 635–642.

30 Gillman PK (2005) Monoamine oxidase inhibitors, opioid analgesics and serotonin toxicity. *British Journal of Anaesthesia.* **95**: 434–441.

31 Gillman PK (2006) A review of serotonin toxicity data: implications for the mechanisms of antidepressant drug action. *Biological Psychiatry.* **59**: 1046–1051.

32 Whyte I (2004) Monoamine oxidase inhibitors. In: RC Dart (ed) *Medical Toxicology.* Lippincott Williams & Wilkins, Baltimore, pp. 823–834.

33 Isbister GK et al. (2003) Moclobemide poisoning: toxicokinetics and occurrence of serotonin toxicity. *British Journal of Clinical Pharmacology.* **56**: 441–450.

34 Isbister GK et al. (2004) Relative toxicity of selective serotonin reuptake inhibitors (SSRIs) in overdose. *Journal of Toxicology: Clinical Toxicology.* **42**: 277–285.

35 Gillman K (2004) Moclobemide and the risk of serotonin toxicity (or serotonin syndrome). *CNS Drug Reviews.* **10**: 83–85; author reply 86–88.

36 FDA (2006) FDA public health advisory. Combined use of 5-hydroxytryptamine receptor agonists (triptans), selective serotonin reuptake inhibitors (SSRIs) or selective serotonin/norepinephrine reuptake inhibitors (SNRIs) may result in life-threatening serotonin syndrome. Food and Drugs Administration. Available from: www.fda.gov/Drugs/DrugSafety/PublicHealthAdvisories/ucm124349.htm

37 Gillman PK (1998) Serotonin syndrome: history and risk. *Fundamental and Clinical Pharmacology.* **12**: 482–491.

38 Gillman PK (1999) The serotonin syndrome and its treatment. *Journal of Psychopharmacology* **13**: 100–109.

39 Boyer EW and Shannon M (2005) The serotonin syndrome. *New England Journal of Medicine.* **352**: 1112–1120.

40 Finley P (1994) Selective serotonin reuptake inhibitors: pharmacologic profiles and potential therapeutic distinctions. *Annals of Pharmacotherapy.* **28**: 1359–1369.

41 Edwards G and Anderson I (1999) Systematic review and guide to selection of selective serotonin reuptake inhibitors. *Drugs.* **57**: 507–533.

42 Bailey J et al. (1995) The 5HT3 antagonist ondansetron reduces gastrointestinal side effects induced by a specific serotonin re-uptake inhibitor in man. *Journal of Psychopharmacology.* **9**: 137–141.

43 Richelson E (1997) Pharmacokinetic drug interactions of new antidepressants: A review of the effects on the metabolism of other drugs. *Mayo Clinic Proceedings.* **72**: 835–847.

44 Max M et al. (1992) Effects of desipramine, amitriptyline, and fluoxetine on pain in diabetic neuropathy. *New England Journal of Medicine.* **326**: 1287–1288.

45 Watson C and Evans R (1985) A comparative trial of amitriptyline and zimelidine in postherpetic neuralgia. *Pain.* **23**: 387–394.

46 Lynch S et al. (1990) Efficacy of antidepressants in relieving diabetic neuropathy pain: amitriptyline vs. desipramine and fluoxetine vs. placebo. *Neurology.* **40**: 437.

47 Sindrup S et al. (1990) The selective serotonin re-uptake inhibitor paroxetine is effective in the treatment of diabetic neuropathy symptoms. *Pain.* **42**: 135–144.

48 Goodnick P et al. (1997) Sertraline in diabetic neuropathy: preliminary results. *Annals of Clinical Psychiatry.* **9**: 255–257.

49 Mayo MJ et al. (2007) Sertraline as a first-line treatment for cholestatic pruritus. *Hepatology.* **45**: 666–674.

50 Vorbach E et al. (1997) Efficacy and tolerability of St John's wort extract LI160 versus imipramine in patients with severe depressive episodes according to ICD10. *Pharmacopsychiatry.* **30**: 81–85.

51 Wheatley D (1997) LI160, an extract of St John's wort versus amitriptyline in mildly to moderately depressed outpatients – a controlled 6-week clinical trial. *Pharmacopsychiatry.* **30**: 77–80.

52 Gaster B and Holroyd J (2000) St John's wort for depression: a systematic review. *Archives of Internal Medicine.* **160**: 152–156.

53 Woelk H (2000) Comparison of St John's wort and imipramine for treating depression: randomised controlled trial. *British Medical Journal.* **321**: 536–539.

54 Linde K and Mulrow C (2001) St. John's wort for depression. *The Cochrane Database of Systematic Reviews.* **2**: CD000448.

55 Lantz M et al. (1999) St John's wort and antidepressant drug interactions in the elderly. *Journal of Geriatric Psychiatry and Neurology.* **12**: 7–10.

56 Anonymous (2000) St. John's wort (Hypericum perforatum) interactions. *Current Problems in Pharmacovigilance.* **26**: 6–7.

57 Barry B (1979) Adverse effects of MAO inhibitors with narcotics reversed with naloxone. *Anaesthesia and Intensive Care.* **7**: 194.

58 Browne B and Linter S (1987) Monoamine oxidase inhibitors and narcotic analgesics. A critical review of the implications for treatment. *British Journal of Psychiatry.* **151**: 210–212.

59 Stockley I (2006) *Drug Interactions* (7e). Pharmaceutical Press, London, pp. 869–870.

60 Robbins B and Reiss RA (1999) Amitriptyline absorption in a patient with short bowel syndrome. *American Journal of Gastroenterology.* **94**: 2302–2304.

61 Thompson D and DiMartini A (1999) Nonenteral routes of administration for psychiatric medications. A literature review. *Psychosomatics.* **40**: 185–192.

62 Davis M et al. (2002) Symptom control in cancer patients: the clinical pharmacology and therapeutic role of suppositories and rectal suspensions. *Supportive Care in Cancer.* **10**: 117–138.

63 Brasseur R (1979) Study of intravenous amitriptyline in acute depressions (author's transl). *Acta Psychiatrica Belgica.* **79**: 96–108.

64 Pollock BG et al. (1989) Acute antidepressant effect following pulse loading with intravenous and oral clomipramine. *Archives of General Psychiatry.* **46**: 29–35.

65 Sallee FR et al. (1989) Intravenous pulse loading of clomipramine in adolescents with depression. *Psychopharmacology Bulletin.* **25**: 114–118.

66 Koelle JS and Dimsdale JE (1998) Antidepressants for the virtually eviscerated patient: options instead of oral dosing. *Psychosomatic Medicine.* **60**: 723–725.

67 Haddad P et al. (1998) Antidepressant discontinuation reactions. *British Medical Journal.* **316**: 1105–1106.

68 Schatzberg A et al. (1997) Serotonin reuptake inhibitor discontinuation syndrome: a hypothetical definition. *Journal of Clinical Psychiatry.* **58**: 5–10.

Guidelines: Depression

Sadness and tears alone, even if associated with transient suicidal thoughts, do not justify the diagnosis of depression or the prescription of an antidepressant. Patients may have an adjustment reaction and/or become demoralized. These do not respond to antidepressants, but may improve with psychosocial support and time.

Evaluation

1 Screening: about 5–10% of patients with advanced cancer develop a major depression. Cases will be missed unless specific enquiry is made of all patients:

'What has your mood been like lately?.... Are you depressed?'

'Have you had serious depression before? Are things like that now?'

2 Assessment interview: if depression is suspected, explore the patient's mood more fully by encouraging the patient to talk further with appropriate prompts. Symptoms overlap with those of cancer (e.g. loss of weight, lack of energy, fatigue) making diagnosis more difficult. The following are suggestive of clinical depression:

- sustained low mood (most of every day for several weeks) ⎱ core symptoms
- sustained loss of pleasure/interest in life (anhedonia) ⎰
- withdrawal from family and friends
- insomnia or hypersomnia
- psychomotor agitation or retardation
- impaired concentration (indecisiveness)
- feelings of worthlessness (or excessive guilt)
- indecisiveness or diminished ability to concentrate
- persistent suicidal ideas, and requests for euthanasia.

3 If in doubt whether the patient is suffering from depression, an adjustment reaction or sadness, review after 1–2 weeks and/or obtain the help of a psychologist/psychiatrist.

4 Medical causes of depression: depression may be the consequence of:
- a medical condition, e.g. hypercalcemia, cerebral metastases
- a reaction to severe uncontrolled physical symptoms
- drugs, e.g. cytotoxics, benodiazepines, antipsychotics, corticosteroids, antihypertensives.

Management

5 Correct the correctable: treat medical causes, particularly severe pain and other distressing symptoms.

6 Non-drug treatment:
- explanation, and assurance that depression generally responds to treatment
- if available, depressed patients generally benefit from attendance at a Palliative Care Day Centre
- specific psychological treatments (via a clinical psychologist, etc.)
- other psychosocial professionals (e.g. chaplain, art therapist) have a therapeutic role but avoid overwhelming the patient with simultaneous multiple referrals.

7 Drug treatment:
- if the patient is expected to live for more than 2–3 weeks, prescribe an antidepressant (see below)
- the initial and continuing doses are generally lower in debilitated patients compared with the physically fit
- antidepressants can cause withdrawal symptoms if stopped abruptly; generally reduce the dose gradually over 2–3 weeks
- except for MAOIs, when switching from one antidepressant class to another, overlap the withdrawal of the old antidepressant with the gradual introduction of the new antidepressant over 2–3 weeks.

continued

PCF preferred antidepressants

First-line antidepressants
Psychostimulant, e.g. methylphenidate
Particularly if prognosis <2–3 months:
- start with 2.5–5mg b.i.d. (on waking/breakfast time and noon/lunchtime)
- if necessary, increase by daily increments of 2.5mg b.i.d. to 20mg b.i.d.
- occasionally higher doses are necessary, e.g. 30mg b.i.d. or 20mg t.i.d.

SSRI, e.g. sertraline
Particularly if prognosis >2–3 months, and if associated anxiety:
- no antimuscarinic effects, but may cause an initial increase in anxiety
- if necessary, prescribe diazepam at bedtime
- start with sertraline 50mg once daily, preferably p.c.
- if no improvement after 2 weeks, increase dose by 50mg every 2–4 weeks
- maximum dose 200mg/24 hours
- low likelihood of a withdrawal (discontinuation) syndrome.
If no response at all after 4 weeks, switch to a second-line antidepressant; but if partial response, wait a further 2 weeks.

Second-line antidepressants
Mirtazapine
A good choice for patients with anxiety/agitation:
- starting dose 15mg at bedtime
- if little or no improvement after 2 weeks, increase to 30mg at bedtime
- concurrent H_1-receptor antagonism leads to sedation but this decreases at the higher dose because of noradrenergic effects.
- fewer undesirable effects than TCAs.
If no response after 4 weeks, switch to a TCA or seek advice from a psychiatrist.

Tricyclic antidepressant (TCA), e.g. amitriptyline or imipramine (SNRI)
- start with 10–25mg at bedtime
- if tolerated, after 3–7 days increase to 25–50mg at bedtime
- if limited improvement, increase dose by 25mg every 4 weeks to 75–150mg at bedtime
- undesirable effects, e.g. dry mouth, sedation, may limit dose escalation.
If no response after 8 weeks, seek advice from a psychiatrist.

AMITRIPTYLINE

Class: Tricyclic antidepressant (TCA), serotonin and norepinephrine re-uptake inhibitor (SNRI).

Indications: Depression, nocturnal enuresis in children, [†]panic disorder, [†]neuropathic pain, [†]urgency of micturition, [†]urge incontinence, [†]bladder spasms, [†]sialorrhea.

Contra-indications: Concurrent administration with an MAOI (see Serotonin toxicity, p.140), recent myocardial infarction, arrhythmias (particularly any degree of heart block), CHF, mania, severe hepatic impairment.

Pharmacology
Amitriptyline blocks the presynaptic re-uptake of serotonin and norepinephrine, and thereby exerts antidepressant and analgesic effects. In addition, it antagonizes muscarinic receptors, H_1-receptors, and α_1-adrenergic receptors.[1] It is these features which account for many of

---

amitriptyline's properties, e.g. antimuscarinic effects (see p.5), drowsiness, and postural hypotension. Amitriptyline may also act as a NMDA-receptor antagonist.[2] Its sedative effect manifests immediately, and improved sleep is often the first benefit of therapy. The analgesic effect may manifest after 3–7 days, whereas the antidepressant effect may not be apparent for 2–4 weeks, or even more.

Amitriptyline (and **imipramine** to a lesser extent) has long been regarded as the main reference TCA, the 'gold standard' against which newer antidepressants are evaluated. After some 40 years and nearly 200 RCTs later, many consider that amitriptyline is still unsurpassed as an antidepressant.[3] However, meta-analysis shows only a 3% efficacy advantage over SSRIs (NNT = 35), and this is probably more than offset by its disadvantages in terms of undesirable effects (NNH = 7).[3,4] Amitriptyline is therefore seldom used as first-line treatment, although it is still used at some centres in severe unresponsive depression. Even so, in practice, about 20% of patients fail to respond, but some of these failures probably relate to a failure to optimize the dose.

On the other hand, amitriptyline is still widely used in the management of neuropathic pain and tension headaches (see p.225). A CADTH Health Technology Assessment concluded that TCAs were a more cost-effective option for neuropathic pain than **gabapentin** and **pregabalin** (antiepileptics) and **duloxetine** and **venlafaxine** (SNRIs).[5]

A dose-response relationship has been shown for the analgesic effect of amitriptyline,[6,7] and there appears to be a 'therapeutic window' in some patients.[8] Patients with post-herpetic neuralgia or painful diabetic neuropathy had good relief with amitriptyline 20–100mg (median 50mg). With this dose the pain was reduced from severe to mild. When the dose was increased, the pain became severe again and, when decreased, the pain became mild again. However, some patients benefit from higher doses.

Amitriptyline frequently causes increased appetite and weight gain; this is a bonus in palliative care, but often an undesirable effect in other circumstances.

Bio-availability no data.
Onset of action 2–4 weeks; <1 week in neuropathic pain.[9]
Time to peak plasma concentration 4h PO; 24–48h IM.
Plasma halflife 9–25h; active metabolite nortriptyline 15–39h.
Duration of action 24h, situation dependent.

Cautions

Suicide risk: the possibility of a suicide attempt is inherent in major depression and persists until remission.

Elderly, cardiac disease (particularly if history of arrhythmia), epilepsy, hepatic impairment, history of mania, psychoses (may aggravate), narrow-angle glaucoma, urinary hesitancy, history of urinary retention. Drowsiness may affect performance of skilled tasks, e.g. driving; effects of alcohol enhanced. Avoid abrupt withdrawal after prolonged use. Also see Stopping antidepressants, p.146 and Cytochrome P450, p.551.

Like other antidepressants, amitriptyline can transform the depressive phase of bipolar disorder (manic depressive psychosis) into the manic phase, and may cause clinically significant hyponatremia, particularly in the elderly.

Undesirable effects

For full list, see manufacturer's Product Monograph.
Antimuscarinic effects, sedation, delirium, postural hypotension, hyponatremia. The use of amitriptyline in the elderly is associated with a doubling of the incidence of femoral fractures.[10]

Dose and use

Because of the potential for undesirable effects, low doses should be used initially, particularly in the frail elderly (Table 4.12). Relatively small doses are often effective in relieving depression in debilitated cancer patients, e.g. amitriptyline 25–50mg at bedtime.

Amitriptyline can be given as a single dose at bedtime for all indications. If a patient experiences early morning drowsiness, or takes a long time to settle at night, amitriptyline should be taken 2h before bedtime.

A small number of patients are stimulated by amitriptyline and experience insomnia, unpleasant vivid dreams, myoclonus and physical restlessness. In these patients, administer amitriptyline each morning or change to an SSRI.

Table 4.12 Dose escalation timetables for amitriptyline

Dose (at bedtime)	Elderly frail/outpatient	Younger patient/inpatient
10mg	Day 1	–
25mg	Day 3	Day 1
50mg	Week 2	Day 3
75mg	Week 3–4	Week 2
100mg	Week 5–6	Week 2
150mg	Week 7–8[a]	Week 3[a]

a. not often necessary in palliative care.

Supply
Amitriptyline (generic)
Tablets 10mg, 25mg, 50mg, 28 days @ 50mg once daily = $2.50.

1 Stahl SM (2000) *Essential Psychopharmacology: Neuroscientific Basis and Practical Applications* (2e). Cambridge University Press, Cambridge, pp. 218–222.
2 Eisenach J and Gebhart G (1995) Intrathecal amitriptyline acts as an N-Methyl-D-Aspartate receptor antagonist in the presence of inflammatory hyperalgesia in rats. *Anesthesiology.* **83**: 1046.
3 Barbui C and Hotopf M (2001) Amitriptyline v. the rest: still the leading antidepressant after 40 years of randomised controlled trials. *British Journal of Psychiatry.* **178**: 129–144.
4 Thompson C (2001) Amitriptyline: still efficacious, but at what cost? *British Journal of Psychiatry.* **178**: 99–100.
5 Iskedjian M et al. (2009) Anticonvulsants, serotonin-norepinephrine reuptake inhibitors and tricyclic antidepressants in management of neuropathic pain: a meta-analysis and economic evaluation (Technology report number 116). Canadian Agency for Drugs and Technologies in Health, Ottawa. Available from: www.cadth.ca/index.php/en/hta/reports-publications/search/publication/870
6 Max M et al. (1987) Amitriptyline relieves diabetic neuropathy pain in patients with normal or depressed mood. *Neurology (Ny).* **37**: 589–596.
7 McQuay HJ et al. (1993) Dose-response for analgesic effect of amitriptyline in chronic pain. *Anaesthesia.* **48**: 281–285.
8 Watson C (1984) Therapeutic window for amitriptyline analgesia. *Canadian Medical Association Journal.* **130**: 105–106.
9 Sindrup SH et al. (2005) Antidepressants in the treatment of neuropathic pain. *Basic & Clinical Pharmacology & Toxicology.* **96**: 399–409.
10 Ray WA et al. (1987) Psychotropic drug use and the risk of hip fracture. *New England Journal of Medicine.* **316**: 363–369.

NORTRIPTYLINE

Class: Tricyclic antidepressant (TCA), norepinephrine re-uptake inhibitor (NRI).

Indications: Depression, †neuropathic pain, †smoking cessation.[1]

Contra-indications: Should not be given with an MAOI or within 2 weeks of its cessation (see Box 4.H, p.141). Avoid in initial recovery period after an acute myocardial infarction.

Pharmacology
Nortriptyline blocks the presynaptic re-uptake of norepinephrine, but not of serotonin. It is the principal active metabolite of **amitriptyline** (see p.150); it is less antimuscarinic, and not so sedating. Nortriptyline undergoes extensive first-pass metabolism to 10-hydroxynortriptyline, which is active.[2] Overall, nortriptyline is as effective as **amitriptyline**.[3] However, compared with

other TCAs, its effects in neuropathic pain have been less extensively studied. Even so, it may be a useful alternative in patients intolerant of other TCAs; e.g. in post-herpetic neuralgia, nortriptyline was as effective as, and better tolerated than, **amitriptyline**.[4]

Although nortriptyline appears to have a therapeutic window at plasma concentrations 50–150nanogram/mL,[5,6] the dose is generally determined by the clinical response. However, in patients who are prescribed >100mg/24h, it is advisable to monitor the plasma concentration. As with **amitriptyline**, it generally takes several weeks for the antidepressant effect to manifest. Given the long plasma halflife of nortriptyline, once daily administration is possible, generally at bedtime.

Bio-availability 60%.
Onset of action 2–6 weeks.
Time to peak plasma concentration 7–8.5h.
Plasma halflife 15–39h.
Duration of action variable, possibly several days.

Cautions

Suicide risk: the possibility of a suicide attempt is inherent in major depression and persists until remission. Alcohol increases the risk of suicide attempts.

Elderly, cardiac disease (particularly if history of arrhythmia), epilepsy, hepatic impairment, history of mania, psychosis (may aggravate), narrow-angle glaucoma, urinary hesitancy. Avoid abrupt withdrawal after prolonged use. Also see Stopping antidepressants, p.146 and Cytochrome P450, p.551.

Nortriptyline is metabolized by CYP2D6. Caution should be used in patients thought to be 'poor metabolizers' and in patients taking other medications known to be metabolized by CYP2D6, e.g. antipsychotics, **carbamazepine**, **cimetidine**, **clarithromycin**, **erythromycin**, **fluconazole**, **fluoxetine**, **gatifloxacin**, **moxifloxacin**, **paroxetine**, **phenytoin**, **quinidine**, **St John's wort**, **sulfamethoxazole**, **tramadol**, **warfarin**.

Like other antidepressants, nortriptyline can transform the depressive phase of bipolar disorder (manic depressive psychosis) into the manic phase, and may cause clinically significant hyponatremia, particularly in the elderly.

Undesirable effects

For full list, see manufacturer's Product Monograph.
Very common (>10%): antimuscarinic effects (see p.5), anorexia, nausea, drowsiness, fatigue, weight gain.
Very rare (<0.01%): arrhythmias, AV conduction changes, heart block.

Dose and use

See general advice for **amitriptyline**, p.151.

Depression
- start with 25mg at bedtime
- if necessary, increase the dose by 25mg every 2–4 weeks up to 150mg/24h
- if no response with 150mg after 4 weeks, switch to an alternative antidepressant
- if effective, continue on the same dose until the patient has been symptom–free for 6–12 months; after this, discontinue over 2–8 weeks.

Neuropathic pain
- start with 10–25mg at bedtime
- increase by 10mg/24h every 3–5 days up to 50mg, or double dose from 25mg to 50mg after 2 weeks[4]
- if necessary and if undesirable effects permit, increase further by 25mg every 2 weeks to 150mg
- if effective, continue on the same dose until the patient has been symptom-free for 6–12 months; after this, discontinue over 2–8 weeks.

Supply
Nortriptyline (generic)
Capsules 10mg, 25mg, 50mg, 75mg, 28 days @ 25mg t.i.d. = $22.

Aventyl HCl Pulvules® (Pharmascience)
Capsules 10mg, 25mg, 28 days @ 25mg t.i.d. = $39.

1 Ranney L et al. (2006) Systematic review: smoking cessation intervention strategies for adults and adults in special populations. Annals of Internal Medicine. **145**: 845–856.
2 Nordin C and Bertilsson L (1995) Active hydroxymetabolites of antidepressants. Emphasis on E–10-hydroxy-nortriptyline. Clinical Pharmacokinetics. **28**: 26–40.
3 Barbui C and Hotopf M (2001) Amitriptyline v. the rest: still the leading antidepressant after 40 years of randomised controlled trials. British Journal of Psychiatry. **178**: 129–144.
4 Watson CP et al. (1998) Nortriptyline versus amitriptyline in postherpetic neuralgia: a randomized trial. Neurology. **51**: 1166–1171.
5 APA (American Psychiatric Association) (1985) Task Force on the Use of Laboratory Tests in Psychiatry: Tricyclic antidepressants-blood level measurements and clinical outcome. American Journal of Psychiatry. **142**: 155–162.
6 Perry PJ (1984) The relationship of free nortriptyline levels to antidepressant response. Drug Intelligence and Clinical Pharmacy. **18**: 510.

DESIPRAMINE

Class: Tricyclic antidepressant (TCA), norepinephrine re-uptake inhibitor (NRI).

Indications: Depression, †chronic pain, †neuropathic pain, †interstitial cystitis, †irritable bowel syndrome.

Contra-indications: Should not be given with an MAOI or within 2 weeks of its cessation, recent myocardial infarction.

Pharmacology
Like **nortriptyline**, desipramine blocks the presynaptic re-uptake of norepinephrine, but not of serotonin. Compared with **amitriptyline**, it is less antimuscarinic, and not so sedating. Like other TCAs, desipramine has been used for treating neuropathic pain as well as depression.[1–4] Desipramine also has an opioid-sparing effect;[5] a property shared by **imipramine**,[6] and almost certainly by TCAs generally. As an analgesic, desipramine probably works mainly by potentiating descending spinal inhibition.

At many centres, desipramine is the preferred TCA for neuropathic pain in elderly and/or debilitated patients because, compared with **amitriptyline**, it causes fewer undesirable effects.[7] Desipramine undergoes extensive first-pass metabolism to a less potent but active metabolite, 2-hydroxydesipramine.[8] Some patients are slow metabolizers, and require lower doses.[9,10] Desipramine is the principal active metabolite of **imipramine**, the first TCA.

Bio-availability 30–50% (high patient variability).
Onset of action 2–4 weeks; <1 week in neuropathic pain.[11]
Time to peak plasma concentration 4–6h.
Plasma halflife 7–77h; mean 20–30h in elderly.[10]
Duration of action 24h, situation dependent.

Cautions

Suicide risk: the possibility of a suicide attempt is inherent in major depression and persists until remission.

Slow metabolizers require much lower doses than normal metabolizers. Failure to recognize this can lead to serious toxicity/overdosage.

Like other antidepressants, desipramine can transform the depressive phase of bipolar disorder (manic depressive psychosis) into the manic phase, and may cause clinically significant hyponatremia, particularly in the elderly.

Undesirable effects

For full list, see manufacturer's Product Monograph.

Common (<10%, >1%): headache, anorexia, dizziness, drowsiness, fatigue, weakness, blurred vision, bloating, nausea, constipation, weight gain.

Dose and use

See general advice for **amitriptyline**, p.151.

Depression

- start with 25mg at bedtime
- if necessary, increase the dose by 25mg every 2–4 weeks up to 150mg/24h
- if no response with 150mg after 4 weeks, switch to an alternative antidepressant
- if effective, continue on the same dose until the patient has been symptom-free for 6–12 months; after this, discontinue over 2–8 weeks.

Neuropathic pain

- start with 10–25mg at bedtime
- increase by 10mg/24h every 3–5 days up to 50mg, or double dose from 25mg to 50mg after 2 weeks
- if necessary and if undesirable effects permit, increase further by 25mg every 2 weeks to 150mg[11]
- if effective, continue on the same dose until the patient has been symptom-free for 6–12 months; after this, discontinue over 2–8 weeks.

Supply

Desipramine (generic)

Tablets 10mg, 25mg, 50mg, 75mg, 100mg, 28 days @ 50mg once daily = $12.

1 Kishore-Kumar R et al. (1990) Desipramine relieves postherpetic neuralgia. *Clinical Pharmacology and Therapeutics.* **47**: 305–312.
2 Max M et al. (1992) Effects of desipramine, amitriptyline, and fluoxetine on pain in diabetic neuropathy. *New England Journal of Medicine.* **326**: 1287–1288.
3 Richeimer SH et al. (1997) Utilization patterns of tricyclic antidepressants in a multidisciplinary pain clinic: a survey. *Clinical Journal of Pain.* **13**: 324–329.
4 Reisner L (2003) Antidepressants for chronic neuropathic pain. *Current Pain and Headache Reports.* **7**: 24–33.
5 Gordon NC et al. (1993) Temporal factors in the enhancement of morphine analgesia by desipramine. *Pain.* **53**: 273–276.
6 Walsh T (1986) Controlled study of imipramine and morphine in advanced cancer. *Proceedings of the American Society of Clinical Oncology.* **5**: 237.
7 Gareri P et al. (1998) Antidepressant drugs in the elderly. *General Pharmacology.* **30**: 465–475.
8 DeVane CL et al. (1981) Desipramine and 2-hydroxy-desipramine pharmacokinetics in normal volunteers. *European Journal of Clinical Pharmacology.* **19**: 61–64.
9 Dahl ML et al. (1993) Polymorphic 2–hydroxylation of desipramine. A population and family study. *European Journal of Clinical Pharmacology.* **44**: 445–450.
10 Sallee FR and Pollock BG (1990) Clinical pharmacokinetics of imipramine and desipramine. *Clinical Pharmacokinetics.* **18**: 346–364.
11 Sindrup S et al. (1990) The selective serotonin re-uptake inhibitor paroxetine is effective in the treatment of diabetic neuropathy symptoms. *Pain.* **42**: 135–144.

SERTRALINE

Class: Selective serotonin re-uptake inhibitor (SSRI).

Indications: Depression (with or without anxiety), obsessive-compulsive disorder, panic disorder (with or without agoraphobia), †neuropathic pain, †post-traumatic stress disorder in women.

Contra-indications: Concurrent administration with an MAOI (see Serotonin toxicity, p.140).

Pharmacology

Sertraline has no affinity for muscarinic, serotoninergic, dopaminergic, adrenergic, histaminergic, or GABA-ergic receptors. Unlike **amitriptyline**, sertraline does not cause weight gain. Discontinuation symptoms are less likely than with **paroxetine**. Sertraline exhibits linear pharmacokinetics in doses up to 200mg, and steady-state plasma concentrations are achieved after 1 week. However, there is no clear relationship between plasma concentrations and therapeutic response.

Manufacturers' information regarding the impact of food on the bio-availability of sertraline, and advice on timing in relation to meals, varies from brand to brand in different countries. The Canadian manufacturer of Zoloft® states that food reduces bio-availability by 40% but, even so, that capsules should be taken with food.

Sertraline's main metabolite is inactive. Metabolites are excreted equally in feces and urine. Sertraline is as effective as **amitriptyline** in treating depression with anxiety; its antidepressant action may be enhanced by **valproic acid**.[1] Sertraline relieves diabetic neuropathic pain.[2] It is also of benefit in cholestatic pruritus (see Box 5.O, p.339).

Bio-availability >44%.
Onset of action 1–4 weeks.
Time to peak plasma concentration 4.5–8.4h.
Plasma halflife 22–36h.
Duration of action several days, situation dependent.

Cautions

Suicide risk: the possibility of a suicide attempt is inherent in major depression and persists until remission.

Epilepsy, hepatic impairment, renal impairment. All SSRIs increase the risk of GI bleeding,[3] particularly in those aged >80 years.[4]

Sertraline (or other SSRI) should not be started until 2 weeks after stopping an MAOI. Treatment should not be discontinued abruptly (see Box 4.K, p.146). Also see Cytochrome P450, p.551.

Like other antidepressants, sertraline can transform the depressive phase of bipolar disorder (manic depressive psychosis) into the manic phase, and may cause clinically significant hyponatremia, particularly in the elderly.

Undesirable effects

For full list, see manufacturer's Product Monograph.
Initial exacerbation of anxiety, restlessness, headache, anorexia, nausea, diarrhea, sexual dysfunction (diminished libido and delayed orgasm).[5]

Dose and use

Sertraline is easy to use because, for most patients, the starting dose does not need to be increased:
- start with 50mg once daily, either with the evening meal or with breakfast
- occasionally necessary to increase the dose by stages to 100–200mg at 2–4 week intervals
- if no response with 200mg after 4 weeks, switch to an alternative antidepressant
- if effective, continue until the patient has been symptom-free for 6 months; after this, discontinue over 2–4 weeks.

Supply

Sertraline (generic)
Capsules 25mg, 50mg, 100mg, 28 days @ 50mg once daily = $29.

Zoloft® (Pfizer)
Capsules 24mg, 50mg, 100mg, 28 days @ 50mg once daily = $49.

1 Dave M (1995) Antidepressant augmentation with valproate. *Depression.* **3**: 157–158.
2 Goodnick P *et al.* (1997) Sertraline in diabetic neuropathy: preliminary results. *Annals of Clinical Psychiatry.* **9**: 255–257.
3 Paton C and Ferrier IN (2005) SSRIs and gastrointestinal bleeding. *British Medical Journal.* **331**: 529–530.
4 vanWalraven C *et al.* (2001) Inhibition of serotonin reuptake by antidepressants and upper gastrointestinal bleeding in elderly patients: retrospective cohort study. *British Medical Journal.* **323**: 655–657.
5 Modell J *et al.* (1997) Comparative sexual side effects of bupropion, fluoxetine, paroxetine, and sertraline. *Clinical Pharmacology and Therapeutics.* **61**: 476–487.

*VENLAFAXINE

Class: Antidepressant; serotonin and norepinephrine re-uptake inhibitor (SNRI).

Indications: Depression, generalized anxiety disorder, social anxiety disorder, panic disorder (with or without agoraphobia), †neuropathic pain, †hot flashes.

Contra-indications: Concurrent use with an MAOI or within 2 weeks of previous treatment with an MAOI (see Serotonin toxicity, p.140). Uncontrolled hypertension, high risk for ventricular arrhythmia.

Pharmacology

Venlafaxine is a bicyclic compound which can be thought of as 'clean' **amitriptyline**. It inhibits the presynaptic re-uptake of serotonin and norepinephrine, and of dopamine to a lesser extent but, unlike **amitriptyline**, it has little or no post-synaptic antagonistic effects at muscarinic, α-adrenergic or H_1-receptors.[1,2] Venlafaxine's inhibition of presynaptic serotonin re-uptake is about 3 times greater than for norepinephrine re-uptake and at least 10 times greater than for dopamine inhibition.

As an antidepressant, venlafaxine is more effective than SSRIs.[3] Venlafaxine also has a faster onset of action, i.e. a mean of 3 weeks compared with 4 weeks for pure SSRIs. It is a good choice for patients with psychomotor retardation. It is also of benefit in the long-term treatment of generalized anxiety disorder.[4]

Venlafaxine has been shown to have an antinociceptive effect in animals.[5,6] Its antinociceptive effect is said to be mainly mediated by κ- and δ-opioid receptors and α_2-adrenergic receptors. Case reports and case series suggest that venlafaxine relieves several types of chronic pain, e.g. headache, fibromyalgia and neuropathic pain.[7] Benefit in diabetic neuropathy and in a mixed group of patients has been confirmed in placebo-controlled RCTs.[8,9] In another RCT (n = 13), benefit appeared to be positively correlated with the plasma concentration of venlafaxine.[10] In an RCT of **imipramine** 75mg daily vs. venlafaxine 112.5mg daily, the two antidepressants were equally effective and both were significantly better than placebo.[11] Dry mouth was more common with **imipramine**, and tiredness more common with venlafaxine.

Venlafaxine is also of benefit in hot flashes associated with the menopause or hormone therapy,[12,13] including androgen ablation therapy for prostate cancer.[14] This is not a specific effect of venlafaxine; SSRIs seem to share this property, e.g. **paroxetine** and **fluoxetine**.[15,16] Venlafaxine is metabolized to a pharmacologically active metabolite, O-desmethylvenlafaxine (ODV) which has a similar pharmacodynamic profile.

Bio-availability 13%; 45% SR.

Onset of action >2 weeks for depression.

Time to peak plasma concentration about 2.5h; 4.5–7.5h SR and 6.5–11h ODV SR.

Plasma halflife 5h; 11h for ODV.

Duration of effect 12–24h, situation dependent.

Cautions

Suicide risk: the possibility of a suicide attempt is inherent in major depression and persists until remission. The risk appears to be greater with venlafaxine than with SSRIs and TCAs, but this may be because patients prescribed venlafaxine (generally not a first-line antidepressant) may already be at greater risk of suicide.[17–19]

In order to reduce the risk from overdose, the Canadian manufacturer advises limiting each prescription to the smallest quantity needed to meet the patient's requirement.

Patients with epilepsy (as with all antidepressants), pre-existing hypertension, established heart disease with risk of ventricular arrhythmia (e.g. recent myocardial infarction),[19] a history of mania (may precipitate further episodes), concurrent **cimetidine** in the elderly, hepatic or renal impairment. Mydriasis has been reported in association with venlafaxine; patients with raised intra-ocular pressure or at risk of narrow-angle glaucoma should be monitored closely.

Concurrent use with drugs which inhibit either CYP2D6 or CYP3A4 may result in higher plasma concentrations (see Cytochrome P450, p.551), and should generally be avoided in order to prevent clinically important interactions in poor metabolizers.[19] May increase concurrent **haloperidol** plasma concentrations (up to 70% increase in AUC and a possible doubling of the maximum plasma concentration). The dose of **warfarin** may need to be reduced.

Blood pressure should be monitored in all patients, and dose reduction or discontinuation considered in those who show a sustained increase;[19] increases in diastolic pressure of 4–7mmHg have been observed in some patients.

Dose reduction required in patients with mild–moderate hepatic impairment, moderate-severe renal impairment (GFR 10–70mL/min) or on hemodialysis. There are no data to support its use or safety in patients with severe hepatic impairment.

Like other antidepressants, venlafaxine can transform the depressive phase of bipolar disorder (manic depressive psychosis) into the manic phase, and may cause clinically significant hyponatremia, particularly in the elderly.

Because an antidepressant withdrawal (discontinuation) syndrome may occur (see Stopping antidepressants, p.146), venlafaxine should not be stopped abruptly. If ≥75mg/24h have been taken for >1 week, taper over at least 1 week; if ≥150mg/24h have been taken for >6 weeks, taper over at least 2 weeks.

Undesirable effects

For full list, see manufacturer's Product Monograph.

Very common (>10%): dizziness, dry mouth, insomnia, nervousness, drowsiness, constipation, nausea, abnormal ejaculation/orgasm, asthenia, headache, sweating.

Common (<10%, >1%): agitation, confusion, hypertonia, paresthesia, tremor, dyspnea, hypertension, palpitations, tachycardia, postural hypotension, vasodilation, anorexia, diarrhea, dyspepsia, vomiting, urinary frequency, ecchymosis, decreased libido, impotence, menstrual disorders, arthralgia, myalgia, weight gain/loss, abdominal pain, abnormal dreams, chills, pyrexia, pruritus, rash, abnormal vision/accommodation, mydriasis, tinnitus, abnormal taste.

Uncommon (<1%): hallucinations, urinary retention, muscle spasm, hyponatremia, increased liver enzymes, angioedema, maculopapular eruptions, urticaria.

Dose and use

Because of concerns about its safety in overdose and cost-effectiveness, venlafaxine is not recommended as a first-line antidepressant.[19–21] A UK regulatory warning states that specialist supervision is required if a dose of ≥300mg is necessary in severely depressed or hospitalized patients.[19]

A CADTH Health Technology Assessment concluded that venlafaxine was less cost-effective for neuropathic pain than TCAs.[22]

Best taken with or after food. *The capsules should be swallowed whole*, not crushed, chewed or dissolved in water because this destroys the SR mechanism. A reduced dose is recommended in:
- mild–moderate hepatic impairment (reduce by 50%; starting dose 37.5mg SR once daily)
- renal impairment (reduce by 25–50%; starting dose 37.5mg SR once daily)
- patients on hemodialysis (reduce by 50%, and give *after* dialysis; starting dose 37.5mg SR once daily).

Depression
- generally start with 75mg SR once daily
- particularly with frail and elderly patients, it may be better to start with 37.5mg once daily for 4–7 days to allow time for adjustment to the new medication
- if necessary, increase the dose progressively in 75mg increments every 2 weeks

- a daily dose of 225mg is generally sufficient for moderately depressed outpatients
- in severely depressed inpatients, higher daily doses may be indicated, e.g. ≤375mg
- if effective, continue until the patient has been symptom-free for 6 months; then discontinue over 2–4 weeks.

Generalized and social anxiety disorders
- start with 37.5mg SR once daily for 4–7 days
- then increase to 75mg SR once daily
- if necessary at intervals of ≥4 days, increase in 75mg increments to a maximum daily dose of 225mg.

Panic disorder
- start with 37.5mg SR once daily for 1 week
- then increase to 75mg SR once daily
- if necessary at intervals of ≥1 week, increase in 75mg increments to a maximum daily dose of 225mg.

Neuropathic pain and hot flashes
- start with 37.5mg SR once daily for 1 week
- then increase to 75mg SR once daily
- if necessary after a further 2 weeks, increase to 150mg SR once daily.

Supply
Sustained-release
Venlafaxine extended-release (generic)
Capsules SR 37.5mg, 75mg, 150mg, 28 days @ 150mg once daily = $35.

Effexor® XR (Wyeth)
Capsules SR 37.5mg, 75mg, 150mg, 28 days @ 150mg once daily = $58.

1 Horst W and Preskorn S (1998) Mechanisms of action and clinical characteristics of three atypical antidepressants: venlafaxine, nefazodone, bupropion. *Journal of Affective Disorders*. **51**: 237–254.
2 Maj J and Rogoz Z (1999) Pharmacological effects of venlafaxine, a new antidepressant, given repeatedly, on the alpha 1-adrenergic, dopamine and serotonin systems. *Journal of Neural Transmission*. **106**: 197–211.
3 Thase M et al. (2001) Remission rates during treatment with venlafaxine or selective serotonin reuptake inhibitors. *British Journal of Psychiatry*. **178**: 234–241.
4 Allgulander C et al. (2001) Venlafaxine extended release (ER) in the treatment of generalised anxiety disorder. *British Journal of Psychiatry*. **179**: 15–22.
5 Lang E et al. (1996) Venlafaxine hydrochloride (Effexor) relieves thermal hyperalgesia in rats with an experimental mononeuropathy. *Pain*. **68**: 151–155.
6 Schreiber S et al. (1999) The antinociceptive effect of venlafaxine in mice is mediated through opioid and adrenergic mechanisms. *Neuroscience Letters*. **273**: 85–88.
7 Grothe DR et al. (2004) Treatment of pain syndromes with venlafaxine. *Pharmacotherapy*. **24**: 621–629.
8 Kunz N et al. (2000) Diabetic neuropathic pain management with venlafaxine XR. In: *CINP* July.
9 Yucel A et al. (2005) The effect of venlafaxine on ongoing and experimentally induced pain in neuropathic pain patients: a double blind, placebo controlled study. *European Journal of Pain*. **9**: 407–416.
10 Tasmuth T et al. (2002) Venlafaxine in neuropathic pain following treatment of breast cancer. *European Journal of Pain*. **6**: 17–24.
11 Sindrup SH et al. (2003) Venlafaxine versus imipramine in painful polyneuropathy: a randomized, controlled trial. *Neurology*. **60**: 1284–1289.
12 Barlow D (2000) Venlafaxine for hot flushes. *Lancet*. **356**: 2025–2026.
13 Loprinzi C et al. (2000) Venlafaxine in management of hot flashes in survivors of breast cancer: a randomised controlled trial. *Lancet*. **356**: 2059–2063.
14 Quella S et al. (1999) Pilot evaluation of venlafaxine for the treatment of hot flashes in men undergoing androgen ablation therapy for prostate cancer. *Journal of Urology*. **162**: 98–102.
15 Stearns V et al. (1997) A pilot trial assessing the efficacy of paroxetine hydrochloride (Paxil) in controlling hot flashes. *Breast Cancer Research Treatment*. **46**: 23–33.
16 Loprinzi C et al. (1999) Preliminary data from a randomized evaluation of fluoxetine (Prozac) for treating hot flashes in breast cancer survivors. *Breast Cancer Research Treatment*. **57**: 34.
17 Cipriani A et al. (2007) Venlafaxine for major depression. *British Medical Journal*. **334**: 215–216.
18 Rubino A et al. (2007) Risk of suicide during treatment with venlafaxine, citalopram, fluoxetine, and dothiepin: retrospective cohort study. *British Medical Journal*. **334**: 242.
19 Duff G (2006) Updated prescribing advice for venlafaxine (Efexor/Effexor XL). Letter from the chairman of the Commission on Human Medicines, 31st May 2006. Available from: www.mhra.gov.uk/Safetyinformation/Safetywarningsalertsandrecalls/Safetywarningsandmessagesformedicines/CON2023846
20 Buckley NA and McManus PR (2002) Fatal toxicity of serotoninergic and other antidepressant drugs: analysis of United Kingdom mortality data. *British Medical Journal*. **325**: 1332–1333.

21 NICE (2004) Depression: Management of depression in primary and secondary care. In: *National Clinical Practice Guideline Number 23*. National Institute for Clinical Excellence. Available from: www.nice.org.uk/page.aspx?o=236667

22 Iskedjian M et al. (2009) Anticonvulsants, serotonin-norepinephrine reuptake inhibitors, and tricyclic antidepressants in mangement of neuropathic pain: a meta-analysis and economic evaluation (Technology report number 116). Canadian Agency for Drugs and Technologies in Health, Ottawa. Available from: www.cadth.ca/index.php/en/hta/reports-publications/search/publication/870

MIRTAZAPINE

Class: Antidepressant, noradrenergic and specific serotoninergic antidepressant (NaSSA).[1,2]

Indications: Depression, †neuropathic pain, †intractable itch, †serotonin toxicity.

Contra-indications: Should not be given with an MAOI or within 2 weeks of its cessation (see Serotonin toxicity, p.140, but see comment below).

Pharmacology

Mirtazapine is a centrally active presynaptic α_2-adrenergic receptor antagonist, which *increases* central noradrenergic and serotoninergic neurotransmission.[3] Enhancement of serotoninergic neurotransmission by mirtazapine is said to be mediated specifically via $5HT_{1A}$-receptors. However, mirtazapine has no demonstrable serotoninergic symptoms or toxicity in overdose, either by itself or when used concurrently with MAOIs (see Serotonin toxicity, p.140). Thus, it has been suggested that it should not be designated a dual-action drug.[4]

Mirtazapine is an antagonist at $5HT_2$- and $5HT_3$-receptors. Thus, unlike SSRIs, it is *not* associated with nausea and vomiting. Both enantiomers of mirtazapine are presumed to contribute to the antidepressant activity; the S(+) enantiomer by blocking α_2 and $5HT_2$-receptors and the R(−) enantiomer by blocking $5HT_3$-receptors. The histamine H_1-antagonistic activity of mirtazapine is responsible for its sedative properties. At lower doses, the antihistaminic effect of mirtazapine predominates, producing sedation. Mirtazapine 15mg at bedtime is equivalent to 15mg of **diazepam** in terms of reducing anxiety.[1] With higher doses, sedation is reduced as noradrenergic neural transmission increases. Mirtazapine is generally well tolerated. It has no significant antimuscarinic activity.

Mirtazapine is an effective antidepressant with a response rate of nearly 70%.[5,6] The antidepressant effects of mirtazapine are equivalent to **amitriptyline, fluoxetine, clomipramine** and **doxepin**.[2] Generally, treatment with an adequate dose results in a positive response within 2–4 weeks, sometimes in <1 week.[7]

There are fewer relapses compared with **amitriptyline**. Mirtazapine is not associated with cardiovascular toxicity or sexual dysfunction.[8] A blockade of $5HT_2$ and $5HT_3$ leads to appetite stimulation as well as reduced nausea.[9]

Some centres use mirtazapine for neuropathic pain,[10,11] and for intractable pruritus.[12] There is an isolated report on its use in serotonin toxicity.[13]

Mirtazapine displays linear pharmacokinetics within the recommended dose range. Food does not affect absorption. Steady-state is reached after 3–4 days of daily administration. Binding to plasma proteins is about 85%. Mirtazapine is extensively metabolized and eliminated via the urine and feces. Major pathways of biotransformation are demethylation and oxidation, followed by conjugation. Cytochrome P450 enzymes CYP2D6 and CYP1A2 are involved in the formation of the 8-hydroxy metabolite of mirtazapine, whereas CYP3A4 is considered to be responsible for the formation of the N-demethyl and N-oxide metabolites (see p.551). Clearance in the elderly may be reduced by ≤40%.

The demethyl metabolite is pharmacologically active and appears to have the same pharmacokinetic profile as the parent compound. Overdose produces disorientation, drowsiness, memory impairment and tachycardia. Mirtazapine has additive undesirable effects on cognition and motor performance when taken with alcohol or **diazepam**.

Bio-availability 50% PO.

Onset of action hours-days (off-label indications); 1–2 weeks (antidepressant).

Time to peak plasma concentration 2h.

Plasma halflife 20–40h; often shorter in men (26h) than women (37h) but can extend up to 65h.
Duration of action variable; up to several days.

Cautions

Suicide risk: the possibility of a suicide attempt is inherent in major depression and persists until remission.

Hepatic or renal impairment. Like other antidepressants, mirtazapine can transform the depressive phase of bipolar disorder (manic depressive psychosis) into the manic phase. May accentuate the effect of alcohol and of benzodiazepines.

Undesirable effects

For full list, see manufacturer's Product Monograph.
Very common (>10%): increase in appetite and weight gain;[14] drowsiness during the first few weeks of treatment. Dose reduction reduces the likelihood of an antidepressant effect and does not necessarily alleviate drowsiness.
Uncommon (<1%, >0.1%): hepatic impairment.

Dose and use
Depression
- start with 15mg at bedtime
- if necessary, increase the dose by 15mg every 2 weeks up to 45mg[1,6]
- if no response after 4 weeks on 45mg, seek specialist advice
- if effective, continue until the patient has been symptom-free for 6 months; then discontinue over 2–4 weeks.

Neuropathic pain and intractable itch
Use as for depression; continue indefinitely.[10,12]

Supply
Mirtazapine (generic)
Tablets 15mg, 30mg, 28 days @ 30mg at bedtime = $22.

Remeron® (Organon)
Tablets 30mg, 28 days @ 30mg at bedtime = $38.

Remeron RD® (Organon)
Tablets orodispersible 15mg, 30mg, 45mg, 28 days @ 30mg at bedtime = $24.

1 Puzantian T (1998) Mirtazapine, an antidepressant. *American Journal of Health System Pharmacy.* **55**: 44–49.
2 Kent J (2000) SnaRIs, NaSSAs and NaRIs: new agents for the treatment of depression. *Lancet.* **355**: 911–918.
3 deBoer T (1996) The pharmacologic profile of mirtazapine. *Journal of Clinical Psychiatry.* **57**: 19–25.
4 Gillman PK (2006) A systematic review of the serotonergic effects of mirtazapine in humans: implications for its dual action status. *Human Psychopharmacology: Clinical and Experimental.* **21**: 117–125.
5 Kasper S (1995) Clinical efficacy of mirtazapine: a review of meta-analyses of pooled data. *International Clinical Research.* **10**: 25–36.
6 Bailer U et al. (1998) Mirtazapine in inpatient treatment of depressed patients. *Wiener Klinische Wochenschrift.* **110**: 646–650.
7 Burrows G and Kremer C (1997) Mirtazapine: clinical advantages in the treatment of depression. *Journal of Clinical Psychopharmacology.* **1**: 34–39.
8 Gelenberg A et al. (2000) Mirtazapine substitution in SSRI-induced sexual dysfunction. *Journal of Clinical Psychiatry.* **61**: 356–360.
9 Davis M et al. (2001) Mirtazapine: Heir apparent to amitriptyline? *American Journal of Hospice and Palliative Care.* **18 (1)**: 42–46.
10 Brannon G and Stone K (1999) The use of mirtazapine in a patient with chronic pain. *Journal of Pain and Symptom Management.* **18**: 382–385.
11 Ritzenthaler B and Pearson D (2000) Efficacy and tolerability of mirtazapine in neuropathic pain. *Palliative Medicine.* **14**: 346.
12 Krajnik M and Zylicz Z (2001) Understanding pruritus in systemic disease. *Journal of Pain and Symptom Management.* **21**: 151–168.
13 Hoes M and Zeijpveld J (1996) Mirtazapine as treatment for serotonin syndrome. *Pharmacopsychiatry.* **29**: 81.
14 Abed R and Cooper M (1999) Mirtazapine causing hyperphagia. *British Journal of Psychiatry.* **174**: 181–182.

TRAZODONE

Class: Antidepressant.

Indications: Depression, †insomnia, †agitation, †behavioural problems in patients with dementia.

Contra-indications: Should not be given with an MAOI or within 2 weeks of its cessation (see Serotonin toxicity, p.140). Avoid use in the initial recovery period after an acute myocardial infarction.

Pharmacology

Although generally as effective as other antidepressants,[1] trazodone is not often used to treat depression in palliative care because of daytime drowsiness. Thus, when used, it is generally for off-label indications.

Trazodone antagonizes central α_1-adrenergic receptors, and post-synaptic $5HT_2$-receptors. At higher doses, trazodone also blocks the presynaptic re-uptake of serotonin, and it could be this action which is mainly responsible for the antidepressant effect. It is devoid of antimuscarinic activity, but has a marked sedative effect. Food increases its alimentary absorption. Trazodone has an active metabolite, m-chlorophenylpiperazine. Excretion is almost entirely as free or conjugated metabolites. Although trazodone has less effect on cardiac function than TCAs, there are sporadic reports of arrhythmias, ranging from heart block to ventricular tachycardia.[2,3]

Trazodone has been used for behavioural problems in patients with dementia (agitation, restlessness, wandering, physical aggression, inappropriate sexual activity, culturally inappropriate behaviours, hoarding, cursing, shadowing, screaming, sleep disorders).[4-6] However, larger studies have not replicated promising earlier results.[7] Such behaviours occur for many reasons, including an appropriate response to a distressing situation. Possible precipitants should be treated or modified. Medication should only be used as a last resort where non-drug measures have failed (see Antipsychotics, p.126).

Trazodone is used as a night sedative, despite the absence of RCT evidence confirming its efficacy in non-depressed patients.[8,9] In a dose of 25–50mg at bedtime, it is reported to be effective and well tolerated.[10-12] Unlike many other antidepressants, trazodone has no demonstrable analgesic effect.[13]

Bio-availability 65%.

Onset of action 1–4 weeks for an antidepressant effect; 30–60min for insomnia or agitation.

Time to peak plasma concentration 1h if taken fasting; 2h if taken after food.

Plasma halflife 7h; may be doubled in the elderly.

Duration of action variable, situation dependent.

Cautions

Suicide risk: the possibility of a suicide attempt is inherent in major depression and persists until remission.

Pre-existing cardiac disease, epilepsy, severe hepatic impairment. Elimination is delayed if given with inhibitors of CYP3A4, e.g. azole antifungals and protease inhibitors, **indinavir** and **ritonavir**. In contrast, inducers of CYP3A4, e.g. **phenytoin**, will accelerate the metabolism of trazodone.

If trazodone is prescribed concurrently, the dose of **warfarin** may need to be increased,[14] and the dose of **digoxin** and **phenytoin** decreased. Trazodone inhibits most of the acute actions of **clonidine** in animals. Thus, although there are no clinical data, the effect of antihypertensive treatment should be monitored if trazodone is prescribed concurrently.

Undesirable effects

For a complete list, see manufacturer's Product Monograph.

Common (<10%, >1%): daytime drowsiness, lethargy, dizziness (orthostatic hypotension), psychomotor impairment.

Uncommon (<1%, >0.1%): nausea, vomiting, sweating.
Rare (<0.1%, >0.01%): increased libido[15,16] and priapism (in 0.01%).[17,18] These have not been reported with low-dose (25–50mg) night sedation.

Dose and use
Depression
- start with 150mg at bedtime (100mg at bedtime in frail elderly patients)
- if necessary, increase dose by 50mg weekly up to 300mg (either as a single night-time dose or in divided doses)
- maximum dose 600mg/24h in divided doses (generally inpatients only).

Insomnia
- 25–50mg at bedtime[12]
- if necessary, increase to 100mg
- occasionally may need 150–200mg.

Agitated delirium, and challenging behaviours in those with dementia
Note: Trazodone is not a first-line choice for either indication (see Antipsychotics, p.126).
- 25mg t.i.d. or 50–100mg at bedtime
- adjust dose if necessary
- unlikely to need >300mg/24h.[4–6]

Supply
Trazodone (generic)
Tablets 50mg, 100mg, 28 days @ 100mg at bedtime = $12.

Desyrel® (Bristol-Myers Squibb)
Tablets 50mg, 100mg, 28 days @ 100mg at bedtime = $12.

Desyrel Dividose® (Bristol-Myers Squibb)
Tablets 150mg, 28 days @ 100mg at bedtime = $17.

1 Haria M et al. (1994) Trazodone. A review of its pharmacology, therapeutic use in depression and therapeutic potential in other disorders. Drugs Aging. 4: 331–355.
2 Vlay SC and Friedling S (1983) Trazodone exacerbation of VT. American Heart Journal. 106: 604.
3 Johnson BA (1985) Trazodone toxicity. British Journal of Hospital Medicine. 33: 298.
4 Lebert F et al. (1994) Behavioral effects of trazodone in Alzheimer's disease. Journal of Clinical Psychiatry. 55: 536–538.
5 Anonymous (1997) American Psychiatric Association: practice guideline for the treatment of patients with Alzheimer's disease and other dementias of late life. American Journal of Psychiatry. 154: 1–39.
6 Sultzer DL et al. (1997) A double-blind comparison of trazodone and haloperidol for treatment of agitation in patients with dementia. American Journal of Geriatric Psychiatry. 5: 60–69.
7 Jeste DV et al. (2007) ACNP White Paper: Update on Use of Antipsychotic Drugs in Elderly Persons with Dementia. Neuropsychopharmacology.
8 James SP and Mendelson WB (2004) The use of trazodone as a hypnotic: a critical review. Journal of Clinical Psychiatry. 65: 752–755.
9 Mendelson WB (2005) A review of the evidence for the efficacy and safety of trazodone in insomnia. Journal of Clinical Psychiatry. 66: 469–476.
10 Lenhart SE and Buysse DJ (2001) Treatment of insomnia in hospitalized patients. Annals of Pharmacotherapy. 35: 1449–1457.
11 Montplaisir J et al. (2003) Zopiclone and zaleplon vs benzodiazepines in the treatment of insomnia: Canadian consensus statement. Human Psychopharmacology. 18: 29–38.
12 Scott MA et al. (2003) Clinical inquiries. What is the best hypnotic for use in the elderly? Journal of Family Practice. 52: 976–978.
13 Lynch ME (2001) Antidepressants as analgesics: a review of randomized controlled trials. Journal of Psychiatry and Neuroscience. 26: 30–36.
14 Small NL and Giamonna KA (2000) Interaction between warfarin and trazodone. Annals of Pharmacotherapy. 34: 734–736.
15 Gartrell N (1986) Increased libido in women receiving trazodone. American Journal of Psychiatry. 143: 781–782.
16 Sullivan G (1988) Increased libido in three men treated with trazodone. Journal of Clinical Psychiatry. 49: 202–203.
17 Patel AG et al. (1996) Priapism associated with psychotropic drugs. British Journal of Hospital Medicine. 55: 315–319.
18 Pescatori ES et al. (1993) Priapism of the clitoris: a case report following trazodone use. Journal of Urology. 149: 1557–1559.

PSYCHOSTIMULANTS

Indications: Attention deficit hyperactivity disorder; daytime drowsiness due to narcolepsy, obstructive sleep apnea or chronic shift work-related sleep disorder; †depression where prognosis <3 months; †opioid-related drowsiness; †fatigue refractory to correction of underlying contributors.

Pharmacology

Wakefulness is regulated by reciprocal interaction between two opposing systems: one promoting arousal and inhibiting sleep, the other promoting sleep, inhibiting arousal and reducing sensory input. These systems originate in the hypothalamus, thalamus and midbrain reticular formation. Most psychostimulants act directly or indirectly via dopamine.[1] Dopamine has a central role in reward, motivation, attention and arousal. It is released in response to stimuli and thoughts perceived as relevant, particularly with regard to 'reward' (the mesocorticolimbic system). These effects are mediated by D_1 and D_2 receptors.[1,2] Psychostimulants (e.g. **cocaine**, **dextroamphetamine**, **methylphenidate**, **modafinil** and **pemoline**) reverse dopamine re-uptake transporters in the pre-synaptic membrane and storage vesicle membrane causing the release of stored dopamine and inhibition of re-uptake.[1,3,4] They increase alertness and motivation, and have antidepressant and mood-elevating properties.[1,5–7] Other neurotransmitters have also been implicated in the action of **modafinil**.[5]

Dopaminergic dysfunction in the mesocorticolimbic system is implicated in several disorders. In attention-deficit hyperactivity disorder, psychostimulants may improve attention by correcting a deficit in dopamine release in response to relevant stimuli.[8] In psychoses, dopamine excess ('over-attention') may cause hallucinations and delusions, and may account for the beneficial effects of D_2 antagonists (see p.121).[2] There is also interest in inhibiting dopamine-mediated 'reward' systems in addiction disorders.

Caffeine is an adenosine type-1 (A_1) receptor antagonist. It blocks the sleep-promoting GABAergic and antidopaminergic effects of adenosine. This breakdown product of the major neuronal energy source, adenosine triphosphate, accumulates during wakefulness and promotes sleep.[1]

Methylphenidate is the most used psychostimulant in palliative care.[9] However, although not so widely available, **dextroamphetamine** has a potential advantage in that it generally needs to be given only once daily.[10] **Modafinil** is used in sleep medicine because fewer problems with tolerability, tolerance and dependence are reported.[5]

Dextroamphetamine is excreted renally largely unchanged; there is thus a theoretical risk of increased toxicity in renal impairment.[9]

Cautions

Cardiovascular disease (e.g. severe hypertension, arrhythmia and angina); psychiatric illness (e.g. anxiety, agitation, psychosis and addiction disorders); epilepsy (possible lowering of seizure threshold); hyperthyroidism and closed-angle glaucoma (not **modafinil**).

Drug interactions

Methylphenidate and **modafinil** may increase plasma concentrations of **phenytoin** and **warfarin** (check INR more often until restabilized) and TCAs. Their action is antagonized by antipsychotics. **Modafinil** induces CYP 3A4/5 (reduced efficacy of **cyclosporine**, HIV-protease inhibitors, **midazolam**, calcium channel blockers, statins and hormonal contraception).

Undesirable effects

For full list, see manufacturer's Product Monograph.
Undesirable effects have been reported in up to 30% of patients.
Neuropsychiatric: insomnia, agitation and anorexia (generally settle in time if the drug is continued or resolve after several days if the drug is discontinued), psychosis, movement disorders.
Cardiovascular: tachyarrhythmias, hypertension and angina (rare).
Other: headache (common and responds to slower dose titration, *but very rarely cerebral arteritis is seen with* **methylphenidate**). Mild rashes are common with **modafinil**; serious skin reactions occur in 1% of children.

Use of psychostimulants in palliative care
Depression
Methylphenidate is the most commonly used psychostimulant-antidepressant in palliative care (see p.168). **Modafinil** can be used if **methylphenidate** is poorly tolerated.

Psychostimulants are used where a prompt response to treatment is required and tolerance to long-term use is irrelevant. A consensus panel concluded that they were the drugs of choice for treating depression in patients with a prognosis of <3 months.[11] It is often possible to achieve a response in a few days, increasing the dose every 1–2 days until there is a response or undesirable effects prevent further escalation (see Guidelines, p.167).[11]

However, trials are generally of poor quality, short duration and with outcome measures of uncertain clinical significance. Thus, conventional antidepressants should be used if the patient has a sufficient prognosis for a response to manifest, e.g. >2–3 months (see p.150).[11–13] Concurrent use with a conventional antidepressant has been reported, and may hasten the response compared with the latter alone, particularly in relation to fatigue.[12]

Fatigue
Psychostimulants are a supplementary treatment when non-drug treatment is insufficient.[14–16] Non-drug measures include the correction, if feasible, of underlying causal factors (e.g. anemia, depression and electrolyte disturbance) and modification to the patient's daily routine (e.g. gentle exercise, energy conservation and practical help to facilitate adjustment to changing circumstances).[14]

Opioid-related drowsiness
Drowsiness is common when opioids are commenced or the dose is increased; it is generally transient. Persistent drowsiness may indicate opioid toxicity; a trial dose reduction should be made and alternative analgesic measures should be considered (see p.234). However, some patients experience persistent drowsiness despite adjusting the opioid dose; in this circumstance, switching to an alternative opioid may be of benefit (see p.294).

Psychostimulants are sometimes used for drowsiness refractory to these measures, particularly **methylphenidate** (see p.168). They improve psychomotor performance and allow opioid dose escalation to a higher level than would otherwise be possible.[17] This can be particularly helpful for patients experiencing break-through (episodic) pain.[18–21]

Supply
Unless indicated otherwise, all products are Schedule III controlled drugs under the Controlled Drugs and Substances Act (CDSA), and in part 1 of schedule G of the Food and Drugs Act. SR formulations are available, but are not appropriate as daytime stimulants in palliative care.

Dextroamphetamine
Dexedrine® (GlaxoSmithKline)
Tablets 5mg, 28 days @ 5mg once daily = $17.

Also see **Methylphenidate**, p.168.

1 Boutrel B and Koob GF (2004) What keeps us awake: the neuropharmacology of stimulants and wakefulness-promoting medications. *Sleep.* **27**: 1181–1194.
2 Kapur S et al. (2005) From dopamine to salience to psychosis–linking biology, pharmacology and phenomenology of psychosis. *Schizophrenia Research.* **79**: 59–68.
3 Sulzer D et al. (2005) Mechanisms of neurotransmitter release by amphetamines: a review. *Progress in Neurobiology.* **75**: 406–433.
4 Fleckenstein AE et al. (2007) New insights into the mechanism of action of amphetamines. *Annual Review of Pharmacology and Toxicology.* **47**: 681–698.
5 Kumar R (2008) Approved and investigational uses of modafinil: an evidence-based review. *Drugs.* **68**: 1803–1839.
6 Qu WM et al. (2008) Dopaminergic D1 and D2 receptors are essential for the arousal effect of modafinil. *Journal of Neuroscience.* **28**: 8462–8469.
7 Volkow ND et al. (2009) Effects of modafinil on dopamine and dopamine transporters in the male human brain: clinical implications. *Journal of the American Medical Association.* **301**: 1148–1154.
8 Volkow ND et al. (2005) Imaging the effects of methylphenidate on brain dopamine: new model on its therapeutic actions for attention-deficit/hyperactivity disorder. *Biological Psychiatry.* **57**: 1410–1415.
9 Dein S and George R (2002) A place for psychostimulants in palliative care? *J Palliat Care.* **18**: 196–199.
10 Burns MM and Eisendrath SJ (1994) Dextroamphetamine treatment for depression in terminally ill patients. *Psychosomatics.* **35**: 80–83.
11 Block S (2000) Assessing and managing depression in the terminally ill patient. *Annals of Internal Medicine.* **132**: 209–218.

12 Orr K and Taylor D (2007) Psychostimulants in the treatment of depression: a review of the evidence. *CNS Drugs.* **21**: 239–257.

13 Candy M *et al.* (2008) Psychostimulants for depression. *Cochrane Database of Systematic Reviews.* **2**: CD006722.

14 Radbruch L *et al.* (2008) Fatigue in palliative care patients – an EAPC approach. *Palliative Medicine.* **22**: 13–32.

15 Minton O *et al.* (2008) A systematic review and meta-analysis of the pharmacological treatment of cancer-related fatigue. *Journal of the National Cancer Institute.* **100**: 1155–1166.

16 NCCN-fatigue (2008) National comprehensive care network clinical practice guidelines in oncology: cancer related fatigue. Available from: www.nccn.org/professionals/physician_gls/PDF/fatigue.pdf

17 Dalal S and Melzack R (1998) Potentiation of opioid analgesia by psychostimulant drugs: a review. *Journal of Pain and Symptom Management.* **16**: 245–253.

18 Bruera E *et al.* (1989) Use of methylphenidate as an adjuvant to narcotic analgesics in patients with advanced cancer. *Journal of Pain and Symptom Management.* **4**: 3–6.

19 Bruera E *et al.* (1992) Neuropsychological effects of methylphenidate in patients receiving a continuous infusion of narcotics for cancer pain. *Pain.* **48**: 163–166.

20 Bruera E *et al.* (1992) The use of methylphenidate in patients with incident cancer pain receiving regular opiates: a preliminary report. *Pain.* **50**: 75–77.

21 Wilwerding M *et al.* (1995) A randomized, crossover evaluation of methylphenidate in cancer patients receiving strong narcotics. *Supportive Care in Cancer.* **3**: 135–138.

Guidelines: Psychostimulants in depressed patients with a short prognosis

A psychostimulant is the drug of choice for treating depression in patients with a prognosis of <3 months because they may not live long enough to maximally benefit from a conventional antidepressant. It is often possible to achieve a response in a few days by increasing the dose steadily until benefit or undesirable effects occur. Psychostimulants are not as effective as conventional antidepressants, and these should be considered instead or concurrently in patients with a sufficient prognosis for a response to manifest, e.g. >2–3 months.

Advantages

Well tolerated and generally effective.
No lag time to effect.
Rapid clearance from the body.
Paradoxically improve appetite in the physically ill.
Pemoline (not Canada) comes in chewable form.

Disadvantages

Can only be given PO.
May precipitate/exacerbate delirium.
Undesirable effects include restlessness, hallucinations, insomnia, tachycardia, hypertension.
Tolerance may develop.
Withdrawal depression if stopped abruptly after prolonged use.

Agents

Dextroamphetamine:
* start with 2.5–5mg each morning
* if necessary, increase progressively every 1–2 days to 20mg each morning.

Methylphenidate
* start with 2.5–5mg b.i.d. (early morning and noon)
* if necessary, increase progressively every 1–2 days to 20mg b.i.d.

Dose titration

Start with recommended doses.
Check response daily.
Increase dose every 1–2 days by the smallest practical amount until:
* the depression resolves *or*
* unacceptable undesirable effects occur *or*
* the maximum recommended dose is reached.

*METHYLPHENIDATE

Class: Psychostimulant.

Indications: Attention-deficit hyperactivity disorder, †narcolepsy, †depression where prognosis <3 months, †opioid-related drowsiness, †fatigue refractory to correction of underlying causal factors,[1] †hypo-active delirium.[2,3]

Contra-indications: Severe anxiety or agitation, motor tics, hyperthyroidism, severe angina, cardiac arrhythmia, glaucoma.

Pharmacology

Methylphenidate is a CNS stimulant structurally related to **dextroamphetamine** but is less potent and has a shorter halflife (2h vs. 10h).[3,4] Both drugs reverse pre-synaptic dopamine re-uptake transporters thus increasing the release, and inhibiting the pre-synaptic re-uptake, of dopamine (see p.164).[5-7] Their action is thus antagonized by antipsychotics.

Methylphenidate is used for depression where a prompt response to treatment is required and tolerance to longer term use is irrelevant. Benefit is often seen in 2–3 days.[4,8] Despite limited evidence, a consensus panel concluded that a psychostimulant is the antidepressant of choice for patients with a prognosis of <3 months.[9]

Methylphenidate is used alongside non-drug measures for fatigue unresponsive to the correction of underlying causal factors (e.g. anemia).[10-12] It is also used to permit higher doses of opioids without excessive drowsiness in patients with break-through (episodic) pain (see Psychostimulants, p.164).

After almost complete oral absorption, it undergoes extensive first-pass hepatic metabolism via a non-P450 carboxylesterase resulting in an absolute bio-availability of 30%. The effect of food on absorption is unlikely to be significant. Although it is absorbed from the buccal mucosa, this route is not used clinically because of the higher risk of undesirable effects.[13] The major metabolite, ritalinic acid, is inactive and excreted mainly in the urine.[14] Like **dextroamphetamine**, little relation exists between plasma levels and behavioural or physiological effects.[15]

Bio-availability 30% (extensive first-pass metabolism).
Onset of action 20–40min.
Time to peak plasma concentration 1–3h.
Plasma halflife 2h.
Duration of action 3–6h.

Cautions

Cardiovascular disease (e.g. severe hypertension, arrhythmia and angina), psychiatric illness (e.g. anxiety, agitation, psychosis and addiction), epilepsy (possible lowering of seizure threshold), hyperthyroidism, closed-angle glaucoma.

Drug interactions

Methylphenidate may inhibit the metabolism of **warfarin**, TCAs and **phenytoin**. Its action is antagonized by antipsychotics.

Undesirable effects

For full list, see manufacturer's Product Monograph.
Very common (>10%): nervousness and insomnia (at the beginning of treatment, but can be controlled by reducing the dose).
Common (<10%, >1%): headache, dizziness, dyskinesia, tachycardia, palpitations, arrhythmias, increase in blood pressure, abdominal pain, nausea, vomiting (when starting treatment, but may be alleviated by concurrent food intake), decreased appetite (transient), dry mouth, rash, pruritus, urticaria, fever, arthralgia, scalp hair loss.

Dose and use

Individual dose titration is necessary to maximize benefit and minimize undesirable effects:
- start with 2.5–5mg b.i.d. (on waking/breakfast time and noon/lunchtime),
- if necessary, increase by daily increments of 2.5–5mg b.i.d.,
- usual maximum 20mg b.i.d. (occasionally, even higher doses are necessary, e.g. 30mg b.i.d. or 20mg t.i.d.[16]

Supply

Unless indicated otherwise, all products are Schedule III controlled drugs under the Controlled Drugs and Substances Act (CDSA), and in part 1 of schedule G of the Food and Drugs Act. SR formulations are available, but are not appropriate as daytime stimulants in palliative care.

Methylphenidate (generic)
Tablets 5mg, 10mg, 20mg, 28 days @ 10mg b.i.d. = $9.

Ritalin® (Novartis)
Tablets 10mg, 20mg, 28 days @ 10mg b.i.d. = $21.

1 Blockmans D et al. (2006) Does methylphenidate reduce the symptoms of chronic fatigue syndrome? American Journal of Medicine. **119**: 167 e123–130.
2 Gagnon B et al. (2005) Methylphenidate hydrochloride improves cognitive function in patients with advanced cancer and hypoactive delirium: a prospective clinical study. Journal of Psychiatry and Neuroscience. **30**: 100–107.
3 Sood A et al. (2006) Use of methylphenidate in patients with cancer. American Journal of Hospice and Palliative Care. **23**: 35–40.
4 Rozans M et al. (2002) Palliative uses of methylphenidate in patients with cancer: a review. Journal of Clinical Oncology. **20**: 335–339.
5 Boutrel B and Koob GF (2004) What keeps us awake: the neuropharmacology of stimulants and wakefulness-promoting medications. Sleep. **27**: 1181–1194.
6 Sulzer D et al. (2005) Mechanisms of neurotransmitter release by amphetamines: a review. Progress in Neurobiology. **75**: 406–433.
7 Fleckenstein AE et al. (2007) New insights into the mechanism of action of amphetamines. Annual Review of Pharmacology and Toxicology. **47**: 681–698.
8 Homsi J et al. (2000) Psychostimulants in supportive care. Supportive Care in Cancer. **8**: 385–397.
9 Block S (2000) Assessing and managing depression in the terminally ill patient. Annals of Internal Medicine. **132**: 209–218.
10 Minton O et al. (2008) A systematic review and meta-analysis of the pharmacological treatment of cancer-related fatigue. Journal of the National Cancer Institute. **100**: 1155–1166.
11 NCCN-fatigue (2008) National comprehensive care network clinical practice guidelines in oncology: cancer related fatigue. Available from: www.nccn.org/professionals/physician_gls/PDF/fatigue.pdf
12 Radbruch L et al. (2008) Fatigue in palliative care patients – an EAPC approach. Palliative Medicine. **22**: 13–32.
13 Pleak R (1995) Adverse effects of chewing methylphenidate. American Journal of Psychiatry. **152**: 811.
14 Challman TD and Lipsky JJ (2000) Methylphenidate: its pharmacology and uses. Mayo Clinic Proceedings. **75**: 711–721.
15 Little K (1993) d-Amphetamine versus methylphenidate effects in depressed inpatients. Journal of Clinical Psychiatry. **54**: 349–355.
16 Orr K and Taylor D (2007) Psychostimulants in the treatment of depression: a review of the evidence. CNS Drugs. **21**: 239–257.

CANNABINOIDS

Cannabis sativa (marihuana) has been used therapeutically and recreationally for thousands of years.[1] Greater understanding of the endocannabinoid system, together with case reports and RCTs,[2–4] suggest a range of potential therapeutic uses. At present cannabinioids are approved for:
- anti-emesis in chemotherapy
- appetite stimulation in AIDS-related anorexia
- refractory pain in multiple sclerosis and advanced cancer.

Currently available cannabinoids are generally poorly tolerated. However, their use as anti-emetics has been largely eclipsed by the introduction of $5HT_3$-receptor antagonists (see below), and they are less effective (and/or less well tolerated) than established analgesics in many settings.[5,6] In the future, it is possible that tolerability will be improved by the development of:
- CB_2 selective agonists[7]
- peripherally-acting cannabinoids
- targeting endocannabinoid metabolism or uptake[8]
- combining cannabinoids with different properties, e.g. Δ^9-tetrahydrocannabinol (Δ^9-THC) with cannabidiol (CBD) (see below).[9]

Cannabinoids may have therapeutic value in other situations including migraine, muscle spasticity, Parkinson's disease, epilepsy and glaucoma; but the evidence for these claims is either scanty or conflicting.[10] Other possible benefits include an antitumour effect, immunomodulation, mood elevation, and relief of insomnia.[11]

The endocannabinoid system

The endocannabinoid system comprises:[12]
- 2 known receptors:
  ▷ CB_1, expressed by central and peripheral neurones
  ▷ CB_2, expressed mainly by immune cells
- several endocannabinoids, mainly fatty acids derived from arachidonic acid (a precursor for many other biochemical mediators including prostaglandins)
- enzymes and uptake systems involved in endocannabinoid metabolism, including COX-2.[8]

CB_1 has an important regulatory role in the synapse. Endocannabinoids are synthesized de novo in post-synaptic neurones in response to rising intracellular calcium. They act upon pre-synaptic CB_1-receptors, inhibiting further neurotransmitter release. In this way, they are thought to play an important modulatory role in the release of GABA and glutamate in cortical, limbic, and other areas associated with pain signaling.[12]

CB_2 is implicated in immune regulation. Located on antigen-presenting cells, and influencing their production of cytokines (e.g. interleukin (IL) 10 and 12), it affects the cytokine profile of T-helper cells.[13,14] This may partly explain its anti-inflammatory and antihyperalgesic effects. Its expression is upregulated in the dorsal root ganglia and spinal cord following sciatic nerve injury. The antihyperalgesic effects of CB_1 and CB_2 activation are distinct and additive.[15]

Endocannabinoids also act at other receptors, including the capsaicin receptor (TRPV1, involved in pain signaling), and perhaps also G protein-coupled receptors (GPR) 55 and 119.[16]

Most endocannabinoids are fatty acids derived from arachidonic acid, produced de novo as required, and then rapidly removed by hydrolysis. Several have been identified, notably anandamide (arachidonylethanolamide) and 2-arachidonyl glycerin (2-AG).[17] The modulatory role of cannabinoids appears to parallel that of the opioid system functionally.[18]

A range of exogenous ligands have been identified, both naturally-occurring cannabinoids from marihuana (Cannabis sativa), e.g. Δ^9-THC (**dronabinol**; see p.175), CBD, and synthetic substances, e.g. **nabilone** (see p.173).

Cannabinoids as anti-emetics

A systematic review of chemotherapy-induced nausea and vomiting found that cannabinoids had some anti-emetic efficacy in moderately emetogenic settings when compared with placebo, similar to that seen with dopamine antagonists.[19] However, in highly emetogenic settings, cannabinoids were indistinguishable from placebo. Most of these studies were performed before the introduction of specific $5HT_3$-receptor antagonists (see p.192), which have a high therapeutic index. Compared with $5HT_3$-receptor antagonists, the undesirable effects of cannabinoids outweigh their benefits (see below).[10,20]

Cannabinoids as analgesics

A systematic review of cannabinoids as analgesics for mainly postoperative and cancer pain showed that cannabinoids are no more effective than **codeine** 60mg in relieving acute and chronic pain but had more undesirable effects.[5,10] Undesirable effects were common and sometimes severe; the most common being drowsiness.

A combination of the 2 phytocannabinoids, Δ^9-THC and CBD, has been investigated in an attempt to improve the efficacy/tolerability profile (Box 4.L). CBD reduced Δ^9-THC-induced anxiety in healthy volunteers, perhaps by inhibiting the metabolism of Δ^9-THC to a more psycho-active metabolite, 11-hydroxyTHC.[21,22] Of 3 RCTs in patients with chronic pain, 2 found modest improvements in tolerability and patient preference compared with Δ^9-THC alone[23,24] whereas the third found no difference.[25] RCTs comparing this combination (Sativex®, see Box 4.L) with placebo for various non-cancer neuropathic pains consistently found a reduction in pain of ~1/10, with 6–18% of subjects withdrawing because of undesirable effects. Although modest, these reductions in pain are seen despite cannabinoids being added to optimized conventional analgesia and for difficult pain syndromes.[23,25–27] Open-label extension studies found that analgesia was maintained without dose escalation for 1–1.5 years.[27,28]

> **Box 4.L** Sativex® (Δ^9-THC 27mg/mL and CBD 25mg/mL) buccal spray (also see Canadian Product Monograph)
>
> **Indications**
> Approved as adjunctive treatment for neuropathic pain in multiple sclerosis and opioid poorly-responsive pain in cancer.
>
> **Contra-indications**
> Children, pregnant and nursing women, a history of psychosis, serious cardiovascular disease, allergy to cannabinoids, alcohol, peppermint oil or propylene glycol.
>
> **Cautions**
> Elderly (may cause postural hypotension), concurrent psycho-active drugs (additive effects with other psychotropics and CNS depressants, e.g. alcohol, sedatives). May reduce seizure threshold.
>
> **Drug interactions**
> Sativex® inhibits numerous P450 enzymes, although generally not at typical therapeutic concentrations. Caution is advised when substrates for CYP2C19, 2D6 (e.g. amitriptyline) and 3A4 (e.g. fentanyl and sufentanil) are used concurrently with Sativex®.
>
> **Undesirable effects**
> Dizziness (30% of patients, dose-dependent).
> Cognitive: disorientation, altered mood, dissociation and paranoia.
> Physical and psychological dependence.
> Cardiovascular: tachycardia, fainting and transient changes in blood pressure. Buccal: 20% of patients, including irritation, taste alteration and dry mouth.
>
> **Dose and use**
> Used for pain relief on a self-titration regimen.
> Start with 1 spray up to q4h (maximum 4 sprays in the first 24h).
> Direct spray beneath the tongue or inside the cheeks (not towards the pharynx).
> Vary the site and inspect buccal mucosa regularly for signs of irritation.
> Titrate up on a daily basis (but more slowly if dizziness occurs).
> Median number of sprays/day = 8 in cancer patients and 5 in multiple sclerosis.
> Most patients required $\leqslant$12/day.

An RCT of Δ^9-THC alone vs. placebo in patients with multiple sclerosis similarly found only a modest reduction in pain (−0.6).[29] An RCT of Sativex® in opioid poorly-responsive cancer pain also showed only modest benefit.[30]

Cannabinoids could have a therapeutic advantage over opioids because, unlike opioid receptors, CB_1-receptors persist in the spinal cord after peripheral nerve injury,[31,32] and there are 10 times more CB_1-receptors in the brain than opioid receptors.[33] Other animal experiments strongly suggest that the CB_2-receptor agonists have a potential role in antinociception (analgesia).[7] Synergy between **dronabinol** and opioids has also been shown.[34] CB_2-receptor agonists have a peripheral site of action and thus do not exhibit CNS effects such as sedation and respiratory depression. This could be a major advantage in pain management.

Cannabinoids and the respiratory system

Studies of the effects of smoking marihuana cigarettes or inhaling **dronabinol** have shown a bronchodilator effect together with either an increase in CO_2 sensitivity[35] or a slight respiratory depressant effect.[36,37] However, the potential benefits that could accrue from these actions are overshadowed by the finding that long-term cannabis smoking is associated with a form of chronic bronchitis (although this is not relevant for most patients receiving palliative care). Compared with smoking tobacco alone, smoking cannabis in addition increases the overall risk of cancer, particularly of the head and neck and the prostate.[38,39]

Undesirable effects

Numerous dose-limiting effects of oral cannabinoids and smoked marihuana have been noted in clinical trials (Box 4.M). Those seen with buccal Sativex® are comparable. Long-term use of cannabis increases the risk of developing schizophrenia, by a factor of 50.[40,41]

Box 4.M Dose-limiting effects of oral cannabinoids and smoked marihuana reported in clinical trials[10,20]

Physiological	**Psychological**
Ataxia	Drowsiness
Dizziness	Dysphoria
Blurred vision	Abnormal thinking
Dry mouth	Depersonalization
Hypotension	Hallucinations
	Psychosis

The psychotomimetic effects develop 30–90min after oral ingestion, are maximal after 2–4h, and may last up to 12h. Abrupt withdrawal after long-term use of high doses may result in withdrawal phenomena, e.g. inner unrest, irritability, insomnia, hot flashes, sweating, rhinorrhea, diarrhea, anorexia and hiccup. These are generally mild and the risk is low.

Supply

Marihuana is a controlled substance in Canada. It is not legal to grow or possess marihuana except with legal permission from Health Canada. The Marihuana Medical Access Regulations allow access to marihuana to people who are suffering from grave and debilitating illnesses (see p.177). Contact Health Canada at 1-866-337-7705 or see the programme information at www.hc-sc.gc.ca/dhp-mps/marihuana/index-eng.php.

Sativex® (GW Pharmaceuticals)
Oromucosal spray Cannabis sativa extract (**dronabinol** 2.92mg and **cannabidiol** 2.7mg per actuation; about 50 actuations/spray), pack of 4 × 5.5mL sprays = $549; *contains 50% alcohol.*

---

1 Mechoulam R (1986) The pharmacohistory of cannabis sativa. In: R Mechoulam (ed) *Cannabinoids as Therapeutic Agents.* CRC Press, Boca Raton, Fla.
2 Guy GW *et al.* (eds) (2004) *The Medicinal Uses of Cannabis and Cannabinoids.* Pharmaceutical Press, London.
3 Williamson EM and Evans FJ (2000) Cannabinoids in clinical practice. *Drugs.* **60**: 1303–1314.
4 Ashton CH (2001) Pharmacology and effects of cannabis: a brief review. *British Journal of Psychiatry.* **178**: 101–106.
5 Campbell F *et al.* (2001) Are cannabinoids an effective and safe treatment option in the management of pain? A qualitative systematic review. *British Medical Journal.* **323**: 13–16.
6 Frank B *et al.* (2008) Comparison of analgesic effects and patient tolerability of nabilone and dihydrocodeine for chronic neuropathic pain: randomised, crossover, double blind study. *British Medical Journal.* **336**: 199–201.
7 Ibrahim MM *et al.* (2006) CB2 cannabinoid receptor mediation of antinociception. *Pain.* **122**: 36–42.
8 Jhaveri MD *et al.* (2007) Endocannabinoid metabolism and uptake: novel targets for neuropathic and inflammatory pain. *British Journal of Pharmacology.* **152**: 624–632.
9 Barnes MP (2006) Sativex: clinical efficacy and tolerability in the treatment of symptoms of multiple sclerosis and neuropathic pain. *Expert Opinion on Pharmacotherpy.* **7**: 607–615.
10 Bagshaw SM and Hagan NA (2002) Medical efficacy of cannabinoids and marijuana: a comprehensive review of the literature. *Journal of Palliative Care.* **18 (2)**: 111–122.
11 Walsh D *et al.* (2003) Established and potential therapeutic applications of cannabinoids in oncology. *Supportive Care in Cancer.* **11**: 137–143.
12 Rea K *et al.* (2007) Supraspinal modulation of pain by cannabinoids: the role of GABA and glutamate. *British Journal of Pharmacology.* **152**: 633–648.
13 Correa F *et al.* (2005) Activation of cannabinoid CB2 receptor negatively regulates IL-12p40 production in murine macrophages: role of IL-10 and ERK1/2 kinase signaling. *British Journal of Pharmacology.* **145**: 441–448.
14 Ziring D *et al.* (2006) Formation of B and T cell subsets require the cannabinoid receptor CB2. *Immunogenetics.* **58**: 714–725.
15 Gutierrez T *et al.* (2007) Activation of peripheral cannabinoid CB1 and CB2 receptors suppresses the maintenance of inflammatory nociception: a comparative analysis. *British Journal of Pharmacology.* **150**: 153–163.
16 Brown AJ (2007) Novel cannabinoid receptors. *British Journal of Pharmacology.* **152**: 567–575.
17 Mechoulam R *et al.* (1998) Endocannabinoids. *European Journal of Pharmacology.* **359**: 1–18.

---

18 Piomelli D et al. (2000) The endocannabinoid system as a target for therapeutic drugs. Trends in Pharmacological Science. **21**: 218–224.

19 Tramer M et al. (2001) Cannabinoids for control of chemotherapy induced nausea and vomiting: quantitative systemic review. British Medical Journal. **323**: 16–21.

20 Institute of Medicine (1999) Marijuana and Medicine. National Academy Press, Washington.

21 Zuardi AW et al. (1982) Action of cannabidiol on the anxiety and other effects produced by delta 9-THC in normal subjects. Psychopharmacology (Berl). **76**: 245–250.

22 Russo EB and McPartland JM (2003) Cannabis is more than simply delta(9)-tetrahydrocannabinol. Psychopharmacology (Berl). **165**: 431–432; author reply 433–434.

23 Wade DT et al. (2003) A preliminary controlled study to determine whether whole-plant cannabis extracts can improve intractable neurogenic symptoms. Clinical Rehabilitation. **17**: 21–29.

24 Notcutt W et al. (2004) Initial experiences with medicinal extracts of cannabis for chronic pain: results from 34 'N of 1' studies. Anaesthesia. **59**: 440–452.

25 Berman JS et al. (2004) Efficacy of two cannabis based medicinal extracts for relief of central neuropathic pain from brachial plexus avulsion: results of a randomised controlled trial. Pain. **112**: 299–306.

26 Rog DJ et al. (2005) Randomized, controlled trial of cannabis-based medicine in central pain in multiple sclerosis. Neurology. **65**: 812–819.

27 Nurmikko TJ et al. (2007) Sativex successfully treats neuropathic pain characterised by allodynia: a randomised, double-blind, placebo-controlled clinical trial. Pain. **133**: 210–220.

28 Wade DT et al. (2006) Long-term use of a cannabis-based medicine in the treatment of spasticity and other symptoms in multiple sclerosis. Multiple Sclerosis. **12**: 639–645.

29 Svendsen KB et al. (2004) Does the cannabinoid dronabinol reduce central pain in multiple sclerosis? Randomised double blind placebo controlled crossover trial. British Medical Journal. **329**: 253.

30 Johnson JR and Wright S (2005) Cannabis-based medicines in the treatment of cancer pain: a randomized, double-blind, parallel group, placebo-controlled, comparative study of the efficacy, safety, and tolerability of Sativex and Tetranabinex in patients with cancer-related pain. Journal of Supportive Oncology. **3 (supp 3)**: 21.

31 Hohmann AG and Herkenham M (1998) Regulation of cannabinoid and mu opioid receptors in rat lumbar spinal cord following neonatal capsaicin treatment. Neuroscience Letters. **252**: 13–16.

32 Farquhar-Smith WP and Rice AS (2001) Administration of endocannabinoids prevents a referred hyperalgesia associated with inflammation of the urinary bladder. Anesthesiology. **94**: 507–513; discussion 506A.

33 Davis M et al. (2007) The emerging role of cannabinoid neuromodulators in symptom management. Supportive Care in Cancer. **15**: 63–71.

34 Cichewicz DL and McCarthy EA (2003) Antinociceptive synergy between delta(9)-tetrahydrocannabinol and opioids after oral administration. Journal of Pharmacology and Experimental Therapeutics. **304**: 1010–1015.

35 Vachon L et al. (1973) Single-dose effect of marihuana smoke. New England Journal of Medicine. **288**: 985–989.

36 Bellville J et al. (1975) Respiratory effects of delta-9-tetrahydrocannabinol. Clinical Pharmacology and Therapeutics. **17**: 541–548.

37 Tashkin D et al. (1977) Bronchial effects of aerosolized 9-tetrahydrocannabinol in healthy and asthmatic subjects. American Review of Respiratory Disease. **115**: 57–65.

38 Hashibe M et al. (2005) Epidemiologic review of marijuana use and cancer risk. Alcohol. **35**: 265–275.

39 Hall W et al. (2005) Cannabinoids and cancer: causation, remediation, and palliation. Lancet Oncology. **6**: 35–42.

40 Zammit S et al. (2002) Self reported cannabis use as a risk factor for schizophrenia in Swedish conscripts of 1969: historical cohort study. British Medical Journal. **325**: 1199.

41 Fergusson DM et al. (2006) Cannabis and psychosis. British Medical Journal. **332**: 172–175.

*NABILONE

Class: Cannabinoid.

Indications: Severe nausea and vomiting associated with cancer chemotherapy, †breathlessness, †spasticity.

Contra-indications: History of psychosis.

Pharmacology

Nabilone is a synthetic cannabinoid which has significant anti-emetic activity in patients receiving moderately emetogenic cytotoxic chemotherapy.[1,2] Its mechanism of action is not fully understood but there are several points where nabilone could act to block emesis.[3] Nabilone is well absorbed orally. The main metabolite, 9-hydroxynabilone, is pharmacologically active with a plasma halflife up to 5 times longer than that of nabilone itself.[4] Like other cannabinoids, nabilone may cause sedation and, less often, hallucinations and other psychotomimetic effects. Undesirable effects on mental state can last 2-3 days after the last dose. Since the advent of specific $5HT_3$-receptor antagonists, used alone or with **dexamethasone**, there is only a limited place for nabilone as an anti-emetic with cancer chemotherapy.[1]

At a typical anti-emetic dose of 2mg b.i.d., nabilone has bronchodilator activity in normal subjects and increases the ventilatory response to CO_2.[5] This respiratory stimulation occurs at the time of maximal cortical sedation. Both the bronchodilation and the ventilatory enhancement may be a reflection of a widespread non-specific sympathetic arousal. Thus subjects taking

nabilone can feel relaxed and drowsy, and may have demonstrable reduction in PO_2 as a result but, paradoxically, sensitivity to CO_2 is increased. This combination of effects has led to its occasional use for the relief of breathlessness in terminally ill patients.[6] In this context, nabilone should be reserved for patients who:
- are frequently or continuously breathless
- exhibit great anxiety
- would be in danger of slipping into hypercapnic respiratory failure with other conventional respiratory sedatives.

Nabilone and other potentially sedative drugs (e.g. benzodiazepines, opioids, alcohol) have additive CNS depressant events.

Bio-availability 85% PO.
Onset of action 60–90min.
Time to peak plasma concentration 2h.
Plasma halflife 2h; active metabolite 9-hydroxynabilone 5–10h; combined metabolites 35h.
Duration of action 8–12h.

Cautions
Because of possible hypotension and reflex tachycardia, nabilone is unsuitable for patients with atrial fibrillation or in heart failure, and possibly the elderly. History of psychoses.

Undesirable effects
For full list, see manufacturer's Product Monograph.

Very common (>10%): drowsiness, vertigo, euphoria, dry mouth, depression, ataxia, sensation disturbance.
Common (<10%, >1%): anorexia, asthenia, headache, orthostatic hypotension, hallucinations.
Uncommon (<1%): tremors, tachycardia, syncope, nightmares, distortion in the perception of time, confusion, dissociation, dysphoria, psychotic reactions, seizures.
Tolerance to CNS effects generally develops after a few days.

Dose and use
Nausea and vomiting
Should be given immediately before, during and for 2 days after each pulse of chemotherapy:
- start with 1mg b.i.d.
- if necessary, increase to 2mg b.i.d.
- the maximum recommended dose is 2mg t.i.d.[7]

Breathlessness
The doses are much lower than those for anti-emesis:
- start with 100microgram b.i.d.
- if necessary, increase to 250microgram q.i.d.[8]

Above this dose, many patients find the sedation unacceptable.

Spasticity
The use of nabilone for spasticity in multiple sclerosis is under investigation.[9]

Supply
Cesamet® (Valiant)
Capsules 250microgram, 500microgram, 1mg, 28 days @ 1mg b.i.d. = \$495.
Doses of <500microgram can be given by compounding with lactose powder, or by preparing a solution.

1 Kris MG *et al.* (2006) American Society of Clinical Oncology guideline for antiemetics in oncology: update 2006. *Journal of Clinical Oncology.* **24**: 2932–2947.
2 Tramer M *et al.* (2001) Cannabinoids for control of chemotherapy induced nausea and vomiting: quantitative systemic review. *British Medical Journal.* **323**: 16–21.
3 Piomelli D *et al.* (2000) The endocannabinoid system as a target for therapeutic drugs. *Trends in Pharmacological Science.* **21**: 218–224.

4 Rubin A et al. (1977) Physiologic disposition of nabilone, a cannabinol derivative, in man. Clinical Pharmacology and Therapeutics. **22**: 85–91.
5 McAlpine L and Thomson N (1989) Lidocaine-induced bronchoconstriction in asthmatic patients. Relation to histamine airway responsiveness and effect of preservative. Chest. **96**: 1012–1015.
6 Ahmedzai S (1988) Respiratory distress in the terminally ill patient. Respiratory Disease in Practice. **5**: 21–29.
7 Mannix K (1997) Palliation of nausea and vomiting. In: D Doyle et al. (eds) Oxford Textbook of Palliative Medicine (2e). Oxford University Press, Oxford, pp. 489–499.
8 Ahmedzai S (1997) Palliation of respiratory symptoms. In: D Doyle et al. (eds) Oxford Textbook of Palliative Medicine (2e). Oxford University Press, Oxford, pp. 583–616.
9 Pertwee RG (2002) Cannabinoids and multiple sclerosis. Pharmacology and Therapeutics. **95**: 165–174.

*DRONABINOL

Class: Cannabinoid.

Indications: Chemotherapy-induced nausea and vomiting, AIDS-related anorexia and weight loss, †spasticity, †tremor and ataxia in multiple sclerosis, cerebral palsy and spinal cord injury,[1] †glaucoma, †pain.

Contra-indications: Children, pregnant and nursing women, women of child-bearing age not on reliable contraception, men intending to father a child, a history of psychosis, serious cardiovascular disease, significant hepatic or renal impairment.

Pharmacology

Dronabinol is synthetic tetrahydrocannabinol (THC). It is probably the most important naturally-occurring psycho-active compound of the plant *Cannabis sativa* (marihuana). *Cannabis sativa* also contains other active compounds, including cannabidiol, cannabigerol, cannabinol, cannabichromene, and olivetol. Pharmacological data from animal studies suggest that not all the observed therapeutic effects can be traced to the THC content or any other single cannabinoid.[2] Thus, *Cannabis sativa* and dronabinol do not have identical pharmacologic effects. Dronabinol has proven efficacy in relieving chemotherapy-induced nausea and vomiting[3,4] and AIDS-related anorexia.[4] However, an RCT showed no benefit in cancer-related anorexia.[5]

Although dronabinol has been used for the treatment of break-through nausea and vomiting associated with chemotherapy, it is not the drug of choice for prophylaxis. First-line prophylactic medication is a $5HT_3$-receptor antagonist (see p.192) and/or **metoclopramide** (see p.185) and/or corticosteroids (see p.381). The effects of cannabinoids on other types of nausea and vomiting are less pronounced.[6]

Although dronabinol 20mg has a weak analgesic effect, comparable to **codeine** in patients with cancer pain,[7] the incidence of undesirable effects precludes its routine use (see Box 4.M, p.172).[8,9] In a trial of dronabinol 10mg daily in patients with multiple sclerosis, a small statistically significant benefit was seen (mean pain intensity 4/10 vs. 5/10 on placebo), and no patient withdrew because of undesirable effects.[10] However, in an open study in 8 patients with refractory neuropathic pain, no benefit was seen with individually titrated doses of dronabinol (increased weekly if tolerated from 2.5mg b.i.d. to a maximum dose of 12.5mg b.i.d.), and 7 patients withdrew because of undesirable effects.[11] With various forms of induced pain, dronabinol 20mg in volunteers did not relieve pain, and there was a suggestion that it partly antagonized **morphine** analgesia.[12] On the other hand, in a case report, a woman with chronic painful cystitis obtained ongoing good relief with dronabinol 2.5mg on alternate days.[13]

Bio-availability 10–30% PO.[2,14]
Onset of action 0.5–2h PO.[14]
Time to peak plasma concentration 2–3h PO.
Plasma halflife 15–18h for the primary active metabolite, 11-hydroxydronabinol; 25–36h for secondary active metabolites.
Duration of action 1–4h PO.

Cautions

Use caution when using dronabinol in patients with cardiac disorders; hypotension, hypertension, syncope, or tachycardia is possible. Concurrent therapy with sedatives, hypnotics, or other psycho-active drugs may potentiate sedative and CNS depressant effects. The elderly may be more sensitive to the psycho-active effects of dronabinol. Caution should be exercised when using dronabinol in patients with a history of substance abuse, mania, depression, schizophrenia, or other mental illness.

Undesirable effects

For full list, see manufacturer's Product Monograph.

A range of feelings described as a 'high' occur in about 80% of patients using dronabinol, including easy laughing, elation, heightened awareness, mild aberrations of fine motor co-ordination, minimal distortion of activities and interactions with others. The most common undesirable effects (3–10%) with dronabinol are CNS effects, including dizziness, euphoria, paranoid thoughts, drowsiness and abnormal thinking. Less common (0.3–1%) are depression, nightmares, speech difficulties and tinnitus.

It may also cause hypotension, hypertension, syncope, tachycardia, palpitations, vasodilation, facial flushing, nausea, vomiting, abdominal pain, dry mouth and rash.

Dose and use

Anti-emetic

5–15mg/m^2 q3–6h.

Appetite stimulation

2.5mg PO b.i.d., generally before lunch and dinner. Reduce dose to 2.5mg before dinner or at bedtime if undesirable effects occur and do not resolve within 3 days of continued use. May gradually increase to a maximum of 20mg daily for greater therapeutic effect if undesirable effects are absent.

Supply

Marinol® (Solvay Pharma)

Capsules (*all contain sesame oil*) 2.5mg, 5mg, 10mg, 28 days @ 2.5mg b.i.d. = $119; 28 days @ 5mg q.i.d. = $473.

1 Killestein J et al. (2004) Cannabinoids in multiple sclerosis: do they have a therapeutic role? *Drugs.* **64**: 1–11.
2 Grotenhermen F (2003) Pharmacokinetics and pharmacodynamics of cannabinoids. *Clinical Pharmacokinetics.* **42**: 327–360.
3 Tramer M et al. (2001) Cannabinoids for control of chemotherapy induced nausea and vomiting: quantitative systemic review. *British Medical Journal.* **323**: 16–21.
4 Walsh D et al. (2003) Established and potential therapeutic applications of cannabinoids in oncology. *Supportive Care in Cancer.* **11**: 137–143.
5 Strasser F et al. (2006) Comparison of orally administered cannabis extract and delta-9-tetrahydrocannabinol in treating patients with cancer-related anorexia-cachexia syndrome: a multicenter, phase III, randomized, double-blind, placebo-controlled clinical trial from the Cannabis-In-Cachexia-Study-Group. *Journal of Clinical Oncology.* **24**: 3394–3400.
6 Williamson EM and Evans FJ (2000) Cannabinoids in clinical practice. *Drugs.* **60**: 1303–1314.
7 Noyes R et al. (1975) The analgesic properties of delta-9-tetrahydrocannabinol and codeine. *Clinical Pharmacology and Therapeutics.* **18**: 84–89.
8 Campbell F et al. (2001) Are cannabinoids an effective and safe treatment option in the management of pain? A qualitative systematic review. *British Medical Journal.* **323**: 13–16.
9 Bagshaw SM and Hagan NA (2002) Medical efficacy of cannabinoids and marijuana: a comprehensive review of the literature. *Journal of Palliative Care.* **18 (2)**: 111–122.
10 Svendsen KB et al. (2004) Does the cannabinoid dronabinol reduce central pain in multiple sclerosis? Randomised double blind placebo controlled crossover trial. *British Medical Journal.* **329**: 253.
11 Attal N et al. (2004) Are oral cannabinoids safe and effective in refractory neuropathic pain? *European Journal of Pain.* **8**: 173–177.
12 Naef M et al. (2003) The analgesic effect of oral delta-9-tetrahydrocannabinol (THC), morphine, and a THC-morphine combination in healthy subjects under experimental pain conditions. *Pain.* **105**: 79–88.
13 Krenn H et al. (2003) A case of cannabinoid rotation in a young woman with chronic cystitis. *Journal of Pain and Symptom Management.* **25**: 3–4.
14 Ashton CH (2001) Pharmacology and effects of cannabis: a brief review. *British Journal of Psychiatry.* **178**: 101–106.

MEDICINAL MARIHUANA

Class: Cannabinoid.

Marihuana is not an approved drug, and has not been issued a Notice of Compliance under the Food and Drug Regulations. Although the federal Controlled Drugs and Substances Act presently permits the *possession* of up to 30g of marihuana,[1] the only allowance for its *use* is contained in the Marihuana Medical Access Regulations (MMAR) 2001; amended 2005.[2,3] The regulations outline two categories of people who can possess marihuana for medical purposes.

Indications: Category 1: †Any symptoms treated within the context of compassionate end-of-life care, or symptoms associated with the specified medical conditions listed in the schedule to the MMAR, namely †severe pain and/or †persistent muscle spasms from multiple sclerosis, spinal cord injury or spinal cord disease; †severe pain, †cachexia, †anorexia, †weight loss and/or †severe nausea from cancer or HIV infection/AIDS; †severe pain from severe forms of arthritis; or †epileptic seizures.
Category 2: †Debilitating symptoms of medical conditions other than those in Category 1.

Contra-indications: History of psychosis.

Pharmacology
Marihuana contains about 65 different cannabinoids, of which Δ^9-tetrahydrocannabinol (Δ^9-THC) is the main source of the pharmacological effects.[4,5] Others identified include Δ^8-tetrahydrocannabinol (Δ^8-THC), cannabinol and cannabidiol, the last having no psycho-active properties. Users of marihuana claim greater symptom relief than with the use of approved THC products such as **dronabinol** or **nabilone**. However, reports of symptom relief from smoked or PO marihuana vary, but claimed benefits include improved appetite (particularly in cachectic HIV/AIDS patients), reduced nausea and vomiting, relief of chronic pain (particularly neuropathic pain), relief of spasticity associated with multiple sclerosis or spinal cord injury, decreased bladder spasms, improved sleep, reduced anxiety, improved mood, and a sense of wellbeing.[5]
Bio-availability 10–35% inhaled.[6]
Onset of action a few seconds inhaled.[6]
Time to peak plasma concentration 3–10min inhaled.[6]
Duration of action 3–4h inhaled.[6]

Cautions
As for the approved oral cannabinoids, **dronabinol** (see p.175) and **nabilone** (see p.173).

Undesirable effects
Chronic cannabis smoking is associated with bronchitis, emphysema, and squamous metaplasia of the tracheobronchial epithelium.[7] There is an increased association with cancer of the oropharynx and tongue, nasal and sinus epithelium, and larynx. It also has dose-related effects on driving and other psychomotor skills.[6] Other undesirable effects include slowed thoughts, fatigue or tiredness, decreased energy, confusion, anxiety, paranoia, tachycardia, and unwanted increases in appetite and weight.[5]

Dose and use
Severe pain, muscle spasm, spasticity, nausea, anorexia/cachexia and epileptic seizures
- generally 1–3g/24h (average 2.5g/24h)
- range: <1g–5g/24h.[4,5,8]

Supply

Marihuana is a controlled substance. Supply and possession are illegal outside the provisions of the MMAR. Physicians are strongly advised to read the information on the Health Canada website before signing the form supporting a patient's application.[4]

Patients wishing to use marihuana for symptom relief must apply in writing to Health Canada for either seeds to grow their own supply (or a person can be designated to grow it for them), or for a supply of dried marihuana. Application forms and guidelines are available from the Health Canada website[4] or by calling Health Canada toll-free at 1-866-337-7705. Applicants must provide a declaration from a medical practitioner to support the application (this form is also available online).

For Category 1 patients, any physician may sign the medical declaration. Under Category 2, patients with debilitating symptoms can apply for an authorization to possess dried marihuana for medical purposes if a specialist confirms:
- the diagnosis *and*
- that conventional treatments have either failed or are judged inappropriate to relieve the applicant's symptoms.

Although an assessment of the applicant's case by a specialist is required, the treating physician, whether or not a specialist, can sign the medical declaration.

The physician is required to indicate the daily dose of marihuana, and the form and route of administration that the applicant intends to use. Applicants have to sign a declaration that they have discussed the risks of using marihuana with their physician. The Canadian Medical Protective Association (CMPA) recommends that physicians who complete the medical declaration ask the applicant to sign a release from liability.[9] This is not a requirement of the MMAR, but the Health Canada website directs applicants to the CMPA website to obtain the release form.

The dried marihuana and seeds provided are from standardized strains of *Cannabis sativa* L. '*Indica*'. The dried marihuana has a Δ^9-THC level of $12.5 \pm 2\%$ and a moisture content of approximately 14%. The seeds have a typical germination rate of 80% and should be stored in a refrigerator until sowing.[4]

1 Department of Justice Canada (1996) Controlled Drugs and Substances Act 1996. Available from: http://laws.justice.gc.ca/en/showdoc/cs/C-38.8///en?page=1

2 Government of Canada (2001) Marihuana Medical Access Regulations. In: Canada Gazette 135 (Number 14, July 4). Available from: http://canadagazette.gc.ca/partII/2001/20010704/html/sor227-e.html

3 Government of Canada (2005) Regulations amending the Marihuana Medical Access Regulations. In: *Canada Gazette 139* (Number 13, June 29). Available from: http://canadagazette.gc.ca/partII/2005/20050629/html/sor177-e.html

4 Health Canada (2007) Medical use of marihuana. Available from: www.hc-sc.gc.ca/dhp-mps/marihuana/index_e.html

5 Grotenhermen F (2004) Pharmacology of cannabinoids. Neuro Endocrinology Letters. **25**: 14–23.

6 Grotenhermen F (2003) Pharmacokinetics and pharmacodynamics of cannabinoids. Clinical Pharmacokinetics. **42**: 327–360.

7 Ashton CH (1999) Adverse effects of cannabis and cannabinoids. British Journal of Anaesthesia. **83**: 637–649.

8 Lynch ME et al. (2006) A case series of patients using medicinal marihuana for management of chronic pain under the Canadian Marihuana Medical Access Regulations. Journal of Pain and Symptom Management. **32**: 497–501.

9 CMPA (2006) Canadian Medical Protective Association website. Available from: www.cmpa-acpm.ca/

ANTI-EMETICS

The use of anti-emetics in palliative care is currently guided by the probable cause of the nausea and vomiting in relation to the mechanism of action of the drug (Figure 4.2; Table 4.13; Table 4.14),[1–6] largely extrapolated from experimental data and RCTs in postoperative and chemotherapy-related nausea and vomiting. Data from RCTs in palliative care are relatively sparse.[7] However, this 'mechanistic approach' is successful in the majority of patients.[5] Other factors to consider include:
- response to anti-emetics already given
- relative merits of alternatives:
  ▷ undesirable effects
  ▷ cost ($5HT_3$-receptor antagonists, **aprepitant** and **octreotide** are expensive)

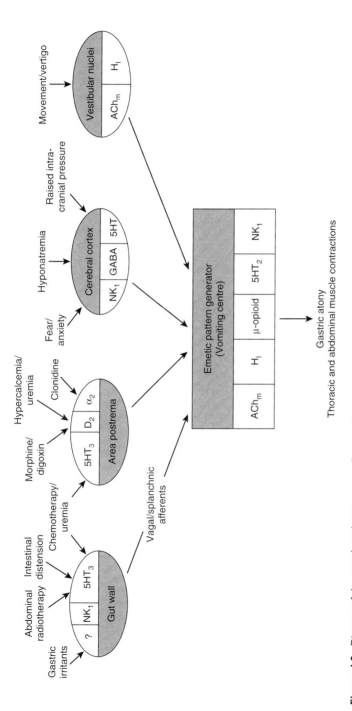

Figure 4.2 Diagram of the neural mechanisms controlling vomiting.

Abbreviations refer to receptor types: ACh_m = muscarinic cholinergic; α_2 = α_2-adrenergic; D_2 = dopamine type 2; 5HT, 5HT$_2$, 5HT$_3$ = 5-hydroxytryptamine (serotonin) type undefined, type 2, type 3; H$_1$ = histamine type 1; NK$_1$ = neurokinin 1. Anti-emetics act as antagonists at these receptors, whereas the central anti-emetic effects of clonidine and opioids are agonistic.

Table 4.13 Classification of drugs used to control nausea and vomiting

Putative site of action	Class	Example
Central nervous system		
Vomiting centre	Antimuscarinic	Scopolamine (hyoscine) hydrobromide
	Antihistaminic antimuscarinic[a]	Dimenhydrinate, hydroxyzine, meclizine, promethazine
	$5HT_2$-receptor antagonist	Methotrimeprazine, olanzapine
	NK_1-receptor antagonist	Aprepitant
Area postrema (chemoreceptor trigger zone)	D_2-receptor antagonist	Haloperidol, metoclopramide, domperidone
	$5HT_3$-receptor antagonist	Granisetron, ondansetron, dolasetron mesylate
	NK_1-receptor antagonist	Aprepitant
Cerebral cortex	Benzodiazepine	Lorazepam
	Cannabinoid	Dronabinol, nabilone
	Corticosteroid	Dexamethasone
	NK_1-receptor antagonist	Aprepitant
GI tract		
Prokinetic	$5HT_4$-receptor agonist	Metoclopramide
	D_2-receptor antagonist	Metoclopramide, Domperidone
	Motilin receptor agonist	Erythromycin
Antisecretory	Antimuscarinic	Hyoscine (scopolamine) butylbromide, Glycopyrrolate
	Somatostatin analogue	Octreotide, lanreotide
Vagal $5HT_3$-receptor blockade	$5HT_3$-receptor antagonist	Granisetron, ondansetron dolasetron mesylate (metoclopramide at high doses)
	NK_1-receptor antagonist	Aprepitant
Anti-inflammatory	Corticosteroid	Dexamethasone

a. antihistamines and phenothiazines both have H_1-receptor antagonistic and antimuscarinic properties (see Table 4.14 below).

Table 4.14 Receptor site affinities of selected anti-emetics[1–3,9]

	D_2-receptor antagonist	H_1-receptor antagonist	Muscarinic antagonist	$5HT_2$-receptor antagonist	$5HT_3$-receptor antagonist	$5HT_4$-receptor agonist
Metoclopramide	++	0	0	0	+	++
Domperidone	++[a]	0	0	0	0	0
Ondansetron, granisetron, dolasetron mesylate	0	0	0	0	+++	0
Meclizine	0	++	++	0	0	0
Dimenhydrinate	0	++	++	0	0	0
Promethazine	+/++	++	++	0	0	0
Haloperidol	+++	0	0	0	0	0
Prochlorperazine	++	+	0	0	0	0
Chlorpromazine	++	++	+	0	0	0
Methotrimeprazine	++	+++	++	+++	0	0
Olanzapine	++	++	++	++	0	0
Scopolamine (hyoscine) hydrobromide	0	0	+++	0	0	0

Pharmacological activity: 0 = none or insignificant; + = slight; ++ = moderate; +++ = marked.
a. domperidone does not normally cross the blood-brain barrier; thus the risk of extrapyramidal effects is negligible (see p.187).

▷ effects on GI motility (i.e. prokinetic (**metoclopramide, domperidone**) or antikinetic (antimuscarinics))
▷ appropriate route or formulation
- when more than one anti-emetic drug is considered:
  ▷ use combinations with different receptor affinities (e.g. **dimenhydrinate** and **haloperidol**)
  ▷ avoid combinations with antagonistic actions (e.g. **meclizine** or **dimenhydrinate** and **metoclopramide**)[8]
  ▷ consider a single broader spectrum drug. **Methotrimeprazine** (see p.130) and **olanzapine** (see p.134)[9] have affinity at many receptors and may well be as effective as, and easier for patients to handle than, two or more different anti-emetics simultaneously
- adjuvant use of:
  ▷ antisecretory drugs (e.g. **hyoscine (scopolamine)** *butylbromide*, **glycopyrrolate, octreotide**)
  ▷ corticosteroids (e.g. **dexamethasone**)
  ▷ benzodiazepines (e.g. **lorazepam, midazolam**)
- non-drug treatments.

Generally, the initial choice of an anti-emetic in palliative care lies between two drugs, namely **metoclopramide** (see p.185) and **haloperidol** (see p.128). These should be prescribed both regularly and as needed (see Guidelines, p.183).

In intestinal obstruction with large-volume vomiting or associated intestinal colic, an antisecretory agent (which acts partly by reducing the volume of GI secretions) may be used either alone as a first-line manoeuvre, e.g. **hyoscine (scopolamine)** *butylbromide* 60–120mg/24h CSCI (occasionally as high as 300mg/24h) or **glycopyrrolate** 600–1200microgram/24h CSCI, or with **dimenhydrinate** or **promethazine**. If this proves inadequate, a trial of **octreotide** should be considered (see p.395).

Corticosteroids and **methotrimeprazine** or **olanzapine** are useful options when first-line anti-emetics fail to relieve nausea and vomiting. **Dexamethasone** is generally added to an existing regimen, whereas **methotrimeprazine** or **olanzapine** is generally substituted. Sometimes it is necessary to use **dexamethasone** and either **methotrimeprazine** or **olanzapine** concurrently.

Other phenothiazines are still often used as anti-emetics, notably **promethazine** (see p.189), **prochlorperazine** and **chlorpromazine**. **Prochlorperazine** (see p.132) is often effective against moderate chemical emetogenic stimuli at a dose of 5–10mg PO t.i.d.; suppositories and injections are also available. However, because it is a potent irritant, bolus SC injection and CSCI should be avoided. **Chlorpromazine** has an even broader spectrum of receptor affinity (Table 4.14) but this does not extend to the $5HT_2$-receptor antagonism of **olanzapine** and **methotrimeprazine**. The latter drugs should be used in preference to **chlorpromazine** when a broad-spectrum drug is indicated.

$5HT_3$-receptor antagonists, developed primarily to control chemotherapeutic vomiting, have a definite but limited role in palliative care (see p.192). Drug-induced nausea and vomiting can be problematic. They may be caused by several different mechanisms (Table 4.15), each of which calls for a distinct therapeutic response.

Aprepitant, a neurokinin 1-receptor antagonist, is approved for the prevention of acute and delayed nausea and vomiting associated with highly emetogenic **cisplatin**-based chemotherapy and moderately emetogenic anthrocycline-cyclophosphamide-based chemotherapy.[10,11] It is given with **dexamethasone** and a $5HT_3$ antagonist.[12]

Table 4.15 Causes of drug-induced nausea and vomiting

Mechanism	Drugs
Gastric irritation	Antibacterials Iron supplements NSAIDs Corticosteroids Tranexamic acid
Gastric stasis	Antimuscarinics Opioids Phenothiazines TCAs
Area postrema stimulation (chemoreceptor trigger zone)	Antibacterials Cytotoxics Digoxin Imidazoles Opioids
$5HT_3$-receptor stimulation	Antibacterials Cytotoxics SSRIs

1 Peroutka SJ and Snyder SH (1982) Antiemetics: neurotransmitter receptor binding predicts therapeutic actions. *Lancet.* **1**: 658–659.
2 Dollery C (1991) *Therapeutic Drugs.* Churchill Livingstone, Edinburgh.
3 Dollery C (1992) *Therapeutic Drugs: Supplement 1.* Churchill Livingstone, Edinburgh.
4 Twycross RG et al. (1997) The use of low dose levomepromazine (methotrimeprazine) in the management of nausea and vomiting. *Progress in Palliative Care.* **5**: 49–53.
5 Bentley A and Boyd K (2001) Use of clinical pictures in the management of nausea and vomiting: a prospective audit. *Palliative Medicine.* **15**: 247–253.
6 Twycross RG and Wilcock A (2001) *Symptom Management in Advanced Cancer* (3e). Radcliffe Medical Press, Oxford, pp. 104–109.
7 Glare P et al. (2004) Systematic review of the efficacy of antiemetics in the treatment of nausea in patients with far-advanced cancer. *Support Care Cancer.* **12**: 432–440.
8 Twycross RG and Back I (1998) Nausea and vomiting in advanced cancer. *European Journal of Palliative Care.* **5**: 39–45.
9 Fleming M and Hawkins C (2005) Use of atypical antipsychotic olanzapine as an anti-emetic. *European Journal of Palliative Care.* **12**: 144–146.
10 Hesketh PJ et al. (2003) Differential involvement of neurotransmitters through the time course of cisplatin-induced emesis as revealed by therapy with specific receptor antagonists. *European Journal of Cancer.* **39**: 1074–1080.
11 Navari RM (2004) Role of neurokinin-1 receptor antagonists in chemotherapy-induced emesis: summary of clinical trials. *Cancer Investigation.* **22**: 569–576
12 Dando TM and Perry CM (2004) Aprepitant: a review of its use in the prevention of chemotherapy-induced nausea and vomiting. *Drugs.* **64**: 777–794.

Guidelines: Management of nausea and vomiting

1 Careful evaluation and documentation of the symptoms, their most likely cause(s), and the response to subsequent treatment are essential for the effective management of nausea and vomiting.

2 Correct correctable causes/exacerbating factors, e.g. drugs, severe pain, infection, cough and hypercalcemia. (*Correction of hypercalcemia is not always appropriate in a dying patient.*) Anxiety exacerbates nausea and vomiting from any cause and may need specific treatment.

3 Prescribe the most appropriate anti-emetic stat, regularly and p.r.n. (see below). Give by SC injection or CSCI if continuous nausea or frequent vomiting occurs.

Commonly used anti-emetics

Prokinetic anti-emetic (about 50% of patients)
For gastritis, gastric stasis, functional intestinal obstruction (peristaltic failure):
metoclopramide 10mg PO stat & q.i.d. or 10mg SC stat & 40–100mg/24 hours CSCI, & 10mg p.r.n. up to q.i.d.

Anti-emetic acting principally in chemoreceptor trigger zone (about 25% of patients)
For most chemical causes of vomiting, e.g. morphine, hypercalcemia and renal failure:
haloperidol 1.5–3mg PO stat & at bedtime or 2.5–5mg SC stat & 2.5–10mg/24 hours CSCI, & 2.5–5mg p.r.n. up to q.i.d.
Metoclopramide also has a central action.

Antispasmodic and antisecretory anti-emetic
If intestinal colic and/or need to reduce GI secretions:
hyoscine (scopolamine) *butylbromide* 20mg SC stat, 60–120mg/24 hours CSCI (occasionally as high as 300mg/24 hours), & 20mg SC hourly p.r.n.

Anti-emetic acting principally in the vomiting centre
For raised intracranial pressure (in conjunction with dexamethasone), motion sickness and in organic intestinal obstruction:
dimenhydrinate 50–100mg PO stat, b.i.d.–t.i.d. & p.r.n., or 50mg SC stat & 100–300mg/24 hours CSCI, & 50mg SC p.r.n. up to q.i.d.

Broad-spectrum anti-emetic
For organic intestinal obstruction and when other anti-emetics are unsatisfactory:
methotrimeprazine 6–12.5mg PO/SC stat, at bedtime & p.r.n. up to q.i.d.

---

4 Review anti-emetic dose daily; take note of p.r.n. use and the patient's symptoms.

5 If little benefit occurs despite optimizing the dose, reconsider the likely cause(s).

6 Anti-emetics for inoperable intestinal obstruction (commonly persistent partial/subacute) can conveniently be given by CSCI, although methotrimeprazine can often be given once daily, e.g. at bedtime:

continued

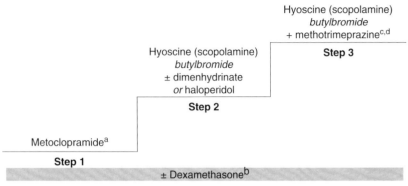

Hyoscine (scopolamine)
butylbromide
+ methotrimeprazine[c,d]

Step 3

Hyoscine (scopolamine)
butylbromide
± dimenhydrinate
or haloperidol

Step 2

Metoclopramide[a]

Step 1

± Dexamethasone[b]

a. if severe colic, omit step 1
b. the place of dexamethasone in inoperable intestinal obstruction is controversial
c. if methotrimeprazine is too sedative, consider using olanzapine 1.25–2.5mg SC at bedtime instead; or revert to step 2 but give both dimenhydrinate and haloperidol
d. see below for further options.

7 In patients who fail to respond to the commonly used anti-emetics, consider:

Other drugs for nausea and vomiting

Corticosteroid
Adjuvant anti-emetic for intestinal obstruction and when all else fails:
dexamethasone 8–16mg PO/SC stat & daily; try reducing the dose after 7 days.

5HT$_3$-receptor antagonist
For chemical causes of nausea and vomiting refractory to haloperidol or methotrimeprazine or when massive release of 5HT/serotonin from enterochromaffin cells or platelets, e.g. chemotherapy, abdominal radiation, intestinal obstruction/distension, renal failure:
e.g. granisetron 1–2mg stat & daily or ondansetron 8mg stat & b.i.d.–t.d.s PO/SC.

Somatostatin analogue
An anti-secretory agent without antispasmodic effects; use in obstruction if hyoscine (scopolamine) butylbromide is inadequate or, initially, if rapid relief is necessary:
octreotide 100microgram SC stat, 250–500microgram/24 hours CSCI or 50–150microgram t.d.s. SC, & 100microgram p.r.n. SC up to q.i.d.

---

8 Some patients with nausea and vomiting need more than one anti-emetic.

9 The prokinetics, metoclopramide and domperidone, act through a cholinergic system which is competitively antagonized by antimuscarinic drugs, e.g. hyoscine (scopolamine), dimenhydrinate; concurrent use is best avoided.

10 Continue anti-emetics unless the cause is self-limiting. Except in organic intestinal obstruction, consider changing to PO after 3 days of good control with parenteral administration.

METOCLOPRAMIDE

Class: Prokinetic anti-emetic.

Indications: Nausea and vomiting, particularly in GI disorders (e.g. gastric irritation and delayed gastric emptying) and with chemotherapy and radiation therapy, dysmotility dyspepsia, heartburn, migraine, hiccups.

Contra-indications: Pheochromocytoma (may induce an acute hypertensive response). GI hemorrhage or perforation. Do not use concurrently with IV 5HT$_3$-receptor antagonists (risk of cardiac arrhythmia,[1] or within <3 days of GI surgery (vigorous contractions may impair healing).

Pharmacology

Metoclopramide is a combined D$_2$-receptor antagonist and 5HT$_4$-receptor agonist. In daily doses above 100mg SC, it manifests 5HT$_3$-receptor antagonism. Metoclopramide is therefore a broad-spectrum anti-emetic but its clinical value mainly resides in its prokinetic properties (see Prokinetics, p.13). As a centrally-acting D$_2$-receptor antagonist, it is second to **haloperidol** (see p.128) and, as a 5HT$_3$-receptor antagonist, it is second to the specific 5HT$_3$-receptor antagonists (see p.192).

Prokinetics act by triggering a cholinergic system in the wall of the GI tract. Opioids impede this action, and antimuscarinics block it competitively.[2] Thus, *ideally, prokinetics and antimuscarinics should not be given concurrently.* However, if they are, metoclopramide will still exert an antagonistic effect at the dopamine receptors in the area postrema. (**Haloperidol** is generally a better choice in this situation because of the advantage of daily administration, see p.128.)

D$_2$-receptor antagonists block the 'dopamine brake' on gastric emptying induced by stress, anxiety and nausea from any cause. In contrast, 5HT$_4$-receptor agonists have a direct excitatory effect which in theory gives them an advantage over the D$_2$-receptor antagonists particularly for patients with gastric stasis or functional intestinal obstruction. However, when used for dysmotility dyspepsia, metoclopramide and **domperidone** are comparable in standard doses.[3]

Along with other drugs which block central dopamine receptors, there is a risk of developing acute dystonic reactions with facial and skeletal muscle spasms and oculogyric crises (see Drug-induced movement disorders, p.561). These are more common in the young (particularly girls and young women), generally occur within a few days of starting treatment, and subside within 24h of stopping the drug. Thus, when possible, use alternatives in patients aged <20 years.

Bio-availability 50–80% PO.
Onset of action 10–15min IM; 15–60min PO.
Time to peak plasma concentration 1–2.5h PO.
Plasma halflife 2.5–5h.
Duration of action 1–2h (data for single dose and relating to gastric emptying).

Cautions

Serious drug interactions: a combination of IV metoclopramide and IV **ondansetron** occasionally causes cardiac arrhythmias.[1] 5HT$_3$-receptors influence various aspects of cardiac function, including inotropy, chronotropy and coronary arterial tone,[4] effects which are mediated by both the parasympathetic and the sympathetic nervous systems. Thus, in any given patient, blockade of 5HT$_3$-receptors will produce effects dependent on the pre-existing serotoninergic activity in both arms of the autonomic nervous system.

Because antimuscarinics competitively block the final common (cholinergic) pathway through which prokinetics act,[2] concurrent prescription with metoclopramide should be avoided if possible.

Metoclopramide enhances the effects of catecholamines in patients with essential hypertension.[5,6] Acute dystonic reactions occur in <5% of patients receiving metoclopramide. The risk is dose-related and greater if also taking other drugs known to cause extrapyramidal effects, e.g. antipsychotics, 5HT$_3$-receptor antagonists and antidepressants (see Drug-induced movement disorders, p.561).

Undesirable effects

For full list, see manufacturer's Product Monograph.
Extrapyramidal effects, neuroleptic (antipsychotic) malignant syndrome (see p.123). Occasionally drowsiness, restlessness, depression, diarrhea.

Dose and use

The use of high-dose IV metoclopramide to treat chemotherapy-induced nausea and vomiting is not considered here.[7] In palliative care, metoclopramide is the most commonly used anti-emetic.[8,9] Although it typically has immediate effect, benefit may increase throughout the first week of use.[10] Metoclopramide is also of benefit in dysmotility dyspepsia, delayed gastric emptying, and chronic nausea.[11,12]

Gastric irritation

- 10mg PO q.i.d. or 40–60mg/24h CSCI and 10mg PO/SC p.r.n.; prescribe appropriate gastroprotective drug and, if possible, discontinue causal drug/substance.

Delayed gastric emptying

- as above, consider increasing to 100mg/24h CSCI.

Nausea and vomiting

- as above, but **haloperidol** is generally more convenient if the cause is stimulation of the chemoreceptor trigger zone/area postrema (see p.180).

For nausea and vomiting associated with 5HT release, a selective $5HT_3$-receptor antagonist should be used rather than high-dose metoclopramide (see p.192).

Hiccup

If caused by delayed gastric emptying, gastric distension, or acid reflux:
- 10mg PO t.i.d.–q.i.d. and p.r.n. $\pm$ an antifoaming agent (see p.3)
- if no response to PO treatment, consider 10–20mg IV stat.

Supply

Metoclopramide (generic)
Tablets 10mg, 28 days @ 10mg q.i.d. = $7.
Oral solution 5mg/5mL, 28 days @ 10mg q.i.d. = $46.
Injection 5mg/mL, 2mL amp = $2.50.

1 Baguley W et al. (1997) Cardiac dysrhythmias associated with the intravenous administration of ondansetron and metoclopramide. *Anesthesia and Analgesia.* **84**: 1380–1381.
2 Schuurkes JAJ et al. (1986) Stimulation of gastroduodenal motor activity: dopaminergic and cholinergic modulation. *Drug Development Research.* **8**: 233–241.
3 Barone J (1999) Domperidone: a peripherally acting dopamine$_2$-receptor antagonist. *Annals of Pharmacotherapy.* **33**: 429–440.
4 Saxena P and Villalon C (1991) 5-Hydroxytryptamine: a chameleon in the heart. *Trends in Pharmacological Sciences.* **12**: 223–227.
5 Kuchel O et al. (1985) Effect of metoclopramide on plasma catecholamine release in essential hypertension. *Clinical Pharmacology and Therapeutics.* **37**: 372–375.
6 Agabiti-Rosei E (1995) Hypertensive crises in patients with phaeochromocytoma given metoclopramide. *Annals of Pharmacology.* **29**: 381–383.
7 Gralla R et al. (1999) Recommendations for the use of antiemetics: evidence-based, clinical practice guidelines. *Journal of Clinical Oncology.* **17**: 2971–2994.
8 Twycross RG and Back I (1998) Nausea and vomiting in advanced cancer. *European Journal of Palliative Care.* **5**: 39–45.
9 Ripamonti C et al. (2001) Clinical-practice recommendations for the management of bowel obstruction in patients with end-stage cancer. *Supportive Care in Cancer.* **9**: 223–233.
10 Bruera E et al. (2004) Dexamethasone in addition to metoclopramide for chronic nausea in patients with advanced cancer: a randomized controlled trial. *Journal of Pain and Symptom Management.* **28**: 381–388.
11 Bruera E et al. (1996) Chronic nausea in advanced cancer patients: a retrospective assessment of a metoclopramide-based antiemetic regimen. *Journal of Pain and Symptom Management.* **11**: 147–153.
12 Bruera E et al. (2000) A double-blind, crossover study of controlled-release metoclopramide and placebo for the chronic nausea and dyspepsia of advanced cancer. *Journal of Pain and Symptom Management.* **19**: 427–435.

DOMPERIDONE

Class: Prokinetic anti-emetic.

Indications: Nausea and vomiting, upper GI dysmotility (due to gastritis and diabetic gastroparesis), gastro-esophageal reflux, vomiting and hypotension associated with antiparkinsonian drugs.

Contra-indications: Prolactinoma, GI hemorrhage or perforation.

Pharmacology

Domperidone is a D_2-receptor antagonist. It is structurally related to the butyrophenones, but does not normally cross the blood-brain barrier.[1] Domperidone has a dual anti-emetic effect. First, it acts on dopamine receptors in the chemoreceptor trigger zone (CTZ) in the area postrema. (Although situated on the surface of the brain stem, the CTZ is outside the physiological blood-brain barrier.) Second, it acts on D_2-receptors at the gastro-esophageal and gastroduodenal junctions, and thereby counteracts the gastric 'dopamine brake' associated with nausea from any cause. Domperidone may also inhibit cholinesterase activity.[2] Because negligible amounts of domperidone penetrate the blood-brain barrier, there is negligible risk of extrapyramidal effects (mediated via the basal ganglia). Domperidone is the prokinetic and anti-emetic of choice in Parkinson's disease; it counteracts the emetic effect of **levodopa** and **bromocriptine** without adversely affecting the antiparkinsonian (dopaminergic) effect of these drugs.[3]

Although almost completely absorbed from the GI tract, bio-availability is relatively poor because of extensive first-pass metabolism in the wall of the GI tract and the liver. Bio-availability in healthy volunteers is nearly doubled if taken *after* a meal.[4] Maximal absorption requires an acid environment; H_2-receptor antagonists, PPIs and antacids all reduce absorption, and bio-availability. Under standard conditions, absorption is linear up to a 40mg single dose.

Following absorption, domperidone is metabolized to inactive compounds via the hepatic CYP450 mixed oxidase system, principally CYP3A4 (see Cautions). The plasma halflife is increased by up to 50% in renal failure but the plasma concentrations do not increase (possibly because of an altered volume of distribution). Further, because renal clearance is a minor route of elimination, accumulation is not a concern.[5] Although rectal bio-availability is almost the same as by mouth, the recommended rectal dose is three times the oral dose. This stems from pharmacodynamic studies, and possibly relates to slower absorption from the rectum.

The effect of domperidone on the lower esophageal sphincter is equivocal.[2] Because domperidone, unlike **metoclopramide**, does not have any $5HT_4$-receptor agonist action, it might be anticipated that domperidone would be less effective in treating gastroparesis. However, the results of a systematic review indicate otherwise (Table 4.16).[6] Domperidone may be effective even when there is no response to **metoclopramide**.[2,7]

Domperidone 20mg q.i.d. causes less frequent and less severe undesirable effects than **metoclopramide** 10mg q.i.d., e.g. less drowsiness and loss of mental acuity.[8] In diabetic patients, the prokinetic effect for solids attenuates after 1–2 months, although the effect on liquid emptying persists.[9,10]

Table 4.16 Comparison of prokinetic drugs[6]

Drug	Erythromycin	Domperidone	Metoclopramide
Mechanism of action			
Motilin agonist	+	−	−
D_2-receptor antagonist	−	+	+
$5HT_4$-receptor agonist	−	−	+
Response to treatment[a]			
Gastric emptying			
(mean % acceleration)	45	30	20
Symptom relief			
(mean % improvement)	50	50	40

a. all percentages rounded to nearest 5%.

The usefulness of domperidone is limited by the absence of a parenteral formulation. It was withdrawn in the early 1980s, after several patients died from ventricular arrhythmias when given IV domperidone.[11] Domperidone does not significantly alter the pharmacokinetics or pharmacodynamics of other drugs. Because the prokinetic effect of domperidone is mediated through a cholinergic final common pathway, its prokinetic effect will be impaired by concurrently administered antimuscarinic drugs.[12]

Bio-availability 12–18% PO (fasting), 24% PO (after food).
Onset of action 30min.
Time to peak plasma concentration 0.5–2h PO.
Plasma halflife 7–16h; increasing up to 21h in severe renal impairment.[2]
Duration of action 12–24h (estimate based on halflife).

Cautions

Renal and hepatic impairment. The concurrent use of an antimuscarinic drug is likely to reduce the prokinetic effect of domperidone (but will not affect its central anti-emetic effect).

The main metabolic pathway of domperidone is CYP3A4-mediated. The concurrent use of CYP3A4 inhibitors (e.g. **erythromycin**, **ritonavir**, SSRIs, macrolide antibiotics and grapefruit juice) may increase the domperidone plasma concentration, increasing the risk of QT prolongation and thus *torsade de pointes*.[13] The AUC and the peak plasma concentration of domperidone are *trebled* when oral **ketoconazole** is administered concurrently. The QT interval is slightly prolonged (<10msec) by this combination, greater than the increase seen with **ketoconazole** alone. QT prolongation is less likely when domperidone is given alone (Unpublished data on file).

Undesirable effects

For full list, see manufacturer's Product Monograph.
Very common (>10%): gynecomastia, galactorrhea, amenorrhea (secondary to increased prolactin secretion), reduced libido, transient colic.[2]
Common (<10%, >1%): pruritus, rash, cramp, headache.[2]
Very rare (<0.01%): extrapyramidal effects (acute dystonias), which resolve rapidly and completely once domperidone is stopped.[14] In two women with polycystic ovaries, hyperestrogenism may have been a predisposing factor.[2]

Dose and use

The manufacturer recommends giving domperidone t.i.d.–q.i.d. although, given its halflife, b.i.d. is likely to be satisfactory:
• starting dose 20mg PO b.i.d. or 10mg PO q.i.d.
• increase if necessary to 40mg PO b.i.d. or 20mg PO q.i.d.
The maximum dose recommended by the CPS is 80mg/24h, although up to 120mg/24h has been used for many years in patients with diabetic gastropathy.[2]

Supply

Domperidone (generic)
Tablets 10mg, 28 days @ 10mg q.i.d. = $17.

1 Barone J (1999) Domperidone: a peripherally acting dopamine₂-receptor antagonist. *Annals of Pharmacotherapy.* **33**: 429–440.
2 Prakash A and Wagstaff AJ (1998) Domperidone. A review of its use in diabetic gastropathy. *Drugs.* **56**: 429–445.
3 Langdon N et al. (1986) Comparison of levodopa with carbidopa, and levodopa with domperidone in Parkinson's disease. *Clinical Neuropharmacology.* **9**: 440–447.
4 Heykants J et al. (1981) On the pharmacokinetics of domperidone in animals and man. IV. The pharmacokinetics of intravenous domperidone and its bioavailability in man following intramuscular, oral and rectal administration. *European Journal of Drug Metabolism and Pharmacokinetics.* **6**: 61–70.
5 Brogden RN et al. (1982) Domperidone. A review of its pharmacological activity, pharmacokinetics and therapeutic efficacy in the symptomatic treatment of chronic dyspepsia and as an antiemetic. *Drugs.* **24**: 360–400.
6 Sturm A et al. (1999) Prokinetics in patients with gastroparesis: a systematic analysis. *Digestion.* **60**: 422–427.
7 Dumitrascu D and Weinbeck M (2000) Domperidone versus metoclopramide in the treatment of diabetic gastroparesis. *American Journal of Gastroenterology.* **95**: 316–317.

8 Patterson D et al. (1999) A double-blind multicenter comparison of domperidone and metoclopramide in the treatment of diabetic patients with symptoms of gastroparesis. American Journal of Gastroenterology. **94**: 1230–1234.

9 Horowitz M et al. (1985) Acute and chronic effects of domperidone on gastric emptying in diabetic autonomic neuropathy. Digestive Diseases and Sciences. **30**: 1–9.

10 Koch KL et al. (1989) Gastric emptying and gastric myoelectrical activity in patients with diabetic gastroparesis: effect of long-term domperidone treatment. American Journal of Gastroenterology. **84**: 1069–1075.

11 Osborne R et al. (1985) Cardiotoxicity of intravenous domperidone. Lancet. **2**: 385–385.

12 Schuurkes JAJ et al. (1986) Stimulation of gastroduodenal motor activity: dopaminergic and cholinergic modulation. Drug Development Research. **8**: 233–241.

13 Health Canada (2007) Domperidone: heart rate and rhythm disorders. Canadian Adverse Reaction Newsletter. **17 (January)**: 2.

14 Casteels-Van Daele M et al. (1984) Refusal of further cancer chemotherapy due to antiemetic drug. Lancet. **1**: 57.

ANTIHISTAMINIC ANTIMUSCARINIC ANTI-EMETICS

Indications: Table 4.17

Table 4.17 Indications for the use of an antihistaminic antimuscarinic anti-emetic

	Dimenhydrinate	Hydroxyzine[a]	Meclizine	Promethazine
Nausea and vomiting due to:				
Motion sickness	+		+	+
Radiation sickness	+		+	
Postoperative nausea and vomiting	+			
Meniere's syndrome, labyrinthitis and other vestibular disturbances	+		+	
Vertigo associated with vestibular disease	+		+	
Anxiety		+		+
Pruritus		+		†+
Allergic reactions				+

a. also used for †alcohol withdrawal symptoms.

Contra-indications:
Dimenhydrinate: glaucoma, chronic lung disease, difficulty in urination due to prostatic hypertrophy.
Promethazine: intra-arterial or SC injection (is a chemical irritant and may cause local necrosis), asthma.

Pharmacology

Antihistaminic antimuscarinic anti-emetics embrace several chemical classes including some phenothiazines (e.g. **promethazine**), piperazines (e.g. **meclizine, hydroxyzine**) and mono-ethanolamines (e.g. **diphenhydramine, dimenhydrinate**). The piperazines and mono-ethanolamines were first marketed as H_1-antihistamines, and are often classed separately as antihistaminic anti-emetics. They decrease excitability of the inner ear labyrinth and block conduction in the vestibular-cerebellar pathways, as well as acting directly on the vomiting centre in the brain stem. However, there is considerable overlap between their receptor site affinity and that of the antipsychotic phenothiazines (see Table 4.14, p.180).

The piperazines and mono-ethanolamines began to be used for the prevention of motion sickness after a patient with urticaria reported relief from car sickness when taking **dimenhydrinate.**[1] After the Second World War, studies were conducted in American servicemen crossing the Atlantic Ocean in the General Ballou, a modified freight ship without stabilizers. Although the drugs differ in antihistaminic potency, they were equally effective,[1,2] suggesting that their anti-emetic effect is the result of multiple receptor site activity.

Antihistaminic anti-emetics are effective in many causes of vomiting, including opioid-induced.[3,4] However, in practice **metoclopramide** (see p.185) and **haloperidol** (see p.128) are often used in preference, sometimes because of more specific indications or to avoid drowsiness and antimuscarinic effects. Drowsiness is increased if antihistaminics are used with other CNS depressants, e.g. benzodiazepines, barbiturates, antipsychotics, and alcohol. Metabolism is mainly hepatic, and the inactive metabolites are excreted in the urine.

Hydroxyzine is a later addition to this group of drugs, and is principally used as an anxiolytic-sedative and antipruritic. Unlike other anthistaminic drugs, **hydroxyzine** inhibits apomorphine-induced vomiting, suggesting that some of its anti-emetic effect is mediated via the chemoreceptor trigger zone. In postoperative patients, **hydroxyzine** 100mg IM has analgesic activity approaching that of **morphine** 8mg,[5] and **morphine** 5mg and **hydroxyzine** 100mg gave comparable relief to **morphine** 10mg alone.[6] The sedative effect of the combination was not significantly different from **morphine** alone. For pharmacokinetic details, see Table 4.18.

Table 4.18 Pharmacokinetic details

	Dimenhydrinate	Hydroxyzine	Meclizine	Promethazine
Bio-availability	40–60% PO	No data	No data	25% PO
Onset of action	15–30min PO, 20–30min IM, 30–45min PR	15–30min	30–60min	About 20min IM, 3–5min IV
Time to peak plasma concentration	1–4h PO	~2h	2h PO	4.5h PO (syrup), 6–9h PR
Plasma halflife	3.5h	3–7h	4–6h	7–14h
Duration of action	4–7h	4–6h	8–24h	2–6h

Cautions

Hepatic and renal impairment, epilepsy. Sedation may affect the ability to perform skilled tasks (e.g. driving), and is enhanced by alcohol. Can precipitate or exacerbate narrow-angle glaucoma and urinary tract obstruction (see Antimuscarinics, p.5). Elderly patients are more susceptible to sedative and central antimuscarinic effects, e.g. postural hypotension, memory impairment and extrapyramidal reactions.

Dimenhydrinate: may interfere with laboratory measurement of serum **theophylline** concentrations.

Hydroxyzine: asthma, COPD, hepatic impairment (give only once daily), moderate-severe renal impairment (reduce dose by 50%). When injected IV, extravasation into the SC tissues can cause a sterile abscess and tissue induration. Give well diluted as a 15–30min IVI only if strictly necessary.

Undesirable effects

For full list, see manufacturer's Product Monograph.

Dry mouth and other antimuscarinic effects (see Antimuscarinics, p.5), drowsiness, headache, fatigue, nervousness, dizziness, thickening of bronchial secretions.

Dose and use

Because of their antimuscarinic properties, the use of this group of drugs tends to be restricted to situations where **metoclopramide** and/or other more specific anti-emetics (e.g. **haloperidol**, 5HT$_3$-receptor antagonists) have failed to relieve, e.g. some patients with mechanical intestinal obstruction, or as the anti-emetic of choice for raised intracranial pressure.

In Canada, **dimenhydrinate** is generally the antihistaminic antimuscarinic anti-emetic of choice. Depending on circumstances, **dimenhydrinate** is generally given PO or SC:

- 50–100mg PO b.i.d.–q.i.d. & p.r.n. or 100mg SR q12h–q8h
- 100–300mg/24h CSCI (typically 100mg) & 50mg SC p.r.n.
- usual maximum daily dose 400mg PO and CSCI.

Dimenhydrinate suppositories are also available.

The manufacturers' approved doses for antihistaminic drugs when used as anti-emetics are shown in Table 4.19, and for other indications in Table 4.20.

Table 4.19 Approved dose recommendations for use as anti-emetics

	Dimenhydrinate	Hydroxyzine	Meclizine	Promethazine
Motion sickness	50–100mg PO q4h p.r.n. maximum 400mg/day		12.5–50mg PO 1h before traveling, repeat q12–24h p.r.n.	25mg PO or PR 30–60min before traveling, repeat q12h p.r.n.
Vomiting	25–50mg IM/IV/SC q4h, maximum 400mg/day	25–100mg IM q4–6h p.r.n.		

Table 4.20 Approved dose recommendations for other indications[a]

	Diphenhydramine	Hydroxyzine	Meclizine	Promethazine
Vertigo			25–100mg/day p.c. in divided doses	
Night-time sedation	50mg PO at bedtime	50–100mg PO at bedtime		
General sedation		50–100mg PO or 25–100mg IM single dose.		25–50mg PO/IM/IV/PR single dose
Anxiety		25–100mg PO q.i.d., maximum 600mg/day.		
Allergic reactions	25–50mg PO q4-6h, maximum 400mg/day	25mg PO t.i.d.–q.i.d.		12.5mg PO/PR t.i.d. & 25mg at bedtime; 25mg IM/IV, repeat q2h p.r.n.
Dystonic reactions	50mg IM/IV, repeat after 20–30min p.r.n.			

a. dimenhydrinate is approved only as an anti-emetic.

Compatibility

Promethazine is compatible when mixed in syringes with various drugs, including **fentanyl**, **hydromorphone**, and **midazolam**. It is also compatible with **hydroxyzine**, and the principal antimuscarinics, i.e. **atropine, glycopyrrolate**, and **scopolamine (hyoscine) hydrobromide**. However, combined use with these latter drugs is either unnecessary or inadvisable. There is no parenteral formulation of **meclizine**.

Supply

Oral products
Dimenhydrinate (generic)
Tablets 50mg, 28 days @ 50mg t.i.d. = $6; *also available OTC @ $7 for 100 tablets.*
Oral liquid 15mg/5mL, 28 days @ 45mg (15mL) t.i.d. = $29; *also available OTC @ $17 for 250mL.*

Gravol® (Church & Dwight)
Capsules (softgel) 50mg, 8 capsules = $5.
Tablets 50mg, 30 tablets = $7.
Tablets chewable 15mg, 12 tablets = $6; *cherry flavour.*
Tablets chewable (adult strength) 50mg, 8 tablets = $6; *orange flavour.*
Caplets SR 100mg, 24 caplets = $13.
Oral liquid 15mg/5mL, 28 days @ 45mg (15mL) t.i.d. = $53; *also available OTC @ $10 for 75mL; mixed fruit flavour.*
All products available OTC.

Hydroxyzine hydrochloride (generic)
Capsules 10mg, 25mg, 50mg, 28 days @ 25mg t.i.d. = $16.
Oral syrup 10mg/5mL, 28 days @ 25mg t.i.d. = $45.

Meclizine hydrochloride
Bonamine® (McNeil)
Tablets chewable 25mg, available OTC @ $9 for 15 tablets; *raspberry flavour.*
Note: at the time of going to press, Bonamine® was temporarily unavailable because of a continuing manufacturer's supply difficulty.

Injectable products
Dimenhydrinate (generic)
Injection 50mg/mL, 5mL amp for IV use = $5.
Injection 50mg/mL, 1mL vial for IM use = $1.50, 5mL vial for IM use = $5.

Gravol® (Church & Dwight)
Injection 50mg/mL, 1mL amp for IV use = $1.50.
Injection 50mg/mL, 5mL vial for IM use = $5.

Hydroxyzine hydrochloride (generic)
Injection 50mg/mL, 1mL amp = $5.

Promethazine hydrochloride (generic)
Injection 25mg/mL, 1mL amp = $1, 2mL amp = $2.

Rectal products
All products available OTC.
Dimenhydrinate (generic)
Suppositories 50mg, 10 = $8; 100mg, 10 = $9.

Gravol® (Church & Dwight)
Suppositories 25mg, 10 = $9; 100mg, 10 = $10.

---

1 Gay L and Carliner P (1949) The prevention and treatment of motion sickness. *Bulletin of John Hopkins Hospital.* **49**: 470–491.
2 Gutner B *et al.* (1952) The effects of potent analgesics upon vestibular function. *Journal of Clinical Investigations.* **31**: 259–266.
3 Dundee J and Jones P (1968) The prevention of analgesic-induced nausea and vomiting by cyclizine. *British Journal of Clinical Practice.* **22**: 379–382.
4 Walder A and Aitkenhead A (1995) A comparison of droperidol and cyclizine in the prevention of postoperative nausea and vomiting associated with patient-controlled analgesia. *Anaesthesia.* **50**: 654–656.
5 Beaver WT and Feise G (1976) Comparison of analgesic effects of morphine sulphate, hydroxyzine and their combination in patients with postoperative pain. In: JJ Bonica and D Albe-Fessard (eds) *Advances in Pain Research and Therapy* Vol 1. Raven Press, New York, pp. 553–557.
6 Hupert C *et al.* (1980) Effect of hydroxyzine on morphine analgesia for the treatment of postoperative pain. *Anesthesia and Analgesia.* **59**: 690–696.

5HT₃-RECEPTOR ANTAGONISTS

Indications: Nausea and vomiting after surgery, chemotherapy and radiation therapy, †intractable vomiting due to chemical, abdominal and cerebral causes when usual approaches have failed, †opioid-induced pruritus,[1,2] †uremic and †cholestasic pruritus.

Contra-indications: Concurrent IV administration with IV **metoclopramide** (risk of arrhythmia: see p.185).

Pharmacology

5HT₃-receptor antagonists were developed specifically to control emesis associated with highly emetogenic chemotherapy, e.g. **cisplatin**. They block the amplifying effect of excess 5HT on vagal nerve fibres, and are thus of particular value in situations when excessive amounts of 5HT are released from the body's stores, i.e. from enterochromaffin cells after chemotherapy or radiation-induced damage of the GI mucosa, or because of intestinal distension, or from leaky platelets when there is severe renal impairment.

In an open RCT, **tropisetron** (not Canada) was shown to be of benefit in patients with far-advanced cancer and nausea and vomiting of indeterminate cause when given either as a sole agent or with a second anti-emetic, particularly **dexamethasone**.[3] 5HT$_3$-receptor antagonists also relieve nausea and vomiting after head injury, brain stem radiation therapy,[4,5] and in multiple sclerosis with brain stem disease;[6] leakage of 5HT from the raphe nucleus probably accounts for the benefit seen in these circumstances. 5HT$_3$-receptor antagonists are also effective in nausea and vomiting associated with acute gastro-enteritis.[7] In one patient who experienced persistent nausea after the insertion of an endo-esophageal tube, a 5HT$_3$-receptor antagonist brought about relief after failure with **metoclopramide** and **cyclizine** (not Canada).[8]

IV **ondansetron** 4–8mg relieves itch induced by spinal opioids in 3–30min.[1,9,10] Although trials have not been conducted with other 5HT$_3$-receptor antagonists, it is likely that the benefit shown with **ondansetron** is a class effect.[11] Good results have also been noted in case reports and open studies of both single and multiple doses of IV or PO **ondansetron** in cholestasis[11–14] and uremia (**ondansetron** 4mg PO b.i.d. resulted in progressive improvement over 2 weeks).[14] However, two RCTs of **ondansetron** in chronic cholestasis showed either no benefit (IV 8mg stat + tablets 8mg b.i.d. for 5 days)[15] or minimal benefit (tablets 8mg t.i.d. for 1 week).[16] Similarly, an RCT in uremic itch showed no benefit with **ondansetron**.[17] For pharmacokinetic details see Table 4.21.

Table 4.21 Pharmacokinetic details of 5HT$_3$-receptor antagonists

		Ondansetron	Granisetron	Dolasetron mesylate
Bio-availability	PO	56–71% (60% PR)	60%	75%
Onset of action	PO	<30min	<30min	
	IV	<5min	<15min	
Plasma halflife		3–5h (6h PR)	10–11h	7h
Time to peak plasma concentration	PO	1.5h	No data	<1h
	IM	10min		n/a
	PR	6h		n/a
Duration of action		12h	24h	

Cautions

5HT$_3$-receptor antagonists reduce colonic motility and can cause or worsen constipation. *Ondansetron*: the dose should be reduced in moderate–severe hepatic impairment. **Ondansetron** reduces the analgesic effect of **tramadol** (possibly by blocking the action of serotonin at presynaptic 5HT$_3$-receptors on primary afferent nociceptive neurones in the spinal dorsal horn).[18] In postoperative pain, the dose of **tramadol** needed by IV PCA was increased 2–3 times in patients receiving **ondansetron** 1mg/h by CIVI. There was also an increase in vomiting (despite the **ondansetron**).[19] *Note: this is probably a class effect for 5HT$_3$-receptor antagonists.*

Undesirable effects

For full list, see manufacturer's Product Monograph.
Very common (>10%): headache.[20]
Common (<10%, >1%): lightheadedness, dizziness, nervousness, tremor, ataxia, asthenia, drowsiness, fever, sensation of warmth or flushing (particularly when given IV), thirst, constipation or diarrhea.
Uncommon (<1%, >0.1%): ondansetron: dystonic reactions, arrhythmia, hypotension, raised LFTs.
Rare (<0.1%, >0.01%): hiccup.
Very rare (<0.01%): ondansetron: transient blindness during IV administration (sight generally returns within 20min).

Dose and use

All 5HT$_3$-receptor antagonists are expensive, and it is important not to use them unnecessarily. In palliative care, their use first-line for nausea and vomiting is rarely appropriate.[21] If a

5HT$_3$-receptor antagonist is prescribed but not definitely effective within 3 days, it should be discontinued.

When used for intractable nausea and vomiting in advanced cancer, 5HT$_3$-receptor antagonists are often more effective when combined with other anti-emetics.[3] They are typically used in combination with an antipsychotic with affinity for multiple receptors (e.g. **methotrimeprazine (levomepromazine)**, **olanzapine**) $\pm$ **dexamethasone**.

Generic **ondansetron** is used at some centres as the cheapest option at heavily discounted hospital contract prices. However, **granisetron** needs to be given only once daily (instead of b.i.d.–t.i.d.). 5HT$_3$-receptor antagonists are equally effective PO and by injection.[22–24] Regimens include:

- **granisetron** 1–2mg PO/SC once daily for 3 days *or*
- **ondansetron** 8mg PO/SC b.i.d.–t.i.d. for 3 days
- if clearly of benefit, continue indefinitely unless the cause is self-limiting
- some patients benefit from higher doses, occasionally as high as **granisetron** 9mg daily[25]
- in patients with moderate-severe hepatic impairment, the dose of **ondansetron** should be limited to 8mg daily, whereas no dose reduction is necessary for **granisetron** (in renal impairment, no dose reduction is necessary with either drug).

Note: to control nausea and vomiting caused by severely emetogenic chemotherapy, **granisetron** (or other 5HT$_3$-receptor antagonist) is used with other anti-emetics, typically **dexamethasone** and **metoclopramide**.[26]

For use in pruritus associated with spinally administered opioids or end-stage renal failure, see discussion in Pharmacology section above.

Supply
Granisetron
Kytril® (Roche)
Tablets 1mg, 28 days @ 1mg once daily = $540.
Injection 1mg/mL, for dilution and use as an injection or infusion, 1mL amp = $75.

Ondansetron (generic)
Tablets 4mg, 8mg, 28 days @ 8mg b.i.d. = $645.
Injection 2mg/mL, 2mL amp = $14, 4mL amp = $27.

Zofran® (GlaxoSmithKline)
Tablets 4mg, 8mg, 28 days @ 8mg b.i.d. = $1,225.
Tablets orodispersible (Zofran ODT®) 4mg, 8mg, 28 days @ 8mg b.i.d. = $1,197.
Oral syrup (sugar-free) 4mg/5mL, 28 days @ 8mg b.i.d. = $1,225; *strawberry flavour.*
Injection 2mg/mL, 2mL amp = $20, 4mL amp = $40.

Dolasetron Mesylate
Anzemet® (Sanofi-Aventis)
Tablets 50mg, single dose = $15; 100mg, single dose = $30; *use restricted to nausea and vomiting caused by chemotherapy.*
Injection 20mg/mL, for IV use, 5mL vial = $12.

1 Borgeat A and Stimemann H-R (1999) Ondansetron is effective to treat spinal or epidural morphine-induced pruritus. *Anesthesiology.* **90**: 432–436.
2 Kyriakides K *et al.* (1999) Management of opioid-induced pruritus: a role for 5HT antagonists? *British Journal of Anaesthesia.* **82**: 439–441.
3 Mystakidou K *et al.* (1998) Comparison of the efficacy and safety of tropisetron, metoclopramide, and chlorpromazine in the treatment of emesis associated with far advanced cancer. *Cancer.* **83**: 1214–1223.
4 Kleinerman K *et al.* (1993) Use of ondansetron for control of projectile vomiting in patients with neurosurgical trauma: two case reports. *Annals of Pharmacotherapy.* **27**: 566–568.
5 Bodis S *et al.* (1994) The prevention of radiosurgery-induced nausea and vomiting by ondansetron: evidence of a direct effect on the central nervous system chemoreceptor trigger zone. *Surgery and Neurology.* **42**: 249–252.
6 Rice G and Ebers G (1995) Ondansetron for intractable vertigo complicating acute brainstem disorders. *Lancet.* **345**: 1182–1183.
7 Cubeddu L *et al.* (1997) Antiemetic activity of ondansetron in acute gastroenteritis. *Alimentary Pharmacology and Therapeutics.* **11**: 185–191.
8 Fair R (1990) Ondansetron in nausea. *Pharmaceutical Journal.* **245**: 514.

9 Arai L et al. (1996) The use of ondansetron to treat pruritus associated with intrathecal morphine in two paediatric patients. *Paediatric Anaesthesia*. **6**: 337–339.

10 Larijani G et al. (1996) Treatment of opioid-induced pruritus with ondansetron: report of four patients. *Pharmacotherapy*. **16**: 958–960.

11 Quigley C and Plowman PN (1996) 5HT3 receptor antagonists and pruritus due to cholestasis. *Palliative Medicine*. **10**: 54.

12 Schworer H and Ramadori G (1993) Improvement of cholestatic pruritus by ondansetron. *Lancet*. **341**: 1277.

13 Raderer M et al. (1994) Ondansetron for pruritus due to cholestasis. *New England Journal of Medicine*. **330**: 1540.

14 Balaskas E et al. (1998) Histamine and serotonin in uremic pruritus: effect of ondansetron in CAPD-pruritic patients. *Nephron*. **78**: 395–402.

15 O'Donohue J et al. (1997) Ondansetron in the treatment of pruritus of cholestasis: a randomised controlled trial. *Gastroenterology*. **112**: A1349.

16 Muller C et al. (1998) Treatment of pruritus in chronic liver disease with the 5-hydroxytryptamine receptor type 3 antagonist ondansetron: a randomized, placebo-controlled, double-blind cross-over trial. *European Journal of Gastroenterology and Hepatology*. **10**: 865–870.

17 Murphy M et al. (2001) A randomised, placebo-controlled, double-blind trial of ondansetron in renal itch. *British Journal of Dermatology*. **145 (suppl 59)**: 20–21.

18 De Witte JL et al. (2001) The analgesic efficacy of tramadol is impaired by concurrent administration of ondansetron. *Anesthesia and Analgesia*. **92**: 1319–1321.

19 Arcioni R et al. (2002) Ondansetron inhibits the analgesic effects of tramadol: a possible 5-HT(3) spinal receptor involvement in acute pain in humans. *Anesthesia and Analgesia*. **94**: 1553–1557, table of contents.

20 Goodin S and Cunningham R (2002) 5-HT3-receptor antagonists for the treatment of nausea and vomiting: a reappraisal of their side-effect profile. *The Oncologist*. **7**: 424–436.

21 Currow D et al. (1997) Use of ondansetron in palliative medicine. *Journal of Pain and Symptom Management*. **13**: 302–307.

22 Gralla R et al. (1997) Can an oral antiemetic regimen be as effective as intravenous treatment against cisplatin: results of a 1054 patient randomized study of oral granisetron versus IV ondansetron. *Proceedings of the American Society of Clinical Oncology*. **16**: 178.

23 Perez E et al. (1997) Efficacy and safety of oral granisetron versus IV ondansetron in prevention of moderately emetogenic chemotherapy-induced nausea and vomiting. *Proceedings of the American Society of Clinical Oncology*. **16**: 149.

24 Perez EA et al. (1997) Efficacy and safety of different doses of granisetron for the prophylaxis of cisplatin-induced emesis. *Support Care Cancer*. **5**: 31–37.

25 Minami M (2003) Granisetron: is there a dose-response effect on nausea and vomiting? *Cancer Chemotherapy and Pharmacology*. **52**: 89–98.

26 Kris MG et al. (2006) American Society of Clinical Oncology guideline for antiemetics in oncology: update 2006. *Journal of Clinical Oncology*. **24**: 2932–2947.

SCOPOLAMINE (HYOSCINE) HYDROBROMIDE

Class: Antimuscarinic.

Indications: Prevention of motion sickness (TD route), drying secretions (including surgical premedication, †sialorrhea, †drooling, †death rattle and †inoperable intestinal obstruction), †paraneoplastic pyrexia and sweating, †smooth muscle spasm (e.g. intestine, bladder).

Contra-indications: Narrow-angle glaucoma, prostatic hyperplasia, pyloric obstruction, paralytic ileus.

Pharmacology

Scopolamine (hyoscine) *hydrobromide* is a naturally occurring belladonna alkaloid with smooth muscle relaxant (antispasmodic) and antisecretory properties. In many countries it is available as both the *hydrobromide* and *butylbromide* salts. **Hyoscine (scopolamine) *butylbromide*** is a quaternary compound which does not cross the blood-brain barrier and, unlike scopolamine *hydrobromide*, the *butylbromide* does not cause drowsiness and does not have a central anti-emetic action (see p.11). In contrast, repeated administration of scopolamine *hydrobromide* SC q4h may result in accumulation leading to sedation and delirium. However, a small number of patients are stimulated rather than sedated.

Despite scopolamine *hydrobromide* having a plasma halflife of several hours, the duration of the antisecretory effect in volunteers after a single dose is only about 2h.[1] However, particularly after repeated injections in moribund patients, a duration of effect of up to 9h has been observed.[2] Scopolamine *hydrobromide* relieves death rattle in 50–60% of patients.[3] However, provided that time is taken to explain the cause of the rattle to the relatives and there is ongoing support, relatives' distress is relieved in >90% of cases.[2] Scopolamine *hydrobromide* can also be used in other situations where an antimuscarinic effect is needed.

A TD patch is available as prophylactic treatment for motion sickness.[4] Off-label uses include the management of sialorrhea and drooling in patients with disorders of the head and neck.[5,6] Features of the patch include:
- an immediate-release priming dose of 140microgram
- a drug reservoir containing 1.5mg
- a rate-controlling membrane allowing the release of 5microgram/h (120microgram/24h)
- steady-state is reached after about 24h, and maintained for 72h[6]
- absorption is best when the patch is applied on hairless skin behind the ear.[4]

Bio-availability 60–80% SL.
Onset of action 3–5min IM, 10–15min SL.
Time to peak effect 20–60min SL/SC; 24h TD.
Plasma halflife 5–6h.
Duration of action IM 15min (spasmolytic), 1–9h (antisecretory).

Cautions

Interacts competitively to block the prokinetic effect of **metoclopramide** and **domperidone**.[7] Increases the antimuscarinic toxicity of antihistamines, phenothiazines and TCAs (see p.5). Wash hands after handling the TD patch (and the application site after removing it) to avoid transfering scopolamine *hydrobromide* into the eyes (may cause mydriasis and exacerbate narrow-angle glaucoma).

Likely to exacerbate acid reflux. Use in hot weather or pyrexia may lead to heatstroke. Use with caution in myasthenia gravis, and in conditions predisposing to tachycardia (e.g. thyrotoxicosis, heart failure and concurrent use with β-adrenergic receptor agonists).

TD patches contain metal in the backing, and must be removed before MRI to avoid burns.[8,9]

Undesirable effects

For full list, see manufacturer's Product Monograph.
Antimuscarinic effects (see p.5), including central antimuscarinic (anticholinergic) syndrome, i.e. agitated delirium, drowsiness, ataxia. Local irritation ± rash occasionally occurs with TD patch.

Dose and use
Sialorrhea and drooling
- scopolamine *hydrobromide* 1mg/72h TD; if necessary, use 2 patches concurrently.

Note: an alternative drug PO with antimuscarinic effects may be preferable in some patients because of convenience or concurrent symptom management, e.g. **amitriptyline** (see p.150).

Death rattle (noisy respiratory secretions)
With death rattle caused by excess secretions pooling in the pharynx, an antisecretory drug is best administered as soon as the rattle becomes evident because the drug cannot dry up the existing secretions (see p.10).
- 400microgram SC stat,
- continue with 1,200microgram/24h CSCI
- if necessary, increase to 2,000microgram/24h CSCI
- repeat 400microgram p.r.n.

Some centres use **hyoscine (scopolamine) butylbromide** instead (see p.11).[10] Other options include **glycopyrrolate** (see p.465) and **atropine** (see p.10).

Supply

Transderm V® (Novartis Pharmaceuticals Canada)
TD (post-auricular) patch 1mg/72h, 1 patch = $7.50.

Scopolamine hydrobromide (generic)
Injection 400microgram/mL, 1mL amp = $2; 600microgram/mL, 1mL amp = $2.

1 Herxheimer A and Haefeli L (1966) Human pharmacology of hyoscine butylbromide. *Lancet*. **ii**: 418–421.
2 Hughes A *et al*. (1997) Management of 'death rattle'. *Palliative Medicine*. **11**: 80–81.
3 Hughes A *et al*. (2000) Audit of three antimuscarinic drugs for managing retained secretions. *Palliative Medicine*. **14**: 221–222.
4 Clissold S and Heel R (1985) Transdermal hyoscine (scopolamine). A preliminary review of its pharmacodynamic properties and therapeutic efficacy. *Drugs*. **29**: 189–207.
5 Gordon C *et al*. (1985) Effect of transdermal scopolamine on salivation. *Journal of Clinical Pharmacology*. **25**: 407–412.
6 Talmi YP *et al*. (1990) Reduction of salivary flow with transdermal scopolamine: a four-year experience. *Otolaryngology – Head and Neck Surgery*. **103**: 615–618.
7 Schuurkes JAJ *et al*. (1986) Stimulation of gastroduodenal motor activity: dopaminergic and cholinergic modulation. *Drug Development Research*. **8**: 233–241.
8 Institute for Safe Medication Practices (2004) Medication Safety Alert. Burns in MRI patients wearing transdermal patches. Available from: www.ismp.org/Newsletters/acutecare/articles/20040408.asp?ptr=y
9 Health Canada (2005) Notice to hospitals. Health Canada endorsed important safety information on magnetic resonance imaging systems. Available from: www.hc-sc.gc.ca/dhp-mps/alt_formats/hpfb-dgpsa/pdf/medeff/mri-irm_patch-timbre_nth-ah_e.pdf
10 Bennett M *et al*. (2002) Using anti-muscarinic drugs in the management of death rattle: evidence based guidelines for palliative care. *Palliative Medicine*. **16**: 369–374.

ANTI-EPILEPTICS

Indications: (Licensed indications vary; see individual drug monographs for details.) Epilepsy, neuropathic pain, mania, anxiety, †sweats and hot flashes, †refractory hiccup, †terminal agitation.

Pharmacology

Anti-epileptic drugs are structurally and functionally diverse. The relationship between clinical activity and mode of action is not fully understood. Further, clinically relevant differences exist between anti-epileptics acting in similar ways, and additional actions contribute to the beneficial and/or undesirable effects of some. Choice of drug thus remains partly empirical.[1]

Anti-epileptic drug actions include (see Figure 4.3, Figure 4.4 and Table 4.22):

• membrane stabilization:
  ▷ sodium channel blockers
• reduced neurotransmitter release:
  ▷ N, P and Q-type calcium channel blockers ($\alpha2\delta$ ligands)
  ▷ SV2A ligands
• increased GABA-mediated inhibition:
  ▷ GABAmimetics.

The accumulation of sodium channels at sites of nerve injury is responsible for seizures or neuropathic pain through ectopic action potential generation (see p.212). Membrane stabilizers

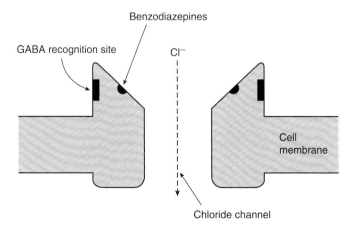

Figure 4.3   Diagram of GABA (inhibitory) receptor-channel complex.

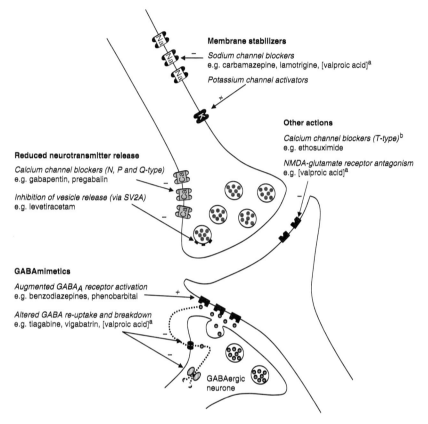

Figure 4.4 Mechanisms of action of anti-epileptics.[1,3,4,6–9] Squared parentheses indicate a contributory, but not predominant, action of the anti-epileptic.

a. although many anti-epileptics have more than one mode of action, valproic acid in particular is thought to have no single predominant action (see p.209)
b. T-type calcium channels are responsible for thalamic burst firing (implicated in absence seizures); they are also found in some nociceptors, where they may influence firing thresholds (see text).

(e.g. **carbamazepine**, **phenytoin** and **lamotrigine**) reduce the excitability of damaged neurones by blocking such channels.

The $\alpha2\delta$ ligands, **gabapentin** and **pregabalin**, block N, P and Q-type calcium channels. This reduces the calcium influx required to trigger neurotransmitter release (see p.219).[2] **Levetiracetam** binds to SV2A, a protein involved in neurotransmitter vesicle release.[5]

GABAmimetic anti-epileptics either affect GABA metabolism (synthesis, re-uptake or breakdown, e.g. **vigabatrin**, **tiagabine**) or act directly on GABA$_A$ receptors (e.g. benzodiazepines, see Fig. 4.3 and Table 4.22). **Vigabatrin** and **tiagabine** have an effect on all GABA transmission, and this may explain their ability to worsen absence seizures (via thalamic GABA$_B$ receptors), a feature not seen with GABA$_A$ selective anti-epileptics.

The broad spectrum of efficacy of **valproic acid** is explained by its multiple actions including blockade of T-type calcium channels, implicated in the burst firing responsible for absence seizures[1] and perhaps also in regulating pain excitation thresholds in a 'T-rich' subset of peripheral nociceptors.[4] The endocannabinoid system is another important inhibitory neurotransmitter system; cannabinoids have been proposed as potential future anti-epileptics.[5]

Table 4.22 Mechanisms of action of anti-epileptics [1,3,4,6-10]

	Membrane stabilizers		↓Neurotransmitter release		GABAmimetics		↓Thalamic burst firing
	Na channel blocker	K channel activator	Ca channel blocker (N, P and Q-type)	↓vesicle release (SV2A)	GABA$_A$ receptor modulation	Altered GABA synthesis and re-uptake	Ca channel blocker (T-type)
Benzodiazepines					++		
Carbamazepine	++						
Ethosuximide		+					++
Gabapentin			++				
Lacosamide	++						
Lamotrigine	++		++				
Levetiracetam				++			
Oxcarbazepine	++	+					
Phenobarbital					++		
Phenytoin	++						
Pregabalin			++				
Tiagabine						++[b]	
Topiramate	++				++		
Valproic acid	+[a]					+[a,b]	+[a]
Vigabatrin						++[b]	
Zonisamide	++		++				++

Key: ++ predominant action, + putative or non-predominant action.

a. although many anti-epileptics have more than one mode of action, valproic acid in particular is thought to have no single predominant mode of action, helping to explain its broad-spectrum of activity (see p.209)

b. tiagabine and vigabatrin inhibit GABA re-uptake and breakdown (via GABA transaminase) respectively. Valproic acid affects both synthesis and re-uptake/breakdown of GABA in selected brain regions.

Genetic variations in anti-epileptic targets have been identified (e.g. sodium and potassium channels, the $GABA_A$ receptor complex). Some cause inherited epilepsy, but there is no straightforward link between the affected channel/receptor and either the epilepsy type or optimal choice of anti-epileptic.[11,12] A polymorphism in the gene (SCN1A) encoding the sodium channel α-subunit has been linked to **carbamazepine**-resistant epilepsy.[13]

The pharmacokinetics of anti-epileptics are summarized in Table 4.23. Whereas absorption is generally unaffected by increasing age, the volume of distribution may change (reduced albumin, total body water and lean:fat mass ratio) and elimination rates slow (altered metabolism, renal function and volume of distribution).[14]

Genetic factors affect both pharmacokinetics and the risk of undesirable effects. Two poor metabolizer CYP2C9 alleles (which occur in 10–20% of Caucasians, 10% of Japanese, and 1–5% of Asians and Africans) reduce the mean effective daily **phenytoin** dose by 20–40%.[12] Human leukocyte antigen (HLA) genes are associated with the risk of Stevens-Johnson syndrome in patients taking **carbamazepine** or **phenytoin**.[15,16] The UK MHRA recommends testing HLA B*1502 status before **carbamazepine** is started in people of Han Chinese, Hong Kong Chinese or Thai origin.[17]

Table 4.23 Pharmacokinetic details of anti-epileptics[14,18–25]

Drug	Bio-availability PO (%)	T_{max} (h)	Plasma binding (%)	Plasma halflife (h)	Fate
Carbamazepine	80	4–8	75	8–24	CYP3A4, CYP2C8[h]
Clonazepam	≥80	1–4	80–90	30–40	CYP3A
Diazepam	≥80	1–3	95–98	24–48 48–120[g]	CYP2C19, CYP3A4[h]
Gabapentin	60[a]	1–4	0	6	Excreted unchanged
Lamotrigine	98	1–4	55	15–30 8–20[d] 30–90[e]	Glucuronidation
Levetiracetam	≥95	1–2	<10	6–8	Non-hepatic hydrolysis (70% excreted unchanged)
Oxcarbazepine[f]	≥95	1–3 3–8[f]	65 40[f]	1–5 7–20[f]	Cytosolic keto-reduction to MHD,[f] which then undergoes glucuronidation[h]
Phenobarbital	≥90	2–12	50	72–144	CYP2C9 (25% excreted unchanged)
Phenytoin	90–95	4–8	90	10–70[a]	CYP2C9
Pregabalin	>90	1	0	5–9[b]	Excreted unchanged
Tiagabine	≥90	1–2	96	4–13 2–5[d]	CYP3A4
Topiramate	≥80	1–4	13	20–30 8–15[d]	Multiple pathways (>60% excreted unchanged)
Valproic acid	95	1–2[c]	90	9–18 5–12[d]	Multiple pathways[h] (see p.209)
Vigabatrin	80–90	1–2	0	6	Excreted unchanged
Zonisamide	≥50	1–4	50	50–70 25–35[d]	CYP3A4 (15–30% excreted unchanged)

a. dose or plasma concentration dependent
b. >2 days in severe renal impairment and hemodialysis patients
c. 3–5h for e/c tablets, 5–10h for m/r tablets
d. with concurrent enzyme-inducers
e. with concurrent sodium valproic acid
f. monohydroxycarbazepine, active metabolite of oxcarbazepine (a pro-drug)
g. nordiazepam, active metabolite
h. metabolites biologically active.

Cautions
For full list, see manufacturer's Product Monograph.

Safety concerns with **vigabatrin** (visual field deficits) and **felbamate** (aplastic anemia and hepatic failure) limit their use to refractory epilepsy under specialist supervision when all other measures have failed.

Driving
Canadian Medical Association guidelines state that patients suffering from epilepsy must not drive a motor vehicle unless they have had a seizure-free period of 6 months (on medication) or, if subject to seizures only while asleep, have had a 1-year period without seizures (with therapeutic drug levels). People suffering from epilepsy must not drive a commercial vehicle unless they have had a seizure-free period of 5 years. Patients affected by drowsiness should not drive or operate machinery.

Skin rashes and cross-reactive hypersensitivity
In relation to skin rashes, cross-reactive hypersensitivity may occur with various anti-epileptics:[26]
- **carbamazepine**: increased risk of skin rash if rash has occurred with a previous anti-epileptic (particularly **phenytoin**, **phenobarbital** or **oxcarbazepine**) or TCA; use alternative if possible
- **phenytoin**: increased risk of skin rash if rash has occurred with a previous anti-epileptic (particularly **carbamazepine** or **phenobarbital**); use alternative if possible
- **oxcarbazepine**: 25–30% risk of cross-reactivity if previous reaction to **carbamazepine**
- **zonisamide** (not Canada): avoid if hypersensitive to sulphonamides
- **lamotrigine**: increased risk of rash if rash has occurred with a previous anti-epileptic, rapidly titrated and/or receiving concurrent **valproic acid**.

Hepatic impairment
With the exception of **gabapentin**, **pregabalin**, and **vigabatrin**, the manufacturers advise caution with all the anti-epileptics listed in Table 4.23 (i.e. lower initial doses, slower titration and careful monitoring). Specific advice is given for **levetiracetam** (halve the dose in severe hepatic impairment because of probable concurrent renal impairment), **lamotrigine** (see Product Monograph), **oxcarbazepine** (usual dose with mild–moderate impairment, no data with severe impairment), **phenytoin** (monitor plasma concentration), **tiagabine** (reduce dose if mild, avoid if severe), and **zonisamide** (not Canada; avoid if possible).

Further, previous or concurrent hepatic disease increases the risk of **valproic acid**- and **carbamazepine**-related hepatic failure. However, no specific information is available about the risks with hepatic metastases. They do not generally affect the hepatic metabolism of drugs unless there is concurrent cirrhosis.[27,28] Increase monitoring or use alternatives.

Renal impairment
With the exception of **phenytoin** and **tiagabine**, the manufacturers advise caution with all the anti-epileptics listed in Table 4.23 (i.e. lower initial doses, slower titration and careful monitoring). Specific advice on dose adjustment is available for **gabapentin** (see Table 4.29, p.222) and **pregabalin** (see Table 4.30, p.225). Further, there are occasional reports of renal failure with **pregabalin** which improved when it was stopped.

Females of child-bearing age
Consider teratogenicity when choosing an anti-epileptic. Enquire about oral contraceptive if using an enzyme-inducing anti-epileptic.

Suicide
Anti-epileptic drugs are associated with suicidal thoughts or behaviour in 1/500 patients from the start of treatment onwards. Monitor for suicidal ideation, and advise patients to get in touch if they experience mood disturbance or suicidal thoughts.[29,30]

Additional cautions with specific anti-epileptics
- atrioventricular block (**carbamazepine** and **oxcarbazepine** may cause complete block)
- previous bone marrow suppression (**carbamazepine**, possible increased risk of bone marrow toxicity)
- heart failure (**oxcarbazepine** and **pregabalin**, fluid retention can cause exacerbation; monitor weight and plasma sodium).

Interactions

For full list, see manufacturer's Product Monograph.
Interactions are described in individual drug monographs:
- **gabapentin** (p.220), **pregabalin** (p.224) and **levetiracetam** have no clinically significant pharmacokinetic interactions
- **phenobarbital** (p.226), **carbamazepine** (p.215) and **phenytoin** (p.213) cause numerous interactions through hepatic enzyme induction.

Undesirable effects

For full list, see manufacturer's Product Monograph.
Despite their diverse actions and structures, anti-epileptics share many undesirable effects. Their relative incidence is often similar.[31,32]

All anti-epileptics cause psychotropic and CNS depressant effects including drowsiness, ataxia, cognitive impairment, agitation, diplopia and dizziness. Cognitive impairment is worst with **phenobarbital** and least with newer anti-epileptics and **valproic acid**.[25,33] Anti-epileptics cause suicidal ideation in 1/500 patients (see Cautions).

Most cause hematological derangements. These are often asymptomatic and may not require discontinuation of the drug (see Product Monographs for specific advice). Severe derangement (e.g. aplastic anemia and agranulocytosis) is also reported particularly with **felbamate** (not Canada) and **carbamazepine** (where symptoms of bone marrow suppression and blood counts should be monitored), but also with many newer anti-epileptics. Folate deficiency occurs with enzyme-inducers (e.g. **phenytoin**).

Biochemical derangements (particularly of LFTs) are also common but are generally asymptomatic. Albeit rarely, hepatic failure is seen with many anti-epileptics, again particularly with **felbamate** (not Canada) and **carbamazepine** (where symptoms of hepatic disease and liver function tests should be monitored), as well as with newer anti-epileptics. The incidence compared with **carbamazepine** is unknown. Pancreatitis affects 1:3,000 users of **valproic acid**.[34] It also occurs with many newer anti-epileptics but the incidence compared with **valproic acid** is unknown.

Transient rashes are particularly associated with **lamotrigine**, **carbamazepine** and **oxcarbazepine**. Risk factors include rashes with previous anti-epileptics, higher starting doses and rapid titration (and, with **lamotrigine**, childhood and concurrent **valproic acid**). Severe rashes such as Stevens-Johnson syndrome are reported with all anti-epileptics, but most commonly with **lamotrigine** (affecting 1:1,000 adults). An HLA type is known to predispose specific groups to **carbamazepine**- and **phenytoin**-related Stevens-Johnson syndrome (see above).

Undesirable effects seen with particular anti-epileptics include: urolithiasis, **topiramate** and **zonisamide** (not Canada); and coarse facies, acne, hirsutism and gingival hypertrophy, **phenytoin**.

Use of anti-epileptics in palliative care

Particularly when prescribing more than one anti-epileptic, it is important to consider:
- pharmacokinetic drug–drug interactions (see below)
- seizure type (generalized seizures may be precipitated by **carbamazepine**, **oxcarbazepine**, **gabapentin**, **tiagabine** and **vigabatrin**)
- additive cognitive impairment.

Neuropathic pain

Gabapentin, **pregabalin**, **carbamazepine** and **valproic acid** are commonly used for central and peripheral neuropathic pain. Their efficacy and tolerability appear comparable to each other and to alternatives (e.g. antidepressants), as judged by NNT and NNH,[35–37] although few have been directly compared.

In some countries, **gabapentin** and **pregabalin** are first-line choices for neuropathic pain because this indication is included in their marketing authorizations. However, the latter differ between countries; for Canada, see individual drug monographs on p.220 and p.224 respectively. **Pregabalin** is more expensive, without evidence of superiority, but its twice daily administration is a possible advantage. Benefit has been confirmed for painful diabetic neuropathy, post-herpetic neuralgia and central neuropathic pain (see p.224).[38–49] **Gabapentin** is also effective for malignant neuropathic pain although the benefit in an RCT was small (see p.220).[50] **Gabapentin** appeared to act more quickly and with less sedation than **carbamazepine** in relation to neuropathic pain in Guillain-Barre syndrome, but neither was used optimally (dose regimens were fixed).[51]

Valproic acid is used in some centres as an alternative first choice where a smaller tablet load, syrup preparation or once daily regimen is required, particularly if a TCA cannot be used. Benefit is reported for cancer-related neuropathic pain,[52,53] but results of RCTs in non-cancer pain are conflicting (see p.209) It appears to be well tolerated in both cancer series and RCTs: rates of discontinuation because of adverse events are low [3–5%][54–57] compared with trials of **gabapentin** [8–19%][38,39] and **pregabalin** [8–32%][40–43,45,46,58] in similar populations.

Carbamazepine is a licensed first-line treatment for trigeminal neuralgia. It has long been used off-label for other neuropathic pains despite few supporting RCTs.[59] It requires slow titration and particular care with regard to drug interactions (see p.215). **Phenytoin** is also effective, at least in the short-term.[60] The important role of sodium channels in neuropathic pain (see above) has led to trials of other membrane stabilizers, particularly **oxcarbazepine** and **lamotrigine**, but results are conflicting (see p.212).

Clonazepam is reported to improve both cancer-related and non-cancer neuropathic pain.[61–64] Its concurrent anxiolytic and muscle-relaxant properties have led to its use for selected palliative care patients despite the absence of supporting RCTs.

Alternatives to anti-epileptics include antidepressants (see p.235) and opioids. They are also often used in combination. **Gabapentin**'s efficacy was similar to TCAs in two RCTs, although one found TCAs to cause more dry mouth, constipation and postural hypotension.[65,66] **Morphine** was as effective as TCAs,[67] whereas the combination of **morphine** and **gabapentin** was superior to either treatment alone.[68] An open-label trial in cancer pain with a neuropathic component also found this combination to be superior to **morphine** alone.[69]

Combinations of ≥2 anti-epileptics are used less commonly. Undesirable effects may be increased and alternative options (e.g. antidepressants, opioids, **ketamine** and interventional anesthesia) are often more appropriate. Where a second anti-epileptic drug is added, the first is generally withdrawn, although examples of combined use are reported. Improvements in efficacy and tolerability have been described in 11 patients with multiple sclerosis whose trigeminal neuralgia had been unsatisfactorily controlled by **carbamazepine** ± **lamotrigine**. The addition of **gabapentin** brought relief in 10 patients. The former were reduced to the minimal effective dose, with improved overall tolerability, but could not be withdrawn completely in any patient, suggesting that both anti-epileptics were contributing to overall relief.[70]

Although generally not used for *nociceptive* pain, **phenytoin**, **lamotrigine**, **gabapentin** and **pregabalin** have an antinociceptive/analgesic effect.[71–74]

Doses are described in individual monographs: (†)**carbamazepine** (p.215); †**clonazepam** (p.117); **gabapentin** (p.220); †**oxcarbazepine** (p.218); **pregabalin** (p.224) and †**valproic acid** (p.209).

Epilepsy

Overtreatment with anti-epileptic drugs is common. Seek specialist advice where the diagnosis of seizures or the dose or choice of anti-epileptic drug is in doubt.

Initiating treatment

In palliative care, an anti-epileptic is generally commenced after a first seizure because the persisting underlying cause (e.g. cerebral tumour, multiple sclerosis) makes further seizures probable. In other settings, this risk is lower and an anti-epileptic is often withheld unless a second seizure occurs.[75] Focal lesions cause seizures of partial onset +/− secondary generalization. True generalized convulsive seizures are generally evident within the first two decades of life, and may be exacerbated by some anti-epileptics (see above). Choice of anti-epileptic is guided by seizure type, potential for drug interactions, co-morbidities, the simplicity of the regimen and teratogenicity where relevant (seek specialist advice when treating females of childbearing age): see Box 4.N[76–78] **Valproic acid**, **levetiracetam**, **gabapentin**, **carbamazepine** and **phenytoin** are among the anti-epileptics examined in trials for seizures secondary to cerebral tumours. Enzyme-inducing anti-epileptics can interfere with chemotherapy.

Anti-epileptics are better tolerated if commenced at lower than recommended doses.[79] Doses can be increased if seizures persist. However, less additional benefit is seen when increasing higher doses. In one observational study, 90% of those responding to a first-line anti-epileptic required:

- **valproic acid** ≤1,500mg/24h
- **lamotrigine** ≤300mg/24h
- **carbamazepine** ≤800mg/24h.[80]

Few patients responded to increases above these doses.[80] In such patients, a change of anti-epileptic is indicated.

For doses, see individual monographs (for **valproic acid** (p.209), **carbamazepine** (p.215), **oxcarbazepine** (p.218), **gabapentin** (p.220) and **pregabalin** (p.224)) or manufacturer's Product Monograph.

Box 4.N   Anti-epileptics for seizures in palliative care[77,78]

First-line alternatives
Oxcarbazepine
Fewer drug interactions than phenytoin and carbamazepine; effective doses achieved more quickly than with lamotrigine and carbamazepine.

Valproic acid[a]
Can be titrated rapidly, IV if necessary.

Phenytoin
Can be rapidly titrated, IV if necessary; but numerous drug interactions can occur.

Second-line
Switch to another first-line choice, or prescribe
Levetiracetam

---

a. despite abnormal *in vitro* hemostasis, valproic acid has not been shown to increase neurosurgical bleeding complications,[81,82] but some surgeons advise caution; discuss with surgeons before starting if neurosurgery is planned.

Switching vs. combining anti-epileptics for epilepsy

If the first choice treatment fails, add a second anti-epileptic (Box 4.N). When the second one is at an adequate or maximally tolerated dose, the first one is slowly withdrawn (see below).[83] Long-term combination therapy is generally avoided unless two trials of monotherapy have proved ineffective because:

- there is an increased likelihood of drug interactions
- toxicity may be enhanced
- evidence of benefit compared with monotherapy is limited.[79,84]

Combinations are guided by the same considerations as those for choosing first- and second-line anti-epileptics. Many successful combinations have been reported,[84,85] but the relative benefits of such combinations have not been established. Studies of older anti-epileptics indicate probable benefit in combining GABAmimetics with sodium channel blockers or possibly with other GABAmimetics, but not in using two sodium channel blockers together.[86] Despite this, combinations of sodium channel blockers are among those used by epileptologists.[84] Combining **valproic acid** and **lamotrigine** increases the risk of skin reactions.

Do not combine three or more anti-epileptics except on specialist advice; additional benefit is rare.[79]

Prophylaxis in patients with cerebral tumours

Although about 20% of patients diagnosed with cerebral tumours will experience seizures, the risk is not reduced by prophylactic anti-epileptics. Sub-therapeutic levels, a potential explanation in some trials, does not adequately account for this lack of effect. Thus anti-epileptics should not generally be commenced in the absence of a history of seizures.[75,87] Peri-neurosurgical use is an exception, but anti-epileptics should generally be slowly tapered after one week. [87]

Status epilepticus

Figure 4.5 is modified from the current Health Canada recommendations.[88] Hypoglycemia should be excluded in all patients. If alcoholism or severely impaired nutrition is suspected, give thiamine 250mg IV. **Phenobarbital** has been given preference over **phenytoin** because it is more likely to be immediately available in many palliative care units.

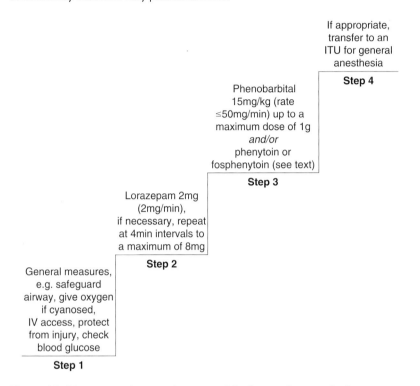

If appropriate,
transfer to an
ITU for general
anesthesia

Step 4

Phenobarbital
15mg/kg (rate
≤50mg/min) up to a
maximum dose of 1g
and/or
phenytoin or
fosphenytoin (see text)

Step 3

Lorazepam 2mg
(2mg/min),
if necessary, repeat
at 4min intervals to
a maximum of 8mg

Step 2

General measures,
e.g. safeguard
airway, give oxygen
if cyanosed,
IV access, protect
from injury, check
blood glucose

Step 1

Figure 4.5   Management of status epilepticus in adults. See text for more detail.

Lorazepam is the benzodiazepine of choice in the control of status epilepticus (see p.119)[89] but, if unavailable, **midazolam** 10mg (see p.115) is an alternative. If venous access cannot be obtained give **midazolam** 10mg †buccally or †SC, or **diazepam** 10–20mg PR (see p.113).

Fosphenytoin is a pro-drug of **phenytoin** (1.5mg of the former is equivalent to 1mg of the latter). The dose is expressed as **phenytoin sodium** equivalent (PE). It can be given more rapidly than **phenytoin**. Ideally, heart rate, blood pressure and respiratory function should be monitored during and for 30min after the administration of **fosphenytoin** 20mg(PE)/kg (100–150mg(PE)/min). IV **phenytoin sodium** 15mg/kg up to a maximum total dose of 1g (≤50mg/min; dilute 500mg with 50mL 0.9% saline) can be used instead, preferably with ECG monitoring.

Terminal agitation

Phenobarbital is sometimes used in the management of intractable agitation in patients who are imminently dying (see p.226).[90]

Mania

Valproic acid is generally added only when the response to an antipsychotic and a benzodiazepine is inadequate, but is an alternative first-line therapy particularly when it has been effective previously. **Carbamazepine** and **lamotrigine** can also be used.[91]

Anxiety

Despite benefit in various anxiety disorders,[92] anti-epileptics are not commonly used. In the UK (but not Canada), **pregabalin** (see p.224) is licensed for generalized anxiety disorder. Its efficacy is similar to **lorazepam**, **alprazolam** and **venlafaxine**. It has a faster rate of onset than **venlafaxine**, and causes less nausea. It has a similar rate of onset to **lorazapam** and **alprazolam**, and causes less drowsiness but more dizziness.[93] It is also effective for social phobia.[94] RCTs also show some benefit with **gabapentin**,[95,96] **tiagabine**[97] and **lamotrigine**.[98]

Sweats and hot flashes

Gabapentin is effective for hot flashes associated with breast cancer or the menopause.[99,100] Benefit is also reported in idiopathic sweating in cancer (see p.220).[101]

Refractory hiccup

Gabapentin is reported to be effective for hiccup (see p.220).

Stopping anti-epileptics

Abrupt cessation of long-term anti-epileptic therapy should be avoided because rebound seizures may be precipitated, even if use is for indications other than epilepsy. If treatment is to be discontinued, particularly barbiturates and benzodiazepines, this is best done *slowly over at least 6 months* (Table 4.24). However, with **gabapentin** and **pregabalin**, withdrawal over 1–2 weeks is generally possible.

Table 4.24 Recommended monthly reductions of selected anti-epileptics[102]

Drug[a]	Reduction
Carbamazepine	100mg
Clobazam	10mg
Clonazepam	0.5mg
Ethosuximide	250mg
Lamotrigine	25mg
Levetiracetam	1,000mg[b]
Phenobarbital	15mg
Phenytoin	50mg
Topiramate	25mg
Valproic acid	250mg
Vigabatrin	500mg

a. gabapentin and pregabalin can be stopped progressively over 1–2 weeks
b. data from Product Monograph.

In adults, the risk of relapse of pre-existing epilepsy on stopping treatment is 40–50%.[103] Caution should also be exercised when switching to an alternative anti-epileptic drug. In contrast to switching opioids (see p.294), the first drug should *not* be withdrawn until the new drug has been titrated up to an anticipated effective dose.

For patients who are imminently dying (i.e. death expected within a few days) and who can no longer swallow medication, consider substituting SC midazolam or SC phenobarbital. However, remember that some anti-epileptics have a long halflife (see Table 4.23) and, in a moribund patient, might continue to be effective for 2–3 days after the last PO dose.

1 Perucca E (2005) An introduction to antiepileptic drugs. *Epilepsia.* **46 (suppl 4)**: 31–37.
2 Taylor CP (2009) Mechanisms of analgesia by gabapentin and pregabalin–calcium channel alpha2-delta [Cavalpha2-delta] ligands. *Pain.* **142**: 13–16.
3 Lynch BA (2004) The synaptic vesicle protein SV2A is the binding site for the antiepileptic drug levetiracetam. *Proceedings of the National Academy of Sciences of the United States of America.* **101 (26)**: 9861–9866.
4 Jevtovic-Todorovic V et al. (2006) The role of peripheral T-type calcium channels in pain transmission. *Cell Calcium.* **40**: 197–203.
5 Bagshaw SM and Hagan NA (2002) Medical efficacy of cannabinoids and marijuana: a comprehensive review of the literature. *Journal of Palliative Care.* **18 (2)**: 111–122.
6 Kochegarov AA (2003) Pharmacological modulators of voltage-gated calcium channels and their therapeutical application. *Cell Calcium.* **33**: 145–162.

7 Shin HS (2006) T-type Ca2+ channels and absence epilepsy. *Cell Calcium*. **40**: 191–196.

8 Loscher W (2002) Basic pharmacology of valproate: a review after 35 years of clinical use for the treatment of epilepsy. *CNS Drugs*. **16**: 669–694.

9 Lee CH et al. (2008) Gabapentin activates ROMK1 channels by a protein kinase A (PKA)-dependent mechanism. *British Journal of Pharmacology*. **154**: 216–225.

10 Sheets PL et al. (2008) Differential block of sensory neuronal voltage-gated sodium channels by lacosamide [(2R)-2-(acetylamino)-N-benzyl-3-methoxypropanamide], lidocaine, and carbamazepine. *Journal of Pharmacology and Experimental Therapeutics*. **326**: 89–99.

11 Mann MW and Pons G (2007) Various pharmacogenetic aspects of antiepileptic drug therapy: a review. *CNS Drugs*. **21**: 143–164.

12 Loscher W et al. (2009) The clinical impact of pharmacogenetics on the treatment of epilepsy. *Epilepsia*. **50**: 1–23.

13 Abe T et al. (2008) Association between SCN1A polymorphism and carbamazepine-resistant epilepsy. *British Journal of Clinical Pharmacology*. **66**: 304–307.

14 Perucca E (2006) Clinical pharmacokinetics of new-generation antiepileptic drugs at the extremes of age. *Clinical Pharmacokinetics*. **45**: 351–363.

15 Chung WH et al. (2004) Medical genetics: a marker for Stevens-Johnson syndrome. *Nature*. **428**: 486.

16 Locharernkul C et al. (2008) Carbamazepine and phenytoin induced Stevens-Johnson syndrome is associated with HLA-B*1502 allele in Thai population. *Epilepsia*. **49**: 2087–2091.

17 MHRA (2008) Drug safety update. 1 (9, April): 5. Available from: www.mhra.gov.uk/Publications/Safetyguidance/DrugSafetyUpdate/CON014505

18 Perucca E (1999) The clinical pharmacokinetics of the new antiepileptic drugs. *Epilepsia*. **40 (suppl 9)**: S7–13.

19 Bang LM and Goa KL (2004) Spotlight on oxcarbazepine in epilepsy. *CNS Drugs*. **18**: 57–61.

20 Kwan P and Brodie MJ (2004) Phenobarbital for the treatment of epilepsy in the 21st century: a critical review. *Epilepsia*. **45**: 1141–1149.

21 Patsalos PN and Patsalos PN (2004) Clinical pharmacokinetics of levetiracetam. *Clinical Pharmacokinetics*. **43**: 707–724.

22 Anderson et al. (2002) *Handbook of clinical drug data* (10e). McGraw Hill.

23 Garnett WR (2000) Clinical pharmacology of topiramate: a review. *Epilepsia*. **41 (suppl 1)**: S61–65.

24 May TW et al. (2003) Clinical pharmacokinetics of oxcarbazepine. *Clinical Pharmacokinetics*. **42**: 1023–1042.

25 Perucca E (2002) Pharmacological and therapeutic properties of valproate: a summary after 35 years of clinical experience. *CNS Drugs*. **16**: 695–714.

26 Hirsch LJ et al. (2008) Cross-sensitivity of skin rashes with antiepileptic drug use. *Neurology*. **71**: 1527–1534.

27 Morgan DJ and McLean AJ (1995) Clinical pharmacokinetic and pharmacodynamic considerations in patients with liver disease. An update. *Clinical Pharmacokinetics*. **29**: 370–391.

28 Ford-Dunn S (2005) Managing patients with cancer and advanced liver disease. *Palliative Medicine*. **19**: 563–565.

29 FDA (2008) Safety information. Antiepileptic drugs. Available from: www.fda.gov/Safety/MedWatch/SafetyInformation/SafetyAlertsforHumanMedicalProducts/ucm074939.htm

30 EMEA (2008) Meeting highlights from the Committee for Medicinal Products for Human Use, 15–18 December 2008. Available from: www.emea.europa.eu/pdfs/human/press/pr/67072408en.pdf

31 Marson AG et al. (2007) The SANAD study of effectiveness of carbamazepine, gabapentin, lamotrigine, oxcarbazepine, or topiramate for treatment of partial epilepsy: an unblinded randomised controlled trial. *Lancet*. **369**: 1,000–1015.

32 Marson AG et al. (2007) The SANAD study of effectiveness of valproate, lamotrigine, or topiramate for generalised and unclassifiable epilepsy: an unblinded randomised controlled trial. *Lancet*. **369**: 1016–1026.

33 Kwan P and Brodie MJ (2001) Neuropsychological effects of epilepsy and antiepileptic drugs. *Lancet*. **357**: 216–222.

34 French JA (2007) First-choice drug for newly diagnosed epilepsy. *Lancet*. **369**: 970–971.

35 Finnerup NB et al. (2005) Algorithm for neuropathic pain treatment: an evidence based proposal. *Pain*. **118**: 289–305.

36 Saarto T and Wiffen PJ (2007) Antidepressants for neuropathic pain. *Cochrane Database of Systematic Reviews*. CD005454. [Update of Cochrane Database Syst Rev. 2005;(3):CD005454; PMID: 16034979].

37 Dworkin RH et al. (2007) Pharmacologic management of neuropathic pain: evidence-based recommendations. *Pain*. **132**: 237–251.

38 Backonja M et al. (1998) Gabapentin for the symptomatic treatment of painful neuropathy in patients with diabetes mellitus: a randomized controlled trial. *Journal of the American Medical Association*. **280**: 1831–1836.

39 Rowbotham M et al. (1998) Gabapentin for the treatment of postherpetic neuralgia: a randomized controlled trial. *Journal of the American Medical Association*. **280**: 1837–1842.

40 Richter RW et al. (2005) Relief of painful diabetic peripheral neuropathy with pregabalin: a randomized, placebo-controlled trial. *Journal of Pain*. **6**: 253–260.

41 Rosenstock J et al. (2004) Pregabalin for the treatment of painful diabetic peripheral neuropathy: a double-blind, placebo-controlled trial. *Pain*. **110**: 628–638.

42 Tolle T et al. (2008) Pregabalin for relief of neuropathic pain associated with diabetic neuropathy: a randomized, double-blind study. *European Journal of Pain*. **12**: 203–213.

43 Freynhagen R et al. (2005) Efficacy of pregabalin in neuropathic pain evaluated in a 12-week, randomised, double-blind, multicentre, placebo-controlled trial of flexible- and fixed-dose regimens. *Pain*. **115**: 254–263.

44 Dworkin RH et al. (2003) Pregabalin for the treatment of postherpetic neuralgia: a randomized, placebo-controlled trial. *Neurology*. **60**: 1274–1283.

45 Sabatowski R et al. (2004) Pregabalin reduces pain and improves sleep and mood disturbances in patients with post-herpetic neuralgia: results of a randomised, placebo-controlled clinical trial. *Pain*. **109**: 26–35.

46 van Seventer R et al. (2006) Efficacy and tolerability of twice-daily pregabalin for treating pain and related sleep interference in postherpetic neuralgia: a 13-week, randomized trial. *Current Medical Research and Opinion*. **22**: 375–384.

47 Levendoglu F et al. (2004) Gabapentin is a first line drug for the treatment of neuropathic pain in spinal cord injury. *Spine*. **29**: 743–751.

48 Vranken JH et al. (2008) Pregabalin in patients with central neuropathic pain: a randomized, double-blind, placebo-controlled trial of a flexible-dose regimen. *Pain*. **136**: 150–157.

49 Siddall PJ et al. (2006) Pregabalin in central neuropathic pain associated with spinal cord injury: a placebo-controlled trial. *Neurology*. **67**: 1792–1800.

50 Caraceni A et al. (2004) Gabapentin for neuropathic cancer pain: a randomized controlled trial from the Gabapentin Cancer Pain Study Group. *Journal of Clinical Oncology*. **22**: 2909–2917.

51 Pandey CK *et al.* (2005) The comparative evaluation of gabapentin and carbamazepine for pain management in Guillain-Barre syndrome patients in the intensive care unit. *Anesthesia and Analgesia.* **101**: 220–225.

52 Snare AJ (1993) Sodium Valproate. Retrospective analysis of neuropathic pain control in patients with advanced cancer. *Journal of Pharmacy Technology.* **9**: 114–117.

53 Hardy JR *et al.* (2001) A phase II study to establish the efficacy and toxicity of sodium valproate in patients with cancer-related neuropathic pain. *Journal of Pain and Symptom Management.* **21**: 204–209.

54 Kochar DK *et al.* (2002) Sodium valproate in the management of painful neuropathy in type 2 diabetes – a randomized placebo controlled study. *Acta Neurologica Scandinavica.* **106**: 248–252.

55 Kochar DK *et al.* (2004) Sodium valproate for painful diabetic neuropathy: a randomized double-blind placebo-controlled study. *Quarterly Journal of Medicine.* **97**: 33–38.

56 Kochar DK *et al.* (2005) Divalproex sodium in the management of post-herpetic neuralgia: a randomized double-blind placebo-controlled study. *Quarterly Journal of Medicine.* **98**: 29–34.

57 Otto M *et al.* (2004) Valproic acid has no effect on pain in polyneuropathy: a randomized, controlled trial. *Neurology.* **62**: 285–288.

58 Dworkin RH *et al.* (2003) Pregabalin for the treatment of postherpetic neuralgia: a randomized, placebo-controlled trial. *Neurology.* **60**: 1274–1283.

59 Wiffen PJ *et al.* (2005) Carbamazepine for acute and chronic pain. *Cochrane Database of Systematic Reviews.* **3**: CD005451.

60 McCleane G (1999) Intravenous infusion of phenytoin relieves neuropathic pain: a randomized, double-blinded, placebo-controlled, crossover study. *Anesthesia and Analgesia.* **89**: 985–988.

61 Swerdlow M and Cundill J (1981) Anticonvulsant drugs used in the treatment of lancinating pain: a comparison. *Anaesthesia.* **36**: 1129–1132.

62 Bouckoms AJ and Litman RE (1985) Clonazepam in the treatment of neuralgic pain syndrome. *Psychosomatics.* **26**: 933–936.

63 Bartusch S *et al.* (1996) Clonazepam for the treatment of lancinating phantom limb pain. *Clinical Journal of Pain.* **12**: 59–62.

64 Hugel H *et al.* (2003) Clonazepam as an adjuvant analgesic in patients with cancer-related neuropathic pain. *Journal of Pain and Symptom Management.* **26**: 1073–1074.

65 Morello C *et al.* (1999) Randomized double-blind study comparing the efficacy of gabapentin with amitriptyline on diabetic peripheral neuropathy pain. *Archives of Internal Medicine.* **159**: 1931–1937.

66 Chandra K *et al.* (2006) Gabapentin versus nortriptyline in post-herpetic neuralgia patients: a randomized, double-blind clinical trial–the GONIP Trial. *International Journal of Clinical Pharmacology and Therapeutics.* **44**: 358–363.

67 Raja SN *et al.* (2002) Opioids versus antidepressants in postherpetic neuralgia: a randomized, placebo-controlled trial. *Neurology.* **59**: 1015–1021.

68 Gilron I *et al.* (2005) Morphine, gabapentin, or their combination for neuropathic pain. *New England Journal of Medicine.* **352**: 1324–1334.

69 Keskinbora K *et al.* (2007) Gabapentin and an opioid combination versus opioid alone for the management of neuropathic cancer pain: a randomized open trial. *Journal of Pain and Symptom Management.* **34**: 183–189.

70 Solaro C *et al.* (2000) Low-dose gabapentin combined with either lamotrigine or carbamazepine can be useful therapies for trigeminal neuralgia in multiple sclerosis. *European Neurology.* **44**: 45–48.

71 Webb J and Kamali F (1998) Analgesic effects of lamotrigine and phenytoin on cold-induced pain: a crossover placebo-controlled study in healthy volunteers. *Pain.* **76**: 357–363.

72 Hill CM *et al.* (2001) Pregabalin in patients with postoperative dental pain. *European Journal of Pain.* **5**: 119–124.

73 Ho KY *et al.* (2006) Gabapentin and postoperative pain – a systematic review of randomized controlled trials. *Pain.* **126**: 91–101.

74 Jokela R *et al.* (2008) A randomized controlled trial of perioperative administration of pregabalin for pain after laparoscopic hysterectomy. *Pain.* **134**: 106–112.

75 Miller LC and Drislane FW (2007) Treatment strategies after a single seizure: rationale for immediate versus deferred treatment. *CNS Drugs.* **21**: 89–99.

76 Schaller B (2006) Brain tumor and seizures: pathophysiology and its implications for treatment revisited (epilepsia 2003; 44:1223–1232). *Epilepsia.* **47**: 661; author reply 661.

77 Vecht C (2006) Otimizing therapy of seizures in patients with brain tumours. *Neurology.* **67**: S10–S13.

78 van Breemen MS *et al.* (2007) Epilepsy in patients with brain tumours: epidemiology, mechanisms, and management. *Lancet Neurology.* **6**: 421–430.

79 Perucca E and Kwan P (2005) Overtreatment in epilepsy: how it occurs and how it can be avoided. *CNS Drugs.* **19**: 897–908.

80 Kwan P and Brodie MJ (2001) Effectiveness of first antiepileptic drug. *Epilepsia.* **42**: 1255–1260.

81 Ward MM *et al.* (1996) Preoperative valproate administration does not increase blood loss during temporal lobectomy. *Epilepsia.* **37**: 98–101.

82 Anderson GD *et al.* (1997) Absence of bleeding complications in patients undergoing cortical surgery while receiving valproate treatment. *Journal of Neurosurgery.* **87**: 252–256.

83 NICE (2004) The epilepsies: the diagnosis and management of the epilepsies in adults and children in primary and secondary care. Available from: www.nice.org.uk/nicemedia/pdf/CG020fullguideline.pdf

84 Karceski S *et al.* (2005) Treatment of epilepsy in adults: expert opinion, 2005. *Epilepsy and Behavior.* **7 (suppl 1)**: S1–64; quiz S65–67.

85 Stephen LJ and Brodie MJ (2002) Seizure freedom with more than one antiepileptic drug. *Seizure.* **11**: 349–351.

86 Deckers CL *et al.* (2000) Selection of antiepileptic drug polytherapy based on mechanisms of action: the evidence reviewed. *Epilepsia.* **41**: 1364–1374.

87 Glantz MJ *et al.* (2000) Practice parameter: anticonvulsant prophylaxis in patients with newly diagnosed brain tumors. Report of the Quality Standards Subcommittee of the American Academy of Neurology. *Neurology.* **54**: 1886–1893.

88 Health Canada (2005) Chapter 8. Central nervous system. Clinical practice guidelines for nurses in primary care. Available from: www.hc-sc.gc.ca/fniah-spnia/pubs/services/_nursing-infirm/2000_clin-guide/chap_08-eng.php

89 Prasad K *et al.* (2005) Anticonvulsant therapy for status epilepticus. *Cochrane Database of Systematic Reviews.* **4**: CD003723.

90 Twycross R *et al.* (2009) *Symptom Management in Advanced Cancer.* palliativedrugs.com, Nottingham, pp. 430–433.

91 NICE (2006) The management of bipolar disorder in adults, children and adolescents, in primary and secondary care. Clinical guideline CG38. Available from: http://guidance.nice.org.uk/CG38

92 Van Ameringen M *et al.* (2004) Antiepileptic drugs in the treatment of anxiety disorders: role in therapy. *Drugs.* **64**: 2199–2220.

93 Frampton JE and Foster RH (2006) Pregabalin: in the treatment of generalised anxiety disorder. *CNS Drugs.* **20**: 685–693; discussion 694–695. [Erratum appears in CNS Drugs. 2007;21(6):481.]

94   Pande AC et al. (2004) Efficacy of the novel anxiolytic pregabalin in social anxiety disorder: a placebo-controlled, multicenter study. Journal of Clinical Psychopharmacology. 24: 141–149.
95   Pande AC et al. (1999) Treatment of social phobia with gabapentin: a placebo-controlled study. Journal of Clinical Psychopharmacology. 19: 341–348.
96   Pande AC et al. (2000) Placebo-controlled study of gabapentin treatment of panic disorder. Journal of Clinical Psychopharmacology. 20: 467–471.
97   Pollack MH et al. (2005) The selective GABA reuptake inhibitor tiagabine for the treatment of generalized anxiety disorder: results of a placebo-controlled study. Journal of Clinical Psychiatry. 66: 1401–1408.
98   Hertzberg MA et al. (1999) A preliminary study of lamotrigine for the treatment of posttraumatic stress disorder. Biological Psychiatry. 45: 1226–1229.
99   Pandya KJ et al. (2005) Gabapentin for hot flashes in 420 women with breast cancer: a randomised double-blind placebo-controlled trial. Lancet. 366: 818–824.
100 Nelson HD et al. (2006) Nonhormonal therapies for menopausal hot flashes: systematic review and meta-analysis. Journal of the American Medical Association. 295: 2057–2071.
101 Porzio G et al. (2006) Gabapentin in the treatment of severe sweating experienced by advanced cancer patients. Supportive Care in Cancer. 14: 389–391.
102 Chadwick D (1995) The withdrawal of antiepileptic drugs. In: A Hopkins et al. (eds) Epilepsy (2e). Chapman and Hall, London, pp. 215–220.
103 Hopkins A and Shorvon S (1995) Definitions and epidemiology of epilepsy. In: A Hopkins et al. (eds) Epilepsy (2e). Chapman and Hall, London, pp. 1–24.

VALPROIC ACID

Class: Anti-epileptic (multimodal action).

Indications: Epilepsy (see Product Monograph for details), †neuropathic pain, †mania associated with bipolar disorder, †migraine prophylaxis.

Contra-indications: active hepatic disease (see text), past or family history of severe hepatic impairment (particularly drug-related), porphyria.

Pharmacology

No single mode of action accounts for the anti-seizure activity of valproic acid. It is a sodium and T-type calcium channel blocker, an NMDA receptor-channel blocker, it increases potassium conductance and alters GABA, dopamine and serotonin transmission, although the relative significance of these actions is unclear. In contrast to other GABAmimetics, its effect is selective (particularly for the midbrain) and involves several mechanisms (altered synthesis, release, reuptake and degradation).[1]

Valproic acid is well absorbed orally. It is ⩾90% plasma protein-bound, and crosses the blood-brain barrier and neuronal membranes via active transporters. It is metabolized by CYP-mediated oxidation (10%: CYP2A6, 2B6, 2C9 and 2C19), mitochondrial β-oxidation (40%) and direct microsomal UDP-mediated glucuronidation (50%). Some metabolites are active, but their cerebral concentrations are too low to contribute to valproic acid's overall effect. Metabolites may be responsible for idiosyncratic hepatic toxicity. CYP enzyme inducers, inhibitors and polymorphisms affect the proportion of CYP-metabolites, perhaps altering this risk.[2,3]

Valproic acid remains a first-line treatment for generalized seizures, its efficacy and tolerability comparing favourably to those of newer anti-epileptics.[4,5] Its main safety concerns are idiosyncratic hepatic damage, affecting 1:3,000–1:20,000 people, and teratogenicity.[3,6] However, the incidence of serious idiosyncratic reactions reported with newer anti-epileptics is unknown.

A beneficial effect is reported for malignant neuropathic pain,[7,8] but the results of RCTs in non-malignant pain are less clear. Three RCTs from one group found significant benefit in painful diabetic neuropathy (n = 43, n = 57)[9,10] and post-herpetic neuralgia (n = 45).[11] However, a fourth RCT (n = 37) found no benefit in peripheral neuropathic pain of mixed cause.[12] The discrepancy is difficult to explain. Although conducted in a mixed group, diabetes accounted for ~50% of patients in the latter study; it was a crossover trial (the others were parallel group designs), but no carry-over effect was found; it was a European population (the others were conducted in India), but the above favourable series are European[8] and Australian;[7] it was shorter (4-week active arm, whereas maximum benefit in the others occurred progressively over 4 to 12 weeks), although case series often report a rapid onset. A fifth RCT in central (spinal cord) neuropathic pain found non-significant trends towards benefit of a comparable magnitude to

those of the first 3 studies.[13] Its size (n = 20) raises the possibility that it was underpowered. Valproic acid was well tolerated in all 5 studies, with fewer patients (≤5%) discontinuing because of undesirable effects compared with **gabapentin** (8–19%) and **pregabalin** (8–32%) (see p.202).
Bio-availability 95% PO.
Onset of action often within 24h (for neuropathic pain).[7]
Peak plasma concentration 1–2h (3–5h for EC, 5–10h for SR).
Plasma halflife 9–18h (5–12h with concurrent enzyme inducers).
Duration of action 12–24h.[3]

Cautions

For full list, see manufacturer's Product Monograph.
Idiosyncratic, potentially fatal, hepatic failure occurs in 1:3,000–1:20,000 patients, usually within the first 6 months of treatment. Risk factors include age <3 years, pre-existing liver disease and deranged LFTs. Chronic hepatitis was the commonest reported liver disease:[14,15] it is unclear whether hepatic metastases affect the risk. Symptoms (drowsiness, fatigue, vomiting, and increased seizure frequency) may precede altered LFTs,[3] but both are common in palliative care populations. Mildly deranged LFTs do not require discontinuation but should prompt increased monitoring. Valproic acid should be stopped if co-existent coagulopathy, severely deranged LFTs or rapidly evolving symptoms occur in the absence of an alternative explanation. Treatment with IV **carnitine** has been proposed; seek specialist advice.

Lower initial doses and slower titration may be required in patients with renal impairment. Alternatives may be preferred in females trying to conceive; seek specialist advice. Harmless ketone metabolites, detected by bedside urinalysis, may cause diagnostic confusion in diabetic patients.

Drug interactions

The clearance of valproic acid is increased by hepatic enzyme inducers such as **carbamazepine**, **phenytoin**, **phenobarbital** and **rifampin**.[3] Its clearance is inhibited by **isoniazid**.

Valproic acid inhibits the metabolism of **carbamazepine**'s active/epoxide metabolite (increasing undesirable effects), **ethosuximide**, **phenytoin**, **phenobarbital**, **lamotrigine** and some antiretrovirals.

Concurrent administration with carbapenem β-lactam antibacterials can decrease the plasma concentration of valproic acid dramatically by 85–90% through the combined impact on intestinal absorption, distribution and metabolism, with consequential loss of therapeutic effect.[16] Because increasing the dose may not overcome this drug-drug interaction, alternative antibacterials should be considered for patients taking valproic acid.

Undesirable effects

For full list, see manufacturer's Product Monograph.
Hepatic failure (see above) and pancreatitis are the most important idiosyncratic effects. Other rare effects include severe skin reactions (e.g. Stevens-Johnson syndrome) and reversible encephalopathy, parkinsonism and dementia.

Common problems include gastric intolerance (particularly nausea: reduced by EC formulations or taking with food), drowsiness and postural tremor (a rarer flapping tremor is seen with hyperammonemia), although the incidence varies markedly between individual studies. Hyperammonemia is usually asymptomatic but can cause nausea, ataxia or encephalopathy.

Dose and use

The manufacturer recommends that LFTs, prothrombin time (PT) and full blood count (FBC) be checked before and during the first 6 months of treatment, although this may not improve the early detection of hepatotoxicity.

Epilepsy

- start with valproic acid 250mg b.i.d.
- if necessary, increase by 250mg b.i.d. every 3 days

- maximum recommended dose = 2.5g/24h
- 90% of those responding to valproic acid first-line require ≤1.5g/24h; few patients respond to increases above this dose.[17]

IV valproic acid is used when the oral route cannot be used. Patients already receiving oral treatment are given the same daily dose in continuous or intermittent (over 3–5min) infusions. Patients starting valproic acid are given 500–800mg (max 10mg/kg) followed by continuous or intermittent infusions of up to 2.5g/24h.

Neuropathic pain
- start with valproic acid 250mg at bedtime
- if necessary, increase by 250mg every 3 days
- response likely at doses lower than those used in epilepsy, e.g. 500–750mg at bedtime/24h
- some patients need 2g/24h.[7,8]

Mania
- start with valproic acid 250mg t.i.d.
- increase as rapidly as possible to achieve the optimal response, to a maximum of 60mg/kg/24h
- patients receiving >45mg/kg/24h should be carefully monitored
- most patients respond to doses <2g/24h.[18,19]
- **Migraine prophylaxis**
- start with valproic acid 250mg b.i.d.[20]
- if necessary, increase progressively to a total daily dose of 1g.[21]

Supply

Valproic acid (generic)
Capsules 250mg, 500mg, 28 days @ 500mg at bedtime = $8.
Capsules EC 500mg, 28 days @ 500mg at bedtime = $15.
Oral solution 250mg/5mL, 28 days @ 500mg at bedtime = $17.
Injection 100mg/mL, 500mg vial; available via the Canadian Special Access Programme.

Depakene® (Abbott)
Capsules 250mg, 28 days @ 500mg at bedtime = $31.
Oral solution 250mg/5mL, 28 days @ 500mg at bedtime = $32.

Sodium valproate
Divalproex sodium (generic)
Tablets 125mg, 250mg, 500mg, 28 days @ 500mg at bedtime = $14.

Epival® (Abbott)
Tablets 125mg, 250mg, 500mg, 28 days @ 500mg at bedtime = $30.

The pharmacokinetics, efficacy, and tolerability of valproic acid and sodium valproate are similar; sodium valproate 579mg is equivalent to valproic acid 500mg.[22]

1 Loscher W (2002) Basic pharmacology of valproate: a review after 35 years of clinical use for the treatment of epilepsy. CNS Drugs. **16**: 669–694.
2 Mann MW and Pons G (2007) Various pharmacogenetic aspects of antiepileptic drug therapy: a review. CNS Drugs. **21**: 143–164.
3 Perucca E (2002) Pharmacological and therapeutic properties of valproate: a summary after 35 years of clinical experience. CNS Drugs. **16**: 695–714.
4 Marson AG et al. (2007) The SANAD study of effectiveness of valproate, lamotrigine, or topiramate for generalised and unclassifiable epilepsy: an unblinded randomised controlled trial. Lancet. **369**: 1016–1026.
5 Karceski S et al. (2005) Treatment of epilepsy in adults: expert opinion, 2005. Epilepsy and Behavior. **7 (suppl 1)**: S1–64; quiz S65–67.
6 French JA (2007) First-choice drug for newly diagnosed epilepsy. Lancet. **369**: 970–971.
7 Snare AJ (1993) Sodium Valproate. Retrospective analysis of neuropathic pain control in patients with advanced cancer. Journal of Pharmacy Technology. **9**: 114–117.
8 Hardy J et al. (2001) A phase II study to establish the efficacy and toxicity of sodium valproate in patients with cancer-related neuropathic pain. Journal of Pain and Symptom Management. **21**: 204–209.
9 Kochar DK et al. (2004) Sodium valproate for painful diabetic neuropathy: a randomized double-blind placebo-controlled study. Quarterly Journal of Medicine. **97**: 33–38.
10 Kochar DK et al. (2002) Sodium valproate in the management of painful neuropathy in type 2 diabetes – a randomized placebo controlled study. Acta Neurologica Scandinavica. **106**: 248–252.

11 Kochar DK et al. (2005) Divalproex sodium in the management of post-herpetic neuralgia: a randomized double-blind placebo-controlled study. Quarterly Journal of Medicine. **98**: 29–34.

12 Otto M et al. (2004) Valproic acid has no effect on pain in polyneuropathy: a randomized, controlled trial. Neurology. **62**: 285–288.

13 Drewes AM et al. (1994) Valproate for treatment of chronic central pain after spinal cord injury. A double-blind cross-over study. Paraplegia. **32**: 565–569.

14 Konig SA et al. (1994) Severe hepatotoxicity during valproate therapy: an update and report of eight new fatalities. Epilepsia. **35**: 1005–1015.

15 Koenig SA et al. (2006) Valproic acid-induced hepatopathy: nine new fatalities in Germany from 1994 to 2003. Epilepsia. **47**: 2027–2031.

16 Mancl EE and Gidal BE (2009) The effect of carbapenem antibiotics on plasma concentrations of valproic acid. Annals of Pharmacotherapy. **43**: 2082–2087.

17 Kwan P and Brodie MJ (2001) Effectiveness of first antiepileptic drug. Epilepsia. **42**: 1255–1260.

18 Keck PE, Jr. et al. (1993) Valproate oral loading in the treatment of acute mania. Journal of Clinical Psychiatry. **54**: 305–308.

19 Macritchie K et al. (2003) Valproate for acute mood episodes in bipolar disorder. Cochrane Database of Systematic Reviews. **1**: CD004052.

20 Kinze S et al. (2001) Valproic acid is effective in migraine prophylaxis at low serum levels: a prospective open-label study. Headache. **41**: 774–778.

21 Freitag FG (2003) Divalproex in the treatment of migraine. Psychopharmacol Bull. **37 (suppl 2)**: 98–115.

22 Fisher (2003) Sodium valproate or valproate semisodium: is there a difference in the treatment of bipolar disorder? Psychiatric Bulletin. **27**: 446–448.

ANTI-EPILEPTIC SODIUM CHANNEL BLOCKERS (MEMBRANE STABILIZERS)

Membrane stabilizers reduce excitability by blocking sodium channels. Such channels are needed in high densities at sites which initiate action potentials (APs), e.g. sensory nerve endings, but lower densities are sufficient to allow APs to propagate along the remainder of the neurone. Neuronal damage interferes with sodium channel transport resulting in such channels accumulating and creating foci of ectopic AP generation.[1] Depending on the site of injury, these can result in seizures or neuropathic pain. Thus, several classes of drug of benefit in these conditions act through sodium channel blockade:

• some anti-epileptics, e.g. **carbamazepine** (see p.215), **oxcarbazepine** (see p.218), **phenytoin** (Box 4.O), **lamotrigine** and **lacosamide** (not Canada)
• local anesthetics, e.g. **lidocaine**
• class I anti-arrhythmics, e.g. **flecainide**.

All have been shown to have antinociceptive and/or anti-neuropathic pain effects.[2–5] However, the duration of blockade before the drug dissociates from the channel varies. This, and effects on targets other than sodium channels, creates important clinical differences between such drugs.

Carbamazepine is a licensed first-line treatment for trigeminal neuralgia. It has long been used for other neuropathic pains despite few supporting RCTs.[2] It requires slow titration and particular care with regard to drug interactions (see p.215). **Phenytoin** is also effective, at least in the short-term (Box 4.O).[6] **Oxcarbazepine** is reported to improve trigeminal neuralgia and post-herpetic neuralgia unresponsive to **carbamazepine** and **carbamazepine** plus **gabapentin** respectively.[7,8] However, the results of 2 RCTs in painful diabetic neuropathy are conflicting (see p.218).[9,10]

Lamotrigine was effective for neuropathic pain in 3 small RCTs (131 patients in total),[11–13] and was comparable to **amitriptyline** in a comparative cross-over study.[14] However, findings from 6 other RCTs, including 4 larger studies (1,040 patients in total), were equivocal or negative.[15–19] Although **lamotrigine** is advocated by some for the specific pains based on the smaller RCTs (HIV neuropathy and central post-stroke pain),[20,21] the 'negative' studies did include both peripheral and central neuropathic (spinal cord) pains. Further, slow titration (over $\geqslant$6 weeks; see Product Monograph) is essential to reduce the risk of skin reactions. **Lacosamide** (not Canada) is less effective for painful diabetic neuropathy than alternatives: NNT for moderate pain relief 8–11 vs. 1.3 for TCAs, 2.1 for **phenytoin**, 2.3 for **carbamazepine**, and 3.8 for **gabapentin**.[3,22–25] Thus, important differences exist between sodium channel blockers, and the routine first-line use of newer sodium channel blockers cannot be recommended at present.

Potential future directions in pain management include reduced blood-brain barrier penetration (reducing undesirable central effects by targeting ectopic foci on damaged peripheral neurones)[1] or subtype-selective sodium channel blockers (inherited abnormalities of one subtype,

$Na_V1.7$, cause congenital insensitivity to pain while leaving other senses unaffected).[26] The opening of potassium channels also has a membrane-stabilizing effect by hyperpolarizing the cell membrane, although it is not thought to be a predominant action of currently available drugs.

Box 4.O   Phenytoin

Pharmacology

Phenytoin is a sodium channel blocker. It has a narrow therapeutic window. It is about 90% bound to plasma albumin and its pharmacological effect is limited to the free, unbound portion. This will be a greater proportion of the total if the patient is hypo-albuminemic (cf. hypercalcemia in the presence of hypo-albuminemia). Those at risk include elderly patients and those with chronic renal failure; they may develop neurotoxicity even when plasma concentrations are reported as being in the therapeutic range.

Further, elimination follows zero-order kinetics (i.e. a constant amount is eliminated per unit of time); thus clearance does *not* increase with increasing plasma concentrations of phenytoin. Thus, what seems like a small increase (e.g. 300mg → 350mg) may lead to a large increase in plasma levels and toxicity.

Phenytoin drug–drug interactions

Phenytoin is a hepatic enzyme inducer with numerous drug interactions (Table 4.25).

Phenytoin toxicity
Clinical features

Phenytoin toxicity generally manifests as a syndrome of cerebellar, vestibular and ocular effects, including some or all of the following:

- nystagmus:
  - ▷ on lateral gaze only (early sign)
  - ▷ spontaneous (more severe toxicity)
- blurred vision/diplopia
- slurred speech
- ataxia.

These may be accompanied by lethargy and/or delirium. Some patients experience break-through seizures (or an increase in the frequency of seizures) when the free phenytoin plasma concentration increases to toxic levels.

Evaluation

If phenytoin toxicity is suspected, check the plasma phenytoin concentration just before the next dose is due to obtain a trough level, and the plasma albumin concentration. The normal therapeutic range with a normal plasma albumin is 40–80micromol/L (10–20microgram/mL). However, toxicity can be present despite a level within this range, particularly if hypoalbuminemic: be prepared to make the diagnosis clinically (e.g. if nystagmus ± other classical symptoms develop), and act accordingly.

Management

There is no specific antidote to phenytoin. If the patient has clinical features suggestive of toxicity, reduce the dose of phenytoin to a known previous non-toxic level. If severe, omit a dose and reduce subsequent doses. Generally, symptoms resolve when the plasma phenytoin concentration falls.[27]

Treat break-through seizures with benzodiazepines (see p.112) because other anti-epileptic drugs may exacerbate the toxicity. If the frequency of seizures increases as the phenytoin toxicity resolves, seek the advice of a neurologist.

Supply

Note: phenytoin *sodium* 55mg is approximately equivalent to phenytoin 50mg; the plasma concentration of phenytoin should be checked after switching from the sodium salt to the free acid form, or vice versa.

continued

Box 4.0 Continued

Phenytoin (generic)
Oral suspension phenytoin 125mg/5mL, 28 days @ 100mg b.i.d. = $7.
Injection phenytoin *sodium* 50mg/mL, 2mL amp = $5, 5mL amp = $11; *contains propylene glycol 40% and alcohol 10% in WFI.*

Dilantin® (Pfizer)
Capsules phenytoin *sodium* 30mg, 100mg, 28 days @ 100mg b.i.d. = $4.
Tablets chewable (Infatabs®) phenytoin 50mg, 28 days @ 100mg b.i.d. = $9.
Oral suspension phenytoin 30mg/5mL, 28 days @ 90mg b.i.d. = $36; 125mg/5mL, 28 days @ 100mg b.i.d. = $12.

Table 4.25 Clinically significant cytochrome P450 interactions with phenytoin resulting in changed drug plasma concentrations

Phenytoin plasma concentration		Drug plasma concentration	
Increased by	Decreased by	Increased by phenytoin	Decreased by phenytoin
Amiodarone	Antiretrovirals[a]	Phenobarbital	Amiodarone
Antifungal azoles[a]	Benzodiazepines[a]		Antifungal and
Azapropazone[b]	Carbamazepine		anthelmintic azoles[a]
Benzodiazepines[a]	Chlorpromazine		Antiretrovirals[a]
Carbamazepine	Dexamethasone		Aprepitant
Celecoxib	Phenobarbital		Benzodiazepines[a]
Chlorpromazine	Rifampin		Calcium channel
Cimetidine	St John's wort		blockers[a]
Dexamethasone	Thioridazine		Carbamazepine
Diltiazem	Valproic acid		Clozapine
Ethosuximide	Vigabatrin		Corticosteroids
Fluoxetine			Disopyramide
Fluvoxamine			Doxycycline
Oxcarbazepine			Ethosuximide
Phenobarbital			Fentanyl
Prochlorperazine			Haloperidol
Stiripentol[b]			Hormonal
Thioridazine			contraceptives
Ticlopidine			Lamotrigine
Topiramate			Methadone
Valproic acid			Mexiletine
			Mirtazapine
			Primidone
			Sertindole
			Theophylline
			Tiagabine[b]
			Topiramate
			Tramadol
			Valproic acid

a. effect not seen with all drug class members
b. not Canada.

---

1 Devor M (2006) Sodium channels and mechanisms of neuropathic pain. *Journal of Pain.* **7**: S3–S12.
2 Wiffen PJ et al. (2005) Carbamazepine for acute and chronic pain. *Cochrane Database of Systematic Reviews.* CD005451.
3 Wiffen PJ et al. (2005) Anticonvulsants for acute and chronic pain. *Cochrane Database of Systematic Reviews.* **3**: CD001133.
4 Challapalli V et al. (2005) Systemic administration of local anesthetic agents to relieve neuropathic pain. *Cochrane Database of Systematic Reviews.* CD003345.
5 von Gunten CF et al. (2007) Flecainide for the treatment of chronic neuropathic pain: a Phase II trial. *Palliative Medicine.* **21**: 667–672.

6 McCleane G (1999) Intravenous infusion of phenytoin relieves neuropathic pain: a randomized, double-blinded, placebo-controlled, crossover study. *Anesthesia and Analgesia.* **89**: 985–988.
7 Gomez-Arguelles JM et al. (2008) Oxcarbazepine monotherapy in carbamazepine-unresponsive trigeminal neuralgia. *Journal of Clinical Neuroscience.* **15**: 516–519.
8 Criscuolo S et al. (2005) Oxcarbazepine monotherapy in postherpetic neuralgia unresponsive to carbamazepine and gabapentin. *Acta Neurologica Scandinavica.* **111**: 229–232.
9 Dogra S et al. (2005) Oxcarbazepine in painful diabetic neuropathy: a randomized, placebo-controlled study. *European Journal of Pain.* **9**: 543–554.
10 Grosskopf J et al. (2006) A randomized, placebo-controlled study of oxcarbazepine in painful diabetic neuropathy. *Acta Neurologica Scandinavica.* **114**: 177–180.
11 Simpson DM et al. (2000) A placebo-controlled trial of lamotrigine for painful HIV-associated neuropathy. *Neurology.* **54**: 2115–2119.
12 Vestergaard K et al. (2001) Lamotrigine for central poststroke pain: a randomized controlled trial. *Neurology.* **56**: 184–190.
13 Eisenberg E et al. (2001) Lamotrigine reduces painful diabetic neuropathy: a randomized, controlled study. *Neurology.* **57**: 505–509.
14 Jose VM et al. (2007) Randomized double-blind study comparing the efficacy and safety of lamotrigine and amitriptyline in painful diabetic neuropathy. *Diabetic Medicine.* **24**: 377–383.
15 Silver M et al. (2007) Double-blind, placebo-controlled trial of lamotrigine in combination with other medications for neuropathic pain. *Journal of Pain and Symptom Management.* **34**: 446–454.
16 Zakrzewska JM et al. (1997) Lamotrigine (lamictal) in refractory trigeminal neuralgia: results from a double-blind placebo controlled crossover trial. *Pain.* **73**: 223–230.
17 Finnerup NB et al. (2002) Lamotrigine in spinal cord injury pain: a randomized controlled trial. *Pain.* **96**: 375–383.
18 McCleane G (1999) 200mg daily of lamotrigine has no analgesic effect in neuropathic pain: a randomised, double-blind, placebo controlled trial. *Pain.* **83**: 105–107.
19 Vinik AI et al. (2007) Lamotrigine for treatment of pain associated with diabetic neuropathy: results of two randomized, double-blind, placebo-controlled studies. *Pain.* **128**: 169–179.
20 Goodyear-Smith F and Halliwell J (2009) Anticonvulsants for neuropathic pain: gaps in the evidence. *Clinical Journal of Pain.* **25**: 528–536.
21 Kumar B et al. (2009) Central poststroke pain: a review of pathophysiology and treatment. *Anesthesia and Analgesia.* **108**: 1645–1657.
22 Saarto T and Wiffen PJ (2007) Antidepressants for neuropathic pain. *Cochrane Database of Systematic Reviews.* CD005454. [Update of Cochrane Database Syst Rev. 2005;(3):CD005454; PMID: 16034979.]
23 Rauck RL et al. (2007) Lacosamide in painful diabetic peripheral neuropathy: a phase 2 double-blind placebo-controlled study. *Clinical Journal of Pain.* **23**: 150–158.
24 Wymer JP et al. (2009) Efficacy and safety of lacosamide in diabetic neuropathic pain: an 18-week double-blind placebo-controlled trial of fixed-dose regimens. *Clinical Journal of Pain.* **25**: 376–385.
25 Shaibani A et al. (2009) Long-term oral lacosamide in painful diabetic neuropathy: a two-year open-label extension trial. *European Journal of Pain.* **13**: 458–463.
26 Cummins TR et al. (2007) The roles of sodium channels in nociception: Implications for mechanisms of pain. *Pain.* **131**: 243–257.
27 Perkin GD (2004) Ch. 24:53. Epilepsy in later childhood and adults. In: DA Warrell et al. (eds) *Oxford Textbook of Medicine* (5e). Oxford University Press, Oxford.

CARBAMAZEPINE

Class: Anti-epileptic (sodium channel blocker).

Indications: Partial seizures ± secondary generalization, trigeminal neuralgia, †neuropathic pain, mania.

Contra-indications: AV block, previous bone marrow depression, concurrent MAOI, hypersensitivity to TCAs (structurally related), porphyria.

Pharmacology

Carbamazepine acts mainly through sodium channel blockade (see p.212). Additional actions of uncertain significance include potassium channel activation, L-type calcium channel blockade, and antagonism of NMDA-glutamate.[1]

Absorption is affected by formulation; slower rates reduce the incidence of undesirable neurological effects.[2] Carbamazepine is mainly metabolized by CYP3A4 to a pharmacologically active epoxide metabolite; this is subsequently inactivated to several renally excreted metabolites. The halflife decreases over the first 1–2 weeks as a result of hepatic enzyme auto-induction.

Carbamazepine is a first-line drug for trigeminal neuralgia and partial seizures ± secondary generalization. In painful diabetic neuropathy it is superior to placebo (n = 30) and comparable to **nortriptyline** (n = 16).[3] Benefit is also reported for paroxysmal nausea associated with meningeal carcinomatosis[4] and itch associated with hematological malignancy.[5]

A polymorphism in the gene (SCN1A) encoding the sodium channel α-subunit has been linked to carbamazepine-resistant epilepsy.[6] Human leukocyte antigen (HLA) genes, known to influence susceptibility to various infections and auto-immune diseases, are closely associated with the risk of carbamazepine-induced Stevens-Johnson syndrome. In Han Chinese, HLA B*1502 was found in 100% of 44 affected individuals compared with 3% of unaffected carbamazepine-treated individuals.[7] The UK MHRA recommends testing HLA B*1502 status before carbamazepine is started in people of Han Chinese, Hong Kong Chinese or Thai origin.[8]

Bio-availability ≥85%.

Onset of action generally delayed by the need for slow titration, but anti-epileptic response is sometimes seen as early as 2 days.

Peak plasma concentration 4–8h (normal-release tablets), 12–26h (SR tablet), 0.5–3h (oral liquid).

Plasma halflife 36h initially, 8–24h after multiple dosing (hepatic auto-induction).

Duration of action No specific data.

Cautions

For full list, see manufacturer's Product Monograph.

Agranulocytosis and aplastic anemia affect about 5 and 2 patients/million/year respectively. Severe hepatic reactions are rare. Mild leukopenia, thrombocytopenia, or cholestatic abnormalities in LFTs should be monitored, and carbamazepine should be discontinued if severe or symptomatic derangement occurs.

Mild skin reactions are common and transient; monitor closely and discontinue carbamazepine if reactions worsen, or if features of Stevens-Johnson syndrome or toxic epidermal necrolysis develop.

Renal, cardiac or hepatic disease; absence seizures (may worsen); previous skin reaction to other anti-epileptic drugs or TCAs.

Drug interactions

Carbamazepine is a hepatic enzyme inducer with numerous drug interactions (Table 4.26).

Table 4.26 Clinically significant cytochrome P450 interactions with carbamazepine resulting in changed drug plasma concentrations

Carbamazepine[a] plasma concentration		Drug plasma concentration	
Increased by	Decreased by	Increased by carbamazepine	Decreased by carbamazepine
Antipsychotics[b]	Efavirenz	Phenytoin	Antipsychotics[b]
Antiretrovirals[b]	Phenobarbital[c]		Antiretrovirals[b]
Azole antifungals[b]	Phenytoin[c]		Azole antifungals[b]
Clarithromycin	Valproic acid[c]		Benzodiazepines[b]
Diltiazem			Calcium channel blockers[b]
Erythromycin			Clozapine
Fluoxetine			Corticosteroids[b]
Fluvoxamine			Coumarin anticoagulants
Haloperidol			Estrogens, progestins
Isoniazid			Ethosuximide
Lamotrigine			Fentanyl
Propoxyphene			Haloperidol
Valproic acid			Indinavir
Verapamil			Lamotrigine
			Levothyroxine
			Methadone
			Phenytoin
			Primidone
			SSRIs[b]
			TCAs[b]
			Tiagabine
			Topiramate
			Tramadol
			Valproic acid

a. or active metabolite
b. effect not seen with all drug class members
c. increase in active metabolite of carbamazepine

Undesirable effects

For full list, see manufacturer's Product Monograph.

Very common (>10%): dizziness, ataxia, drowsiness, fatigue, nausea, mild LFT derangement (see above), urticaria, leukopenia.

Common (<10%, >1%): headache, diplopia, blurred vision, edema, dry mouth, thrombocytopenia, eosinophilia, hyponatremia, (suppositories: rectal irritation).

Uncommon (<1%, >0.1%): include suicidal ideation 0.2% (1/500; advise patients to report mood or thought disturbance).

Rare (<0.1%): aseptic meningitis, movement disorders, neuroleptic malignant syndrome, arrhythmias and cardiac conduction disorders, pancreatitis, hepatitis, jaundice, renal failure, interstitial nephritis, a delayed-onset multi-organ vasculitic hypersensitivity disorder, severe skin reactions (see above).

Dose and use

Starting dose and titration rate will depend on seizure or pain severity. Undesirable effects are minimized by a low starting dose, slow upward titration, and the use of SR products.
* check
    ▷ HLA B*1502 status in people of Han Chinese, Hong Kong Chinese or Thai origin[8]
    ▷ baseline FBC, U+Es, LFTs, and repeat every few months
* start with 50–100mg PO b.i.d. (use SR product for doses ≥100mg)
* increase in 50–100mg increments every 1–2 weeks
* maximum daily dose 2g. In one observational study, 90% of those responding required ≤800mg/day. Few patients responded to increases above this dose.[9]

Supply

SR carbamazepine tablets in Canada, both generic and proprietary, are 'bisected' on both sides to permit splitting into halves.

Carbamazepine (generic)
Tablets 200mg, 400mg, 28 days @ 200mg b.i.d. = $9.
Tablets chewable 100mg, 200mg, 28 days @ 200mg b.i.d. = $9.

Tegretol® (Novartis)
Tablets 100mg, 200mg, 400mg, 28 days @ 200mg b.i.d. = $23.
Tablets chewable 100mg, 200mg, 28 days @ 200mg b.i.d. = $18.
Oral liquid 100mg/5mL, 28 days @ 200mg b.i.d. = $43.

Sustained-release
Carbamazepine (generic)
Tablets SR 200mg, 400mg, 28 days @ 200mg b.i.d. = $11.

Tegretol CR® (Novartis)
Tablets SR 200mg, 400mg, 28 days @ 200mg b.i.d. = $23.

1 Schmidt D and Elger CE (2004) What is the evidence that oxcarbazepine and carbamazepine are distinctly different antiepileptic drugs? *Epilepsy and Behaviour.* **5**: 627–635.
2 Tothfalusi L et al. (2008) Exposure-response analysis reveals that clinically important toxicity difference can exist between bioequivalent carbamazepine tablets. *British Journal of Clinical Pharmacology.* **65**: 110–122.
3 Wiffen PJ et al. (2005) Carbamazepine for acute and chronic pain. *Cochrane Database of Systematic Reviews.* **3**: CD005451.
4 Strohscheer I and Borasio GD (2006) Carbamazepine-responsive paroxysmal nausea and vomiting in a patient with meningeal carcinomatosis. *Palliative Medicine.* **20**: 549–550.
5 Korfitis C and Trafalis DT (2008) Carbamazepine can be effective in alleviating tormenting pruritus in patients with hematologic malignancy. *Journal of Pain and Symptom Management.* **35**: 571–572.
6 Abe T et al. (2008) Association between SCN1A polymorphism and carbamazepine-resistant epilepsy. *British Journal of Clinical Pharmacology.* **66**: 304–307.
7 Chung WH et al. (2004) Medical genetics: a marker for Stevens-Johnson syndrome. *Nature.* **428**: 486.
8 MHRA (2008) Drug safety update. 1 (9, April): 5. Available from: www.mhra.gov.uk/Publications/Safetyguidance/DrugSafetyUpdate/CON014505
9 Kwan P and Brodie MJ (2001) Effectiveness of first antiepileptic drug. *Epilepsia.* **42**: 1255–1260.

OXCARBAZEPINE

Class: Anti-epileptic (sodium channel blocker).

Indications: Monotherapy or adjunctive therapy for partial seizures, †neuropathic pain.

Pharmacology

Oxcarbazepine is structurally related to **carbamazepine**. Both act through sodium channel blockade (see p.212) but differ in tolerability and propensity for drug interactions. Additional actions of uncertain significance include potassium channel activation, N, P and R- type calcium channel blockade and antagonism of NMDA-glutamate receptors.[1]

Oxcarbazepine is a pro-drug which is activated by reduction to its monohydroxy derivative. This is inactivated by glucuronidation and oxidation, and the metabolites are renally excreted.[2] Oxcarbazepine has fewer drug interactions than **carbamazepine** because it is a weaker inducer of hepatic enzymes.

In an RCT, oxcarbazepine was as effective as, but better tolerated than, **carbamazepine**; 14% vs. 25% of patients withdrew because of undesirable effects.[3] Oxcarbazepine is reported to improve trigeminal neuralgia and post-herpetic neuralgia unresponsive to **carbamazepine** and **carbamazepine** + **gabapentin** respectively.[4,5] However, the results of 2 RCTs in painful diabetic neuropathy are conflicting. A dose of 1,200mg daily was ineffective.[6] Titration to a maximum of 1,800mg daily (mean 1,450mg daily) reduced the mean pain VAS score by 1 (NNT = 6 for > 50% reduction in pain).[7]

Bio-availability ≥95%.
Onset of action pain improved ≤1 week, maximum response ≤4 weeks.[7]
Peak plasma concentration 1–3h.
Plasma halflife 1–5h; 7–20h monohydroxy derivative.
Duration of action no specific data.

Cautions

For full list, see manufacturer's Product Monograph.
Previous hypersensitivity to **carbamazepine** (25–30% cross-reactivity), predisposition to hyponatremia, cardiac insufficiency (fluid retention), abnormal cardiac conduction (arrhythmias and AV block occur rarely).

Drug interactions

Oxcarbazepine can induce CYP3A4 and inhibit CYP2C19 but not often to a clinically significant extent. Oral hormonal contraception may become ineffective. **Lamotrigine** and **phenytoin** may require dose adjustment.

Undesirable effects

For full list, see manufacturer's Product Monograph.
Suicidal ideation (1/500; advise patients to report mood or thought disturbance).
Very common (>10%): drowsiness, dizziness, fatigue, headache, diplopia, nausea and vomiting.
Common (<10%, >1%): confusion, agitation, amnesia, altered mood, vertigo, ataxia, tremor, nystagmus, reduced attention, diarrhea, constipation, abdominal pain, rash, alopecia, acne, asymptomatic hyponatremia.
Uncommon (<1%, >0.1%): include suicidal ideation 0.2% (1/500; advise patients to report mood or thought disturbance).
Rare (<0.1%): AV block, arrhythmia, pancreatitis, hepatitis, multi-organ hypersensitivity, systemic lupus erythematosus, angioedema, Stevens-Johnson syndrome, toxic epidermal necrolysis, bone marrow depression.

Dose and use

Many palliative care patients have risk factors for hyponatremia; monitor sodium at baseline, after 2 weeks, then monthly for 3 months. Doses lower than recommended by the manufacturer have been proposed:[2]
- start with 300mg at bedtime
- increase the dose every 3 days by 300mg/24h, up to 900mg/24h

- if necessary, increase to 2,400mg/24h (maximum recommended dose)
- halve the initial dose if creatinine clearance is ≤30mL/min.

Supply
Oxcarbazepine (generic)
Tablets 150mg, 300mg, 600mg, 28 days @ 300mg b.i.d. = $63.

Trileptil® (Novartis)
Tablets 150mg, 300mg, 600mg, 28 days @ 300mg b.i.d. = $100.
Oral liquid 300mg/5mL, 28 days @ 300mg b.i.d. = $100.

1 Schmidt D and Elger CE (2004) What is the evidence that oxcarbazepine and carbamazepine are distinctly different antiepileptic drugs? *Epilepsy and Behaviour.* **5**: 627–635.
2 May TW *et al.* (2003) Clinical pharmacokinetics of oxcarbazepine. *Clinical Pharmacokinetics.* **42**: 1023–1042.
3 Dam M *et al.* (1989) A double-blind study comparing oxcarbazepine and carbamazepine in patients with newly diagnosed, previously untreated epilepsy. *Epilepsy Research.* **3**: 70–76.
4 Gomez-Arguelles JM *et al.* (2008) Oxcarbazepine monotherapy in carbamazepine-unresponsive trigeminal neuralgia. *Journal of Clinical Neuroscience.* **15**: 516–519.
5 Criscuolo S *et al.* (2005) Oxcarbazepine monotherapy in postherpetic neuralgia unresponsive to carbamazepine and gabapentin. *Acta Neurologica Scandinavica.* **111**: 229–232.
6 Grosskopf J *et al.* (2006) A randomized, placebo-controlled study of oxcarbazepine in painful diabetic neuropathy. *Acta Neurologica Scandinavica.* **114**: 177–180.
7 Dogra S *et al.* (2005) Oxcarbazepine in painful diabetic neuropathy: a randomized, placebo-controlled study. *European Journal of Pain.* **9**: 543–554.

ANTI-EPILEPTIC PRE-SYNAPTIC CALCIUM CHANNEL BLOCKERS

Gabapentin and **pregabalin** bind to the $\alpha 2\delta$ type 1 regulatory subunit of pre-synaptic (N, P/Q-type) voltage-gated calcium channels, reducing the calcium influx responsible for triggering neurotransmitter release.[1] Both the spinal dorsal horn and brainstem/forebrain are important sites of action. Calcium channel $\alpha 2\delta$ subunits are upregulated in the spinal dorsal horn during neuropathic pain,[2] and **gabapentin** and **pregabalin** counteract the effect of this. Brainstem/forebrain actions influence descending pain inhibitory pathways and pain processing.[1,3,4] Spinal calcium channels are also targeted by **ziconotide** (not Canada).

Both **gabapentin** and **pregabalin** cause redistribution of calcium channels away from the cell surface, rather than blocking them directly. Effects on sodium and potassium channels have also been shown.[5,6] Despite being GABA analogues, neither **gabapentin** nor **pregabalin** is GABAmimetic.[1] They are unrelated to the L-type calcium channel blockers, **nifedipine**, **diltiazem** and **verapamil** (Table 4.27). L-type channels are also found on neurones, but the

Table 4.27 Classification of calcium channels

Type	Location (function)	Blocked by
L-type ($Ca_V1.1-1.4$)	Cardiovascular and GI tissues (smooth muscle tone, conductivity)	Verapamil, diltiazem, nifedipine (see p.56)
N-, P/Q-type ($Ca_V2.1-2.2$)	Pre-synaptic neurones (calcium influx triggers neurotransmitter release; over-expressed in neuropathic pain)	Gabapentin and pregabalin (N- and P/Q-type), ziconotide (N-type)[1]
T-type ($Ca_V3.1-3.3$)	Thalamic and nociceptive neurones (excitability, threshold setting, pacemaker activity. Thalamic T-type channel dysregulation responsible for absence seizures)	Ethosuximide, valproic acid (see p.209)[7]
R-type ($Ca_V2.3$)	Cerebellum (function unknown)	

significance of anti-epileptics blocking these neuronal L-type channels (e.g. **carbamazepine**) is unclear.

In some countries, **gabapentin** and **pregabalin** are first-line choices for neuropathic pain because this indication is included in their marketing authorizations. However, the latter differ between countries; for Canada, see individual drug monographs on p.220 and p.224 respectively. **Pregabalin** is more expensive, without evidence of superiority, but its twice daily administration is a possible advantage. Both drugs are free of significant pharmacokinetic drug–drug interactions.

1 Taylor CP (2009) Mechanisms of analgesia by gabapentin and pregabalin–calcium channel alpha2-delta [Cavalpha2-delta] ligands. *Pain*. **142**: 13–16.

2 Boroujerdi A *et al.* (2008) Injury discharges regulate calcium channel alpha-2-delta-1 subunit upregulation in the dorsal horn that contributes to initiation of neuropathic pain. *Pain*. **139**: 358–366.

3 Bee LA and Dickenson AH (2008) Descending facilitation from the brainstem determines behavioural and neuronal hypersensitivity following nerve injury and efficacy of pregabalin. *Pain*. **140**: 209–223.

4 Hayashida K *et al.* (2008) Gabapentin acts within the locus coeruleus to alleviate neuropathic pain. *Anesthesiology*. **109**: 1077–1084.

5 Lee CH *et al.* (2008) Gabapentin activates ROMK1 channels by a protein kinase A (PKA)-dependent mechanism. *British Journal of Pharmacology*. **154**: 216–225.

6 Yang RH *et al.* (2009) Gabapentin selectively reduces persistent sodium current in injured type-A dorsal root ganglion neurons. *Pain*. **143**: 48–55.

7 Loscher W (2002) Basic pharmacology of valproate: a review after 35 years of clinical use for the treatment of epilepsy. *CNS Drugs*. **16**: 669–694.

GABAPENTIN

Class: Anti-epileptic (pre-synaptic calcium channel blocker).

Indications: Adjunctive use in epilepsy when conventional treatment is unsatisfactory, †neuropathic pain,[1–10] †intractable itch, †hot flashes,[11,12] †sweating,[13] †refractory hiccup.

Pharmacology

The mode and site of action of gabapentin is described on p.219. Absorption is by a saturable mechanism and bio-availability is more than halved as the dose increases from 100mg to 1,200mg. Gabapentin is not protein-bound and freely crosses the blood-brain barrier. It is excreted unchanged by the kidneys and accumulates in renal impairment. The halflife increases to 50h when creatinine clearance is < 30mL/min, and to over 5 days in anuria. Initial drowsiness or dizziness occurs in 50% of patients and generally resolves over 7–10 days of use.[9] Gabapentin's pharmacokinetic drug interactions are of doubtful clinical significance; **cimetidine** marginally impairs the renal excretion of gabapentin, and antacids containing **aluminum** or **magnesium** reduce gabapentin's bio-availability by 10–25%.

Gabapentin is effective for peripheral and central neuropathic pain.[1–6,8–10,14] Overall efficacy and tolerability are comparable to those of TCAs and other anti-epileptics,[15–17] but TCAs cause more dry mouth, constipation and postural hypotension.[18,19]

Gabapentin, individually titrated to 300–1,800mg/24h, has been reported to improve cancer-related neuropathic pain when given in addition to opioids.[3,20] This reflects the positive benefit of this combination in non-cancer neuropathic pain.[21] However, in an RCT, although the percentage of patients whose pain reduced by ≥1/3 was significantly higher during the first 5 days in those receiving gabapentin, after 10 days there was no difference; and, again after 10 days, the daily mean global and dysesthesia pain scores differed by <1/10 (mean global pain 4.6 on gabapentin vs. 5.5 on placebo), and there was no significant difference in the scores for stabbing (lancinating) and burning pain.[22] The doses of opioids and other analgesics remained unchanged during the study, although the higher 'as needed' opioid use by the placebo group may have obscured the benefit from gabapentin. Further, the lower doses used compared with non-cancer pain trials (≤1,800mg/24h vs. ≤3,600mg/24h) may also have contributed to the negative results in cancer-related neuropathic pain.[23]

Gabapentin is effective in fibromyalgia[24] and may be of benefit in malignant bone pain,[25] postoperative pain[26] and chronic masticatory myalgia.[27] The use of gabapentin for neuropathic itch is based on extrapolation from neuropathic pain management.[28] Gabapentin is effective for uremic itch.[29,30] Benefit is also reported for intractable idiopathic itch.[31,32]

Gabapentin has been reported to be of benefit in generalized anxiety disorder,[33] hot flashes associated with breast cancer or the menopause,[11,12] and paraneoplastic sweating.[13] It reduces spasticity and muscle spasm in multiple sclerosis.[34,35] On the other hand, gabapentin occasionally causes myoclonus (a central phenomenon).[36,37] Paradoxically, it has also been used successfully to abolish opioid-related myoclonus.[38]

Gabapentin has also been reported to be of benefit in refractory hiccup.[39,40] In one series, 'burst gabapentin' relieved persistent hiccup in patients with a history of brain stem stroke.[41] Patients received 400mg t.i.d. for 3 days, 400mg once daily for 3 days, and then stopped. Only 1/15 patients needed a second treatment.

Bio-availability PO 100mg, 74%; *but decreases as dose increases*: 300mg, 60%; 600mg, 49%; 1,200mg, 33%.

Onset of action 1–3h.

Time to peak plasma concentration 2–3h PO.

Plasma halflife 5–7h; 2 days or more in moderate–severe renal impairment, 5 days in anuria, 3–4h during hemodialysis.

Duration of action probably 8–12h, much longer in severe renal impairment/failure.

Cautions

Renal impairment; absence seizures (may worsen); psychotic illness (may precipitate psychotic episodes, generally resolving on dose reduction or discontinuation); false positive readings for urinary protein with Ames N-Multistix SG®.

Drug interactions

Aluminum and **magnesium**-containing compounds reduce bio-availability. **Morphine** and **naproxen** may increase gabapentin levels. High doses of gabapentin may decrease **hydrocodone** levels (mechanisms unknown).

Undesirable effects

For full list, see manufacturer's Product Monograph.

Suicidal ideation (1/500; advise patients to report mood or thought disturbance). Possible causal association with acute pancreatitis.

Very common (>10%): drowsiness, dizziness.

Common (<10%, >1%): amnesia, anxiety, fatigue, amblyopia, diplopia, nystagmus, dysarthria, ataxia, tremor, arthralgia, myalgia, peripheral edema, weight gain, dry mouth, pharyngitis, dyspepsia, diarrhea.

Uncommon (<1%, >0.1%): leucopenia, impotence, gynecomastia.[42]

Dose and use

Gabapentin should *not* be given at the same time as antacids containing **aluminum** or **magnesium**; *give at least 2h apart*.

Neuropathic pain

Although rapid upward titration is suggested in the Product Monograph, a slower titration of the initial dose of gabapentin over several weeks is advisable in debilitated and elderly patients, those with renal impairment (see below) or if receiving other CNS-depressant drugs (Table 4.28).[9,43] In patients with normal renal function it has been suggested that a total daily dose of 1,800mg is necessary to relieve neuropathic pain.[44]

Table 4.28 Dose schedules for gabapentin in neuropathic pain (normal renal function)

Rapid		Slow	
Day 1	300mg at bedtime	Day 1	100mg t.i.d.
Day 2	300mg b.i.d	Day 7	Begin progressive increase to 300mg t.i.d.
Day 3	300mg t.i.d.	Day 14	Continue progressive increase to 600mg t.i.d.
Then increase by 300mg/day every 3 days as needed up to 1,200mg t.i.d.			

The dose of gabapentin should be reduced in adults with renal impairment and those on hemodialysis (Table 4.29).[43] As creatinine clearance declines with age, the maximum tolerated dose is likely to be lower in the elderly, e.g. 1,200mg/24h. If required the capsules can be opened and the contents mixed with water, fruit juice, apple sauce, etc.[45]

Table 4.29 Impact of renal function on the dose of gabapentin (also see Product Monograph)

Creatinine clearance (mL/min)	Starting dose[a]	Maximum dose
>60	300mg t.i.d.	1,200mg t.i.d.
30–59	200mg b.i.d.	700mg b.i.d.
15–29	200mg once daily	700mg once daily
14	100mg once daily	300mg once daily
<14	Reduce dose proportionately (e.g. if creatinine clearance is 7.5mL/min, give half the 15mL/min dose)	
After every 4h of hemodialysis	Supplementary single dose of 125–350mg[b]	

a. smaller starting dose is advisable in elderly patients and those receiving other CNS-depressant drugs (see text)
b. in practice, round dose up or down to convenient capsule/tablet size.

Hot flashes
- start with a low dose, as for neuropathic pain
- if necessary, increase to 300mg t.i.d.[11]

Hiccup
- in relatively robust patients, consider a 6-day 'burst' of gabapentin', e.g.:
  ▷ 300–400mg t.i.d. for 3 days
  ▷ 300–400mg once daily for 3 days
  ▷ if necessary, re-treat long-term if hiccup recurs after a 'burst'
- in frail elderly patients, proceed slowly as for neuropathic pain:
  ▷ start with a low dose, e.g. 100mg t.i.d.
  ▷ if necessary, titrate upwards
  ▷ if successful, consider reducing/stopping gabapentin
  ▷ if necessary, re-treat long-term if hiccup recurs after a 'burst'.[41]

Neuropathic pruritus
- as for neuropathic pain.

Stopping gabapentin
To avoid precipitating seizures or pain, gabapentin should be withdrawn gradually over ≥1 week.

Supply
Gabapentin (generic)
Capsules 100mg, 300mg, 400mg, 28 days @ 300mg t.i.d. = $52.
Tablets 600mg, 800mg, 28 days @ 600mg t.i.d. = $110.

Neurontin® (Pfizer)
Capsules 100mg, 300mg, 400mg, 28 days @ 300mg t.i.d. = $91.
Tablets 600mg, 800mg, 28 days @ 600mg t.i.d. = $163.

1 Backonja M et al. (1998) Gabapentin for the symptomatic treatment of painful neuropathy in patients with diabetes mellitus: a randomized controlled trial. Journal of the American Medical Association. **280**: 1831–1836.
2 Rowbotham M et al. (1998) Gabapentin for the treatment of postherpetic neuralgia: a randomized controlled trial. Journal of the American Medical Association. **280**: 1837–1842.
3 Caraceni A et al. (1999) Gabapentin as an adjuvant to opioid analgesia for neuropathic cancer pain. Journal of Pain and Symptom Management. **17**: 441–445.

4 Rice AS and Maton S (2001) Gabapentin in postherpetic neuralgia: a randomised, double blind, placebo controlled study. *Pain.* **94**: 215–224.

5 Bone M et al. (2002) Gabapentin in postamputation phantom limb pain: a randomized, double-blind, placebo-controlled, cross-over study. *Regional Anesthesia and Pain Medicine.* **27**: 481–486.

6 Pandey CK et al. (2002) Gabapentin for the treatment of pain in guillain-barre syndrome: a double-blinded, placebo-controlled, crossover study. *Anesthesia and Analgesia.* **95**: 1719–1723, table of contents.

7 Pelham A et al. (2002) Gabapentin for coeliac plexus pain. *Palliative Medicine.* **16**: 355–356.

8 Serpell MG (2002) Gabapentin in neuropathic pain syndromes: a randomised, double-blind, placebo-controlled trial. *Pain.* **99**: 557–566.

9 Backonja M and Glanzman RL (2003) Gabapentin dosing for neuropathic pain: evidence from randomized, placebo-controlled clinical trials. *Clinical Therapeutics.* **25**: 81–104.

10 Levendoglu F et al. (2004) Gabapentin is a first line drug for the treatment of neuropathic pain in spinal cord injury. *Spine.* **29**: 743–751.

11 Pandya KJ et al. (2005) Gabapentin for hot flashes in 420 women with breast cancer: a randomised double-blind placebo-controlled trial. *Lancet.* **366**: 818–824.

12 Nelson HD et al. (2006) Nonhormonal therapies for menopausal hot flashes: systematic review and meta-analysis. *Journal of the American Medical Association.* **295**: 2057–2071.

13 Porzio G et al. (2006) Gabapentin in the treatment of severe sweating experienced by advanced cancer patients. *Supportive Care in Cancer.* **14**: 389–391.

14 Gordh TE et al. (2008) Gabapentin in traumatic nerve injury pain: a randomized, double-blind, placebo-controlled, cross-over, multi-center study. *Pain.* **138**: 255–266.

15 Collins S et al. (2000) Antidepressants and anticonvulsants for diabetic neuropathy and postherpetic neuralgia: a quantitative systematic review. *Journal of Pain and Symptom Management.* **20**: 449–458.

16 Wiffen P et al. (2000) Anticonvulsant drugs for acute and chronic pain. *Cochrane Database of Systematic Reviews.* **3**: CD001133.

17 Vinik A (2005) Clinical review: Use of antiepileptic drugs in the treatment of chronic painful diabetic neuropathy. *Journal of Clinical Endocrinology and Metabolism.* **90**: 4936–4945.

18 Morello C et al. (1999) Randomized double-blind study comparing the efficacy of gabapentin with amitriptyline on diabetic peripheral neuropathy pain. *Archives of Internal Medicine.* **159**: 1931–1937.

19 Chandra K et al. (2006) Gabapentin versus nortriptyline in post-herpetic neuralgia patients: a randomized, double-blind clinical trial–the GONIP Trial. *International Journal of Clinical Pharmacology and Therapeutics.* **44**: 358–363.

20 Ross JR et al. (2005) Gabapentin is effective in the treatment of cancer-related neuropathic pain: a prospective, open-label study. *Journal of Palliative Medicine.* **8**: 1118–1126.

21 Gilron I et al. (2005) Morphine, gabapentin, or their combination for neuropathic pain. *New England Journal of Medicine.* **352**: 1324–1334.

22 Caraceni A et al. (2004) Gabapentin for neuropathic cancer pain: a randomized controlled trial from the Gabapentin Cancer Pain Study Group. *Journal of Clinical Oncology.* **22**: 2909–2917.

23 Bennett MI (2005) Gabapentin significantly improves analgesia in people receiving opioids for neuropathic cancer pain. *Cancer Treatment Reviews.* **31**: 58–62.

24 Hauser W et al. (2009) Treatment of fibromyalgia syndrome with gabapentin and pregabalin – a meta-analysis of randomized controlled trials. *Pain.* **145**: 69–81.

25 Caraceni A et al. (2008) Gabapentin for breakthrough pain due to bone metastases. *Palliative Medicine.* **22**: 392–393.

26 Ho KY et al. (2006) Gabapentin and postoperative pain – a systematic review of randomized controlled trials. *Pain.* **126**: 91–101.

27 Kimos P et al. (2007) Analgesic action of gabapentin on chronic pain in the masticatory muscles: a randomized controlled trial. *Pain.* **127**: 151–160.

28 Zylicz Z et al. (eds) (2004) *Pruritus in Advanced Disease.* Oxford University Press, Oxford.

29 Gunal AI et al. (2004) Gabapentin therapy for pruritus in haemodialysis patients: a randomized, placebo-controlled, double-blind trial. *Nephrology Dialysis Transplantation.* **19**: 3137–3139.

30 Naini AE et al. (2007) Gabapentin: a promising drug for the treatment of uremic pruritus. *Saudi Journal of Kidney Diseases and Transplantation.* **18**: 378–381.

31 Kanitakis J (2006) Brachioradial pruritus: report of a new case responding to gabapentin. *European Journal of Dermatology.* **16**: 311–312.

32 Yesudian PD et al. (2005) Efficacy of gabapentin in the management of pruritus of unknown origin. *Archives of Dermatology.* **141**: 1507–1509.

33 Pollack MH et al. (1998) Gabapentin as a potential treatment for anxiety disorders. *American Journal of Psychiatry.* **155**: 992–993.

34 Cutter NC et al. (2000) Gabapentin effect on spasticity in multiple sclerosis: a placebo-controlled, randomized trial. *Archives of Physical Medicine and Rehabilitation.* **81**: 164–169.

35 Paisley S et al. (2002) Clinical effectiveness of oral treatments for spasticity in multiple sclerosis: a systematic review. *Multiple Sclerosis.* **8**: 319–329.

36 Asconape J et al. (2000) Myoclonus associated with the use of gabapentin. *Epilepsia.* **41**: 479–481.

37 Scullin P et al. (2003) Myoclonic jerks associated with gabapentin. *Palliative Medicine.* **17**: 717–718.

38 Mercadante S et al. (2001) Gabapentin for opioid-related myoclonus in cancer patients. *Supportive Care in Cancer.* **9**: 205–206.

39 Jatzko A et al. (2007) Alpha-2-delta ligands for singultus (hiccup) treatment: three case reports. *Journal of Pain and Symptom Management.* **33**: 756–760.

40 Alonso-Navarro H et al. (2007) Refractory hiccup: successful treatment with gabapentin. *Clinical Neuropharmacology.* **30**: 186–187.

41 Moretti R et al. (2004) Gabapentin as a drug therapy of intractable hiccup because of vascular lesion: a three-year follow up. *Neurologist.* **10**: 102–106.

42 Zylicz Z (2000) Painful gynecomastia: an unusual toxicity of gabapentin? *Journal of Pain and Symptom Management.* **20**: 2–3.

43 Dworkin R et al. (2003) Advances in neuropathic pain. Diagnosis, mechanisms and treatment recommendations. *Archives of Neurology.* **60**: 1524–1534.

44 Tremont-Lukats IW et al. (2000) Anticonvulsants for neuropathic pain syndromes: mechanisms of action and place in therapy. *Drugs.* **60**: 1029–1052.

45 Gidal B et al. (1998) Gabapentin absorption: effect of mixing with foods of varying macronutrient composition. *Annals of Pharmacotherapy.* **32**: 405–409.

PREGABALIN

Class: Anti-epileptic (pre-synaptic calcium channel blocker).

Indications: Neuropathic pain (diabetic and post-herpetic; with provisional licensing for central neuropathic pain), fibromyalgia, †adjunctive treatment for partial seizures with or without secondary generalization, †generalized anxiety disorder.[1–4]

Pharmacology

The mode and site of action of pregabalin is described on p.219. Pregabalin has a binding affinity 6 times greater than that of **gabapentin**, competitively displacing the latter from the $\alpha 2\delta$ subunit.[5] Individual variability in pharmacokinetics is low ($<20\%$). Bio-availability is high and independent of dose. Pregabalin is not protein-bound and undergoes negligible metabolism. More than 90% is excreted unchanged by the kidneys and it thus accumulates in renal impairment.[6] Half of the drug is removed after 4h of hemodialysis. It has no known pharmacokinetic drug interactions (but see Drug interactions below).[7]

Pregabalin has been shown in RCTs to be effective in painful diabetic neuropathy, post-herpetic neuralgia and central pain due to spinal cord injury.[8–16] Response is dose-related; 1/4 of patients on 150mg/24h and up to 1/2 of patients receiving 300–600mg/24h obtain $\geqslant$50% reduction in pain. In relation to pain and sleep, a slower flexible escalation schedule (dose escalation based on a patient's individual response and tolerability, over a period of $\leqslant$4 weeks) ultimately produces similar benefit to a fixed escalation schedule, and is better tolerated. However, the onset of analgesia is delayed with flexible escalation because of the lower daily dose (75mg b.i.d. compared with 150mg b.i.d.) during the first week.[11]

In six RCTs, the NNT to achieve at least 50% pain relief ranged from 3.3 to 5.6. Patients who had previously failed to respond to **gabapentin** were excluded from three of these trials.[8–10] There are no studies of pregabalin in cancer-related neuropathic pain, nor direct comparisons with **gabapentin** or other neuropathic pain treatments. Although not generally used for other pains, pregabalin is of benefit in post-dental extraction pain,[17] fibromyalgia,[18,19] and postoperative pain.[20]

Pregabalin is as effective as **lorazepam**, **alprazolam** and **venlafaxine** in generalized anxiety disorder. Compared with **venlafaxine**, pregabalin has a faster rate of onset and causes less nausea; it has a similar rate of onset to **lorazapam** and **alprazolam** and causes less drowsiness but more dizziness.[1–4]

Bio-availability $\geqslant$90% PO.
Onset of action 24min post-dental extraction pain; $<$24h neuropathic pain; 2 days epilepsy.[8,17,21]
Time to peak plasma concentration 1h.
Plasma halflife 5–9h, increasing to $>$2 days in severe renal impairment (creatinine clearance $<$15mL/min) and in hemodialysis patients.[6]
Duration of action $>$12h.

Cautions

Renal impairment (dose adjustment required; renal failure reported which resolved on discontinuation), CHF (exacerbation reported).

Drug interactions

Concurrent use with thiazolidinedione antidiabetic drugs (e.g. **pioglitazone**, **rosiglitazone**) may cause weight gain and peripheral edema.

Undesirable effects

For full list, see manufacturer's Product Monograph.
Suicidal ideation (1/500; advise patients to report mood or thought disturbance).
Very common (>10%): dizziness (about 1/3 of patients), drowsiness (about 1/4); these generally resolve spontaneously after a median of 5–8 weeks.[8–10]
Common (<10%, >1%): confusion, irritability, euphoria, amnesia, reduced attention, blurred vision, diplopia, dysarthria, tremor, ataxia, increased appetite, weight gain, dry mouth, decreased libido, impotence, edema.
Uncommon (<1%, >0.1%): painful gynecomastia.[22]

Dose and use for neuropathic pain
- start with 75mg b.i.d.
- if necessary, at intervals of 3–7 days, increase to 150mg b.i.d. → 225mg b.i.d. → 300mg b.i.d. (maximum recommended dose)
- in debilitated patients, start with 25–50mg b.i.d.; and, if necessary, increase the dose correspondingly cautiously.

The intervals between dose increases are pragmatic rather than pharmacokinetic. In one RCT, the effective doses were:
- 150mg b.i.d. in about 1/4 of patients
- 225mg b.i.d. in about 1/3
- 300mg b.i.d. in another 1/3.[11]

Dose reduction is necessary in renal impairment (Table 4.30). For patients on hemodialysis, the regular dose should be adjusted according to the creatinine clearance and a supplementary single dose given after each dialysis (Table 4.31).

Because epileptic seizures are often sporadic, more time is needed to evaluate the initial response, i.e. a minimum of 1 week.

Table 4.30 Impact of renal impairment on starting and maximum doses (manufacturer's recommendations)

Creatinine clearance (mL/min)	Starting dose	Maximum dose
>60	75mg b.i.d.	300mg b.i.d.
31–60	25mg t.i.d.[a]	150mg b.i.d.
15–30	25–50mg once daily	150mg once daily
<15	25mg once daily	75mg once daily

a. 37.5mg capsules not available, necessitating t.i.d. regimen.

Table 4.31 Post-hemodialysis supplementary doses

Daily dose	Supplementary single dose after every 4h of hemodialysis
25mg	25–50mg
50mg	50–75mg
75mg	100–150mg

Stopping pregabalin
To avoid precipitating pain or seizures, pregabalin should be withdrawn gradually over several weeks.

Supply
Lyrica® (Pfizer)
Capsules 25mg, 50mg, 75mg, 150mg, 300mg, 28 days @ 25mg, 50mg t.i.d. = $70 and $110 respectively; 28 days @ 75mg, 150mg, 300mg b.i.d. = $95, $142 and $142 respectively.

Because of unit costs, the overall daily cost is generally less if given b.i.d. rather than t.i.d.

1 Feltner DE et al. (2003) A randomized, double-blind, placebo-controlled, fixed-dose, multicenter study of pregabalin in patients with generalized anxiety disorder. Journal of Clinical Psychopharmacology. **23**: 240–249.
2 Pande AC et al. (2003) Pregabalin in generalized anxiety disorder: a placebo-controlled trial. American Journal of Psychiatry. **160**: 533–540.
3 Rickels K et al. (2005) Pregabalin for treatment of generalized anxiety disorder: a 4-week, multicenter, double-blind, placebo-controlled trial of pregabalin and alprazolam. Archives of General Psychiatry. **62**: 1022–1030.
4 Montgomery SA et al. (2006) Efficacy and safety of pregabalin in the treatment of generalized anxiety disorder: a 6-week, multicenter, randomized, double-blind, placebo-controlled comparison of pregabalin and venlafaxine. Journal of Clinical Psychiatry. **67**: 771–782.

5 Jones DL and Sorkin LS (1998) Systemic gabapentin and S(+)-3-isobutyl-gamma-aminobutyric acid block secondary hyperalgesia. *Brain Research.* **810**: 93–99.

6 Randinitis EJ *et al.* (2003) Pharmacokinetics of pregabalin in subjects with various degrees of renal function. *Journal of Clinical Pharmacology.* **43**: 277–283.

7 Ben-Menachem E (2004) Pregabalin pharmacology and its relevance to clinical practice. *Epilepsia.* **45 (suppl 6)**: 13–18.

8 Dworkin RH *et al.* (2003) Pregabalin for the treatment of postherpetic neuralgia: a randomized, placebo-controlled trial. *Neurology.* **60**: 1274–1283.

9 Rosenstock J *et al.* (2004) Pregabalin for the treatment of painful diabetic peripheral neuropathy: a double-blind, placebo-controlled trial. *Pain.* **110**: 628–638.

10 Sabatowski R *et al.* (2004) Pregabalin reduces pain and improves sleep and mood disturbances in patients with post-herpetic neuralgia: results of a randomised, placebo-controlled clinical trial. *Pain.* **109**: 26–35.

11 Freynhagen R *et al.* (2005) Efficacy of pregabalin in neuropathic pain evaluated in a 12-week, randomised, double-blind, multicentre, placebo-controlled trial of flexible- and fixed-dose regimens. *Pain.* **115**: 254–263.

12 Richter RW *et al.* (2005) Relief of painful diabetic peripheral neuropathy with pregabalin: a randomized, placebo-controlled trial. *Journal of Pain.* **6**: 253–260.

13 van Seventer R *et al.* (2006) Efficacy and tolerability of twice-daily pregabalin for treating pain and related sleep interference in postherpetic neuralgia: a 13-week, randomized trial. *Current Medical Research and Opinion.* **22**: 375–384.

14 Siddall PJ *et al.* (2006) Pregabalin in central neuropathic pain associated with spinal cord injury: a placebo-controlled trial. *Neurology.* **67**: 1792–1800.

15 Vranken JH *et al.* (2008) Pregabalin in patients with central neuropathic pain: a randomized, double-blind, placebo-controlled trial of a flexible-dose regimen. *Pain.* **136**: 150–157.

16 Tolle T *et al.* (2008) Pregabalin for relief of neuropathic pain associated with diabetic neuropathy: a randomized, double-blind study. *European Journal of Pain.* **12**: 203–213.

17 Hill CM *et al.* (2001) Pregabalin in patients with postoperative dental pain. *European Journal of Pain.* **5**: 119–124.

18 Hauser W *et al.* (2009) Treatment of fibromyalgia syndrome with gabapentin and pregabalin-a meta-analysis of randomized controlled trials. *Pain.* **145**: 69–81.

19 Crofford LJ *et al.* (2008) Fibromyalgia relapse evaluation and efficacy for durability of meaningful relief (FREEDOM): a 6-month, double-blind, placebo-controlled trial with pregabalin. *Pain.* **136**: 419–431.

20 Jokela R *et al.* (2008) A randomized controlled trial of perioperative administration of pregabalin for pain after laparoscopic hysterectomy. *Pain.* **134**: 106–112.

21 Perucca E *et al.* (2003) Pregabalin demonstrates anticonvulsant activity onset by second day. *Neurology.* **60 (suppl. 1)**: A145 [abstract P102. 122].

22 Malaga I and Sanmarti FX (2006) Two cases of painful gynecomastia and lower extremity pain in association with pregabalin therapy. *Epilepsia.* **47**: 1576–1579.

PHENOBARBITAL

Class: Anti-epileptic (GABAmimetic).

Indications: Control of generalized tonic-clonic and partial complex seizures, status epilepticus, †terminal agitation.

Pharmacology

Phenobarbital enhances the post-synaptic inhibitory action of GABA by prolonging the opening of the chloride channel in the GABA receptor-channel complex (see Figure 4.3, p.197).[1] Phenobarbital also inhibits the post-synaptic actions of the excitatory neurotransmitter, glutamate, at non-NMDA-receptor-channels. These actions depress CNS activity, and high doses result in general anesthesia. There is considerable interindividual variation in the pharmacokinetics of phenobarbital. Peak CNS concentrations occur some 15–20min after peak plasma concentrations. About 25% is excreted unchanged by the kidney; the rest is converted in the liver, mainly to inactive oxidative metabolites via several enzymes including CYP2C9. Phenobarbital is a strong inducer of CYP3A and glucuronidation, thus reducing plasma concentrations of many concurrently administered drugs.[1–3] The Compendium of Pharmaceutical Specialties advises dose reduction in renal and hepatic impairment but gives no specific guidance.

Phenobarbital's efficacy in epilepsy is comparable to alternatives but concerns about its cognitive and behavioural effects have led to a decline in its use in developed countries, other than for status epilepticus (see p.205).[1]

Phenobarbital is used at some centres for agitation in the imminently dying which fails to respond to the combined use of **midazolam** and an antipsychotic.[4,5] It can also be used as an alternative to **midazolam** in patients in whom there is a potential or actual problem with myoclonus or seizures, e.g. in end-stage renal failure.

Bio-availability 70–90% PO; no data IM.[2,6]

Onset of action 5min IV, maximum effect achieved within 30min, onset after SC or IM administration is slightly slower; 2–3 *weeks* PO (= the time to achieve a therapeutic anti-seizure plasma concentration with a once daily dose of 100–200mg).[6]

Time to peak plasma concentration 2–4h IM,[7,8] 2h PO (some authorities report up to 12h).[6–9]

Plasma halflife 2–6 *days*;[6] 1–3 *days* in children.[7]

Duration of action situation dependent; chronic administration >24h.

Cautions

Elderly, children, debilitated, hepatic impairment, renal impairment, respiratory depression. Avoid sudden withdrawal.

Drug interactions

Concurrent use with other CNS depressants, e.g. alcohol, benzodiazepines and opioids, may produce additive or synergistic sedation or respiratory depression.

Phenobarbital induces various enzymes involved in drug metabolism, including CYP1A2, CYP2C9, CYP2C19 and CYP3A4 (manufacturer's data), and thus reduces plasma concentrations of many drugs.[3] Table 4.32 lists selected drugs which have clinically important interactions with phenobarbital.

Table 4.32 Clinically significant cytochrome P450 interactions with phenobarbital resulting in changed drug plasma concentrations[3]

Phenobarbital plasma concentration		Drug plasma concentration	
Increased by	Decreased by	Increased by phenobarbital	Decreased by phenobarbital
Influenza vaccine Phenytoin[a] Valproic acid[a]	Carbamazepine[a] Chlorpromazine Folic acid St John's wort	Hepatotoxic metabolites of acetaminophen (possibly) Phenytoin (sometimes)[a]	Acetaminophen Some azole antifungals (itraconazole, ketoconazole) Some calcium-channel blockers (felodipine, nifedipine, nimodipine, verapamil) Carbamazepine[a] Chlorpromazine Clonazepam Corticosteroids (dexamethasone, methylprednisolone, prednisone) Coumarins (oral anticoagulants) Cyclosporine Disopyramide Doxycycline Ethosuximide (sometimes)[a] IV fentanyl (significance not known for TD) Haloperidol Lamotrigine Methadone Metronidazole Oral contraceptives Phenytoin (generally)[a] Quinidine Rifampin TCAs Theophylline Valproic acid

a. interactions between anti-epileptic drugs are complex and unpredictable; plasma concentrations may be increased, decreased or unchanged.

Undesirable effects

For full list, see manufacturer's Product Monograph.
Respiratory depression (high doses), drowsiness, lethargy, ataxia, skin reactions (1–3%). Paradoxical excitement, irritability, restlessness/hyperactivity and delirium, particularly in the elderly and children.

Long-term treatment is occasionally complicated by folate-responsive megaloblastic anemia, or by osteomalacia because of changes in vitamin D metabolism.

Dose and use

Because of its long plasma halflife, phenobarbital sodium injection can theoretically be administered by SC bolus b.i.d. or t.i.d. A 60mg/mL product previously imported through the Special Access Programme was successfully used by this route with no site reaction problems. However, the 120mg/mL injection now marketed for IM/IV use in Canada is very alkaline (pH 9.2–10.2) and is formulated in a vehicle containing 60% propylene glycol. Local tissue damage, sometimes leading to necrosis, has been reported after IV extravasation (manufacturer's data), and there are anecdotal reports of site reactions after SC bolus injection of the undiluted product. However, these can be overcome by diluting with an equal volume of 0.9% saline. If well diluted with WFI or 0.9% saline, the injection can generally be given safely *on its own* by IV injection or CSCI; it should never be mixed with another drug (see p.511).[16]

Epilepsy

Phenobarbital is sometimes used as maintenance anti-epileptic therapy in patients who cannot swallow but for whom a benzodiazepine (e.g. **lorazepam**, **diazepam** or **midazolam**) is too sedative. In Canada, it is sometimes given by SC bolus (see note above):[11]
• generally 60–80mg SC b.i.d.–t.i.d., occasionally up to 120mg t.i.d.; administer at a separate site from other drugs.
Alternatively, because of the irritant nature of the undiluted injection and the volume after dilution, stat doses can be given by slow IV injection, followed by CSCI:
• dilute each 120mg (1mL) ampoule with 5mL of WFI or 0.9% saline (i.e. total volume 6mL)
• give 100mg (i.e. 5mL) IV stat
• then 200–400mg/24h CSCI, i.e. total volume 10–20mL.
For use in status epilepticus, see p.205.

Terminal agitation

Phenobarbital is one of several sedative drugs used to treat refractory agitation in the imminently dying (Table 4.33).[12,13] It is generally second- or third-line treatment for patients who, for example, fail to respond to **midazolam** 60–120mg/24h and either **haloperidol** 30mg/24h or **methotrimeprazine** 200mg/24h.[4]

In Canada, it is sometimes given by SC bolus (see note above) as an adjunct to **midazolam** CSCI:[11]
• generally 60–80mg SC b.i.d.–t.i.d., occasionally up to 120mg t.i.d.; administer at a separate site from other drugs.
Alternatively, because of the irritant nature of the injection (and the volume after dilution), stat doses can be given IM/IV, followed by CSCI:
• start with loading dose of 200mg by IM injection (use 2 × 120mg in 1mL ampoules and give 1.7mL *undiluted*) *or*
• dilute 2 × 120mg in 1mL ampoules with 10mL of WFI or 0.9% saline (i.e. total volume 12mL) and give 200mg (10mL) as an IV bolus over 2min
• maintain with 800mg/24h CSCI (= total volume 40mL)
• if agitation recurs, give a further dose of 200mg IM/IV q1h p.r.n.
• if necessary, increase the dose progressively to 1,600mg/24h, i.e. 800 → 1,200 → 1,600mg (= total volume 80mL)
• occasionally it may be necessary to increase to 2,400mg (= total volume 120mL)
• median maximum dose = 1,600mg/24h (= total volume 80mL).[9]
Some centres use **propofol** (see p.473) instead.[14–16]

Table 4.33 Mean, median and range of sedative and antipsychotic doses in final 48h of life (mg/day)[a,17]

Drug	Mean dose	Median dose	Reported range	References
Midazolam	22–70	30–45	3–1,200	18–29
Haloperidol	5	4	5–50	23,26,28
Chlorpromazine	21	50	13–900	23,28,30–33
Levomepromazine	64	100	25–250	23,28,30,33
Phenobarbital	–	800–1,600	200–2,500	23,28,30,33,34
Propofol	1,100	500	400–9,600	23,33,35,36

a. mean, median and range may be derived from different studies.

Stopping phenobarbital

Abrupt cessation of long-term anti-epileptic therapy, particularly barbiturates and benzodiazepines, should be avoided because rebound seizures may be precipitated. If it is decided to discontinue anti-epileptic therapy, it should be done *slowly over 6 months or more*. For phenobarbital, the recommended monthly reduction in dose is *15mg*.[37]

In adults the risk of relapse on stopping treatment is 40–50%.[38] Substituting one anti-epileptic drug regimen for another should also be done cautiously, withdrawing the first drug only when the new regimen has been introduced.

Supply

Unless indicated otherwise, all preparations are Schedule IV controlled drugs under the Controlled Drugs and Substances Act (CDSA).

Phenobarbital (generic)
Tablets 15mg, 30mg, 60mg, 100mg, 28 days @ 60mg t.i.d. = $10.
Oral solution (elixir) 5mg/mL, 28 days @ 60mg t.i.d. = $93.

Phenobarbital sodium (generic)
Injection 30mg/mL, 1mL amp = $4.50; *vehicle contains 60% propylene glycol.*
Injection 120mg/mL, 1mL amp = $5; *vehicle contains 60% propylene glycol.*

1 Kwan P and Brodie MJ (2004) Phenobarbital for the treatment of epilepsy in the 21st century: a critical review. *Epilepsia*. **45**: 1141–1149.
2 Dollery C (1999) Phenobarbital. In: C Dollery (ed) *Therapeutic Drugs Release 1*. Harcourt Brace Company, Edinburgh, UK.
3 Baxter K (ed) (2008) *Stockley's Drug Interactions* (8e). Pharmaceutical Press, London.
4 de Graeff A and Dean M (2007) Palliative sedation therapy in the last weeks of life: a literature review and recommendations for standards. *Journal of Palliative Medicine*. **10**: 67–85.
5 Twycross R et al. (2009) *Symptom Management in Advanced Cancer*. Palliativedrugs.com, Nottingham, pp. 430–433.
6 AHFS (2009) AHFS Drug Information (online edition). Available from: www.medicinescomplete.com/mc/ahfs/current/
7 Sweetman S (ed) (2009) Martindale: the Complete Drug Reference (online edition). Available from: www.medicinescomplete.com/mc/martindale/current/
8 Holford N (ed) (1998) *Clinical Pharmacokinetics: Drug Data Handbook* (3e). Adis International, Auckland.
9 Stirling LC et al. (1999) The use of phenobarbitone in the management of agitation and seizures at the end of life. *Journal of Pain and Symptom Management*. **17**: 363–368.
10 Dickman A et al. (2005) *The Syringe Driver: Continuous Subcutaneous Infusions in Palliative Care* (2e). Oxford University Press, Oxford, p. 80.
11 palliativedrugs com Bulletin Board (2007) Phenobarbital infusion. Available from: www.palliativedrugs.com/forum-read?&f=1&i=12715&t=12715
12 Greene WR and Davis WH (1991) Titrated intravenous barbiturates in the control of symptoms in patients with terminal cancer. *Southern Medical Journal*. **84**: 332–337.
13 Truog R et al. (1992) Barbiturates in the care of the terminally ill. New England *Journal of Medicine*. **327**: 1672–1682.
14 Gertler R et al. (2001) Dexmedetomidine: a novel sedative-analgesic agent. Proceedings (Baylor University Medical Center). **14**: 13–21.
15 Soares L et al. (2002) Dexmedetomidine: a new option for intractable distress in the dying. *Journal of Pain and Symptom Management*. **24**: 6–8.
16 Jackson KC, 3rd et al. (2006) Dexmedetomidine: a novel analgesic with palliative medicine potential. *Journal of Pain and Palliative Care Pharmacotherapy*. **20**: 23–27.
17 Wilcock A et al. (Unpublished work) Sedation Consensus: Drug selection, dosing and titration
18 DeSousa E and Jepson B (1988) Midazolam in terminal care. *Lancet*. **1**: 67–68.
19 Amesbury BDW and Dunphy KP (1989) The use of subcutaneous midazolam in the home care setting. *Palliative Medicine*. **3**: 299–301.

20 Bottomley DM and Hanks GW (1990) Subcutaneous midazolam infusion in palliative care. *Journal of Pain and Symptom Management.* **5**: 259–261.

21 Burke A *et al.* (1991) Terminal restlessness – its management and the role of midazolam. *The Medical Journal of Australia.* **155**: 485–487.

22 McNamara P *et al.* (1991) Use of midazolam in palliative care. *Palliative Medicine.* **5**: 244–249.

23 Morita T *et al.* (1996) Sedation for symptom control in Japan: the importance of intermittent use and communication with family members. *Journal of Pain and Symptom Management.* **12**: 32–38.

24 Fainsinger RL (1998) Use of sedation by a hospital palliative care support team. *Journal of Palliative Care.* **14**: 51–54.

25 Fainsinger R *et al.* (2000) Sedation for delirium and other symptoms in terminally ill patients in Edmonton. *Journal of Palliative Care.* **16 (2)**: 5–10.

26 Fainsinger RL *et al.* (2000) A multicentre international study of sedation for uncontrolled symptoms in terminally ill patients. *Palliative Medicine.* **14**: 257–265.

27 Chiu TY *et al.* (2001) Sedation for refractory symptoms of terminal cancer patients in Taiwan. *Journal of Pain and Symptom Management.* **21**: 467–472.

28 Morita T *et al.* (2002) Definition of sedation for symptom relief: a systematic literature review and a proposal of operational criteria. *Journal of Pain and Symptom Management.* **24**: 447–453.

29 Muller-Busch HC *et al.* (2003) Sedation in palliative care – a critical analysis of 7 years experience. *BMC Palliative Care.* **2**: 2.

30 Roy DJ (1990) Need they sleep before they die? *Journal of Palliative Care.* **6**: 3–4.

31 Cowan J and Walsh D (2001) Terminal sedation in palliative medicine – definition and review of the literature. *Supportive Care in Cancer.* **9**: 403–407.

32 Kohara H *et al.* (2005) Sedation for terminally ill patients with cancer with uncontrollable physical distress. *Journal of Palliative Medicine.* **8**: 20–25.

33 Miccinesi G *et al.* (2006) Continuous deep sedation: physicians' experiences in six European countries. *Journal of Pain and Symptom Management.* **31**: 122–129.

34 Mount B (1996) Morphine drips, terminal sedation, and slow euthanasia: definitions and facts, not anecdotes. *Journal of Palliative Care.* **12**: 31–37.

35 Cherny NI and Portenoy RK (1994) Sedation in the management of refractory symptoms: guidelines for evaluation and treatment. *Journal of Palliative Care.* **10**: 31–38.

36 Braun TC *et al.* (2003) Development of a clinical practice guideline for palliative sedation. *Journal of Palliative Medicine.* **6**: 345–350.

37 Chadwick D (1995) The withdrawal of antiepileptic drugs. In: A Hopkins *et al.* (eds) *Epilepsy* (2e). Chapman and Hall, London, pp. 215–220.

38 Hopkins A and Shorvon S (1995) Definitions and epidemiology of epilepsy. In: A Hopkins *et al.* (eds) *Epilepsy* (2e). Chapman and Hall, London, pp. 1–24.

5: ANALGESICS

PRINCIPLES OF USE OF ANALGESICS

Analgesics can be divided into three classes:
• non-opioid
• opioid
• adjuvant (Figure 5.1).

The principles governing their use have been summarized in the WHO Method for Relief of Cancer Pain:[1,2]
• 'By the mouth'
• 'By the clock'
• 'By the ladder' (Figure 5.2)
• 'Individual dose titration'
• 'Use adjuvant drugs'
• 'Attention to detail'.

Drugs from different categories are used alone or in combination according to the type of pain and response to treatment (Figure 5.1). Because cancer pain typically has an inflammatory component, it is generally appropriate to optimize treatment with an NSAID (or corticosteroid) and an opioid before introducing adjuvant analgesics.[3] However, with treatment-related pains (e.g. chemotherapy-induced neuropathic pain, chronic postoperative scar pain) and concurrent pains (e.g. post-herpetic neuralgia, muscle spasm pain), an adjuvant may be an appropriate first-line treatment. For example, an antidepressant or an anti-epileptic for non-cancer neuropathic pain, or a benzodiazepine for muscle spasm. Pain management in children is comparable with adults.[4]

Genetic variation involving CYP2D6 (see p.551) has been shown to be important for **codeine** (see p.278), and **tramadol** (see p.283).[5] The clinical significance of polymorphism for other opioids metabolized by CYP2D6 is unclear (**dihydrocodeine** (not Canada), **hydrocodone**, **methadone**, **oxycodone**, **propoxyphene**).

Polymorphism is rare for CYP3A4 and of unknown clinical significance.[6] Opioids potentially affected are **buprenorphine** (not available as an analgesic in Canada) and the fentanils. Dosing differences may be partly attributable to interindividual variation in CYP3A4 activity, which varies up to 10 times.[7] Genetic variations have also been shown for opioid receptors and transporters for **alfentanil, morphine** and **pentazocine**.[8]

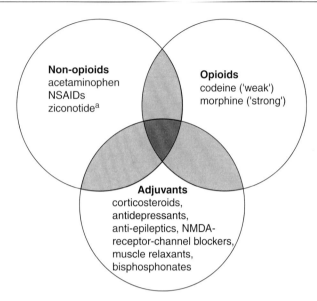

Figure 5.1 Broad-spectrum analgesia; drugs from different categories are used alone or in combination according to the type of pain and response to treatment.

a. ziconotide is an N-type calcium-channel blocker, the first of a new type of non-opioid (not available in Canada). Its place in palliative care remains to be determined.[10,11]

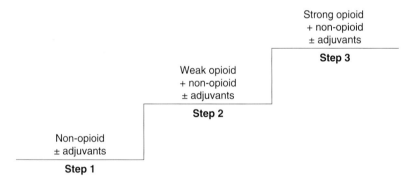

Figure 5.2 The World Health Organization 3-step analgesic ladder.[1]

In relation to the WHO analgesic ladder, there is continuing debate about the need for Step 2.[9] Certainly, there is no absolute pharmacological need for starting with a weak opioid before progressing to a strong opioid. Some pediatric palliative care services omitted Step 2 many years ago. However, in most countries, access to a strong opioid remains difficult (e.g. only as a hospital inpatient, and then sparingly by injection) and sometimes impossible. Further, even where strong opioids can be readily prescribed, they often remain stigmatized, and some patients undoubtedly find the 3-step approach more acceptable than progressing directly from **acetaminophen** (or an NSAID) to a strong opioid. In countries where palliative care is well established, it is perhaps practical to skip Step 2.

If Step 2 is omitted, patients will generally start on a lower dose of **morphine** (20–30mg/24h or the equivalent dose of an alternative strong opioid), and be titrated upwards as necessary.

Several RCTs indicate that **morphine** 60mg/24h is often too high a starting dose in this circumstance.[9]

Break-through (episodic) pain

Some patients require p.r.n. doses for break-through (episodic) pain, a term used to describe a transient exacerbation or recurrence of pain in someone who has mainly stable and/or adequately relieved background pain.[12,13] Patients with inadequately relieved background pain are excluded because this suggests overall poor pain relief, and is an indication for an increase in regular analgesia.

Except for end-of-dose-interval pain (i.e. pain recurring shortly before the next dose of regular analgesic is due), there are two main types of break-through pain:

- *predictable (incident) pain*, related to movement (the majority) or activity, e.g. swallowing, defecation and coughing
- *unpredictable (spontaneous) pain*, unrelated to movement or activity.

Break-through pain is often a resurgence of the background pain, and thus may be either nociceptive or neuropathic. Equally, it could be unrelated to the background pain, e.g. tension headache. Some patients experience two or more different break-through pains.

Various strategies are used to reduce the impact of break-through pain (Figure 5.3).[14,15] A common strategy is to give an extra dose of the regular analgesic, e.g. a p.r.n. dose of normal-release **morphine** for patients taking **morphine** regularly round-the-clock (see p.303). However, at some centres, painful procedures are timed to coincide with the peak plasma concentration after a regular dose of a strong opioid, e.g. 1–2h for **morphine**, and thus obviate the need for additional medication.

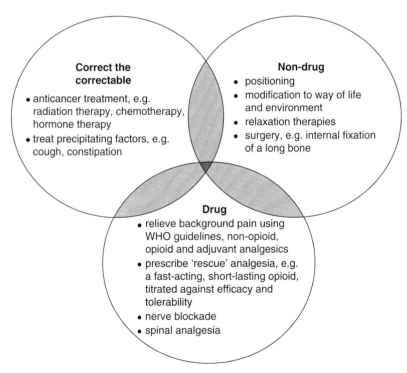

Correct the correctable
- anticancer treatment, e.g. radiation therapy, chemotherapy, hormone therapy
- treat precipitating factors, e.g. cough, constipation

Non-drug
- positioning
- modification to way of life and environment
- relaxation therapies
- surgery, e.g. internal fixation of a long bone

Drug
- relieve background pain using WHO guidelines, non-opioid, opioid and adjuvant analgesics
- prescribe 'rescue' analgesia, e.g. a fast-acting, short-lasting opioid, titrated against efficacy and tolerability
- nerve blockade
- spinal analgesia

Figure 5.3 A multimodal approach to managing break-through (episodic) pain.

In the past, when SR opioid products were unavailable, an extra dose of the regular q4h dose of oral **morphine** was given (i.e. 1/6 of the total daily dose). This was straightforward for the patient. However, many break-through pains are short-lived and this approach effectively doubles the patient's opioid intake for the next 4h. Increasingly, now that SR formulations are available, a more measured approach has been adopted. Thus, many centres now recommend that the patient initially takes, as a normal-release formulation, 10% of the total daily regular dose as the p.r.n. dose.[16,17]

A standard fixed-dose is unlikely to suit all patients and all pains, particularly because the intensity and the impact of break-through pain vary considerably. Thus, when patients are encouraged to optimize their p.r.n. dose, the chosen dose varies from 5 to 20% of the total daily dose.[12,18] Generally, break-through pain has a relatively rapid onset and short duration (e.g. 20–30min, but ranging from 1min to 2–3h), whereas oral **morphine** has a relatively slow onset of action (30min) and long duration of effect (3–6h). This possibly explains why, in one survey, only 1/2 the patients with incident pain took extra medication, and only 3/4 of patients with spontaneous break-through pain did so.[13]

Other measures include oral transmucosal **fentanyl** (using the injection or compounded sprays SL or buccally) (see p.318) and PO/SC **ketamine** (see p.468). With transmucosal **fentanyl**, there is no correlation between the dose of TD **fentanyl** (or of other regularly administered strong opioid) and p.r.n **fentanyl** requirements.

1 WHO (1986) *Cancer Pain Relief.* World Health Organisation, Geneva.
2 WHO (1996) *Cancer Pain Relief: with a Guide to Opioid Availability* (2e). World Health Organisation, Geneva.
3 Twycross R et al. (2009) *Symptom Management in Advanced Cancer* (4e). palliativedrugs.com, Nottingham, pp.27–34.
4 Zernikow B et al. (2006) Paediatric cancer pain management using the WHO analgesic ladder-results of a prospective analysis from 2265 treatment days during a quality improvement study. *European Journal of Pain.* **10**: 587–595.
5 Lotsch J and Geisslinger G (2006) Current evidence for a genetic modulation of the response to analgesics. *Pain.* **121**: 1–5.
6 Pirmohamed M and Park BK (2003) Cytochrome P450 enzyme polymorphisms and adverse drug reactions. *Toxicology.* **192**: 23–32.
7 Haddad A et al. (2007) The pharmacological importance of cytochrome CYP3A4 in the palliation of symptoms: review and recommendations for avoiding adverse drug interactions. *Supportive Care in Cancer.* **15**: 251–257.
8 Somogyi AA et al. (2007) Pharmacogenetics of opioids. *Clinical Pharmacology & Therapeutics.* **81**: 429–444.
9 Mercadante S (2007) Opioid titration in cancer pain: a critical review. *European Journal of Pain.* **11**: 823–830.
10 Prommer EE (2005) Ziconotide: can we use it in palliative care? *American Journal of Hospice and Palliative Care.* **22**: 369–374.
11 Narayana AK (2005) Elan: ziconotide review focused on off-label uses. *American Journal of Hospice and Palliative Care.* **22**: 408.
12 Portenoy K and Hagen N (1990) Breakthrough pain: definition, prevalence and characteristics. *Pain.* **41**: 273–281.
13 Gomez-Batiste X et al. (2002) Breakthrough cancer pain: prevalence and characteristics in Catalonia. *Journal of Pain and Symptom Management.* **24**: 45–52.
14 Zeppetella G and Ribeiro MD (2002) Episodic pain in patients with advanced cancer. *American Journal of Hospice and Palliative Care.* **19**: 267–276.
15 Zeppetella G and Ribeiro MD (2003) Pharmacotherapy of cancer-related episodic pain. *Expert Opinion on Pharmacotherapy.* **4**: 493–502.
16 Davis MP (2003) Guidelines for breakthrough pain dosing. *American Journal of Hospice and Palliative Care.* **20**: 334.
17 Davis MP et al. (2005) Controversies in pharmacotherapy of pain management. *Lancet Oncology.* **6**: 696–704.
18 Mercadante S et al. (2002) Episodic (breakthrough) pain: consensus conference of an expert working group of the EAPC. *Cancer.* **94**: 832–839.

ADJUVANT ANALGESICS

Generally speaking, adjuvant analgesics are drugs which are primarily marketed for indications other than pain but which, in certain circumstances, relieve pain. Consequently, they are *not* primarily classified as analgesics – even though they may relieve pain which has proved to be resistant to 'primary' analgesics such as NSAIDs and/or strong opioids. Adjuvant analgesics include:

- corticosteroids
- antidepressants
- anti-epileptics
- NMDA-receptor-channel blockers
- smooth muscle relaxants (antispasmodics)
- skeletal muscle relaxants
- bisphosphonates.

Unfortunately, the term 'adjuvant analgesic' is misleading if interpreted to mean that such drugs work only when used together with a primary analgesic. In many situations, adjuvant analgesics *alone* provide pain relief ± a reduction in undesirable drug effects. For example, although opioids have been shown in RCTs to at least partly relieve neuropathic pain,[1,2] an antidepressant and/or an anti-epileptic may be preferable long-term, particularly when the pain is non-malignant in origin.

Systemic corticosteroids

Systemic corticosteroids can be helpful for various types of pain (see Box 7.B, p.381), but are used particularly for pain and weakness associated with:
- nerve root/nerve trunk compression, e.g. **dexamethasone** 4–8mg/24h
- spinal cord compression, e.g. **dexamethasone** 12–16mg/24h.[3,4]

Systemic corticosteroids do not help in pure non-cancer nerve injury pain, e.g. chronic postoperative scar pain, post-herpetic neuralgia. However, in cancer-related nerve injury pain, a 5–7 day trial of **dexamethasone** may be beneficial.

Antidepressants and anti-epileptics

Comparing drugs in neuropathic pain: a useful statistic is the NNT, i.e. the *number* of patients *needed* to *treat* in order to achieve ⩾50% improvement in one patient compared with placebo. Thus an NNT of 3 means that 1 in 3 (or 33%) of patients will achieve such a benefit. However, in clinical practice, one hopes to 'capture' the placebo response as well as the pharmacological one. This means that an NNT of 3 in an RCT is likely to become an NNT of 2 in practice (50% of patients achieving a good response). Further, if a 30% improvement is used as the 'bench mark' of useful improvement, then an even greater number will be deemed to have benefited, maybe as many as 70–80%.

The opposite of the NNT is the NNH, namely the *number* of patients *needed* to be treated in order to *harm* one patient sufficiently to cause withdrawal from the trial. This gives a useful measure of comparative drug toxicity.[5]

Antidepressants and anti-epileptics are often of benefit when used as single agents in 'pure' nerve injury pain, e.g. chronic surgical incision pain, painful diabetic neuropathy, and post-herpetic neuralgia.[6–10] However, if the nerve injury pain is associated with an infiltrating cancer, **morphine** and an NSAID should be tried first before *adding* an antidepressant or an anti-epileptic.[11–13]

About 90% of patients with nerve injury pain respond to the use of non-opioids, opioids and adjuvant analgesics.[14] The remainder require spinal analgesia (e.g. **morphine + bupivacaine ± clonidine**) or a neurolytic procedure to obtain adequate relief. Some patients derive benefit from other non-drug measures, e.g. transcutaneous electrical nerve stimulation (TENS).

Antidepressants are not equally effective in relieving neuropathic pain. It is debatable how effective SSRIs are. Two small trials (n ⩽ 20) showed a small but significant effect for **paroxetine** and **citalopram** in painful diabetic neuropathy.[15,16] However, **fluoxetine** in a larger trial (n = 46) had no effect.[17] Together these results give an NNT for SSRIs of 7.

For **venlafaxine**, a mixed serotonin and norepinephrine re-uptake inhibitor (SNRI), the NNT is 5.5 overall, and 4.6 if only those who received at least 150mg/24h are included.[18–20] On the other hand, this could be an underestimate because in a head-to-head comparison with **imipramine** (see below) it was not possible to distinguish between the two drugs.[18] **Duloxetine**, another SNRI, has also yielded promising results.[21] However, a health technology assessment by the Canadian Agency for Drugs and Technologies in Health (CADTH) concluded that SNRIs (**duloxetine** and **venlafaxine**) were less cost-beneficial in neuropathic pain than TCAs and anti-epileptics (**gabapentin** and **pregabalin**). Although the differences in effectiveness between drug classes were not statistically significant, NNTs were always lowest with TCAs and highest with non-TCA SNRIs, regardless of the design of the comparison and whether a response was classed as a 50% or a 30% reduction in pain. Further, switching all patients from TCAs to **duloxetine** would increase government health costs by $171 million per year.[10]

Excluding that associated with HIV (where TCAs are *not* beneficial),[22] in peripheral neuropathy the NNT for TCAs is 2.3.[20] For TCAs with 'balanced' inhibition of neuronal re-uptake of serotonin and norepinephrine (SNRIs), the NNT is 2.2, and for TCAs which are mainly inhibitors of norepinephrine re-uptake (NRIs), the NNT is 2.5.[20] This suggests that inhibition of norepinephrine re-uptake is more important than inhibition of serotonin re-uptake. Remarkably, in a trial in which the dose of **imipramine** was titrated to achieve a combined plasma concentration of >400nmol for **imipramine** and **desipramine** (the active metabolite), the NNT was 1.4.[9]

Central pain is generally harder to relieve than peripheral neuropathic pain. Even so, in central post-stroke pain, **amitriptyline** has an NNT of 1.7, despite having no measurable effect in spinal cord injury pain. Overall, the NNT for **amitriptyline** in central pain is 4.[20]

The analgesic effect of TCAs probably depends on several pharmacological mechanisms. These could include:

- inhibition of pre-synaptic re-uptake of serotonin and norepinephrine (Figure 5.4)
- post-synaptic receptor antagonism:
  - ▷ α-adrenergic
  - ▷ histamine type 1 (H₁)
  - ▷ μ-opioid (low affinity)
- channel blockade:
  - ▷ NMDA-receptor
  - ▷ sodium
  - ▷ calcium.[9]

Response may also depend on the duration of the pain. Thus, in post-herpetic neuralgia, if **amitriptyline** is initiated within 6 months of onset, the response rate is about 75%, but if delayed >2 years the response rate drops to 25%.[23,24]

TCAs also have an opioid-sparing effect when used in cancer pain generally. In one RCT, the patients who received **imipramine** 50mg PO at bedtime in addition to **morphine** PO q4h needed 20% less **morphine** than the control group.[25]

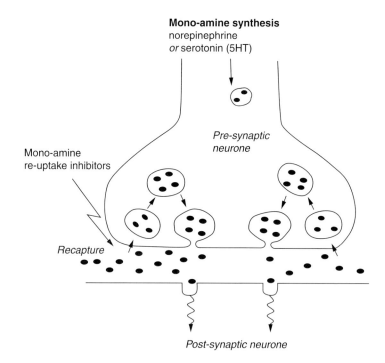

Mono-amine synthesis
norepinephrine
or serotonin (5HT)

Pre-synaptic neurone

Mono-amine re-uptake inhibitors

Recapture

Post-synaptic neurone

Figure 5.4 Mono-amine re-uptake inhibitors, comprising mainly SNRIs, SSRIs, and NRIs (see Box 4.F, p.139), facilitate one or both of the two descending spinal inhibitory pathways by blocking presynaptic re-uptake (one serotoninergic, the other noradrenergic). SNRIs and SSRIs also potentiate opioid analgesia by a serotoninergic mechanism in the brain stem.

Bupropion, a unique antidepressant chemically related to the central stimulant **diethylpropion**, is a weak inhibitor of neuronal re-uptake of serotonin and norepinephrine and, in addition, inhibits the re-uptake of dopamine. In a trial in 41 patients with neuropathic pain from differing causes, **bupropion** had an NNT of 1.6.[26] However, such a remarkable result needs confirmation. **Trazodone**, another unique antidepressant which antagonizes α_1-noradrenergic and $5HT_2$-receptors, is *not* recommended for use as an adjuvant analgesic.[27]

For anti-epileptics, the NNT for **carbamazepine** in painful neuropathies is 2.5.[28] However, other than for trigeminal neuralgia, **carbamazepine** is often disappointing in clinical practice.[8] For **gabapentin** (approved for neuropathic pain in some countries but only as an anti-epileptic agent in Canada), the combined NNT is 3.7.[28] However, specifically in painful diabetic neuropathy, the NNT is 4.3, and in post-herpetic neuralgia it is 4.3.[20] **Lamotrigine**, another anti-epileptic, has an NNT of 4. In contrast, **valproic acid** has an NNT of 2–2.5.[5,29–32]

Clonazepam has also been used successfully in some patients with neuropathic pain, including phantom limb,[33] post-herpetic,[34] diabetic,[35] and cancer-related[36] (see p.117), although there is no supporting RCT evidence.

The mechanisms by which anti-epileptics relieve pain differ from the antidepressants (Figure 5.5).[37] Some anti-epileptics act as peripheral sodium-channel blockers. Others impact mainly on the dorsal horn by inhibiting the glutamate (excitatory) system or activating the GABA (inhibitory) system, or both, in one of several ways. **Gabapentin** and **pregabalin**, although structural analogues of GABA, act principally as $\alpha_2\delta$-type calcium-channel blockers.[38] Thus, it makes sense to combine an antidepressant with an anti-epileptic in those patients who fail to achieve satisfactory relief with either class of drug individually. Although benefit may well be seen in clinical practice, combining two different types of adjuvant analgesic is not generally based on RCT evidence.[39] However, adding **venlafaxine** to **gabapentin** in painful diabetic neuropathy results in significant additional benefit.[40] Further, in both diabetic neuropathy and post-herpetic neuralgia, combining **morphine** and **gabapentin** results in better pain relief at lower doses than when either drug is used as a single agent.[41]

It is important to establish a practical protocol for neuropathic pain management, selecting only one or two drugs from each category of drugs (Figure 5.6).[42,43] For example, in Steps 2 and 3, although now less often used to treat depression, **amitriptyline** 25–75mg at bedtime is still widely used as an adjuvant analgesic.[44] For an anti-epileptic, some centres still use **valproic acid** 400–1,000mg at bedtime. However, **gabapentin** and **pregabalin** are increasingly used;[44,45] **pregabalin** is approved in Canada for treating neuropathic pain. When considering combining adjuvant analgesics, the following combinations should be avoided:

- two different antidepressants
- an antidepressant with **tramadol** (see Serotonin toxicity, p.140).

Relief is not an 'all or none' phenomenon. The crucial first step in many cases is to help the patient obtain a good night's sleep. The second is to reduce pain intensity and allodynia associated with nerve injury pain to a bearable level during the day. Initially there may be marked diurnal variation in relief, with more prolonged periods with less or no pain rather than a decrease in worst pain intensity round the clock. The patient should be warned that major benefit often takes a week or more to manifest, although improvement in sleep should occur immediately. Undesirable drug effects are often a limiting therapeutic factor.

NMDA-receptor-channel blockers

NMDA-receptor-channel blockers are most commonly used when neuropathic pain does not respond well to standard analgesics together with an antidepressant and an anti-epileptic. They have also been used in inflammatory pain, e.g. severe mucositis.[46] NMDA-receptor-channel blockers include:

- **ketamine** (see p.468)[47–49]
- **methadone** (see p.327)[50,51]
- **amantadine**.[52,53]

As with other classes of drugs, NMDA-receptor-channel blockers are not always beneficial. Controlled data show only modest benefit with **amantadine** 200mg IV over 3h, whereas earlier case reports indicated dramatic benefit.[53,54] *PCF does not recommend **amantadine**.*

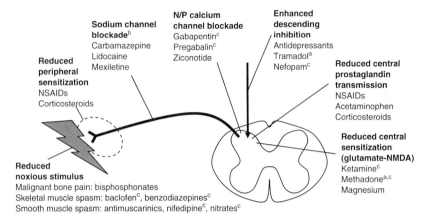

Figure 5.5 Overview of the peripheral and spinal non-opioid sites of action of analgesics.

a. also acts as a μ-opioid receptor agonist

b. reduces ectopic nerve signal transmission by damaged neurones (see p.212); the higher concentrations of lidocaine used in local/regional anesthesia completely inhibit nerve signal transmission

c. additional actions (see individual monographs).

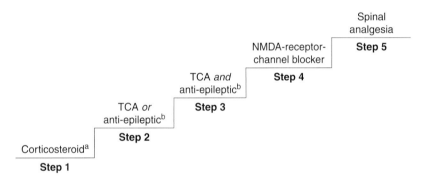

Figure 5.6 Adjuvant analgesics for neuropathic pain. If caused by cancer, use only if the pain does not respond to the combined use of an NSAID and a strong opioid.

a. important when neuropathic pain is associated with limb weakness

b. some centres use mexiletine, a local anesthetic congener and cardiac anti-arrhythmic drug which blocks sodium channels, as an alternative to an anti-epileptic.[42,43]

Smooth muscle relaxants (antispasmodics)

This is a heterogeneous group of drugs encompassing antimuscarinics, **nitroglycerin** (see p.53), and calcium-channel blockers (e.g. **nifedipine**; see p.56). Antimuscarinics are used to relieve visceral distension pain and colic. In advanced cancer, there is little place for 'weak' antispasmodics such as **dicyclomine**. In the UK and Canada, **hyoscine (scopolamine)** *butylbromide* (see p.11) and **glycopyrrolate** (see p.465), quaternary drugs which do not cross the blood–brain barrier, are widely regarded as the antispasmodics of choice. **Atropine** and **scopolamine (hyoscine)** *hydrobromide* have comparable peripheral effects but also have central effects, either stimulation or sedation, and may precipitate delirium.

Nitroglycerin and calcium channel blockers can be used for the same range of indications, but tend to be reserved for painful spasm of the esophagus, rectum and anus.

Skeletal muscle relaxants

These include **baclofen**, **diazepam**, **tizanidine**, and **quinine** (see p.436). However, non-drug treatment is generally preferable for painful skeletal muscle spasm (cramp) and myofascial pain, e.g. physical therapy (local heat, massage, acupuncture).[55] Some patients also benefit from relaxation therapy ± **diazepam** (see p.113). Myofascial trigger points often benefit from direct injection of local anesthetic.[56] *However severe, **morphine** is ineffective for the relief of cramp and trigger point pains.*

Bisphosphonates

Bisphosphonates (see p.371) are osteoclast inhibitors and are used to relieve metastatic bone pain which persists despite analgesics and radiation therapy ± orthopedic surgery. Published data relate mainly to breast cancer and myeloma; benefit is also seen with other cancers. About 50% of patients benefit, typically in 1–2 weeks, and this may last for 2–3 months. Benefit may be seen only after a second treatment but, if there is no response after two treatments, nothing is gained by further use.[57] In those who respond, continue to treat p.r.n. for as long as there is benefit.

1 Eisenberg E et al. (2005) Efficacy and safety of opioid agonists in the treatment of neuropathic pain of nonmalignant origin: systematic review and meta-analysis of randomized controlled trials. *Journal of the American Medical Association.* **293**: 3043–3052.

2 Eisenberg E et al. (2006) Efficacy of mu-opioid agonists in the treatment of evoked neuropathic pain: Systematic review of randomized controlled trials. *European Journal of Pain.* **10**: 667–676.

3 Vecht C et al. (1989) Initial bolus of conventional versus high-dose dexamethasone in metastatic spinal cord compression. *Neurology.* **39**: 1255–1257.

4 Loblaw D and Laperriere N (1998) Emergency treatment of malignant extradural spinal cord compression: an evidence-based guideline. *Journal of Clinical Oncology.* **16**: 1613–1624.

5 Finnerup NB et al. (2005) Algorithm for neuropathic pain treatment: an evidence based proposal. *Pain.* **118**: 289–305.

6 DTB (2000) Drug treatment of neuropathic pain. *Drug and Therapeutics Bulletin.* **38**: 89–93.

7 Collins SL et al. (2000) Antidepressants and anticonvulsants for diabetic neuropathy and postherpetic neuralgia: a quantitative systematic review. *Journal of Pain and Symptom Management.* **20**: 449–458.

8 Backonja M (2001) Anticonvulsants and antiarrhythmics in the treatment of neuropathic pain syndromes. In: PT Hansson et al. (eds) *Neuropathic pain: pathophysiology and treatment.* IASP, Seattle, pp. 185–201.

9 Sindrup S and Jensen T (2001) Antidepressants in the treatment of neuropathic pain. In: PT Hansson et al. (eds) *Neuropathic pain: pathophysiology and treatment.* IASP, Seattle, pp. 169–183.

10 Iskedjian M et al. (2009) Anticonvulsants, serotonin–norepinephrine reuptake inhibitors and tricyclic antidepressants in management of neuropathic pain: a meta-analysis and economic evaluation (Technology report number 116). Canadian Agency for Drugs and Technologies in Health, Ottawa. Available from: www.cadth.ca/index.php/en/hta/reports-publications/search/publication/870

11 Dellemijn P et al. (1994) Medical therapy of malignant nerve pain. A randomised double-blind explanatory trial with naproxen versus slow-release morphine. *European Journal of Cancer.* **30A**: 1244–1250.

12 Ripamonti C et al. (1996) Continuous subcutaneous infusion of ketorolac in cancer neuropathic pain unresponsive to opioid and adjuvant drugs. A case report. *Tumori.* **82**: 413–415.

13 Dellemijn P (1999) Are opioids effective in relieving neuropathic pain? *Pain.* **80**: 453–462.

14 Grond S et al. (1999) Assessment and treatment of neuropathic cancer pain following WHO guidelines. *Pain.* **79**: 15–20.

15 Sindrup SH et al. (1992) Lack of effect of mianserin on the symptoms of diabetic neuropathy. *European Journal of Clinical Pharmacology.* **43**: 251–255.

16 Sindrup SH et al. (1992) The selective serotonin reuptake inhibitor citalopram relieves the symptoms of diabetic neuropathy. *Clinical Pharmacology and Therapeutics.* **52**: 547–552.

17 Max M et al. (1992) Effects of desipramine, amitriptyline, and fluoxetine on pain in diabetic neuropathy. *New England Journal of Medicine.* **326**: 1287–1288.

18 Sindrup SH et al. (2003) Venlafaxine versus imipramine in painful polyneuropathy: a randomized, controlled trial. *Neurology.* **60**: 1284–1289.

19 Rowbotham MC et al. (2004) Venlafaxine extended release in the treatment of painful diabetic neuropathy: a double-blind, placebo-controlled study. *Pain.* **110**: 697–706.

20 Sindrup SH et al. (2005) Antidepressants in the treatment of neuropathic pain. *Basic & Clinical Pharmacology & Toxicology.* **96**: 399–409.

21 Detke M et al. (2003) Efficacy of duloxetine in the treatment of pain associated with diabetic neuropathy. *Diabetologia.* **46 (suppl 2)**: A315.

22 Attal N et al. (2006) EFNS guidelines on pharmacological treatment of neuropathic pain. *European Journal of Neurology.* **13**: 1153–1169.

23 Bowsher D (1997) The effects of pre-emptive treatment of postherpetic neuralgia with amitriptyline: a randomized, double-blind, placebo-controlled trial. *Journal of Pain and Symptom Management.* **13**: 327–331.

24 Bowsher D (2000) The important time parameter is missing. Comment on Sindrup and Jensen 1999. *Pain.* **88**: 313.

25 Walsh T (1986) Controlled study of imipramine and morphine in advanced cancer. *Proceedings of the American Society of Clinical Oncology.* **5**: 237.

26 Semenchuk MR et al. (2001) Double-blind, randomized trial of bupropion SR for the treatment of neuropathic pain. *Neurology.* **57**: 1583–1588.

27 Ansari A (2000) The efficacy of newer antidepressants in the treatment of chronic pain: a review of current literature. *Harvard Review of Psychiatry.* **7**: 257–277.

28 Wiffen PJ et al. (2005) Anticonvulsants for acute and chronic pain. Cochrane Database of Systematic Reviews. **3**: CD001133.
29 Kochar DK et al. (2002) Sodium valproate in the management of painful neuropathy in type 2 diabetes – a randomized placebo controlled study. Acta Neurologica Scandinavica. **106**: 248–252.
30 Kochar DK et al. (2004) Sodium valproate for painful diabetic neuropathy: a randomized double-blind placebo-controlled study. Quarterly Journal of Medicine. **97**: 33–38.
31 Kochar DK et al. (2005) Divalproex sodium in the management of post-herpetic neuralgia: a randomized double-blind placebo-controlled study. Quarterly Journal of Medicine. **98**: 29–34.
32 Otto M et al. (2004) Valproic acid has no effect on pain in polyneuropathy: a randomized, controlled trial. Neurology. **62**: 285–288.
33 Bartusch S et al. (1996) Clonazepam for the treatment of lancinating phantom limb pain. Clinical Journal of Pain. **12**: 59–62.
34 Mamdani FS (1994) Pharmacologic management of herpes zoster and postherpetic neuralgia. Canadian Family Physician. **40**: 321–326, 329–332.
35 Young JP and Clarke BF (1985) Pain relief in diabetic neuropathy: the effectiveness of imipramine and related drugs. Diabetic Medicine. **2**: 363–366.
36 Hugel H et al. (2003) Clonazepam as an adjuvant analgesic in patients with cancer-related neuropathic pain. Journal of Pain and Symptom Management. **26**: 1073–1074.
37 Vinik A (2005) Clinical review: use of antiepileptic drugs in the treatment of chronic painful diabetic neuropathy. Journal of Clinical Endocrinology and Metabolism. **90**: 4936–4945.
38 Stahl SM (2004) Anticonvulsants and the relief of chronic pain: pregabalin and gabapentin as alpha(2)delta ligands at voltage-gated calcium channels. Journal of Clinical Psychiatry. **65**: 596–597.
39 Raja SN and Haythornthwaite JA (2005) Combination therapy for neuropathic pain–which drugs, which combination, which patients? New England Journal of Medicine. **352**: 1373–1375.
40 Simpson DA (2001) Gabapentin and venlafaxine for the treatmetn of painful diabetic neuropathy. Journal of Clinical Neuromuscular Diseases. **3**: 53–62.
41 Gilron I et al. (2005) Morphine, gabapentin, or their combination for neuropathic pain. New England Journal of Medicine. **352**: 1324–1334.
42 Chabal C et al. (1992) The use of oral mexiletine for the treatment of pain after peripheral nerve injury. Anaesthesiology. **76**: 513–517.
43 Chong S et al. (1997) Pilot study evaluating local anesthetics administered systemically for treatment of pain in patients with advanced cancer. Journal of Pain and Symptom Management. **13**: 112–117.
44 McQuay H et al. (1996) A systematic review of antidepressants in neuropathic pain. Pain. **68**: 217–227.
45 McQuay H et al. (1995) Anticonvulsant drugs for the management of pain: a systematic review. British Medical Journal. **311**: 1047–1052.
46 Jackson K et al. (2001) 'Burst' ketamine for refractory cancer pain: an open-label audit of 39 patients. Journal of Pain and Symptom Management. **22**: 834–842.
47 Enarson M et al. (1999) Clinical experience with oral ketamine. Journal of Pain and Symptom Management. **17**: 384–386.
48 Fine P (1999) Low-dose ketamine in the management of opioid nonresponsive terminal cancer. Journal of Pain and Symptom Management. **17**: 296–300.
49 Finlay I (1999) Ketamine and its role in cancer pain. Pain Reviews. **6**: 303–313.
50 Gannon C (1997) The use of methadone in the care of the dying. European Journal of Palliative Care. **4**: 152–158.
51 Morley J and Makin M (1998) The use of methadone in cancer pain poorly responsive to other opioids. Pain Reviews. **5**: 51–58.
52 Kornhuber J et al. (1995) Therapeutic brain concentration of the NMDA receptor antagonist amantadine. Neuropharmacology. **34**: 713–721.
53 Pud D et al. (1998) The NMDA receptor antagonist amantadine reduces surgical neuropathic pain in cancer patients: a double blind, randomized, placebo controlled trial. Pain. **75**: 349–354.
54 Eisenberg E and Pud D (1998) Can patients with chronic neuropathic pain be cured by acute administration of the NMDA receptor antagonist amantadine? Pain. **74**: 337–339.
55 Twycross R et al. (2009) Symptom Management in Advanced Cancer (4e). palliativedrugs.com, Nottingham.
56 Sola A and Bonica J (1990) Myofascial pain syndromes. In: J Bonica (ed) The Management of Pain (2e). Lea and Febiger, Philadelphia, pp. 352–367.
57 Mannix K et al. (2000) Using bisphosphonates to control the pain of bone metastases: evidence-based guidelines for palliative care. Palliative Medicine. **14**: 455–461.

ACETAMINOPHEN

Class: Non-opioid analgesic.

Indications: Mild–moderate pain, migraine, headache, pyrexia.

Pharmacology

Acetaminophen (rINN paracetamol) is a synthetic centrally-acting non-opioid analgesic. Although some studies have suggested a peripheral action,[1,2] most evidence points to a purely central effect.[3] Like NSAIDs, acetaminophen is antipyretic; unlike NSAIDs, it has no peripheral anti-inflammatory effect.

Acetaminophen reduces the production of prostanoids in the CNS by inhibiting cyclo-oxygenase (COX).[4] It is possible that acetaminophen reduces the active oxidized form of COX to an inactive form. Thus, the mechanism by which acetaminophen inhibits COX activity could be different from that of NSAIDs. Acetaminophen also interacts with the l-arginine-nitric oxide, serotonin and opioid systems.[5,6] Animal studies suggest that there may be synergy between acetaminophen and NSAIDs.[7]

The metabolism of acetaminophen is age and dose-dependent. Only 2–5% of a therapeutic dose of acetaminophen is excreted unchanged in the urine; the remainder is metabolized mainly by the liver. At therapeutic doses, >80% of acetaminophen is metabolized to glucuronide and sulfate conjugates. About 10% is converted by cytochrome P450-dependent hepatic mixed-function oxidase to a highly reactive metabolite. In turn, this metabolite is rapidly inactivated by conjugation with glutathione and excreted in the urine after further metabolism.

The recommended dose limit for acetaminophen of 4g/24h is more traditional than scientific. However, although a single therapeutic dose of 1.5–2g is not harmful, the effects of taking acetaminophen at >4g/24h over a long period could be dangerous in debilitated patients.[8,9] Little is known about the relationship between acetaminophen dose and body weight; 1g equates to 25mg/kg in a 40kg person, but only 12.5mg/kg in someone weighing 80kg; however, the clinical significance of this is uncertain.

Factors which place a patient at increased risk of hepatotoxicity from an overdose include:
- old age
- poor nutritional status } lower glutathione stores[10]
- fasting/anorexia
- concurrent use of enzyme-inducing drugs, e.g. **phenobarbital**
- chronic alcohol abuse.[11]

Acute alcohol intake does not increase the risk of hepatotoxicity. In fact, because alcohol and acetaminophen compete for the same oxidative enzymes, acute alcohol consumption at the time of an acetaminophen overdose may be protective.

In alcoholics, and possibly others at increased risk, acute hepatic failure can occur with the regular ingestion of 7–8g/24h.[8] Acute hepatic failure has also been reported in patients treating themselves for dental pain, notably in a 21-year-old man who took >9g/24h for 4 days.[12] Animal data suggest that a high dose may be more toxic when divided than when given as a single dose.

A single overdose of acetaminophen below 125mg/kg (7.5g in a 60kg person) is unlikely to result in liver damage. At twice this dose, the probability of liver damage is around 50%, but the individual may remain well. A dose of 500mg/kg (30g in a 60kg person) is almost certain to produce life-threatening liver damage. Hepatotoxicity results from the production of a toxic metabolite, N-acetyl-p-benzoquinoneimine (NAPQI; Figure 5.7). Normally this is detoxified by conjugation with glutathione but, in acetaminophen overdose, the body's glutathione store becomes exhausted and the resulting large quantity of NAPQI reacts with liver parenchymal cells, leading to cell death. Overdose can be treated using the glutathione precursor, IV **acetylcysteine**. This should ideally be given within 15h of the overdose, when it prevents NAPQI from reacting with liver cell proteins, but may well help for up to 3 days because it has a protective effect against apoptosis (programmed cell death).[13]

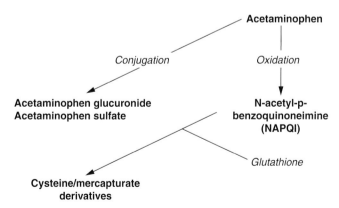

Figure 5.7 Metabolism of acetaminophen.

In patients undergoing molar dental extraction, compared with 1g, 2g of acetaminophen gave 50% more relief for 50% more time (5h vs. 3.2h).[14] Thus, there may be a place for an initial loading dose when prescribing acetaminophen. However, chronic administration of doses of 2g cannot be recommended because of the danger of hepatotoxicity.[9]

RCTs have yielded conflicting results regarding the benefit of acetaminophen in cancer patients receiving strong opioids. In one, no benefit was seen with acetaminophen (vs. placebo)[15] whereas, in the second, a small but clinically important additive effect was seen in about 1/3 of patients despite the fact that 1/2 were already taking an NSAID or a corticosteroid as well as a strong opioid.[16]

Thus, a pragmatic solution would be:

- to limit the long-term use of acetaminophen to patients in whom definite benefit is seen within 48h of starting treatment
- if already taking acetaminophen with definite past benefit but increasing pain now necessitates the *addition* of a strong opioid, to review the need for continued acetaminophen by stopping it after a few days of satisfactory pain relief with both drugs; if the pain returns, re-instate the acetaminophen, otherwise do not.

Bio-availability 60% after 500mg PO, 90% after 1g PO; PR is about 2/3 of PO, but is higher with two 500mg suppositories than with one 1g suppository.

Onset of action 15–30min PO; delayed if administered with food, particularly carbohydrates.[17]

Time to peak plasma concentration widely variable PO, e.g. 20min in fasting state but 1–2h if delayed gastric emptying, and if SR.[18,19]

Plasma halflife 1.25–3h PO.[18,19]

Duration of action 4–6h PO (normal-release); ⩾8h PO SR.[19]

Cautions

Concurrent use of $5HT_3$-receptor antagonists may completely block the analgesic effect of acetaminophen.[20]

Renal impairment. Severe hepatic impairment, particularly when associated with alcohol dependence and malnutrition. Overdose causes liver damage and, less frequently, renal damage.[21]

Concurrent administration with **warfarin**: a regular total *daily* intake of acetaminophen ⩾1,300mg for one week may increase the INR to >6,[22,23] but a total *weekly* dose of acetaminophen of ⩽2g has no effect. The underlying mechanism is not clear, but may relate to interference with the hepatic synthesis of factors II, VII, IX and X.

Metoclopramide speeds the absorption of acetaminophen. **Cholestyramine** reduces its absorption; separate administration by ⩾1h.[24]

There is no definite evidence that acetaminophen precipitates asthma in asthmatics.[25,26] Acetaminophen can be taken by at least 2/3 of patients who are hypersensitive to **aspirin** or other NSAID.[27,28] In people with a history of **aspirin**/NSAID-induced asthma, give a test dose of 250mg and observe for 2–3h. If no undesirable effects occur, acetaminophen can safely be used in standard doses.[26]

Undesirable effects

For full list, see manufacturer's Product Monograph.

Rare (<0.1%, >0.01%): cholestatic jaundice,[29,30] acute pancreatitis, thrombocytopenia, agranulocytosis, anaphylaxis.[31–33]

Dose and use

In patients already receiving strong opioids (± an NSAID), if definite added benefit is not seen within 2 days of starting regular acetaminophen, it should be discontinued.[15]

Typical PO doses for adults range from 500mg–1g q6h–q4h: the latter dose exceeds the 4g maximum recommended for daily use but is often given with normal-release **morphine** q4h.[16] In children, the standard dose is 15mg/kg q.i.d. Given the lower bio-availability of PR acetaminophen, 1.5g q.i.d. would seem to be a reasonable and safe dose in adults.

Supply

Acetaminophen (generic)
Tablets 325mg, 28 days @ 650mg q.i.d. = $6.
Tablets 500mg, 28 days @ 1g q.i.d. = $17.
Caplets (capsule-shaped tablets) and **Geltabs** 500mg are available OTC; many patients find these easier to swallow.
Oral suspension 160mg/5mL, 28 days @ 1g q.i.d. = $169; *cherry, grape or bubble gum flavour.*

Tylenol® (McNeil)
Tablets regular strength 325mg, 28 days @ 650mg q.i.d. = $30.
Tablets extra strength 500mg, 28 days @ 1g q.i.d. = $34.
Caplets (capsule-shaped tablets) 325mg and 500mg, and **rapid-release capsules (Gelcaps)** 500mg are available OTC; many patients find these easier to swallow.
Oral suspension 160mg/5mL, 28 days @ 1g q.i.d. = $353; *grape or bubble gum flavour.*

Sustained-release
Tylenol® Arthritis Pain (McNeil)
Caplets ER 650mg, 28 days @ 1.3g t.i.d. = $35; *the caplets are biphasic, releasing 325mg immediately and 325mg in a timed-release manner over 8h.*

Rectal products
Acetaminophen (generic)
Suppositories 325mg, 650mg, 28 days @ 1 q.i.d. = $139 and $160 respectively.

Acetaminophen is also available in several combination products with weak opioids or **oxycodone.**

1 Lim R *et al.* (1964) Site of action of narcotic and non-narcotic analgesics determined by blocking bradykinin-evoked visceral pain. *Archives Internationales de Pharmacodynamie et de Therapie.* **152**: 25–58.
2 Moore U *et al.* (1992) The efficacy of locally applied aspirin and acetaminophen in postoperative pain after third molar surgery. *Clinical Pharmacology and Therapeutics.* **52**: 292–296.
3 Twycross RG *et al.* (2000) Paracetamol. *Progress in Palliative Care.* **8**: 198–202.
4 Flower RJ and Vane JR (1972) Inhibition of prostaglandin synthetase in brain explains the anti-pyretic activity of paracetamol. *Nature.* **240**: 410–411.
5 Bjorkman R *et al.* (1994) Acetaminophen (paracetamol) blocks spinal hyperalgesia induced by NMDA and substance P. *Pain.* **57**: 259–264.
6 Pini L *et al.* (1997) Naloxone-reversible antinociception by paracetamol in the rat. *Journal of Pharmacology and Experimental Therapeutics.* **280**: 934–940.
7 Miranda HF *et al.* (2006) Synergism between paracetamol and nonsteroidal anti-inflammatory drugs in experimental acute pain. *Pain.* **121**: 22–28.
8 Larson AM *et al.* (2005) Acetaminophen-induced acute liver failure: results of a United States multicenter, prospective study. *Hepatology.* **42**: 1364–1372.
9 Watkins PB *et al.* (2006) Aminotransferase elevations in healthy adults receiving 4 grams of acetaminophen daily: a randomized controlled trial. *Expert Opinion on Pharmacotherapy.* **296**: 87–93.
10 Horsmans Y *et al.* (1998) Paracetamol-induced liver toxicity after intravenous administration. *Liver.* **18**: 294–295.
11 Zimmerman H and Maddrey W (1995) Acetaminophen (paracetamol) hepatotoxicity with regular intake of alcohol: analysis of instances of therapeutic misadventure. *Hepatology.* **22**: 767–773.
12 Sivaloganathan K *et al.* (1993) Pericoronitis and accidental paracetamol overdose: a cautionary tale. *British Dental Journal.* **174**: 69–71.
13 BNF (2008) Emergency treatment of poisoning. In: *British National Formulary* (No. 55). British Medical Association and Royal Pharmaceutical Society of Great Britain, London. Current BNF available from: www.bnf.org/bnf/bnf/current/
14 Juhl GI *et al.* (2006) Analgesic efficacy and safety of intravenous paracetamol (acetaminophen) administered as a 2g starting dose following third molar surgery. *European Journal of Pain.* **10**: 371–377.
15 Axelsson B and Christensen S (2003) Is there an additive analgesic effect of paracetamol at step 3? A double-blind randomized controlled study. *Palliative Medicine.* **17**: 724–725.
16 Stockler M *et al.* (2004) Acetaminophen (paracetamol) improves pain and well-being in people with advanced cancer already receiving a strong opioid regimen: a randomized, double-blind, placebo-controlled cross-over trial. *Journal of Clinical Oncology.* **22**: 3389–3394.
17 Divoll M *et al.* (1982) Effect of food on acetaminophen absorption in young and elderly subjects. *Journal of Clinical Pharmacology.* **22**: 571–576.
18 Prescott LF (1996) *Paracetamol (Acetaminophen) A Critical Bibliographic Review.* Taylor & Francis, London.
19 AHFS (2009) Acetaminophen AHFS Drug Information (online edition). American Society of Health-System Pharmacists. Bethesda. Available from: www.ahfsdruginformation.com
20 Pickering G *et al.* (2006) Analgesic effect of acetaminophen in humans: first evidence of a central serotonergic mechanism. *Clinical Pharmacology and Therapeutics.* **79**: 371–378.
21 D'Arcy P (1997) Paracetamol. *Adverse Drug Reaction Toxicology Review.* **16**: 9–14.
22 Bell W (1998) Acetaminophen and warfarin: undesirable synergy. *Journal of the American Medical Association.* **279**: 702–703.
23 Hylek E *et al.* (1998) Acetaminophen and other risk factors for excessive warfarin in anticoagulation. *Journal of the American Medical Association.* **279**: 657–662.

24 Baxter K (ed) (2008) *Stockley's Drug Interactions* (8e). Pharmaceutical Press, London.
25 Shaheen S *et al.* (2000) Frequent paracetamol use and asthma in adults. *Thorax.* **55**: 266–270.
26 Shin G *et al.* (2000) Paracetamol and asthma. *Thorax.* **55**: 882–884.
27 Szczeklik A (1986) Analgesics, allergy and asthma. *Drugs.* **32**: 148–163.
28 Settipane R *et al.* (1995) Prevalence of cross-sensitivity with acetaminophen in aspirin-sensitive asthmatic subjects. *Journal of Allergy and Clinical Immunology.* **96**: 480–485.
29 Waldum H *et al.* (1992) Can NSAIDs cause acute biliary pain and cholestasis? *Journal of Clinical Gastroenterology.* **14**: 328–330.
30 Wong V *et al.* (1993) Paracetamol and acute biliary pain with cholestasis. *Lancet.* **342**: 869.
31 Leung R *et al.* (1992) Paracetamol anaphylaxis. *Clinical and Experimental Allergy.* **22**: 831–833.
32 Mendizabal S and Gomez MD (1998) Paracetamol sensitivity without aspirin intolerance. *Allergy.* **53**: 457–458.
33 Morgan S and Dorman S (2004) Paracetamol (acetaminophen) allergy. *Journal of Pain and Symptom Management.* **27**: 99–101.

NON-STEROIDAL ANTI-INFLAMMATORY DRUGS (NSAIDS)

Non-steroidal anti-inflammatory drugs (NSAIDs) are essential drugs for cancer pain management.[1,2] They prevent or reverse inflammation-induced hyperalgesia, not only locally but also in the CNS.[3]

However, many NSAIDs have been linked with an increased risk of thrombotic events.[4] The risk is established with the coxibs and this led to the withdrawal of **rofecoxib** and **valdecoxib**.[5–11] Consequently, *PCF* does not, at present, feature any of the coxibs in an individual drug monograph.

The situation with non-selective NSAIDs is more variable.[11,12] There appears to be no risk with **naproxen** (even with doses ≥1g/24h),[13] an increased risk with **diclofenac** and high-dose **ibuprofen**, but not low-dose **ibuprofen** (see p.265).[4,14] Thus, thrombosis is *not* a class effect of non-selective NSAIDs. However, as yet, no study has examined cancer patients receiving NSAIDs.

The increased risk must be kept in perspective: even for coxibs, the number of additional thrombotic events (mainly myocardial infarctions) is only 3/1,000 patients per year of use.[4] It is not clear how many of these are fatal. If 1/6–1/3, this would give a death rate of about 1 in 1,000–2,000 patients *per year of use* from thrombosis.

Strictly comparable data are not available for serious GI morbidity and mortality. However, derived from cohort studies, in patients taking an NSAID for *at least 2 months* the risk of a bleeding ulcer or perforation is of the order of 1 in 500.[15] Further, on average, 1 in 1,200 patients taking NSAIDs for *at least 2 months* will die from gastroduodenal complications.[15]

The relevance of these figures obviously varies according to the patient-group concerned. In those with terminal illness, the benefit associated with greater physical comfort may far outweigh the potential harm from thrombotic or GI complications, even foreshortened survival.

Indeed, despite their potential for harm, *PCF* regards NSAIDs as essential analgesics for most patients with cancer pain, and for other pains with an inflammatory component. Even so, it is important to heed the official warnings which have been issued and, as a general rule, to use the lowest effective dose for the shortest possible length of time.[6,7,10,14,16]

In the midst of the current uncertainty, we would like to draw the attention of prescribers to **nabumetone** (see p.273). Although available for several decades, it is still widely overlooked (and thus there is a dearth of data about its use in palliative care). It is known to have low GI toxicity,[17,18] and it does not affect bleeding time.

NSAIDs are, by definition, anti-inflammatory analgesics. They are also antipyretic.[19] NSAIDs are of particular benefit for pains associated with inflammation, and thus are essential analgesics for most forms of pain caused by cancer, including neuropathic pain.[1,2,20–26] It is generally accepted that inhibition of cyclo-oxygenase is the main mechanism of action of NSAIDs.[27]

Cyclo-oxygenase

There are two distinct cyclo-oxygenase (COX) isoforms; COX-1 is 'constitutive', i.e. is part of the body's normal physiological constitution with near constant levels and activity in most tissues, including the CNS.[28,29] In contrast, COX-2 expression is generally low or non-existent but is 'inducible', i.e. is massively produced within a few hours by inflammation. The main exceptions to this are parts of the CNS, the kidneys, and the seminal vesicles, all of which contain constitutively high levels of COX-2 (Figure 5.8).[30]

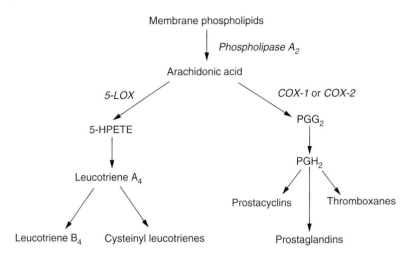

Figure 5.8 Products of arachidonic acid metabolism involved in inflammation.

Key: COX = cyclo-oxygenase; 5-HPETE = hydroperoxyeicosatetraenoic acid; LOX = lipoxygenase; PG = prostaglandin.

A third isoform, COX-3, has been postulated.[31] On the basis of animal studies, it was suggested that this was a variant of COX-1, made from the COX-1 gene, and that it was most abundant in the cerebral cortex and heart. It was thought by some to explain both the antipyretic and analgesic effects of **acetaminophen** (see p.240).[31] However, the present majority view is that COX-3 does *not* exist, certainly not in humans.[32–34]

Cyclo-oxygenase inhibition
Inflammation is associated with increased prostaglandin (PG) production both in the peripheral tissues and in the CNS.[35] The peripheral free nerve endings responsive to noxious stimuli become hypersensitive in the presence of inflammatory substances. Increased sensitivity of the nerve endings leads to increased transduction and thus to increased pain. Inflammation also leads to the increased production of PGs in the CNS, triggered hormonally, which leads to central sensitization of neurones in the dorsal horn, with further magnification of the noxious stimulus and more severe pain.[36,37]

By inhibiting the production of COX, NSAIDs block the synthesis of PGs both peripherally in the tissues and in the CNS. The relative peripheral and central contributions to the total analgesic effect depends, *inter alia*, on the NSAID in question, its pharmacokinetic characteristics, and the route of administration.[27]

Classification
Most commonly, NSAIDs are classified on the basis of their relative ability to inhibit COX-1 and COX-2. However, the degree of COX-2 selectivity varies according to the assay used[38,39] and whether the result is expressed in terms of 50% or 80% inhibition of the enzyme.[40,41] Although 80% inhibition is theoretically a better comparator, most studies use 50% (Table 5.1). Further, the

results of *in vitro* assays may not reliably reflect *in vivo* reality because of the potential impact of pharmacokinetic factors.[42]

Table 5.1 COX-2 selectivity ratio of IC_{50} COX-1/COX-2 (human whole blood assays)[41]

Drug	COX-2 selectivity ratio
Etoricoxib[a]	106
Rofecoxib[b]	35
Valdecoxib[c]	30
Celecoxib	7.6
Nimesulide[a]	7.3
Diclofenac	3.0
Etodolac	2.4
Meloxicam	2.0
Indomethacin	0.4
Ibuprofen	0.2
Piroxicam	0.08

a. not Canada
b. withdrawn worldwide
c. withdrawn in Europe, the USA and Canada.

Although it is more correct to think of a spectrum of selectivity,[38,40] it is customary to divide NSAIDs into several seemingly disparate categories (Table 5.2). Inevitably, there will be differences of opinion as to where the cut off between categories should come, particularly because selectivity can be dose-dependent.[38] For example, with **meloxicam** 7.5mg/24h, there is 70% COX-2 and 7% COX-1 inhibition but, with 15mg/24h, there is 80% COX-2 and 25% COX-1 inhibition.[43] Further, thromboxane B_2 production is reduced 66% by **meloxicam** 15mg/24h; the result of COX-1 inhibition (this compares with 95% inhibition by **indomethacin** 25mg t.i.d.).[44]

Table 5.2 Classification of NSAIDS

Preferential COX-1 inhibitors	Non-selective COX inhibitors	Preferential COX-2 inhibitors	Selective COX-2 inhibitors
Indomethacin	Aspirin	Celecoxib[a]	Coxibs
Ketorolac	Fenamates,	Diclofenac	
	e.g. mefenamic acid	Etodolac	
	Flurbiprofen	Meloxicam	
	Ibuprofen	Nabumetone	
	Naproxen	Nimesulide (not Canada)	
	Salicylates		

a. see Table 5.1 above for the rationale for this designation.

Additional sites of action

NSAIDs have other actions apart from inhibiting COX.[45–47] For example, NSAIDs affect brain concentrations of kynurenic acid, an endogenous antagonist which acts on the glycine recognition site of the NMDA-receptor-channel complex.[48] **Diclofenac** and **indomethacin** (dual COX inhibitors) increase brain kynurenic acid concentrations, whereas **meloxicam** and **parecoxib** (preferential and selective COX-2 inhibitors respectively; **parecoxib** is not available in Canada) cause a decrease. It is possible that at least some NSAIDs tonically modulate kynurenic acid metabolism, and thereby impact on central nociceptive mechanisms.

Other laboratory studies have shown that, under comparable conditions to those used in studies for **retigabine** (a novel anti-epileptic, not Canada), **diclofenac** and **meclofenamic acid** (not Canada) are effective openers of the potassium channels KCNQ2/3, and are thus facilitators of inhibitory M-currents.[49] The kinetics and effective concentrations of this effect were comparable to that shown for **retigabine**.[49] The clinical significance of these findings remains to be determined.

It is possible that non-selective NSAIDs are intrinsically more broad-spectrum in their central effects than COX-2 selective NSAIDs.[50] However, clinically, COX-2 selective inhibitors appear to be equally effective when compared with non-selective NSAIDs in inflammatory, dental and postoperative pain.[51] On the other hand, in dental pain, there is a tendency for weak COX inhibitors to be superior to **aspirin** and for strong inhibitors to be inferior, emphasizing the importance of not adopting too simplistic a view of the mode of action of these drugs (Table 5.3).

Table 5.3 Analgesic efficacy of oral NSAIDs in dental pain compared with aspirin 650mg[52]

Significantly superior	Not significantly different	Significantly inferior
Azapropazone (3)[a,b]	Diclofenac (1)	Fenbufen (1)[b]
Diflunisal (3)[b]	Etodolac (1)	Nabumetone (1)
Flurbiprofen (1)	Sulindac (1)	Ketoprofen (2)
Ketorolac (3)	Naproxen (3)	Tolmetin (3)[b]

a. numbers indicate capacity to inhibit PG synthesis: 1 = strong; 2 = moderate; 3 = weak
b. not Canada.

Animal studies suggest that there may be analgesic synergy between **acetaminophen** and NSAIDs.[53]

NSAIDs and pyrexia

All NSAIDs, including coxibs, are antipyretic.[54] In mice, deletion of the COX-2 gene blunts pyresis. In relation to paraneoplastic pyrexia in humans, it has been claimed that **naproxen** is the NSAID of choice.[55] However, an RCT of **naproxen** 250mg b.i.d. with **diclofenac** 25mg t.i.d. and **indomethacin** 25mg t.i.d. failed to detect a significant difference between the three drugs, although the mean time to response was much shorter for **naproxen** than for the other drugs (8h compared with >20h).[56] However, this could reflect the relatively low doses of **diclofenac** and **indomethacin** used. Although the antipyretic effect of all three NSAIDs tended to wear off after a few months, further benefit was obtained by switching to an alternative NSAID. However, the duration of benefit with second- and third-line drugs was generally shorter. Coxibs appear to be equally effective.[54]

For guidance on the use of drugs for treating paraneoplastic pyrexia and sweating, see Box 5.A.

Box 5.A Symptomatic drug treatment of paraneoplastic pyrexia and sweating

Begin by prescribing an antipyretic:
- acetaminophen 500mg–1g q.i.d. or p.r.n. (generally less toxic than an NSAID)
- NSAID, e.g. ibuprofen 200–400mg t.i.d. or p.r.n. (or the locally preferred alternative).

If the sweating des not respond to an NSAID, prescribe an antimuscarinic:
- amitriptyline 25–50mg at bedtime (may cause sedation, dry mouth and other antimuscarinic effects)
- scopolamine (hyoscine) *hydrobromide* 1mg/3days TD[57]
- glycopyrrolate up to 2mg PO t.i.d.

If an antimuscarinic fails, other options include:
- propranolol 10–20mg b.i.d.–t.i.d.
- cimetidine 400–800mg b.i.d.[58]
- olanzapine 5mg b.i.d.[59]
- thalidomide 100mg at bedtime.[60,61]

Thalidomide is generally seen as the last resort even though the response rate appears to be high.[61] This is because it can cause an irreversible painful peripheral neuropathy, and may also cause drowsiness (see p.405).

NSAIDs and platelet function

NSAIDs differ in their effect on platelet function (Table 5.4).

Table 5.4 NSAIDs and impairment of platelet function

Drug	Effect	Comment
Aspirin	+	Irreversible platelet dysfunction as a result of acetylation of platelet COX-1
Non-acetylated salicylates e.g. choline magnesium trisalicylate[a], diflunisal, salsalate[a]	–	No effect at recommended doses
Classical NSAIDs except diclofenac	+	Reversible platelet dysfunction e.g. ibuprofen, flurbiprofen, ketorolac, naproxen
Diclofenac	–	Although diclofenac inhibits platelet aggregation in laboratory tests, typical doses of diclofenac do not affect platelet function[62]
Etodolac	no data	
Meloxicam[63]	–	
Nabumetone	–	Has a dose-related effect on platelet aggregation, but no effect on bleeding time
Nimesulide[64,a]	–	
Coxibs[43,65]	–	

a. not Canada.

Undesirable effects

The undesirable effects have been categorized as type A ('augmented' effects) and type B ('bizarre' effects). Type A effects are predictable and dose-dependent, whereas type B are unpredictable and dose-independent (Table 5.5 and Table 5.6). GI toxicity is by far the most serious undesirable class effect of NSAIDs (see below).[66,67]

Table 5.5 Type A ('predictable') reactions to NSAIDs[68]

Organ/system	Clinical reaction
Blood	Decreased platelet aggregation (see Table 5.4)
GI tract	Dyspepsia Peptic ulceration Hemorrhage Perforation
Kidney	Salt and water retention Interstitial nephritis
Lung	Bronchospasm (asthma)

NSAIDs and the stomach

The incentive for developing selective COX-2 inhibitors was the need to reduce NSAID-induced gastroduodenal toxicity. RCT data indicate that coxibs reduce the incidence of serious GI events by at least 50%.[69–74] On the other hand, a case-control study involving nearly 100,000 patients suggests that there is no gastroprotective benefit to be gained by using a coxib.[75] However, a case-control study cannot negate the earlier more specific results of several RCTs.

Table 5.6 Type B ('unpredictable') reactions to NSAIDs[68]

Organ/system	Clinical reaction	NSAIDs
Immunological	Anaphylaxis	Most NSAIDs
Skin	Morbilliform rash Angioedema	Fenbufen (not Canada) Ibuprofen Azapropazone (not Canada) Piroxicam
Blood	Thrombocytopenia	Diclofenac Ibuprofen Piroxicam
	Hemolytic anemia	Mefenamic acid Diclofenac
GI tract	Diarrhea	Fenamates, e.g. mefenamic acid
Liver	Reye's syndrome (in children) Hepatotoxicity	Aspirin Diclofenac Sulindac
CNS	Aseptic meningitis	Ibuprofen

How much of the benefit relates to COX-2 selectivity is uncertain. Gastroduodenal toxicity depends on multiple factors (Box 5.B). **Ibuprofen** (a non-selective COX inhibitor)[76,77] and **nabumetone** (a preferential COX-2 inhibitor)[18] also have a low propensity for causing serious GI events, i.e. perforation, ulceration, bleeding (PUB). **Diclofenac** (a preferential COX-2 inhibitor) and **naproxen** (a non-selective COX inhibitor) would seem to be the next safest from this point of view.[76,77] In fact, when used for >6 months in patients with osteo-arthritis and rheumatoid arthritis, **diclofenac** caused no more gastrotoxicity than **celecoxib**.[78,79]

Box 5.B Factors intrinsic to NSAIDs which result in low gastroduodenal toxicity[80]

Competitive masking of COX-1 by inactive forms, e.g. R-ibuprofen, R-etodolac.

Weak/no uncoupling of oxidative phosphorylation
Low disruption of phospholipids in protective mucus and mucous membranes } non-acidic compounds, e.g. nabumetone, coxibs.

High protein-binding (less available).

Weak/no inhibition of platelet aggregation, e.g. non-acetylated salicylates, diclofenac, meloxicam, coxibs.

The situation may change when dual LOX/COX inhibitors come onto the market. Such drugs inhibit lipoxygenase (LOX) as well as both COX-1 and COX-2 and, compared with placebo, are said to cause no excess GI toxicity.[81]

Helicobacter pylori infection is also important in relation to NSAID-induced gastropathy. The infection-associated type B chronic atrophic gastritis mainly affects the antrum, and makes the extracellular matrix in that part of the stomach wall vulnerable to the back-diffusion of acid. Ionized NSAID molecules, circulating in the plasma, are transported passively through leaky capillary walls into the inflamed matrix where they become unionized in the acidic environment. In this state, the molecules are lipid-soluble and they move freely into the mucosal cells where, at a higher pH, the molecules become ionized again and consequently trapped. The local high concentration of NSAID leads to inhibition of the production of gastroprotective COX-1 in the stomach mucosa. Eradication of *H. pylori* infection (see p.367) will correct the atrophic gastritis and end the sequence of events initiated by acid back-diffusion. Eradication of *H. pylori* thus renders all COX-1-inhibiting NSAIDs safer to use.[82–86]

Risk factors for an NSAID-induced serious GI event (PUB) are listed in Box 5.C. For example, concurrent administration of a classical NSAID with coumarin anticoagulants increases the risk of bleeding >10 times. In rheumatoid arthritis, the risk of hospitalization and/or death increases progressively from 50 years.[87] Thus, compared with those under 50, the risk is twice as great in patients aged 50–65 years, 6 times greater in patients aged 65–75, and some 14 times greater in the over 75s. However, in rheumatoid arthritis there may well be concurrent risk factors which may confound the impact of aging. Thus, 65 years is widely considered to be the appropriate point for regarding age as a risk factor.

Box 5.C Risk factors for NSAID-induced serious gastro-intestinal event[66,87]

Age >65 years (see text).

Gastric infection with *H. pylori*.

Acid dyspepsia with an NSAID despite concurrent use of a gastroprotective agent, now or in the past.

Peptic ulcer ± GI hemorrhage in the last year confirmed by endoscopy, or strong clinical suspicion, e.g. hematemesis, melena.

Long-term use of maximum recommended doses of an NSAID.

Serious morbidity, e.g. cancer, diabetes mellitus, hypertension, cardiovascular disease, hepatic impairment, renal impairment.

Concurrent use of a corticosteroid, low-dose aspirin, or anticoagulant (warfarin or heparin).

Concurrent use of a serotonin re-uptake inhibitor (see text).

Platelets $<50 \times 10^9$/L.

Antidepressants which inhibit presynaptic serotonin re-uptake, notably SSRIs, **clomipramine**, **amitriptyline**, **venlafaxine**, decrease serotonin uptake from the blood by platelets.[88] Because platelets do not synthesize serotonin, serotonin re-uptake inhibitors decrease the platelet serotonin concentration which may adversely affect platelet aggregation. Particularly in those over 80, serotonin re-uptake inhibitors are an independent risk factor for GI bleeding.[89]

Patients with a high risk of serious gastropathy are best treated with an NSAID with a low propensity for causing gastrotoxicity (Box 5.D). Concurrent prophylaxis with a gastroprotective agent also helps to prevent serious gastric complications.[90–92] However, in one study, only 30% of patients with ≥2 risk factors received a gastroprotective agent.[93]

Note: even in high-risk patients, there is no evidence of additional benefit from a coxib combined with a gastroprotective drug compared with a traditional non-selective NSAID and a gastroprotective drug.[94,95]

Box 5.D Risk of NSAID-related gastroduodenal toxicity (see individual monographs)

Low	Average	High
Coxibs	Flurbiprofen	Aspirin
Diclofenac	Indomethacin	Ketorolac
Ibuprofen	Ketoprofen	
Meloxicam	Naproxen	
Nabumetone	Piroxicam	
Nimesulide (not Canada)		

Misoprostol, PPIs, and *double-dose* H_2-receptor antagonists are all effective at preventing chronic NSAID-related endoscopic gastric and duodenal ulcers.[91] **Misoprostol** 400microgram/24h is less effective than 800microgram and is still associated with diarrhea. Of all these treatments, only

misoprostol 800microgram/24h has been definitely shown to reduce the overall incidence of ulcer complications (perforation, hemorrhage or obstruction).[91] In addition, PPIs definitely reduce the incidence of re-bleeding from endoscopically confirmed peptic ulcers,[96] and may reduce the incidence of ulcer complications.[92]

NSAIDs and the cardiovascular system

Activated platelets synthesize thromboxane A_2 (TXA_2) which is COX-1-mediated (potent platelet aggregant and vasoconstrictor, i.e. prothrombotic). In contrast, endothelial cells synthesize PGI_2 which is COX-2-mediated (inhibits platelet activation and induces vasodilation, i.e. antithrombotic). **Aspirin**, via COX-1 and COX-2 inhibition, reduces both TXA_2 production and PGI_2 production, i.e. produces a balanced reduction of prostanoids with opposing actions. In contrast, coxibs (selective COX-2 inhibitors) will block PGI_2 production but have no impact on TXA_2 production, i.e. will lead to an imbalance between antithrombotic and prothrombotic states (favouring thrombosis).

In a study comparing long-term **rofecoxib** with **naproxen**, the rate of serious thrombotic events was significantly higher in the patients who received **rofecoxib**.[97] Subsequent confirmation of this tendency in a trial of **rofecoxib** in patients with a history of colorectal adenoma, manifesting after 18 months treatment, led to the worldwide withdrawal of **rofecoxib** in 2004.[98–100]

Other reports suggest that all coxibs may be prothrombotic,[67,101,102] particularly where there is a predisposition to thrombosis, e.g. in connective tissue disorders.[103] Because cancer is often associated with a prothrombotic tendency,[104–106] caution should be exercised if a coxib is prescribed for a cancer patient.

Celecoxib was not implicated initially, but more recent data suggest a dose-related hazard risk.[107–109] Thus, although there is no significant increased risk of a serious cardiovascular event with 400mg once daily, the hazard ratio is approximately doubled with 200mg b.i.d., and trebled with 400mg b.i.d.[109]

After the withdrawal of **rofecoxib**, and an increase in myocardial infarctions and strokes in patients given **parecoxib** or **valdecoxib** after coronary artery bypass grafting, the regulatory agencies in several countries launched enquiries into the cardiovascular safety of coxibs and other NSAIDs.[5–11] Health Canada concluded that:
- when *high* doses are used for *long* periods, all NSAIDs (whether or not COX-2 selective) are associated with an increased risk of cardiovascular events, including myocardial infarction and stroke. However:
  ▷ the exact nature of that increased risk may differ from one product to another
  ▷ it is not possible to identify precisely which patients are at higher risk.[8–11]

Further, Health Canada:
- restricted the licensed indications for COX-2-selective NSAIDs to osteo-arthritis, rheumatoid arthritis and short-term treatment of acute pain, e.g. sprains, tooth extraction
- advised patients with significant risk factors for myocardial infarction or stroke to consult their physician with a view to finding alternatives to COX-2-selective NSAIDs, and contra-indicated the use of **celecoxib** in such patients
- advised other patients on COX-2-selective NSAIDs to discuss the benefits and risks of other treatment options with their physician, based on their personal risk profile
- advised that NSAIDs should be prescribed for the shortest possible duration of treatment and used at the lowest effective dose.

In relation to non-selective NSAIDs, published data indicate:[4,13,14,110]
- no risk with **naproxen** (even with doses ⩾1g/24h),[13]
- a small thrombotic risk with **diclofenac** 150mg/24h[110]
- a small thrombotic risk with high doses of **ibuprofen** (e.g. 2,400mg/24h), but not at low doses (e.g. ⩽1,200mg/24h).

Thus, thrombosis should *not* be regarded as a class effect of non-selective NSAIDs.

NSAIDs and the kidneys

All NSAIDs cause an increase in Cl^- resorption from the proximal tubules, and enhance ADH activity, leading to salt (Na^+) and water retention. Thus NSAIDs antagonize the action of diuretics, and can exacerbate existing hypertension or lead to new onset hypertension.[111]

The proximal passive resorption of Na^+ leads to increased resorption of K^+ in the distal tubules; this can result in hyperkalemia. The renal risks of different NSAIDs (including coxibs) are similar, and thus are not a factor in determining choice.[112] Early studies which suggested that **sulindac** has little or no effect on renal PG synthesis have not been substantiated by subsequent reports.[113]

NSAIDs may also cause acute or acute-on-chronic renal failure particularly in patients with hypovolemia from any cause, e.g. diuretics, fever, dehydration, vomiting, diarrhea, hemorrhage, surgery. Thus, except in patients expected to die in a few days, dehydrated patients should be rehydrated when starting treatment with an NSAID. The risk of NSAID-induced renal failure is increased in situations where the plasma concentrations of vasoconstrictor substances such as angiotensin II, norepinephrine and vasopressin are increased, e.g. in heart failure, cirrhosis and nephrotic syndrome. The inhibition of renal PG production by NSAIDs prevents the protective vasodilatory mechanism for safeguarding renal blood flow from functioning effectively.[114,115]

Sporadic cases of interstitial nephritis ($\pm$ nephrotic syndrome or $\pm$ papillary necrosis) have been reported with most NSAIDs. However, acute renal failure necessitating discontinuation of treatment is uncommon ($<1\%$ of patients prescribed an NSAID).[116] Patients with multiple myeloma are at particular risk, although this is rare in the absence of Bence-Jones (light chain) proteinuria.[117–119]

NSAIDs and bronchospasm

Some patients, with or without a history of atopic asthma, give a history of **aspirin-** or NSAID-induced asthma. The prevalence, derived from oral provocation testing studies, is about 20% in the general adult population, and 5% in children.[120] Those who experience **aspirin**-induced asthma possibly differ from other people with asthma by depending more on the bronchodilating activity of PGE_2 than on the β-adrenergic receptor system.[121] **Aspirin** and other NSAIDs inhibit the production of PGE_2 with the result that more arachidonic acid is available as a substrate for leukotriene production; leukotrienes C4 and D4 are potent bronchoconstrictors and mucus secretagogues. Other unidentified bronchoconstrictors could also be involved.[122]

Aspirin-induced asthma typically occurs 30min–3h after ingestion of **aspirin**. Half of those affected react to even low-dose **aspirin** (80mg). Cross-sensitivity with other NSAIDs is normal, e.g. **diclofenac** (93%), **ibuprofen** (98%), **naproxen** (100%).[120] A history of allergic-type reactions (asthma, acute rhinitis, nasal polyps, angioedema, urticaria) with **aspirin** or other NSAID calls for extreme caution in prescribing a further NSAID (Table 5.7). Although previously considered safe in this respect, there are now reports of bronchospasm associated with the use of **benzydamine** oral rinse and **celecoxib** (manufacturers' data on file).

In contrast, the incidence of cross-sensitivity to **acetaminophen** is only 7%, and $<2\%$ of asthmatic patients are sensitive to both **aspirin** and **acetaminophen**.[123] Further, reactions to **acetaminophen** are generally less severe. Thus, **acetaminophen** should always be the initial non-opioid of choice for asthmatic patients.

Table 5.7 Use of NSAIDs in asthmatic patients

Patient characteristics	Recommendation
Anyone who has ever had an asthmatic reaction to aspirin or other NSAID; or anyone with high risk features of aspirin-induced asthma (severe asthma, nasal polyps, urticaria, or chronic rhinitis)	Avoid all products containing aspirin or other NSAID indefinitely; use acetaminophen instead unless also contra-indicated
Asthmatic patient >40 years old	Because aspirin-induced asthma may develop late in life, inform of risks of aspirin and other NSAIDs, and recommend acetaminophen. If NSAIDs are necessary, the first dose should be taken under medical supervision
All other asthmatic patients	Any NSAID, including aspirin, may be considered; but if any respiratory reaction is experienced, treatment should be stopped and medical advice obtained

NSAIDs and the liver

Patients with hepatic impairment are more susceptible to NSAID-induced renal impairment. Hence most Product Monographs for NSAIDs include active liver disease or significant hepatic impairment as a contra-indication.

In patients with cirrhosis it is difficult to obtain an accurate measure of renal function because the plasma creatinine concentrations tends to be low. This may relate to a reduced muscle mass and reduced conversion of creatine to creatinine.[124] NSAID-induced impairment of platelet function may increase the risk of bleeding from esophageal varices.

Cholestasis may reduce the elimination of NSAIDs excreted in bile (**indomethacin**, **sulindac**), and may reduce or delay absorption of fat-soluble NSAIDs, e.g. **ibuprofen**.[125]

Hepatotoxicity is a rare and unpredictable effect seen with most NSAIDs, including COX-2-selective ones. **Diclofenac** and **sulindac** may have the highest risk, and **ibuprofen** the least.[125]

NSAIDs and bone healing

There is strong evidence in animals that, after a fracture, NSAIDs (including coxibs) and corticosteroids prolong bone healing time and impair the mechanical strength of the new bone.[126] In contrast, in humans, there is a relative dearth of clinical data. However, high-dose and long-term NSAIDs (e.g. >2 weeks) probably have a similar effect, and increase the incidence of non-union.[127] On the other hand, even when used for only 2–5 days, NSAIDs decrease heterotopic (ectopic) bone formation, such as that commonly seen after major hip surgery.[127,128]

Thus, after a fracture, the use of an NSAID should ideally be limited to about 10 days, and then discontinued until healing is complete. However, in patients with other risk factors for delayed union or non-union (e.g. smoking, diabetes mellitus, corticosteroids), use **acetaminophen** instead.[126] On the other hand, if pain relief is inadequate despite the combined use of **acetaminophen** and an opioid, an NSAID should be prescribed despite its potential negative effect.

Contra-indications for NSAIDs

Although the Product Monographs for NSAIDs are not wholly consistent in this respect, the following is a general list of contra-indications for NSAIDs: active GI ulceration, bleeding, perforation or inflammation, hypersensitivity to **aspirin** or other NSAID (urticaria, rhinitis, asthma, angioedema), severe heart failure, active liver disease or significant hepatic impairment, severe renal impairment (creatinine clearance <30mL/min; CPS advises avoiding use if creatinine clearance <50mL/min), deteriorating renal function, hyperkalemia (>5mmol/L).

The listed contra-indications are not necessarily absolute. Depending on individual circumstances, there may well be occasions when 'contra-indication' means 'use but only with great caution and in the absence of a safer alternative'.

Important NSAID–other drug interactions

Patients on **warfarin** should have their INR closely monitored during the first week after starting an NSAID; increases of up to 60% have been reported (Table 5.8).[129,130]

Drug interactions are summarized in Table 5.8 and Table 5.9 (also see Cytochrome P450, p.000). Of particular importance is the interaction with **methotrexate** which is 60–80% excreted unchanged by the kidney. *Concurrent administration of* **methotrexate** *and an NSAID decreases the excretion of* **methotrexate** *and increases its toxicity.*[131] Two deaths have occurred with **aspirin**, three with **ketoprofen** and one with **naproxen**. Fatal or severe renal failure has also developed when intermediate-dose or high-dose **methotrexate** was combined with **ibuprofen** or **indomethacin**, and life-threatening neutropenia has been reported with several other NSAIDs.[131,132] Toxicity is related to dose and renal function; it is much less likely with chronic low-dose **methotrexate** in psoriasis or rheumatoid arthritis than with high-dose pulses of cancer chemotherapy, and in patients without pre-existing renal impairment.[131]

Table 5.8 Pharmacokinetic interactions: NSAIDs affecting other drugs [131,133]

Drug affected	NSAIDs implicated	Effect	Clinical implications
Aminoglycosides	All NSAIDs	Reduce renal function in susceptible individuals, reducing aminoglycoside clearance and increasing plasma concentration	Monitor plasma concentration and adjust dose
Baclofen	Ibuprofen ?other NSAIDs	Reduced excretion of baclofen with increased risk of toxicity	Reduce dose of baclofen
Chlorpropamide	Aspirin ?other salicylates	?Inhibits renal tubular excretion of chlorpropamide, increasing plasma concentration and hypoglycemic effects	Reduce chlorpropamide dose if necessary
Cyclosporine	Mefenamic acid Piroxicam ?Sulindac	?Inhibit the renal prostacyclin synthesis needed to maintain glomerular filtration and renal blood flow in patients on cyclosporine. Increase cyclosporine plasma concentrations and risk of renal toxicity	Monitor renal function
Corticosteroids	Indomethacin Naproxen	Displace corticosteroids from plasma protein-binding sites, increasing free corticosteroid levels and possibly therapeutic effect	Possible steroid-sparing effect
Digoxin	All NSAIDs (?except ketoprofen, meloxicam, piroxicam)	In heart failure, NSAIDs may precipitate renal failure, reducing digoxin excretion with increased risk of toxicity	In heart failure, avoid NSAIDs if possible; if not, check digoxin and creatinine plasma concentrations and reduce digoxin dose if necessary
Indomethacin	Diflunisal	Inhibits glucuronidation, increasing indomethacin plasma concentration (by about 50%) and risk of toxicity	Avoid combination
Lithium	All NSAIDs (?except salicylates; sulindac unpredictable)	?Inhibit renal excretion of lithium and increase plasma concentration with increased risk of severe toxicity	Halve dose of lithium and monitor lithium concentration

continued

Table 5.8 Continued

Drug affected	NSAIDs implicated	Effect	Clinical implications
Methotrexate	Salicylates All NSAIDs	Competitively inhibit the tubular excretion of methotrexate. Inhibit PGE_2 synthesis, reducing renal perfusion. Increase methotrexate plasma concentration with risk of severe toxicity	Avoid aspirin and other salicylates during chemotherapy; probably safe between pulses. Use other NSAIDs with caution. Much lower risk with low-dose chronic methotrexate therapy used in psoriasis or rheumatoid arthritis and if no pre-existing renal impairment
Phenytoin	?All NSAIDs	Displace phenytoin from plasma proteins	Clinical significance uncertain because the excess free phenytoin may be metabolized by the liver. However, phenytoin toxicity can develop even when the plasma concentration is still within the therapeutic range
Valproic acid	Aspirin ?other NSAIDS	Displaces from plasma proteins, inhibits valproic acid metabolism and increases plasma concentration	Avoid aspirin; with other NSAIDs reduce the dose of valproic acid if toxicity suspected
Warfarin	Celecoxib Flurbiprofen	Inhibits metabolism of warfarin and increases INR	Isolated cases also reported with several other NSAIDs, including diclofenac, ibuprofen, ketoprofen, sulindac, tiaprofenic acid, tolmetin and etoricoxib (not Canada); reduce dose of warfarin and check INR
Zidovudine	All NSAIDs	Increased hematological toxicity	Monitor blood count

Table 5.9 Pharmacokinetic interactions: other drugs affecting NSAIDs[131,133]

Drug implicated	NSAIDs affected	Effect	Clinical implications
Antacids	All EC NSAIDs	Destruction of enteric coating	Administer at different times
Antacids	Aspirin	Decreased absorption and reduced plasma concentration	Use an alternative NSAID
Antacids	Diflunisal	Aluminum- and magnesium-containing antacids reduce absorption unless taken with food, ?because of adsorption in the GI tract	
Antacids	Fenamates, e.g. mefenamic acid	Variable effects: aluminum hydroxide reduces rate but not extent of absorption, magnesium hydroxide increases rate and extent of absorption, sodium bicarbonate has no effect	Avoid aluminum-containing antacids
Antacids	Indomethacin Naproxen	Variable effects: aluminum-containing antacids reduce rate and extent of absorption of indomethacin and naproxen; magnesium-containing antacids reduce rate and extent of absorption of naproxen; sodium bicarbonate increases rate and extent of absorption of indomethacin and naproxen	Check NSAID remains effective
Barbiturates	Possibly all NSAIDs	Increased metabolic clearance of NSAID	May need higher dose of NSAID
Cyclosporine	Diclofenac	Increased plasma concentration of diclofenac	Halve the dose of diclofenac
Cholestyramine	Diclofenac Ibuprofen ?other NSAIDs	Anion exchange resin binds NSAIDs in the GI tract, reducing absorption	Separate administration by 4h; may need higher dose of NSAID
Cholestyramine	Meloxicam Piroxicam Tenoxicam Sulindac	Binding in GI tract prevents enterohepatic recycling and increases fecal loss, even if NSAID administered IV	Increase NSAID dose if necessary or use alternative NSAID; cholestyramine may be used to speed removal of NSAID after overdose

continued

Table 5.9 Continued

Drug implicated	NSAIDs affected	Effect	Clinical implications
Fluconazole	Celecoxib	Reduced celecoxib metabolism	Halve the dose of celecoxib
Ketoconazole	Etoricoxib (not Canada)	Reduced etoricoxib metabolism	Reduce the dose of etoricoxib
Metoclopramide	Aspirin	Increased rate and extent of absorption of aspirin in patients with migraine	Can be used therapeutically to speed onset of action of aspirin
Metoclopramide	Ketoprofen ?other poorly soluble NSAIDs	Reduced absorption, ?because faster gastric transit carries poorly soluble NSAIDs past their absorption site	Take NSAID 1–2h before metoclopramide
Probenecid	Probably all NSAIDs	Reduced metabolism and renal clearance of NSAIDs and glucuronide metabolite which are hydrolyzed back to parent drug; NSAIDs also reduce the uricosuric effect of probenecid	Consider a reduction in the dose of NSAID but could be used therapeutically to increase the response
Rifampin	Diclofenac Etoricoxib (not Canada)	Plasma concentration reduced because of CYP3A4 induction	Increase NSAID dose if pain returns
Ritonavir	Piroxicam ?other NSAIDs	Increased plasma concentration with increased risk of toxicity	Avoid concurrent use

Choice of NSAID

In practice, the choice of NSAID depends on several factors, including availability, efficacy, safety, and cost. In Canada, **nabumetone** (the safest NSAID from a GI point of view) costs more than **ibuprofen** and **naproxen**, but less than **diclofenac**. However, the ability to use **nabumetone** without gastric protection makes it comparable to **ibuprofen** or **naproxen** plus **misoprostol** 200microgram b.i.d., and considerably cheaper than any of these three NSAIDs plus either **misoprostol** 200microgram q.i.d. or a PPI. The renal risks of different NSAIDs, including coxibs, are similar, and thus are not a factor in determining choice.[112]

It is unclear if some cancer patients obtain more benefit from one particular NSAID as is anecdotally reported in rheumatoid arthritis, or if apparent differences simply relate to a relative increase in inhibition of PG synthesis. Patients with hypertension[134] and with cardiac, hepatic or renal impairment may deteriorate, and should be monitored appropriately.

Taking the various relevant factors into account, the following pragmatic approach is recommended:

- pain relief is a priority in palliative care, and even high-risk patients should not be denied the benefit of an NSAID if its use provides definitely better relief than, say, **acetaminophen** and **morphine**
- weigh up the risks and benefits for each patient before prescribing an NSAID
- generally avoid coxibs
- reserve **celecoxib** for patients with particularly high GI risk but with low cardiovascular risk
- as first-line NSAID, generally use:
  ▷ **nabumetone** (see p.273) and *no* gastroprotection *or*
  ▷ **ibuprofen** (see p.265) or **naproxen** (see p.271) plus **misoprostol** or a PPI as gastroprotection.

Ketorolac is the only parenteral NSAID available in Canada. It is not widely used in palliative care because of concerns about GI toxicity. Some centres prescribe it from time to time (either PO or SC) for patients with nociceptive pain which is not relieved by another NSAID combined with a strong opioid (see p.267).

For patients who have been taking an NSAID PO but now can no longer swallow, there are several options other than parenteral **ketorolac**:

- **naproxen** suppositories 500mg b.i.d.
- **diclofenac** suppositories 50mg b.i.d.–t.i.d.
- **indomethacin** suppositories 50–100mg b.i.d.
- **acetaminophen** suppositories 650mg q.i.d.

However, in someone expected to die within a day or so, it is generally possible to discontinue the NSAID without provoking a resurgence of pain.

In patients undergoing chemotherapy or with thrombocytopenia from other causes, it is better to use an NSAID which has no effect on bleeding time, e.g. **nabumetone** (see p.273) or **diclofenac** (see p.262).

Topical Nsaids

Topical NSAIDs are of value for the relief of pain associated with soft tissue trauma, e.g. strains and sprains.[135] Topically applied salicylates and some other NSAIDs can achieve local high SC concentrations, and therapeutically effective concentrations within synovial fluid and peri-articular tissues similar to those seen after PO administration.[136–138] Topical **ibuprofen** has been shown in an RCT to be better than placebo, but a trial with **piroxicam** showed no additional benefit.[139,140] Large quantities of topical NSAIDs have been associated with systemic effects, e.g. hypersensitivity, rash, asthma and renal impairment.[141] Topical **diclofenac** *sodium* 1.5% (Pennsaid®) and **diclofenac** *diethylamine* 1.16% (Voltaren Emulgel®) are marketed in Canada. A wound dressing impregnated with **ibuprofen** (Biatain-Ibu®) is also available. Locally compounded topical NSAIDs include **diclofenac** 2–5%, **ibuprofen** 5–10%, and **ketoprofen** 5–20%, generally formulated in pluronic lecithin organogel (PLO).

1 Mercadante S (2001) The use of anti-inflammatory drugs in cancer pain. *Cancer Treatment Reviews*. **27**: 51–61.
2 McNicol E et al. (2004) Nonsteroidal anti-inflammatory drugs, alone or combined with opioids, for cancer pain: a systematic review. *Journal of Clinical Oncology*. **22**: 1975–1992.
3 Koppert W et al. (2004) The cyclooxygenase isozyme inhibitors parecoxib and paracetamol reduce central hyperalgesia in humans. *Pain*. **108**: 148–153.

4   Kearney PM et al. (2006) Do selective cyclo-oxygenase-2 inhibitors and traditional non-steroidal anti-inflammatory drugs increase the risk of atherothrombosis? Meta-analysis of randomised trials. *British Medical Journal.* **332**: 1302–1308.

5   CHM (2004) Cardiovascular safety of COX-2 inhibitors and non-selective NSAIDs. Commission on Human Medicines. Available from: www.mhra.gov.uk/home/idcplg?IdcService=SS_GET_PAGE&nodeId=227

6   FDA (2005) Decision memo- Analysis and recommendations for agency action- COX-2 selective and non-selective NSAIDs. Food and Drugs Administration. Available from: www.fda.gov/downloads/Drugs/DrugSafety/PostmarketDrugSafetyInformationforPatientsandProviders/ucm106201.pdf

7   FDA (2005) FDA public health advisory. FDA announces important changes and additional warnings for COX-2 selective and non-selective non-steroidal anti-inflammatory drugs (NSAIDs). Food and Drugs Administration. Available from: www.fda.gov/Drugs/DrugSafety/PostmarketDrugSafetyInformationforPatientsandProviders/ucm150314.htm

8   Health Canada (2004) Safety and regulatory information regarding Celebrex® (celecoxib), Bextra™ (valdecoxib), and meloxicam subsequent to the withdrawl of Vioxx® (rofecoxib). Available from: www.hc-sc.gc.ca/ahc-asc/media/advisories-avis/_2004/2004_50bk1-eng.php

9   Health Canada (2004) Safety information regarding selective COX-2 inhibitor NSAIDs: Vioxx®, (rofecoxib), Celebrex® (celecoxib), Bextra™ (valdecoxib), Mobicox® (meloxicam) and generic forms of meloxicam. Available from: www.hc-sc.gc.ca/ahc-asc/media/advisories-avis/_2004/2004_69-eng.php

10 Health Canada (2005) Health Canada has asked Pfizer to suspend sales of its drug Bextra™ and informs Canadians of new restrictions on the use of Celebrex®. Available from: www.hc-sc.gc.ca/ahc-asc/media/advisories-avis/_2005/2005_17-eng.php

11 Health Canada (2005) Health Canada prohibits sale of Bextra in Canada. Available from: www.hc-sc.gc.ca/ahc-asc/media/advisories-avis/_2005/2005_134-eng.php

12 Patrignani P et al. (2008) NSAIDs and cardiovascular disease. *Heart.* **94**: 395–397.

13 Ray WA et al. (2009) Cardiovascular risks of nonsteroidal anti-inflammatory drugs in patients after hospitalization for serious coronary heart disease. *Circulation Cardiovascular Quality and Outcomes.* **2**: 155–163.

14 Duff G (2006) Safety of selective and non-selective NSAIDs. In: *Letter to health professionals from the Chairman of the Commission on Human Medicines, 24th October 2006.* Available from: www.mhra.gov.uk/Safetyinformation/Safetywarningsalertsandrecalls/Safetywarningsandmessagesformedicines/CON2025040

15 Tramer M et al. (2000) Quantitative estimation of rare adverse events which follow a biological progression: a new model applied to chronic NSAID use. *Pain.* **85**: 169–182.

16 EMEA (2006) Questions and answers on the review of non-selective NSAIDs. European Agency for the Evaluation of Medicinal Products. Available from: www.emea.europa.eu/pdfs/human/opiniongen/nsaidsq&a.pdf

17 Huang JQ et al. (1999) Gastrointestinal safety profile of nabumetone: a meta-analysis. *American Journal of Medicine.* **107 (suppl)**: 55S–61S; discussion 61S–64S.

18 Hedner T et al. (2004) Nabumetone: Therapeutic use and safety profile in the management of osteoarthritis and rheumatoid arthritis. *Drugs.* **64**: 2315–2343; discussion 2344–2345.

19 Turini ME and DuBois RN (2002) Cyclooxygenase-2: a therapeutic target. *Annual Review of Medicine.* **53**: 35–57.

20 Minotti V et al. (1998) Double-blind evaluation of short-term analgesic efficacy of orally administered diclofenac, diclofenac plus codeine, and diclofenac plus imipramine in chronic cancer pain. *Pain.* **74**: 133–137.

21 Yalcin S et al. (1998) A comparison of two nonsteroidal antiinflammatory drugs (diflunisal versus dipyrone) in the treatment of moderate to severe cancer pain: a randomized crossover study. *American Journal of Clinical Oncology.* **21**: 185–188.

22 Jenkins C and Bruera E (1999) Nonsteroidal anti-inflammatory drugs as adjuvant analgesics in cancer patients. *Palliative Medicine.* **13**: 183–196.

23 Mercadante S et al. (1999) Analgesic effects of nonsteroidal anti-inflammatory drugs in cancer pain due to somatic or visceral mechanisms. *Journal of Pain and Symptom Management.* **17**: 351–356.

24 Caraceni A et al. (2001) More on the use of nonsteroidal anti-inflammatories in the management of cancer pain. *Journal of Pain and Symptom Management.* **21**: 89–91.

25 Shah S and Hardy J (2001) Non-steroidal anti-inflammatory drugs in cancer pain: a review of the literature as relevant to palliative care. *Progress in Palliative Care.* **9**: 3–7.

26 Mercadante S et al. (2002) A randomised controlled study on the use of anti-inflammatory drugs in patients with cancer pain on morphine therapy: effects on dose-escalation and a pharmacoeconomic analysis. *European Journal of Cancer.* **38**: 1358–1363.

27 Burian M and Geisslinger G (2005) COX-dependent mechanisms involved in the antinociceptive action of NSAIDs at central and peripheral sites. *Pharmacology and Therepeutics.* **107**: 139–154.

28 Yermakova AV et al. (1999) Cyclooxygenase-1 in human Alzheimer and control brain: quantitative analysis of expression by microglia and CA3 hippocampal neurons. *Journal of Neuropathology and Experimental Neurology.* **58**: 1135.

29 Steven TD (2003) Similar enzymes, different mechanisms: COX-1 and COX-2 enzymes in neurologic disease. *Archives of Neurology.* **60**: 632.

30 Zha S et al. (2004) Cyclooxygenases in cancer: progress and perspective. *Cancer Letters.* **215**: 1–20.

31 Chandrasekharan N et al. (2002) COX-3, a cyclooxygenase-1 variant inhibited by acetaminophen and other analgesic/antipyretic drugs: cloning, structure, and expression. *Proceedings of the National Academy of Sciences of the United States of America.* **99**: 13926–13931.

32 Warner TD and Mitchell JA (2002) Cyclooxygenase-3 (COX-3): filling in the gaps toward a COX continuum? *Proceedings of the National Academy of Science USA.* **99**: 13371–13373.

33 Kis B et al. (2003) Putative cyclooxygenase-3 expression in rat brain cells. *Journal of Cerebral Blood Flow and Metabolism.* **23**: 1287–1292.

34 Kis B et al. (2004) Regional distribution of cyclooxygenase-3 mRNA in the rat central nervous system. *Brain Research Molecular Brain Research.* **126**: 78–80.

35 Schwab JM and Schluesener HJ (2003) Cyclooxygenases and central nervous system inflammation: conceptual neglect of cyclooxygenase 1. *Archives of Neurology.* **60**: 630–632.

36 Baba H et al. (2001) Direct activation of rat spinal dorsal horn neurons by prostaglandin E2. *Journal of Neuroscience.* **21**: 1750–1756.

37 Samad T et al. (2001) Interleukin-1B-mediated induction of COX-2 in the CNS contributes to inflammatory pain hypersensitivity. *Nature.* **410**: 471–475.

38 Churchill L et al. (1996) Selective inhibition of human cyclo-oxygenase-2 by meloxicam. *Inflammopharmacology.* **4**: 125–135.

39 Brooks P et al. (1999) Interpreting the clinical significance of the differential inhibition of cyclooxygenase-1 and cyclooxygenase-2. *Rheumatology.* **38**: 779–788.

40 Warner T *et al.* (1999) Nonsteroidal drug selectivities for cyclo-oxygenase-1 rather than cyclo-oxygenase-2 are associated with human gastrointestinal toxicity: a full *in vitro* analysis. *Proceedings of the National Academy of Science USA.* **96**: 7563–7568.

41 Riendeau D *et al.* (2001) Etoricoxib (MK-0663): Preclinical profile and comparison with other agents that selectively inhibit cyclooxygenase-2. *Journal of Pharmacology and Experimental Therapeutics.* **296**: 558–566.

42 Blain H *et al.* (2002) Limitation of the *in vitro* whole blood assay for predicting the COX selectivity of NSAIDs in clinical use. *British Journal of Clinical Pharmacology.* **53**: 255–265.

43 vanHecken A *et al.* (2000) Comparative inhibitory activity of rofecoxib, meloxicam, diclofenac, ibuprofen and naproxen on COX-2 versus COX-1 in healthy volunteers. *Journal of Clinical Pharmacology.* **40**: 1109–1120.

44 deMeijer A *et al.* (1999) Meloxicam, 15mg/day, spares platelet function in healthy volunteers. *Clinical Pharmacology and Therapeutics.* **66**: 425–430.

45 Abramson S *et al.* (1991) Non-steroidal anti-inflammatory drugs: effects on a GTP binding protein within the neutrophil plasma membrane. *Biochemical Pharmacology.* **41**: 1567–1573.

46 McCormack K (1994) Nonsteroidal anti-inflammatory drugs and spinal nociceptive processing. *Pain.* **59**: 9–43.

47 Svensson CI and Yaksh TL (2002) The spinal phospholipase-cyclooxygenase-prostanoid cascade in nociceptive processing. *Annual Review of Pharmacology and Toxicology.* **42**: 553–583.

48 Schwieler L *et al.* (2005) Prostaglandin-mediated control of rat brain kynurenic acid synthesis – opposite actions by COX-1 and COX-2 isoforms. *Journal of Neural Transmission.* **112**: 863–872.

49 Peretz A *et al.* (2005) Meclofenamic acid and diclofenac, novel templates of KCNQ2/Q3 potassium channel openers, depress cortical neuron activity and exhibit anticonvulsant properties. *Molecular Pharmacology.* **67**: 1053–1066.

50 McCormack K and Twycross RG (2001) Are COX-2 selective inhibitors effective analgesics. *Pain Review.* **8**: 13–26.

51 Dougados M *et al.* (2001) Evaluation of the structure-modifying effects of diacerein in hip osteoarthritis: ECHODIAH, a three-year, placebo-controlled trial. Evaluation of the Chondromodulating Effect of Diacerein in OA of the Hip. *Arthritis and Rheumatism.* **44**: 2539–2547.

52 McCormack K and Brune K (1991) Dissociation between the antinociceptive and anti-inflammatory effects of the nonsteroidal anti-inflammatory drugs: a survey of their analgesic efficacy. *Drugs.* **41**: 533–547.

53 Miranda HF *et al.* (2006) Synergism between paracetamol and nonsteroidal anti-inflammatory drugs in experimental acute pain. *Pain.* **121**: 22–28.

54 Kathula SK *et al.* (2003) Cyclo-oxygenase II inhibitors in the treatment of neoplastic fever. *Support Care Cancer.* **11**: 258–259.

55 Chang J (1988) Antipyretic effect of naproxen and corticosteroids on neoplastic fever. *Journal of Pain and Symptom Management.* **3**: 141–144.

56 Tsavaris N *et al.* (1990) A randomized trial of the effect of three nonsteroidal anti-inflammatory agents in ameliorating cancer-induced fever. *Journal of Internal Medicine.* **228**: 451–455.

57 Mercadante S (1998) Hyoscine in opioid-induced sweating. *Journal of Pain and Symptom Management.* **15**: 214–215.

58 Pittelkow M and Loprinzi C (2003) Pruritus and sweating in palliative medicine. In: D Doyle *et al.* (eds) *Oxford Textbook of Palliative Medicine* (3e). Oxford University Press, Oxford, pp. 573–587.

59 Zylicz Z and Krajnik M (2003) Flushing and sweating in an advanced breast cancer patient relieved by olanzapine. *Journal of Pain and Symptom Management.* **25**: 494–495.

60 Calder K and Bruera E (2000) Thalidomide for night sweats in patients with advanced cancer. *Palliative Medicine.* **14**: 77–78.

61 Deaner P (2000) The use of thalidomide in the management of severe sweating in patients with advanced malignancy: trial report. *Palliative Medicine.* **14**: 429–431.

62 Todd P and Sorkin E (1988) Diclofenac sodium: a reappraisal of its pharmacodynamic and pharmacokinetic properties, and therapeutic efficacy. *Drugs.* **35**: 244–285.

63 Guth B *et al.* (1996) Therapeutic doses of meloxicam do not inhibit platelet aggregation in man. *Rheumatology in Europe.* **25**: Abstract 443.

64 Cullen L *et al.* (1997) Selective suppression of cyclooxygenase-2 during chronic administration of nimesulide in man. In: *the Fourth International Congress on essential fatty acids and eicosanoids*; Edinburgh.

65 Clemett D and Goa K (2000) Celecoxib: a review of its use in osteoarthritis, rheumatoid arthritis and acute pain. *Drugs.* **59**: 957–980.

66 Hawkins C and Hanks G (2000) The gastroduodenal toxicity of nonsteroidal anti-inflammatory drugs. A review of the literature. *Journal of Pain and Symptom Management.* **20**: 140–151.

67 Ray WA *et al.* (2004) Cardiovascular toxicity of valdecoxib. *New England Journal of Medicine.* **351**: 2767.

68 Rawlins M (1997) Non-opioid analgesics. In: D Doyle *et al.* (eds) *Oxford Textbook of Palliative Medicine* (2e). Oxford University Press, Oxford, pp. 355–361.

69 Laine L *et al.* (1999) A randomized trial comparing the effect or rofecoxib, a cyclooxygenase 2-specific inhibitor, with that of ibuprofen on the gastroduodenal mucosa of patients with osteoarthritis. *Gastroenterology.* **117**: 776–783.

70 Lanza F *et al.* (1999) Specific inhibition of cyclooxygenase-2 with MK-0966 is associated with less gastroduodenal damage than either aspirin or ibuprofen. *Alimentary Pharmacology and Therapeutics.* **13**: 761–767.

71 Hawkey C *et al.* (2000) Comparison of the effect of rofecoxib (a cyclooxygenase 2 inhibitor), ibuprofen, and placebo on the gastroduodenal mucosa of patients with osteoarthritis. *Arthritis and Rheumatism.* **43**: 370–377.

72 Deeks J *et al.* (2002) Efficacy, tolerability, and upper gastrointestinal safety of celecoxib for treatment of osteoarthritis and rheumatoid arthritis; systematic review of randomised controlled trials. *British Medical Journal.* **325**: 619–623.

73 Laine L *et al.* (2002) Upper gastrointestinal event risk with COX-2 inhibitors depended on known risk factors. *Gastroenterology.* **123**: 1006–1012.

74 Mamdani M *et al.* (2002) Observational study of upper gastrointestinal haemorrhage in elderly patients given selective cyclo-oxygenase-2 inhibitors or conventional non-steroidal anti-inflammatory drugs. *British Medical Journal.* **325**: 624–627.

75 Hippisley-Cox J and Coupland C (2005) Risk of myocardial infarction in patients taking cyclo-oxygenase-2 inhibitors or conventional non-steroidal anti-inflammatory drugs: population based nested case-control analysis. *British Medical Journal.* **330**: 1366.

76 Laporte JR *et al.* (2004) Upper gastrointestinal bleeding associated with the use of NSAIDs: newer versus older agents. *Drug Safety.* **27**: 411–420.

77 Lanas A *et al.* (2006) Risk of upper gastrointestinal ulcer bleeding associated with selective cyclo-oxygenase-2 inhibitors, traditional non-aspirin non-steroidal anti-inflammatory drugs, aspirin and combinations. *Gut.* **55**: 1731–1738.

78 Bombardier C (2002) An evidence-based evaluation of the gastrointestinal safety of coxibs. *American Journal of Cardiology.* **89 (suppl 6)**: 3d–9d.

79 Juni P et al. (2002) Risk of myocardial infarction associated with selective COX-2 inhibitors: questions remain. *Archives of Internal Medicine.* **162**: 2639–2640.

80 Rainsford K (1999) Profile and mechanisms of gastrointestinal and other side effects of nonsteroidal anti-inflammatory drugs (NsAIDs). *American Journal of Medicine.* **107 (suppl 6A)**: 27s–36s.

81 Bias P et al. (2004) The gastrointestinal tolerability of the LOX/COX inhibitor, licofelone, is similar to placebo and superior to naproxen therapy in health volunteers: Results from a randomized, controlled trial. *American Journal of Gastroenterology.* **99**: 611–618.

82 McCormack K (1989) Mathematical model for assessing risk of gastrointestinal reactions to NSAIDs. In: K Rainsford (ed) *Azapropazone–over two decades of clinical use.* Kluwer Academic Publishers, Boston, pp. 81–93.

83 Becker JC et al. (2004) Current approaches to prevent NSAID-induced gastropathy–COX selectivity and beyond. *British Journal of Clinical Pharmacology.* **58**: 587–600.

84 Sung JJ (2004) Should we eradicate *Helicobacter pylori* in non-steroidal anti-inflammatory drug users? *Alimentary Pharmacology and Therapeutics.* **20 (suppl 2)**: 65–70.

85 Chang CC et al. (2005) Eradication of *Helicobacter pylori* significantly reduced gastric damage in nonsteroidal anti-inflammatory drug-treated Mongolian gerbils. *World Journal of Gastroenterology.* **11**: 104–108.

86 Di Leo V et al. (2005) Effect of *Helicobacter pylori* and eradication therapy on gastrointestinal permeability. Implications for patients with seronegative spondyloarthritis. *Journal of Rheumatology.* **32**: 295–300.

87 Fries J et al. (1991) Nonsteroidal anti-inflammatory drug-associated gastropathy: incidence and risk factor models. *American Journal of Medicine.* **91**: 213–222.

88 Ross S et al. (1980) Inhibition of 5-hydroxytryptamine uptake in human platelets by antidepressant agents *in vivo*. *Psychopharmacology.* **67**: 1–7.

89 van Walraven C et al. (2001) Inhibition of serotonin reuptake by antidepressants and upper gastrointestinal bleeding in elderly patients: retrospective cohort study. *British Medical Journal.* **323**: 655–657.

90 Hollander D (1994) Gastrointestinal complications of nonsteroidal anti-inflammatory drugs: prophylactic and therapeutic strategies. *American Journal of Medicine.* **96**: 274–281.

91 Rostom A et al. (2002) Prevention of NSAID-induced gastroduodenal ulcers. *Cochrane Database Systematic Review.* **10**: CD002296.

92 Hooper L et al. (2004) The effectiveness of five strategies for the prevention of gastrointestinal toxicity induced by non-steroidal anti-inflammatory drugs: systematic review. *British Medical Journal.* **329**: 948.

93 Smalley W et al. (2002) Underutilization of gastroprotective measures in patients receiving nonsteroidal antiinflammatory drugs. *Arthritis and Rheumatism.* **46**: 2195–2200.

94 Cryer B (2006) A COX-2-specific inhibitor plus a proton-pump inhibitor: is this a reasonable approach to reduction in NSAIDs' GI toxicity? *American Journal of Gastroenterology.* **101**: 711–713.

95 Scheiman JM et al. (2006) Prevention of ulcers by esomeprazole in at-risk patients using non-selective NSAIDs and COX-2 inhibitors. *American Journal of Gastroenterology.* **101**: 701–710.

96 Leontiadis GI et al. (2005) Systematic review and meta-analysis of proton pump inhibitor therapy in peptic ulcer bleeding. *British Medical Journal.* **330**: 568.

97 Bombardier C et al. (2000) Comparison of upper gastrointestinal toxicity of rofecoxib and naproxen in patients with rheumatoid arthritis. *New England Journal of Medicine.* **343**: 1520–1528.

98 Dieppe PA et al. (2004) Lessons from the withdrawal of rofecoxib. *British Medical Journal.* **329**: 867–868.

99 Fitzgerald GA (2004) Coxibs and cardiovascular disease. *New England Journal of Medicine.* **351**: 1709–1711.

100 Topol EJ (2004) Failing the public health–rofecoxib, Merck, and the FDA. *New England Journal of Medicine.* **351**: 1707–1709.

101 Finckh A and Aronson MD (2005) Cardiovascular risks of cyclooxygenase-2 inhibitors: where we stand now. *Annals of Internal Medicine.* **142**: 212–214.

102 Topol EJ (2005) Arthritis medicines and cardiovascular events–'house of coxibs'. *Journal of the American Medical Association.* **293**: 366–368.

103 Crofford L et al. (2000) Thrombosis in patients with connective tissue diseases treated with specific cyclooxygenase 2 inhibitors. A report of four cases. *Arthritis and Rheumatism.* **43**: 1891–1896.

104 Levine M and Hirsh J (1990) The diagnosis and treatment of thrombosis in the cancer patient. *Seminars in Oncology.* **17**: 160–171.

105 Piccioli A et al. (1996) Cancer and venous thromboembolism. *American Heart Journal.* **132**: 850–855.

106 Blom JW et al. (2005) Malignancies, Prothrombotic Mutations, and the Risk of Venous Thrombosis. *Journal of the American Medical Association.* **293**: 715.

107 Caldwell B et al. (2006) Risk of cardiovascular events and celecoxib: a systematic review and meta-analysis. *Journal of the Royal Society of Medicine.* **99**: 132–140.

108 Singh G et al. (2006) Celecoxib versus naproxen and diclofenac in osteoarthritis patients: SUCCESS-I Study. *American Journal of Medicine.* **119**: 255–266.

109 Solomon SD et al. (2008) Cardiovascular risk of celecoxib in 6 randomized placebo-controlled trials: the cross trial safety analysis. *Circulation.* **117**: 2104–2113.

110 Cannon CP et al. (2006) Cardiovascular outcomes with etoricoxib and diclofenac in patients with osteoarthritis and rheumatoid arthritis in the Multinational Etoricoxib and Diclofenac Arthritis Long-term (MEDAL) programme: a randomised comparison. *Lancet.* **368**: 1771–1781.

111 Cheng HF and Harris RC (2004) Cyclooxygenases, the kidney, and hypertension. *Hypertension.* **43**: 525–530.

112 Schneider V et al. (2006) Association of selective and conventional nonsteroidal antiinflammatory drugs with acute renal failure: A population-based, nested case-control analysis. *American Journal of Epidemiology.* **164**: 881–889.

113 Eriksson L-O et al. (1990) Effects of sulindac and naproxen on prostaglandin excretion in patients with impaired renal function and rheumatoid arthritis. *American Journal of Medicine.* **89**: 313–321.

114 MacDonald T (1994) Selected side-effects: 14. Non-steroidal anti-inflammatory drugs and renal damage. *Prescribers' Journal.* **34**: 77–80.

115 Patrono C and Dunn MJ (1987) The clinical significance of inhibition of renal prostaglandin synthesis. *Kidney International.* **32**: 1–12.

116 Venturini C et al. (1998) Nonsteroidal anti-inflammatory drug-induced renal failure: a brief review of the role of cyclooxygenase isoforms. *Current Opinion in Nephrology and Hypertension.* **7**: 79–82.

117 Winearls C (1995) Acute myeloma kidney. *Kidney International.* **48**: 1347–1361.

118 Iggo N et al. (1997) The development of cast nephropathy in multiple myeloma. *QJM: Monthly Journal of the Association of Physicians.* **90**: 653–656.

119 Irish AB et al. (1997) Presentation and survival of patients with severe renal failure and myeloma. QJM: Monthly Journal of the Association of Physicians. 90: 773–780.

120 Jenkins C et al. (2004) Systematic review of prevalence of aspirin induced asthma and its implications for clinical practice. British Medical Journal. 328: 434.

121 Szczeklik A and Sanak M (2000) Genetic mechanisms in aspirin-induced asthma. American Journal of Respiratory and Critical Care Medicine. 161: S142–146.

122 Capron A et al. (1985) New functions for platelets and their pathological implications. International Archives of Allergy and Applied Immunology. 77: 107–114.

123 Settipane R et al. (1995) Prevalence of cross-sensitivity with acetaminophen in aspirin-sensitive asthmatic subjects. Journal of Allergy and Clinical Immunology. 96: 480–485.

124 Delco F et al. (2005) Dose adjustment in patients with liver disease. Drug Safety. 28: 529–545.

125 North-Lewis P (ed) (2008) Drugs and the Liver. Pharmaceutical Press, London, pp. 178–187.

126 Boursinos LA et al. (2009) Do steroids, conventional non-steroidal anti-inflammatory drugs and selective Cox-2 inhibitors adversely affect fracture healing? Journal of Musculoskeletal Neuronal Interactions. 9: 44–52.

127 Pountos I et al. (2008) Pharmacological agents and impairment of fracture healing: what is the evidence? Injury. 39: 384–394.

128 Vuolteenaho K et al. (2008) Non-steroidal anti-inflammatory drugs, cyclooxygenase-2 and the bone healing process. Basic & Clinical Pharmacology and Toxicology. 102: 10–14.

129 Brown A et al. (2003) An interaction between warfarin and COX-2 inhibitors: two case studies. The Pharmaceutical Journal. 271: 782.

130 Verrico M et al. (2003) Adverse drug events involving COX-2 inhibitors. Annals of Pharmacotherapy. 37: 1203–1213.

131 Baxter K (ed) (2006) Stockley's Drug Interactions (7e). London.

132 Patrignani P et al. (1997) Differential inhibition of human prostaglandin endoperoxide synthase-1 and -2 by nonsteroidal anti-inflammatory drugs. Journal of Physiology and Pharmacology. 48: 623–631.

133 Tonkin A and Wing L (1988) Interactions of nonsteroidal anti-inflammatory drugs. In: P Brooks (ed) Bailliere's Clinical Rheumatology Anti-rheumatic Drugs Vol 2. Bailliere Tindall, London, pp. 455–483.

134 Whelton A et al. (2002) Effects of celecoxib and rofecoxib on blood pressure and edema in patients >65 years of age with systemic hypertension and osteoarthritis. American Journal of Cardiology. 90: 959–963.

135 Moore R et al. (1998) Quantitative systematic review of topically applied non-steroidal anti-inflammatory drugs. British Medical Journal. 316: 333–338.

136 Mondino A et al. (1983) Kinetic studies of ibuprofen on humans. Comparative study for the determination of blood concentrations and metabolites following local and oral administration. Med Welt. 34: 1052–1054.

137 Chlud K and Wagener H (1987) Percutaneous nonsteroidal anti-inflammatory drug (NSAID) therapy with particular reference to pharmacokinetic factors. EULAR Bulletin. 2: 40–43.

138 Peters H et al. (1987) Percutaneous kinetics of ibuprofen (German). Aktuelle Rheumatologie. 12: 208–211.

139 Kageyama T (1987) A double blind placebo controlled multicenter study of piroxicam 0.5% gel in osteoarthritis of the knee. European Journal of Rheumatology and Inflammation. 8: 114–115.

140 DTB (1990) More topical NSAIDs: worth the rub? Drugs and Therapeutics Bulletin. 28: 27–28.

141 O'Callaghan C et al. (1994) Renal disease and use of topical NSAIDs. British Medical Journal. 308: 110–111.

DICLOFENAC

Class: Non-opioid analgesic, NSAID, non-selective COX inhibitor.

Indications: Pain and inflammation in arthritic conditions (diclofenac *sodium*), †acute gout, musculoskeletal and soft tissue disorders and trauma (diclofenac *potassium*), dysmenorrhea (diclofenac *potassium*), postoperative pain after dental extraction (diclofenac *potassium*), †neoplastic fever.

Contra-indications: Active GI ulceration, bleeding, perforation or inflammation, hypersensitivity to **aspirin** or other NSAID (urticaria, rhinitis, asthma, angioedema), severe heart failure, active liver disease or significant hepatic impairment, severe renal impairment (creatinine clearance <30mL/min; CPS advises avoiding use if creatinine clearance <50mL/min), deteriorating renal function.

Pharmacology

Diclofenac is an acetate NSAID.[1] It is traditionally classed as a dual COX inhibitor although in some assays it appears to be COX-1-sparing.[2] Although diclofenac is a potent reversible inhibitor of platelet aggregation *in vitro*, typical oral doses have no effect on platelet adhesiveness or bleeding time.[3] Further, although IV diclofenac (not Canada) has a measurable effect on bleeding time, most subjects remain within the normal range. About 10% of patients experience undesirable effects (mainly gastric intolerance) which are generally mild and transient; diclofenac needs to be withdrawn in only 2%.[3] Age and renal or hepatic impairment do not have any significant effect on plasma concentrations of diclofenac, although metabolite concentrations increase in severe renal impairment. The principal metabolite, hydroxydiclofenac, possesses little anti-inflammatory effect.

Diclofenac has other actions in addition to inhibiting COX.[4-6] For example, it affects brain concentrations of kynurenic acid, an endogenous antagonist which acts on the glycine recognition site of the NMDA-receptor-channel complex.[7] Diclofenac and **indomethacin** (dual COX inhibitors) increase brain kynurenic acid concentrations, whereas **meloxicam** (a preferential COX-2 inhibitor) and **parecoxib** (a selective COX-2 inhibitor; not Canada) cause a decrease. It is possible that diclofenac (and **indomethacin**) tonically modulate kynurenic acid metabolism, and thus impact on central nociception by a non-COX inhibitory mechanism.

Other laboratory studies have shown that, under comparable conditions to those used in studies of **retigabine** (a novel anti-epileptic), diclofenac and **meclofenamic acid** (not Canada) are effective openers of the potassium channels KCNQ2/3, and are thus facilitators of inhibitory M-currents.[8] The kinetics and effective concentrations of this effect were comparable to that shown for **retigabine**. The clinical significance of these findings remains to be determined.[8] It is possible that diclofenac (and **meclofenamic acid**) are intrinsically more broad-spectrum in their central effects than COX-2 selective NSAIDs.[9] On the other hand, COX-2 selective inhibitors seem to be equally effective when compared with non-selective NSAIDs in inflammatory, dental and postoperative pain.[10]

When used for > 6 months in patients with osteo-arthritis and rheumatoid arthritis, diclofenac causes no more gastrotoxicity than **celecoxib**.[11,12] Diclofenac is only rarely associated with certain sporadic undesirable effects seen with many other NSAIDs, e.g. acute pancreatitis, aseptic meningitis, serious cutaneous reactions and photosensitivity. However, severe local necrosis has been described anecdotally after IM and SC use.[13] Diclofenac is available as the *sodium* and *potassium* salts; diclofenac *potassium* is absorbed more quickly and peak plasma concentration is reached sooner.

Bio-availability almost 100% diclofenac *sodium* EC, diclofenac *sodium* SR and diclofenac *potassium* PO; suppositories 2/3 of EC.

Onset of action 20–30min.

Time to peak plasma concentration diclofenac *sodium*: 2.5h EC (fasting), 6h EC (taken with food), ≥4h SR, 1h suppositories; diclofenac *potassium* PO 20–60min (not significantly affected by food).

Plasma halflife 1–2h.

Duration of action 8h.

Cautions

Also see NSAIDs, p.244.

To minimize the potential for serious undesirable effects, use the lowest effective dose for the shortest treatment duration possible.

Published data show an increased risk of thrombotic events with many NSAIDs (see p.251).[14] There appears to be no risk with **naproxen** (even with doses ≥1g/24h),[15] an increased risk with diclofenac (particularly at 150mg/24h) and high-dose **ibuprofen** (2,400mg/24h), but not low-dose **ibuprofen** (≤1,200mg/24h).[14,16,17] The risk of serious thrombotic events may increase with duration of treatment; use with caution in patients with pre-existing cardiovascular disease, risk factors for cardiovascular disease or fluid retention. No study to date has examined patients with cancer receiving NSAIDs.

Diclofenac is a substrate of CYP1A2, 3A4, 2B6, 2C8/9, 2C19 and 2D6, and inhibits CYP1A2, 2C8/9 and 2E1. It can increase the effects of **aspirin**, **digoxin**, **insulin**, **lithium**, **methotrexate**, potassium-sparing diuretics, and sulfonylureas.

Because an increase in INR is occasionally seen when diclofenac and **warfarin** are taken concurrently, if diclofenac is prescribed for a patient already taking **warfarin**, monitor the INR weekly for 3–4 weeks and adjust the dose of **warfarin** accordingly.[18]

Undesirable effects

For full list, see manufacturer's Product Monograph.

Also see NSAIDs, p.248. Because it causes sodium and fluid retention, diclofenac may decrease the effect of thiazides and **furosemide**.

Common (<10%, >1%): headache, dizziness, edema, nausea, indigestion, abdominal distension, pain or cramp, flatulence, diarrhea, constipation, pruritus, rash.

Dose and use

Diclofenac *sodium* is the NSAID of choice at some centres:
- 50mg b.i.d.–t.i.d.
- SR 75mg b.i.d. or 100mg once daily.

Some patients obtain greater benefit with no increase in undesirable effects from 200mg/24h, e.g. SR 100mg b.i.d. However, doses >150mg/24h are off-label and may be associated with an increased cardiovascular risk (see Cautions).

Diclofenac is available in some countries as an injection (but not Canada) and is used primarily to relieve biliary and renal colic (75mg IM p.r.n.).[19,20] If given by CSCI, it must be given via a separate syringe driver (or other delivery device) because it is incompatible with other drugs. A typical regimen is 75mg SC/IM stat and 150mg/24h CSCI.

Supply

Diclofenac *sodium* (generic)
Tablets EC 25mg, 50mg, 28 days @ 50mg t.i.d. = $34.
Suppositories 50mg, 10 = $7; 100mg, 10 = $9.

Voltaren® (Novartis)
Tablets EC 25mg, 50mg, 28 days @ 50mg t.i.d. = $75.
Suppositories 50mg, 10 = $14; 100mg, 10 = $18.

Diclofenac *potassium* (generic)
Tablets 50mg, 28 days @ 50mg t.i.d. = $34.

Voltaren® Rapide (Novartis)
Tablets 50mg, 28 days @ 50mg t.i.d. = $72.

Sustained release
Diclofenac *sodium* (generic)
Tablets SR 75mg, 100mg, 28 days @ 75mg b.i.d. = $32 and 100mg b.i.d. = $46.

Voltaren® SR (Novartis)
Tablets SR diclofenac *sodium* 75mg, 100mg, 28 days @ 75mg b.i.d. = $70 and 100mg b.i.d. = $99.

With **misoprostol**
Arthrotec® 50 (Pfizer)
Tablets EC diclofenac *sodium* 50mg + **misoprostol** 200microgram, 28 days @ 1 t.i.d. = $52.

Arthrotec® 75 (Pfizer)
Tablets EC diclofenac *sodium* 75mg + **misoprostol** 200microgram, 28 days @ 1 b.i.d. = $71.

Topical
Pennsaid® (Squire Pharmaceuticals)
Topical solution diclofenac *sodium* 1.5%, 60mL bottle = $42.

Voltaren Emulgel® (Novartis Consumer Health Canada)
Gel diclofenac *diethylamine* 1.16%, 50g = $11, 100g = $15, available OTC.

1 John V (1979) The pharmacokinetics and metabolism of diclofenac sodium (Voltarol) in animals and man. *Rheumatology and Rehabilitation.* **(suppl 2)**: 22–37.
2 Patrignani P et al. (1997) Differential inhibition of human prostaglandin endoperoxide synthase-1 and -2 by nonsteroidal anti-inflammatory drugs. *Journal of Physiology and Pharmacology.* **48**: 623–631.
3 Todd P and Sorkin E (1988) Diclofenac sodium: a reappraisal of its pharmacodynamic and pharmacokinetic properties, and therapeutic efficacy. *Drugs.* **35**: 244–285.
4 Abramson S et al. (1991) Non-steroidal anti-inflammatory drugs: effects on a GTP binding protein within the neutrophil plasma membrane. *Biochemical Pharmacology.* **41**: 1567–1573.
5 McCormack K (1994) Nonsteroidal anti-inflammatory drugs and spinal nociceptive processing. *Pain.* **59**: 9–43.
6 Svensson CI and Yaksh TL (2002) The spinal phospholipase-cyclooxygenase-prostanoid cascade in nociceptive processing. *Annual Review of Pharmacology and Toxicology.* **42**: 553–583.
7 Schwieler L et al. (2005) Prostaglandin-mediated control of rat brain kynurenic acid synthesis – opposite actions by COX-1 and COX-2 isoforms. *Journal of Neural Transmission.* **112**: 863–872.
8 Peretz A et al. (2005) Meclofenamic acid and diclofenac, novel templates of KCNQ2/Q3 potassium channel openers, depress cortical neuron activity and exhibit anticonvulsant properties. *Molecular Pharmacology.* **67**: 1053–1066.
9 McCormack K and Twycross RG (2001) Are COX-2 selective inhibitors effective analgesics? *Pain Review.* **8**: 13–26.

10 Dougados M et al. (2001) Evaluation of the structure-modifying effects of diacerein in hip osteoarthritis: ECHODIAH, a three-year, placebo-controlled trial. Evaluation of the Chondromodulating Effect of Diacerein in OA of the Hip. *Arthritis and Rheumatism.* **44**: 2539–2547.

11 Bombardier C (2002) An evidence-based evaluation of the gastrointestinal safety of coxibs. *American Journal of Cardiology.* **89 (suppl 6)**: 3d–9d.

12 Juni P et al. (2002) Risk of myocardial infarction associated with selective COX-2 inhibitors: questions remain. *Archives of Internal Medicine.* **162**: 2639–2640.

13 Kirkpatrick G (2003) SC diclofenac. In: *Bulletin Board Discussion.* Palliativedrugs.com. Available from: www.palliativedrugs.org/forum/read.php?f=1&i=3710&t=3710

14 Kearney PM et al. (2006) Do selective cyclo-oxygenase-2 inhibitors and traditional non-steroidal anti-inflammatory drugs increase the risk of atherothrombosis? Meta-analysis of randomised trials. *British Medical Journal.* **332**: 1302–1308.

15 Ray WA et al. (2009) Cardiovascular risks of nonsteroidal anti-inflammatory drugs in patients after hospitalization for serious coronary heart disease. *Circulation Cardiovascular Quality and Outcomes.* **2**: 155–163.

16 Duff G (2006) Safety of selective and non-selective NSAIDs. In: *Letter to health professionals from the Chairman of the Commission on Human Medicines, 24th October 2006.* Available from: www.mhra.gov.uk/Safetyinformation/Safetywarningsalertsandrecalls/Safetywarningsandmessagesformedicines/CON2025040

17 Patrignani P et al. (2008) NSAIDs and cardiovascular disease. *Heart.* **94**: 395–397.

18 Baxter K (ed) (2006) *Stockley's Drug Interactions* (7e). Pharmaceutical Press, London, p. 298.

19 Lundstam SOA et al. (1982) Prostaglandin-synthetase inhibition with diclofenac sodium in treatment of renal colic: comparison with use of a narcotic analgesic. *Lancet.* **1**: 1096–1097.

20 Thompson JF et al. (1989) Rectal diclofenac compared with pethidine injection in acute renal colic. *British Medical Journal.* **299**: 1140–1141.

IBUPROFEN

Class: Non-opioid analgesic, NSAID, non-selective COX inhibitor.

Indications: Pain and inflammation in arthritic conditions, musculoskeletal disorders and trauma, dental pain, dysmenorrhea, headache, migraine, postoperative analgesia, fever.

Contra-indications: Active GI ulceration, bleeding, perforation or inflammation, hypersensitivity to **aspirin** or other NSAID (urticaria, rhinitis, asthma, angioedema), severe heart failure, active liver disease or significant hepatic impairment, severe renal impairment (creatinine clearance <30mL/min; CPS advises avoiding use if creatinine clearance <50mL/min), deteriorating renal function, hyperkalemia, systemic lupus erythematosus.

Pharmacology

Ibuprofen acts predominantly as an analgesic in doses up to 1,200mg/24h, its anti-inflammatory properties becoming more evident at higher doses. Doses of 2,400mg/24h are well tolerated by most patients. Ibuprofen is 3 times more potent than **aspirin**, i.e. 200mg is equivalent to 600mg of **aspirin**. Higher doses of ibuprofen have a greater analgesic effect than standard doses of **aspirin**.

Although a non-selective COX inhibitor, ibuprofen has a low propensity for causing serious GI events, i.e. perforation, ulceration and bleeding (PUB). In consequence, ibuprofen can be purchased OTC.[1] It is also safe in overdose; only 2 deaths attributable to ibuprofen alone have been reported, involving overdoses of 36g and 105g respectively.[2,3]

Ibuprofen can be used topically (as a compounded preparation), particularly for sprains, strains and arthritis.[4] Although application to the skin produces plasma concentrations which are only 5% of those obtained with oral administration, the underlying muscle and fascial concentrations are 25 times greater.[5,6] An RCT showed that patients with sprains and bruises treated with TD ibuprofen did significantly better in relation to speed of resolution, relief of pain, reduction in swelling and return of function.[7]

A Health Technology Assessment found that topical and PO ibuprofen were equally effective for chronic knee pain in patients aged ⩾50 years, although those with more severe or widespread pain preferred PO treatment. Major undesirable effect rates were similar, but topical treatment led to fewer minor undesirable effects and less treatment discontinuation. Based on the cost per quality-adjusted life-year, topical ibuprofen was more cost–effective over the first year, whereas PO treatment was more cost-effective over 2 years.[8]

Bio-availability 90% PO.
Onset of action 20–30min.
Time to peak plasma concentration 1–2h.
Plasma halflife 2h.[9]
Duration of action 4–6h.

Cautions
Also see NSAIDs, p.244.
To minimize the potential for serious undesirable effects, use the lowest effective dose for the shortest treatment duration possible.

Published data show an increased risk of thrombotic events with many NSAIDs (see p.251).[10] There appears to be no risk with **naproxen** (even with doses ≥1g/24h),[11] an increased risk with **diclofenac** (particularly at 150mg/24h) and high-dose ibuprofen (2,400mg/24h), but not low-dose ibuprofen (≤1,200mg/24h).[10,12,13] The risk of serious thrombotic events may increase with duration of treatment; use with caution in patients with pre-existing cardiovascular disease, risk factors for cardiovascular disease or fluid retention. No study to date has examined patients with cancer receiving NSAIDs.

Ibuprofen is metabolized by CYP2C8/9 and 2C19, and inhibits CYP2C8/9. It may increase serum concentrations of **digoxin**, **lithium** and **methotrexate**, and decrease the effects of ACE inhibitors, angiotensin antagonists and diuretics. Its serum concentrations may be reduced by **aspirin**.
    Because an increase in INR is occasionally seen when ibuprofen and **warfarin** are taken concurrently, if ibuprofen is prescribed for a patient already taking **warfarin**, monitor the INR weekly for 3–4 weeks and adjust the dose of **warfarin** accordingly.[14]

Patients taking low-dose **aspirin** once daily as cardiovascular prophylaxis need to take the **aspirin** 1–2h before taking ibuprofen. Otherwise, the ibuprofen blocks the docking site for aspirin and thus blocks the effect of the **aspirin**.[15] However, patients prescribed regular round-the-clock ibuprofen will have continuous (or fairly continuous) impairment of platelet function, and thus there is no real need for concurrent **aspirin** administration. Thus, **aspirin** as prophylaxis can be stopped when regular ibuprofen is prescribed.

Undesirable effects
For full list, see manufacturer's Product Monograph.
Also see NSAIDs, p.248.
Common (<10%, >1%): headache, nervousness, fatigue, tinnitus, edema, heartburn, indigestion, nausea, vomiting, abdominal pain/cramp, flatulence, diarrhea, constipation, pruritus, urticaria, rash.

Dose and use
Ibuprofen is the NSAID of choice at many centres:
• start with 400mg t.i.d.
• if necessary, increase to 800mg t.i.d.

Supply
Ibuprofen (generic)
Capsules (liqui-gel) 200mg, 28 days @ 400mg t.i.d. = $31; available OTC.
Tablets 200mg, 400mg, 28 days @ 400mg t.i.d. = $15; available OTC.
Tablets 600mg, 28 days @ 600mg t.i.d. = $4; prescription-only medicine.
Oral suspension 100mg/5mL, 28 days @ 400mg t.i.d. = $110; available OTC.

Advil® (Wyeth)
Capsules (liqui-gel) 200mg, 400mg, 28 days @ 400mg t.i.d. = $36; available OTC.
Tablets 200mg, 28 days @ 400mg t.i.d. = $26; available OTC.
Caplets (capsule-shaped tablets) 200mg, 28 days @ 400mg t.i.d. = $20; available OTC.
Tablets extra strength 400mg, 28 days @ 400mg t.i.d. = $25; available OTC.
Oral syrup 100mg/5mL, 28 days @ 400mg t.i.d. = $249; *dye-free; grape, fruit and blue raspberry flavours*; available OTC.

Topical formulations can be compounded; 5–10% is generally suitable.

1 Rainsford K (1999) *Ibuprofen: a Critical Bibliographic Review*. Taylor and Francis, London.
2 Krenova M and Pelclova D (2005) Fatal poisoning with ibuprofen. *Clinical Toxicology.* **43**: 537.
3 Wood DM *et al.* (2006) Fatality after deliberate ingestion of sustained-release ibuprofen: a case report. *Critical Care.* **10**: R44.
4 Chlud K and Wagener H (1987) Percutaneous nonsteroidal anti-inflammatory drug (NSAID) therapy with particular reference to pharmacokinetic factors. *EULAR Bulletin.* **2**: 40–43.
5 Mondino A *et al.* (1983) Kinetic studies of ibuprofen on humans. Comparative study for the determination of blood concentrations and metabolites following local and oral administration. *Medizinische Welt.* **34**: 1052–1054.
6 Kageyama T (1987) A double blind placebo controlled multicenter study of piroxicam 0.5% gel in osteoarthritis of the knee. *European Journal of Rheumatology and Inflammation.* **8**: 114–115.
7 Peters H *et al.* (1987) Percutaneous kinetics of ibuprofen (German). *Aktuelle Rheumatologie.* **12**: 208–211.
8 Underwood M *et al.* (2008) Topical or oral ibuprofen for chronic knee pain in older people. The TOIB study. Available from: www.hta.ac.uk/project/1302.asp
9 Brocks D and Jamali F (1999) The pharmacokinetics of ibuprofen. In: K Rainsford (ed) *Ibuprofen: A Critical Bilbiographic Review.* Taylor and Francis, London.
10 Kearney PM *et al.* (2006) Do selective cyclo-oxygenase-2 inhibitors and traditional non-steroidal anti-inflammatory drugs increase the risk of atherothrombosis? Meta-analysis of randomised trials. *British Medical Journal.* **332**: 1302–1308.
11 Ray WA *et al.* (2009) Cardiovascular risks of nonsteroidal anti-inflammatory drugs in patients after hospitalization for serious coronary heart disease. *Circulation Cardiovascular Quality and Outcomes.* **2**: 155–163.
12 Duff G (2006) Safety of selective and non-selective NSAIDs. In: *Letter to health professionals from the Chairman of the Commission on Human Medicines, 24th October 2006.* Available from: www.mhra.gov.uk/Safetyinformation/Safetywarningsalertsand recalls/Safetywarningsandmessagesformedicines/CON2025040
13 Patrignani P *et al.* (2008) NSAIDs and cardiovascular disease. *Heart.* **94**: 395–397.
14 Baxter K (ed) (2006) *Stockley's Drug Interactions* (7e). Pharmaceutical Press, London, p. 298.
15 Catella-Lawson F *et al.* (2001) Cyclooxygenase inhibitors and the antiplatelet effects of aspirin. *New England Journal of Medicine.* **345**: 1809–1817.

*KETOROLAC TROMETHAMINE

Class: Non-opioid analgesic, NSAID, non-selective COX inhibitor.

Indications: Short-term management of moderate–severe acute pain.

Contra-indications: Active peptic ulceration or history of peptic ulceration, GI bleeding, suspected or confirmed cerebrovascular bleeding, hemorrhagic diatheses or other high-risk factor for bleeding, inflammatory GI disease, hypersensitivity to **aspirin** or other NSAID (urticaria, rhinitis, asthma, angioedema), moderate–severe renal impairment (creatinine >170micromol/L), hypovolemia, active liver disease or significant hepatic impairment. Concurrent prescription with **warfarin, heparin, aspirin**, other NSAID, **pentoxifylline, probenecid.** Because of the risk of bleeding, ketorolac is unsuitable for use as a prophylactic analgesic before major surgery. Epidural or intrathecal administration (injection contains alcohol).

Pharmacology

Ketorolac is a cyclic propionate structurally related to the acetate NSAIDs, **tolmetin** and **indomethacin**.[1,2] Ketorolac tromethamine is more water-soluble than the parent substance. Over 99% of the oral dose is absorbed and about 75% of a dose is excreted in the urine within 7h, and over 90% within 2 days, over 1/2 as unmodified ketorolac.[3] The rest is excreted in the feces. The analgesic and anti-inflammatory activity of ketorolac resides mainly in the levorotatory $(S(-))$ isomer. The analgesic effect is far greater than the antipyretic and anti-inflammatory properties. In animal studies, ketorolac is about 350 times more potent than **aspirin** as an analgesic but only 20 times more potent as an antipyretic.[4] As an anti-inflammatory ketorolac is about 1/2 as potent as **indomethacin** and twice as potent as **naproxen**. Like most NSAIDs, ketorolac inhibits platelet aggregation.

Of all the NSAIDs, ketorolac (PO or parenteral) appears to carry the highest risk for upper GI bleeding or perforation.[5,6] However, reports are contradictory; for example, one study gives a 5-fold increase in risk[7] whereas another found no excess risk when compared with either **diclofenac** or **ketoprofen**.[8]

Other postoperative studies indicate that, compared with opioids, the short-term use of ketorolac is associated with only a small increased risk of GI and operative site bleeding.[9,10] The risk is largely related to old age and increases significantly if treatment is continued for >1 week.[9,11] Because of the early reports of fatal GI bleeding, approval for ketorolac is restricted to short-term use, generally in a postoperative setting.[12,13] In some countries, approval has been withdrawn, e.g. France (1998) and Germany (1999). However, ketorolac is also used in emergency departments for post-traumatic pain.[10]

In palliative care, ketorolac has been used for extended periods but always with a gastroprotective drug.[4,14–16] Anecdotal clinical experience suggests that parenteral ketorolac may be effective in some patients, notably with bone pain, who fail to obtain relief with NSAIDs PO, including PO ketorolac.[4,14–16]

Bio-availability 100% PO.
Onset of action 30min PO, 10–30min IM/IV.
Time to peak plasma concentration 35min.[17]
Plasma halflife 5h; 7h in the elderly;[18] 6–19h with renal impairment.[11]
Duration of action 6h PO, 4–6h IM.

Cautions

Mild renal impairment (dose limitation required, see below). Interacts with **furosemide** (decreased diuretic response), ACE inhibitors (increased risk of renal impairment), **methotrexate** and **lithium** (decreased clearance), **probenecid** (increased ketorolac levels and halflife), **warfarin**, **heparin** and **pentoxifylline** (increased bleeding tendency). Also see NSAIDs, p.244.

Undesirable effects

For full list, see manufacturer's Product Monograph.
Also see NSAIDs, p.248.

Very common (>10%): headache, dyspepsia, nausea, abdominal pain.

Common (<10%, >1%): dizziness, drowsiness, tinnitus, edema, hypertension, anemia, stomatitis, vomiting, bloating, flatulence, GI ulceration, diarrhea, constipation, abnormal renal function, pruritus, purpura, rash, bleeding and pain at injection site (less with CSCI).

Dose and use

Moderate–severe acute pain

- approved in Canada for a maximum of 5 days PO for postoperative patients or 7 days PO for patients with musculoskeletal pain. Approved for no more than 2 days by IM injection; combined IM and PO use should not exceed 5 days
- usual dose:
  ▷ 30mg IM/IV *or*
  ▷ 20mg PO stat, then 10mg PO q6h–q4h
- maximum recommended daily dose 120mg IM/IV and 40mg PO (Note: latter dose smaller than parenteral dose, possibly because being given postoperatively at a time when analgesic requirements are tailing off).

For those aged >65 years, patients with mild renal impairment and those weighing <50kg:
- 15mg IM/IV *or*
- 10mg PO q6h–q4h (maximum recommended daily dose 60mg IM/IV; 40mg PO).

Cancer pain

Ketorolac is used at some centres when a parenteral NSAID is indicated. Ketorolac can be given by intermittent injections 15–30mg SC t.i.d. but these are uncomfortable; it is better given by CSCI. It is generally given for a short period (≤3 weeks) while arranging and awaiting benefit from more definitive therapy, e.g. radiation therapy. However, when all other options have been exhausted, ketorolac has been used for 6 months without undesirable effects:[16]

- start with 60mg/24h by CSCI; also the recommended maximum dose in people over 65 and those <50kg
- if necessary, increase by 15mg/24h to 90mg/24h
- prescribe a gastroprotective drug concurrently, preferably either **misoprostol** 200microgram t.i.d.–q.i.d,[14] or a PPI once daily.

CSCI: because ketorolac is irritant, dilute to the largest volume possible (e.g. for a Graseby syringe driver, 18mL in a 30mL luerlock syringe given over 12–24h) and use 0.9% saline as the diluent (see p.515).

Ketorolac is alkaline in solution and there is a high risk of incompatibility when mixed with acidic drugs. Incompatibility has been reported with **glycopyrrolate, haloperidol, hydroxyzine, meperidine, midazolam, morphine**, and **promethazine** (see CSCI, p.511).[3] There are 2-drug compatibility data for ketorolac in 0.9% saline with **oxycodone**.[19] For more details and 3-drug compatibility data, see Charts A4.1–A4.4, p.591. Information on compatibility in WFI can be found on www.palliativedrugs.com Syringe Driver Survey Database (SDSD).

Supply

Ketorolac tromethamine (generic)
Tablets 10mg, 5 days @ 10mg q.i.d. = $51.
Injection 30mg/mL, 1mL vial = $4, 10mL vial = $37; *vehicle contains 10% alcohol.*

Toradol® (Roche)
Tablets 10mg, 5 days @ 10mg q.i.d. = $82.
Injection 10mg/mL, 1mL vial = $2.50; 30mg/mL, 1mL vial = $5; *vehicle contains 10% alcohol.*

1 Buckley MM-T and Brogden R (1990) Ketorolac: a review of its pharmacodynamic and pharmacokinetic properties, and therapeutic potential. *Drugs.* **39**: 86–109.
2 Gillis J and Brogden R (1997) Ketorolac: A reappraisal of its pharmacodynamic and pharmacokinetic properties and therapeutic use in pain management. *Drugs.* **53**: 139–188.
3 Litvak K and McEvoy G (1990) Ketorolac: an injectable nonnarcotic analgesic. *Clinical Pharmacy.* **9**: 921–935.
4 Blackwell N et al. (1993) Subcutaneous ketorolac – a new development in pain control. *Palliative Medicine.* **7**: 63–65.
5 Lanas A et al. (2006) Risk of upper gastrointestinal ulcer bleeding associated with selective cyclo-oxygenase-2 inhibitors, traditional non-aspirin non-steroidal anti-inflammatory drugs, aspirin and combinations. *Gut.* **55**: 1731–1738.
6 Laporte JR et al. (2004) Upper gastrointestinal bleeding associated with the use of NSAIDs: newer versus older agents. *Drug Safety.* **27**: 411–420.
7 Garcia Rodriguez LA et al. (1998) Risk of hospitalization for upper gastrointestinal tract bleeding associated with ketorolac, other nonsteroidal anti-inflammatory drugs, calcium antagonists, and other antihypertensive drugs. *Archives of Internal Medicine.* **158**: 33–39.
8 Forrest JB et al. (2002) Ketorolac, diclofenac, and ketoprofen are equally safe for pain relief after major surgery. *British Journal of Anaesthesia.* **88**: 227–233.
9 Strom B et al. (1996) Parenteral ketorolac and risk of gastrointestinal and operative site bleeding. A postmarketing surveillance study. *Journal of the American Medical Assocation.* **275**: 376–382.
10 Rainer T et al. (2000) Cost effectiveness analysis of intravenous ketorolac and morphine for treating pain after limb injury: double blind randomised controlled trial. *British Medical Journal.* **321**: 1247–1251.
11 Reinhart D (2000) Minimising the adverse effects of ketorolac. *Drug Safety.* **22**: 487–497.
12 Choo V and Lewis S (1993) Ketorolac doses reduced. *Lancet.* **342**: 109.
13 Lewis S (1994) Ketorolac in Europe. *Lancet.* **343**: 784.
14 Myers K and Trotman I (1994) Use of ketorolac by continuous subcutaneous infusion for the control of cancer-related pain. *Postgraduate Medical Journal.* **70**: 359–362.
15 Middleton RK et al. (1996) Ketorolac continuous infusion: a case report and review of the literature. *Journal of Pain and Symptom Management.* **12**: 190–194.
16 Hughes A et al. (1997) Ketorolac: continuous subcutaneous infusion for cancer pain. *Journal of Pain and Symptom Management.* **13**: 315–317.
17 Gordon M et al. (1995) Ketorolac tromethamine bioavailability via tablet, capsule, and oral solution dosage forms. *Drug Development and Industry Pharmacy.* **21**: 1143–1155.
18 Greenwald R (1992) Ketorolac: an innovative nonsteroidal analgesic. *Drugs of Today.* **28**: 41–61.
19 Dickman A et al. (2005) *The Syringe Driver: Continuous Subcutaneous Infusions in Palliative Care* (2e). Oxford University Press, Oxford.

MELOXICAM

Class: Non-opioid analgesic, NSAID, preferential COX-2 inhibitor.

Indications: Osteo-arthritis, rheumatoid arthritis, †cancer pain.

Contra-indications: Active GI ulceration, bleeding, perforation or inflammation, recent cerebrovascular bleeding or other bleeding disorders, hypersensitivity to **aspirin** or other NSAID (urticaria, rhinitis, asthma, angioedema), severe heart failure, recent coronary artery bypass graft surgery, active liver disease or severe hepatic impairment, severe renal impairment (creatinine clearance < 30mL/min; CPS advises avoiding use if creatinine clearance < 50mL/min), deteriorating renal function, known hyperkalemia, age < 18 years.

Pharmacology

Meloxicam preferentially inhibits COX-2; with a dose of 7.5mg/24h, there is 70% COX-2 and 7% COX-1 inhibition but, with 15mg/24h, there is 80% COX-2 and 25% COX-1 inhibition.[1,2] In volunteers, meloxicam 15mg/24h led to a reduction in platelet thromboxane B_2 production of 66% (indicative of COX-1 inhibition).[3] However, thromboxane B_2 formation has to be inhibited by > 90% before there is significant impairment of platelet function.[4] Thus, in practice, there is only a minor increase in bleeding time with meloxicam.[3]

In post-marketing surveillance studies,[5,6] compared with **celecoxib** and **rofecoxib**, patients who had received meloxicam had fewer cerebrovascular thrombotic events, *but a similar number of cardiovascular thrombotic events*. The number of peripheral venous thrombotic events associated with meloxicam was comparable with **celecoxib** but significantly more than with **rofecoxib**. However, it should be noted that, with all three drugs, the incidence of the different types of thrombotic events was ≤0.5%.

GI safety was evaluated in RCTs of meloxicam 7.5mg/24h and **piroxicam** 20mg/24h, a chemically-related enolic acid derivative (the SELECT trial),[7] and of meloxicam 7.5mg/24h and SR **diclofenac** 100mg/24h (the MELISSA trial).[8] In both trials, each involving > 8,000 patients, there were significantly fewer undesirable GI effects with meloxicam; 10% vs. 15%, and 13% vs. 19% respectively. The number of serious GI events, i.e. perforation, ulceration, bleeding (PUB) was also significantly less with meloxicam compared with **piroxicam** (7 vs. 16). But there was no difference in this respect between meloxicam and **diclofenac** (5 vs. 7). The relatively favourable GI profile with meloxicam was subsequently confirmed by a meta-analysis of 12 trials,[9] and by post-marketing surveillance.[10]

In patients with osteo-arthritis, meloxicam 7.5mg/24h is less effective than both **piroxicam** 20mg/24h and SR **diclofenac** 100mg/24h, but probably not to a clinically important degree.[7,8] Withdrawal because of lack of relief in both the SELECT and MELISSA trials was < 2% for all three drugs.[7,8]

Meloxicam is well absorbed from the GI tract. It undergoes extensive biotransformation in the liver to inactive metabolites. Transformation to the main metabolite (accounts for 60% of the dose) is mediated principally by CYP2C9, with a minor contribution from CYP3A4. Neither hepatic nor moderate renal impairment have a substantial effect on the pharmacokinetics of meloxicam.

Bio-availability 89–93% PO.[11]

Onset of action 1–2h.

Time to peak plasma concentration < 2h suspension (not Canada); 4–6h tablets (with a second peak at 12–14h suggesting enterohepatic circulation).

Plasma halflife 15–20h.

Duration of action >24h.

Cautions

Also see NSAIDs, p.244.

To minimize the potential for serious undesirable effects, use the lowest effective dose for the shortest treatment duration possible. The risk of serious thrombotic events may increase with duration of treatment; use with caution in patients with pre-existing cardiovascular disease, risk factors for cardiovascular disease or fluid retention (see Pharmacology above).

Although studies have not shown an increase in INR when given concurrently with **warfarin**, it is still advisable to monitor the INR for 3–4 weeks if meloxicam is prescribed for a patient already taking **warfarin**.[12]

Undesirable effects

For full list see manufacturer's Product Monograph.

Also see NSAIDs, p.248.

Common (<10%, >1%): dizziness, headache, paresthesia, drowsiness, tinnitus, flu-like symptoms, edema, nausea, dyspepsia, abdominal pain, flatulence, diarrhea.

Dose and use
Can be taken without regard to mealtimes, but taking with or after food or milk reduces GI symptoms.

Osteo-arthritis and rheumatoid arthritis
* start with 7.5mg once daily
* if necessary, increase to 15mg once daily
* maximum recommended dose 15mg once daily.

Cancer pain
* generally start with 15mg once daily
* in the very frail and very old, start with 7.5mg once daily, and increase if necessary.[13]

Supply
Meloxicam (generic)
Tablets 7.5mg, 15mg, 28 days @ 7.5 mg and 15mg once daily = $14 and $16 respectively.

Mobicox® (Boehringer Ingelheim)
Tablets 7.5mg, 15mg, 28 days @ 7.5 mg and 15mg once daily = $24 and $28 respectively.

1 Churchill L et al. (1996) Selective inhibition of human cyclo-oxygenase-2 by meloxicam. Inflammopharmacology. **4**: 125–135.
2 vanHecken A et al. (2000) Comparative inhibitory activity of rofecoxib, meloxicam, diclofenac, ibuprofen and naproxen on COX-2 versus COX-1 in healthy volunteers. Journal of Clinical Pharmacology. **40**: 1109–1120.
3 deMeijer A et al. (1999) Meloxicam, 15mg/day, spares platelet function in healthy volunteers. Clinical Pharmacology and Therapeutics. **66**: 425–430.
4 Reilly IA and FitzGerald GA (1987) Inhibition of thromboxane formation in vivo and ex vivo: implications for therapy with platelet inhibitory drugs. Blood. **69**: 180–186.
5 Layton D et al. (2003) Comparison of the incidence rates of thromboembolic events reported for patients prescribed rofecoxib and meloxicam in general practice in England using prescription-event monitoring (PEM) data. Rheumatology (Oxford). **42**: 1342–1353.
6 Layton D et al. (2003) Comparison of the incidence rates of thromboembolic events reported for patients prescribed celecoxib and meloxicam in general practice in England using Prescription-Event Monitoring (PEM) data. Rheumatology (Oxford). **42**: 1354–1364.
7 Dequeker J et al. (1998) Improvement in gastrointestinal tolerability of the selective cyclooxygenase (COX)-2 inhibitor, meloxicam, compared with piroxicam: results of the Safety and Efficacy Large-scale Evaluation of COX-inhibiting Therapies (SELECT) trial in osteoarthritis. British Journal of Rheumatology. **37**: 946–951.
8 Hawkey C et al. (1998) Gastrointestinal tolerability of meloxicam compared to diclofenac in osteoarthritis patients. International MELISSA Study Group. Meloxicam Large-scale International Study Safety Assessment. British Journal of Rheumatology. **37**: 937–945.
9 Schoenfeld P (1999) Gastrointestinal safety profile of meloxicam: a meta-analysis and systematic review of randomized controlled trials. American Journal of Medicine. **107**: 48s–54s.
10 Zeidler H et al. (2002) Prescription and Tolerability of Meloxicam in Day-to-Day Practice. Journal of Clinical Rheumatology. **8**: 305–315.
11 Davies NM and Skjodt NM (1999) Clinical pharmacokinetics of meloxicam. A cyclo-oxygenase-2 preferential nonsteroidal anti-inflammatory drug. Clinical Pharmacokinetics. **36**: 115–126.
12 Baxter K (ed) (2008) Stockley's Drug Interactions (8e). Pharmaceutical Press, London.
13 Smith HS and Baird W (2003) Meloxicam and selective COX-2 inhibitors in the management of pain in the palliative care population. American Journal of Hospice and Palliative Care **20**: 297–306.

NAPROXEN

Class: Non-opioid analgesic, NSAID, non-selective COX inhibitor.

Indications: Pain and inflammation in arthritic conditions, musculoskeletal disorders and trauma, dysmenorrhea, †acute gout, †cancer pain, †neoplastic fever.

Contra-indications: Active GI ulceration, bleeding, perforation or inflammation, cerebro-vascular bleeding or other bleeding disorders hypersensitivity to **aspirin** or other NSAID (urticaria, rhinitis, asthma, angioedema), severe heart failure, active liver disease or severe hepatic impairment, severe renal impairment (creatinine clearance < 30mL/min; CPS advises avoiding use if creatinine clearance < 50mL/min); deteriorating renal function, hyperkalemia.

Pharmacology

Naproxen is a propionic acid derivative. Absorption is not affected by food or antacids. A steady-state is achieved after 3 days of b.i.d. administration. Excretion is almost entirely urinary, mainly as conjugated naproxen, with some unchanged drug. Plasma concentrations do not increase with doses >500mg b.i.d. because of rapid urinary excretion.[1]

Naproxen *sodium* 550mg is equivalent to 500mg naproxen. Naproxen *sodium* is more rapidly absorbed, resulting in plasma concentrations about 1.5–2 times higher than those of naproxen over the first hour, and better analgesia from 4h onwards.[2] However, it is approximately 3 times more expensive than naproxen. Although generally given b.i.d., a single dose of 500mg at bedtime was equal in efficacy to 250mg b.i.d. in patients with osteo-arthritis[3,4] and with rheumatoid arthritis.[5]

Bio-availability 99–100% PO.
Onset of action 20–30min.
Time to peak plasma concentration 1.5–5h depending on dose and formulation.[6,7]
Plasma halflife 12–15h.
Duration of action 6–8h with single dose; >12h with multiple doses.

Cautions

Also see NSAIDs, p.244.
To minimize the potential for serious undesirable effects, use the lowest effective dose for the shortest treatment duration possible.

Published data show an increased risk of thrombotic events with many NSAIDs (see p.251).[8] There appears to be no risk with naproxen (even with doses ≥1g/24h),[9] an increased risk with **diclofenac** (particularly at 150mg/24h) and high-dose **ibuprofen** (2,400mg/24h), but not low-dose **ibuprofen** (≤1,200mg/24h).[8,10,11] The risk of serious thrombotic events may increase with duration of treatment; use with caution in patients with pre-existing cardiovascular disease, risk factors for cardiovascular disease or fluid retention. No study to date has examined patients with cancer receiving NSAIDs.

Because of their Na^+ content (see Supply), naproxen *sodium* products and naproxen suspension should be used with caution in patients on a salt-restricted diet.

Naproxen is metabolized by CYP1A2 and CYP2C8/9. Thus, it may increase serum concentrations of **lithium** and **methotrexate** and slightly increase **warfarin** levels. Naproxen serum concentrations are also increased by **probenecid**.

Although studies have not shown any increase in INR when given concurrently with **warfarin**, it is still advisable to monitor the INR for 3–4 weeks if naproxen is prescribed for a patient already taking **warfarin**.[12]

Undesirable effects

For full list, see manufacturer's Product Monograph.
Also see NSAIDs, p.248.
Very common (>10%): headache.
Common (<10%, >1%): nervousness, malaise, drowsiness, tinnitus, edema, hemolysis, dyspnea, stomatitis, heartburn, nausea, abdominal pain/cramp, GI perforation, ulceration or bleeding (PUB), diarrhea, constipation, pruritus, rash, ecchymosis.

Dose and use

Naproxen is the NSAID of choice at some centres:
- typically 250–500mg b.i.d.
- can be taken as a single daily dose, either each morning or each evening with food
- occasionally, with careful monitoring, it may be worth titrating up to a total daily dose of 1.5g (e.g. 500mg t.i.d.); this is higher than the manufacturer's recommended maximum daily doses of 1–1.25g (depending on indication) and should normally be done for only a limited period. This is comparable to doses used in the UK for severe rheumatoid arthritis.

Supply

Naproxen (generic)
Tablets 125mg, 250mg, 375mg 500mg, 28 days @ 500mg b.i.d. = $12.
Tablets EC 250mg, 375mg, 500mg, 28 days @ 500mg b.i.d. = $39.
Suppositories 500mg, 28 days @ 500mg b.i.d. = $47.

Naprosyn® (Hoffman-La Roche)
Tablets EC 250mg, 375mg, 500mg, 28 days @ 500mg b.i.d. = $59.
Oral suspension 25mg/mL, 28 days @ 500mg b.i.d. = $74; *contains sodium chloride 20mg/mL, equivalent to Na+ 8mg/mL.*

Sustained-release
Naprosyn® (Hoffman-La Roche)
Tablets SR 750mg, 28 days @ 750mg once daily = $39.

Naproxen *sodium* (generic)
Tablets 275mg, 550mg, 28 days @ 550mg b.i.d. = $38; *275mg tablets contain Na+ 25mg per tablet, 550mg tablets contain Na+ 50mg per tablet.*
(Note: 275mg naproxen *sodium* is equivalent to 250mg naproxen.)

Anaprox® (Hoffman-La Roche)
Tablets 275mg, 550mg, 28 days @ 550mg b.i.d. = $71; *275mg tablets contain Na+ 25mg per tablet, 550mg tablets contain Na+ 50mg per tablet.*
(Note: 275mg naproxen *sodium* is equivalent to 250mg naproxen.)

Naproxen *sodium* 220mg tablets are also available OTC as Aleve® (Bayer Inc. Consumer Care Division).

---

1   Simon L and Mills J (1980) Nonsteroidal anti-inflammatory drugs. Part 2. *New England Journal of Medicine.* **302**: 1237–1243.
2   Sevelius H *et al.* (1980) Bioavailability of naproxen sodium and its relationship to clinical analgesic effects. *British Journal of Clinical Pharmacology.* **10**: 259–263.
3   Brooks P *et al.* (1982) Evaluation of a single daily dose of naproxen in osteoarthritis. *Rheumatology and Rehabilitation.* **21**: 242–246.
4   Mendelsohn s (1991) Clinical efficacy and tolerability of naproxen in osteoarthritis patients using twice-daily and once-daily regimens. *Clinical Therapy.* **13 (suppl A)**: 8–15.
5   Graziano F (1991) Once-daily or twice-daily administration of naproxen in patients with rheumatoid arthritis. *Clinical Therapy.* **13 (suppl A)**: 20–25.
6   Kelly J *et al.* (1989) Pharmacokinetic properties and clinical efficacy of once-daily sustained-release naproxen. *European Journal of Clinical Pharmacology.* **36**: 383–388.
7   Davies N and Anderson K (1997) Clinical pharmacokinetics of naproxen. *Clinical Pharmacokinetics.* **32**: 268–293.
8   Kearney PM *et al.* (2006) Do selective cyclo-oxygenase-2 inhibitors and traditional non-steroidal anti-inflammatory drugs increase the risk of atherothrombosis? Meta-analysis of randomised trials. *British Medical Journal.* **332**: 1302–1308.
9   Ray WA *et al.* (2009) Cardiovascular risks of nonsteroidal anti-inflammatory drugs in patients after hospitalization for serious coronary heart disease. *Circulation Cardiovascular Quality and Outcomes.* **2**: 155–163.
10 Duff G (2006) Safety of selective and non-selective NSAIDs. In: *Letter to health professionals from the Chairman of the Commission on Human Medicines, 24th October 2006.* Available from: www.mhra.gov.uk/Safetyinformation/Safetywarningsalertsand recalls/Safetywarningsandmessagesformedicines/CON2025040
11 Patrignani P *et al.* (2008) NSAIDs and cardiovascular disease. *Heart.* **94**: 395–397.
12 Baxter K (ed) (2008) *Stockley's Drug Interactions* (8e). Pharmaceutical Press, London.

NABUMETONE

Class: Non-opioid analgesic, NSAID, preferential COX-2 inhibitor.

Indications: Pain in osteo-arthritis and rheumatoid arthritis, †cancer pain.

Contra-indications: Active GI ulceration, bleeding, perforation or inflammation, hypersensitivity to **aspirin** or other NSAID (urticaria, rhinitis, asthma, angioedema), active liver disease or severe hepatic impairment, severe renal impairment (creatinine clearance <30mL/min; CPS advises avoiding use if creatinine clearance <50mL/min), deteriorating renal function (but see Dose and use below).

Pharmacology

World-wide, nabumetone is one of the most commonly prescribed NSAIDs.[1] It is a unique NSAID in that it is both a pro-drug and non-acidic. Absorption is mainly unaffected by food, and is increased if taken with milk.[1] It undergoes rapid and extensive first-pass metabolism in the liver to mainly 6-methoxy-2-naphthylacetic acid (6-MNA), which is further metabolized by O-methylation and conjugation to inactive compounds.[2] Less than 1% of a dose is excreted as 6-MNA. Steady-state plasma concentrations of 6-MNA are not altered in patients with reduced renal function even though the renal excretion of 6-MNA is reduced.[1] This could relate to non-linear protein-binding or increased excretion by other routes. Thus, the dose of nabumetone does not need to be adjusted in patients with mild–moderate renal impairment (but see Dose and use below).

6-MNA preferentially inhibits COX-2.[1] Nabumetone has a dose-related effect on platelet aggregation, but no effect on bleeding time in clinical studies.[1,3–5] In most patients, nabumetone can be given once daily.

In a dose of 1g/24h, it is as effective as other NSAIDs in rheumatoid and osteo-arthritis, and after acute soft tissue injury; RCTs include comparisons with **diclofenac**, **ibuprofen**, **indomethacin**, **naproxen**, and **piroxicam**.[6–8] In patients with osteo-arthritis, nabumetone is significantly less gastrotoxic than **diclofenac** and **piroxicam**; the incidence of serious GI events, i.e. perforation, ulceration, bleeding (PUB) over 6 months = 1.1% vs. 4.3%, and no hospitalizations vs. 1.4%.[9] Nabumetone produces fewer endoscopic ulcers over 12 weeks than **ibuprofen**, and is comparable to **ibuprofen**+**misoprostol** 800microgram/24h.[10] It is less gastrotoxic than **naproxen** (endosopic monitoring for 5 years).[11]

Meta-analysis of 13 studies, incorporating some 50,000 patients, showed that PUBs were 10–36 times less likely than with the comparator NSAIDs. Hospitalization for NSAID-related events was also less frequent (odds ratio 3.7, 95% CI 1.3–10.7).[12] Over some 30 years on the ARAMIS database (for patients with rheumatoid arthritis; www.aramis.stanford.edu), nabumetone has had the least hospitalizations for PUBs of all the NSAIDs. In a population-based cohort following up 18,500 patients on NSAIDs for 6 months, **diclofenac**+**misoprostol** (as Arthrotec®) and nabumetone resulted in significantly less hospitalizations than **naproxen**, or **diclofenac**+**misoprostol** (given separately); there was one bleed in the nabumetone group vs. 10 with Arthrotec® (although this was not significant at the 5% probability level).[13] The same sample of patients showed significantly fewer deaths from all causes in the nabumetone group compared with Arthrotec®, **diclofenac**+**misoprostol** separately, or **naproxen**, despite comparable patient characteristics.[14]

In practice this means that, except when there is very high risk of gastrotoxicity, a gastroprotective drug need not be prescribed with nabumetone. The decreased propensity for causing gastroduodenal toxicity is related to the fact that nabumetone:
- is non-acidic
- has only a weak uncoupling effect on oxidative phosphorylation, and thus causes only low level disruption (and inactivation) of phospholipids in the gastric protective mucus and mucous membranes
- undergoes no enterohepatic recirculation of its active metabolite.

In patients with treated hypertension, compared with **ibuprofen**, fewer on nabumetone had a significant increase in blood pressure (17% vs. 6%).[15] There are no comparative data available for cardiovascular and cerebrovascular morbidity. However, the number of serious adverse events reported for nabumetone (0.5%) and the number of withdrawals from RCTs (<4%) are no greater than with placebo.[1]

Bio-availability of 6-MNA 38% (increased by administration with milk).[1,16]
Onset of action 1–2h.
Time to peak plasma concentration for 6-MNA 3–6h.[2]
Plasma halflife of 6-MNA about 24h.
Duration of action ≥24h.

Cautions

Also see NSAIDs, p.244.

To minimize the potential for serious undesirable effects, use the lowest effective dose for the shortest treatment duration possible.

No data are available for risk of cardiovascular events. Use with caution in patients with pre-existing cardiovascular disease, risk factors for cardiovascular disease or fluid retention.

6-MNA is highly protein-bound and may displace other highly bound drugs from plasma proteins, e.g. **phenytoin**, sulfonylureas. Although nabumetone does not normally alter platelet aggregation or affect the INR in anticoagulated patients, there is an isolated report of hemarthrosis and raised INR in a patient taking **warfarin**.[17] Thus, if nabumetone is prescribed to a patient already taking **warfarin**, monitor the INR weekly for 3–4 weeks and adjust the dose of **warfarin** if necessary.[18]

Undesirable effects

For full list, see manufacturer's Product Monograph.
Also see NSAIDs, p.248.
Very common (>10%): dyspepsia, abdominal pain, diarrhea (dose-dependent).[19]
Common (<10%, >1%): headache, nausea.
Uncommon (<1%, >0.1%): GI ulcers.

Dose and use

- start with 1g each evening
- if necessary, increase to 500mg each morning and 1g each evening
- if necessary, increase further to 1g b.i.d.
- in very elderly (80+ years) frail patients, start with 500mg, and limit to 1g once daily.

Dose reduction is not necessary in patients with mild–moderate renal impairment.[1] However, the Canadian manufacturers suggest considering dose reduction for patients with moderate renal impairment (creatinine clearance 30–49mL/min).

Further, although the Product Monograph states that nabumetone is contra-indicated in severe renal impairment (creatinine clearance <30mL/min), the warnings and precautions section advises that reduced doses may be considered provided that renal function is closely monitored and the drug is discontinued if deterioration occurs. This is consistent with the advice given in the UK, where nabumetone is *not* contra-indicated in severe renal impairment.

Supply

Nabumetone (generic)
Tablets 500mg, 750mg, 28 days @ 1g once daily = $29.

The higher cost of nabumetone compared with **diclofenac**, **ibuprofen** or **naproxen** is largely offset by not needing to prescribe a gastroprotective drug (e.g. a PPI or **misoprostol**) concurrently.

1 Hedner T et al. (2004) Nabumetone: Therapeutic use and safety profile in the management of osteoarthritis and rheumatoid arthritis. Drugs. **64**: 2315–2343; discussion 2344–2345.
2 Davies NM (1997) Clinical pharmacokinetics of nabumetone. The dawn of selective cyclo-oxygenase-2 inhibition? Clinical Pharmacokinetics. **33**: 404–416.
3 Hilleman DE et al. (1993) Nonsteroidal antiinflammatory drug use in patients receiving warfarin: emphasis on nabumetone. American Journal of Medicine. **95** (suppl): 30S–34S.
4 Cipollone F et al. (1995) Effects of nabumetone on prostanoid biosynthesis in humans. Clinical Pharmacology and Therapeutics. **58**: 335–341.
5 Knijff-Dutmer EA et al. (1999) Effects of nabumetone compared with naproxen on platelet aggregation in patients with rheumatoid arthritis. Annals of the Rheumatic Diseases. **58**: 257–259.
6 Friedel HA et al. (1993) Nabumetone. A reappraisal of its pharmacology and therapeutic use in rheumatic diseases. Drugs. **45**: 131–156.
7 Lister BJ et al. (1993) Efficacy of nabumetone versus diclofenac, naproxen, ibuprofen, and piroxicam in osteoarthritis and rheumatoid arthritis. American Journal of Medicine. **95** (suppl): 2S–9S.
8 Morgan GJ et al. (1993) Efficacy and safety of nabumetone versus diclofenac, naproxen, ibuprofen, and piroxicam in the elderly. American Journal of Medicine. **95** (suppl): 19S–27S.
9 Scott DL and Palmer RH (2000) Safety and efficacy of nabumetone in osteoarthritis: emphasis on gastrointestinal safety. Alimentary Pharmacology and Therapeutics. **14**: 443–452.
10 Roth SH et al. (1993) A controlled study comparing the effects of nabumetone, ibuprofen, and ibuprofen plus misoprostol on the upper gastrointestinal tract mucosa. Archives of Internal Medicine. **153**: 2565–2571.
11 Roth SH et al. (1994) A longterm endoscopic evaluation of patients with arthritis treated with nabumetone vs naproxen. Journal of Rheumatology. **21**: 1118–1123.
12 Huang JQ et al. (1999) Gastrointestinal safety profile of nabumetone: a meta-analysis. American Journal of Medicine. **107** (suppl): 55S–61S; discussion 61S–64S.
13 Ashworth NL et al. (2005) Risk of hospitalization with peptic ulcer disease or gastrointestinal hemorrhage associated with nabumetone, Arthrotec, diclofenac, and naproxen in a population based cohort study. Journal of Rheumatology. **32**: 2212–2217.

14 Ashworth NL et al. (2004) A population based historical cohort study of the mortality associated with nabumetone, Arthrotec, diclofenac, and naproxen. Journal of Rheumatology. **31**: 951–956.

15 Palmer R et al. (2003) Effects of nabumetone, celecoxib, and ibuprofen on blood pressure control in hypertensive patients on angiotensin converting enzyme inhibitors. American Journal of Hypertension. **16**: 135–139.

16 Dollery C (1999) Therapeutic Drugs (2e). Churchill Livingstone, Edinburgh.

17 Dennis VC et al. (2000) Potentiation of oral anticoagulation and hemarthrosis associated with nabumetone. Pharmacotherapy. **20**: 234–239.

18 Baxter K (ed) (2006) Stockley's Drug Interactions (7e). Pharmaceutical Press, London.

19 Willkens RF (1990) An overview of the long-term safety experience of nabumetone. Drugs. **40 (suppl 5)**: 34–37.

WEAK OPIOIDS

There is no pharmacological need for Step 2 of the WHO Analgesic Ladder. Low doses of **morphine**, or an alternative strong opioid, can be used instead.[1,2] Moving directly from Step 1 to Step 3 is now the preferred option at some centres. However, from an international perspective, Step 2 remains a practical necessity because of the highly restricted availability (or even non-availability) of oral **morphine**, and other strong opioids, in many countries.

Codeine is the archetypical weak opioid (and **morphine** the archetypical strong opioid).[3] However, the division of opioids into 'weak' and 'strong' is to a certain extent arbitrary. In reality, opioids manifest a range of strengths which is not fully reflected in two discrete categories.

High-dose **codeine** (or alternative) is comparable to low-dose **morphine** (or alternative), and vice versa. Further, a strong opioid may be formulated with a non-opioid in such a way that they can be used only as a weak opioid, e.g. **hydrocodone** combined with **ibuprofen**.

By IM injection, weak opioids can all provide analgesia equivalent, or almost equivalent, to **morphine** 10mg but, generally, weak opioids are not marketed as injections. Weak opioids are said to have a 'ceiling' effect for analgesia. This is an oversimplification; whereas mixed agonist–antagonists such as **pentazocine** have a true ceiling effect, the maximum effective dose of weak opioid agonists is arbitrary. At higher doses, there are progressively more undesirable effects, e.g. nausea and vomiting, which outweigh any additional analgesic effect.

There is little to choose between the weak opioids in terms of efficacy (Table 5.10) but, at present, there is no consensus in Canada about which is the weak opioid of choice. The following should be noted:

- **pentazocine** should not be used; it often causes psychotomimetic effects (dysphoria, depersonalization, frightening dreams, hallucinations)[4]
- **codeine** is more constipating than **propoxyphene** and **tramadol**.[5] It has little or no analgesic effect until metabolized to **morphine** mainly via CYP2D6; it is thus essentially ineffective in poor metabolizers (see p.278). Although widely prescribed, there is only limited RCT data on the efficacy and tolerability of fixed-dose **acetaminophen-codeine** combinations in cancer pain. A Cochrane review comparing these combinations with **acetaminophen** alone in cancer pain is in progress[6]
- **propoxyphene** has effectively been withdrawn in the UK, and withdrawal has been recommended throughout Europe.[7] Further, the FDA has strengthened safety warnings in product literature while considering its withdrawal in the USA.[8,9] This action has been taken because of **propoxyphene's** relatively common use in intentional overdose, and its potential fatal toxicity in accidental overdose (see p.280).[10] There are no plans to withdraw **propoxyphene** for safety reasons in Canada, although only one product remains available
- if used with another drug which affects serotonin metabolism/availability, the use of **tramadol** can lead to serotonin toxicity, particularly in the elderly (see p.140); it also lowers seizure threshold. Further, it has significantly reduced analgesic effect unless metabolized to O-desmethyltramadol (M1) via CYP2D6; it is thus practically ineffective in poor metabolizers (see p.283)
- **hydrocodone** products available in Canada are marketed specifically as cough suppressants (see Antitussives, p.105).

On balance, **codeine** and **tramadol** are probably the best current choices for a weak opioid in Canada. In addition, **codeine** is cheap, widely available through provincial formularies and government and third party health insurance, and comes in a range of formulations and strengths as a single agent (see p.278). **Tramadol** is licensed for moderate–severe pain, whereas other

Table 5.10 Weak opioids

Drug	Bio-availability (%)	Time to peak plasma concentration (h)	Plasma halflife (h)	Duration of analgesia (h)[a]	Approximate potency ratio with codeine
Codeine	40 (12–84)	1–2	2.5–3.5	4–6	1
Hydrocodone	25	1.7	4	4–8	6–10
Pentazocine	20	1	3	2–3	1[b]
Propoxyphene	40	2–2.5	6–12[c]	6–8	7/8[d]
Tramadol	75[e]	2	6[f]	4–6	1[b]

a. when used in usual doses for mild–moderate pain
b. estimated on basis of potency ratio with morphine
c. increased > 50% in elderly
d. multiple doses; single dose = 1/2–2/3
e. multiple doses > 90%
f. active metabolite (M1) 7.4h; both figures double in cirrhosis and severe renal failure.

weak opioids are licensed only for mild–moderate pain. It is not as constipating as **codeine**, and is not currently a controlled drug, which makes prescribing more straightforward. However, it is expensive and not always covered by provincial formularies or health insurance. Further, the only normal-release formulation is an **acetaminophen-tramadol** combination, so doses for breakthrough (episodic) pain are limited by the **acetaminophen** content.

The following general rules should be observed:
- a weak opioid should be added to, not substituted for, a non-opioid
- generally it is inappropriate to switch from one weak opioid to another weak opioid
- if a weak opioid is inadequate when given regularly, change to **morphine** (or an alternative strong opioid).

As with all opioids, patients must be monitored for undesirable effects, particularly nausea and vomiting, and constipation (see Box 5.F, p.289). Depending on individual circumstances, an anti-emetic should be prescribed for regular or p.r.n. use (see p.183) and, routinely, a laxative prescribed (see p.26).

1 Marinangeli F et al. (2004) Use of strong opioids in advanced cancer pain: a randomized trial. *Journal of Pain and Symptom Management*. **27**: 409–416.
2 Maltoni M et al. (2005) A validation study of the WHO analgesic ladder: a two-step vs three-step strategy. *Support Care Cancer*. **13**: 888–894.
3 WHO (1986) *Cancer Pain Relief*. World Health Organisation, Geneva.
4 Woods A et al. (1974) Medicines evaluation and monitoring group: central nervous system effects of pentazocine. *British Medical Journal*. **1**: 305–307.
5 Wilder-Smith C et al. (2001) Treatment of severe pain from osteoarthritis with slow-release tramadol or dihydrocodeine in combination with NSAID's: a randomised study comparing analgesia, antinociception and gastrointestinal effects. *Pain*. **91**: 23–31.
6 Jackson KC and Wiffen PJ (2007) Codeine, alone and with paracetamol (acetaminophen), for cancer pain (Protocol). *Cochrane Database of Systematic Reviews*. **3**: CD006601.
7 European Medicines Agency (2009) Press Release. European Medicines Agency recommends withdrawal of dextropropoxyphene-containing medicines. Available from: www.emea.europa.eu/pdfs/human/press/pr/40106209en.pdf
8 FDA Joint Advisory Committee (2009) Final summary minutes. Joint meeting of the Anesthetic and Life Support Drugs Advisory Committee and the Drug Safety and Risk Management Committee. January 30th 2009. Available from: www.fda.gov/ohrms/dockets/ac/09/minutes/2009-4411m1-final.pdf
9 FDA (2009) Propoxyphene questions and answers. Available from: www.fda.gov/Drugs/DrugSafety/PostmarketDrugSafety InformationforPatientsandProviders/ucm170268.htm
10 Hawton K et al. (2003) Co-proxamol and suicide: a study of national mortality statistics and local non-fatal self poisonings. *British Medical Journal*. **326**: 1006–1008.

CODEINE PHOSPHATE

Class: Opioid analgesic.

Indications: Mild–moderate pain, cough, diarrhea.

Contra-indications: None absolute if titrated carefully to effect.

Pharmacology

Codeine (methylmorphine) is an opium alkaloid, about 1/10 as potent as **morphine**. An increasing analgesic response has been reported with IM doses up to 360mg.[1] However, in practice, codeine is generally used PO in doses of 15–60mg, often in combination with a non-opioid. Although widely prescribed, there is only limited RCT information on the efficacy and tolerability of fixed-dose **acetaminophen**-codeine combinations in cancer pain. A Cochrane review comparing these combinations with **acetaminophen** alone in cancer pain is in progress.[2] Codeine is metabolized mainly by conjugation to codeine-6-glucuronide, but also by O-demethylation to **morphine** (via CYP2D6) and by N-demethylation (via CYP3A3/4).

It is unclear how much of the analgesic effect of codeine is a direct one.[3] Codeine is at least partly a pro-drug, with 2–10% of codeine biotransformed to **morphine**.[4,5] The major metabolite (80%) is codeine-6-glucuronide, and this may also contributes to the overall analgesic effect.[6,7]

Codeine lacks significant analgesic activity when the biotransformation to **morphine** is blocked by CYP2D6 inhibitors such as **fluoxetine**, **paroxetine** and **quinidine** (see p.551). Further, genetic polymorphism of the CYP2D6 enzyme results in significant interindividual variation in the production of **morphine**, which may lead to differences in patient response.[8–10] In one study, nearly 50% of children and nearly 40% of adults had genotypes associated with reduced enzyme activity.[11] In contrast, ultra-rapid CYP2D6 metabolism can occasionally lead to an increased amount of **morphine**, and life-threatening opioid intoxication.[12,13]

Like **morphine**, codeine is antitussive and also slows GI transit.[14] Given that opioids can cause pruritus, it is noteworthy that a patient with primary biliary cirrhosis obtained relief with regular oral codeine (also see Opioid antagonists, p.338).[15] Because of constipation, codeine was stopped and the pruritus returned. When codeine was restarted, together with a laxative, the patient again obtained relief.

Bio-availability 40% (12–84%) PO.[4]
Onset of action 30–60min for analgesia; 1–2h for antitussive effect.
Time to peak plasma concentration 1–2h.
Plasma halflife 2.5–3.5h.[4]
Duration of action 4–6h.

Cautions and undesirable effects

For full list, see manufacturer's Product Monograph.
Also see Strong opioids, p.288.
Driving ability may be impaired by a dose of 50mg.[16,17]

Dose and use

*It is bad practice to prescribe codeine to patients already taking **morphine** or any other strong opioid; if a greater effect is needed, the dose of **morphine** (or other strong opioid) should be increased.*

Pain relief

Codeine is often given in a combination product with a non-opioid. The codeine content of these products is generally 15mg, 30mg or 60mg (lower strengths, e.g. 8mg, are present in some OTC **acetaminophen**-codeine products). Thus patients with inadequate relief may benefit by changing to a higher strength product. When given alone, the dose is generally 30–60mg q4h. Higher doses can be given but equivalent analgesic doses of **morphine** (1/10 the dose of codeine) are probably less constipating.

Cough

Codeine an antitussive by any route. The dose is tailored to the patient's need, e.g. 15–30mg p.r.n., up to q4h. Administration as an oral liquid or syrup is *not* necessary.

Diarrhea

To control diarrhea, a dose of 30–60mg is used both p.r.n. and regularly up to q4h. However, **loperamide** may be preferable (see p.22).

As with all opioids, patients must be monitored for undesirable effects, particularly nausea and vomiting, and constipation (see Box 5.F, p.289). Depending on individual circumstances, an anti-emetic should be prescribed for regular or p.r.n. use (see p.183) and, routinely, a laxative prescribed (see p.26).

Supply

Unless indicated otherwise, all products are Schedule I controlled drugs under the Controlled Drugs and Substances Act, and are subject to the Narcotic Control Regulations of the act. Combination products containing codeine and **guaifenesin** are available OTC for cough.

Codeine phosphate (generic)
Tablets 15mg, 30mg, 28 days @ 30mg q.i.d. = $9.
Oral syrup 5mg/mL, 28 days @ 30mg q.i.d. = $20.
Injections are available but are not recommended.

Sustained-release
Codeine Contin® (Purdue Pharma)

Note: doses of Codeine Contin® are expressed as codeine *base*, whereas those of codeine phosphate formulations are expressed as the *phosphate* salt. Codeine phosphate contains approximately 75% codeine base. Thus, when transferring from normal-release codeine phosphate to Codeine Contin®, the total daily dose should be reduced to 3/4 of the previous codeine phosphate total daily dose.

Tablets SR Codeine Contin® 50, codeine *monohydrate* and codeine *sulfate trihydrate* equivalent to a total of 50mg of codeine base, 28 days @ 50mg b.i.d. = $18.
Tablets SR Codeine Contin® 100, codeine *monohydrate* and codeine *sulfate trihydrate* equivalent to a total of 100mg of codeine base, 28 days @ 100mg b.i.d. = $36.
Tablets SR Codeine Contin® 150, codeine *monohydrate* and codeine *sulfate trihydrate* equivalent to a total of 150mg of codeine base, 28 days @ 150mg b.i.d. = $55.
Tablets SR Codeine Contin® 200, codeine *monohydrate* and codeine *sulfate trihydrate* equivalent to a total of 200mg of codeine base, 28 days @ 200mg b.i.d. = $72.

With **acetaminophen** (selected list)
Codeine and **acetaminophen** 30/300 (generic)
Tablets codeine phosphate 30mg + **acetaminophen** 300mg, 28 days @ 2 t.i.d. = $22.

Codeine and **acetaminophen** 60/300 (generic)
Tablets codeine phosphate 60mg + **acetaminophen** 300mg, 28 days @ 1 t.i.d. = $14.

Tylenol® with codeine No 4 (Janssen-Ortho)
Tablets codeine phosphate 60mg + **acetaminophen** 300mg, 28 days @ 1 t.i.d. = $16.

1 Beaver W (1966) Mild analgesics: a review of their clinical pharmacology (Part II). *American Journal of Medical Science.* **251**: 576–599.
2 Jackson KC and Wiffen PJ (2007) Codeine, alone and with paracetamol (acetaminophen), for cancer pain (Protocol). *Cochrane Database of Systematic Reviews.* **3**: CD006601.
3 Quiding H et al. (1993) Analgesic effect and plasma concentrations of codeine and morphine after two dose levels of codeine following oral surgery. *European Journal of Clinical Pharmacology.* **44**: 319–323.
4 Persson K et al. (1992) The postoperative pharmacokinetics of codeine. *European Journal of Clinical Pharmacology.* **42**: 663–666.
5 Findlay JWA et al. (1978) Plasma codeine and morphine concentrations after therapeutic oral doses of codeine-containing analgesics. *Clinical Pharmacology and Therapeutics.* **24**: 60–68.
6 Vree TB et al. (2000) Codeine analgesia is due to codeine-6-glucuronide, not morphine. *International Journal of Clinical Practice.* **54**: 395–398.
7 Lotsch J et al. (2006) Evidence for morphine-independent central nervous opioid effects after administration of codeine: contribution of other codeine metabolites. *Clinical Pharmacology & Therapeutics.* **79**: 35–48.
8 Sindrup SH and Brosen K (1995) The pharmacogenetics of codeine hypoalgesia. *Pharmacogenetics.* **5**: 335–346.
9 Caraco Y et al. (1996) Pharmacogenetic determination of the effects of codeine and prediction of drug interactions. *Journal of Pharmacology and Experimental Therapeutics.* **278**: 1165–1174.

10 Lurcott G (1999) The effects of the genetic absence and inhibition of CYP2D6 on the metabolism of codeine and its derivatives, hydrocodone and oxycodone. *Anesthesia Progress.* **45**: 154–156.

11 Williams DG *et al.* (2002) Pharmacogenetics of codeine metabolism in an urban population of children and its implications for analgesic reliability. *British Journal of Anaesthesia.* **89**: 839–845.

12 Gasche Y *et al.* (2004) Codeine intoxication associated with ultrarapid CYP2D6 metabolism. *New England Journal of Medicine.* **351**: 2827–2831.

13 Koren G *et al.* (2006) Pharmacogenetics of morphine poisoning in a breastfed neonate of a codeine-prescribed mother. *Lancet.* **368**: 704.

14 Anonymous (1989) Drugs in the management of acute diarrhoea in infants and young children. *Bulletin of the World Health Organization.* **67**: 94–96.

15 Zylicz Z and Krajnik M (1999) Codeine for pruritus in primary biliary cirrhosis. *Lancet.* **353**: 813.

16 Linnoila M and Mattila MJ (1973) Proceedings: Drug interaction on driving skills as evaluated by laboratory tests and by a driving simulator. *Pharmakopsychiatric Neuro-Psychopharmakologie.* **6**: 127–132.

17 Linnoila M and Hakkinen S (1974) Effects of diazepam and codeine, alone and in combination with alcohol, on simulated driving. *Clinical Pharmacology and Therapeutics.* **15**: 368–373.

PROPOXYPHENE (DEXTROPROPOXYPHENE)

Class: Opioid analgesic.

Indications: Mild–moderate pain.

Contra-indications: **Acetaminophen**-propoxyphene should not be prescribed to the following groups: age <18 years, alcohol-dependent, unwilling to abstain from alcohol while taking **acetaminophen**-propoxyphene, addiction-prone, thought to be suicidal, severe renal impairment (creatinine clearance <10mL/min).

Pharmacology

Propoxyphene (rINN dextropropoxyphene) is a synthetic derivative of **methadone**. It is a μ-opioid receptor agonist with affinity similar to that of **codeine**. However, whereas **codeine** is mainly a pro-drug (see p.278), propoxyphene itself is responsible for most of its analgesic effect. It is also a weak NMDA-receptor-channel blocker[1] but this is unlikely to be clinically relevant. Propoxyphene undergoes extensive dose-dependent first-pass hepatic metabolism; systemic availability increases with increasing doses.[2] The principal metabolite, norpropoxyphene, is also analgesic but crosses the blood–brain barrier to a lesser extent.

In *single-dose* RCTs in patients with postoperative pain, arthritis and musculoskeletal pain, no added benefit is seen when propoxyphene combined with **acetaminophen** is compared with **acetaminophen** alone.[3] Such reports have led to doubts about the efficacy of propoxyphene. However, propoxyphene *hydrochloride* 65mg (not Canada) has been shown to have a definite analgesic effect in several placebo-controlled trials,[4] and a dose-response curve for both propoxyphene *hydrochloride* and propoxyphene *napsylate* has been established (Figure 5.9).[4,5] Placebos do not have a dose-response curve.

Because of the long halflife of both propoxyphene and norpropoxyphene in elderly patients, it takes about 1 week to achieve a steady-state when propoxyphene is taken regularly t.i.d.–q.i.d., and plasma concentrations are some 5 and 7 times greater than after a single dose.[6,7] Thus, rather like **methadone** (see p.327), the effect of multiple doses cannot be estimated from single-dose studies.[8,9] Further, whereas the NNT in single-dose studies for a 50% reduction in moderate or severe postoperative pain for propoxyphene *hydrochloride* 65mg is 8, for 130mg the NNT is only 3. Because of accumulation when given regularly round the clock, the latter NNT is likely to more closely reflect the response with multiple doses of 65mg.

The relative potency of a *single* dose of propoxyphene is 1/2–2/3 that of **codeine**.[2] However, because of accumulation with multiple doses, when given regularly t.i.d.–q.i.d., it is reasonable to assume that it is at least as potent as **codeine**, i.e. is about 1/10 as potent as PO **morphine** on a weight-for-weight basis. Propoxyphene causes less nausea and vomiting, drowsiness and dry mouth than low-dose **morphine**, particularly during initial treatment.[10]

Bio-availability 40% PO.

Onset of action 20–30min.

Time to peak plasma concentration 2–2.5h.

Plasma halflife 6–12h, norpropoxyphene 30–36h; increasing in the elderly to 36h, norpropoxyphene to >50h.[6]

Duration of action single dose 4–6h; longer in the elderly and when taken regularly.

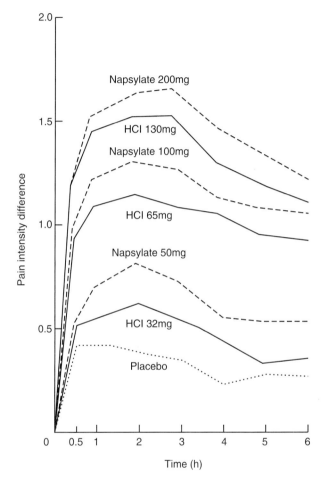

Figure 5.9 Incremental pain relief with increasing doses of propoxyphene *hydrochloride* and propoxyphene *napsylate*.[5]

Cautions

May impair the ability to perform skilled tasks, e.g. driving. In elderly patients prescribed a standard dose regimen, because of increased plasma halflife, accumulation leading to drowsiness, delirium and respiratory depression is possible after 7–10 days.

Hepatic or renal impairment.[11,12] Propoxyphene may enhance the effect of **warfarin**, **carbamazepine**[13] and CNS depressants, including alcohol. Patients should be advised to severely restrict or abstain from alcohol when taking propoxyphene. Propoxyphene prolongs the plasma halflife of **alprazolam** by 50% (12h → 18h); it has no effect on the metabolism of **lorazepam** and a clinically unimportant effect on **diazepam**.[14]

Subacute painful myopathy has occurred after chronic ingestion of larger-than-recommended doses. Chronic ingestion of propoxyphene *napsylate* doses exceeding 800mg/24h has caused toxic psychoses and seizures.

In 2007, **acetaminophen**-propoxyphene was withdrawn from general availability in the UK.[15,16] This was primarily because of its relatively common use in intentional overdose and its potential fatal toxicity in accidental overdose.[17] The withdrawal of propoxyphene products has now been recommended throughout Europe,[18] and the FDA has strengthened product warnings while considering its withdrawal in the USA.[19,20] There are no plans to withdraw propoxyphene on safety grounds in Canada, although only one product remains available. The UK, European and US authorities stated that there is no good evidence that **acetaminophen**-propoxyphene is superior to **acetaminophen** alone as an analgesic.[15,18,19] However, although this may be true for single doses, it is *not* true for chronic regular use (see Pharmacology).

Undesirable effects

For full list, see manufacturer's Product Monograph.
The most frequently reported undesirable effects of propoxyphene *napsylate* are dizziness, drowsiness, nausea and vomiting. Others include lightheadedness, headache, weakness, euphoria, dysphoria, sleep disturbances (drowsiness or insomnia), paradoxical excitement, minor visual disturbances, constipation, abdominal pain and rashes.

Propoxyphene *napsylate* has also been associated with hypoglycemia, abnormal LFTs and, more rarely, with reversible jaundice (both hepatocellular and cholestatic).

Dose and use

Around the world, propoxyphene is marketed as either the *hydrochloride* salt (discontinued in Canada in 2008) or as the *napsylate*; propoxyphene *napsylate* 100mg is equivalent to propoxyphene *hydrochloride* 65mg, the difference relating to the different molecular weights of the two salts. For propoxyphene *napsylate*:
* start with 100mg t.i.d.–q.i.d.
* if satisfactory pain relief, consider reducing the total daily dose in the elderly after 5–7 days by increasing the interval between doses, e.g. reducing from q.i.d. to t.i.d.
* maximum total daily dose 600mg; exceeding this dose increases the risk of toxic effects
* a lower maximum maintenance daily dose would seem advisable in the elderly, e.g. 300mg (100mg t.i.d.).

As with all opioids, patients must be monitored for undesirable effects, particularly nausea and vomiting, and constipation (see Box 5.F, p.239). Depending on individual circumstances, an anti-emetic should be prescribed for regular or p.r.n. use (see p.183) and, routinely, a laxative prescribed (see p.26).

Overdose

The manufacturer's Product Monograph contains detailed instructions for managing an overdose of propoxyphene napsylate.

Supply

Propoxyphene is a Schedule I controlled drug under the Controlled Drugs and Substances Act (CDSA), and is subject to the CDSA Narcotic Control Regulations.

Darvon-N® (Paladin)
Capsules propoxyphene *napsylate* 100mg (equivalent to propoxyphene *hydrochloride* 65mg), 28 days @ 100mg q4h = $66.

1 Ebert B et al. (1998) Dextropropoxyphene acts as a noncompetitive N-methyl d-aspartate antagonist. *Journal of Pain and Symptom Management.* **15**: 269–274.
2 Perrier D and Gibaldi M (1972) Influence of first-pass effect on the systemic availability of propoxyphene. *The Journal of Clinical Pharmacology.* **Nov/Dec**: 449–452.
3 Li-Wan-Po A and Zhang W (1997) Systematic overview of co-proxamol to assess analgesic effects of addition of dextropropoxyphene to paracetamol. *British Medical Journal.* **315**: 1565–1571.

4 Collins SL et al. (1998) Single-dose dextropropoxyphene in post-operative pain: a quantitative systematic review. European Journal of Clinical Pharmacology. **54**: 107–112.
5 Beaver WT (1984) Analgesic efficacy of dextropropoxyphene and dextropropoxyphene-containing combinations: a review. Human Toxicology. **3 (suppl)**: 191s–220s.
6 Crome P et al. (1984) Pharmacokinetics of dextropropoxyphene and nordextropropoxyphene in elderly hospital patients after single and multiple doses of distalgesic. Preliminary analysis of results. Human Toxicology. **3 (suppl)**: 41s–48s.
7 Twycross RG (1984) Plasma concentrations of dextropropoxyphene and norpropoxyphene. Human Toxicology. **3 (suppl)**: 58s–59s.
8 Sykes JV et al. (1996) Coproxamol revisited. Lancet. **348**: 408.
9 Hanks GW and Forbes K (1998) Co-proxamol is effective in chronic pain. British Medical Journal. **316**: 1980–.
10 Mercadante S et al. (1998) Dextropropoxyphene versus morphine in opioid-naive cancer patients with pain. Journal of Pain and Symptom Management. **15**: 76–81.
11 Gibson T et al. (1980) Propoxyphene and norpropoxyphene plasma concentrations in the anephric patient. Clinical Pharmacology and Therapeutics. **27**: 665–670.
12 Giacomini KM et al. (1980) Effect of hemodialysis on propoxyphene and norpropoxyphene concentrations in blood of anephric patients. Clinical Pharmacology and Therapeutics. **27**: 508–514.
13 Bergendal L et al. (1997) The clinical relevance of the interaction between carbamazepine and dextropropoxyphene in elderly patients in Gothenburg, Sweden. European Journal of Clinical Pharmacology. **53**: 203–206.
14 Abernethy D et al. (1985) Interaction of propoxyphene with diazepam, alprazolam and lorazepam. British Journal of Clinical Pharmacology. **19**: 51–57.
15 Anonymous (2006) The withdrawal of co-proxamol: alternative analgesics for mild to moderate pain. MeReC Bulletin. **16**: 13–16.
16 CHM (2006) Withdrawal of co-proxamol (Distalgesic, Cosalgesic, Dolgesic). Current Problems in Pharmacovigilance. **31 (May)**: 11.
17 Hawton K et al. (2003) Co-proxamol and suicide: a study of national mortality statistics and local non-fatal self poisonings. British Medical Journal. **326**: 1006–1008.
18 European Medicines Agency (2009) Press Release. European Medicines Agency recommends withdrawal of dextropropoxyphene-containing medicines. Available from: www.emea.europa.eu/pdfs/human/press/pr/40106209en.pdf
19 FDA Joint Advisory Committee (2009) Final summary minutes. Joint meeting of the Anesthetic and Life Support Drugs Advisory Committee and the Drug Safety and Risk Management Committee. January 30th 2009. Available from: www.fda.gov/ohrms/dockets/ac/09/minutes/2009-4411m1-final.pdf
20 FDA (2009) Propoxyphene questions and answers. Available from: www.fda.gov/Drugs/DrugSafety/PostmarketDrugSafetyInformationforPatientsandProviders/ucm170268.htm

TRAMADOL

Class: Opioid analgesic.

Indications: Moderate–severe pain.

Contra-indications: Use of MAO inhibitors concurrently or within 14 days. Severe renal impairment (creatinine clearance < 30mL/min), severe hepatic impairment (Child-Pugh Class C), age < 18 years.

Pharmacology

Tramadol is a synthetic centrally acting analgesic with both opioid and non-opioid properties.[1,2] It stimulates neuronal serotonin release and inhibits the presynaptic re-uptake of both norepinephrine and serotonin. In animal models, tramadol also has an anti-inflammatory effect which is independent of PG inhibition.[3] A comparison of opioid receptor site affinities and mono-amine re-uptake inhibition illustrates the unique combination of properties which underlie the action of tramadol (Table 5.11 and Table 5.12); it is necessary to invoke synergism to explain its analgesic effect.[2]

Table 5.11 Opioid receptor affinities: K_i (micromol) values[a,4]

	μ	δ	κ
Morphine	0.0003	0.09	0.6
Propoxyphene	0.03	0.38	1.2
Codeine	0.2	5	6
Tramadol	2	58	43

a. the lower the K_i value, the greater the receptor affinity.

Table 5.12 Inhibition of mono-amine uptake: K_i (micromol) values[a,4]

	Norepinephrine	Serotonin
Imipramine	0.0066	0.021
Tramadol	0.78	0.99
Codeine		
Propoxyphene }	IA[b]	IA[b]
Morphine		

a. the lower the K_i value, the greater the receptor affinity
b. IA = inactive at 10micromol.

Although **naloxone** can only partially reverse the effects of tramadol,[4,5] in a series of 11 patients with a tramadol overdose, seven had a good response to **naloxone**, and only one had no response.[6]

Tramadol is converted in the liver mainly via CYP2D6 to O-desmethyltramadol (M1). This is an active metabolite which, in animals, is 6 times more potent than tramadol.[7] Further biotransformation results in many inactive metabolites which are excreted by the kidneys.

Poor metabolizers, comprising 7–10% of the Caucasian population in Europe, lack CYP2D6.[8,9] Poor metabolizers have a decreased response to tramadol.[10–12] A reduced effect has also been reported when tramadol and **paroxetine**, a CYP2D6 inhibitor, have been prescribed concurrently.[13]

Tramadol has a negligible antihyperalgesic effect.[14] However, in a short-term experimental pain study in volunteers, when combined with **acetaminophen** (a non-opioid with known antihyperalgesic properties), the combination manifested greater analgesia and greater antihyperalgesia, even when the dose of both drugs was halved.[14]

In placebo-controlled trials, tramadol significantly improves neuropathic pain (e.g. diabetic neuropathy, post-herpetic neuralgia, polyneuropathy), with an NNT of 3.8.[15] This is comparable with several anti-epileptics, but not as good as the TCAs (NNT = 2.3, see p.235) Further, **oxycodone** has an NNT of 2.5 in post-herpetic neuralgia[16] and, in an RCT of cancer and non-cancer patients with and without neuropathic pain, tramadol was indistinguishable from **morphine**.[17]

Tramadol is as effective as **codeine** as a cough suppressant.[18] Tramadol causes less constipation and respiratory depression than equi-analgesic doses of **morphine**.[19–21] In contrast to **morphine**, tramadol reduces the basal pressure in the Sphincter of Oddi (for less than 20min after IM administration) and does not increase the pressure in the common bile duct.[22] Its dependence liability is also considerably less,[23] and it is not a controlled drug in Canada, although this is currently under review.[24] As with other opioids, physical dependence develops with chronic use.[25]

By injection (not Canada), tramadol is generally regarded as 1/10 as potent as **morphine** (e.g. tramadol 100mg is equivalent to **morphine** 10mg).[26] In fact, various pre- and postoperative studies give a range of potency ratios, from 1:11–1:19,[27,28] suggesting that the figure of 1:10 is more of a 'convenient to remember' ratio than a scientifically precise one. Some of the postoperative studies also suggest that, to produce adequate analgesia, tramadol needs to be administered more frequently than **morphine** over the first few hours (by IV PCA), after which doses become less frequent. The need for the equivalent of a loading dose with tramadol may reflect its different mode of action from **morphine**. A delayed maximum effect has also been reported in an RCT of oral tramadol and **morphine**.[17]

By mouth compared with **morphine**, RCTs indicate a potency ratio of 1:5 and 1:4 respectively (i.e. tramadol 100mg PO = **morphine** 20–25mg).[29,30] However, extensive clinical experience has led many physicians to regard the potency ratio for PO tramadol and PO **morphine** to be 1:10 (i.e. tramadol 100mg PO = **morphine** 10mg PO), i.e. the same as by injection.[31,32]

Bio-availability 65–75% PO; 90% with multiple doses;[33] 77% PR.[34,35]
Onset of action 30min–1h.
Time to peak plasma concentration 2h; 4–8h SR.
Plasma halflife 6h; active metabolite 7.4h; these more than double in cirrhosis and severe renal failure.
Duration of action 4–9h.

Cautions

Epilepsy, head trauma or raised intracranial pressure, mild–moderate renal or hepatic impairment, suicide-prone patients.

Tramadol has been associated with seizures, notably when the total daily dose exceeds 400mg or when tramadol is used concurrently with other medications which lower the seizure threshold, e.g. TCAs, SSRIs, antipsychotics, and other opioids.[6,36,37] Seizures have also been reported in patients after rapid IV injection of tramadol. Treat with standard measures, i.e. IV benzodiazepines (see p.112). Resolution generally occurs in <1 day.[6] Fatalities resulting from tramadol-induced seizures are extremely rare.[7]

Serotonin toxicity has occasionally occurred when tramadol has been taken concurrently with a second drug which also interferes with presynaptic serotonin re-uptake (see p.140). Caution is necessary in patients with a history of substance abuse because of the risk of tramadol-dependence in such individuals.[32]

The analgesic effect of tramadol is reduced by **ondansetron** (possibly by blocking the action of serotonin at presynaptic $5HT_3$-receptors on primary afferent nociceptive neurones in the spinal dorsal horn).[38] In postoperative pain, the dose of tramadol needed by IV PCA was 2–3 times greater in patients also receiving **ondansetron** 1mg/h by CIVI. There was also an increase in vomiting (despite the **ondansetron**).[39] This is probably a class effect for $5HT_3$-receptor antagonists.

Carbamazepine also decreases the effect of tramadol. CYP2D6 inhibitors, e.g. **quinidine** and **paroxetine**, decrease analgesia by inhibiting the conversion of tramadol to its active metabolite.[13] Tramadol occasionally and unpredictably prolongs the INR of patients taking **warfarin**;[40,41] monitor the INR closely and adjust the **warfarin** dose if necessary.[41]

Undesirable effects

For full list, see manufacturer's Product Monograph.

Very common (>10%): headache, drowsiness, dizziness. nausea, vomiting, constipation.

Common (<10%, >1%): asthenia, seizures (dose-dependent, see Cautions above), sweating, dry mouth, diarrhea.

Also see Strong opioids, p.288.

Dose and use

- With cancer pain in patients already taking a non-opioid, generally start with 200mg SR once daily (100–150mg in very frail patients or those with hepatic or renal impairment)[1]
- if necessary, increase the dose in stages to a maximum recommended total daily dose of 400mg (less in very frail patients or those with hepatic or renal impairment)
- higher doses have been given, e.g. 600mg/24h, and sometimes more[31,32,42]
- for break-through (episodic) pain when taking SR tramadol, consider tramadol and **acetaminophen** in combination (Tramacet®), or normal-release **morphine** (see p.301).

As with all opioids, patients must be monitored for undesirable effects, particularly nausea and vomiting, and constipation (see Box 5.F, p.289). Depending on individual circumstances, an anti-emetic should be prescribed for regular or p.r.n. use (see p.183) and, routinely, a laxative prescribed (see p.26).

If tramadol becomes inadequate, the patient will generally be switched to a strong opioid. It has been suggested that the dose of tramadol should be tapered over several days, rather than being stopped abruptly.[2] However, this is not necessary when switching to **morphine** (or other strong opioid); an abrupt switch from tramadol does *not* result in an antidepressant type discontinuation/withdrawal syndrome.[43]

Supply

Tramadol is not currently a controlled drug. However, the Canadian government is considering applications for it to be made a Schedule I or Schedule IV drug under the Controlled Drugs and

Substances Act to establish consistency with the scheduling of other opioids, and to reflect the potential for abuse.[24]

Sustained-release
Ralivia® (Biovail Pharmaceuticals Canada)
Tablets SR 100mg, 200mg, 300mg, 28 days @ 300mg once daily = $92.

Tridural® (Labopharm)
Tablets SR 100mg, 200mg, 300mg, 28 days @ 300mg once daily = $92.

Zytram XL® (Purdue Pharma)
Tablets SR 150mg, 200mg, 300mg, 400mg, 28 days @ 300mg once daily = $92.

With **acetaminophen**
Tramacet® (Janssen-Ortho)
Tablets tramadol hydrochloride 37.5mg, **acetaminophen** 325mg, 28 days @ 2 q.i.d. = $167.

1 Grond S and Sablotzki A (2004) Clinical pharmacology of tramadol. *Clinical Pharmacokinetics*. **43**: 879–923.
2 Dickman A (2007) Tramadol: a review of this atypical opioid. *European Journal of Palliative Care*. **14**: 181–185.
3 Buccellati C et al. (2000) Tramadol anti-inflammatory activity is not related to a direct inhibitory action on prostaglandin endoperoxide synthases. *European Journal of Pain*. **4**: 413–415.
4 Raffa RB et al. (1992) Opioid and nonopioid components independently contribute to the mechanism of action of tramadol, an 'atypical' opioid analgesic. *Journal of Pharmacology and Therapeutics*. **260**: 275–285.
5 Shipton EA (2000) Tramadol – present and future. *Anaesthesia and Intensive Care*. **28**: 363–374.
6 Marquardt KA et al. (2005) Tramadol exposures reported to statewide poison control system. *Annals of Pharmacotherapy*. **39**: 1039–1044.
7 Close BR (2005) Tramadol: does it have a role in emergency medicine? *Emergency Medicine Australasia*. **17**: 73–83.
8 Sachse C et al. (1997) Cytochrome P450 2D6 variants in a Caucasian population: allele frequencies and phenotypic consequences. *American Journal of Human Genetics*. **60**: 284–295.
9 Zanger UM et al. (2004) Cytochrome P450 2D6: overview and update on pharmacology, genetics, biochemistry. *Naunyn Schmiedeberg's Archives of Pharmacology*. **369**: 23–37.
10 Collart L et al. (1993) [Duality of the analgesic effect of tramadol in humans]. *Schweizerische Medizinische Wochenschrift*. **123**: 2241–2243.
11 Poulsen L et al. (1996) The hypoalgesic effect of tramadol in relation to CYP2D6. *Clinical Pharmacology and Therapeutics*. **60**: 636–644.
12 Stamer UM et al. (2003) Impact of CYP2D6 genotype on postoperative tramadol analgesia. *Pain*. **105**: 231–238.
13 Laugesen S et al. (2005) Paroxetine, a cytochrome P450 2D6 inhibitor, diminishes the stereoselective O-demethylation and reduces the hypoalgesic effect of tramadol. *Clinical Pharmacology and Therapeutics*. **77**: 312–323.
14 Filitz J et al. (2007) Supra-additive effects of tramadol and acetaminophen in a human pain model. *Pain*.
15 Hollingshead J et al. (2006) Tramadol for neuropathic pain. *Cochrane Database Syst Rev*. **3**: CD003726.
16 Watson C and Babul N (1998) Efficacy of oxycodone in neuropathic pain: a randomized trial in postherpetic neuralgia. *Neurology*. **50**: 1837–1841.
17 Leppert W (2001) Analgesic efficacy and side effects of oral tramadol and morphine administered orally in the treatment of cancer pain. *Nowotwory*. **51**: 257–266.
18 Szekely SM and Vickers MD (1992) A comparison of the effects of codeine and tramadol on laryngeal reactivity. *European Journal of Anaesthesiology*. **9**: 111–120.
19 Wilder-Smith C and Bettiga A (1997) The analgesic tramadol has minimal effect on gastrointestinal motor function. *British Journal of Clinical Pharmacology*. **43**: 71–75.
20 Wilder-Smith CH et al. (1999) Effect of tramadol and morphine on pain and gastrointestinal motor function in patients with chronic pancreatitis. *Digestive Diseases and Sciences*. **44**: 1107–1116.
21 Houmes R et al. (1992) Efficacy and safety of tramadol versus morphine for moderate and severe postoperative pain with special regard to respiratory depression. *Anesthesia and Analgesia*. **74**: 510–514.
22 Wu SD et al. (2004) Effects of narcotic analgesic drugs on human Oddi's sphincter motility. *World Journal of Gastroenterology*. **10**: 2901–2904.
23 Preston K et al. (1991) Abuse potential and pharmacological comparison of tramadol and morphine. *Drug and Alcohol Dependency*. **27**: 7–18.
24 Edwards R (2008) Notice to interested parties – proposal regarding the regulation of tramadol under the Controlled Drugs and Substances Act (CDSA) and its Regulations. In: *Canada Gazette part I, 2nd February 2008*. Available from: www.gazette.gc.ca/rp-pr/p1/2008/2008-02-02/pdf/g1-14205.pdf
25 Soyka M et al. (2004) Tramadol use and dependence in chronic noncancer pain patients. *Pharmacopsychiatry*. **37**: 191–192.
26 Vickers M et al. (1992) Tramadol: pain relief by an opioid without depression of respiration. *Anaesthesia*. **47**: 291–296.
27 Naguib M et al. (1998) Perioperative antinociceptive effects of tramadol. A prospective, randomized, double-blind comparison with morphine. *Canadian Journal of Anesthesia*. **45**: 1168–1175.
28 Pang WW et al. (1999) Comparison of patient-controlled analgesia (PCA) with tramadol or morphine. *Canadian Journal of Anesthesia*. **46**: 1030–1035.
29 Tawfik MO et al. (1990) Tramadol hydrochloride in the relief of cancer pain: a double blind comparison against sustained release morphine. *Pain*. **(suppl. 5)**: S377.
30 Wilder-Smith CH et al. (1994) Oral tramadol, a mu-opioid agonist and monoamine reuptake-blocker, and morphine for strong cancer-related pain. *Annals of Oncology*. **5**: 141–146.
31 Grond S et al. (1999) High-dose tramadol in comparison to low-dose morphine for cancer pain relief. *Journal of Pain and Symptom Management*. **18**: 174–179.
32 Leppert W and Luczak J (2005) The role of tramadol in cancer pain treatment–a review. *Support Care Cancer*. **13**: 5–17.

33 Gibson T (1996) Pharmacokinetics, efficacy, and safety of analgesia with a focus on tramadol HCl. *American Journal of Medicine.* **101 (suppl 1A)**: 47s–53s.

34 Lintz W et al. (1998) Pharmacokinetics of tramadol and bioavailability of enteral tramadol formulations. 3rd Communication: suppositories. *Arzneimittelforschung.* **48**: 889–899.

35 Mercadante S et al. (2005) Randomized double-blind, double-dummy crossover clinical trial of oral tramadol versus rectal tramadol administration in opioid-naive cancer patients with pain. *Support Care Cancer.* **13**: 702–707.

36 Spiller HA et al. (1997) Prospective multicenter evaluation of tramadol exposure. *Journal of Toxicology and Clinical Toxicology.* **35**: 361–364.

37 Boyd IW (2005) Tramadol and seizures. *Medical Journal of Australia.* **182**: 595–596.

38 De Witte JL et al. (2001) The analgesic efficacy of tramadol is impaired by concurrent administration of ondansetron. *Anesthesia and Analgesia.* **92**: 1319–1321.

39 Arcioni R et al. (2002) Ondansetron inhibits the analgesic effects of tramadol: a possible 5-HT(3) spinal receptor involvement in acute pain in humans. *Anesthesia and Analgesia.* **94**: 1553–1557, table of contents.

40 Sabbe JR et al. (1998) Tramadol–warfarin interaction. *Pharmacotherapy.* **18**: 871–873.

41 Baxter K (ed) (2008) *Stockley's Drug Interactions* (8e). Pharmaceutical Press, London.

42 Osipova N et al. (1991) Analgesic effect of tramadol in cancer patients with chronic pain: A comparison with prolonged-action morphine sulfate. *Current Therapeutic Research.* **50**: 812–815.

43 Leppert W (2008) Personal communication.

STRONG OPIOIDS

Strong opioids exist to be given, not merely to be withheld; their use should be dictated by therapeutic need and response, not by brevity of prognosis.[1,2]

Contra-indications: Provided the dose of an opioid is carefully titrated against the patient's pain, there are generally no absolute contra-indications to the use of strong opioids in palliative care. However, there are circumstances, e.g. renal impairment, when it may be better to avoid the use of certain opioids and/or positively choose certain other ones (see p.295; also see Guidance about prescribing in palliative care, p.477).

Opioid receptors

There are four opioid receptors (μ, κ, δ, and ORL-1) distributed in varying densities throughout the body, particularly in nervous tissue. Their naturally-occurring ligands are peptides which function as neural transmitters. Like other peptides, they are synthesized as large inactive precursors in the neuronal cell body, and are then cleaved while being transported to the nerve terminals. The active fragment is released into the synapse and binds to one or more receptors. All opioid receptors are inhibitory (Table 5.13).

Opioid receptors are found both pre- and post-synaptically, with the former predominating. Presynaptic receptor activation controls the release of several neurotransmitters. Endogenous peptides are rapidly degraded, and have a relatively short duration of action. In contrast, exogenous opioids such as **morphine** have a prolonged effect. They produce analgesia primarily by interacting with μ-opioid receptors in the CNS. In the presence of local inflammation, opioids also have a peripheral analgesic action because inflammation activates otherwise dormant opioid receptors in the peripheral nerve terminals. Undesirable effects relate to both central and peripheral receptors, mainly in the CNS and GI tract.

All clinically important opioid analgesics act as agonists at the μ-opioid receptor (Table 5.13), and some may also have significant effects on δ-opioid receptors (e.g. **methadone**, see p.327) and κ-opioid receptors (e.g. **oxycodone**, see p.335). Some opioids are mixed agonist–antagonists (e.g. **buprenorphine** is a partial μ-opioid receptor *agonist*, an opioid-receptor-like (ORL-1) *agonist*, and a κ- and δ-opioid receptor *antagonist*.)[3–6] Note: there are no **buprenorphine** products available in Canada for analgesic use.

Clinical use

Morphine is the strong opioid of choice for cancer pain management (see p.300).[9–11] Other strong opioids are used mainly when:
- **morphine** is not readily available
- the TD route is preferable
- the patient has unacceptable undesirable effects with **morphine**.[12]

Table 5.13   Opioid receptors, ligands,[7,8] and effects[a]

Receptors	Mu (μ)	Delta (δ)	Kappa (κ)	ORL-I
Endogenous opioid	β-Endorphin Endormorphins	Enkephalins	Dynorphins	Nociceptin
Exogenous agonist	Morphine Buprenorphine[b] Codeine Fentanils Hydromorphone Meperidine Methadone Oxycodone	DSTBULET Methadone (?)	U50488H Oxycodone (?)	Buprenorphine
Antagonists	Naloxone Naltrexone	Buprenorphine Naloxone	Buprenorphine Naloxone	
Effector mechanism	G protein opens K$^+$ channel	G protein opens K$^+$ channel	G protein closes Ca^{++} channel	G protein opens K$^+$ channel
Effects	*Hyperpolarisation of neurones, inhibition of neurotransmitter release* Analgesia Euphoria Nausea Constipation Cough suppression Dependence Respiratory depression Miosis	Similar to μ but less marked	Analgesia Aversion Diuresis	Mixed analgesia (spinal) and anti-opioid (brain)

a. see also individual drug monographs
b. partial agonist.

Differences between opioids relate in part to differences in receptor affinity (see Table 5.13). Improved pain relief should not be expected if a patient is switched to another opioid of similar opioid-receptor affinity. However, the pattern and severity of undesirable effects may be altered, e.g. when switching from **morphine** to **oxycodone** (see p.335) or TD **fentanyl** (see p.315).

Strong opioids are not the panacea for cancer pain; effective analgesia generally requires the use of both a strong opioid and a non-opioid. Further, even combined use does not guarantee success, particularly with neuropathic pain or if the psychosocial dimension of suffering is ignored. Other reasons for poor relief include:

- underdosing (failure to titrate the dose upwards or dose at the correct interval)
- poor patient adherence (patient not taking medication)
- poor alimentary absorption, e.g. because of vomiting.

Pentazocine should *not* be used; it is a weak opioid by mouth,[13,14] and often causes psychotomimetic effects (dysphoria, depersonalization, frightening dreams, hallucinations).[15] **Meperidine** also should *not* be used (Box 5.E).

Undesirable effects
For full list, see manufacturer's Product Monograph.
Strong opioids tend to cause the same range of undesirable effects (Box 5.F), although to a varying degree. It is necessary to develop strategies to deal with the undesirable effects of **morphine** and other strong opioids, particularly nausea and vomiting (see p.183), and constipation (see p.26).[21]

Respiratory depression
Pain is a physiological antagonist to the central depressant effects of opioids.
When appropriately titrated against the patient's pain, strong opioids do not cause clinically important respiratory depression in patients in pain.[22,23,24] **Naloxone**, a specific opioid

---

Box 5.E Meperidine

The use of meperidine (pethidine) is actively discouraged in palliative care.
By mouth, in typical doses, it is little more than a weak opioid (see Table 5.15, p.295). It has a relatively short duration of action (2–3h) and is thus a bad choice for round-the-clock analgesia.

Meperidine has a toxic metabolite, normeperidine, which accumulates when meperidine is given regularly. Particularly in renal impairment, normeperidine causes tremors, multifocal myoclonus, agitation, and occasionally seizures.[16]

Meperidine:
- is not antitussive
- is less constipating than morphine but causes more vomiting
- causes less smooth muscle spasm (e.g. sphincter of Oddi)
- is antimuscarinic (anticholinergic)
- does not cause constriction of the pupils.[17]

Drug–drug interaction with:
phenobarbital ⎱
chlorpromazine ⎰ increase production of normeperidine.
MAOIs ⎱

Serotonin toxicity
Meperidine must not be given concurrently with an MAOI because of the risk of serotonin toxicity.[18–20] Within minutes of administration of an injection of meperidine, if a critical level of serotonin is exceeded in the CNS, the patient manifests:
agitation (may become violent)
multifocal myoclonus
sweating
cyanosis
hypertension
increased tendon reflexes and clonus
extensor plantar responses
Cheyne-Stokes respirations.

Overdose and effect of naloxone
Overdose is a mixed picture of CNS depression (meperidine) and excitation (normeperidine), with both stupor and seizures.
Naloxone will reverse the meperidine-induced stupor but not the stimulant effects of normeperidine. Seizures should be treated with a benzodiazepine (see p.112).

Box 5.F Undesirable effects of opioids when used for analgesia

Common initial
Nausea and vomiting
Drowsiness
Lightheadedness/unsteadiness
Delirium (acute confusional state)

Common ongoing
Constipation
Nausea and vomiting
Dry mouth

Possible ongoing
Suppression of hypothalamic-pituitary axis
Suppression of immune system

Less common
Neurotoxicity:
myoclonus
allodynia
hyperalgesia
cognitive failure/delirium
hallucinations
Sweating
Pruritus

Rare
Respiratory depression
Psychological dependence

---

antagonist, is rarely needed in palliative care (see p.343). In contrast to postoperative patients, cancer patients with pain:
- have generally been receiving a weak opioid for some time, i.e. are not opioid-naïve
- take medication PO (slower absorption, lower peak concentration)
- titrate the dose upwards step by step (less likelihood of an excessive dose being given).

The relationship of the therapeutic dose to the lethal dose of a strong opioid (the therapeutic ratio) is greater than commonly supposed. For example, patients who take a double dose of **morphine** at bedtime are no more likely to die during the night than those who do not.[25]

The *belief* that the lethal dose of **morphine** is the weight of the patient in kg given as mg of **morphine** is *false*, and, in any case, is irrelevant to palliative care practice. Patients receiving an individually titrated dose of PO **morphine** on a regular basis to relieve pain are not the same physiologically as people without pain who receive *de novo* **morphine** 40–80mg by injection.

Tolerance and dependence

Tolerance to strong opioids is not a practical problem.[26,27] Psychological dependence (addiction) to **morphine** is rare in patients.[24,28,29] Caution in this respect should be reserved for patients with a present or past history of substance abuse (Box 5.G); but even then strong opioids should be used when there is clinical need.[30,31] Physical dependence does not prevent a reduction in the dose of **morphine** if the patient's pain ameliorates, e.g. as a result of radiation therapy or a nerve block.[32]

Opioid-induced pruritus

Pruritus occurs in about 1% of those who receive an opioid agonist systemically but in up to 90% of patients who receive spinal opioids.[34] The incidence depends on which opioid is used and whether the patient is opioid-naïve.[35,36] After spinal injection, pruritus spreads rostrally through the thorax from the level of the injection and is characteristically maximal in the face and, in some patients, limited just to the nose.[37]

Pruritus induced by clinical doses of opioids administered spinally or systemically is *not* caused by histamine release from mast cells in the skin. The pruritus is relieved by **naloxone** but *not* by H_1-antihistamines.[38] Indeed, *in vitro* studies indicate that the dose of **morphine** or **methadone** needed to release histamine from mast cells is some 10,000 times greater than the dose needed for μ-opioid receptor-mediated agonist effects.[39] Thus, a central opioid receptor-mediated mechanism is the likely cause for generalized pruritus associated with spinal or systemic opioids.[37,40] In animals, administration of small amounts of **morphine** into the CNS causes intense scratching behaviour.[41] Subsequent IM **morphine** reduces the scratching, suggesting that the dose-response curve for opioid-induced pruritus may be bell-shaped.[42]

On the other hand, it has recently been suggested that the μ-opioid receptors mediate pruritus, whereas the κ-opioid receptors may suppress pruritus.[43] In keeping with this hypothesis is the observation that a κ-opioid receptor agonist, TRK-820, reduces scratching in a mouse model.[44] Further, in hemodialysis patients with pruritus, the expression of all opioid receptors on lymphocytes is lower than that in healthy volunteers, with μ-opioid receptors being less affected than κ-opioid receptors. This imbalance in the expression of μ- and κ-opioid receptors could contribute to the pathogenesis of uremic pruritus.[43]

Other neurotransmitter systems interact with the opioid system in relation to the mediation of pruritus, notably the serotonin system, and this possibly explains why **ondansetron**, a specific $5HT_3$-receptor antagonist, relieves pruritus caused by spinal **morphine** (see p.521).[45–47]

Opioid-induced pruritus is uncommon in palliative care; few patients receive spinal opioids and those who do are not opioid-naïve. Further, such patients almost always receive **bupivacaine** concurrently, and this tends to restrict pruritus to just the face.[48] When pruritus is induced by a systemic opioid, switching to an alternative opioid may help.[36,49,50] H_1-antihistamines are ineffective for generalized opioid-induced pruritus. However, opioid antagonists (see p.338) and some other drugs are effective, notably **ondansetron** (see p.192).[51,52]

Opioid-related serotonin toxicity

Serotonin toxicity results from the ingestion of drug(s) which increase brain serotonin above a critical level (see p.140).[53] Toxicity manifests as a triad of neuro-excitatory features:
- *autonomic hyperactivity*; sweating, fever, mydriasis, tachycardia, hypertension, tachypnea, sialorrhea, diarrhea
- *neuromuscular hyperactivity*; tremor, clonus, myoclonus, hyperreflexia, and pyramidal rigidity (advanced stage)
- *altered mental status*; agitation, hypomania, and delirium (advanced stage).

Box 5.G Example of a contract for controlled substance prescriptions with addicts[a]

Controlled substance medications (narcotics, tranquillizers and barbiturates) are very useful, but have high potential for misuse and are therefore closely controlled by the local, state, and federal government. They are intended to relieve pain, to improve function and/or ability to work, not simply to feel good. Because my physician is prescribing such medication for me to help manage my condition, I agree to the following conditions:

1 I am responsible for my controlled substance medications. If the prescription of medication is lost, misplaced, or stolen, or if I use it up sooner than prescribed, I understand that it will not be replaced.

2 I will not request or accept controlled substance medication from any other physicians or individual while I am receiving such medication from Dr._____. Besides being illegal to do so, it may endanger my health. The only exception is if it is prescribed while I am admitted in a hospital.

3 Refills of controlled substance medication:

- Will be made only during Dr._____ regular office hours, in person, once each month during a scheduled office visit. Refills will not be made at night, on holidays, or weekends.
- Will not be made if I "run out early". I am responsible for taking the medication in the dose prescribed and for keeping track of the amount remaining.
- Will not be made as an "emergency", such as on Friday afternoon because I suddenly realize I will "run out tomorrow". I will call at least seventy-two hours ahead if I need assistance with a controlled substance medication prescription.

4 I will bring in the containers of all medications prescribed by Dr. _____ each time I see him even if there is no medication remaining. These will be in the original containers from the pharmacy for each medication.

5 I understand that if I violate any of the above conditions, my controlled substances prescription and/or treatment with Dr._____ may be ended immediately. If the violation involves obtaining controlled substances from another individual, as described above, I may also be reported to my physician, medical facilities, and other authorities.

6 I understand that the main treatment goal is to improve my ability to function and/or work. In consideration of that goal and the fact that I am being given potent medication to help me reach that goal, I agree to help myself by the following better health habits: exercise, weight control, and the non-use of tobacco and alcohol. I understand that only through following a healthier life-style can I hope to have the most successful outcome to my treatment.

I have been fully informed by Dr._____ and his staff regarding psychological dependence (addiction) of a controlled substance, which I understand is rare. I know that some persons may develop a tolerance, which is the need to increase the dose of the medication to achieve the same effect of pain control, and I do know that I will become physically dependent on the medication. This will occur if I am on the medication for several weeks, and, when I stop the medication, I must do so slowly and under medical supervision or I may have withdrawal symptoms.

I have read this contract and it has been explained to my by Dr._____ and/or his staff. In addition, I fully understand the consequences of violating said contract.

_____	_____	_____	_____
Patient's Signature	Date	Witness	Date

a. reproduced with permission from Hansen 1999.[33] ©Southern Medical Association.

Clonus (inducible, spontaneous or ocular), agitation, sweating, tremor and hyperreflexia are essential features. Spontaneous clonus, in the presence of a serotoninergic drug, is the most reliable indicator of serotonin toxicity.[54]

Opioids are relatively weak serotonin re-uptake inhibitors and only cause symptoms in higher doses or susceptible individuals, or when used concurrently with a second drug with serotoninergic potency, notably an MAOI but also with many other antidepressants and some psychostimulants (see Box 4.H, p.141).

Fatalities from serotonin toxicity have occurred with **dextromethorphan**, **meperidine** (see Box 5.E, p.289), **tramadol**, and possibly **fentanyl**.[55] Non-fatal serotonin toxicity has also been observed with **propoxyphene**, other **fentanils**, **methadone**, and **pentazocine**. It has *not* been observed with other opioids, and the 'blanket' warning against the concurrent use of an MAOI and other opioids is misplaced (Box 5.H).

Box 5.H   A misleading report about morphine and MAOIs[56]

A patient who regularly took an MAOI and trifluoperazine 20mg/24h was given pre-operative promethazine 50mg IM and morphine 1mg IV followed by two doses of morphine 2.5mg IV. About 3min later she became unresponsive and hypotensive (systolic pressure 40mmHg); responding within 2min to IV naloxone.

Although repeatedly referenced as such, this was *not* MAOI-related serotonin toxicity; it was a hypotensive response to IV morphine in someone chronically taking trifluoperazine, an α-adrenergic antagonist.

The onset of toxicity is generally rapid and progressive, typically as the second drug reaches effective blood levels (one or two doses). Occasionally, recurrent mild symptoms may occur for weeks before the development of severe toxicity. The patient is often alert or agitated, with tremor (sometimes severe), myoclonus and hyperreflexia. Ankle clonus is generally demonstrable or, in severe toxicity, occurs spontaneously. Neuromuscular signs are initially greater in the lower limbs, then become more generalized as toxicity increases. Other symptoms include shaking, shivering (often including chattering of the teeth), and sometimes trismus. Pyramidal rigidity is a late development in severe cases, and can impair respiration. Rigidity, a fever of $>38.5°C$ or deteriorating blood gases indicate life-threatening toxicity.

Opioids and hypothalamic–pituitary function

Chronic administration of opioids can interfere with hypothalamic-pituitary function:
- inhibition of hypothalamic gonadotrophin-releasing hormone from the hypothalamus:
  - ▷ ↓ luteinizing hormone (LH) release from the pituitary → ↓ production of testosterone (testes) or estrogen (ovaries)
  - ▷ ↓ follicle-stimulating hormone (FSH) release from the pituitary → ↓ production of sperm or ovarian follicles
  - ▷ associated with loss of libido, impotence, irregular menses or amenorrhea, subfertility and other consequences of hypogonadism, e.g. reduced muscle mass, osteoporosis
- inhibition of adrenocorticotrophic hormone (ACTH) from the pituitary:
  - ▷ ↓ cortisol production and release (adrenals)
  - ▷ associated with symptoms such as fatigue, weight loss, anorexia, vomiting, diarrhea, abdominal pain, hypoglycemia, hypotension
- inhibition of growth hormone from the pituitary:
  - ▷ associated with decreased exercise tolerance, decreased mood and general wellbeing, reduced bone remodelling activity, altered body fat distribution (increased central adiposity), hyperlipidemia and increased predisposition to atherogenesis.[57]

In patients with chronic non-cancer pain, hormone suppression is evident after 1 week of opioid administration and appears dose-related; in one study, abnormally low levels of sex hormones were found in 3/4 of men receiving opioids by mouth equivalent to <150mg **morphine**/24h and in all receiving >150mg/24h.[58] IT **morphine** (mean doses 5–12mg/24h) produced hypogonadism in most subjects, both men and women.[59–61] In one study, 1/3 of patients also developed hypocortisolism ± growth hormone deficiency, leading to an Addisonian crisis in one patient.[59] Thus, particularly for patients receiving long-term opioids for non-cancer pain, who have symptoms suggestive of hypothalamic dysfunction, it may be necessary to refer to an endocrinologist for investigation and possible replacement hormone therapy.[59]

Opioids and immune function

Opioids modulate immune cell function directly and indirectly via activation of the hypothalamic–pituitary-adrenal axis (HPA) and the autonomic nervous system. Lymphocytes and mononuclear phagocytes express μ-, κ- and δ-opioid receptors, which when activated trigger cellular apoptosis. Immune function is suppressed by the opioid-induced release of glucocorticoids and catecholamines (e.g. epinephrine, norepinephrine and dopamine) from the adrenal medulla and the release of catecholamines from sympathetic nerve fibres which innervate lymphoid tissue (e.g. lymph nodes, spleen).[62] Thus, **morphine** depresses natural killer cell activity, T-lymphocyte proliferation, monocyte/macrophage function and cytokine function (e.g. interleukin (IL)-2, interferon (IFN)-γ), potentially reducing host resistance to bacterial, fungal and viral infections.[63–65] Compared with **morphine**, other opioids are less immunosuppressive and **buprenorphine**, **hydromorphone**, **oxycodone**, **oxymorphone** and **tramadol** have little or no effect.[66–68] The clinical implications of these effects are uncertain. However, they may help to explain the increased susceptibility to infection seen in opioid abusers.[69] On the other hand, because pain is immunosuppressive, opioid analgesia may improve immune function in patients with pain.[70]

Opioid-induced hyperalgesia

Opioid-induced hyperalgesia (OIH) appears important in both acute and chronic pain. Although poorly understood, it appears to result from sustained sensitization of the nervous system in which the excitatory amino acid neurotransmitter system and the NMDA-receptor-channel complex play important roles.[71] Possible causes include:

- opioid-induced activation of glial cells, which play a role in inflammation, pain signal transmission, pain hypersensitivity and opioid tolerance[72,73]
- alteration in the G protein coupling of opioid receptors, i.e. G_s rather than $G_{i/o}$; the G_s variant has an excitatory rather than an inhibitory effect[74]
- in the case of **morphine**, accumulation of M3G.[75]

Genetic make-up probably plays an important part in its development.

Clinical features

In surgical pain, OIH may contribute to exaggerated levels of pain in the immediate postoperative period and the development of a chronic pain state. In patients with cancer, OIH may manifest in various ways:

- rapidly developing tolerance to opioids
- short-lived benefit from increased doses
- a change of pain pattern (Table 5.14).

Table 5.14 Opioid-induced hyperalgesia.[76]

What the patient says	What the doctor finds
Increased sensitivity to pain stimulus (hyperalgesia)	Any dose of any opioid, but particularly with high-dose morphine or hydromorphone, and in renal failure
Worsening pain despite increasing doses of opioids	Pain elicited from ordinary non-painful stimuli, e.g. stroking skin with cotton (allodynia)
Pain which becomes more diffuse, extending beyond the distribution of the pre-existing pain	Presence of other manifestations of opioid-induced neural hyperexcitability: myoclonus, seizures, delirium

The extreme upper end of the spectrum may be those patients who manifest evidence of severe neural hyperexcitability (myoclonus, allodynia, and/or hyperalgesia), particularly when taking high doses of **morphine** or an alternative strong opioid. This may be accompanied by sedation and delirium (when it is often described as opioid neurotoxicity). However, OIH:

- is *not* limited to very high doses, or to any one opioid
- is probably under-diagnosed
- is more common than generally thought.

Severe pain which does not respond to increasing doses of opioids, or is complicated by severe undesirable effects, should raise the *possibility* of OIH.[76]

Evaluation

A diagnosis of OIH is generally made on the basis of a high level of clinical suspicion, probability, and pattern recognition. OIH must be differentiated from increased pain caused by disease progression or the development of opioid tolerance, both of which may be managed by increasing the opioid dose.

Management

Management is based largely on theoretical grounds and clinical observation.

Prophylaxis

Use a multimodal approach to analgesia, e.g.:

- an NSAID may help to reduce the production of excitatory amino acid neurotransmitters which activate the pronociceptive and anti-opioid systems
- **gabapentin** may block calcium channels which may contribute to hyperalgesia in nerve pain.

Treatment

- progressively and rapidly reduce the dose of the causal opioid to about 25% of the peak dose
- switch to an opioid with less risk of OIH, i.e. **fentanyl** (highest) → **morphine → methadone → buprenorphine** (lowest)[77]
- (rarely) if occurring at very low doses (<10mg/24h), discontinue the opioid completely
- use a multimodal approach to analgesia, i.e. use non-opioids, e.g. **acetaminophen** or an NSAID, and adjuvant analgesics, e.g. **gabapentin**
- start oral or parenteral **ketamine** (an NMDA-receptor-channel blocker).[78]

Note that when switching from **morphine** because of severe neural hyperexcitability, a lower than expected dose of the alternative opioid is likely to be needed unless the dose of **morphine** has been much reduced (as suggested above).[79,80] If these steps do not lead to a resolution of the OIH:

- consider spinal, regional or local analgesia (with local anesthetics), and tail off systemic opioids completely
- check for hypomagnesemia because this can aggravate OIH.[81,82]
- consider treatment with ultralow doses of an opioid antagonist.[83–85]

Opioid switching ('rotation')

Some patients need to be switched from **morphine** (or other strong opioid) to an alternative, about 20% according to one published prospective survey.[86] Changes from **morphine** to TD **fentanyl** (or vice versa) are included in this figure. Higher figures have been published elsewhere, e.g. 44%.[87] The lower figure better reflects clinical experience in the UK.[88] The main reasons for switching opioids are:

- poor adherence (→ TD **fentanyl**)
- intractable constipation (→ TD **fentanyl**)
- poor response to **morphine** plus an NSAID (→ **methadone**)[89]
- hyperalgesia or other manifestations of neurotoxicity (cognitive failure/delirium, hallucinations, myoclonus, allodynia)
- significant decline in the patient's renal function (**morphine → methadone**, TD **fentanyl** or **hydromorphone**)
- non-availability of a suitable formulation when a change of route is necessary (e.g. because parenteral **oxycodone** is not available in Canada → parenteral **morphine** or **hydromorphone** if a patient no longer able to take PO **oxycodone**).

Hydromorphone, oxycodone and **methadone** have all been substituted successfully for **morphine** in cases of neurotoxicity.[90–92]

When converting from an alternative strong opioid to oral **morphine**, the initial dose depends on the relative potency of the two drugs (Table 5.15). For most drugs at typical doses, these conversion ratios are generally safe for switching in both directions, except perhaps for **hydromorphone**. Some sources suggest a conversion ratio of about 5:1 if switching from

Table 5.15 Approximate PO opioid potency ratios (morphine = 1)[a]

Analgesic	Potency ratio with morphine	Duration of action (h)[b]
Codeine		
Dihydrocodeine (not Canada) }	1/10	3–6
Propoxyphene		
Tramadol	1/10	4–6
Meperidine	1/8	2–4
Hydrocodone	2/3	4–8
Papaveretum (not Canada)	2/3[c]	3–5
Oxycodone	1.5 (2)[d]	3–4
Methadone	5–10[e]	8–12
Hydromorphone	4–5 (5–7.5)[d]	4–5
Buprenorphine (SL) (not Canada)	80	6–8
Buprenorphine (TD) (not Canada)	100 (75–115)[d]	Formulation dependent
Fentanyl (TD)	100 (150)[d]	72

a. multiply dose of opioid by its potency ratio to determine the equivalent dose of morphine sulfate/hydrochloride

b. dependent in part on severity of pain and on dose; often longer lasting in very elderly and those with renal impairment

c. papaveretum (strong opium) is standardized to contain 50% morphine base; potency expressed in relation to morphine sulfate

d. the numbers in parenthesis are the manufacturers' preferred ratios; for explanation of divergence, see individual drug monographs

e. a single 5mg dose of methadone is equivalent to morphine 7.5mg, but a variable long plasma halflife and broad-spectrum receptor affinity result in a much higher than expected potency ratio when administered regularly, sometimes much higher than the range given above (see p.327).[79,96]

morphine to **hydromorphone** but only 1:4 if switching from **hydromorphone** to **morphine**.[93,94]

However, potency and thus conversion ratios are approximations and can vary from source to source. For example, the UK manufacturer considers **hydromorphone** PO to be about 7.5 times more potent than **morphine** PO, while the Canadian Product Monograph states 5–7.5 times.

Switching opioids always requires caution and careful monitoring (see Opioid dose conversion ratios, p.497).[95]

Switching (rotating) at high doses

The recommended equivalent doses of the strong opioids are an approximate guide only; they cannot be exact for everybody.[93,94,97] They are based on typical **morphine** doses. As the dose of **morphine** escalates, e.g. >2g/24h, the recommended equivalent doses will become progressively more erroneous. Any error will be further increased in the presence of opioid-induced neurotoxicity/hyperalgesia.[98] Thus, when converting at high dose levels it is best to adopt a cautious approach and give 1/4–1/2 the calculated equivalent dose (see also Opioid dose conversion ratios, p.497.). A separate strategy is necessary for **methadone** (see p.327).

Combining opioids

It is generally considered to be bad practice to prescribe two or more opioids for simultaneous use. Thus, for example, regular **morphine** is best backed up by p.r.n **morphine** for break-through (episodic) pain. However, there are circumstances when the p.r.n. opioid differs from the regular opioid, for example TD **fentanyl** backed up by p.r.n. **morphine** (see p.322). Also, someone with good pain relief from a regular weak opioid may have a supply of **morphine** for back-up use in case of severe break-through (episodic) pain. However, there are reports of two strong opioids being used successfully in combination, i.e. better pain relief at relatively lower doses and reduced undesirable effects.[99] Despite such reports, it is important to re-state that, as a general rule, patients should not have two opioids prescribed concurrently on a regular basis.[100,101]

Opioids in end-stage renal failure

In end-stage renal failure, extra caution is required regardless of the opioid used, whether or not the patient is on dialysis.

Table 5.16 Opioid analgesia and renal impairment (modified from Dean 2004)[103]

Opioid	Main metabolites[a,b]	Impact of renal impairment[c]	Dialysability	Comment
Not recommended for chronic use				
Codeine	C6G[d] (80%), morphine (10%) → M3G, M6G	Accumulation of C6G, M3G, M6G (prolonged effects)	±	M3G is implicated in morphine neurotoxicity (see p.293)
Morphine	M3G (55%), *M6G* (10%)	Accumulation of M3G (may cause neurotoxicity) and M6G (prolonged effect)	±	Plasma concentration reduced to 40% during dialysis.[104] H3G may be implicated in hydromorphone neurotoxicity
Use cautiously				
Hydromorphone	H3G (35%)	AUC increases ×4; accumulation of H3G	+	Oxycodone, noroxycodone and oxymorphone all removed during hemodialysis[105]
Oxycodone	Noroxycodone *Oxymorphone* (10%)	Plasma halflife prolonged and clearance reduced (prolonged effect)	+	
Tramadol	O-desmethyltramadol		+	30% excreted unchanged in urine
Generally safe with close monitoring				
Buprenorphine (not Canada)	NB, BG, NBG[e]	Accumulation of NB	−	70% excreted in feces after glucuronidation in the wall of the GI tract; accumulation of NB probably irrelevant because little or no central effect[106,107]
Fentanyl	Norfentanyl (>99%)	Clearance may be reduced	−	Possibly removed by certain dialysis membranes, e.g. polysulphone (Fresenius filter F10HPS, low flux 2.4),[108,109] cellulose triacetate 190[110]
Methadone	Methadone pyrolidine		±	Fecal excretion increases in anuria; <5% unchanged[111]

a. *italicized* metabolites are those which are active as analgesics
b. percentages rounded to nearest 5%
c. renal impairment may cause a slowing of hepatic metabolism
d. C6G = codeine-6-glucuronide, etc.
e. NB = norbuprenorphine; BG = buprenorphine glucuronide; NBG = norbuprenorphine glucuronide.

Pharmacokinetics, and consequently pharmacodynamics, are altered by renal impairment (see p.477).[102] Active drugs which undergo renal excretion unchanged and renally-excreted active metabolites accumulate leading to increased and more prolonged effects, and thus a greater risk of toxicity. Although with extra care **morphine** can be used in end-stage renal failure, switching to a 'renally safer' drug may be preferable; some centres routinely avoid the use of morphine in patients with renal impairment (Table 5.16).

Figure 5.10 provides an analgesic ladder for use in patients on dialysis based on clinical practice in centres in the UK.[112] New UK guidelines for analgesia in patients at the end of life with severe renal failure (GFR <30mL/min) opt for **fentanyl** as the preferred strong opioid.[113] However, some centres prefer the cautious use of a familiar opioid, rather than switching to an unfamiliar (albeit 'renally safer') one.

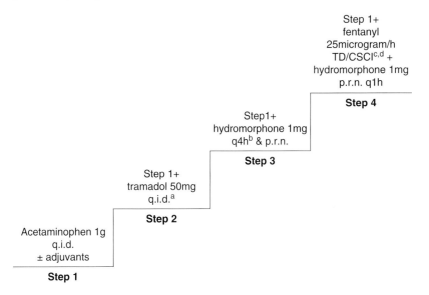

Figure 5.10 An example of an analgesic ladder for patients on dialysis based on clinical experience at several renal centres in the UK; doses PO unless stated otherwise.

a. equivalent to about morphine 20mg/24h PO
b. equivalent to about morphine 30mg/24h PO
c. equivalent to about morphine 60mg/24h PO; generally use only when total daily dose of hydromorphone ≥12mg
d. CSCI alfentanil can be substituted for CSCI fentanyl; it is about 1/4 as potent as fentanyl

Buprenorphine (like **fentanyl**) also has no active metabolite and is not removed by hemodialysis. Although norbuprenorphine has similar opioid receptor-binding affinities to **buprenorphine**, it does not readily cross the blood–brain barrier and thus has little, if any, central effect.[106,107] Given the resurgence of interest in **buprenorphine**, it could well become a popular choice in patients with renal impairment.[114] However, in Canada, **buprenorphine** is only available in a combination product containing **naloxone**, and this is not a practical option.

Ketamine may also have a role to play in some patients with renal impairment (see p.468).[115]

1 Portenoy RK et al. (2006) Opioid use and survival at the end of life: a survey of a hospice population. *Journal of Pain and Symptom Management.* **32**: 532–540.
2 Ballantyne JC (2007) Regulation of opioid prescribing. *British Medical Journal.* **334**: 811–812.
3 Rothman R (1995) Buprenorphine: a review of the binding literature. In: A Cowan and J Lewis (eds) *Buprenorphine: Combatting Drug Abuse with A Unique Opioid.* Wiley-Liss, New York, pp. 19–29.

4 Zaki P et al. (2000) Ligand-induced changes in surface mu-opioid receptor number: relationship to G protein activation? *Journal of Pharmacology and Experimental Therapeutics.* **292**: 1127–1134.

5 Lutfy K et al. (2003) Buprenorphine-induced antinociception is mediated by mu-opioid receptors and compromised by concomitant activation of opioid receptor-like receptors. *Journal of Neuroscience.* **23**: 10331–10337.

6 Lewis JW and Husbands SM (2004) The orvinols and related opioids–high affinity ligands with diverse efficacy profiles. *Current Pharmaceutical Design.* **10**: 717–732.

7 Hill RG (1992) Multiple opioid receptors and their ligands. *Frontiers of Pain.* **4**: 1–4.

8 Corbett AD et al. (1993) Selectivity of ligands for opioid receptors. In: A Herz (ed) *Opioids.* Springer-Verlag, London, pp. 657–672.

9 WHO (1986) *Cancer Pain Relief.* World Health Organisation, Geneva.

10 Hanks G et al. (2001) Morphine and alternative opioids in cancer pain: the EAPC recommendations. *British Journal of Cancer.* **84**: 587–593.

11 Quigley C (2005) The role of opioids in cancer pain. *British Medical Journal.* **331**: 825–829.

12 Cherny N (1996) Opioid analgesics: comparative features and prescribing guidelines. *Drugs.* **51**: 713–737.

13 Hoskin P and Hanks G (1991) Opioid agonist–antagonist drugs in acute and chronic pain states. *Drugs.* **41**: 326–344.

14 Twycross RG (1994) Pentazocine. In: *Pain Relief in Advanced Cancer.* Churchill Livingstone, Edinburgh, pp. 247–248.

15 Woods A et al. (1974) Medicines evaluation and monitoring group: central nervous system effects of pentazocine. *British Medical Journal.* **1**: 305–307.

16 Plummer JL et al. (2001) Norpethidine toxicity. *Pain Reviews.* **8**: 159–170.

17 Sweetman SC (ed) (2005) *Martindale: The Complete Drug Reference* (34e). Pharmaceutical Press, London, pp. 80–82.

18 Shee JC (1960) Dangerous potentiation of pethidine by iproniazid, and its treatment. *British Medical Journal.* **ii**: 507–509.

19 Taylor D (1962) Alarming reaction to pethidine in patients on phenelzine. *Lancet.* **2**: 401–402.

20 Rogers KJ and Thornton JA (1969) The interaction between monoamine oxidase inhibitors and narcotic analgesics in mice. *British Journal of Pharmacology.* **36**: 470–480.

21 Cherny N et al. (2001) Strategies to manage the adverse effects of oral morphine: an evidence-based report. *Journal of Clinical Oncology.* **19**: 2542–2554.

22 Borgbjerg FM et al. (1996) Experimental pain stimulates respiration and attenuates morphine-induced respiratory depression: a controlled study in human volunteers. *Pain.* **64**: 123–128.

23 Estfan B et al. (2007) Respiratory function during parenteral opioid titration for cancer pain. *Palliative Medicine.* **21**: 81–86.

24 Sykes NP (2007) Morphine kills the pain, not the patient. *Lancet.* **369**: 1325–1326.

25 Regnard CFB and Badger C (1987) Opioids, sleep and the time of death. *Palliative Medicine.* **1**: 107–110.

26 Collin E et al. (1993) Is disease progression the major factor in morphine 'tolerance' in cancer pain treatment? *Pain.* **55**: 319–326.

27 Portenoy RK (1994) Tolerance to opioid analgesics: clinical aspects. *Cancer Surveys.* **21**: 49–65.

28 Passik S and Portenoy R (1998) Substance abuse issues in palliative care. In: A Berger (ed) *Principles and Practice of Supportive Oncology.* Lippincott-Raven, Philadelphia, pp. 513–529.

29 Joranson D et al. (2000) Trends in medical use and abuse of opioid analgesics. *Journal of the American Medical Association.* **283**: 1710–1714.

30 Passik S et al. (1998) Substance abuse issues in cancer patients. Part 1: prevalence and diagnosis. *Oncology.* **12**: 517–521.

31 Passik S et al. (1998) Substance abuse issues in cancer patients. Part 2: evaluation and treatment. *Oncology.* **12**: 729–734.

32 Twycross RG and Wald SJ (1976) Longterm use of diamorphine in advanced cancer. In: JJ Bonica and D Albe-Fessard (eds) *Advances in Pain Research and Therapy* Vol 1. Raven Press, New York, pp. 653–661.

33 Hansen H (1999) Treatment of chronic pain with antiepileptic drugs. *Southern Medical Journal.* **92**: 642–649.

34 Ballantyne J et al. (1989) The incidence of pruritus after epidural morphine. *Anaesthesia.* **44**: 863.

35 Woodham M (1988) Pruritus with sublingual buprenorphine. *Anaesthesia.* **43**: 806–807.

36 Katcher J and Walsh D (1999) Opioid-induced itching: morphine sulfate and hydromorphone hydrochloride. *Journal of Pain and Symptom Management.* **17**: 70–72.

37 Ballantyne J et al. (1988) Itching after epidural and spinal opiates. *Pain.* **33**: 149–160.

38 Kuraishi Y et al. (2000) Itch-scratch responses induced by opioids through central mu opioid receptors in mice. *Journal of Biomedicine and Science.* **7**: 248–252.

39 Barke K and Hough L (1993) Opiates, mast cells and histamine release. *Life Sciences.* **53**: 1391–1399.

40 Reisine T and Pasternak G (1996) Opioid analgesics and antagonists. In: J Hardman et al. (eds) *Goodman and Gilman's The Pharmacological Basis of Therapeutics* (9e). McGraw-Hill, London, pp. 521–1555.

41 Koenigstein H (1948) Experimental study of itch in animals. *Archives de dermatologie et de syphiligraphie.* **57**: 828–849.

42 Thomas D et al. (1993) Multiple effects of morphine on facial scratching in monkeys. *Anesthesia and Analgesia.* **77**: 933–935.

43 Kumagai H et al. (2000) Endogenous opioid system in uraemic patients. In: *Joint Meeting of the Seventh World Conference on Clinical Pharmacology and IUPHAR – Division of Clinical Pharmacology and the Fourth Congress of the European Association for Clinical Pharmacology and Therapeutics.*

44 Okano K et al. (2000) Anti-pruritic effect of opioid kappa receptor agonist TRK-820. *British Journal of Clinical Pharmacology; abstracts of the joint meeting of VII World Conference on Clinical Pharmacology and Therapeutics IUPHAR.* 283.

45 Arai L et al. (1996) The use of ondansetron to treat pruritus associated with intrathecal morphine in two paediatric patients. *Paediatric Anaesthesia.* **6**: 337–339.

46 Borgeat A and Stimemann H-R (1999) Ondansetron is effective to treat spinal or epidural morphine-induced pruritus. *Anesthesiology.* **90**: 432–436.

47 Kyriakides K et al. (1999) Management of opioid-induced pruritus: a role for 5HT antagonists? *British Journal of Anaesthesia.* **82**: 439–441.

48 Asokumar B et al. (1998) Intrathecal bupivacaine reduces pruritus and prolongs duration of fentanyl analgesia during labor: a prospective, randomized, controlled trial. *Anaesthesia and Analgesia.* **87**: 1309–1315.

49 Gunter J et al. (2000) Continuous epidural butorphanol relieves pruritus associated with epidural morphine infusions in children. *Paediatric Anaesthesia.* **10**: 167–172.

50 Franco J (1999) Pruritus. *Current Treatment Options in Gastroenterology.* **2**: 451–456.

51 Kjellberg F and Tramer M (2001) Pharmacological control of opioid-induced pruritus: a quantitative systematic review of randomized trials. *European Journal of Anaesthesiology.* **18**: 346–357.

52 Twycross RG and Zylicz Z (2004) Systemic therapy: making rational choices. In: Z Zylicz et al. (eds) *Pruritus in advanced disease.* Oxford University Press, London, pp. 161–178.

53 Gillman P (2006) Serotonin toxicity, serotonin syndrome: 2006 update, overview and analysis. Available from: www.psychotropical.com
54 Dunkley EJ et al. (2003) The Hunter Serotonin Toxicity Criteria: simple and accurate diagnostic decision rules for serotonin toxicity. Quarterly Journal of Medicine. 96: 635–642.
55 Gillman PK (2005) Monoamine oxidase inhibitors, opioid analgesics and serotonin toxicity. British Journal of Anaesthesia. 95: 434–441.
56 Barry B (1979) Adverse effects of MAO inhibitors with narcotics reversed with naloxone. Anaesthesia and Intensive Care. 7: 194.
57 The Society for Endocrinology and the Royal College of Physicians (2002) Health Technology Appraisal of Human Growth Hormone Replacement in Adults. In: National Institute for Clinical Excellence. Available from: www.endocrinology.org/SFE/GHAppraisal.pdf
58 Daniell HW (2002) Hypogonadism in men consuming sustained-action oral opioids. The Journal of Pain. 3: 377–384.
59 Abs R et al. (2000) Endocrine consequences of long-term intrathecal administration of opioids. Journal of Clinical Endocrinology and Metabolism. 85: 2215–2222.
60 Finch PM et al. (2000) Hypogonadism in patients treated with intrathecal morphine. Clinical Journal of Pain. 16: 251–254.
61 Roberts LJ et al. (2002) Sex hormone suppression by intrathecal opioids: a prospective study. Clinical Journal of Pain. 18: 144–148.
62 Vallejo R et al. (2004) Opioid therapy and immunosuppression: a review. American Journal of Therapeutics. 11: 354–365.
63 Sacerdote P et al. (1997) Antinociceptive and immunosuppressive effects of opiate drugs: a structure-related activity study. British Journal of Pharmacology. 121: 834–840.
64 Risdahl JM et al. (1998) Opiates and infection. Journal of Neuroimmunology. 83: 4–18.
65 McCarthy L et al. (2001) Opioids, opioid receptors, and the immune response. Drug and Alcohol Dependence. 62: 111–123.
66 Sacerdote P et al. (2000) The effects of tramadol and morphine on immune responses and pain after surgery in cancer patients. Anesthesia and Analgesia. 90: 1411–1414.
67 Budd K and Shipton E (2004) Acute pain and the immune system and opioimmunosuppression. Acute Pain. 6: 123–135.
68 Budd K and Raffa R (eds) (2005) Buprenorphine – the unique opioid analgesic. Georg Thieme Verlag, Stuttgart, Germany, p. 134.
69 Alonzo NC and Bayer BM (2002) Opioids, immunology, and host defenses of intravenous drug abusers. Infectious Disease Clinics of North America. 16: 553–569.
70 Page GG (2005) Immunologic effects of opioids in the presence or absence of pain. Journal of Pain and Symptom Management. 29: S25–31.
71 Simonnet G (2008) Preemptive antihyperalgesia to improve preemptive analgesia. Anesthesiology. 108: 352–354.
72 Ren K and Dubner R (2008) Neuron-glia crosstalk gets serious: role in pain hypersensitivity. Current Opinion in Anesthesiology. 21: 570–579.
73 Romero-Sandoval EA et al. (2008) Neuroimmune interactions and pain: focus on glial-modulating targets. Current Opinion in Investigational Drugs. 9: 726–734.
74 Crain S and Shen K (2000) Antagonists of excitatory opioid receptor functions enhance morphine's analgesic potency and attenuate opioid tolerance/dependence liability. Pain. 84: 121–131.
75 Bartlett S et al. (1994) Pharmacology of morphine and morphine-3-glucuronide at opioid, excitatory amino acid, GABA and glycine binding sites. Pharmacology and Toxicology. 75: 73–81.
76 Zylicz Z and Twycross R (2008) Opioid-induced hyperalgesia may be more frequent than previously thought. Journal of Clinical Oncology. 26: 1564; author reply 1565.
77 Filitz J et al. (2008) Supra-additive effects of tramadol and acetaminophen in a human pain model. Pain. 136: 262–270.
78 Walker SM and Cousins MJ (1997) Reduction in hyperalgesia and intrathecal morphine requirements by low-dose ketamine infusion. Journal of Pain and Symptom Management. 14: 129–133.
79 Bruera E et al. (1996) Opioid rotation in patients with cancer pain. Cancer. 78: 852–857.
80 Lawlor P et al. (1998) Dose ratio between morphine and methadone in patients with cancer pain. Cancer. 82: 1167–1173.
81 Dubray C et al. (1997) Magnesium deficiency induces an hyperalgesia reversed by the NMDA receptor antagonist MK801. Neuroreport. 8: 1383–1386.
82 Begon S et al. (2002) Magnesium increases morphine analgesic effect in different experimental models of pain. Anesthesiology. 96: 627–632.
83 Gan T et al. (1997) Opioid-sparing effects of a low-dose infusion of naloxone in patient-administered morphine sulfate. Anesthesiology. 87: 1075–1081.
84 Chindalore VL et al. (2005) Adding ultralow-dose naltrexone to oxycodone enhances and prolongs analgesia: a randomized, controlled trial of Oxytrex. Journal of Pain. 6: 392–399.
85 Rauck RL et al. (2006) A randomized, double-blind, placebo-controlled study of intrathecal ziconotide in adults with severe chronic pain. Journal of Pain and Symptom Management. 31: 393–406.
86 Sarhill N et al. (2001) Parenteral opioid rotation in advanced cancer: A prospective study. Abstracts of the MASCC/ISOO 13th International Symposium Supportive Care in Cancer, Copenhagen, Denmark, June 14–16. Support Care Cancer. 9: 307.
87 Cherny NJ et al. (1995) Opioid pharmacotherapy in the management of cancer pain: a survey of strategies used by pain physicians for the selection of analgesic drugs and routes of administration. Cancer. 76: 1283–1293.
88 Twycross RG, Unpublished work.
89 Morley J and Makin M (1998) The use of methadone in cancer pain poorly responsive to other opioids. Pain Reviews. 5: 51–58.
90 Ashby M et al. (1999) Opioid substitution to reduce adverse effects in cancer pain management. Medical Journal of Australia. 170: 68–71.
91 Sjogren P et al. (1994) Disappearance of morphine-induced hyperalgesia after discontinuing or substituting morphine with other opioid agonists. Pain. 59: 313–316.
92 Hagen N and Swanson R (1997) Strychnine-like multifocal myoclonus and seizures in extremely high-dose opioid administration: treatment strategies. Journal of Pain and Symptom Management. 14: 51–58.
93 Anderson R et al. (2001) Accuracy in equianalgesic dosing: conversion dilemmas. Journal of Pain and Symptom Management. 21: 397–406.
94 Pereira J et al. (2001) Equianalgesic dose ratios for opioids: a critical review and proposals for long-term dosing. Journal of Pain and Symptom Management. 22: 672–687.
95 Fine PG and Portenoy RK (2009) Establishing 'best practices' for opioid rotation: conclusions of an expert panel. Journal of Pain and Symptom Management. 38: 418–425.
96 Nixon AJ (2005) Methadone for cancer pain: a case report. American Journal of Hospice and Palliative Care. 22: 337.

97 Pasternak G (2001) Incomplete cross tolerance and multiple mu opioid peptide receptors. *Trends in Pharmacological Sciences.* **22**: 67–70.

98 Twycross R *et al.* (2009) *Symptom Management in Advanced Cancer* (4e). palliativedrugs.com, Nottingham.

99 Mercadante S *et al.* (2004) Addition of a second opioid may improve opioid response in cancer pain: preliminary data. *Support Care Cancer.* **12**: 762–766.

100 Davis MP *et al.* (2005) Look before leaping: combined opioids may not be the rave. *Supportive Care in Cancer.* **13**: 769–774.

101 Strasser F (2005) Promoting science in a pragmatic world: not (yet) time for partial opioid rotation. *Supportive Care in Cancer.* **13**: 765–768.

102 Schug SA and Morgan J (2004) Treatment of cancer pain: special considerations in patients with renal disease. *American Journal of Cancer.* **3**: 247–256.

103 Dean M (2004) Opioids in renal failure and dialysis patients. *Journal of Pain and Symptom Management.* **28**: 497–504.

104 Durnin C *et al.* (2001) Pharmacokinetics of oral immediate-release hydromorphone (Dilaudid IR) in subjects with renal impairment. *Proceedings of the Western Pharmacology Society.* **44**: 81–82.

105 Lee MA *et al.* (2005) Measurements of plasma oxycodone, noroxycodone and oxymorphone levels in a patient with bilateral nephrectomy who is undergoing haemodialysis. *Palliative Medicine.* **19**: 259–260.

106 Hand CW *et al.* (1990) Buprenorphine disposition in patients with renal impairment: single and continuous dosing, with special reference to metabolites. *British Journal of Anaesthesia.* **64**: 276–282.

107 Elkader A and Sproule B (2005) Buprenorphine: clinical pharmacokinetics in the treatment of opioid dependence. *Clinical Pharmacokinetics.* **44**: 661–680.

108 Hardy JR *et al.* (2007) Opioids in patients on renal dialysis. *Journal of Pain and Symptom Management.* **33**: 1–2.

109 Hardy JR (2006) Personal communication.

110 Joh J *et al.* (1998) Nondialyzability of fentanyl with high-efficiency and high-flux membranes. *Anesthesia & Analgesia.* **86**: 447.

111 Kreek MJ *et al.* (1980) Methadone use in patients with chronic renal disease. *Drug Alcohol Dependence.* **5**: 197–205.

112 Ferro CJ *et al.* (2004) Management of pain in renal failure. In: EJ Chambers *et al.* (eds) *Supportive Care for the Renal Patient.* Oxford University Press, Oxford, UK, pp. 105–153.

113 Marie Curie Palliative Care Institute (2008) Liverpool Care Pathway for the Dying Patient (LPC), National LCP Rental Project Group Guidelines for LCP Drug Presribing in Advanced Chronic Kidney Disease. Available from: http://www.mcpcil.org.uk/about_the_institute/news/june_2008/06_june_2008

114 Murtagh FE *et al.* (2007) The use of opioid analgesia in end-stage renal disease patients managed without dialysis: recommendations for practice. *Journal of Pain & Palliative Care Pharmacotherapy.* **21**: 5–16.

115 Murphy EJ (2005) Acute pain management pharmacology for the patient with concurrent renal or hepatic disease. *Anaesthesia and Intensive Care.* **33**: 311–322.

MORPHINE

Class: Opioid analgesic.

Indications: Moderate–severe pain, †breathlessness, †diarrhea, †cough.

Contra-indications: None absolute if titrated carefully against a patient's pain (also see Strong opioids, p.287).

Pharmacology

Morphine is the main pharmacologically active constituent of opium. Its effects are mediated by specific opioid receptors both within the CNS and peripherally. Under normal circumstances, its main peripheral action is on smooth muscle. However, in the presence of inflammation, normally silent peripheral receptors become activated.[1] The liver is the principal site of morphine metabolism.[2] Metabolism also occurs in other organs,[3] including the CNS.[4] Glucuronidation is rarely impaired except in severe hepatic impairment,[5] and morphine is well tolerated in patients with mild–moderate hepatic impairment.[6] However, with impairment severe enough to prolong the prothrombin time, the plasma halflife of morphine may be increased[3] and the dose of morphine may need to be reduced or given less often, i.e. q8h–q6h. The major metabolites of morphine are morphine-3-glucuronide (M3G) and morphine-6-glucuronide (M6G);[7] the latter binds to opioid receptors whereas M3G does not. M6G contributes substantially to the analgesic effect of morphine,[8,9] and can cause nausea and vomiting, sedation and respiratory depression.[10] In renal failure, the plasma halflife of M6G increases from 2.5h up to 7.5h, and is likely to lead to cumulative toxicity unless the frequency of administration and/or the dose of morphine is reduced.

Morphine is administered by a range of routes. Systemic absorption from topical application to ulcers or inflamed surfaces varies with the amount and concentration of the gel used; bio-availability ranges from negligible (with 0.06–0.125% gel) to almost the same as SC (0.125–0.5% gel applied to large ulcers).[11-14]

Bio-availability 35% PO, ranging from 15–64%; 25% PR.
Peak effect ≤60min PO (normal-release tablets); 20min IV; 30–60min IM; 50–90min SC.[15]
Time to peak plasma concentration 15–60min PO (normal-release tablets), 30min–10h SR (product dependent); 10–20min IM; 30min SC; 45–60min PR.[15,16]
Plasma halflife 1.5–4.5h PO; 1.5h IV.
Duration of action 3–6h; 12–24h SR (product dependent).

Undesirable effects

For full list, see manufacturer's Product Monograph.
Also see Table 5.17 and Strong opioids, p.238.

Dose and PO use

The oral to SC potency ratio of morphine is between 1:2 and 1:3 (i.e. the SC dose is 1/3 to 1/2 of the oral dose), the same ratio holds true for IM and IV injections.[5,18] In practice, many centres divide the PO dose by 2, and re-titrate as necessary. However, Health Canada now recommends dividing the PO dose by 3.[19]

Morphine should generally be given with a non-opioid. It is administered as tablets (normal-release), aqueous solutions, and SR tablets and capsules. Because the pharmacokinetic profiles of SR products differ,[20,21] it is best to keep individual patients on the same brand. Most are administered b.i.d., some once daily. Patients can be started on either an ordinary (normal-release) or an SR formulation (Box 5.I). The time to peak plasma concentration is significantly shorter with an aqueous solution of morphine compared with a normal-release tablet (0.5h vs. 1.5h),[22] suggesting that morphine solutions are a better option than tablets for p.r.n. use.

Traditionally, to make things easier for patients, morphine q4h has been given on waking, 1000h, 1400h, 1800h with a double dose at bedtime. Although clinically this seems satisfactory, one non-blind RCT concluded that patients who take a single dose at bedtime plus a regular 0200h dose need significantly fewer p.r.n. doses during the night and have less pain on waking in the morning.[23] However, pending confirmation from a double-blind trial, the traditional approach is still recommended.

When adjusting the dose of morphine, generally increase by 33–50%.[24] Two-thirds of patients never need > 30mg q4h (or SR morphine 100mg q12h); the rest need up to 200mg q4h (or SR morphine 600mg q12h), and occasionally more.[25] Instructions must be clear: extra p.r.n. morphine does not mean that the next regular dose is omitted. As a proportion of the total daily dose, p.r.n. doses vary, but 1/6 or 1/10 of the total daily dose are the commonest amounts. Some patients benefit by titration of the p.r.n. dose, which in a few will be either greater or less than these two 'standard' proportions.[26] *As a general rule, the p.r.n. dose must be increased when the regular dose is increased.*

A laxative should be prescribed routinely unless there is a definite reason for not doing so, e.g. the patient has an ileostomy (see Guidelines: Opioid-induced constipation, p.26). An antiemetic, e.g. **haloperidol** 1–2mg stat and at bedtime, should be supplied for p.r.n. use during the first week or prescribed regularly if the patient has had nausea with a weak opioid. Laxative suppositories and enemas continue to be necessary in about 1/3 of patients.[27] *Constipation may be more difficult to manage than the pain.* Warn patients about the possibility of initial drowsiness. If swallowing is difficult or vomiting persists, give 1/2 the oral dose of morphine as CSCI morphine. Alternatively, morphine may be given PR (same dose as PO).

Rapid IV/SC titration of morphine dose for severe pain

Although rapid IV/SC titration of morphine is generally *not* necessary, it can be useful in patients with severe acute pain, whether already taking opioids ('opioid-tolerant') or 'opioid-naïve'.[28] Further, because of difficulties in relation to follow-up, rapid IV titration is the norm at some centres in India for new patients presenting with pain of ≥5/10. Several methods have been reported (Box 5.J, Box 5.K, Box 5.L).[28–32] The recommended time interval between IV boluses varies from 1min to 30min. Although these methods have all been used safely in many patients, **naloxone** should be readily available (see p.343).

Table 5.17 Potential intolerable effects of morphine

Type	Effects	Initial action	Comment
For general undesirable effects of opioid analgesics, see Box 5.F, p.289.			
Gastric stasis	Epigastric fullness, flatulence, anorexia, hiccup, persistent nausea	Metoclopramide 10–20mg q4h	If the problem persists, change to an alternative opioid, with less impact on the GI tract
Sedation	Intolerable persistent sedation	Reduce dose of morphine; consider methylphenidate 5–10mg once daily–b.i.d.	Sedation may be caused by other factors; stimulant rarely appropriate
Cognitive failure	Agitated delirium with hallucinations	Prescribe haloperidol 1–5mg stat & p.r.n.; reduce dose of morphine and, if no improvement, switch to an alternative opioid	Some patients develop intractable delirium with one opioid but not with an alternative opioid
Myoclonus	Multifocal twitching ± jerking of limbs	Prescribe diazepam/midazolam 5mg or lorazepam 500microgram stat & p.r.n.; reduce dose of morphine but increase again if pain recurs	Uncommon with typical oral doses; more common with high dose IV and spinal morphine
Neurotoxicity	Abdominal muscle spasms, symmetrical jerking of legs; whole-body allodynia, hyperalgesia (manifests as excruciating pain)	Prescribe diazepam/midazolam 5mg or lorazepam 500microgram stat & p.r.n.; reduce dose of morphine; consider changing to an alternative opioid	A rare syndrome in patients receiving intrathecal or high dose IV morphine; occasionally seen with typical oral and SC doses
Vestibular stimulation	Movement-induced nausea and vomiting	Prescribe meclizine, dimenhydrinate or promethazine 25–50mg q8h–q6h	If intractable, try methotrimeprazine or switch to an alternative opioid
Pruritus	Whole-body itch with systemic morphine; localized to upper body or face/nose with spinal morphine	Ondansetron 8mg IV stat and 8mg PO b.i.d. for 3–5 days	This is a central phenomenon and does not respond to H$_1$-antihistamines; centrally-acting opioid antagonists also relieve the itch but antagonize analgesia[17]
Histamine release	Bronchoconstriction → dyspnea	Prescribe IV/IM antihistamine (e.g. diphenhydramine 25–50mg) and a bronchodilator; change to a chemically distinct opioid immediately; e.g. methadone	Rare

Box 5.1   Starting a patient on PO morphine

Oral morphine is indicated in patients with pain which does not respond to the optimized combined use of a non-opioid and a weak opioid.

The starting dose of morphine is calculated to give a greater analgesic effect than the medication already in use:
- if the patient was previously receiving a weak opioid regularly (e.g. codeine 240mg/24h or equivalent), give 10mg q4h or SR 20–30mg q12h
- if changing from an alternative strong opioid (e.g. fentanyl, methadone) a much higher dose of morphine may be needed
- if the patient is frail and elderly, a lower dose helps to reduce initial drowsiness, confusion and unsteadiness, e.g. 5mg q4h
- because of accumulation of an active metabolite, a lower and/or less frequent regular dose may suffice in mild–moderate renal impairment, e.g. 5–10mg q6h (but the use of a 'renally safer' opioid is generally advisable with moderate–severe renal impairment, e.g. hydromorphone, fentanyl, see p.295).

If the patient needs 2–3 p.r.n. doses in 24h, the regular dose should be increased by 30–50% every 2–3 days.

As with all opioids, patients must be monitored for undesirable effects, particularly nausea and vomiting, and constipation (see Box 5.F, p.289). Depending on individual circumstances, an anti-emetic should be prescribed for regular or p.r.n. use (see p.183) and, routinely, a laxative prescribed (see p.26).

Upward titration of the dose of morphine stops when either the pain is relieved or intolerable undesirable effects supervene. In the latter case, it is generally necessary to consider alternative measures. The aim is to have the patient free of pain and mentally alert.

Because of poor absorption, SR morphine may not be satisfactory in patients troubled by frequent vomiting or those with diarrhea or an ileostomy.

Scheme 1: ordinary (normal-release) morphine tablets or solution
- morphine given q4h 'by the clock' with p.r.n. doses 50–100% of the q4h dose
- after 1–2 days, recalculate q4h dose by dividing the total used in previous 24h (regular +p.r.n. use) by 6
- continue q4h and p.r.n. doses
- increase the regular dose until there is adequate relief throughout each 4h period, taking p.r.n. use into account
- a double dose at bedtime obviates the need to wake the patient for a dose during the night.

Scheme 2: ordinary (normal-release) morphine and sustained-release (SR) morphine
- begin as for Scheme 1
- when the q4h dose is stable, replace with SR morphine q12h, or once daily if a 24h product is prescribed
- the q12h dose will be three times the previous q4h dose; a q24h dose will be six times the previous q4h dose, rounded to a convenient number of tablets or capsules
- continue to provide ordinary morphine tablets or solution for p.r.n. use; give the equivalent of a q4h dose, i.e. 1/6 of the total daily dose (some centres use 1/10).

Scheme 3: SR morphine and ordinary (normal-release) morphine
- generally start with SR morphine 20–30mg q12h
- use ordinary morphine tablets or solution for p.r.n. medication; give about 1/6 of the daily dose (some centres use 1/10)
- if necessary, increase the dose of SR morphine every 2–3 days until there is adequate relief throughout each 12h period, guided by p.r.n. use.

Box 5.J Rapid titration of morphine dose in 'opioid-naïve' patients (Institute of Palliative Medicine, India)[29]

Prerequisites
Pain ≥5/10 on a numerical scale.
Probability of a partial or complete response to morphine.[a]

Method
Obtain venous access with a butterfly cannula.
Give metoclopramide 10mg IV routinely.
Dilute the contents of 15mg morphine ampoule in a 10mL syringe.[b]
Inject 1.5mg (1mL) every 10min until the patient is pain-free or complains of undue sedation.[c]
If patients experience nausea, give additional metoclopramide 5mg IV.

Results
Dose required (with approximate percentages):
  1.5–4.5mg (40%); 6–9mg (40%)
  10.5–15mg (15%); >15mg (5%).
Complete relief in 80%; none in 1%.
Drop outs 2%.
Undesirable effects: sedation 32%; other 3%.

Ongoing treatment
Prescribe a dose of oral morphine q4h which is similar to the IV requirement, rounded to the nearest 5mg, i.e. relief with morphine 3–6mg IV → 5mg PO etc.; the minimum dose is 5mg q4h.
Instruct patients to take p.r.n. doses and to adjust the dose the next day according to need. In practice, 20% of patients need a dose increase within 3 days.

a. most patients will already be taking an NSAID
b. ampoule strengths varies from country to country; use local standard
c. if ampoule = 10mg/mL (diluted to 10mg in 10mL), a bolus dose of 2mg would be reasonable.

Box 5.K Rapid titration of morphine dose in both 'opioid-tolerant' and 'opioid-naïve' patients (based on practice at Cleveland Clinic, Ohio, USA)[28,30,31]

Sequence	IV	SC
Dose	1mg/min up to 10mg	2mg q5min up to 10mg
Pause	5min	10min
Dose	1mg/min up to 10mg	2mg q5min up to 10mg
Pause	5min	10min
Dose	1mg/min up to 10mg[a]	2mg q5min up to 10mg[a]

Maintenance IV/SC dose
Regard cumulative effective dose as the equivalent of a q4h dose, and prescribe accordingly.

Example
Cumulative effective IV dose = 9mg.
If giving intermittent injections, dose = 9mg q4h, rounded to 10mg.
If CIVI, total daily IV dose = 9mg×6 = 54mg/24h.
Round this up or down to convenient number of ampoules, i.e. 50mg or 60mg.
P.r.n. dose = 5–10mg q1h.

a. review cause if relief inadequate after a total of 30mg.

Box 5.L Rapid IV titration of morphine dose in cancer patients already on regular PO morphine[33,34]

Prerequisites

An increase of pain from ≤4/10 to ≥8/10 on a numerical scale lasting several hours, unresponsive to ≥2 doses of the patient's normal rescue medication.

If no previous dose-limiting effects with PO morphine, proceed with IV morphine but, if previous unacceptable effects with morphine, consider an alternative strong opioid.

Context

In the published case series, the median age was 47 years (range 31–70), and the median baseline PO 'morphine equivalents' was >3.3g/24h (range 48mg–16.8g), i.e. the patients were relatively young and most were taking high/very high doses of PO opioid medication.

Caution

Used appropriately, IV morphine (or other strong opioid) for a pain emergency is generally low risk. However, naloxone should be readily accessible and given:
- if the respiratory rate falls to ≤6/min (or ≤12/min in a patient with moderate–severe COPD) *and*
- oxygen saturation falls below 90% despite oxygen via nasal prongs.

If using naloxone, to avoid a complete reversal of analgesia, dilute contents of a standard ampoule (400microgam) to 10mL, and give 0.5–1mL (20–40microgram) IV every 2min until respiratory status satisfactory. Give oxygen and, if necessary, assist ventilation, e.g. with Ambubag.

Method

Give 10mg IV morphine over 15min; but if the previous total daily PO morphine dose was high (e.g. ≥1g/24h) give 20mg.

Pause for a further 15min, and then re-evaluate.

If pain is still ≥6/10, double the initial dose and infuse over 15min.

Pause for a further 15min, and then re-evaluate.

If pain is still >6/10 and there is no evidence of opioid toxicity, give further doses over 15min followed by pauses of 15min, *doubling the dose each time.*

When re-evaluated, if the pain has reduced to 5–6/10, repeat the same dose or increase the next dose by only 50%.

Note:
- extend the pauses to 30min in patients with cognitive impairment or reduced level of consciousness
- the maximum recommended bolus dose of IV morphine is 320mg (reached after 4–5 doublings of the dose).

Results from a series of 10 pain emergencies in 9 patients

All responded within a median of 90min (range 4min to <4h).

Number of 15min infusions needed:

   1 = 4 patients (highest dose given = 10–20mg)
   2 = 2 (highest dose = 20–40mg)
   3 = 2 (highest dose = 40–80mg)
   4 = 2 (highest dose = 80–160mg).

Ongoing treatment

Subsequent maintenance analgesia is based on the dose of IV morphine needed to control the pain, and is given either by CIVI (e.g. per 24h, 4–6 times the final IV dose) or regularly PO (e.g. per 24h, 10 times the final IV dose).

Rescue medication for break-through (episodic) pain (pain ≥5/10) over the next 24h = the final IV morphine dose.

In India, a single IV dose is given, followed immediately by PO medication (Box 5.J). About 80% of patients obtain relief with 10mg or less.[29] At the Cleveland Clinic (USA), patients are maintained on CIVI for several days before conversion to PO medication (Box 5.K).

A third method was developed for occasional use in patients already on regular PO morphine, when there is a marked increase in pain which is unresponsive to 2–3 doses of the patient's normal rescue medication. The cause of the exacerbation is generally cancer-related, e.g. pathological fracture, hemorrhage into an intra-hepatic metastasis, infection around a cancer (Box 5.L).[33]

IV patient-controlled analgesia (PCA) can also be used, but is more costly, requires inpatient admission and may take >10h to achieve relief.[35] Some centres use a more rapidly acting strong opioid, e.g. IV **fentanyl**, with subsequent doses given after pauses of only 5–10min.[36]

Note: patients who have required a rapid escalation in opioid requirements must be monitored closely. The underlying cause may be transient, e.g. hemorrhage into a liver metastasis, and a subsequent reduction in dose will be necessary.

CSCI: There are 2-drug compatibility data for morphine sulfate in 0.9% saline with **dexamethasone, haloperidol, scopolamine** *hydrobromide*, **ketamine, metoclopramide**, and **midazolam**.

Morphine sulfate is incompatible with **ketorolac** and may be incompatible with higher concentrations of **haloperidol** or **midazolam**.

For more details and 3-drug compatibility data, see Charts A4.1 (p.594) and A4.4 (p.600). Information on compatibility in WFI can be found on www.palliativedrugs.com Syringe Driver Survey Database.

Alternative routes

Buccal morphine

Morphine is slowly absorbed through the buccal mucosa.[37] However, most of a morphine solution given sublingually or into the gingival gutter will be swallowed and absorbed from the GI tract. Nonetheless, in the past, this route was successfully used in moribund patients.

Rectal morphine

Morphine is absorbed from suppositories.[38] From the lower and middle rectum, it will enter the systemic circulation bypassing the liver. From the upper rectum, it will undergo hepatic first-pass metabolism after it enters the portal circulation. However, there are extensive anastomoses between the rectal veins which make it impossible to predict how much will enter the portal circulation.[39,40] Despite the uncertainty, in practice the same dose is given PR as PO.

Although not approved for this route and not generally recommended, SR morphine tablets have been used PR to provide emergency analgesia in moribund patients while organizing a more reliable delivery method.[41]

Spinal morphine

This route of administration (see p.521) is normally undertaken by an anesthetist. Particularly with neuropathic pain, morphine is generally combined with a local anesthetic (e.g. **bupivacaine**), and sometimes with **clonidine**.

Topical morphine

Nociceptive afferent nerve fibres contain peripheral opioid receptors which are silent except in the presence of local inflammation.[1,11,42] This property is exploited in joint surgery where morphine is given intra-articularly at the end of the operation.[43] Topical morphine has also been used successfully to relieve otherwise intractable pain associated with cutaneous ulceration, often decubitus ulcers.[44–47] It is often given as a 0.1% (1mg/mL) gel, using IntraSite®. If prepared under sterile conditions, morphine sulfate is stable for at least 28 days when mixed with IntraSite® gel at a concentration of 0.125% (1.25mg/mL). This preparation can be made by thoroughly mixing 1mL of morphine sulfate 10mg/mL injection with an 8g sachet of IntraSite® gel.[48]

Higher concentrations, namely 0.3–0.5%, have been used when managing pain associated with:
- oral mucositis
- vaginal inflammation associated with a fistula
- rectal ulceration.[45]

The amount of gel applied varies according to the size and the site of the ulcer, but is typically 5–10mL applied b.id.–t.i.d. The topical morphine is kept in place with either a non-absorbable pad or dressing, e.g. Opsite® or Tegaderm®, or gauze coated with petroleum jelly.

Morphine for breathlessness

Morphine and other opioids reduce the ventilatory response to hypercapnia, hypoxia and exercise, decreasing respiratory effort and breathlessness.[49] Improvements are seen at doses that *do not* cause respiratory depression.[50–54] A systematic review supports the use of opioids by the oral and parenteral but *not* the nebulized route, and the latter should not be used outside of a clinical trial.[55–59]

Generally, opioids are more beneficial in patients who are breathless at rest than in those who are breathless only on exertion. Even with maximal exertion, breathlessness generally recovers within a few minutes, much quicker than the time it takes to locate, administer and obtain benefit from an opioid. Thus, non-drug measures are of primary importance in this circumstance.[49]

Patients often fear suffocating to death and a positive approach to the patient, their family and colleagues about the relief of terminal breathlessness is important. Because of the distress, inability to sleep and exhaustion, patients and their carers generally accept that drug-related drowsiness may need to be the price paid for greater comfort. However, unless there is overwhelming distress, sedation is not the primary aim of treatment and some patients become mentally brighter when their breathlessness is reduced. Even so, because increasing drowsiness also generally reflects the deteriorating clinical condition, it is important to stress the gravity of the situation and the aim of treatment to the relatives.

In opioid-naïve patients:[50,51,53,54,60–63]
- start with small doses of morphine, e.g. 2.5–5mg PO p.r.n.; larger doses can be poorly tolerated
- if ≥2 doses/24h are needed, prescribe morphine regularly and titrate the dose according to response, duration of effect and undesirable effects
- relatively small doses may suffice, e.g. 20–60mg/24h.

In patients already taking morphine for pain and with:
- severe breathlessness (i.e. ≥7/10), a dose that is 100% or more of the q4h analgesic dose may be needed
- moderate breathlessness (i.e. 4–6/10), a dose equivalent to 50–100% of the q4h analgesic dose may suffice
- mild breathlessness (i.e. ≤3/10), a dose equivalent to 25–50% of the q4h analgesic dose may suffice.

Clinical experience suggests that in some patients, morphine by CSCI is better tolerated and provides greater relief, possibly by avoiding the peaks (with undesirable effects) and troughs (with loss of effect) of oral medication.

Severe breathlessness in the last days of life:[64]
- no patient should die with distressing breathlessness
- failure to relieve terminal breathlessness is a failure to utilize drug treatment correctly
- give an opioid with a sedative-anxiolytic parenterally, e.g. morphine and **midazolam** or **lorazepam** by CSCI and p.r.n.
- if the patient becomes agitated or confused (sometimes aggravated by a benzodiazepine), **haloperidol** should be added.

If using an alternative opioid to morphine, adopt the same approach as above.

Supply

Unless indicated otherwise, all products are Schedule I controlled drugs under the Controlled Drugs and Substances Act, and are subject to the Narcotic Control Regulations of the act.

Normal-release oral products
Morphine *hydrochloride* (generic)
Oral syrup 1mg/mL, 5mg/mL, 10mg/mL, 20mg/mL, 20mg dose = $0.40, $0.35, $0.40 and $0.60 respectively.

M.O.S.® (Valeant)
Tablets 10mg, 20mg, 40mg, 60mg, 20mg dose = $0.50.
Oral syrup 1mg/mL, 5mg/mL, 10mg/mL, 20mg dose = $0.50.
Concentrated oral syrup 20mg/mL, 50mg/mL, 20mg dose = $0.50.

Morphine *sulfate*
M.O.S. Sulphate® (Valeant)
Tablets 5mg, 10mg, 25mg, 50mg, 25mg dose = $0.25.

MS IR® (Purdue Pharma)
Tablets 5mg, 10mg, 20mg, 30mg, 20mg dose = $0.35.

Statex® (Pharmascience)
Tablets 5mg, 10mg, 25mg, 50mg, 25mg dose = $0.25.
Oral syrup 1mg/mL, 5mg/mL, 10mg/mL, 20mg dose = $0.40.
Oral liquid drops 20mg/mL, 50mg/mL, 20mg dose = $0.40.

Sustained-release oral products
Morphine *hydrochloride*
M.O.S.® (Valeant)
Tablets SR 30mg, 60mg, 28 days @ 60mg b.i.d. = $51.

Morphine *sulfate* (generic)
Tablets SR 15mg, 30mg, 60mg, 100mg, 200mg, 28 days @ 60mg b.i.d. = $54.

Kadian® (Mayne Pharma International)
Capsules SR 10mg, 20mg, 50mg, 100mg, 28 days @ 50mg daily = $39.

M-Eslon® (Ethypharm)
Capsules SR 10mg, 15mg, 30mg, 60mg, 100mg, 200mg, 28 days @ 30mg bid = $30.

MS Contin® (Purdue Pharma)
Tablets SR 15mg, 30mg, 60mg, 100mg, 200mg, 28 days @ 30mg b.i.d. = $59.

Normal-release rectal products
Morphine *sulfate*
Statex® (Pharmascience)
Suppositories 5mg, 10mg, 20mg, 30mg, 10mg dose = $2.

Parenteral products
Morphine *sulfate* (generic)
Injection (for epidural use) 500microgram/mL, 10mL amp = $10; 1mg/mL, 5mL amp = $10.
Injection 1mg/mL, 5mL amp = $2.50, 10mL amp = $3, 30mL amp = $14.
Injection 2mg/mL, 1mL amp = $1, 50mL amp = $12.
Injection 5mg/mL, 30mL amp = $12.
Injection 10mg/mL, 1mL amp = $1.
Injection 15mg/mL, 1mL amp = $1, 30mL amp = $28.
Injection 25mg/mL, 1mL amp = $3, 4mL amp = $11.
Injection 50mg/mL, 1mL amp = $4, 5mL amp = $17, 10mL amp = $33, 50mL amp = $161.

1 Krajnik M et al. (1998) Opioids affect inflammation and the immune system. *Pain Reviews.* 5: 147–154.
2 Hasselstrom J et al. (1986) The metabolism and bioavailability of morphine in patients with severe liver cirrhosis. *British Journal of Clinical Pharmacology.* 29: 289–297.
3 Mazoit J-X et al. (1987) Pharmacokinetics of unchanged morphine in normal and cirrhotic subjects. *Anesthesia and Analgesia.* 66: 293–298.
4 Sandouk P et al. (1991) Presence of morphine metabolites in human cerebrospinal fluid after intracerebroventricular administration of morphine. *European Journal of Drug Metabolism and Pharmacology.* 16: 166–171.
5 Max MB et al. (1992) *Principles of Analgesic Use in the Treatment of Acute Pain and Cancer Pain* (3e). American Pain Society, Skokie, Illinois, p. 12.
6 Regnard CFB and Twycross RG (1984) Metabolism of narcotics (letter). *British Medical Journal.* 288: 860.
7 McQuay HJ et al. (1990) Oral morphine in cancer pain: influences on morphine and metabolite concentration. *Clinical Pharmacology and Therapeutics.* 48: 236–244.
8 Thompson P et al. (1992) Mophine-6-glucuronide: a metabolite of morphine with greater emetic potency than morphine in the ferret. *British Journal of Pharmacology.* 106: 3–8.
9 Buetler TM et al. (2000) Analgesic action of i.v. morphine-6-glucuronide in healthy volunteers. *British Journal of Anaesthesia.* 84: 97–99.
10 Osborne RJ et al. (1986) Morphine intoxication in renal failure: the role of morphine-6-glucuronide. *British Medical Journal.* 292: 1548–1549.
11 Ribeiro MD et al. (2004) The bioavailability of morphine applied topically to cutaneous ulcers. *J Pain Symptom Manage.* 27: 434–439.
12 Watterson G et al. (2004) Peripheral opioids in inflammatory pain. *Archives of Disease in Childhood.* 89: 679–681.
13 Jansen M (2006) Morphine gel. Palliativedrugs.com bulletin board message. Available from: http://www.palliativedrugs.com/forum/read.php?f=1&i=9271&t=9189
14 Westerling D et al. (1994) Transdermal administration of morphine to healthy subjects. *British Journal of Clinical Pharmacology.* 37: 571–576.
15 AHFS (American Hospital Formulary Service) (2009) Morphine sulfate: In: AHFS Drug Information (online version). *American Society of Health-System Pharmacists, Bethesda.* Section 28.08.08.

16 Micromedex (2009) Morphine. Available from: www.micromedex.com
17 Twycross RG et al. (2003) Itch: scratching more than the surface. Quarterly Journal of Medicine. **96**: 7–26.
18 Hanks G et al. (2001) Morphine and alternative opioids in cancer pain: the EAPC recommendations. British Journal of Cancer. **84**: 587–593.
19 Health Canada (2010) Available from: http://www.hc-sc.gc.ca/dhp-mps/medeff/advisories-avis/prof/_2010/fentanyl_2_hpc-cps-eng.php
20 Bloomfield S et al. (1993) Analgesic efficacy and potency of two controlled-release morphine preparations. Clinical Pharmacology and Therapeutics. **53**: 469–478.
21 Gourlay G et al. (1993) A comparison of Kapanol (a new sustained-release morphine formulation), MST Continus and morphine solution in cancer patients: pharmacokinetic aspects. In: The Seventh World Congress on Pain; Seattle. IASP Press.
22 Boehringer Ingelheim GmbH Data on file.
23 Todd J et al. (2001) An assessment of the efficacy and tolerability of a 'double dose' of immediate-release morphine at bedtime. In: Seventh Congress of EAPC; Palermo, Italy.
24 Carver AC and Foley KM (2001) Symptom assessment and management. Neurologic Clinics. **19**: 921–947.
25 Schug SA et al. (1992) A long-term survey of morphine in cancer pain patients. Journal of Pain and Symptom Management. **7**: 259–266.
26 Donnelly S et al. (2002) Morphine in cancer pain management: a practical guide. Supportive Care in Cancer. **10**: 13–35.
27 Twycross RG and Harcourt JMV (1991) The use of laxatives at a palliative care centre. Palliative Medicine. **5**: 27–33.
28 Davis MP et al. (2004) Opioid dose titration for severe cancer pain: a systematic evidence-based review. Journal of Palliative Medicine. **7**: 462–468.
29 Kumar K et al. (2000) Intravenous morphine for emergency treatment of cancer pain. Palliative Medicine. **14**: 183–188.
30 Davis MP (2004) Acute pain in advanced cancer: an opioid dosing strategy and illustration. American Journal of Hospice and Palliative Care. **21**: 47–50.
31 Davis MP (2005) Rapid opiod titration in severe cancer pain. European Journal of Palliative Care. **12**: 11–14.
32 Hagen N et al. (1997) Cancer pain emergencies: a protocol for management. Journal of Pain and Symptom Management. **14**: 45–50.
33 Hagen NA et al. (1997) Cancer pain emergencies: a protocol for management.[see comment]. Journal of Pain and Symptom Management. **14**: 45–50.
34 Hagen (2009) Personal communication.
35 Radbruch L et al. (1999) Intravenous titration with morphine for severe cancer pain: report of 28 cases. Clinical Journal of Pain. **15**: 173–178.
36 Soares LG et al. (2003) Intravenous fentanyl for cancer pain: a 'fast titration' protocol for the emergency room. Journal of Pain and Symptom Management. **26**: 876–881.
37 Coluzzi P (1998) Sublingual morphine: efficacy reviewed. Journal of Pain and Symptom Management. **16**: 184–192.
38 deBoer AG et al. (1982) Rectal drug administration: clinical pharmacokinetic considerations. Clinical Pharmacokinetics. **7**: 285–311.
39 Johnson AG and Lux G (1988) Progress in the Treatment of Gastrointestinal Motility Disorder. The role of cisapride. Excerpta Medica, Amsterdam.
40 Ripamonti C and Bruera E (1991) Rectal, buccal and sublingual narcotics for the management of cancer pain. Journal of Palliative Care. **7 (1)**: 30–35.
41 Wilkinson T et al. (1992) Pharmacokinetics and efficacy of rectal versus oral sustained-release morphine in cancer patients. Cancer Chemotherapy and Pharmacology. **31**: 251–254.
42 Krajnik M and Zylicz Z (1997) Topical opioids – fact or fiction? Progress in Palliative Care. **5**: 101–106.
43 Likar R et al. (1999) Dose-dependency of intra-articular morphine analgesia. British Journal of Anaesthesia. **83**: 241–244.
44 Back NI and Finlay I (1995) Analgesic effect of topical opioids on painful skin ulcers. Journal of Pain and Symptom Management. **10**: 493.
45 Krajnik M et al. (1999) Potential uses of topical opioids in palliative care – report of 6 cases. Pain. **80**: 121–125.
46 Twillman R et al. (1999) Treatment of painful skin ulcers with topical opioids. Journal of Pain and Symptom Management. **17**: 288–292.
47 Zeppetella G et al. (2003) Analgesic efficacy of morphine applied topically to painful ulcers. Journal of Pain and Symptom Management. **25**: 555–558.
48 Zeppetella G and Ribeiro MD (2005) Morphine in intrasite gel applied topically to painful ulcers. Journal of Pain and Symptom Management. **29**: 118–119.
49 Twycross RG and Wilcock A (2001) Symptom Management in Advanced Cancer (3e). Radcliffe Medical Press, Oxford, pp. 141–154.
50 Bruera E et al. (1990) Effects of morphine on the dyspnea of terminal cancer patients. Journal of Pain and Symptom Management. **5**: 341–344.
51 Bruera E et al. (1993) Subcutaneous morphine for dyspnoea in cancer patients. Annals of Internal Medicine. **119**: 906–907.
52 Mazzocato C et al. (1999) The effects of morphine on dyspnoea and ventilatory function in elderly patients with advanced cancer: A randomized double-blind controlled trial. Annals of Oncology. **10**: 1511–1514.
53 Abernethy AP et al. (2003) Randomised, double blind, placebo controlled crossover trial of sustained release morphine for the management of refractory dyspnoea. British Medical Journal. **327**: 523–528.
54 Allen S et al. (2005) Low dose diamorphine reduces breathlessness without causing a fall in oxygen saturation in elderly patients with end-stage idiopathic pulmonary fibrosis. Palliative Medicine. **19**: 128–130.
55 Davis C (1999) Nebulized opioids should not be prescribed outside a clinical trial. American Journal of Hospice and Palliative Care. **16**: 543.
56 Jennings A et al. (2002) A systematic review of the use of opioids in the management of dyspnoea. Thorax. **57**: 939–944.
57 Foral PA et al. (2004) Nebulized opioids use in COPD. Chest. **125**: 691–694.
58 Brown SJ et al. (2005) Nebulized morphine for relief of dyspnea due to chronic lung disease. Annals of Pharmacotherapy. **39**: 1088–1092.
59 Bruera E et al. (2005) Nebulized versus subcutaneous morphine for patients with cancer dyspnea: a preliminary study. Journal of Pain and Symptom Management. **29**: 613–618.
60 Cohen M et al. (1991) Continuous intravenous infusion of morphine for sever dyspnoea. Southern Medical Journal. **84**: 229–234.
61 Boyd K and Kelly M (1997) Oral morphine as symptomatic treatment of dyspnoea in patients with advanced cancer. Palliative Medicine. **11**: 277–281.

62 Poole PJ et al. (1998) The effect of sustained-release morphine on breathlessness and quality of life in severe chronic obstructive pulmonary disease. American Journal of Respiratory and Critical Care Medicine. **157**: 1877–1880.

63 Allard P et al. (1999) How effective are supplementary doses of opioids for dyspnea in terminally ill cancer patients? A randomized continuous sequential clinical trial. Journal of Pain and Symptom Management. **17**: 256–265.

64 Navigante AH et al. (2006) Midazolam as adjunct therapy to morphine in the alleviation of severe dyspnea perception in patients with advanced cancer. Journal of Pain and Symptom Management. **31**: 38–47.

*ALFENTANIL

Class: Opioid analgesic.

Indications: Intra-operative analgesia, analgesia and procedure-related pain in mechanically ventilated patients on intensive care units, †an alternative in cases of intolerance to other strong opioids, particularly in renal failure,[1] †procedure-related pain in non-ventilated patients,[2,3] †break-through (episodic) pain.[4,5]

Contra-indications: None absolute if titrated carefully against a patient's pain (see also Strong opioids, p.287).

Pharmacology

Alfentanil is a synthetic derivative of **fentanyl** with distinct properties: a more rapid onset of action, a shorter duration of action, and a potency approximately 1/4 that of **fentanyl**[6] (and about 20 times more than parenteral **morphine**). Alfentanil is less lipophilic than **fentanyl** and is 90% bound to mainly α_1-acid glycoprotein.[7] However, because most of the unbound alfentanil is unionized, it rapidly enters the CNS. It is metabolized in the liver by CYP3A4 to inactive metabolites that are excreted in the urine. Alfentanil can accumulate with chronic administration, particularly when clearance is reduced, e.g. in the elderly, the obese, patients with burns or with hepatic impairment. It has been suggested that analgesic tolerance occurs rapidly with alfentanil, but this appears not to be a problem in palliative care practice (Table 5.18).[8–10]

Although dose reductions may be necessary in patients with severe hepatic impairment, this is not necessary in renal failure. Consequently, alfentanil is used at some centres as the parenteral opioid of choice in end-stage renal failure (see p.295).[11] Alfentanil is available in a more concentrated form (500microgram/mL) than **fentanyl** (50microgram/mL), reducing the dose volume and facilitating its administration CSCI using a standard syringe driver or SL (see p.000). For similar reasons, **sufentanil**, which is 10 times more potent than **fentanyl**, is also used SL (see Table 5.19);[12] it is often preferred to **fentanyl** and alfentanil for SL administration in Canada.

Alfentanil has been used successfully by short-term PCA or CSCI for dressing changes in burns or trauma patients.[2,3] It is used SL (and occasionally nasally) for cancer-related break-through (episodic) pain.[4] In the UK, a spray bottle containing alfentanil 5mg in 5mL is manufactured from alfentanil powder, delivering 140microgram/0.14mL spray. Details and instructions for use can be downloaded from www.palliativedrugs.com.[5] In an audit of patients already on regular strong opioids, about 3/4 benefited from SL alfentanil in doses of 560–1680microgram (4–12 sprays; titrated as necessary). Pain relief was seen within 10min, with more consistent benefit obtained for the prevention of predictable incident compared with unpredictable break-through (episodic) pain, possibly reflecting greater natural variation in the latter. This suggests that the p.r.n. dose for unpredictable break-through pain should be a range rather than a fixed dose. As with all fentanils, there is little point in spinal administration because of the rapid clearance into the systemic circulation.[13,14]

Table 5.18 Pharmacokinetics of single IV doses of fentanyl congeners[15–17]

	Alfentanil	Sufentanil	Fentanyl
Onset of action (min)	0.75	1	1.5
Time to peak effect (min)	1.5	2.5	4.5
Plasma halflife (min)	95	165	220
Duration of action (min)	30	60	60

Onset of action <1min IV; <5min IM.
Time to peak plasma concentration 15min IM.
Plasma halflife 95min.
Duration of action 30min IV; 1h IM.

Cautions
As for **morphine** (see p.300). Alfentanil levels are increased by inhibitors of CYP3A4, e.g. **cimetidine**, **diltiazem**, **erythromycin**, **fluconazole**, **itraconazole**, **ketoconazole**, **ritonavir**, **troleandomycin**, and decreased by inducers of CYP3A4, e.g. **rifampin** (see Cytochrome P450, p.551).

Undesirable effects
For full list, see manufacturer's Product Monograph.
Also see Strong opioids, p.289.

Dose and use
Alternative to morphine
Used mostly for patients in renal failure in whom there is evidence of **morphine** neurotoxicity. The following are safe practical conversion ratios:
- PO **morphine** to SC alfentanil, give 1/30–1/40 of the 24h dose, e.g. **morphine** 60mg/24h PO = alfentanil 2mg/24h SC
- SC **morphine** to SC alfentanil, give 1/15–1/20 of the 24h dose, e.g. **morphine** 30mg/24h SC = alfentanil 2mg/24h SC.

Conventionally, SC p.r.n. doses are 1/6–1/10 of the total 24h CSCI dose.

Procedure-related pain (see Guidelines, p.313)
- 250–500microgram SL (from ampoule for injection) or SC/IV.

Break-through (episodic) pain, SL administration
There is a poor relationship between the effective p.r.n. dose and regular background opioid dose. Individual dose titration is necessary starting with 250–500microgram. For **fentanyl** and **sufentanil** see Table 5.19. Retaining even 2mL in the mouth (sublingually or buccally) for 5–10min is difficult. Thus, the smaller the volume, the easier it is for the patient.

Table 5.19 Equivalent volumes of parenteral formulations of alfentanil, sufentanil and fentanyl for SL use[a,b]

Alfentanil (500microgram/mL)		Sufentanil (50microgram/mL)		Fentanyl (50microgram/mL)	
Dose (microgram)	Volume (mL)	Dose (microgram)	Volume (mL)	Dose (microgram)	Volume (mL)
100	0.2	2.5	N/A	25	0.5
200	0.4	5	0.1	50	1
300	0.6	7.5	0.15	75	1.5
400	0.8	10	0.2	100	2
500	1	12.5	0.25	125	N/O
600	1.2	15	0.3	150	N/O
800	1.6	20	0.4	200	N/O
1,000	2	25	0.5	250	N/O
2,000	N/O	50	1	500	N/O
3,000	N/O	75	1.5	750	N/O
4,000	N/O	100	2	1,000	N/O

a. this is not a true dose conversion chart. Alfentanil, sufentanil and fentanyl have differing properties and, although bio-availability and onset of effect are broadly similar, duration of effect differs (fentanyl > sufentanil > alfentanil). As always with analgesics, individual patient dose titration is required
b. N/O = not optimal, because >2mL.

As with all opioids, patients must be monitored for undesirable effects, particularly nausea and vomiting, and constipation (see p.289). Depending on individual circumstances, an anti-emetic should be prescribed for regular or p.r.n. use, (see p.183) and, routinely, a laxative prescribed (see p.26).

CSCI: There are 2-drug compatibility data for alfentanil in 0.9% saline with **haloperidol**, **ketamine**, **midazolam** and **ondansetron**.

For more details, and 3-drug compatibility data, see Charts A4.1 (p.594) and A4.2 (p.596). Information on compatibility in WFI can be found on www.palliativedrugs.com Syringe Driver Survey Database.

Supply

Unless indicated otherwise, all products are Schedule I controlled drugs under the Controlled Drugs and Substances Act, and are subject to the Narcotic Control Regulations of the act.

Alfentanil (generic)
Injection 500microgram/mL, 2mL amp = $7.

1 Kirkham SR and Pugh R (1995) Opioid analgesia in uraemic patients. *Lancet.* **345**: 1185.
2 Sim KM *et al.* (1996) Use of patient-controlled analgesia with alfentanil for burns dressing procedures: a preliminary report of five patients. *Burns.* **22**: 238–241.
3 Gallagher G *et al.* (2001) Target-controlled alfentanil analgesia for dressing change following extensive reconstructive surgery for trauma. *Journal of Pain and Symptom Management.* **21**: 1–2.
4 Duncan A (2002) The use of fentanyl and alfentanil sprays for episodic pain. *Palliative Medicine.* **16**: 550.
5 Palliativedrugs.com (2003) Hot Topics: alternatives to sublingual fentanyl. In: *August Newsletter.* Available from: www.palliativedrugs.com
6 Larijani G and Goldberg M (1987) Alfentanil hydrochloride: a new short acting narcotic analgesic for surgical procedures. *Clinical Pharmacy.* **6**: 275–282.
7 Bernards C (1999) Clinical implications of physicochemical properties of opioids. In: C Stein (ed) *Opioids in Pain Control: basic and Clinical Aspects.* Cambridge University Press, Cambridge, pp. 166–187.
8 Hill HF *et al.* (1992) Patient-controlled analgesia infusions: alfentanil versus morphine. *Pain.* **49**: 301–310.
9 Kissin I *et al.* (2000) Acute tolerance to continuously infused alfentanil: the role of cholecystokinin and N-methyl-d-aspartate-nitric oxide systems. *Anesthesia and Analgesia.* **91**: 110–116.
10 Urch CE *et al.* (2004) A retrospective review of the use of alfentanil in a hospital palliative care setting. *Palliative Medicine.* **18**: 516–519.
11 Chambers EJ *et al.* (eds) (2004) *Supportive Care for the Renal Patient.* Oxford University Press, Oxford, pp. 122, 262–265.
12 Gardner-Nix J (2001) Oral transmucosal fentanyl and sufentanil for incident pain. *Journal of Pain and Symptom Management.* **22**: 627–630.
13 Burm A *et al.* (1994) Pharmacokinetics of alfentanil after epidural administration. Investigation of systemic absorption kinetics with a stable isotope method. *Anesthesiology.* **81**: 308–315.
14 Ummenhofer W *et al.* (2000) Comparative spinal distribution and clearance kinetics of intrathecally administered morphine, fentanyl, alfentanil, and sufentanil. *Anesthesiology.* **92**: 739–953.
15 Willens JS and Myslinski NR (1993) Pharmacodynamics, pharmacokinetics, and clinical uses of fentanyl, sufentanil, and alfentanil. *Heart Lung.* **22**: 239–251.
16 Scholz J *et al.* (1996) Clinical pharmacokinetics of alfentanil, fentanyl and sufentanil. An update. *Clinical Pharmacokinetics.* **31**: 275–292.
17 Hall A and Hardy JR (2009) The lipophilic opioids: fentanyl, alfentanil, sufentanil, and remifentanil. In: MP Davis *et al.* (eds) *Opioids in Cancer Pain* (2e). Oxford University Press, Oxford, pp. 175–192.

Guidelines: Management of procedure-related pain

I Palliative care patients may experience pain while undergoing procedures, e.g.:

- position change
- investigation, e.g. MRI
- wound dressing change
- venous cannulation
- urethral catheterization
- removing impacted feces
- insertion of nasogastric tube
- insertion/removal of central line
- insertion/removal of spinal line
- drainage of chest/abdomen
- treatment, e.g. radiation therapy

2 The goal is adequate pain relief without undesirable effects. What is appropriate depends on the anticipated pain severity, procedure duration, current opioid use, and the patient's past personal experience. Thus, severe procedure-related pain may necessitate parenteral analgesia and sedation as first-line therapy.

3 Always include non-drug approaches:

- discuss past experiences of procedure-related pain, identify what was helpful or unhelpful, and clarify present concerns
- explain the procedure thoroughly before starting
- assure that you will stop immediately if requested
- as far as possible, choose the most comfortable position for the patient
- distract and relax, e.g. through talking, music, hypnosis and other relaxation techniques.

4 Use a local anesthetic when a cannula, urinary catheter or tube is inserted transdermally, e.g.:
- if needle phobic or if requested, EMLA® cream for venous cannulation (wait 60 minutes)
- lidocaine gel 2% for urethral catheterization (wait 5 minutes)
- lidocaine injection 1% 5mL infiltrated into the tissues for chest aspiration (wait 5 minutes).

5 If available, consider nitrous oxide-oxygen (Entonox®) inhalation if the procedure is short and the patient is able to use the mask or mouthpiece effectively.

6 Give analgesia from the appropriate step of the ladder. (General anesthetic approaches are beyond the scope of these guidelines.)

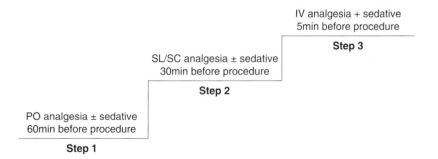

IV analgesia + sedative
5min before procedure

Step 3

SL/SC analgesia ± sedative
30min before procedure

Step 2

PO analgesia ± sedative
60min before procedure

Step 1

7 If pain relief inadequate, give a repeat dose and wait again; if still inadequate, move to the next step.

8 When a sedative or sedative analgesic is used, practitioners must be competent in airway management. Monitor the patient to ensure that the airway remains patent, and consider intervention if the patient becomes cyanosed because of severely depressed respiration.

continued

> **Examples of analgesia for procedure-related pain**
>
> **Step 1: If anticipating mild–moderate pain**
> *Give 60 minutes before the procedure:*
> PO morphine, give the patient's usual rescue dose for break-through (episodic) pain.
> If necessary, combine with:
> - PO diazepam 5mg *or*
> - SL lorazepam 500microgram–1mg *or*
> - an alternative sedative.
>
> **Step 2: If anticipating moderate–severe pain**
> *Give 30 minutes before procedure:*
> SC morphine, give 50% of the patient's usual PO morphine rescue dose.
> If necessary, combine with:
> - SL/SC midazolam 2.5–5mg *or*
> - SL lorazepam 500microgram–1mg *or*
> - an alternative sedative.
>
> **Step 3: If anticipating severe–excruciating pain**
> *Give 5 minutes before procedure:*
> IV morphine, give 50% of the patient's usual PO morphine rescue dose *or*
> IV ketamine 0.5–1mg/kg (typically 25–50mg). Combine with:
> - IV midazolam 2.5–5mg *or*
> - an alternative sedative.
>
> Note: there is a risk of marked sedation when ketamine and a sedative such as midazolam are combined in this way; use only if competent in airway management.
>
> **Alternatives to SC/IV morphine**
> - alfentanil 250–500microgram SL (*from ampoule for injection*) or SC/IV
> - fentanyl 50–100microgram SL (*from ampoule for injection*) or SC/IV
> - sufentanil 12.5–25microgram SL (*from ampoule for injection*) or SC/IV.

9 An opioid antagonist (naloxone) and a benzodiazepine antagonist (flumazenil) should be available in case of need. To prevent the complete reversal of any background regular opioid analgesic therapy, use naloxone 20–100microgram IV, repeated every 2 minutes until the respiratory rate and cyanosis have improved. The initial dose of flumazenil is 200microgram IV over 15 seconds; if the desired level of consciousness is not obtained after 1 minute, further 100microgram doses can be given at 1 minute intervals p.r.n. up to a maximum total dose of 1mg.

10 If the procedure is to be repeated, give analgesia based on previous experience, e.g. drugs used and the patient's comments.

FENTANYL

Class: Strong opioid analgesic.

Indications: *Transdermal (TD)* moderate–severe chronic (persistent, long-term) pain, including cancer, †AIDS,[1] †**morphine** intolerance.[2] *Injection* †SL use for procedure-related pain and also break-through (episodic) pain in patients on regular strong opioid treatment.

Contra-indications: TD fentanyl should not be used for acute (transient, intermittent or short-term) pain, e.g. postoperative, or when there is need for rapid dose titration for severe uncontrolled pain. In Canada and the USA, TD fentanyl is contra-indicated in opioid-naïve patients because of reports of unintentional overdoses, with serious (sometimes fatal) consequences.[3] However, in the UK, TD fentanyl is licensed for first-line use (see Dose and use).

Pharmacology

Fentanyl (*like* **morphine**) is a strong μ-opioid receptor agonist. It has a relatively low molecular weight and (*unlike* **morphine**) is lipophilic. This makes it suitable for TD and oral transmucosal administration. Fentanyl is sequestered in body fats, including epidural fat and the white matter of the CNS.[4,5] Thus, by any route (including spinally), after systemic redistribution, fentanyl acts supraspinally mainly in the thalamus (white matter). Any effect in the dorsal horn (grey matter) is probably minimal.[4] This may account for the clinical observation that patients with poor pain relief despite using very high doses (e.g. 600microgram/h TD) sometimes obtain good relief with relatively smaller doses of **morphine**, e.g. 10–20mg SC.[6] The lipophilic nature of fentanyl also provides one explanation for differences compared with **morphine** in the undesirable effects profile (Figure 5.11).[7] Converting from PO or parenteral **morphine** to TD or parenteral fentanyl results in a massive decrease in opioid molecules outside the CNS with, in consequence:

- less constipation (probably always)
- less nausea and vomiting (possibly often)
- peripherally-mediated withdrawal symptoms in physically-dependent subjects (sometimes).

TD fentanyl is used in the management of chronic severe pain,[8–10] particularly in cancer.[11–18] Steady-state plasma concentrations of fentanyl are generally achieved after 36–48 hours[1] but may take 6–12 days. Elimination mainly involves biotransformation in the liver by CYP3A4 to inactive norfentanyl which is excreted in the urine. Less than 7% is excreted unchanged. If effective analgesia does not last for 3 days, the correct response is to increase the patch strength. Even so, a small percentage of patients do best if the patch is changed every 2 days.[18,19] The manufacturer recommends a dose conversion ratio for **morphine** and fentanyl of 150:1. However, one RCT suggested a ratio of only 70:1 and another 125:1.[11,20] Consequently, *PCF* has opted for 100:1; this is also the ratio used in the Product Monograph in Germany.

Because fentanyl is less constipating than **morphine**,[11,19,21,22] when converting from **morphine** to fentanyl, the dose of laxative should be halved and subsequently adjusted according to need. Some patients experience withdrawal symptoms (e.g. diarrhea, colic, nausea, sweating, restlessness) when changed from PO **morphine** to TD fentanyl despite satisfactory pain relief. This is probably related to differences between the two opioids in relation to their relative impact on peripheral and central μ-opioid receptors (Figure 5.11). Such symptoms generally resolve after a few days but are easily treatable by using rescue doses of **morphine** (or alternative strong opioid) or **loperamide**.

Pharmacokinetic data for TD fentanyl are summarized below. Bio-availability is irrelevant in relation to TD patches; the stated delivery rates reflect the mean amount of drug delivered to patients throughout the patch's recommended duration of use. Inevitably, there will be interindividual variation in the amount absorbed, e.g. for the 100microgram/h patch, the mean ($\pm$SD) delivery is 92 ($\pm$26) microgram/h,[23] and the amount of unused fentanyl in the patch after 3 days can vary from 30 to 85% of the original contents.[24]

In cachectic patients, plasma concentrations of fentanyl are reduced by 1/3 to 1/2, presumably because of reduced absorption.[25] The reason for this is unclear; it probably does not relate to loss of subcutaneous adipose tissue,[26] but loss of skin hydration is one possibility.[25]

Onset of action 3–23h.[27]

Time to peak plasma concentration 24–72h.

Plasma halflife 13–22h (after a patch has been removed and not replaced).[28]

Duration of action 72h; for some patients, 48h.[29]

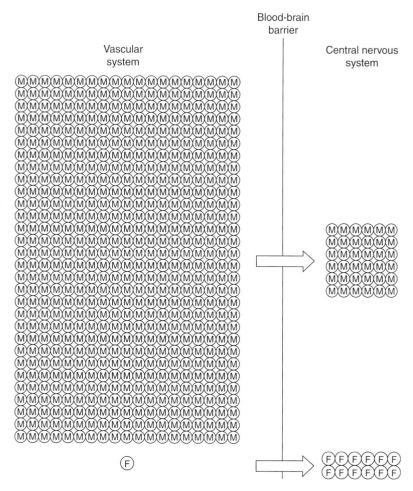

Figure 5.11 Distribution of equipotent doses of morphine and fentanyl in the vascular and central nervous systems based on animal data.[7] For clinical relevance, see p.315.

Cautions

The reservoir patches should not be cut because damage to the rate-controlling membrane can lead to a rapid release of fentanyl and overdose. Although cutting matrix patches is theoretically safer, some strongly discourage it because of similar concerns.[30] However, cutting has become unnecessary with the introduction of a 12microgram/h patch.

After reports of serious adverse events (overdoses and deaths), regulatory authorities in Canada and the USA have issued safety warnings about the use of TD fentanyl.[3,31] Factors which contributed to the adverse drug events included:

- lack of appreciation that fentanyl is a strong opioid analgesic
- inappropriate use for short-term, intermittent or postoperative pain in patients who had not previously been receiving a strong opioid
- lack of patient education regarding directions for safe use, storage and disposal
- lack of awareness of the signs of an overdose and when to seek attention

- lack of awareness that the rate of absorption of fentanyl may be increased if the skin under the patch becomes vasodilated, e.g. in febrile patients, or by an external heat source, e.g. electric blanket, heat lamps, saunas, hot tubs
- lack of awareness of drug interactions which can increase fentanyl levels.

Fentanyl is metabolized by CYP3A4. Potent CYP3A4 inhibitors which may increase fentanyl plasma concentrations include **cimetidine, clarithromycin, fluconazole, itraconazole, ketoconazole, nefazodone** (not Canada), **nelfinavir, ritonavir, troleandomycin** (not Canada). A probable case of fatal interaction between **fluconazole** and TD fentanyl has been reported.[32]

In contrast, concentrations are decreased by potent CYP3A4 inducers (e.g. **carbamazepine, phenytoin, rifampin**) and this may lead to a loss of analgesia.[33–36]

Fentanyl acts as a weak serotonin re-uptake inhibitor and there are rare case reports of probable serotonin toxicity resulting from its combined use with other serotoninergic drugs, e.g. SSRIs (see p.142).[37–40] Fentanyl should not be used concurrently with an MAOI or within two weeks of stopping an MAOI.

Although fentanyl analgesia is generally unaffected by hemodialysis,[41] there are rare reports of pain recurring in patients on TD fentanyl during and after hemodialysis.[42] This probably relates only to certain dialysis membranes and may reflect loss of fentanyl through membrane adsorption rather than loss into the dialysate solution.[41]

Undesirable effects

For full list, see manufacturer's Product Monograph.
TD Occasional skin irritation.
Also see Strong opioids, p.289.

Dose and use
TD fentanyl

The use of TD fentanyl patches is summarized in the Guidelines, p.322. These and the comments in this section are based on a dose conversion ratio with **morphine** of 1:100. Prescribers using the manufacturer's preferred ratio of 1:150 should follow the dose conversion guidelines in the Product Monograph, which are also outlined in a Health Canada-endorsed letter to health professionals.[43]

Under no circumstances should a *reservoir* patch be cut in an attempt to reduce the dose. Leakage from the cut reservoir could result in either the patient receiving minimal or no fentanyl, or, alternatively, an overdose from the rapid absorption of fentanyl through the surrounding skin.

Two different TD formulations are currently available, although reservoir patches are being phased out:

- *reservoir* patch (generic made by Ranbaxy; expected to be discontinued during 2010) the fentanyl is contained within a reservoir, and the release of fentanyl is controlled by a rate-limiting membrane
- *matrix* patch (Durogesic MAT®, generics made by Novopharm, Pharmascience, Ranbaxy, ratiopharm and Sandoz) the fentanyl is evenly distributed throughout a drug-in-adhesive matrix, and the release of fentanyl is controlled by the physical characteristics of the matrix.

Absorption of the fentanyl through the skin and into the systemic circulation is influenced by both the stratum corneum of the skin and blood flow. Thus, if the skin is warm and vasodilated, the rate of absorption will be increased. The *reservoir* and *matrix* patches are bio-equivalent with similar pharmacokinetic profiles, and patients can be switched from one to the other with no loss of efficacy or increase in undesirable effects.[44–46] The matrix patch is thinner (because there is no reservoir) and, for ratiopharm patches, about 25% smaller. Consequently, to avoid confusing the patients and carers, it is generally better if one formulation is prescribed consistently for any one individual.

Health Canada and the Canadian manufacturer[3,43] stress that TD fentanyl should not be used in opioid-naïve patients, and should be commenced only in patients who have been receiving strong opioids in a dose at least equivalent to a 25microgram/h patch for ≥1 week, e.g.:

- **morphine** 60mg/24h PO
- **oxycodone** 30mg/24h PO
- **hydromorphone** 8mg/24h PO.

In contrast, in the UK, TD fentanyl is licensed for use as a *first-line strong opioid* and has been used satisfactorily in, for example, patients with severe dysphagia, renal failure or who are living in social circumstances where there is a high risk of diversion and tablet misuse. (Note: it is possible to extract fentanyl, particularly from the *reservoir* patch, and misuse it.).

TD fentanyl is also used in *totally opioid-naïve patients* at centres which skip Step 2 of the WHO analgesic ladder.[47–49] Licensed starting doses for TD fentanyl as a *first-line strong opioid* in the UK are 12microgram/h and 25microgram/h, depending on the individual product, equivalent to **morphine** 30mg and 60mg PO respectively. Thus, the 12microgram/h dose will be a safer starting dose for *totally opioid-naïve* patients and for some *strong* (but not weak) *opioid-naïve* patients, e.g. frail patients using low doses of weak opioid with moderate pain. Undesirable effects are more frequent in strong opioid-naïve patients and, in one study, resulted in 2%, 6% and 8% of patients discontinuing TD fentanyl 25microgram/h depending on whether they had previously been receiving strong opioids, weak opioids or non-opioids respectively.[49]

Although not recommended by the manufacturers, when using the 25microgram/h patch to initiate TD treatment, some practitioners cover part of the underside of the patch (*reservoir*) or cut patches (*matrix*) so as to decrease the initial dose. These practices have become unnecessary since the introduction of the 12microgram/h patch.

It should be noted that, unless patients have been taking several rescue doses per day of **morphine** (or other strong opioid) for break-through (episodic) pain, escalating in one step from 25 to 50microgram/h (a dose increase of 100%) can cause a marked (but temporary) increase in undesirable effects.[50]

It is important to give adequate rescue doses of **morphine** (see Guidelines, p.322) or other strong opioid (see p.497). Adjusting the patch strength on a daily basis is not recommended.[51] With inpatients, the use of a fentanyl patch chart is recommended (Box 5.M). If the manufacturer's recommended potency ratio with PO morphine of 150:1 is used, 50% of patients will need an increase in patch strength after the first 3 days.[52]

Fentanyl solution

In some countries, rapid-acting formulations of fentanyl (e.g. oral transmucosal lozenges, buccal tablets, nasal sprays) are commercially available for the treatment of break-through (episodic) pain. Because these are not available in Canada, some palliative care services use the parenteral formulation for SL administration, e.g. fentanyl (50microgram/mL), **sufentanil** (50microgram/mL) or **alfentanil** (500microgram/mL and 5mg/mL).[53–55] Onset of analgesic effect may be broadly similar (5–10 minutes) but duration of effect is likely to differ (fentanyl > **sufentanil** > **alfentanil**) (see Alfentanil, p.310). Several small doses can be given until pain relief is obtained. Drawing up the correct amount of the parenteral formulation into a syringe is inconvenient; this can be overcome by the use of a spray bottle.[55,56] Use a 1mL graduated oral syringe:

- start with 25–50microgram (0.5–1mL of 50microgram/mL)
- if necessary, increase to 50–100microgram; many patients do not need more than this
- doses >100microgram are impractical because 2mL is the maximum volume that can be reliably kept in the mouth for transmucosal absorption[54]
- if >75microgram SL is required, some centres switch to SL **sufentanil** to reduce volume (see Table 5.19, p.311 and http://palliative.info/IncidentPain.htm).

Supply

Unless indicated otherwise, all products are Schedule I controlled drugs under the Controlled Drugs and Substances Act (CDSA), and are subject to the CDSA Narcotic Control Regulations.

Transdermal products
Fentanyl transdermal (generic)
Reservoir patches (for 3 days) 25microgram/h, 1 = $6; 50microgram/h, 1 = $12; 75microgram/h, 1 = $16; 100microgram/h, 1 = $20.
Matrix patches (for 3 days) 12microgram/h, 1 = $4; 25microgram/h, 1 = $6; 37microgram/h, 1 = $10; 50microgram/h, 1 = $12; 75microgram/h, 1 = $16; 100microgram/h, 1 = $20.

Duragesic MAT® (Janssen-Ortho)
Matrix patches (for 3 days) 25microgram/h, 1 = $12; 50microgram/h, 1 = $22; 75microgram/h, 1 = $30; 100microgram/h, 1 = $37. *A 12microgram/h patch is expected to be released in the near future.*

Box 5.M Fentanyl patch chart: example of a nursing record

Fentanyl Patch Chart

Patient's name:
Date of birth:

Hospital No:

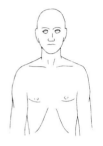

Generally apply to dry, flat, non-hairy skin on the trunk or upper arm.

Press firmly in place with the hand for 30 seconds to ensure good contact.

Mark the patch with the date and time it was applied, and record the site of application on the chart.

Rotate sites.

General Information

- Fentanyl patches need to be prescribed on the inpatient medicine chart; sign the administration box as usual, and also complete this chart.
- A nurse should check that each patch is still in place twice daily, e.g. 10am and 10pm, and sign below.
- Comments should be made about any problems, stating the action taken, e.g. patch lifted, secured with Tegaderm.
- Fentanyl patches are normally replaced every 72 hours.
- When removed, fold patches in half with the adhesive side inwards and discard in the sharps bin. A second nurse should witness this and countersign below.

Date & time patch applied	Strength (microgram/h) No. of patches Site	Signature	12 hourly observation				Comments Removal & discarding Date & Time Signatures
			10am	Sig	10pm	Sig	
23/2/10 10am	25 × 1	S Thorp			23/2 ✓	AS	
	Left arm		24/2 ✓	ST	24/2 ✓	MB	
			25/2 ✓	ST	25/2 ✓	MB	
			26/2 ✓	AS			26/2/07 10am A Smith S Thorp

Injections
Fentanyl citrate (generic)
Injection (for epidural, IM or IV use) fentanyl (as citrate) 50microgram/mL, 2mL amp = $4, 5mL amp = $7, 10mL amp = $14, 20mL amp = $27, 50mL amp = $70; *preservative-free.*

1 Newshan G and Lefkowitz M (2001) Transdermal fentanyl for chronic pain in AIDS: a pilot study. *Journal of Pain and Symptom Management.* **21**: 69–77.
2 Morita T *et al.* (2005) Opioid rotation from morphine to fentanyl in delirious cancer patients: an open-label trial. *Journal of Pain and Symptom Management.* **30**: 96–103.
3 Health Canada (2008) Fentanyl transdermal patch and fatal adverse reactions. *Canadian Adverse Reaction Newsletter.* **18 (3)**: 1–2.
4 Bernards C (1999) Clinical implications of physicochemical properties of opioids. In: C Stein (ed) *Opioids in Pain Control: basic and clinical aspects.* Cambridge University Press, Cambridge, pp. 166–187.
5 Ummenhofer W *et al.* (2000) Comparative spinal distribution and clearance kinetics of intrathecally administered morphine, fentanyl, alfentanil, and sufentanil. *Anesthesiology.* **92**: 739–953.
6 Zylicz Z (2001) Personal communication.
7 Herz A and Teschemacher H-J (1971) Activities and sites of antinociceptive action of morphine-like analgesics and kinetics of distribution following intravenous, intracerebral and intraventricular application. *Advances in Drug Research.* **6**: 79–119.
8 Simpson R *et al.* (1997) Transdermal fentanyl as treatment for chronic low back pain. *Journal of Pain and Symptom Management.* **14**: 218–224.
9 Milligan K and Campbell C (1999) Transdermal fentanyl in patients with chronic, nonmalignant pain: a case study series. *Advances in Therapy.* **16**: 73–77.
10 Allan L *et al.* (2001) Randomised crossover trial of transdermal fentanyl and sustained release oral morphine for treating chronic non-cancer pain. *British Medical Journal.* **322**: 1154–1158.
11 Ahmedzai S and Brooks D (1997) Transdermal fentanyl versus sustained-release oral morphine in cancer pain: preference, efficacy and quality of life. *Journal of Pain and Symptom Management.* **13**: 254–261.
12 Wong J-N *et al.* (1997) Comparison of oral controlled-release morphine with transdermal fentanyl in terminal cancer pain. *Acta Anaesthesiologica Singapore.* **35**: 25–32.
13 Yeo W *et al.* (1997) Transdermal fentanyl for severe cancer-related pain. *Palliative Medicine.* **11**: 233–239.
14 Kongsgaard U and Poulain P (1998) Transdermal fentanyl for pain control in adults with chronic cancer pain. *European Journal of Pain.* **2**: 53–62.
15 Payne R *et al.* (1998) Quality of life and cancer pain: satisfaction and side effects with transdermal fentanyl versus oral morphine. *Journal of Clinical Oncology.* **16**: 1588–1593.
16 Sloan P *et al.* (1998) A clinical evaluation of transdermal therapeutic system fentanyl for the treatment of cancer pain. *Journal of Pain and Symptom Management.* **16**: 102–111.
17 Nugent M *et al.* (2001) Long-term observations of patients receiving transdermal fentanyl after a randomized trial. *Journal of Pain and Symptom Management.* **21**: 385–391.
18 Radbruch L *et al.* (2001) Transdermal fentanyl for the management of cancer pain: a survey of 1005 patients. *Palliative Medicine.* **15**: 309–321.
19 Donner B *et al.* (1998) Long-term treatment of cancer pain with transdermal fentanyl. *Journal of Pain and Symptom Management.* **15**: 168–175.
20 Donner B *et al.* (1996) Direct conversion from oral morphine to transdermal fentanyl: a multicenter study in patients with cancer pain. *Pain.* **64**: 527–534.
21 Grond S *et al.* (1997) Transdermal fentanyl in the long-term treatment of cancer pain: a prospective study of 50 patients with advanced cancer of the gastrointestinal tract or the head and neck region. *Pain.* **69**: 191–198.
22 Megens A *et al.* (1998) Comparison of the analgesic and intestinal effects of fentanyl and morphine in rats. *Journal of Pain and Symptom Management.* **15**: 253–258.
23 Varvel JR *et al.* (1989) Absorption characteristics of transdermally administered fentanyl. *Anesthesiology.* **70**: 928–934.
24 Marquardt KA *et al.* (1995) Fentanyl remaining in a transdermal system following three days of continuous use. *Annals of Pharmacotherapy.* **29**: 969–971.
25 Heiskanen T *et al.* (2009) Transdermal fentanyl in cachectic cancer patients. *Pain.* **144**: 218–222.
26 Hadgraft J and Lane ME (2005) Skin permeation: the years of enlightenment. *International Journal of Pharmaceutics.* **305**: 2–12.
27 Gourlay GK *et al.* (1989) The transdermal administration of fentanyl in the treatment of post-operative pain: pharmacokinetics and pharmacodynamic effects. *Pain.* **37**: 193–202.
28 Portenoy RK *et al.* (1993) Transdermal fentanyl for cancer pain. *Anesthesiology.* **78**: 36–43.
29 Smith J and Ellershaw J (1999) Improvement in pain control by change of fentanyl patch after 48 hours compared with 72 hours. *Poster EAPC Congress, Geneva.* PO1/1376.
30 Anonymous (2007) Safe use of fentanyl (Duragesic) patches. *Pharmacist's Letter/Prescriber's Letter.* **23(10, detail document 231010)**: 1–5.
31 FDA (2007) Fentanyl transdermal system (marketed as Duragesic) Information. Available from: www.fda.gov/Drugs/DrugSafety/PostmarketDrugSafetyInformationforPatientsandProviders/ucm114961.htm
32 Hallberg *et al.* (2006) Possible fluconazole-fentanyl interaction: a case report. *European Journal of Clinical Pharmacology.* **62**: 491–492.
33 Kharasch *et al.* (2004) Influence of hepatic and intestinal cytochrome P4503A activity on the acute disposition and effects of oral transmucosal fentanyl citrate. *Anesthesiology.* **101**: 729–737.
34 Baxter K (ed) (2006) *Stockley's Drug Interactions* (7e), London.
35 Sasson M and Shvartzman P (2006) Fentanyl patch sufficient analgesia for only one day. *Journal of Pain and Symptom Management.* **31**: 389–391.
36 Morii H *et al.* (2007) Failure of pain control using transdermal fentanyl during rifampicin treatment. *Journal of Pain and Symptom Management.* **33**: 5–6.
37 Gillman PK (2005) Monoamine oxidase inhibitors, opioid analgesics and serotonin toxicity. *British Journal of Anaesthesia.* **95**: 434–441.
38 Rang ST *et al.* (2008) Serotonin toxicity caused by an interaction between fentanyl and paroxetine. *Canadian Journal of Anaesthesia.* **55**: 521–525.

39 Kirschner R and Donovan JW (2008) Serotonin syndrome precipitated by fentanyl during procedural sedation. *Journal of Emergency Medicine.*

40 Alkhatib AA *et al.* (2009) Serotonin Syndrome as a Complication of Fentanyl Sedation During Esophagogastroduodenoscopy. *Digestive Diseases and Sciences.*

41 Dean M (2004) Opioids in renal failure and dialysis patients. *Journal of Pain and Symptom Management.* **28**: 497–504.

42 Hardy JR *et al.* (2007) Opioids in patients on renal dialysis. *Journal of Pain and Symptom Management.* **33**: 1–2.

43 Janssen-Ortho *et al.* (2009) Health Canada endorsed important safety information on fentanyl transdermal systems. Available from: www.hc-sc.gc.ca/dhp-mps/medeff/advisories-avis/prof/_2009/fentanyl_hpc-cps-eng.php

44 Janssen-Cilag Ltd *Data on file.*

45 Freynhagen R *et al.* (2005) Switching from reservoir to matrix systems for the transdermal delivery of fentanyl: a prospective, multicenter pilot study in outpatients with chronic pain. *Journal of Pain and Symptom Management.* **30**: 289–297.

46 Marier JF *et al.* (2006) Pharmacokinetics, tolerability, and performance of a novel matrix transdermal delivery system of fentanyl relative to the commercially available reservoir formulation in healthy subjects. *Journal of Clinical Pharmacology.* **46**: 642–653.

47 Vielvoye-Kerkmeer A *et al.* (2000) Transdermal fentanyl in opioid-naive cancer pain patients: an open trial using transdermal fentanyl for the treatment of chronic cancer pain in opioid-naive patients and a group using codeine. *Journal of Pain and Symptom Management.* **19**: 185–192.

48 van Seventer R *et al.* (2003) Comparison of TTS-fentanyl with sustained-release oral morphine in the treatment of patients not using opioids for mild-to-moderate pain. *Current Medical Research and Opinion.* **19**: 457–469.

49 Tawfik MO *et al.* (2004) Use of transdermal fentanyl without prior opioid stabilization in patients with cancer pain. *Current Medical Research and Opinion.* **20**: 259–267.

50 Mercadante S *et al.* (2001) Clinical problems with transdermal fentanyl titration from 25 to 50mcg/hr. *Journal of Pain and Symptom Management.* **21**: 448–449.

51 Korte W *et al.* (1996) Day-to-day titration to initiate transdermal fentanyl in patients with cancer pain: short and long term experiences in a prospective study of 39 patients. *Journal of Pain and Symptom Management.* **11**: 139–146.

52 Muijsers RB and Wagstaff AJ (2001) Transdermal fentanyl: an updated review of its pharmacological properties and therapeutic efficacy in chronic cancer pain control. *Drugs.* **61**: 2289–2307.

53 Gardner-Nix J (2001) Oral transmucosal fentanyl and sufentanil for incident pain. *Journal of Pain and Symptom Management.* **22**: 627–630.

54 Zeppetella G (2001) Sublingual fentanyl citrate for cancer-related breakthrough pain: a pilot study. *Palliative Medicine.* **15**: 323–328.

55 Palliativedrugs.com (2003) Hot Topics: alternatives to sublingual fentanyl. In: *August Newsletter.* Available from: www.palliativedrugs.com

56 Duncan A (2002) The use of fentanyl and alfentanil sprays for episodic pain. *Palliative Medicine.* **16**: 550.

Guidelines: Use of transdermal fentanyl patches

These guidelines differ from the recommendations in the Canadian fentanyl patch Product Monographs. Instead of using a dose conversion ratio for PO morphine to TD fentanyl of 150:1, they use 100:1 (as in the German Product Monograph); they also include recommendations from the USA Package Insert.

Note: pain not relieved by morphine will generally not be relieved by fentanyl. If in doubt, seek specialist advice before prescribing TD fentanyl.

1 Indications for using TD fentanyl include:
- intolerable undesirable effects with morphine or other oral strong opioid, e.g. nausea and vomiting, constipation, hallucinations, dysphagia
- renal failure (fentanyl has no active metabolite)
- 'tablet phobia' or poor compliance with oral medication
- high risk of tablet misuse/diversion.

2 TD fentanyl is contra-indicated in patients with acute (short-term) pain, and in those who need rapid dose titration for severe uncontrolled pain. In Canada and the USA (but not in the UK), it is also contra-indicated in opioid-naïve patients; TD fentanyl is authorized for use only when a patient has been receiving a strong opioid in a dose equivalent to a 25microgram/h patch for ⩾1 week.

3 TD fentanyl patches are available in 6 strengths: 12, 25, 37, 50, 75 and 100microgram/h for 3 days. The 12microgram/h patch is to aid titration; it can also be used as the starting dose for TD fentanyl when the 25microgram/h patch is considered excessive, e.g. for elderly, frail patients.

4 Use the table below to decide a safe starting dose for TD fentanyl, and an appropriate rescue dose of morphine.

5 For patients taking a dose of morphine that is not the exact equivalent of a fentanyl patch, it will be necessary to opt for a patch which is either slightly more or slightly less than the morphine dose. Thus, if the patient still has pain, round up to a higher patch strength; if pain-free and frail, round down.

Table Comparative doses of PO morphine and TD fentanyl (using dose ratio 100:1)

PO Morphine[a]		SC/IV Morphine[a]		TD Fentanyl	
mg/24h	p.r.n mg[b]	mg/24h[c]	p.r.n mg[b]	microgram/h	mg/24h
30	3	15	1.5	12	0.3
60	6	30	3	25	0.6
120	12	60	6	50	1.2
180	18	90	9	75	1.8
240	24	120	12	100[d]	2.4

a. if an alternative strong opioid is used, the dose is calculated by using the appropriate conversion factor
b. using 1/10 of total daily dose; round to a convenient tablet size or volume
c. assuming potency ratio of morphine SC/IV to PO of 2:1
d. for combinations of patches, add the p.r.n. doses together, e.g. 100 + 75microgram/h patches = 12 + 9mg morphine SC/IV = 21mg morphine SC/IV, rounded down to 20mg for convenience.

6 The date of application and/or the date for renewal should be written in a consistent manner on the patch. Apply to dry, non-inflamed, non-irradiated, hairless skin on the upper trunk or arm. Body hair may be clipped with scissors but not shaved. If the skin is washed beforehand, use only water; do not use soap and do not apply oils, cream or ointment to the area. Press patch firmly in place for at least 30sec. Micropore® or Tegaderm® can be used to ensure adherence. Careful removal of the patch helps to minimize local skin irritation.

continued

www.palliativedrugs.com

7 Effective systemic analgesic concentrations are generally reached within 12 hours. When converting from:
- 4-hourly PO morphine, give regular doses for the first 12h after applying the patch
- 12-hourly SR morphine, apply the patch and the final SR dose at the same time
- 24-hourly SR morphine, apply the patch 12h after the final SR dose
- CSCI/CIVI, continue the infusion for about 12h after applying the patch.

8 When starting TD fentanyl, patients should use p.r.n. doses liberally, particularly during the first 24h. Safe rescue doses of PO morphine are given in the table above. The maximum clinical effect of TD fentanyl is generally achieved in 36–48h.

9 After 48 hours, if a patient still needs ≥3 rescue doses of morphine/day, the strength of the next patch to be applied should be increased by 12–25microgram/h. (Note: with the manufacturer's recommended starting doses, about 50% of patients need to increase the patch strength after the first 3 days.)

10 About 10% of patients experience opioid withdrawal symptoms when changed from morphine to TD fentanyl. These manifest with symptoms like gastric flu and last for a few days; p.r.n. doses of morphine will relieve troublesome symptoms.

11 Fentanyl is less constipating than morphine; halve the dose of laxatives when starting fentanyl and re-titrate. Some patients develop diarrhea; if persistent, stop the laxatives completely. If necessary, use p.r.n. loperamide or morphine.

12 Fentanyl probably causes less nausea and vomiting than morphine but, if necessary, prescribe haloperidol 1mg stat & at bedtime.

13 In febrile patients, the rate of absorption of fentanyl increases, and may cause toxicity, e.g. drowsiness. Absorption is also enhanced by an external heat source over the patch, e.g. electric blanket or hot-water bottle; patients should be warned about this. Patients may shower with a patch but should not soak in a hot bath.

14 Remove patches after 72h; change the position of the new patches so as to rest the underlying skin for 3–6 days.

15 A reservoir of fentanyl accumulates in the body and significant blood levels generally persist for at least 24h after discontinuing TD fentanyl.

16 TD fentanyl is unsatisfactory in <5% of patients.

17 In moribund patients, continue TD fentanyl and give additional SC morphine p.r.n. (see Table). If ≥3 rescue doses are required/day, give morphine by CSCI, starting with a dose equal to the sum of the p.r.n. doses over the preceding 24h. If necessary, adjust the p.r.n. dose taking into account the total opioid dose (i.e. TD fentanyl + CSCI morphine).

18 Used patches still contain fentanyl; after removal, fold the patch with the adhesive side inwards and discard preferably in a sharps container or, at home, a childproof tamperproof container or trash can, and wash hands. Ultimately, any unused patches should be returned to a pharmacy.

HYDROMORPHONE

Class: Opioid analgesic.

Indications: Moderate–severe pain, particularly when a high-dose, small-volume opioid injection is required; †an alternative in cases of intolerance to other strong opioids, †cough.

Contra-indications: None absolute if titrated carefully against a patient's pain (see also Strong opioids, p.287).

Pharmacology

Hydromorphone is an analogue of **morphine** with similar pharmacokinetic and pharmacodynamic properties.[1–3] According to the UK manufacturer, hydromorphone PO and SC/IM is about 7.5 times more potent than **morphine**.[4,5] Canadian Product Monographs consider PO hydromorphone to be 5–7.5 times more potent than PO **morphine**, and give a wide range of parenteral conversion ratios based on use in acute pain (see Product Monographs). Others suggest that when switching from **morphine** to hydromorphone, the conversion ratio is approximately 5:1 (i.e. the hydromorphone dose should be 1/5 of the **morphine** dose)[6,7] and when switching from hydromorphone to **morphine** a ratio of 1:4 should be used (i.e. the **morphine** dose should be 4 times the hydromorphone dose).[8,9] Also see Opioid switching, p.294.

Normal-release hydromorphone provides useful analgesia for about 4h. It also has an antitussive effect. As with **morphine**, there is wide interindividual variation in bio-availability. Caution should be exercised in severe hepatic impairment because metabolism may be impaired, and result in an increase in plasma hydromorphone concentration. The main metabolite is hydromorphone-3-glucuronide (H3G); hydromorphone-6-glucuronide is not formed.[10,11] Two minor metabolites, dihydro-isomorphine and dihydromorphine, are pharmacologically active; they are metabolized to 6-glucuronides. Hydromorphone clearance is unchanged in renal impairment but glucuronide metabolites will accumulate. Opioid neurotoxicity (see Box 5.F, p.289) has been reported in patients with renal failure taking hydromorphone.[10,11] Normal H3G to hydromorphone plasma ratio is 27:1 but in renal failure it can increase to 100:1.[12] By the spinal route in opioid-naïve subjects, hydromorphone causes less pruritus than **morphine** (11% vs. 44%).[13]

Bio-availability 37–62% PO.[9]
Onset of action 15min SC/IM; 30min PO.
Time to peak plasma concentration 1h PO.
Plasma halflife 2.5h early phase, with a prolonged late phase.
Duration of action 4–5h.

Undesirable effects

For full list, see manufacturer's Product Monograph.
Also see Strong opioids, p.289.

Dose and use

Analgesia

PO hydromorphone is used in the same way as PO **morphine**, generally q4h as normal-release tablets or liquid, or q12h as SR capsules; the SR capsules can be swallowed whole, or opened and the contents sprinkled on soft food, e.g. yoghurt. Note:

- the SR granules should not be crushed or chewed because this could lead to a rapid release of an overdose
- hydromorphone can be given PR as a 3mg suppository q4–8h p.r.n.
- when converting from PO to SC, divide the dose of hydromorphone by 2
- if given by CSCI, high-potency ampoules can be used (Box 5.N).

Box 5.N Summary of compatibility reports for hydromorphone

Note: Entries in *italics* indicate *incompatibility*.
Diluent = 5% glucose unless otherwise stated (see footnotes).

Chemical and physical laboratory data[14–20]
Hydromorphone+
Bupivacaine[a]
Clonidine[b]
Dimenhydrinate[b]
Methotrimeprazine[c]
Lorazepam[b]
Metoclopramide[c]
Ondansetron[a]
Prochlorperazine[b]
Dexamethasone sodium phosphate[d] (incompatible at high concentrations of both drugs)
Haloperidol[c] (incompatible at high concentrations of both drugs)

Physical laboratory data only[17,21–23]
Hydromorphone+
Atropine
Diazepam
Diphenhydramine
Glycopyrrolate[d]
Hydroxyzine
Scopolamine (hyoscine) hydrobromide
Midazolam
Phenobarbital
Promethazine[a]
Ketorolac[c] (incompatible at high concentrations of both drugs)

Observational data only[24,25]
Hydromorphone+
Cyclizine[c] (not Canada) (one report of incompatibility)

Hydromorphone + 2 other drugs
Cyclizine (not Canada) and octreotide[c]
Glycopyrrolate and metoclopramide[a]
Haloperidol and scopolamine (hyoscine) hydrobromide
Haloperidol and metoclopramide[a]
Haloperidol and midazolam[c]
Haloperidol and octreotide[a]
Hyoscine (scopolamine) butylbromide and midazolam[a]
Scopolamine (hyoscine) hydrobromide and octreotide
Ketamine and metoclopramide[a]
Ketamine and midazolam[a]
Methotrimeprazine and octreotide[a]
Metoclopramide and midazolam[a]
Metoclopramide and ondansetron
Haloperidol and ketorolac[c] (incompatible)

Hydromorphone + 3 other drugs
Cyclizine (not Canada), haloperidol and midazolam[c]
Glycopyrrolate, haloperidol and promethazine
Glycopyrrolate, haloperidol and octreotide
Glycopyrrolate, metoclopramide and octreotide
Scopolamine (hyoscine) hydrobromide, methotrimeprazine and midazolam[a]

continued

> **Box 5.N** Continued
>
> Scopolamine (hyoscine) hydrobromide, metoclopramide and octreotide
> Ketamine, metoclopramide and midazolam[a]
> *Haloperidol, promethazine and scopolamine (hyoscine) hydrobromide (incompatible)*
>
> More details can be found on www.palliativedrugs.com Syringe Driver Survey Database.
> Also see Chart A4.1 (p.594).

a. diluent = 0.9% saline
b. diluent = none
c. diluent = water for injection
d. diluent = unknown.

Cough
- in opioid-naïve patients, give 1mg PO q3–4h p.r.n., either in tablet or liquid form.

As with all opioids, patients must be monitored for undesirable effects, particularly nausea and vomiting, and constipation (see p.289). Depending on individual circumstances, an anti-emetic should be prescribed for regular or p.r.n. use (see p.183) and, routinely, a laxative prescribed (see p.26).

Supply
Unless indicated otherwise, all products are Schedule I controlled drugs under the Controlled Drugs and Substances Act, and are subject to the Narcotic Control Regulations of the act.

Normal-release oral products
Hydromorphone hydrochloride (generic)
Tablets 1mg dose = $0.10, 2mg dose = $0.15, 4mg dose = $0.23, 8mg dose = $0.36.
Oral syrup 1mg/mL, 28 days @ 1mg q4h = $13.

Dilaudid® (Purdue)
Tablets 1mg dose = $0.10, 2mg dose = $0.15, 4mg dose = $0.23, 8mg dose = $0.36.
Oral solution 1mg/mL, 28 days @ 1mg q4h = $14.

Sustained-release oral products
Hydromorph Contin® (Purdue)
Capsules enclosing SR granules 3mg, 6mg, 12mg, 18mg, 24mg, 30mg, 28 days @ 3mg, 12mg or 30mg q12h = $39, $100 and $220 respectively.

Normal-release rectal products
Hydromorphone hydrochloride (generic)
Suppositories 3mg, 28 days @ 3mg q6h = $258.

Parenteral products
Hydromorphone hydrochloride (generic)
Injection 2mg/mL, 1mL amp = $1.50.
Injection high potency 10mg/mL, 1mL amp = $3, 5mL amp = $14, 50mL amp = $120.
Injection high potency 20mg/mL, 50mL amp = $226.
Injection high potency 50mg/mL, 1mL amp = $14, 50mL amp = $525.
Injection forte 100mg/mL, 10mL amp = $350.

Dilaudid® (Purdue)
Injection 2mg/mL, 1mL amp = $1.50.
Injection (powder for reconstitution) 250mg vial = $72.

Dilaudid-HP® (Purdue)
Injection high potency 10mg/mL, 1mL amp = $3, 5mL amp = $15, 50mL amp = $142.

Dilaudid-HP Plus® (Purdue)
Injection high potency 20mg/mL, 50mL amp = $230.

Dilaudid-XP® (Purdue)
Injection high potency 50mg/mL, 50mL amp = $534.

1 Sarhill N et al. (2001) Hydromorphone: pharmacology and clinical applications in cancer patients. Supportive Care in Cancer. **9**: 84–96.
2 Murray A and Hagen NA (2005) Hydromorphone. Journal of Pain and Symptom Management. **29 (suppl 5)**: s57–s66.
3 Quigley C and Glare P (2009) Hydromorphone. In: M Davis et al. (eds) Opioids in Cancer Pain (2e). Oxford University Press, Oxford, pp. 245–252.
4 McDonald C and Miller A (1997) A comparative potency study of a controlled release tablet formulation of hydromorphone with controlled release morphine in patients with cancer pain. European Journal of Palliative Care Abstracts of the Fifth Congress.
5 Moriarty M et al. (1999) A randomised crossover comparison of controlled release hydromorphone tablets with controlled release morphine tablets in patients with cancer pain. Journal of Clinical Research. **2**: 1–8.
6 Wallace MS and Thipphawong J (2007) Clinical Trial Results with OROS(R) Hydromorphone. Journal of Pain and Symptom Management. **33**: S25–32.
7 Palangio M et al. (2002) Dose conversion and titration with a novel, once-daily, OROS osmotic technology, extended-release hydromorphone formulation in the treatment of chronic malignant or nonmalignant pain. Journal of Pain and Symptom Management. **23**: 355–368.
8 Anderson R et al. (2001) Accuracy in equianalgesic dosing: conversion dilemmas. Journal of Pain and Symptom Management. **21**: 397–406.
9 Pereira J et al. (2001) Equianalgesic dose ratios for opioids: a critical review and proposals for long-term dosing. Journal of Pain and Symptom Management. **22**: 672–687.
10 Babul N and Darke AC (1992) Putative role of hydromorphone metabolites in myoclonus. Pain. **51**: 260–261.
11 Davis M and Wilcock A (2001) Modified-release opioids. European Journal of Palliative Care. **8**: 142–146.
12 Babul N et al. (1995) Hydromorphone metabolite accumulation in renal failure. Journal of Pain and Symptom Management. **10**: 184–186.
13 Chaplan SR et al. (1992) Morphine and hydromorphone epidural analgesia. Anesthesiology. **77**: 1090–1094.
14 Storey P et al. (1990) Subcutaneous infusions for control of cancer symptoms. Journal of Pain and Symptom Management. **5**: 33–41.
15 Walker SE et al. (1991) Compatibility of dexamethasone sodium phosphate with hydromorphone hydrochloride or diphenhydramine hydrochloride. American Journal of Hospital Pharmacy. **48**: 2161–2166.
16 Walker S et al. (1993) Stability and compatibility of combinations of hydromorphone and dimenhydrinate, lorazepam or prochlorperazine. Canadian Journal of Hospital Pharmacy. **46**: 61–65.
17 Huang E and Anderson RP (1994) Compatibility of hydromorphone hydrochloride with haloperidol lactate and ketorolac tromethamine. American Journal of Hospital Pharmacy. **51**: 2963.
18 Trissel LA et al. (1994) Compatibility and stability of ondansetron hydrochloride with morphine sulfate and with hydromorphone hydrochloride in 0.9% sodium chloride injection at 4, 22, and 32 degrees C. American Journal of Hospital Pharmacy. **51**: 2138–2142.
19 Christen C et al. (1996) Stability of bupivacaine hydrochloride and hydromorphone hydrochloride during simulated epidural coadministration. American Journal of Health System Pharmacy. **53**: 170–173.
20 Rudich Z et al. (2004) Stability of clonidine in clonidine-hydromorphone mixture from implanted intrathecal infusion pumps in chronic pain patients. Journal of Pain and Symptom Management. **28**: 599–602.
21 Ingallinera TS et al. (1979) Compatibility of glycopyrrolate injection with commonly used infusion solutions and additives. American Journal of Hospital Pharmacy. **36**: 508–510.
22 Chandler S et al. (1996) Combined administration of opioids with selected drugs to manage pain and other cancer symptoms: initial safety screening for compatibility. Journal of Pain and Symptom Management. **12**: 168–171.
23 Henderson F (1996) 21-day compatibility of hydromorphone hydrochloride and promethazine hydrochloride in a cassette. American Journal of Health System Pharmacy. **53**: 2338–2339.
24 Dickman A et al. (2002) The Syringe Driver: Continuous Subcutaneous Infusions in Palliative Care. Oxford University Press, Oxford.
25 Anonymous (2006) Syringe Driver Compatibility. Available from: www.pallcare.info

*METHADONE

Class: Opioid analgesic.

Methadone should be used as a strong opioid analgesic only by those fully conversant with its pharmacology. In Canada, the prescriber must also be authorized by the federal government before prescribing, supplying or administering methadone (see Supply). Methadone is generally best reserved for patients who fail to respond well to **morphine** or other μ-opioid receptor agonists. Important facts about methadone include:
- a widely variable plasma halflife
- dosing which is more complicated than for other strong opioids
- metabolism which is modified to a clinically important extent by other drugs which may be used in palliative and hospice care

- an association with a potentially fatal cardiac arrhythmia (see Cautions below and, Prolongation of the QT interval in palliative care, p.547).

In addition, because methadone is used to treat opioid addiction, there is a social stigma attached to its use.

Indications: Severe pain, †cough, †an alternative in cases of intolerance to other strong opioids, †morphine poorly-responsive pain, †pain relief in severe renal failure.[1,2] Also †treatment of opioid addiction.

Contra-indications: None absolute if titrated carefully against a patient's pain (see also Strong opioids, p.287).

Pharmacology

Methadone is a synthetic strong opioid with mixed properties.[3,4] Thus, it is a μ-opioid receptor agonist, possibly a δ-opioid receptor agonist,[5] an NMDA-receptor-channel blocker,[6,7] and a presynaptic blocker of serotonin re-uptake.[8] Methadone is a racemic mixture; L-methadone is responsible for most of the analgesic effect, whereas D-methadone is antitussive. Methadone is a non-acidic and lipophilic drug which is absorbed well from all routes of administration.

Partly because of its lipid-solubility methadone has a high volume of distribution with only about 1% of the drug in the blood.[9] Methadone accumulates in tissues when given repeatedly, creating an extensive reservoir.[10] Protein-binding (principally to a glycoprotein) is 60–90%;[11] this is double that of **morphine**. Both volume of distribution and protein-binding contribute to the long plasma halflife, and accumulation is a potential problem. Methadone is metabolized mainly in the liver to several inactive metabolites.[12] About 1/2 of the drug and its metabolites are excreted by the intestines and 1/2 by the kidneys, most of the latter unchanged.[13] Renal and hepatic impairment do not affect methadone clearance.[14,15] However, in renal and hepatic failure (see p.477), it is generally best to reduce the starting dose, e.g. by at least 50%, and titrate according to response.

In single doses, methadone PO is about 1/2 as potent as IM,[16] and IM a single dose of methadone is marginally more potent than **morphine**. With repeated doses, methadone is several times more potent and longer-acting; analgesia lasts 8–12h and sometimes more.[17,18] There is no single potency ratio between methadone and **morphine**. When patients with inadequate pain relief or undesirable effects with **morphine** are switched, the eventual 24h dose of methadone *is typically 5–10 times smaller than the previous dose of **morphine**, sometimes 20–30 times smaller, and occasionally even smaller.*[19–22] The potency ratio tends to increase as the dose of **morphine** increases, i.e. proportionately less methadone is required as the **morphine** dose increases.[19,23] When considering the use of methadone, the difficulty of subsequently switching from methadone to another opioid should also be borne in mind.[24]

Methadone is used in several different settings. A systematic review of methadone for cancer pain identified nine RCTs but, because different methods were used, meta-analysis was not possible.[25] First-line, methadone provides similar analgesia to **morphine** but more undesirable effects. In an RCT, 20% of patients allocated to methadone 7.5mg b.i.d. discontinued treatment compared with 5% of those who received **morphine** 15mg b.i.d. Half of the withdrawals occurred in the first week, and most were because of sedation or nausea. For patients remaining in the study, there was no difference in efficacy or undesirable effects.[18] This suggests that a smaller starting dose of methadone (e.g. 2.5–5mg b.i.d., or even 1–2 mg b.i.d.[26] would have been more appropriate.

Second-line, patients who experience inadequate analgesia with **morphine**, with or without unacceptable undesirable effects such as nausea, vomiting, hallucinations or sedation, can obtain good relief with relatively low-dose methadone with few undesirable effects.[19,21,27] Patients who experience more specific neurotoxicity with **morphine**, e.g. hyperalgesia, allodynia and/or myoclonus±sedation and delirium, generally also benefit by switching (rotating) to methadone. However, switching to other opioids, e.g. **fentanyl**, **oxycodone**, also helps.[28–31] Thus, when switching from **morphine**, it would seem sensible to choose an opioid which is easier and safer to use than methadone, e.g. **oxycodone**, **hydromorphone**, **fentanyl**.

Methadone is an alternative strong opioid for patients with chronic renal failure who would be at risk of excessive drowsiness ± delirium with **morphine** because of accumulation of morphine-6-glucuronide.[2] Methadone is poorly removed by hemodialysis.[32] However, for moribund patients, **alfentanil** or **fentanyl** are probably better choices. Methadone can also be used as a strong opioid analgesic in former opioid addicts who are being maintained on methadone.[33]

Bio-availability 80% (range 40–100%) PO.

Onset of action <30min PO, 15min IM.

Time to peak plasma concentration 4h PO; 1h IM.

Plasma halflife highly variable, mean 20–35h (range 5–130h);[34] longer in older patients; acidifying the urine results in a shorter halflife (20h) and raising the pH with sodium bicarbonate a longer halflife (>40h).[35]

Duration of action 4–5h PO and 3–5h IM single dose; 8–12h repeated doses.

Cautions

In 2006, after a review of deaths and life-threatening adverse events (e.g. respiratory depression, cardiac arrhythmia) associated with unintentional overdose, drug interactions, and prolongation of the QT interval, the FDA issued a safety warning about the use of methadone. This highlighted the need for:
- physicians to be fully aware of the pharmacology of methadone
- close monitoring of the patient when starting methadone, particularly when switching from a high dose of another opioid
- slow dose titration, and close monitoring of the patient when changing the dose of methadone
- warning the patient not to exceed the prescribed dose.

Because methadone generally has a long plasma halflife, accumulation to a variable extent should be anticipated, particularly in the elderly. Drowsiness and respiratory depression may develop after several days/weeks on a steady dose. *PCF* recommends p.r.n. dose titration to minimize the risk of this occurring (see below).[36]

QT interval prolongation and, rarely, a serious ventricular arrhythmia (*torsade de pointes*) have been observed during treatment with methadone. Generally, the latter is associated with, but not limited to, higher dose treatment (>200mg/24h) (see Prolongation of the QT interval in palliative care, p.543).[37] The Product Monograph recommends that methadone is administered with caution to patients at risk of developing QT prolongation, e.g. those with:
- a history of cardiac conduction abnormalities
- a family history of sudden death
- advanced heart disease or ischemic heart disease
- liver disease
- electrolyte abnormalities
- concurrent treatment with drugs which:
  ▷ may cause electrolyte abnormalities
  ▷ have a potential to prolong QT
  ▷ inhibit cytochrome P450 3A4.

Note: the IV formulation of methadone imported from the USA (but *not* the UK), contains a preservative chlorobutanol, which has an additive QT prolonging effect.[38]

The risk this rare but potentially fatal cardiac complication poses must be considered in the context of the patient's circumstances. A commonsense approach should prevail, and ECG monitoring will be largely irrelevant in the last days of life. On the other hand, for a patient with a reasonable prognosis, it may be more appropriate to identify any risk factors for QT prolongation and consider ECG ± electrolyte monitoring (see p.547). A USA expert panel has drawn up guidelines for monitoring patients receiving parenteral methadone.[39] Even so, research is needed to establish the magnitude of the risk of *torsade de pointes* with methadone and the overall value of monitoring in the palliative care setting.[37]

Drug interactions

Methadone is metabolized by several cytochrome P450 enzymes, mainly CYP3A4 with CYP2B6, CYP2D6, CYP2C9, CYP2C19, and CYP1A2 also involved to varying degrees. Clinically relevant and well-established CYP-related drug–drug interactions are listed in Table 5.20. Note particularly that **carbamazepine**, **phenobarbital**, **phenytoin**, **rifampin** and **St John's wort** increase the

Table 5.20 Cytochrome P450 interactions with methadone resulting in changed drug plasma concentrations[41,42]

Methadone plasma concentrations increased by	Methadone plasma concentrations decreased by	Drug plasma concentrations increased by methadone	Drug plasma concentrations decreased by methadone
TCAs	Carbamazepine	Desipramine	Amprenavir
SSRIs	Phenobarbital	Zidovudine (AZT)	
MAOIs	Phenytoin		
Cimetidine	Rifampin		
Ciprofloxacin	St John's wort		
Diazepam	Antiretroviral drugs,		
(high-dose)	e.g. abacavir,		
Fluconazole	amprenavir, efavirenz,		
Voriconazole	lopinavir, nelfinavir,		
	nevirapine, ritonavir,		
	tipranavir		

metabolism of methadone, and may reverse previously satisfactory pain relief, or even precipitate withdrawal sysptoms.

Undesirable effects

For full list, see manufacturer's Product Monograph.
As for all strong opioids (see p.289). Local erythema and induration when given by CSCI.[43] Methadone occasionally causes neurotoxicity, e.g. myoclonus,[44] or more florid opioid-induced hyperalgesia.[45,46]

Dose and use

Dose titration is different from **morphine** because of the wide interindividual variation in the pharmacokinetics of methadone. Several guidelines exist for switching from **morphine** to methadone, but all require practitioners to be experienced in the use of methadone and close observation of the patient, generally as an inpatient.[2,19–21,27,47–51] Some have reported carefully controlled outpatient regimens, but pain relief can take weeks rather than days to achieve.[48,51] When using methadone, the implication of its large volume of distribution must be considered. During the first few days, while the body tissues become saturated, a greater daily dose of methadone will be required for satisfactory analgesia than subsequently; once saturation is complete, a smaller daily dose of methadone is then sufficient. Continuing on the initial daily dose is likely to result in sedation within a few days, and possibly respiratory depression and even death.[52,53]

PCF favours a 'stop and go' approach, i.e. the abrupt cessation of the **morphine** and introduction of methadone p.r.n. (see Guidelines, p.333). These guidelines are an evolution from earlier ones, incorporating feedback to www.palliativedrugs.com from clinicians.[2,20,54] A single loading dose aids tissue saturation and helps to reduce the number of p.r.n. doses required in the first 48h.[20] The recommendations may be overcautious but are safer, particularly in the elderly and for those switching from large doses of **morphine**.

Several other methods for switching from **morphine** or from another strong opioid have been published.[19,50,55–59] Regardless of the method used, the importance of close supervision cannot be overemphasized. Caution is also required when there has been rapid dose escalation of the pre-switch opioid; in these circumstances it is probably safer to calculate the initial dose of methadone using the pre-escalation dose.[60] Maintenance doses vary considerably, but most are <80mg/24h.[49] *Subsequent switching from methadone to other opioids can be difficult. In one series 12/13 patients experienced increased pain ± dysphoria.*[24]

Injectable methadone is not commercially available in Canada, but can be imported (see Supply). Methadone SC (generally doses >25mg) or CSCI can cause marked local inflammation necessitating site rotation, and possibly other measures (see Guidelines, p.333).[61,62,63] When switching from methadone PO to SC, a safe conversion is to halve the methadone PO dose. However, for some patients, particularly those receiving a small dose of methadone (<80mg/24h), a 1:1 conversion ratio may be more appropriate and subsequent upwards dose titration may be required.[62] Methadone can also be given SL, PR, IV, CIVI ± PCA.[3,55,64,65] It has also been used as a topical analgesic for mouth ulcers (as a mouthwash),[66] and for open wounds and ulcers (in powder form mixed with Stomahesive®).[67]

As with all opioids, patients must be monitored for undesirable effects, particularly nausea and vomiting, and constipation (see p.289). Depending on individual circumstances, an anti-emetic should be prescribed for regular or p.r.n. use (see p.183) and, routinely, a laxative prescribed (see p.26).

Supply

Unless indicated otherwise, all products are Schedule I controlled drugs under the Controlled Drugs and Substances Act, and are subject to the Narcotic Control Regulations of the act.

Physicians must obtain a Federal Ministerial Exemption under section 56 of the Controlled Drugs and Substances Act before prescribing, supplying or administering methadone for analgesia. The exemption must be renewed annually. Details of the application procedure and training requirements can be obtained from the provincial Colleges of Physicians. A separate exemption is required to prescribe methadone for addiction management.

Metadol® (Pharmascience)
Tablets 1mg, 5mg, 10mg, 25mg, 28 days @ 25mg b.i.d. = $96.
Oral solution 1mg/mL, 10mg/mL, 28 days @ 25mg b.i.d. (using 10mg/mL solution) = $53.

Methadone injection is not commercially available in Canada, but can be imported from the UK or USA through the Special Access Programme (see p.xx).

1 Gannon C (1997) The use of methadone in the care of the dying. *European Journal of Palliative Care.* **4**: 152–158.
2 Morley J and Makin M (1998) The use of methadone in cancer pain poorly responsive to other opioids. *Pain Reviews.* **5**: 51–58.
3 Davis M and Walsh D (2001) Methadone for relief of cancer pain: a review of pharmacokinetics, pharmacodynamics, drug interactions and protocols of administration. *Supportive Care in Cancer.* **9**: 73–83.
4 Watanabe S (2001) Methadone the renaissance. *Journal of Palliative Care.* **17** (2): 117–120.
5 Raynor K et al. (1994) Pharmacological characterization of the cloned kappa-, delta-, and mu-opioid receptors. *Molecular Pharmacology.* **45**: 330–334.
6 Ebert B et al. (1995) Ketobemidone, methadone and pethidine are noncompetitive N-methyl-d-aspartate (NMDA) antagonists in the rat cortex and spinal cord. *Neuroscience Letters.* **187**: 165–168.
7 Gorman A et al. (1997) The d- and l- isomers of methadone bind to the non-competitive site on the N-methyl-d-aspartate (NMDA) receptor in rat forebrain and spinal cord. *Neuroscience Letters.* **223**: 5–8.
8 Codd E et al. (1995) Serotonin and norepinephrine uptake inhibiting activity of centrally acting analgesics: structural determinants and role in antinociception. *Journal of Pharmacology and Experimental Therapeutics.* **274**: 1263–1270.
9 Ferrari A et al. (2004) Methadone—metabolism, pharmacokinetics and interactions. *Pharmacological Research.* **50**: 551–559.
10 Robinson AE and Williams FM (1971) The distribution of methadone in man. *Journal of Pharmacy and Pharmacology.* **23**: 353–358.
11 Eap CB et al. (1990) Binding of d-methadone, l-methadone and dl-methadone to proteins in plasma of healthy volunteers: role of variants of X1-acid glycoprotein. *Clinical Pharmacology and Therapeutics.* **47**: 338–346.
12 Fainsinger R et al. (1993) Methadone in the management of cancer pain: clinical review. *Pain.* **52**: 137–147.
13 Inturrisi CE and Verebely K (1972) The levels of methadone in the plasma in methadone maintenance. *Clinical Pharmacology and Therapeutics.* **13**: 633–637.
14 Kreek MJ et al. (1980) Methadone use in patients with chronic renal disease. *Drug Alcohol Dependence.* **5**: 197–205.
15 Novick DM et al. (1981) Methadone disposition in patients with chronic liver disease. *Clinical Pharmacology and Therapeutics.* **30**: 353–362.
16 Beaver WT et al. (1967) A clinical comparison of the analgesic effects of methadone and morphine administered intramuscularly, and of orally and parenterally administered methadone. *Clinical Pharmacology and Therapeutics.* **8**: 415–426.
17 Sawe J et al. (1981) Patient-controlled dose regimen of methadone for chronic cancer pain. *British Medical Journal.* **282**: 771–773.
18 Bruera E et al. (2004) Methadone versus morphine as a first-line strong opioid for cancer pain: a randomized, double-blind study. *Journal of Clinical Oncology.* **22**: 185–192.
19 Mercadante S et al. (2001) Switching from morphine to methadone to improve analgesia and tolerability in cancer patients: a prospective study. *Journal of Clinical Oncology.* **19**: 2898–2904.
20 Cornish CJ and Keen JC (2003) An alternative low-dose ad libitum schedule for conversion of other opioids to methadone. *Palliative Medicine.* **17**: 643–644.
21 Tse DM et al. (2003) An ad libitum schedule for conversion of morphine to methadone in advanced cancer patients: an open uncontrolled prospective study in a Chinese population. *Palliative Medicine.* **17**: 206–211.
22 Nixon AJ (2005) Methadone for cancer pain: a case report. *American Journal of Hospice and Palliative Care.* **22**: 337.
23 Ripamonti C et al. (1998) Switching from morphine to oral methadone in treating cancer pain: what is the equianalgesic dose ratio? *Journal of Clinical Oncology.* **16**: 3216–3221.

24 Moryl N et al. (2002) Pitfalls of opioid rotation: substituting another opioid for methadone in patients with cancer pain. Pain. 96: 325–328.

25 Nicholson AB (2007) Methadone for cancer pain. Cochrane Database of Systematic Reviews. 4: CD003971.

26 Gallagher R (2009) Methadone: an effective, safe drug of first choice for pain management in frail older adults. Pain Medicine. 10: 319–326.

27 Mercadante S et al. (1999) Rapid switching from morphine to methadone in cancer patients with poor response to morphine. Journal of Clinical Oncology. 17: 3307–3312.

28 Sjogren P et al. (1994) Disappearance of morphine-induced hyperalgesia after discontinuing or substituting morphine with other opioid agonists. Pain. 59: 313–316.

29 Hagen N and Swanson R (1997) Strychnine-like multifocal myoclonus and seizures in extremely high-dose opioid administration: treatment strategies. Journal of Pain and Symptom Management. 14: 51–58.

30 Ashby M et al. (1999) Opioid substitution to reduce adverse effects in cancer pain management. Medical Journal of Australia. 170: 68–71.

31 Morita T et al. (2005) Opioid rotation from morphine to fentanyl in delirious cancer patients: an open-label trial. Journal of Pain and Symptom Management. 30: 96–103.

32 Furlan V et al. (1999) Methadone is poorly removed by haemodialysis. Nephrology, Dialysis, Transplantation. 14: 254–255.

33 Manfredi P et al. (2001) Methadone analgesia in cancer pain patients on chronic methadone maintenance therapy. Journal of Pain and Symptom Management. 21: 169–174.

34 Lugo RA et al. (2005) Pharmacokinetics of methadone. Journal of Pain and Palliative Care Pharmacotherapy. 19: 13–24.

35 Nilsson MI et al. (1982) Pharmacokinetics of methadone during maintenance treatment: adaptive changes during the induction phase. European Journal of Clinical Pharmacology. 22: 343–349.

36 Hendra T et al. (1996) Fatal methadone overdose. British Medical Journal. 313: 481–482.

37 Wilcock A and Beattie JM (2009) Prolonged QT interval and methadone: implications for palliative care. Current Opinion in Supportive and Palliative Care. 3: 252–257.

38 Kornick CA et al. (2003) QTc interval prolongation associated with intravenous methadone. Pain. 105: 499–506.

39 Shaiova L et al. (2008) Consensus guideline on parenteral methadone use in pain and palliative care. Palliative and Supportive Care. 6: 165–176.

40 Kreek MJ et al. (1976) Rifampin-induced methadone withdrawal. New England Journal of Medicine. 294: 1104–1106.

41 Baxter K (ed) (2008) Stockley's Drug Interactions (8e). Pharmaceutical Press, London.

42 Leavitt SB (2006) Methadone-drug interactions. Available from: www.pain-topics.org/opioid_rx/methadone.php#methintr

43 Bruera E et al. (1991) Local toxicity with subcutaneous methadone. Experience of two centers. Pain. 45: 141–143.

44 Sarhill N et al. (2001) Methadone-induced myoclonus in advanced cancer. American Journal of Hospice and Palliative Care. 18 (1): 51–53.

45 El Osta B et al. (2007) Intractable pain: intoxication or undermedication? Journal of Palliative Medicine. 10: 811–814.

46 Davis MP et al. (2007) When opioids cause pain. Journal of Clinical Oncology. 25: 4497–4498.

47 Ripamonti C et al. (1997) An update on the clinical use of methadone cancer pain. Pain. 70: 109–115.

48 Hagen N and Wasylenko E (1999) Methadone: outpatient titration and monitoring strategies in cancer patients. Journal of Pain and Symptom Management. 18: 369–375.

49 Scholes C et al. (1999) Methadone titration in opioid-resistant cancer pain. European Journal of Cancer Care. 8: 26–29.

50 Nauck F et al. (2001) A German model for methadone conversion. American Journal of Hospice and Palliative Care. 18 (3): 200–202.

51 Soares LG (2005) Methadone for cancer pain: what have we learned from clinical studies? American Journal of Hospice and Palliative Care. 22: 223–227.

52 Twycross RG (1977) A comparison of diamorphine with cocaine and methadone. British Journal of Clinical Pharmacology. 4: 691–692.

53 Lipman AG (2005) Methadone: effective analgesia, confusion, and risk. Journal of Pain and Palliative Care Pharmacotherapy. 19 (2): 3–5.

54 Palliativedrugs.com (2005) Hot Topics: new draft methadone monograph. In: September Newsletter. Available from: www.palliativedrugs.com

55 Santiago-Palma J et al. (2001) Intravenous methadone in the management of chronic cancer pain: safe and effective starting doses when substituting methadone for fentanyl. Cancer. 92: 1919–1925.

56 Blackburn D et al. (2002) Methadone: an alternative conversion regime. European Journal of Palliative Care. 9: 93–96.

57 Benitez-Rosario MA et al. (2004) Opioid switching from transdermal fentanyl to oral methadone in patients with cancer pain. Cancer. 101: 2866–2873.

58 Blackburn D (2005) Methadone: the analgesic. European Journal of Palliative Care. 12: 188–191.

59 Bruera E et al. (1996) Opioid rotation in patients with cancer pain. Cancer. 78: 852–857.

60 Zimmermann C et al. (2005) Rotation to methadone after opioid dose escalation: How should individualization of dosing occur? Journal of Pain and Palliative Care Pharmacotherapy. 19 (2): 25–31.

61 Mathew P and Storey P (1999) Subcutaneous methadone in terminally ill patients: manageable local toxicity. Journal of Pain and Symptom Management. 18: 49–52.

62 Centeno C and Vara F (2005) Intermittent subcutaneous methadone administration in the management of cancer pain. Journal of Pain and Palliative Care Pharmacotherapy. 19: 7–12.

63 Hum A et al. (2007) Subcutaneous methadone—an issue revisited. Journal of Pain and Symptom Management. 34: 573–575.

64 Fitzgibbon D and Ready L (1997) Intravenous high-dose methadone administered by patient controlled analgesia and continuous infusion for the treatment of cancer pain refractory to high-dose morphine. Pain. 73: 259–261.

65 Manfredi PL and Houde RW (2003) Prescribing methadone, a unique analgesic. Journal of Supportive Oncology. 1: 216–220.

66 Gallagher R (2004) Methadone mouthwash for the management of oral ulcer pain. Journal of Pain and Symptom Management. 27: 390–391.

67 Gallagher RE et al. (2005) Analgesic effects of topical methadone: a report of four cases. Clinical Journal of Pain. 21: 190–192.

Guidelines: Use of methadone for cancer pain

Methadone has both opioid and non-opioid properties, and a long variable halflife (approximately 5–130h vs. 2.5h for morphine). Thus there is no single potency ratio for methadone and other opioids. When switching from morphine, the eventual 24h dose of methadone is typically 5–10 times smaller than the dose of morphine, sometimes 20–30 times smaller, and occasionally even smaller. Inevitable accumulation is the reason for the week-long intervals between dose adjustments. Switching must be closely supervised, generally as an inpatient. If in doubt, seek specialist advice.

Indications for use
- neuropathic or mixed nociceptive-neuropathic pain not responding to an NSAID + morphine + adjuvant analgesics, e.g. an antidepressant ± an anti-epileptic
- neurotoxicity with morphine at any dose (e.g. myoclonus, allodynia, hyperalgesia) which does not respond to a reduction in morphine dose, and switching to another easier-to-use opioid (e.g. fentanyl, hydromorphone, oxycodone) is not possible
- the strong opioid of choice, instead of morphine
- end-stage renal failure.

Dose titration
1 When prescribing PO methadone as first-line strong opioid:
- start with methadone 5mg (1–2.5mg in the elderly) q12h regularly and q3h p.r.n.
- if necessary, titrate the regular dose upwards once a week, guided by p.r.n. use
- continue with 5mg p.r.n., or 1–2.5mg in the elderly
- with doses ≥30mg q12h, increase the p.r.n. dose to 1/10 of the q24h dose, rounded to a convenient tablet size or volume.

2 If the patient is already receiving morphine, use the following method.

PO morphine to PO methadone

Morphine is stopped abruptly when methadone is started.
If switching from:
- normal-release morphine, give the first dose of methadone ≥2h (pain present) or 4h (pain-free) after last dose of morphine
- SR morphine, give the first dose of methadone ≥6h (pain present) or 12h (pain-free) after the last dose of a 12h product, or ≥12h (pain present) or 24h (pain-free) after the last dose of a 24h product.

Give a single loading dose of PO methadone 1/10 of the previous total 24h PO morphine dose, up to a maximum of 30mg.

Give q3h p.r.n. doses of methadone 1/3 of the loading dose (i.e. 1/30 of the previous total 24h PO morphine dose) rounded to a convenient tablet size or volume, up to a maximum of 30mg per dose.

Example 1: Morphine 300mg/24h PO = loading dose of methadone 30mg PO, and 10mg q3h p.r.n.

Example 2: Morphine 1,200mg/24h PO = loading dose of methadone 120mg PO, and 40mg q3h p.r.n.; however, both are limited to the maximum of 30mg.

For patients in severe pain who need more analgesia in <3h, see point 6 below.

On Day 6, the amount of methadone taken over the previous 2 days is noted and divided by 4 to give a regular q12h dose, with 1/10 of the 24h dose q3h p.r.n., e.g. *methadone 80mg PO in previous 48h → 20mg q12h and 5mg PO q3h p.r.n.*

If ≥2 doses/day of p.r.n. methadone continue to be needed, the dose of regular methadone should be increased once a week, guided by p.r.n. use.

---

3 If using another strong opioid, calculate the morphine equivalent daily dose and then follow the guidelines for morphine.

4 If converting from PO methadone to SC/IV methadone, or from another CSCI/CIVI opioid, see the respective boxes below. Methadone injection can be imported through the Special Access Programme.

5 If there has been recent rapid escalation of the pre-switch opioid dose, calculate the initial dose of methadone using the pre-escalation dose of the opioid.

6 For patients in severe pain and who need more analgesia in < 3h, options include:
- taking the previously used opioid q1h p.r.n. (50–100% of the p.r.n. dose used before switching)
- if neurotoxicity with the pre-switch opioid, use an appropriate dose of an alternative strong opioid
- ketamine.

7 The switch to methadone is successful (i.e. improved pain relief and/or reduced toxicity) in about 75% of patients.

8 If a patient:
- becomes oversedated, reduce the dose generally by 33–50% (some centres monitor the level of consciousness and respirations q4h for 24h)
- develops opioid abstinence symptoms, give p.r.n. doses of the previous opioid to control these.

PO methadone to SC/IV or CSCI/CIVI methadone

To convert PO methadone to SC/IV methadone, halve the PO dose, e.g. methadone 10mg/24h PO = 5mg/24h SC/IV.
This is a safe conversion ratio; for some patients the SC/IV dose = PO dose.

Due to its long halflife, methadone (10mg/mL) can be given SC q12h–q8h. If SC injection is painful or causes local inflammation, give by CSCI/CIVI instead.

If CSCI methadone causes a skin reaction:
- administer as a more dilute solution
- change the site daily
- consider applying hydrocortisone cream 1% topically around the needle entry site (under an occlusive dressing)
- consider adding dexamethasone 1mg to the diluted combination of drugs (compatibility data permitting).

For additional rescue doses of methadone SC/IV, give 1/10 of the 24h SC/IV dose q3h p.r.n., e.g. methadone 20mg CIVI/24h = 2mg q3h p.r.n. SC/IV.

If ≥2 p.r.n doses/day continue to be needed, the 24h SC/IV dose should be increased once a week, guided by p.r.n. use.

For patients in severe pain who need more analgesia in < 3h, see point 6 above.

Other CSCI/CIVI opioids to CSCI/CIVI methadone

The safest approach is to follow the method for PO switching, using bolus injections of SC/IV methadone instead of PO doses.

Convert the opioid 24h CSCI/CIVI dose to its PO equivalent and determine the PO methadone dose (Dose titration, point 2).

The SC/IV dose of methadone is half the PO dose; the maximum initial dose of SC/IV methadone will be 15mg. This is a safe conversion ratio; for some patients the SC/IV dose = PO dose.

OXYCODONE

Class: Opioid analgesic.

Indications: Moderate–severe pain, †an alternative in cases of intolerance to other strong opioids.

Contra-indications: None absolute if titrated carefully against a patient's pain (also see Strong opioids, p.287).

Pharmacology

Oxycodone is a strong opioid with similar properties to **morphine**.[1–5] However, its opioid receptor site affinities remain a matter of controversy.[6,7] Studies with selective opioid antagonists suggest that oxycodone and **morphine** produce analgesia through different populations of opioid receptors.[8] Thus, in rats, naloxonazine (a selective μ-opioid receptor antagonist) completely blocks **morphine**-induced antinociception but does not attenuate the effect of oxycodone.[9] In contrast, norbinaltorphimine (a selective κ-opioid receptor antagonist) completely blocks oxycodone-induced antinociception but does not attenuate the effect of **morphine**. On the other hand, in other studies (rats, mice, and humans), oxycodone showed definite μ-opioid receptor activity.[10–12] However, some of this activity could have been mediated by active metabolites, e.g. **oxymorphone**.[10] Although synergy between **morphine** and oxycodone has been shown in rats,[13] no synergy is seen in humans.[14]

Oxycodone is metabolized principally to noroxycodone via CYP3A and 10% to **oxymorphone** via CYP2D6[15,16] Parenteral **oxymorphone** is 10 times more potent than parenteral **morphine**.[17] However, after blocking CYP2D6 with **quinidine**, the non-analgesic effects of oxycodone in volunteers are unchanged.[15] Thus it is unlikely that, in most people, **oxymorphone** contributes significantly to the analgesic effect of oxycodone. However, CYP2D6 ultra-rapid metabolizers may be at risk of undesirable CNS effects even with low-dose oxycodone.[18] This is probably due to an enhanced production of the more potent **oxymorphone** (also see Cytochrome P450, p.551).

By mouth, oxycodone is more potent than **morphine** (i.e. *fewer* mg of oxycodone are needed than **morphine** to have a comparable analgesic effect).[19–24] The PO potency ratio for oxycodone to **morphine** is about 1.5:1, and thus the dose of oxycodone by mouth is about 2/3 that of **morphine** (i.e. oxycodone 10mg is equivalent to **morphine** 15mg). Hence, the dose conversion table in the Canadian manufacturers' Product Monograph, which indicates that the dose of PO **morphine** should be halved when converting to PO oxycodone, although reasonable in terms of caution and safety, almost certainly exaggerates the actual potency of oxycodone.

Oxycodone hydrochloride is available in 10mg and 20mg suppositories. Traditionally, oxycodone PO and oxycodone PR have been regarded as equipotent. The recommendation by the manufacturer to give q8h–q6h is questionable in the absence of comparative pharmacokinetic data.

Parenterally, a short-term (2h) postoperative PCA study suggested that **morphine** is less potent than oxycodone (i.e. *more* mg of **morphine** will be needed).[25] However, earlier single-dose studies and two more recent longer PCA studies (1–2 days) suggest that by injection **morphine** is more potent than oxycodone, in the region of 4:3 (*fewer* mg of **morphine** will be needed, e.g. **morphine** 10mg is approximately equivalent to oxycodone 13mg).[17,19,26] If it is accepted that longer studies are likely to be more reliable, on balance it would seem that **morphine** by injection is more potent than oxycodone. Earlier single-dose studies, in fact, gave similar results to the more recent 1–2 day studies. However, given the modest difference in potency, together with the constraints of ampoule size, it is reasonable in clinical practice to use a parenteral potency ratio of 1:1 when converting from one drug to the other (i.e. regard IV/SC oxycodone 10mg as equivalent to IV/SC **morphine** 10mg).

About 20% of oxycodone is excreted unchanged in the urine. In mild–moderate hepatic impairment, oxycodone and noroxycodone concentrations increase (but the **oxymorphone** concentration decreases) and the elimination halflife increases by about 2h. In renal impairment the clearance of oxycodone, noroxycodone and conjugated **oxymorphone** are reduced. Oxycodone plasma concentration increases by 50% and the halflife lengthens by 1h.[20,27]
Bio-availability 75% PO, ranging from 60 to 87%; 61% rectal.[28,29]
Onset of action 20–30min PO; 45min rectal.
Time to peak plasma concentration 1–1.5h PO; 3h SR; 2.5–3h rectal.

Plasma halflife 3.5h; 4.5h in renal failure.
Duration of action 4–6h; 12h SR.

Cautions

SR products should be swallowed whole; crushing or chewing them may lead to a rapid release of an overdose of oxycodone.

Inhibitors of CYP3A4 (e.g. **ketoconazole** and **erythromycin**) can inhibit oxycodone metabolism, and may enhance its effects. However, current evidence suggests pharmacokinetic changes resulting from inhibition of CYP2D6 (e.g. with **quinidine**) are not clinically relevant.

Hepatic impairment, mild–moderate renal impairment; dose reduction is advisable (see Dose and use).

Concern about concurrent prescription with an MAOI is misplaced (see p.143).

Undesirable effects

For full list, see manufacturer's Product Monograph.

Essentially the same as **morphine**, but constipation may be more common and vomiting and hallucinations less common with oxycodone.[20] Also see Strong opioids, p.289.

Dose and use

Because oxycodone is more expensive, it should generally be reserved for patients who cannot tolerate **morphine**.

Oral

Normal-release oxycodone is generally given q4h but, in some patients, q6h is satisfactory.[30] SR tablets are biphasic in their release of oxycodone, i.e. there is an initial fast release which leads to the early onset of analgesia and a slow release which provides a prolonged duration of action.

For strong opioid-naïve patients:
* starting dose 5mg q6h–q4h for normal-release tablets
* starting dose 10mg q12h for SR tablets
* titrate as necessary to optimize analgesia.

For patients transferring from oral **morphine**:
* use an initial dose conversion ratio of 1.5:1 (e.g. replace **morphine** 15mg by oxycodone 10mg)
* titrate as necessary to optimize analgesia.

Note: this recommendation differs from the conversion ratio of 2:1 indicated by the data in the dose conversion tables in the manufacturers' Product Monographs (see Pharmacology above; also see Opioid dose conversion ratios, p.497).

Canadian manufacturers give no guidance regarding dose reductions in hepatic and renal impairment. UK and US manufacturers recommend that the initial dose is reduced by 1/3–1/2 in patients with hepatic impairment or mild–moderate renal impairment.
* start at 2.5mg q6h for normal-release tablets or 5mg q12h for SR tablets.

Rectal

Recommended dose = 10–20mg q8h–q6h.[31] However, given that the available suppositories (like the normal-release tablets) contain oxycodone hydrochloride, it may be necessary to administer q4h. Further, given the lower rectal bio-availability, it is reasonable to convert from PO to PR on a 1:1 basis, and titrate the dose upwards as necessary. There is no pharmacological reason for limiting the rectal dose to 10–20mg.

As with all opioids, patients must be monitored for undesirable effects, particularly nausea and vomiting, and constipation (see p.289). Depending on individual circumstances, an anti-emetic should be prescribed for regular or p.r.n. use (see p.183) and, routinely, a laxative prescribed (see p.26).

Supply

Unless indicated otherwise, all products are Schedule I controlled drugs under the Controlled Drugs and Substances Act, and are subject to the Narcotic Control Regulations of the act.

Oxy.IR® (Purdue)
Tablets 5mg dose = $0.28, 10mg dose = $0.41, 20mg dose = $0.71.

Supeudol® (Sandoz Canada)
Tablets 5mg dose = $0.18, 10mg dose = $0.28, 20mg dose = $0.44.
Suppositories 10mg, box of 12 = $25; 20mg, box of 12 = $32.

Sustained-release
OxyContin® (Purdue)
Tablets SR 5mg, 10mg, 20mg, 40mg, 80mg, 28 days @ 10mg, 20mg and 80mg b.i.d. = $51, $77 and $245 respectively.

Oxycodone is also available in combination products with **acetaminophen** and **aspirin**.

1 Glare PA and Walsh TD (1993) Dose-ranging study of oxycodone for chronic pain in advanced cancer. *Journal of Clinical Oncology.* **11**: 973–978.

2 Poyhia R *et al.* (1993) Oxycodone: an alternative to morphine for cancer pain. A review. *Journal of Pain and Symptom Management.* **8**: 63–67.

3 Shah S and Hardy J (2001) Oxycodone: a review of the literature. *European Journal of Palliative Care.* **8**: 93–96.

4 Davis MP *et al.* (2003) Normal-release and controlled-release oxycodone: pharmacokinetics, pharmacodynamics, and controversy. *Supportive Care in Cancer.* **11**: 84–92.

5 Kalso E (2005) Oxycodone. *Journal of Pain and Symptom Management.* **29 (suppl 5)**: s47–s56.

6 Poyhia R and Kalso EA (1992) Antinociceptive effects and central nervous system depression caused by oxycodone and morphine in rats. *Pharmacology and Toxicology.* **70**: 125–130.

7 Poyhia R *et al.* (1993) A review of oxycodone's clinical pharmacokinetics and pharmacodynamics. *Journal of Pain and Symptom Management.* **8**: 63–67.

8 Smith M *et al.* (2001) Oxycodone has a distinctly different pharmacology from morphine. *European Journal of Pain.* **15 (suppl A)**: 135–136.

9 Ross F and Smith M (1997) The intrinsic antinociceptive effects of oxycodone appear to be kappa-opioid receptor mediated. *Pain.* **73**: 151–157.

10 Kalso E *et al.* (1990) Morphine and oxycodone in the management of cancer pain: plasma levels determined by chemical and radioreceptor assays. *Journal of Pharmacology and Toxicology.* **67**: 322–328.

11 Chen ZR *et al.* (1991) Mu receptor binding of some commonly used opioids and their metabolites. *Life Sciences.* **48**: 2165–2171.

12 Yoburn B *et al.* (1995) Supersensitivity to opioid analgesics following chronic opioid antagonist treatment: relationship to receptor selectivity. *Pharmacology, Biochemistry and Behavior.* **51**: 535–539.

13 Ross FB *et al.* (2000) Co-administration of sub-antinociceptive doses of oxycodone and morphine produces marked antinociceptive synergy with reduced CNS side-effects in rats. *Pain.* **84**: 421–428.

14 Grach M *et al.* (2004) Can coadministration of oxycodone and morphine produce analgesic synergy in humans? An experimental cold pain study. *British Journal of Clinical Pharmacology.* **58**: 235–242.

15 Heiskanen T *et al.* (1998) Effects of blocking CYP2D6 on oxycodone. *Clinical Pharmacology and Therapeutics.* **64**: 603–611.

16 Lalovic B *et al.* (2006) Pharmacokinetics and pharmacodynamics of oral oxycodone in healthy human subjects: role of circulating active metabolites. *Clinical Pharmacology and Therapeutics.* **79**: 461–479.

17 Beaver WT *et al.* (1978) Analgesic studies of codeine and oxycodone in patients with cancer. II. Comparisons of intramuscular oxycodone with intramuscular morphine and codeine. *Journal Pharmacology and Experiemental Therapeutics.* **207**: 101–108.

18 de Leon J *et al.* (2003) Adverse drug reactions to oxycodone and hydrocodone in CYP2D6 ultrarapid metabolizers. *Journal of Clinical Psychopharmacology.* **23**: 420–421.

19 Kalso E and Vainio A (1990) Morphine and oxycodone in the management of cancer pain. *Clinical Pharmacology and Therapeutics.* **47**: 639–646.

20 Heiskanen T and Kalso E (1997) Controlled-release oxycodone and morphine in cancer related pain. *Pain.* **73**: 37–45.

21 Bruera E *et al.* (1998) Randomized, double-blind, cross-over trial comparing safety and efficacy of oral controlled-release oxycodone with controlled-release morphine in patients with cancer pain. *Journal of Clinical Oncology.* **16**: 3222–3229.

22 Mucci-LoRusso P *et al.* (1998) Controlled-release oxycodone compared with controlled-release morphine in the treatment of cancer pain: a randomized, double-blind, parallel-group study. *European Journal of Pain.* **2**: 239–249.

23 Curtis GB *et al.* (1999) Relative potency of controlled-release oxycodone and controlled-release morphine in a postoperative pain model. *European Journal of Clinical Pharmacology.* **55**: 425–429.

24 Lauretti GR *et al.* (2003) Comparison of sustained-release morphine with sustained-release oxycodone in advanced cancer patients. *British Journal of Cancer.* **89**: 2027–2030.

25 Kalso E *et al.* (1991) Intravenous morphine and oxycodone for pain after abdominal surgery. *Acta Anaesthesiologica Scandinavica.* **35**: 642–646.

26 Silvasti M *et al.* (1998) Comparison of analgesic efficacy of oxycodone and morphine in postoperative intravenous patient-controlled analgesia. *Acta Anaesthesiologica Scandinavica.* **42**: 576–580.

27 Glare P and Davis MP (2009) Oxycodone. In: MP Davis *et al.* (eds) *Opioids in Cancer Pain* (2e). Oxford University Press, Oxford, pp. 155–173.

28 Leow K *et al.* (1992) Single-dose and steady-state pharmacokinetics and pharmacodynamics of oxycodone in patients with cancer. *Clinical Pharmacology and Therapeutics.* **52**: 487–495.

29 Poyhia R *et al.* (1992) The pharmacokinetics and metabolism of oxycodone after intramuscular and oral administration to healthy subjects. *British Journal of Clinical Pharmacology.* **33**: 617–621.

30 Lugo RA and Kern SE (2004) The pharmacokinetics of oxycodone. *Journal of Pain and Palliative Care Pharmacotherapy.* **18 (4)**: 17–30.

31 Sweetman S (ed) (2007) *Martindale: the Complete Drug Reference* (35e). Pharmaceutical Press, London, p. 91.

OPIOID ANTAGONISTS

Pharmacology

Naloxone, **naltrexone**, **nalmefene** (not Canada) and **methylnaltrexone** are generally classed as pure antagonists. They possess a high affinity for opioid receptors but no intrinsic activity. They block access to the opioid receptors by opioid agonists/opioid analgesics; and, if administered after a strong opioid, they displace the latter because of their higher receptor affinity.[1]

However, the discovery that ultra-low doses of **naloxone** and **nalmefene** given post-operatively either potentiate the analgesic effect of **morphine** (and presumably of other agonist opioids) or reduce undesirable effects (nausea and vomiting, and pruritus), or both, means that the full reality is more complex.[2,3] In fact, it is 30 years since **naloxone** was shown in rodents to have low-order antinociceptive activity.[4] Subsequently in humans, in post-dental extraction pain, it was shown that **naloxone** could produce either analgesia (low-dose) or hyperalgesia (high-dose).[5] Further, in the same circumstances, **naloxone** 400microgram neutralizes the analgesic effect of **morphine** 8mg IV (as expected) but more than doubles the analgesic effect of **pentazocine** 60mg IV.[6] (**Pentazocine** is a partial μ and κ agonist and δ antagonist.)[7]

Various putative explanations have been put forward to explain these phenomena. It has been suggested that these findings can be explained if the μ, δ and κ opioid receptors respond to ligands in a bimodal way.[8] If this is the case, opioid receptors would have an excitatory as well as an inhibitory mode. Excitation would produce hyperalgesia (and possibly tolerance), whereas inhibition would produce typical opioid analgesic and other effects. This theory can also be used to explain why high doses of **morphine** sometimes cause hyperalgesia.[9]

Opioid antagonists have a role to play in the management of pruritus associated with chronic disease, notably in cholestasis.[10,11] Pruritus in cholestasis is a central phenomenon caused by increased opioidergic tone secondary to an increase in plasma enkephalin concentration.[12,13] Opioid antagonists are effective in counterbalancing the increased tone, and thereby relieve the pruritus.[14-17] Unfortunately, an opioid-like withdrawal syndrome may be precipitated.[12,18] This can be avoided by using small incremental doses of the opioid antagonist (see p.344 and p.346).

As a general rule, patients with cholestatic jaundice and both pruritus and severe pain should not be treated with an opioid antagonist. Instead, an alternative treatment for pruritus, such as **rifampin** or **danazol** should be used (Box 5.O and Table 5.21), and the pain treated appropriately with both non-opioid and opioid analgesics. However, in specialist clinics, it is occasionally possible to treat both the pruritus and the pain with low doses of **naloxone** or **naltrexone**.[19]

In uremic pruritus, the situation is more complex because there are several causal mechanisms, both peripheral (cutaneous) and central (neural).[20,21] The opioid system is involved, but in uremia there is no increase in opioidergic tone (and thus no danger of a withdrawal syndrome if an opioid antagonist is given). Instead, the ratio between μ-opioid receptors (pruritus-inducing; relative increase in number) and κ-opioid receptors (pruritus-suppressing; relative decrease in number) alters in favour of the former.[22,23] This predisposes to the development of pruritus. It also suggests that both κ-opioid *agonists* and μ-opioid receptor *antagonists* could bring relief. Thus, in an RCT lasting 2–4 weeks of **nalfurafine**, a novel κ-agonist, 36% of subjects receiving **nalfurafine** responded (at least 50% reduction in worst itching) compared with 15% in the placebo group.[24] However, two RCTs of **naltrexone** have given conflicting results. Benefit was seen in uremic patients with very severe pruritus[25] but not in those with moderately severe pruritus.[26]

Methylnaltrexone (see Box 5.P, p.341) and **alvimopan** (not Canada) are quaternary compounds which do not readily cross the blood–brain barrier. They are peripheral opioid receptor antagonists which improve opioid-induced constipation.[27-30]

Uses

Naloxone is used principally to reverse life-threatening respiratory depression (see p.344). **Naloxone** and **naltrexone** are both used to:
- prevent relapse in opioid ex-addicts
- relieve pruritus associated with cholestasis[31,32]

Note: pruritus associated with chronic diseases other than cholestasis generally requires alternative specific measures (Box 5.O and Table 5.21) However, in an open study of patients

---

Box 5.O Management of pruritus in non-skin diseases[a]

Non-drug treatment

Dry skin	Emollient cream (moisturizer) daily–b.i.d.
Malignant extrahepatic cholestasis	Stenting of common bile duct
Uremia	Modify dialysis regimen UVB phototherapy **A**[35]
Hodgkin's lymphoma	Curative radiation therapy and/or chemotherapy

Specific drug treatment

Cholestasis	Naltrexone 12.5–250mg once daily **A**[36]
	Rifampin 75–300mg once daily **A**[37]
	Sertraline 50–100mg each morning **A**[38]
	Cholestyramine 4g×2 once daily–b.i.d. **B**[b,39]
	17α-alkyl androgen, e.g.:[40,41]
	    methyltestosterone 25mg once daily *sublingual*
	    (not Canada)[41]
	    danazol 200mg once daily–t.i.d.
	    fluoxymesterone (not Canada)

Hodgkin's lymphoma	Corticosteroids ± palliative chemotherapy (e.g. vinblastine) Cimetidine 800mg/24h **B**[42]
Paraneoplasia	Paroxetine 5–20mg once daily **A**[43] Thalidomide 100mg at bedtime[44]
Uremia	Thalidomide 100mg at bedtime **A**[45] Naltrexone 50mg once daily[c,25,26]

Spinal opioids	Bupivacaine intrathecal **A**[46]
	NSAID:
	    diclofenac 100mg PR **A**[47]
	    tenoxicam 20mg IV (injection not Canada) **A**[48]
	Butorphanol intranasal[49] or epidural
	(injection not Canada)[50]
	Ondansetron 8mg IV **A**[51]
	Propofol IV **A**[52]

Consider when specific treatments fail

Paroxetine 5–20mg once daily Mirtazapine 7.5–15mg at bedtime }	*add* mirtazapine if paroxetine loses its effect

a. strength of recommendations: grade A is based on evidence from ≥1 RCTs, and grade B on well-designed non-randomized studies;[53] where no grade is given, recommendation based on case reports and/or expert opinion
b. not of value in complete large duct biliary obstruction
c. controlled trials give diametrically opposite results (much benefit vs. no benefit).

---

with various skin and systemic disorders, good relief of pruritus was obtained in 70% of the patients with PO **naltrexone**.[10] In the absence of controlled data, the results should be interpreted with caution.

• correct opioid-induced GI disorder (i.e. delayed gastric emptying and constipation).[33,34]
This last indication is likely to shift to the quaternary opioid antagonists (Box 5.P).

Table 5.21 Suggested management of pruritus in non-skin diseases and strength of recommendation[a,b]

Condition	Step 1	Step 2	Step 3
Uremia[c]	UVB phototherapy A[35] or capsaicin cream 0.025–0.075% once daily–b.i.d. (if localized) A[54]	Naltrexone 50mg once daily A[d,25,26]	Thalidomide 100mg at bedtime A[e,45]
Cholestasis[f]	Naltrexone 12.5–250mg once daily A[36]	Rifampin 75–300mg once daily A[37] or sertraline 50–100mg once daily A[38]	Methyltestosterone 25mg SL once daily (not Canada) A[40,41] or danazol 200mg once daily–t.i.d.[g]
Lymphoma[h]	Prednisolone 10–20mg t.i.d.	Cimetidine 800mg/24h A[42]	Mirtazapine 15–30mg at bedtime or carbamazepine 200mg b.i.d.
Polycythemia vera[h]	Aspirin 100–300mg once daily A[55]	Paroxetine 5–20mg once daily A[56]	Sedative, e.g. benzodiazepine
Spinal opioid-induced pruritus[i]	Give spinal bupivacaine concurrently A[46]	Ondansetron 8mg IV stat A[51,57]	Switch opioid, e.g. morphine→hydromorphone B[58]
Systemic opioid-induced pruritus[j]	Stat dose of H₁-antihistamine, e.g. chlorphenamine 4–12mg; if after 2–3h there is definite benefit, prescribe 4mg t.i.d.; if not, proceed to Step 2	Switch opioid[k], e.g. morphine→oxycodone[59]	Ondansetron 8mg b.i.d.
Paraneoplastic pruritus[h]	Paroxetine 5–20mg once daily A[43]	Mirtazapine 15–30mg at bedtime	Thalidomide 100mg at bedtime[e] or carbamazepine 200mg b.i.d.
Other causes or origin unknown	Paroxetine 5–20mg once daily	Mirtazapine 15–30mg at bedtime	Thalidomide 100mg at bedtime[e]

a. strength of recommendations: grade A is based on evidence from ≥1 RCTs, and grade B on well-designed non-randomized studies;[53] where no grade is given, recommendation based on case reports and/or expert opinion
b. given PO unless stated otherwise
c. after the hemodialysis regimen has been optimized
d. controlled trials give contradictory results (much benefit vs. no benefit)
e. thalidomide is off-label and may cause severe neuropathy if used long-term
f. in total bile obstruction, where bile duct stenting is impossible or unwanted
g. androgens may be hepatotoxic and may increase cholestasis while reducing pruritus
h. assuming that cytoreductive/anticancer treatment is impossible or unwanted
i. other postoperative options include diclofenac 100mg PR A[47] or tenoxicam 20mg IV (injection not Canada) A[48] but any benefit may relate to the lower dose of opioid needed when these NSAIDs are given concurrently
j. pruritus after systemic opioids is uncommon, and poorly documented. Although some cases may be caused by cutaneous histamine release[60] and may be self-limiting (see main text), the most distressing cases are long-lasting and antihistamine-resistant[59]
k. methylnaltrexone has been used but the large doses required make it impractical and inordinately expensive.[61]

Box 5.P Methylnaltrexone

SC methylnaltrexone is approved for use in patients with 'advanced illness' suffering from opioid-induced constipation despite usual laxative therapy. Constipation is common in advanced disease, even in patients not taking opioids. Thus, so-called 'opioid-induced constipation' is often multifactorial in origin;[62,63] and methylnaltrexone will normally augment laxatives rather than replace them. It is important that laxative therapy (see p.26) should be optimized before using methylnaltrexone.

About 1/2 of patients defecate within 4h of a dose, without impairment of analgesia or the development of withdrawal symptoms.[64,65] Common undesirable effects include abdominal pain, diarrhea, flatulence, and nausea.

Methylnaltrexone is marketed as an SC injection (see manufacturer's Product Monograph):
- for patients weighing 38–62kg, start with 8mg on alternate days
- for patients weighing 62–114kg, start with 12mg on alternate days
- if outside this range, give 150*microgram/kg* and round up to the nearest 0.1mL.

The interval between doses of methylnaltrexone can be adjusted according to individual need, but it should be given more than once daily.

The dose of methylnaltrexone should be halved in severe renal impairment, i.e. when creatinine clearance is < 30mL/min. Methylnaltrexone is contra-indicated in the presence of known or suspected bowel obstruction.

Methylnaltrexone (Relistor®) costs $41 per 12mg (0.6mL) vial.

---

1 Choi YS and Billings JA (2002) Opioid antagonists: a review of their role in palliative care, focusing on use in opioid-related constipation. *Journal of Pain and Symptom Management.* **24**: 71–90.

2 Gan T et al. (1997) Opioid-sparing effects of a low-dose infusion of naloxone in patient-administered morphine sulfate. *Anesthesiology.* **87**: 1075–1081.

3 Joshi G et al. (1999) Effects of prophylactic nalmefene on the incidence of morphine-related side effects in patients receiving intravenous patient-controlled analgesia. *Anesthesiology.* **90**: 1007–1011.

4 Sewell RD and Spencer PS (1976) Antinociceptive activity of narcotic agonist and partial agonist analgesics and other agents in the tail-immersion test in mice and rats. *Neuropharmacology.* **15**: 683–688.

5 Levine JD et al. (1979) Naloxone dose dependently produces analgesia and hyperalgesia in postoperative pain. *Nature.* **278**: 740–741.

6 Levine J and Gordon N (1988) Synergism between the analgesic actions of morphine and pentazocine. *Pain.* **33**: 369–372.

7 Hill RG (1992) Multiple opioid receptors and their ligands. *Frontiers of Pain.* **4**: 1–4.

8 Crain S and Shen K (2000) Antagonists of excitatory opioid receptor functions enhance morphine's analgesic potency and attenuate opioid tolerance/dependence liability. *Pain.* **84**: 121–131.

9 Sjogren P et al. (1994) Disappearance of morphine-induced hyperalgesia after discontinuing or substituting morphine with other opioid analgesics. *Pain.* **59**: 313–316.

10 Metze D et al. (1999) Efficacy and safety of naltrexone, an oral opiate receptor antagonist, in the treatment of pruritus in internal and dermatological diseases. *Journal of the American Academy of Dermatology.* **41**: 533–539.

11 Zylicz Z (2004) Terminal sedation in the Netherlands. *Annals of Internal Medicine.* **141**: 966; author reply 966–967.

12 Thornton J and Losowksy M (1988) Opioid peptides and primary biliary cirrhosis. *British Medical Journal.* **297**: 1501–1504.

13 Swain M et al. (1992) Endogenous opioids accumulate in plasma in a rat model of acute cholestasis. *Gastroenterology.* **103**: 630–635.

14 Bergasa N et al. (1992) A controlled trial of naloxone infusions for the pruritus of chronic cholestasis. *Gastroenterology.* **102**: 544–549.

15 Bergasa N et al. (1995) Effects of naloxone infusions in patients with the pruritus of cholestasis. *Annals of internal medicine.* **123**: 161–167.

16 Bergasa N et al. (1998) Open-label trial of oral nalmefene therapy for the pruritus of cholestasis. *Hepatology.* **27**: 679–684.

17 Bergasa N et al. (1999) Oral nalmefene therapy reduces scratching activity due to the pruritus of cholestasis: a controlled study. *Journal of the American Academy of Dermatology.* **41**: 431–434.

18 Jones E and Dekker L (2000) Florid opioid withdrawal-like reaction precipitated by naltrexone in a patient with chronic cholestasis. *Gastroenterology.* **118**: 431–432.

19 Jones EA and Zylicz Z (2005) Treatment of pruritus caused by cholestasis with opioid antagonists. *Journal of Palliative Medicine.* **8**: 1290–1294.

20 Urbonas A et al. (2001) Uremic pruritus–an update. *American Journal of Nephrology.* **21**: 343–350.

21 Szepietowski J (2004) Uraemic pruritus. In: Z Zylicz et al. (eds) *Pruritus in advanced disease.* Oxford University Press, Oxford, pp. 69–83.

22 Kumagai H et al. (2000) Endogenous opioid system in uraemic patients. In: *Joint Meeting of the Seventh World Conference on Clinical Pharmacology and IUPHAR–Division of Clinical Pharmacology and the Fourth Congress of the European Association for Clinical Pharmacology and Therapeutics.*

23 Odou P et al. (2001) A hypothesis for endogenous opioid peptides in uraemic pruritus: role of enkephalin. *Nephrology Dialysis Transplantation.* **16**: 1953–1954.

---

24 Wikstrom B *et al.* (2005) Kappa-opioid system in uremic pruritus: multicenter, randomized, double-blind, placebo-controlled clinical studies. *Journal of the American Society of Nephrology.* **16**: 3742–3747.

25 Peer G *et al.* (1996) Randomised crossover trial of naltrexone in uraemic pruritus. *Lancet.* **348**: 1552–1554.

26 Pauli-Magnus C *et al.* (2000) Naltrexone does not relieve uremic pruritus. *Journal of the American Society of Nephrology.* **11**: 514–519.

27 Yuan CS *et al.* (2002) Effects of subcutaneous methylnaltrexone on morphine-induced peripherally mediated side effects: a double-blind randomized placebo-controlled trial. *Journal of Pharmacology and Experimental Therapeutics.* **300**: 118–123.

28 Paulson DM *et al.* (2005) Alvimopan: an oral, peripherally acting, mu-opioid receptor antagonist for the treatment of opioid-induced bowel dysfunction–a 21-day treatment-randomized clinical trial. *Journal of Pain.* **6**: 184–192.

29 Yuan C-S (2007) Methylnaltrexone mechanisms of action and effects on opioid bowel dysfunction and other opioid adverse effects. *Annals of Pharmacotherapy.* **41**: 984–993.

30 Shaiova L *et al.* (2007) A review of methylnaltrexone, a peripheral opioid receptor antagonist, and its role in opioid-induced constipation. *Palliative & Supportive Care.* **5**: 161–166.

31 Jones E and Bergasa N (1999) The pruritus of cholestasis. *Hepatology.* **29**: 1003–1006.

32 Jones E and Bergasa N (2004) The pruritus of cholestasis and the opioid neurotransmitter system. In: Z Zylicz *et al.* (eds) *Pruritus in advanced desease.* Oxford University Press, Oxford, pp. 56–68.

33 Sykes N (1991) Oral naloxone in opioid-associated constipation. *Lancet.* **337**: 1475.

34 Culpepper-Morgan J *et al.* (1992) Treatment of opioid-induced constipation with oral naloxone: a pilot study. *Clinical Pharmacology and Therapeutics.* **52**: 90–95.

35 Gilchrest B *et al.* (1997) Relief of uremic pruritus with ultraviolet phototherapy. *New England Journal of Medicine.* **297**: 136–138.

36 Wolfhagen F *et al.* (1997) Oral naltrexone treatment for cholestatic pruritus: A double-blind, placebo-controlled study. *Gastroenterology.* **113**: 1264–1269.

37 Ghent C and Carruthers S (1988) Treatment of pruritus in primary biliary cirrhosis with rifampin. Results of a double-blind crossover randomized trial. *Gastroenterology.* **94**: 488–493.

38 Mayo MJ *et al.* (2007) Sertraline as a first-line treatment for cholestatic pruritus. *Hepatology.* **45**: 666–674.

39 Datta D and Sherlock S (1966) Cholestyramine for long term relief of the pruritus complicating intrahepatic cholestasis. *Gastroenterology.* **50**: 323–332.

40 Ahrens E *et al.* (1950) Primary biliary cirrhosis. *Medicine.* **29**: 299–364.

41 Lloyd-Thomas H and Sherlock S (1952) Testosterone therapy for the pruritus of obstructive jaundice. *British Medical Journal.* **ii**: 1289–1291.

42 Aymard J *et al.* (1980) Cimetidine for pruritus in Hodgkin's disease. *British Medical Journal.* **280**: 151–152.

43 Zylicz Z *et al.* (2003) Paroxetine in the treatment of severe non-dermatological pruritus: a randomized, controlled trial. *Journal of Pain and Symptom Management.* **26**: 1105–1112.

44 Smith J *et al.* (2002) Use of thalidomide in the treatment of intractable itch. In: International Journal of Palliative Nursing (ed) *Palliative Care Congress*; Sheffield. Mark Allen.

45 Silva S *et al.* (1994) Thalidomide for the treatment of uremic pruritus: a crossover randomized double-blind trial. *Nephron.* **67**: 270–273.

46 Asokumar B *et al.* (1998) Intrathecal bupivacaine reduces pruritus and prolongs duration of fentanyl analgesia during labor: a prospective, randomized, controlled trial. *Anaesthesia and Analgesia.* **87**: 1309–1315.

47 Colbert S *et al.* (1999) The effect of rectal diclofenac on pruritus in patients receiving intrathecal morphine. *Anaesthesia.* **54**: 948–952.

48 Colbert S *et al.* (1999) The effect of intravenous tenoxicam on pruritus in patients receiving epidural fentanyl. *Anaesthesia.* **54**: 76–80.

49 Dunteman E and Karanikolas M (1996) Transnasal butorphanol for the treatment of opioid-induced pruritus unresponsive to antihistamines. *Journal of Pain and Symptom Management.* **12**: 255–260.

50 Gunter J *et al.* (2000) Continuous epidural butorphanol relieves pruritus associated with epidural morphine infusions in children. *Paediatric Anaesthesia.* **10**: 167–172.

51 Borgeat A and Stimemann H-R (1999) Ondansetron is effective to treat spinal or epidural morphine-induced pruritus. *Anesthesiology.* **90**: 432–436.

52 Borgeat A *et al.* (1992) Subhypnotic doses of propofol relieve pruritus induced by epidural and intrathecal morphine. *Anesthesiology.* **76**: 510–512.

53 BMJ Publishing Group (2009) Resources for authors. Checklists and forms: clinical management guidelines. Available from: http://resources.bmj.com/bmj/authors/checklists-forms/clinical-management-guidelines

54 Breneman D *et al.* (1992) Topical capsaicin for treatment of hemodialysis-related pruritus. *Journal of the American Academy of Dermatology.* **26**: 91–94.

55 Fjellner B and Hagermark O (1979) Pruritus in polycythemia vera: treatment with aspirin and possibility of platelet involvement. *Acta Dermato-Venereologica (Stockholm).* **59**: 505–512.

56 Tefferi A and Fonseca R (2002) Selective serotonin reuptake inhibitors are effective in the treatment of polycythemia vera-associated pruritus. *Blood.* **99**: 2627.

57 Charuluxananan S *et al.* (2000) Ondansetron for treatment of intrathecal morphine-induced pruritus after cesarean delivery. *Regional Anesthesia and Pain Medicine.* **25**: 535–539.

58 Chaplan SR *et al.* (1992) Morphine and hydromorphone epidural analgesia. *Anesthesiology.* **77**: 1090–1094.

59 Tarcatu D *et al.* (2007) Are we still scratching the surface? A case of intractable pruritus following systemic opioid analgesia. *Journal of Opioid Management.* **3**: 167–170.

60 Krajnik M (2004) Opioid-induced pruritus. In: Z Zylicz *et al.* (eds) *Pruritus in advanced disease.* Oxford University Press, London, pp. 84–96.

61 Yuan CS *et al.* (1998) Efficacy of orally administered methylnaltrexone in decreasing subjective effects after intravenous morphine. *Drug and Alcohol Dependence.* **52**: 161–165.

62 Sykes N (1998) The relationship between opioid use and laxative use in terminally ill cancer patients. *Palliative Medicine.* **12**: 375–382.

63 Davis MP (2008) Cancer constipation: Are opioids really the culprit? *Supportive Care in Cancer.* **16**: 427–429.

64 Portenoy RK *et al.* (2008) Subcutaneous methylnaltrexone for the treatment of opioid-induced constipation in patients with advanced illness: a double-blind, randomized, parallel group, dose-ranging study. *Journal of Pain and Symptom Management.* **35**: 458–468.

65 Thomas J *et al.* (2008) Methylnaltrexone for opioid-induced constipation in advanced illness. *New England Journal of Medicine.* **358**: 2332–2343.

NALOXONE

Class: Opioid antagonist.

Indications: Reversal of opioid-induced respiratory depression, treatment of acute opioid overdose, diagnosis of suspected acute opioid overdose, †adjunctive treatment of septic shock, †cholestatic pruritus. Also, in combination with **buprenorphine** (Suboxone®), prevention of relapse in opioid ex-addicts.

Pharmacology

Naloxone is a potent opioid antagonist. It has a high affinity for opioid receptors and reverses the effect of opioid analgesics by displacement in a dose-related manner. Partial antagonism may be obtained by using small doses. Activity after oral administration is low; it is only 1/15 as potent by mouth as by injection. Naloxone is rapidly metabolized by the liver, primarily to naloxone glucuronide which is excreted by the kidneys.

The most important clinical property of naloxone is reversal of opioid-induced respiratory depression (and other opioid effects) caused by either an overdose of an opioid (including **codeine** and **propoxyphene**) or an exaggerated response to conventional doses. Naloxone has been reported to be only partially effective in reversing the effects of **tramadol**.[1] However, in a series of 11 patients with a **tramadol** overdose, 7 had a good response to naloxone, and 1 had no response.[2] Because of its high receptor affinity, antagonism of **buprenorphine** (not available for analgesic use in Canada) requires much higher doses of naloxone. *Naloxone is not effective against respiratory depression caused by non-opioids, e.g. barbiturates.*

Combined naloxone and **buprenorphine** SL tablets are used for the treatment of opioid dependency. Naloxone is also of benefit in patients with †chronic idiopathic constipation,[3] †septic shock,[4] †**morphine**-induced peripheral vasodilation,[5] †ischemic central neurological deficits[6,7] and †post-stroke central pain.[8]

Postoperative pain studies indicate that low-dose naloxone reduces the undesirable effects of **morphine**.[9,10] Naloxone 400microgram/70kg/24h CIVI reduced **morphine** requirements and halved the incidence of nausea and vomiting (about 80% to 40%) and of pruritus (50% to 25%).[9] Whether this benefit from naloxone can be utilized in palliative care is not clear. These findings can be explained if the μ, δ and κ-opioid receptors respond to ligands in a bimodal way, and have both an excitatory and an inhibitory mode.[11] Excitation would produce hyperalgesia (and possibly tolerance), whereas inhibition would produce typical opioid analgesic and other effects. This theory can also be used to explain why high doses of **morphine** sometimes cause hyperalgesia.[12]

Naloxone by CIVI decreases scratching activity by patients with cholestatic pruritus (see p.344).[13,14] Thus, naloxone has a potential place in the emergency treatment of acute exacerbations of cholestatic pruritus. **Naltrexone** (see p.345),[15,16] which has better oral bio-availability, can then be used long-term. However, opioid antagonists can precipitate an opioid withdrawal-like reaction in patients with cholestasis, including hallucinations and dysphoria.[17,18] To avoid or minimize such a reaction, treatment must be started with a cautious low-dose infusion of naloxone (see p.344), or low-dose **naltrexone** (see p.345).

Bio-availability 6% PO.
Onset of action 1–2min IV; 2–5min SC/IM.
Plasma halflife about 1h.
Duration of action IV 15–90min.

Cautions

In patients receiving opioids for pain relief, naloxone should *not* be used for drowsiness and/or delirium which is not life-threatening because of the danger of reversing the opioid analgesia, and precipitating a major physical withdrawal syndrome.

Undesirable effects

For full list, see manufacturer's Product Monograph.
Nausea and vomiting. Occasionally severe hypertension, pulmonary edema, tachycardia, arrhythmias, cardiac arrest;[19] doses as small as 100–400microgram of naloxone have been

implicated.[20] The mechanism of these sporadic events may be related to the centrally-mediated catecholamine responses to opioid reversal.[21]

Dose and use
Naloxone is best given IV but, if not practical, may be given IM or SC.

Opioid overdose
- give 400microgram–2mg IV every 2–3min p.r.n., up to a total of 10mg
- if the overdose is associated with a long-acting opioid (particularly **methadone** or **propoxyphene**) or an SR formulation, the duration of action of the opioid will exceed that of naloxone. Even if there is an initial response to naloxone, further IV doses may be required later, or it may be necessary to continue treatment with a closely monitored IV infusion of naloxone for up to 24h, sometimes longer.

Reversal of respiratory depression caused by the medicinal use of opioids
- give 100–200microgram IV stat
- give further doses of 100microgram every 2min until respiratory function is satisfactory.

Further IV doses should be given after 1–2h if there is concern that further absorption of the opioid will result in delayed respiratory depression. Even lower doses have been recommended (Box 5.Q). It is important to titrate dose against respiratory function and *not* the level of consciousness because total antagonism will cause a return of severe pain with hyperalgesia and, if physically dependent, severe physical withdrawal symptoms and marked agitation.[22]

Box 5.Q Naloxone for iatrogenic opioid overdose (based on the recommendations of the American Pain Society)[23]

If respiratory rate ≥8 breaths/min, and the patient easily rousable and not cyanosed, adopt a policy of 'wait and see'; consider reducing or omitting the next regular dose of morphine.

If respiratory rate <8 breaths/min, and the patient comatose/unconscious and/or cyanosed:
- dilute a standard 1mL ampoule containing naloxone 400microgram/mL to 10mL with 0.9% saline for injection
- administer 0.5mL (20microgram) IV every 2min until the patient's respiratory status is satisfactory
- further boluses may be necessary because naloxone is shorter-acting than morphine (and other opioids).

Cholestatic pruritus
- to avoid or minimize an opioid withdrawal-like syndrome, start with a sub-optimal dose of naloxone by CIVI, e.g. 0.002microgram/kg/min (about 160–200microgram/24h[18]
- provided no withdrawal-like symptoms occur, the rate can be doubled every 3–4h
- after 18–24h, when a rate known to be associated with opioid antagonistic effects is reached (0.2microgram/kg/min), the infusion is stopped and **naltrexone** 12.5mg t.i.d. or 25mg b.i.d. is started[17,18]
- the dose is escalated over a few days until a satisfactory clinical response is obtained; at this stage the effective dose should be consolidated into a single daily maintenance dose
- the effective dose range for **naltrexone** is 25–250mg daily.[18]

Supply
Naloxone hydrochloride (generic)
Injection 400microgram/mL, 1mL amp = $14, 10mL amp = $128; 1mg/mL, 2mL amp = $39.

---

1 Shipton EA (2000) Tramadol–present and future. *Anaesthesia and Intensive Care.* **28**: 363–374.
2 Marquardt KA *et al.* (2005) Tramadol exposures reported to statewide poison control system. *Annals of Pharmacotherapy.* **39**: 1039–1044.
3 Kreek MJ *et al.* (1983) Naloxone, a specific opioid antagonist, reverses chronic idiopathic constipation. *Lancet.* **i**: 261–262.
4 Peters WP *et al.* (1981) Pressor effect of naloxone in septic shock. *Lancet.* **i**: 529–532.
5 Cohen RA and Coffman JD (1980) Naloxone reversal of morphine-induced peripheral vasodilatation. *Clinical Pharmacology and Therapeutics.* **28**: 541–544.
6 Baskin DS and Hosobuchi Y (1981) Naloxone reversal of ischaemic neurological deficits in man. *Lancet.* **ii**: 272–275.
7 Bousigue J-Y *et al.* (1982) Naloxone reversal of neurological deficit. *Lancet.* **ii**: 618–619.
8 Ray D and Tai Y (1988) Infusions of naloxone in thalamic pain. *British Medical Journal.* **296**: 969–970.
9 Gan T *et al.* (1997) Opioid-sparing effects of a low-dose infusion of naloxone in patient-administered morphine sulfate. *Anesthesiology.* **87**: 1075–1081.
10 Joshi G *et al.* (1999) Effects of prophylactic nalmefene on the incidence of morphine-related side effects in patients receiving intravenous patient-controlled analgesia. *Anesthesiology.* **90**: 1007–1011.
11 Crain S and Shen K (2000) Antagonists of excitatory opioid receptor functions enhance morphine's analgesic potency and attenuate opioid tolerance/dependence liability. *Pain.* **84**: 121–131.
12 Sjogren P *et al.* (1994) Disappearance of morphine-induced hyperalgesia after discontinuing or substituting morphine with other opioid agonists. *Pain.* **59**: 313–316.
13 Bergasa N *et al.* (1992) A controlled trial of naloxone infusions for the pruritus of chronic cholestasis. *Gastroenterology.* **102**: 544–549.
14 Bergasa N *et al.* (1995) Effects of naloxone infusions in patients with the pruritus of cholestasis. *Annals of Internal Medicine.* **123**: 161–167.
15 Carson K *et al.* (1996) Pilot study of the use of naltrexone to treat the severe pruritus of cholestatic liver disease. *American Journal of Gastroenterology.* **91**: 1022–1023.
16 Wolfhagen F *et al.* (1997) Oral naltrexone treatment for cholestatic pruritus: A double-blind, placebo-controlled study. *Gastroenterology.* **113**: 1264–1269.
17 Jones E and Dekker L (2000) Florid opioid withdrawal-like reaction precipitated by naltrexone in a patient with chronic cholestasis. *Gastroenterology.* **118**: 431–432.
18 Jones E *et al.* (2002) Opiate antagonist therapy for the pruritus of cholestasis: the avoidance of opioid withdrawal-like reactions. *Quarterly Journal of Medicine.* **95**: 547–552.
19 Partridge BL and Ward CF (1986) Pulmonary oedema following low-dose naloxone administration. *Anesthesiology.* **65**: 709–710.
20 Pallasch TJ and Gill CJ (1981) Naloxone associated morbidity and mortality. *Oral Surgery.* **52**: 602–603.
21 Smith G and Pinnock C (1985) Editorial: naloxone–paradox or panacea? *British Journal of Anaesthesia.* **57**: 547–549.
22 Cleary J (2000) Incidence and characteristics of naloxone administration in medical oncology patients with cancer pain. *Journal of Pharmaceutical Care in Pain and Symptom Control.* **8**: 65–73.
23 Max MB *et al.* (1992) *Principles of Analgesic Use in the Treatment of Acute Pain and Cancer Pain* (3e). American Pain Society, Skokie, Illinois, p. 12.

NALTREXONE

Class: Opioid antagonist.

Indications: Prevention of relapse in opioid ex-addicts, treatment of alcohol dependence, †pruritus associated with cholestasis[1,2] and, possibly, chronic renal failure.[3,4]

Contra-indications: Patients currently dependent on opioids; acute hepatitis or hepatic failure.

Pharmacology

Naltrexone is a specific opioid antagonist with actions similar to those of **naloxone**.[5] Thus, it reversibly blocks the pharmacological effects of opioids at μ, κ and δ-opioid receptors. Compared with **naloxone**, naltrexone has a higher PO bio-availability, and a longer duration of action. Naltrexone is well absorbed from the GI tract but undergoes extensive first-pass metabolism.[6,7] It is extensively metabolized in the liver and the major metabolite, 6-β-naltrexol, may also possess weak antagonist activity. Naltrexone and its metabolites are excreted mainly in the urine. Less than 1% of an oral dose of naltrexone is excreted unchanged.[8]

In former drug addicts, naltrexone 100mg blocks the effect of a challenge of IV **diamorphine** (**heroin**; not available medicinally in Canada) 25mg:
- 96% at 24h
- 86% at 48h
- 46% at 72h.[9]

Thus, naltrexone is primarily used to prevent relapse in opioid ex-addicts by blocking the opioid 'high'. It is given PO, generally once daily or three times a week. In the USA and UK, naltrexone is also available as a long-acting depot IM injection with a duration of action of >1 month; this is approved for use only in alcoholics. In the UK, it is also available as an unlicensed SC pellet implant in private addiction clinics; the pellet has a duration of action of weeks to months.[10,11]

Naltrexone is also used to treat cholestatic pruritus (see below).[1,2] However, orally administered opioid antagonists can precipitate a transient opioid withdrawal-like reaction in patients with cholestasis, including hallucinations and dysphoria.[12,13] To avoid or minimize such a reaction, treatment must be started cautiously with a sub-optimal low dose. In an open study of patients with various skin and systemic disorders associated with pruritus, good relief was obtained with naltrexone in 70% of patients.[14] However, in the absence of controlled data, the results should be interpreted with caution. The use of naltrexone to relieve cholestatic jaundice may sometimes unmask or exacerbate underlying pain, necessitating discontinuation of naltrexone.[15]

The use of naltrexone will severely impede opioid analgesia.[16] The long-term use of naltrexone also increases the concentration of opioid receptors in the CNS and results in a temporary enhanced response to the subsequent administration of opioid analgesics.[17] The management of acute pain or postoperative pain in patients receiving long-term naltrexone requires careful consideration and detailed planning (Box 5.R).[16] Conversely, ultra-low-dose naltrexone has been shown to potentiate the analgesic effect of **methadone**, and decrease undesirable effects.[18] Although of considerable interest, such use can at present be recommended only within a formal study.

Bio-availability 5–40% PO.

Onset of action may start to precipitate withdrawal symptoms in <5min in opioid-dependent patients.

Time to peak plasma concentration 1–2h PO, IM.

Plasma halflife 4h; 13h for 6-β-naltrexol.[19]

Duration of action 1–3 days.

Cautions

Opioid withdrawal-like syndrome in patients with cholestatic pruritus. Hepatic and renal impairment. Occasional hepatotoxicity;[20] the manufacturers advises checking LFTs before and at intervals during treatment.

Undesirable effects

For full list, see manufacturer's Product Monograph.

Very common (>10% in detoxifying opioid addicts): insomnia, anxiety, nervousness, intestinal colic, nausea and vomiting, low energy, joint and muscle pain, headaches.

Dose and use
Cholestatic pruritus

If administered after initial naloxone infusion, see p.344.

If *de novo*:
- start with 12.5mg b.i.d. (some centres start with 1mg daily)
- increase after 3 days to 25mg b.i.d./50mg daily
- escalate slowly over several weeks
- the effective dose range is 25–250mg daily.[13]

Uremic pruritus
- start with 50mg daily[3,4]
- if ineffective after 1 week, consider increasing dose to 100mg daily.

Supply

ReVia® (Apotex)

Tablets 50mg scored, 28 days @ 50mg daily = $156.

Box 5.R Management of acute pain in patients receiving naltrexone

Elective surgery

The use of naltrexone must be identified well before the operation.

Ensure effective liaison between the substance misuse and acute pain teams.

Discontinue PO naltrexone 72h before the operation.[a]

When possible use non-opioid analgesics, e.g. acetaminophen and/or an NSAID.

Anticipate that greater than usual doses of opioid may be required; conversely be aware of the potential for an increased response.

Unexpected severe acute pain, e.g. trauma, emergency surgery

If possible use non-opioid analgesics, e.g.:

- acetaminophen and/or an NSAID
- ketamine 100microgram/kg IV every 5min until satisfactory analgesia obtained, plus a single dose of midazolam 20–40microgram/kg IV to minimize dysphoria; may be repeated after 30min; give further midazolam only if dysphoria present
- clonidine 1microgram/kg IV every 5min until satisfactory analgesia is obtained, up to a total dose of 4microgram/kg; may be repeated after 4h. (Note: in Canada, clonidine injection is available only through the Special Access Programme).

Note: there is a risk of marked sedation when ketamine and midazolam are combined in this way; to be used only by those competent in airway management.

In patients with no veins, clonidine and ketamine can be given SC; use the same doses as for IV but allow 15min between doses.

The above are generally used to achieve rapid pain relief until other measures can be instituted, e.g.:

- local anesthetic blocks
- epidural analgesia (local anesthetic ± clonidine).

---

a. in countries where depot injections and SC pellet implants are available, patients on depot injections can be switched to PO naltrexone before elective surgery, so that discontinuation is easier. SC pellet implants can be removed 72h before major surgery. For minor surgery, an implant can be left in place if it is anticipated that non-opioids will adequately relieve any postoperative pain.

---

1 Carson K et al. (1996) Pilot study of the use of naltrexone to treat the severe pruritus of cholestatic liver disease. *American Journal of Gastroenterology.* **91**: 1022–1023.
2 Wolfhagen F et al. (1997) Oral naltrexone treatment for cholestatic pruritus: A double-blind, placebo-controlled study. *Gastroenterology.* **113**: 1264–1269.
3 Peer G et al. (1996) Randomised crossover trial of naltrexone in uraemic pruritus. *Lancet.* **348**: 1552–1554.
4 Pauli-Magnus C et al. (2000) Naltrexone does not relieve uremic pruritus. *Journal of the American Society of Nephrology.* **11**: 514–519.
5 Verebey K et al. (1976) Naltrexone: disposition, metabolism and effects after acute and chronic dosing. *Clinical Pharmacology and Therapeutics.* **20**: 315–328.
6 Gonzalez J and Brogden R (1988) Naltrexone: a review of its pharmacodynamic and pharmacokinetic properties and therapeutic efficacy in the management of opioid dependence. *Drugs.* **35**: 192–213.
7 Crabtree B (1984) Review of naltrexone: a long-acting opiate antagonist. *Clinical Pharmacy.* **3**: 273–280.
8 Wall M et al. (1981) Metabolism and disposition of naltrexone in man after oral and intravenous administration. *Drug Metabolism and Disposition.* **9**: 369–375.
9 Verebey K (1981) The clinical pharmacology of naltrexone: pharmacology and pharmacodynamics. *NIDA Research Monograph.* **28**: 147–158.
10 Volpicelli JR et al. (1992) Naltrexone in the treatment of alcohol dependence. *Archives of General Psychiatry.* **49**: 876–880.
11 Swift RM et al. (1994) Naltrexone-induced alterations in human ethanol intoxication. *American Journal of Psychiatry.* **151**: 1463–1467.
12 Jones E and Dekker L (2000) Florid opioid withdrawal-like reaction precipitated by naltrexone in a patient with chronic cholestasis. *Gastroenterology.* **118**: 431–432.
13 Jones E et al. (2002) Opiate antagonist therapy for the pruritus of cholestasis: the avoidance of opioid withdrawal-like reactions. *Quarterly Journal of Medicine.* **95**: 547–552.

---

14 Metze D *et al.* (1999) Efficacy and safety of naltrexone, an oral opiate receptor antagonist, in the treatment of pruritus in internal and dermatological diseases. *Journal of the American Academy of Dermatology.* **41**: 533–539.

15 McRae CA *et al.* (2003) Pain as a complication of use of opiate antagonists for symptom control in cholestasis. *Gastroenterology.* **125**: 591–596.

16 Vickers AP and Jolly A (2006) Naltrexone and problems in pain management. *British Medical Journal.* **332**: 132–133.

17 Yoburn BC *et al.* (1988) Upregulation of opioid receptor subtypes correlates with potency changes of morphine and DADLE. *Life Sciences.* **43**: 1319–1324.

18 Cruciani RA *et al.* (2003) Ultra-low dose oral naltrexone decreases side effects and potentiates the effect of methadone. *Journal of Pain and Symptom Management.* **25**: 491–494.

19 Gutstein H and Akil H (2001) Opioid analgesics. In: J Hardman *et al.* (eds) *Goodman & Gilman's The Pharmacological Basis of Therapeutics* (10e). McGraw-Hill, New York; London.

20 Mitchell J (1986) Naltrexone and hepatotoxicity. *Lancet.* **I**: 1215.

6: INFECTIONS

ANTIBACTERIALS IN PALLIATIVE CARE

Many hospitals have antibacterial policies which govern local infection control practice and treatment, e.g. the prevention of methicillin-resistant *Staphylococcus aureus* (MRSA) infection. When in doubt, obtain advice from a microbiologist or infection control clinician.

Infections with strains of *Escherichia coli* and other Gram-negative bacilli which are resistant to several antibacterials are increasing. Some are resistant to **gentamicin**, quinolones and cephalosporins, as well as other antibacterials.[1]

This possibility should be considered in patients with recurrent urinary or biliary tract sepsis. Appropriate specimens (including blood cultures) should be taken and any previous microbiology reviewed. If a multiresistant isolate has been identified previously, e.g. a **gentamicin**-resistant coliform in urine, treatment must be discussed with a microbiologist because the usual first-line treatment may not be appropriate.

The information given in this chapter is limited to several common situations in palliative care, or to occasional events which demand decisive immediate action, such as:
- local infection causing severe pain (see below)
- acute inflammatory episodes (AIEs) in patients with lymphedema (see p.358)
- ascending cholangitis associated with a biliary stent (see p.364).

General considerations
Stop and think! In a moribund patient with progressive incurable disease, are you justified in giving antibacterials for an intercurrent infection which may be a natural part of the dying process?

In one survey, 25% of patients with advanced cancer and definite infection died within 1 week of starting antibacterials, and a further 25% died within a week of completing a course of antibacterials.[2] Other surveys give comparable short survival times.[3,4]

It has been claimed that the use of antibacterials for *symptomatic* infection (which implies a conscious patient) does *not* prolong survival (and thereby prolong the process and distress of dying).[5] Antibacterials are seen as offering the possibility of ameliorating distressing symptoms (including fever and malaise), and thus can be seen as an integral part of symptom management. Even so, it is important *to stop and think.* If there is an automatic 'reflex' to prescribe antibacterials when infection is diagnosed, it is possible that antibacterials will be overprescribed, and dying prolonged.[6]

Several surveys give similar prevalence rates for symptomatic infection in *conscious* palliative care/hospice patients, namely about 40%,[5] and show that the response to antibacterials varies according to the site of infection (Table 6.1). Provided a patient does not have an indwelling urinary catheter, UTIs should generally be treated routinely unless there is an overriding reason for not doing so (see p.357).[2,5] Cough caused by infection is also significantly reduced by antibacterials.[2] On the other hand, the use of antibacterials to treat bacteremia in a patient with *end-stage* progressive disease would appear to be futile (Table 6.1).

Table 6.1 Response to antimicrobials[a] in >600 home care patients[5]

Type of infection	Number	Response (%)[b]
UTI	265	79
RTI	221	43
Oral cavity[a]	63	46
Skin or SC	59	41
Bacteremia	25	0

a. includes the use of antibacterials for infections at all sites, and of antifungals for oropharyngeal candidosis
b. reduction of fever ± amelioration of site-specific symptoms within 3 days.

> The choice of antibacterials to treat infections tends to be governed by local guidelines. Any specific recommendations about antibacterials in *PCF* should be reviewed at least annually with a local infectious disease specialist.

Antibacterials to relieve infection-related pain

Antibacterials are essential in some patients for the relief of severe pain associated with infection around a malignant tumour in, for example, the neck, the gluteal muscles underlying an ulcerated malignancy, or the perineum.[7] Sometimes there is a history of a rapid increase in pain intensity over several days which is poorly responsive to escalating doses of a strong opioid. The pain is often associated with fever and malaise, and may be complicated by delirium. Commonly, there will be a mixture of more superficial aerobic infection with deeper anaerobic infection. Treatment is similar to that recommended for ascending cholangitis (see p.364).

Respiratory tract infection in the imminently dying patient

Occasionally, death rattle (noisy respiratory secretions) is caused by profuse purulent sputum from a chest infection, and an antibacterial is prescribed in the hope that it will reduce the copious purulent malodorous discharge from the mouth.[8] In this circumstance, a straightforward regimen is needed.

Some centres use single doses of **ceftriaxone**; either 1–2g IV or 1g IM mixed with **lidocaine** 1% (total injection volume 4mL).[8] **Ceftriaxone** is a broad-spectrum antibiotic and has a long duration of action. Patients who responded did so within hours (marked reduction in purulent sputum and resolution of associated halitosis). Non-responders appeared not to benefit from a second dose after 24h.

Other centres give **ceftriaxone** by SC injection[9,10] and administer multiple doses if a patient survives >1 day, e.g. **ceftriaxone** 1g mixed with **lidocaine** 1% 2.2mL (a total of 2.8mL) 250mg–1g SC once daily. If a larger volume of **lidocaine** is added, e.g. 3.3mL (a total of 4mL), the mixture can be administered as a divided dose, given at the same time but using two or more separate SC/IM sites[11] (see manufacturer's Product Monograph for additional information and guidance).

A study in volunteers has shown that the bio-availability of **cefepime** SC is comparable with the IM route.[12] Further, when 1g is infused over 30min, pain at the injection site is absent or minimal. Thus, **cefepime** could be a better option. Concern about the safety of **cefepime**[13] has so far been shown to be groundless.[14]

1 D'Agata EM (2004) Rapidly rising prevalence of nosocomial multidrug-resistant, Gram-negative bacilli: a 9-year surveillance study. *Infection Control and Hospital Epidemiology.* **25**: 842–846.
2 Mirhosseini M *et al.* (2006) The role of antibiotics in the management of infection-related symptoms in advanced cancer patients. *Journal of Palliative Care.* **22**: 69–74.
3 Clayton J *et al.* (2003) Parenteral antibiotics in a palliative care unit: prospective analysis of current practice. *Palliative Medicine.* **17**: 44–48.
4 Brabin E and Allsopp L (2008) How effective are parenteral antibiotics in hospice patients? *European Journal of Palliative Care.* **15**: 115–117.
5 Reinbolt RE *et al.* (2005) Symptomatic treatment of infections in patients with advanced cancer receiving hospice care. *Journal of Pain and Symptom Management.* **30**: 175–182.
6 Lam PT *et al.* (2005) Retrospective analysis of antibiotic use and survival in advanced cancer patients with infections. *Journal of Pain and Symptom Management.* **30**: 536–543.
7 Bruera E and MacDonald N (1986) Intractable pain in patients with advanced head and neck tumors: a possible role of local infection. *Cancer Treatment Reports.* **70**: 691–692.

8 Spruyt O and Kausae A (1998) Antibiotic use for infective terminal respiratory secretions. *Journal of Pain and Symptom Management.* **15**: 263–264.

9 Borner K et al. (1985) Comparative pharmacokinetics of ceftriaxone after subcutaneous and intravenous administration. *Chemotherapy.* **31**: 237–245.

10 Bricaire F et al. (1988) [Pharmacokinetics and tolerance of ceftriaxone after subcutaneous administration]. *Pathologie Biologie (Paris).* **36**: 702–705.

11 Tahmasebi M (2005) Is there any possibility for injecting antibiotics subcutaneously? In: *Bulletin board.* Palliativedrugs.com Ltd. Available from: www.palliativedrugs.org/forum/read.php?f=1&i=8124&t=8016

12 Walker P et al. (2005) Subcutaneous administration of cefepime. *Journal of Pain and Symptom Management.* **30**: 170–174.

13 Yahav D et al. (2007) Efficacy and safety of cefepime: a systematic review and meta-analysis. *The Lancet Infectious Diseases.* **7**: 338–348.

14 FDA (2009) Cefepime (marketed as Maxipime) update of ongoing safety review. Available from: www.fda.gov/Safety/MedWatch/SafetyInformation/SafetyAlertsforHumanMedicalProducts/ucm167427.htm

OROPHARYNGEAL CANDIDOSIS

Invasive (systemic) fungal disease is a complication of cytotoxic chemotherapy. However, its treatment is not dealt with here.[1]

Oral yeast carriage is present in about 1/3 of the general population. The prevalence in patients with advanced cancer is higher, sometimes nearly 90%.[2] Thus, it is not surprising that oropharyngeal candidosis is a common fungal infection in the palliative care population of patients.[3] In fact, almost all patients with AIDS have symptomatic oropharyngeal candidosis.[4]

Most cancer and AIDS patients with oropharyngeal candidosis also have concurrent esophageal infection.[5]

Oral candidosis is associated with:
• poor physical performance status
• dry mouth
• dentures.[6,7]
• in AIDS with CD4 cell count < 200cells/mm^3.[8]

In relation to antibacterials (both topical and systemic) and corticosteroids (both inhaled and systemic), published data are equivocal.[6,7]

Candida albicans probably accounts for about 75% of the infections, and *Candida glabrata* for most of the rest.[3] *C. albicans* is inherently sensitive to antifungal drugs, but can acquire resistance to the azoles, whereas *C. glabrata* is inherently resistant to azoles.

Management strategy
Correct the correctable
Underlying causal factors must be considered and corrected if possible, particularly dry mouth and poor denture hygiene.

Dentures must be thoroughly cleaned at least once daily using an appropriate antiseptic, e.g. 0.12% **chlorhexidine**, or 0.5% **sodium hypochlorite** (Dakin's solution). They should also be soaked overnight in antiseptic, e.g. dilute **sodium hypochlorite**; failure to do this leads to treatment failure.

Dentures can also be sterilized by boiling in water in a domestic microwave oven for 5–10min.[9] However, some dentures contain metal, and some plastics are hardened by microwaves and thus may become deformed. Accordingly, *PCF* does *not* recommend the use of microwaves for this purpose.

Chlorhexidine inactivates **nystatin**[10] and, if used with **nystatin**, the dentures must be thoroughly rinsed before re-insertion. In other circumstances, **chlorhexidine** mouthwashes can be used as an adjunctive antimicrobial treatment.[11]

Drug treatment
Oral candidosis generally responds to topical treatment, e.g. with **nystatin**. A systematic review concluded that there is no difference in efficacy between topical and systemic treatments.[12] When efficacy, lack of resistance, and cost are all taken into account, **nystatin** is clearly the antifungal drug of choice for oral candidosis in non-immunocompromised patients.

On the other hand, because they are more convenient (once daily administration), many patients are treated systemically with an azole antifungal, e.g. **fluconazole** or **ketoconazole**. Further, in AIDS, azoles are generally regarded as the treatment of choice.[8,13] However, organisms resistant to one or more azole do occur. The prevalence of resistant organisms in one group of palliative care patients has been reported as:

- **itraconazole** 22%
- **fluconazole** 8%
- **ketoconazole** 7%
- **amphotericin** 2%
- **nystatin** 0%.[2]

In practice, patients who have *not* received multiple courses of azoles will probably be sensitive to this group of drugs *unless the causal yeast is C. glabrata*.[14] However, cross-resistance and cross-infection do occur and, if there is a high prevalence of azole resistance within the local patient population, then even azole-naïve patients may be infected with azole-resistant organisms. Local treatment protocols must take such factors into account.

Relapse is more common with **ketoconazole** and **clotrimazole** (PO formulation not Canada) than with **fluconazole** and **itraconazole**, but the latter two drugs are more expensive.[15]

Fluconazole achieves a higher clinical and mycological response rate than **ketoconazole** in AIDS patients.[8,13] Even with the most intractable forms of AIDS-associated *Candida*, a response is generally seen in <10 days with 50mg/day or <5 days with 100–200mg/day.[16,17] In cases of **fluconazole** resistance, **itraconazole** is recommended.[18] Response rates in HIV+ patients are 97% for **itraconazole** solution and 87% for **fluconazole**.[19]

Because azole antifungals act by inhibiting cytochrome P450-dependent production of the main fungal cell membrane component, ergosterol, they also have an inhibitory effect on human cytochrome P450 enzymes (see p.551). This results in inhibition of adrenal steroid synthesis (cortisol, testosterone, estrogens and progesterone) and of the metabolism of many drugs. Drug interactions are most likely with **ketoconazole** and **itraconazole**. They are generally less likely and less pronounced with **fluconazole** (a weaker CYP inhibitor), although several clinically important interactions have been reported with all three drugs.[20]

Topical oral **nystatin** 5mL q.i.d. is necessary in patients with azole-resistant infections. Other potential topical treatments include gentian violet[21] (e.g. 0.5–1%, 1.5mL applied twice daily) and tea tree oil.[22]

Cautions

Serious drug interactions: through inhibition of various cytochrome P450 enzymes (particularly CYP3A4), azoles produce clinically important increases in the serum levels of many drugs (see Cytochrome P450, p.551). Avoid concurrent administration of **itraconazole** or **ketoconazole** with **pimozide** or **quinidine** because of a risk of fatal cardiac arrhythmias.

Fluconazole, **itraconazole** or **ketoconazole** increases the toxic/undesirable effects of **alfentanil, carbamazepine, dexamethasone, digoxin, glipizide, glyburide, methylprednisolone, midazolam, nifedipine, phenytoin, theophylline**, TCAs, and **warfarin**.

Strong CYP3A4 inducers, e.g. **carbamazepine, phenytoin** and **rifampin**, reduce **fluconazole**, **itraconazole**, and **ketoconazole** serum levels, which may result in antifungal treatment failure.

Itraconazole may cause or worsen left ventricular dysfunction or CHF.

Renal impairment: reduce dose of **fluconazole** by 50% if creatinine clearance is <50mL/min; do not use **itraconazole** if creatinine clearance is <30mL/min.

Hepatic impairment: serious or fatal hepatotoxicity has very rarely occurred with **fluconazole**, **itraconazole**, and **ketoconazole**, sometimes in patients with no obvious risk factors for liver disease. With **itraconazole** and **ketoconazole**, some cases have arisen within 1 week–1 month of starting treatment, and with **ketoconazole** the risk increases with duration of treatment. Accordingly, the UK manufacturer has restricted its recommended indications for **ketoconazole**, and advises that courses longer than 10 days should be given only after fully considering the likely benefit-risk ratio. With prolonged courses, both the UK and Canadian manufacturers advise monitoring liver function before starting treatment, 2 and 4 weeks after starting treatment, and monthly thereafter. The UK manufacturers of **fluconazole** and **itraconazole** advise further monitoring if raised LFTs are detected during treatment. With all 3 drugs, treatment should be discontinued if symptoms suggestive of hepatotoxicity develop, e.g. jaundice, dark urine.

The systemic absorption of **ketoconazole** is markedly reduced in hypochlorhydric states. Thus, absorption is impaired in patients with AIDS-related hypochlorhydria, and in those taking antacids, an H_2-receptor antagonist or a PPI. Likewise with **sucralfate** (has a weak antacid effect) or buffered **didanosine** (a nucleoside reverse transcriptase inhibitor used in AIDS);[22] separating the time of administration of these two drugs by $\geq$2h from **ketoconazole** reduces the interaction.[20]

In hypochlorhydria, absorption from **itraconazole** capsules is variable but from the oral solution absorption is reliable and bio-availability is higher. Absorption is improved by taking **itraconazole** or **ketoconazole** with an acidic drink, e.g. cola. The absorption of **fluconazole** is not affected by antacids, H_2-receptor antagonists or **sucralfate**.[20]

Undesirable effects

For full list, see manufacturer's Product Monograph.

Common (<10%, >1%): headache (azole antifungals), dizziness (**fluconazole** and **itraconazole**), GI symptoms, i.e. dyspepsia, nausea and vomiting, abdominal pain, diarrhea (**fluconazole** and **itraconazole**), rashes, pruritus, hypokalemia (**fluconazole** and **itraconazole**).

Uncommon, rare or very rare (<1%): anaphylaxis, hepatitis, cholestasis, hepatic failure, adrenal suppression (**itraconazole**), reduced libido, gynecomastia, impotence, menstrual disturbances.

Dose and use

Most patients respond to a 10-day course but some need continuous treatment. Symptomatic relief often occurs within 2–3 days. In AIDS, particularly if the infection extends to the esophagus, higher doses for a longer period are generally necessary (Table 6.2).

Table 6.2 Summary of antifungal treatment recommendations[a]

Class	Drug	Recommended regimen	Comments
Polyene group	Nystatin	Oral suspension 100,000 units/mL; 5mL q.i.d. held in the mouth for 1min, and then swallowed	Necessary to remove dentures before each dose, and clean before re-insertion
Azole group (Tiazoles)	Fluconazole	Capsules 150mg; tablets 50mg, 100mg; oral suspension 50mg/5mL; recommendations vary, e.g. 50mg once daily for 1 week, *but 2 weeks if dentures are worn*, or 100mg once daily for 2–4 weeks if immunocompromised (sometimes 100–200mg daily indefinitely is needed).	Best absorbed on an empty stomach
		Some regimens include a stat (loading) dose of 200mg, followed by 100mg once daily for $\geq$2 weeks. If debilitated and short prognosis, consider a single dose of 150mg	
	Itraconazole	Capsules 100mg; oral solution 10mg/mL; 100mg once daily for 2 weeks but 200mg once daily if immunocompromised	
Azole group (Imidazoles)	Ketoconazole	Tablets 200mg; 1 tablet once daily for 1–2 weeks; if response inadequate, increase to 2 tablets once daily and continue until 1 week after cultures become negative	Suspension can be compounded[23]

a. see relevant manufacturer's Product Monograph.

The use of locally prepared **nystatin** popsicles is sometimes helpful; 5mL of **nystatin** suspension is mixed with blackcurrant or other fruit juice concentrate and frozen in an ice tray with small rounded cups.

Systemic agents are more convenient than **nystatin**, more suitable when candidosis involves the esophagus, and obviate the need for denture removal at each administration (although denture cleaning remains important; see Correct the correctable above).

To help reduce the tablet burden in patients with a prognosis of 1–2 weeks, consider **fluconazole** 150mg stat or **ketoconazole** 200mg once daily for 5 days. If not immuno-suppressed, most patients respond *clinically* but about 1/3 relapse.[24] (Note: the study on which these recommendations are based did not include microbiological tests.)

At some centres, extended courses of **fluconazole** 50mg once daily are given for patients with a major risk factor.

Supply

Nystatin (generic)
Oral suspension 100,000 units/mL, 14 days @ 5mL q.i.d. = $15.

Fluconazole (generic)
Capsules 150mg, single dose 150mg = $10.
Tablets 50mg, 100mg, 7 days @ 100 mg once daily = $39.

Diflucan® (Pfizer Canada)
Capsules 150mg, single dose 150mg = $16.
Oral solution (powder for reconstitution) 50mg/5mL, single dose 150mg = $37; 7 days @ 100mg once daily = $73.

Ketoconazole (generic)
Tablets 200mg, 7 days @ 200mg once daily = $9.
Oral suspension can be compounded from crushed tablets.[23]

Itraconazole
Sporanox® (Janssen-Ortho)
Capsules 100mg, 14 days @ 100mg once daily = $60.
Oral solution 10mg/mL, 14 days @ 100mg once daily = $124.

1 Leather H and Wingard J (2001) Infections following hematopoietic stem cell transplantation. *Infectious Disease Clinics of North America.* **15**: 483–520.
2 Davies A et al. (2002) Resistance amongst yeasts isolated from the oral cavities of patients with advanced cancer. *Palliative Medicine.* **16**: 527–531.
3 Finlay I and Davies A (2005) Fungal Infections. In: A Davies and I Finlay (eds) *Oral Care in Advanced Disease.* Oxford University Press, Oxford, pp. 55–71.
4 Patton LL et al. (2002) Prevalence and classification of HIV-associated oral lesions. *Oral Diseases.* **8 (suppl 2)**: 98–109.
5 Samonis G et al. (1998) Oropharyngeal candidiasis as a marker for esophageal candidiasis in patients with cancer. *Clinical Infectious Diseases.* **27**: 283–286.
6 Davies AN et al. (2006) Oral candidosis in patients with advanced cancer. *Oral Oncology.* **42**: 698–702.
7 Davies AN et al. (2008) Oral candidosis in community-based patients with advanced cancer. *Journal of Pain and Symptom Management.* **35**: 508–514.
8 Greenspan D (1994) Treatment of oropharyngeal candidiasis in HIV-positive patients. *Journal of the American Academy of Dermatology.* **31**: S51–S55.
9 Silva MM et al. (2006) Effectiveness of microwave irradiation on the disinfection of complete dentures. *International Journal of Prosthodontics.* **19**: 288–293.
10 Barkvoll P and Attramadal A (1989) Effect of nystatin and chlorhexidine digluconate on Candida albicans. *Oral Surgery Oral Medicine and Oral Pathology.* **67**: 279–281.
11 Ellepola AN and Samaranayake LP (2001) Adjunctive use of chlorhexidine in oral candidoses: a review. *Oral Diseases.* **7**: 11–17.
12 Worthington HV et al. (2007) Interventions for treating oral candidiasis for patients with cancer receiving treatment. *Cochrane Database Systematic Reviews.* **1**: CD001972.pub 001972.
13 DeWit S et al. (1989) Comparison of fluconazole and ketoconazole for oropharyngeal candidiasis in AIDS. *Lancet.* **1**: 746–748.
14 Bagg J et al. (2003) High prevalence of non-albicans yeasts and detection of anti-fungal resistance in the oral flora of patients with advanced cancer. *Palliative Medicine.* **17**: 477–481.
15 Vazquez J (1999) Options for the management of mucosal candidiasis in patients with AIDS and HIV infection. *Pharmacotherapy.* **19**: 76–87.
16 Hay R (1990) Overview of studies of fluconazole in oropharyngeal candidiasis. *Reviews of Infectious Diseases.* **2 (suppl 3)**: S334–S337.
17 Darouiche R (1998) Oropharyngeal and esophageal candidiasis in immunocompromised patients: treatment issues. *Clinical Infectious Diseases.* **26**: 259–274.

18 Martin M (1999) The use of fluconazole and itraconazole in the treatment of *Candida albicans* infections: a review. *Journal of Antimicrobial Chemotherapy*. **44**: 429–437. [Erratum (2000). 45:555.]

19 Graybill J et al. (1998) Randomized trial of itraconazole oral solution for oropharyngeal candidiasis in HIV/AIDS patients. *American Journal of Medicine*. **104**: 33–39.

20 Baxter K (ed) (2008) *Stockley's Drug Interactions* (8e). Pharmaceutical Press, London.

21 Nyst MJ et al. (1992) Gentian violet, ketoconazole and nystatin in oropharyngeal and esophageal candidiasis in Zairian AIDS patients. *Annales de la Societe Belge de Medecine Tropicale*. **72**: 45–52.

22 Piscitelli S et al. (1996) Drug interactions in patients infected with human immuno-deficiency virus. *Clinical Infectious Diseases*. **23**: 685–693.

23 Allen L (1993) Ketoconazole oral suspension. *US Pharmacist*. **18**: 98 & 101.

24 Regnard C (1994) Single dose fluconazole versus five day ketoconazole in oral candidiasis. *Palliative Medicine*. **8**: 72–73.

METRONIDAZOLE

Class: Antibacterial and antiprotozoal.

Indications: Anaerobic and protozoal infections, *Helicobacter pylori* gastritis (see p.367), †malodour caused by anaerobic infection, †pseudomembranous colitis (see *Clostridium difficile* diarrhea, p.364).

Pharmacology
Metronidazole is highly active against anaerobic bacteria and protozoa. Although it has no activity against aerobic organisms *in vitro*, in mixed infections *in vivo* both aerobes and anaerobes appear susceptible. Unlike most other antibacterials, resistance to metronidazole among anaerobes is uncommon. Metronidazole can be applied topically to malodorous fungating cancers and decubitus ulcers.[1,2] The malodour is caused by volatile fatty acids produced by anaerobic bacteria.
Tinidazole (not Canada) is similar to metronidazole with a longer duration of action; it causes less GI disturbance but costs more.[3]
Bio-availability 100% PO; 60–80% PR; 20% PV.
Onset of action 20–60min PO; 5–12h PR.
Time to peak plasma concentration 1–2h PO; 3h PR.
Plasma halflife 6–11h.
Duration of action 8–12h.

Cautions
Metronidazole precipitates a **disulfiram**-like reaction with alcohol in ≤24% of patients.[4,5] Like **disulfiram**, metabolites of metronidazole inhibit alcohol dehydrogenase, xanthine oxidase and aldehyde dehydrogenase. Inhibition of alcohol dehydrogenase leads to activation of microsomal enzyme oxidative pathways, generating ketones and lactate which may cause acidosis.[6] Xanthine oxidase inhibition can lead to norepinephrine excess.[6] Accumulation of acetaldehyde is probably responsible for most of the symptoms, e.g. flushing of the face and neck, headaches, epigastric discomfort, nausea and vomiting, and a fall in blood pressure.

Patients should be warned that if they drink alcohol when taking metronidazole they may have an unpleasant reaction, although generally this is little more than mild anorexia. However, the occasional patient may vomit profusely. In one patient, nausea and vomiting occurred during concurrent treatment with PO metronidazole and an alcohol-containing mouthwash, some of which the patient swallowed rather than spitting out.[7] The risk of a reaction with metronidazole PV is small because absorption is low.[8]

Undesirable effects
For full list, see manufacturer's Product Monograph.
Nausea and vomiting, unpleasant taste, furred tongue, GI disturbance. May cause darkening of urine; anaphylaxis has been reported.

Dose and use
Tablets should be taken with or after food.

Anaerobic infections

Metronidazole 500mg PO t.i.d. for 2 weeks; 500mg PO b.i.d. in elderly debilitated patients; 500mg PO once daily if significant hepatic impairment.

Re-treat for 2 weeks if malodour or other symptoms and signs of infection recur, then continue indefinitely with 250mg b.i.d.

Ascending cholangitis (see p.364)

Metronidazole 500mg PO q8h and **cefuroxime** 1,500mg IV q8h. Generally taken by mouth, but if the patient is not able to take tablets may need to be given IV (with **cefuroxime**).

Fungating tumours

Metronidazole 0.75 and 1% gel is commercially available and should be applied topically liberally.[1,2,9,10] Some centres use a crushed 250mg tablet in lubricating gel.[11] The dose from a crushed tablet is several times greater than that from commercial products. The higher dose may have an observable impact (reduced odour) within 1 day compared with several days for commercial products, and is significantly cheaper. However, the lower concentration has been shown to be effective.[12,13]

Clostridium difficile infection (see p.364)
Helicobacter pylori gastritis (see p.367)

Supply

Metronidazole (generic)
Capsules 500mg, 7 days @ 500mg t.i.d. = $13.
Tablets 250mg, 7 days @ 500mg t.i.d. = $2.50.
IV infusion 5mg/mL, 100mL = $2.

Flagyl® 500 S-Pak (Sanofi-Aventis Canada)
Capsules 500mg, 7 days @ 500mg t.i.d. = $22.

Topical products
MetroGel® (Galderma)
Gel 0.75%, 60g = $39; 1%, 60g = $39.

Nidagel® (Graceway)
Vaginal gel 0.75%, 70g = $21.

Flagyl (Sanofi-Aventis Canada)
Vaginal cream 10%, 60g = $15.

1 Newman V et al. (1989) The use of metronidazole gel to control the smell of malodorous lesions. Palliative Medicine. **3**: 303–305.
2 Editorial (1990) Management of smelly tumours. Lancet. **335**: 141–142.
3 Carmine AA et al. (1982) Tinidazole in anaerobic infections: a review of its antibacterial activity, pharmacological properties and therapeutic efficacy. Drugs. **24**: 85–117.
4 deMattos H (1968) Relations between alcoholism and the gastrointestinal system. Experience using metronidazole. [In Portuguese]. Hospital (Rio J). **74**: 1669–1676.
5 Penick S et al. (1969) Metronidazole in the treatment of alcoholism. American Journal of Psychiatry. **125**: 1063–1066.
6 Harries D et al. (1990) Metronidazole and alcohol: potential problems. Scottish Medical Journal. **35**: 179–180.
7 Dickman A (2007) Personal communication.
8 Plosker G (1987) Possible interaction between ethanol and vaginally administered metronidazole. Clinical Pharmacy. **6**: 189–193.
9 Ashford R et al. (1984) Double-blind trial of metronidazole in malodorous ulcerating tumours. Lancet. **1**: 1232–1233.
10 Thomas S and Hay N (1991) The antimicrobial properties of two metronidazole medicated dressings used to treat malodorous wounds. Pharmaceutical Journal. **246**: 264–266.
11 Twycross R et al. (2009) Symptom Management in Advanced Cancer (4e). palliativedrugs.com, Nottingham, p. 344.
12 Bower M et al. (1992) A double-blind study of the efficacy of metronidazole gel in the treatment of malodorous fungating tumours. European Journal of Cancer. **28A**: 888–889.
13 Finlay IG et al. (1996) The effect of topical 0.75% metronidazole gel on malodorous cutaneous ulcers. Journal of Pain and Symptom Management. **11**: 158–162.

URINARY TRACT INFECTIONS

Infections with strains of *Escherichia coli* and other Gram-negative bacilli which are resistant to several antibacterials are increasing. Some are resistant to **gentamicin**, quinolones and cephalosporins, as well as other antibacterials.[1]

This possibility should be considered in patients with recurrent urinary sepsis. Appropriate specimens (including blood cultures) should be taken and any previous microbiology reviewed. If a multiresistant isolate has been identified previously, e.g. a **gentamicin**-resistant coliform in urine, treatment must be discussed with a microbiologist because the usual first-line treatment may not be appropriate.

Urinary tract infections (UTIs) are more common in women than in men. *E. coli* is the most common cause of UTI. Less common causes include *Proteus* and *Klebsiella spp. Pseudomonas aeruginosa* infections are generally associated with functional or anatomical abnormalities of the renal tract. *Staphylococcus epidermidis* and *Enterococcus faecalis* infection may complicate catheterization or instrumentation. Whenever possible, a specimen of urine should be collected for culture and sensitivity testing before starting antibacterial treatment.

Management strategy

Use a urine testing strip for nitrite and leucocytes to decide if a patient has a UTI. This is cost-effective and the result is available immediately (Box 6.A). If a UTI is suspected clinically and supported by the urine testing strip results:

- send a urine sample for culture and sensitivity (C&S)
- start empirical treatment with **trimethoprim** 100mg PO b.i.d.
- if systemically unwell, consider IV **cefuroxime** and/or IV **gentamicin** (see Product Monographs for dose regimens).

Recommendations vary in relation to duration of antibacterial treatment from 3 days for an uncomplicated UTI in a woman to 10–14 days for children, men, and women with fever and/or loin pain.

Bacterial colonization is normal in catheterized patients and is not necessarily harmful; it should *not* be investigated unless symptomatic.

Box 6.A   Using urine testing strips to diagnose urinary tract infections

Use urine testing strips that measure urinary pH and specific gravity, and the presence and amount of:

- glucose
- ketone
- blood
- protein
- nitrite, a bacterial metabolite
- leucocytes, produced by inflammation/infection

How to do the test

- take a mid-stream specimen of urine
- dip the strip into the urine and remove immediately
- after 60sec read nitrite result   the colours on the strips should be
- after 2min read the leucocyte result   compared with the bottle colours.

Late readings are of no value

Significance of the results

- nitrite and leucocyte positive: infection probable; send urine specimen for C&S
- nitrite only or leucocyte only positive: infection possible; urine specimen for C&S advisable
- nitrite and leucocyte negative: infection unlikely; no need to send urine specimen for C&S unless definite urinary tract symptoms.

For patients who are about to be decatheterized, antibacterial treatment for 2 days before removal significantly reduces the risk of post-catheter bacteriuria.[2]

Trimethoprim 300mg as a single-dose treatment is useful in debilitated patients, resulting in a 74 and 71% cure rate when re-tested 1 and 6 weeks later.[3,4]

Alternative approaches
These include the use of urinary antiseptics, i.e. **methenamine mandelate** (see p.412), **nitrofurantoin** (see p.412) and **cranberry juice** (see p.415).

Supply
Trimethoprim (generic)
Tablets 100mg, 200mg, 10 days @ 100mg b.i.d. = $6.

Cefuroxime (generic)
Injection (powder for reconstitution) 750mg, 1.5g, 2 days @ 1.5g t.i.d. = $192.

1 D'Agata EM (2004) Rapidly rising prevalence of nosocomial multidrug-resistant, Gram-negative bacilli: a 9-year surveillance study. *Infection Control and Hospital Epidemiology.* **25**: 842–846.
2 Hustinx W *et al.* (1991) Impact of concurrent antimicrobial therapy on catheter-associated urinary tract infection. *Journal of Hospital Infection.* **18**: 45–56.
3 Bailey R and Abbott G (1978) Treatment of urinary tract infection with a single dose of trimethoprim-sulfamethoxazole. *Canadian Medical Association Journal.* **118**: 551–552.
4 Brumfitt W *et al.* (1982) Comparative trial of trimethoprim and co-trimoxazole in recurrent urinary infections. *Infection.* **10**: 280–284.

ACUTE INFLAMMATORY EPISODES IN A LYMPHEDEMATOUS LIMB

Acute inflammatory episodes (AIEs), often called cellulitis, are common in lymphedema:
- mild: pain, increased swelling, erythema (well-defined or blotchy)
- severe: extensive erythema with well-defined margins, increased swelling, blistering and weeping skin; often accompanied by fever, nausea and vomiting, pain and, when the leg is affected, difficulty in walking.[1]

Management strategy
Preventive measures
Patients should be educated about:
- why they are susceptible to AIEs, i.e. skin crevices harbour bacteria, stagnant fluid, reduced immunity[2]
- the consequences of AIEs, i.e. increased swelling, more fibrosis, decreasing response to treatment for reducing limb size
- the importance of daily skin care, i.e. to improve and maintain skin integrity. Risk factors include cracked or macerated interdigital skin, dermatitis, limb wounds (including leg ulcers), and weeping lymphangiectasia (leaking lymph blisters on the skin surface)
- reducing risk, for example, by reducing the swelling, protecting hands when gardening, cleaning cuts, treating fungal infections (**terbinafine** cream once daily for 2 weeks) and ingrowing toenails[3]
- the importance of seeking prompt medical attention and treatment; in situations when accessing medical care may be difficult, e.g. vacations, provide a 2-week supply of **amoxicillin** 500mg q8h (**clindamycin** 300mg q6h for those allergic to penicillin) to patients who had had an AIE in the past.

Non-drug treatment
- compression garments should not be worn until the limb is comfortable
- daily skin hygiene should be continued; washing and gentle drying

- emollients should not be used in the affected area if the skin is broken
- if severe, bed rest is essential with the affected limb elevated in a comfortable position and supported on pillows.[3,4]

Drug treatment

It is often difficult to isolate the responsible pathogen, and AIEs should be treated promptly with 'best guess' antibacterials to prevent increased morbidity from increased swelling and accelerated fibrosis (see Guidelines, p.362).

Although cellulitis in a non-lymphedematous limb is commonly caused by *Staphylococcus aureus*, most AIEs are probably caused by Group A *Streptococci*.[1,5-7] Recommendations about the choice of antibacterials based on those of the British Lymphology Society are summarized in Table 6.3. Similar recommendations have been published elsewhere.[8,9]

Regardless of variation in drug availability, antibacterial resistance, and local prescribing policies, it is essential that all centres treating patients with lymphoedema establish local guidelines for managing AIEs which are easily accessible for all relevant health professionals It is crucial that policy makers are aware that the most likely pathogen is *Streptococcus*, and not *Staphylococcus*.[10] However, *Staphylococcus aureus* should be suspected if there is folliculitis, pus formation, and crusted dermatitis.

The advice of a microbiologist or other local expert should be obtained in unusual circumstances, e.g. an AIE developing shortly after an animal lick or bite, and when the inflammation fails to respond to the recommended antibacterials.

Remember: AIEs are painful: analgesics should be prescribed regularly and p.r.n.

Supply

Amoxicillin (generic)
Capsules 250mg, 500mg, 14 days @ 500mg t.i.d. = $15.
Tablets (chewable) 125mg, 250mg, 14 days @ 500mg t.i.d. = $69.
Oral suspension 125mg/5mL, 250mg/5mL, 14 days @ 500mg t.i.d. = $23.

Penicillin G (benzylpenicillin) sodium
Crystapen® (Alveda Pharmaceuticals)
Injection (powder for reconstitution) (5,000,000 units/vial), 7 days @ 1.2g (2,000,000 units) q6h = $57; *contains* Na^+ 250mg/5 million units vial.

Penicillin V (phenoxymethylpenicillin) potassium (generic)
Tablets 300mg (500,000 units), 14 days @ 600mg q.i.d. = $8.
Oral solution (powder for reconstitution) 300mg (500,000 units)/5mL, 14 days @ 600mg q.i.d. = $35.

Gentamicin (generic)
Injection gentamicin (as sulfate) 10mg/mL, 2mL amp = $4; 40mg/mL, 2mL amp = $5.

Cloxacillin (generic)
Capsules 250mg, 500mg, 14 days @ 500mg t.i.d. = $31.
Oral suspension 125mg/5mL, 14 days @ 500mg t.i.d. = $38.

Clindamycin (generic)
Capsules clindamycin (as hydrochloride) 150mg, 300mg 14 days @ 150mg daily or 300mg q.i.d. = $7 and $55 respectively.
Injection clindamycin (as phosphate) 150mg/mL, 2mL amp, 4mL amp, 6mL amp, 7 days @ 600mg q.i.d. = $373.

Dalacin C® (Pfizer Canada)
Capsules clindamycin (as hydrochloride) 150mg, 300mg, 14 days @ 150mg daily or 300mg q.i.d. = $14 and $113 respectively.
Oral solution (granules for reconstitution) clindamycin (as 2-palmitate hydrochloride) 75mg/5mL, 14 days @ 300mg q.i.d. = $149.
Injection clindamycin (as phosphate) 150mg/mL, 2mL amp, 4mL amp, 6mL amp, 7 days @ 600mg q.i.d. = $482.

Table 6.3 Antibacterials for AIEs[a] (based on the recommendations of the British Lymphology Society, www.lymphoedema.org/bls)

Situation	First-line antibacterials	If allergic to penicillin	Second-line antibacterials	Comments
Acute AIE + septicemia (inpatient admission)	Cloxacillin 2g IV q8h[b] or penicillin G 1.2–2.4g (2–4 million units) IV q6h[c]	Clindamycin 600mg IV q8h[11]	Clindamycin 600mg IV q8h (if poor or no response by 48h)[12]	Switch to cloxacillin 500mg q8h or clindamycin 300mg q6h when: • temperature down for 2 days • inflammation much resolved • falling CRP. Then continue as below
Acute AIE (home care)	Amoxicillin or cloxacillin 500mg q8h	Clindamycin 300mg q6h	Clindamycin 300mg q6h. If fails to resolve, convert to IV regimen in row 1 above	Give for a minimum of 2 weeks. Continue antibacterials until the acute inflammation has completely resolved; this may take 1–2 months
Prophylaxis if 2+ AIEs per year	Penicillin V potassium 600mg once daily for 2 years (1.2g if weight >75kg)	Erythromycin or clarithromycin 250mg once daily	Clindamycin 150mg once daily or clarithromycin 250mg once daily	After 1 year, halve the dose of penicillin V; if an AIE develops after discontinuation, treat the acute episode and then commence life-long prophylaxis
Emergency supply of antibacterials in case of need when away from home	Amoxicillin or cloxacillin 500mg q8h	Clindamycin 300mg q6h	If fails to resolve, or patient becomes generally unwell (e.g. fever, malaise, nausea), convert to IV regimen in row 1 above	

a. administered PO unless stated otherwise
b. UK guidelines recommend IV amoxicillin, but this is not available in Canada
c. add gentamicin 5mg/kg IV once daily for 1 week if the anogenital region is involved; dose adjusted according to renal function.

Erythromycin (generic)
***Capsules enclosing EC granules* erythromycin** 250mg, 14 days @ 250mg once daily = $6.
***Tablets* erythromycin** (as stearate) 250mg, 500mg, 14 days @ 250mg once daily = $3.
***Tablets* erythromycin** 250mg, 14 days @ 250mg once daily = $3.
***Oral suspension* erythromycin** (as ethyl succinate) 200mg/5mL, 400mg/5mL, 14 days @ 250mg once daily = $6.

EryC® (Pfizer Canada)
***Capsules enclosing EC granules* erythromycin** 250mg, 14 days @ 250mg once daily = $8.

Novo-Rythro® Estolate (Novopharm)
***Oral suspension* erythromycin** (as estolate) 125mg/5mL, 250mg/5mL, 14 days @ 250mg once daily = $5.

Clarithromycin (generic)
Tablets 250mg, 500mg, 14 days @ 250mg once daily = $16.

Biaxin® (Abbott)
Tablets 250mg, 500mg, 14 days @ 250mg once daily = $25.
Oral suspension (granules for reconstitution) 125mg/5mL, 250mg/5mL, 14 days @ 250mg once daily = $64.

Terbinafine
Lamisil® (Novartis Pharmaceuticals Canada)
Cream 1%, 30g tube = $17.

1 Mortimer P (2000) Acute inflammatory episodes. In: RG Twycross et al. (eds) Lymphoedema. Radcliffe Medical Press, Oxford, pp. 130–139.
2 Mallon E et al. (1997) Evidence for altered cell-mediated immunity in postmastectomy lymphoedema. British Journal of Dermatology. **137**: 928–933.
3 Twycross R et al. (2000) Lymphoedema. Radcliffe Medical Press, Oxford.
4 Twycross R et al. (2009) Symptom Management in Advanced Cancer (4e). palliativedrugs.com, Nottingham, pp. 312–316.
5 Sabouraud R (1892) Sur la parasitologie de l'elephantiasis nostras. Annales de dermatologie et de syphiligraphie. **3**: 592.
6 Stevens FA (1954) The behavior of local foci causing recurrent streptococcal infections of the skin, subcutaneous tissues, and lymphatics. Surgery, Gynecology and Obstetrics. **99**: 268–272.
7 Chambers J and McGovern K (2004) Dental work as a cause of acute inflammation of a lymphoedematous limb. Palliative Medicine. **18**: 667–668.
8 Harris SR et al. (2001) Clinical practice guidelines for the care and treatment of breast cancer: 11. Lymphedema. Canadian Medical Association Journal. **164**: 191–199.
9 CREST (Clinical Resource Efficiency Support Team) (2008) Guidelines for the diagnosis, assessment and management of lymphoedema. Available from: www.crestni.org.uk/crest_guidelines_on_the_diagnosis__assessment_and_management_of_lymphoedema.pdf
10 Badger C et al. (2004) Antibiotics/anti-inflammatories for reducing acute inflammatory episodes in lymphoedema of the limbs. Cochrane Database Systematic Reviews. CD003143.
11 Bisno AL and Stevens DL (1996) Streptococcal infections of skin and soft tissues. New England Journal of Medicine. **334**: 240–245.
12 Blondel-Hill E and Fryters S (eds) (2006) Bugs & Drugs (online edition) Capital Health. Edmonton. Available from: www.bugsanddrugs.ca/bugs_drugs_website/web-content/COMBINED_BandD2006_certified.pdf

Guidelines: Acute inflammatory episodes (AIEs) in lymphedema

AIEs, often called cellulitis, are common in lymphedema. They are often associated with septicemia (e.g. fever, flu-like symptoms, hypotension, tachycardia, delirium, nausea and vomiting). It may be difficult to identify the infective agent, but *Streptococcus* is the mostly likely pathogen.

Evaluation

1 Clinical features
- mild: pain, increased swelling, erythema (well-defined or blotchy)
- severe: extensive erythema with well-defined margins, increased swelling, blistering and weeping skin; often accompanied by fever, nausea and vomiting, pain and, when the leg is affected, difficulty in walking.

2 Diagnosis is based on pattern recognition and clinical judgement. The following information should be solicited:
- present history: date of onset, precipitating factor (e.g. insect bite or trauma), treatment received to date
- past history: details of previous AIEs, precipitating factors, antibacterials taken
- examination: include sites of lymphatic drainage to and from inflamed area.

3 Establish a baseline
- extent and severity of rash: if well demarcated outline with pen and date
- level of systemic upset: temperature, pulse, BP, CRP, white cell count
- swab cuts or breaks in skin for microbiology before starting antibacterials.

4 Arrange admission to hospital for patients with septicemia or who deteriorate or fail to improve despite antibacterials.

Antibacterials

5 It is often difficult to isolate the causal pathogen. However, to prevent increased swelling and accelerated fibrosis, AIEs should be treated promptly with antibacterials *for a minimum of 2 weeks*. Continue antibacterials until the acute inflammation has completely resolved; this may take 1–2 months.

6 The advice of a microbiologist should be obtained when the inflammation fails to respond to the recommended antibacterials, or in unusual circumstances, e.g. an AIE developing shortly after an animal bite.

7 Standard treatment at home (PO):

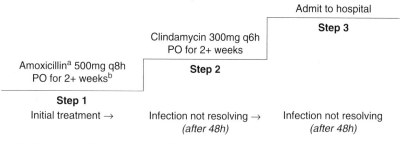

a. if a history of penicillin allergy, start on Step 2
b. add cloxacillin 500mg q6h if features suggest *Staphylococcus aureus* infection, e.g. folliculitis, pus, crusted dermatitis.

continued

8 Standard treatment in hospital (IV): choice of antibacterials may vary with local policy. Switch to PO amoxicillin or clindamycin when no fever for 2 days, inflammation settling and CRP falling (see **7** above).

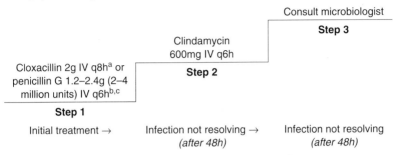

Consult microbiologist

Step 3

Clindamycin
600mg IV q6h

Step 2

Cloxacillin 2g IV q8h[a] or
penicillin G 1.2–2.4g (2–4
million units) IV q6h[b,c]

Step 1

Initial treatment →   Infection not resolving →   Infection not resolving
                   (after 48h)   (after 48h)

a. UK guidelines recommend IV amoxicillin, but this is not available in Canada
b. if a history of penicillin allergy, start on Step 2
c. add gentamicin 5mg/kg IV daily for 1 week if the anogenital region is involved; dose adjusted according to renal function.

9 If ⩾2 AIEs/year, review skin condition and skin care regimen, and consider further steps to reduce limb swelling. Start antibacterial prophylaxis with:
- penicillin V potassium 600mg (1.2g in those >75kg) once daily for 2 years; halve the dose after 1 year if no recurrence
- if allergic to penicillin, use erythromycin or clarithromycin 250mg once daily
- if an AIE develops despite antibacterials, switch to clindamycin 150mg or clarithromycin 250mg once daily
- if an AIE develops after discontinuation of antibacterials after 2 years, treat the acute episode, and then commence life-long prophylaxis.

General

10 Remember:
- if severe, bed rest and elevation of the affected limb on pillows is essential
- AIEs are painful; analgesics should be prescribed regularly and p.r.n.
- because of a possible association between skin infections, NSAIDs and necrotizing fasciitis, acetaminophen and opioids are the preferred analgesics
- compression garments should not be worn until limb is comfortable
- daily skin hygiene should be continued; washing and gentle drying
- emollients should not be used in the affected area if the skin is broken.

11 Patients should be educated about:
- why they are susceptible to AIEs, i.e. skin crevices harbour bacteria, stagnant fluid, reduced immunity
- the consequence of AIEs, i.e. increased swelling, more fibrosis, decreased response to treatment
- the importance of daily skin care, i.e. to improve and maintain skin integrity
- reducing risk, for example, by reducing the swelling, protecting hands when gardening, cleaning cuts, treating fungal infections (terbinafine cream once daily for 2 weeks) and ingrowing toenails
- obtaining prompt medical attention if an AIE occurs and, if a history of AIEs, taking a 2-week supply of amoxicillin 500mg q8h (clindamycin 300mg q6h if allergic to penicillin) for emergency use when away from home.

ASCENDING CHOLANGITIS

Infections with strains of *Escherichia coli* and other Gram-negative bacilli which are resistant to several antibacterials are increasing. Some are resistant to **gentamicin**, quinolones and cephalosporins, as well as other antibacterials.[1]

This possibility should be considered in patients with recurrent biliary tract sepsis. Appropriate specimens (including blood cultures) should be taken and any previous microbiology reviewed. If a multiresistant isolate has been identified previously, treatment must be discussed with a microbiologist as the usual first-line treatment may not be appropriate.

Ascending cholangitis may occur in patients with a partially obstructed or stented common bile duct. It often causes severe systemic disturbance and should be treated promptly with antibacterials.

Treatment

Ascending cholangitis should be treated with a combination of an appropriate cephalosporin and **metronidazole** (see p.355):
- **cefuroxime** 1,500mg IV q8h for 2 days (volume of injection = 6mL)
- **metronidazole** 500mg IV q8h (or PO with or after food).

If IV administration is difficult, alternatives include:
- **ceftazidime** 1g IM q8h, diluted in 3mL WFI or 0.5–1% **lidocaine hydrochloride** solution
- **cefepime** 1g SC q8h diluted in 2.4mL of either 0.9% saline, 5% glucose (dextrose), WFI, or 0.5–1% **lidocaine hydrochloride** solution (see p.350).

In addition:
- if the patient is in septic shock, give a single dose of **gentamicin** 5mg/kg (maximum dose 500mg) IV over 20–30min
- if severe infection,; consider **ciprofloxacin** 400mg IV b.i.d. instead of **cefuroxime**, but reduce the dose by 50% in severe renal impairment (GFR < 20mL/min); discuss with a microbiologist.

Supply

Cefuroxime (generic)
Injection (powder for reconstitution) 750mg, 1.5g, 2 days @ 1.5g t.i.d. = $192.

Cefepime
Maxipime® (Bristol-Myers Squibb Canada)
Injection (powder for reconstitution) 1g, 2g, 2 days @ 1g q8h = $101.

Ceftazidime (generic)
Injection (powder for reconstitution) 1g, 2g, 6g, 2 days @ 1g t.i.d. = $149.

Fortaz® (GSK)
Injection (powder for reconstitution) 1g, 2g, 6g, 2 days @ 1g t.i.d. = $145.

Also see **Metronidazole**, p.355.

---

1 D'Agata EM (2004) Rapidly rising prevalence of nosocomial multidrug-resistant, Gram-negative bacilli: a 9-year surveillance study. *Infection Control and Hospital Epidemiology.* **25**: 842–846.

CLOSTRIDIUM DIFFICILE INFECTION

Clostridium difficile infection is a complication of antibacterial treatment, particularly broad-spectrum antibacterials. A pseudomembranous colitis develops in severe cases (Box 6.B), with sloughing of the inflamed colonic epithelium. This manifests as foul-smelling diarrhea mingled with mucus and blood. *C. difficile* infection has a mortality of up to 25% in elderly frail patients.[1]

Box 6.B *Clostridium difficile* infection

Causal antibacterials[2]

Highest risk
Cephalosporins (second/third generation)
Clindamycin
Fluoroquinolones

Medium risk
Amoxicillin/ampicillin
Co-amoxiclav
Macrolides

Low risk
Aminoglycosides
Benzylpenicillin
Piptazobactam
Tetracyclines
Trimethoprim
Vancomycin

Clinical features
Watery diarrhea + mucus ± blood
Abdominal pain and tenderness ± tenesmus
Fever and malaise
± Nausea, vomiting, and anorexia
± Dehydration and delirium
± Leukocytosis

Symptoms generally begin within 1 week of starting antibacterial treatment or shortly after stopping, but may occur up to 2 months later.[3] It is caused by colonization of the GI tract by *C. difficile* and the production of toxins A and B which cause the mucosal damage. A failure to mount an immune response is associated with colonization and toxin production. The main risk factors for *C. difficile* infection are:
• old age
• long inpatient stay in hospital (1% incidence if <1 week; 50% if >4 weeks)[4]
• antibacterial use, particularly prolonged treatment or multiple antibacterials.
These and other risk factors are listed in Box 6.C.

Box 6.C Risk factors for *Clostridium difficile* infection

Patient-related factors
Age >65 years
Previous infection with *C. difficile*

Underlying disease states
Cancer
COPD
Renal failure
Immunosuppression

Treatment-related factors
Prolonged hospitalization
GI procedures (non-surgical or surgical)
Nasogastric tubes
PPIs
Radiation therapy

Antibacterial use
Prolonged duration of antibacterial therapy
Use of high and medium risk antibacterials (see Box 6.B)

C. difficile is spread indirectly by the fecal-oral route by spores left on surfaces:
• asymptomatic colonization in the general population is about 5%
• asymptomatic colonization in hospital and nursing home populations may be ≤30%[3]
• in about 33% of those colonized, *C. difficile* produces diarrhea-producing toxins.[5]

Diagnosis

- a high level of suspicion in high-risk patients who develop diarrhea, e.g. > 300mL of liquid feces in 1 day or two to six loose stools in 36h; however, the use of opioids, including **diphenoxylate** and **loperamide**, may modify the clinical picture, particularly in mild–moderate cases
- *C. difficile* is strongly anaerobic and difficult to culture; most laboratories no longer attempt to culture it
- diagnosis is confirmed by the detection in the feces of toxins produced by *C. difficile*
- if in doubt, endoscopy and rectal biopsy may be of value, but endoscopy identifies pseudomembranous colitis in only about 50% of cases confirmed by laboratory criteria (a positive culture for *C difficile* and a positive fecal cytotoxin test)[6]
- a trial of therapy may be the most practical way of confirming the diagnosis.

Management strategy

Preventive measures

Spread of *C. difficile* is by the ingestion of spores from the environment around symptomatic patients. Environmental controls ('universal precautions') will generally prevent the spread of outbreaks:

- patients should be isolated while they have diarrhea, and have their own dedicated commode
- carers should use gloves and gowns, and thoroughly wash their hands after patient contact using antibacterial soap and water
- areas where there are patients with *C. difficile* should be thoroughly cleaned using chlorine disinfectants.[7]

Antibacterial prescribing policies should aim to minimize the use of broad-spectrum antibacterials, and to regulate treatment duration.[2,7]

Drug treatment

Metronidazole PO is the treatment of choice; it is as effective as **vancomycin**[8,9] for mild-moderate infections, and much cheaper.[10] IV **metronidazole** has been used in patients unable to take oral formulations, but treatment failures have occurred.[3]

Vancomycin must be given PO or PR, because it is not secreted into the GI tract after IV administration.[11] It is generally reserved for:

- patients with an ileus
- patients more severely ill, e.g. WBC > 20,000[10]
- patients unable to tolerate **metronidazole** or being treated with alcohol-containing solutions (see p.355)
- non-responders to **metronidazole**.

Most patients show some symptom improvement in <2 days, e.g. reduction of fever. However, resolution of diarrhea may take ⩽6 days.[12] Other antibacterials are sometimes used.[11]

About 20% of patients relapse, most ⩽3 weeks.[10] This may be caused by germination of residual spores within the colon, re-infection with *C. difficile* (50% of recurrences are caused by infection with a new strain)[13] or further antibacterial treatment:

- mild relapses often resolve spontaneously, but repeat treatment with **metronidazole** is recommended[10,14]
- repeated relapses require prolonged treatment with a slowly decreasing dose of **vancomycin**, e.g. over 6 weeks:[13]
  ▷ week 1, 125mg q.i.d.
  ▷ week 2, 125mg b.i.d.
  ▷ week 3, 125mg once daily
  ▷ week 4, 125mg every other day
  ▷ week 5 and 6, 125mg every 3 days
- this latter intermittent therapy allows spores to germinate on 'antibiotic −' days with subsequent destruction on 'antibiotic +' days
- some centres add rifampicin 300mg PO b.i.d. for 10–14 days.[12]

Relapse because of resistance of *C. difficile* to antibacterial treatment is rare.[15] Probiotics may reduce the incidence of relapse, but are not used routinely.[16,17]

Dose and use
- **metronidazole** 500mg PO t.i.d. for 10–14 days[10,13]
- **vancomycin**:
  - ▷ PO 125mg q.i.d. for 10–14 days[10,12] *or*
  - ▷ if very severe (e.g. toxic megacolon), administer by intracolonic (rectal) route: dissolve 500mg–1g in 1L 0.9% saline, administer 250mL via a rectal tube and clamp for 3h, repeat q6h.[12,13]

Supply
See **Metronidazole**, p.356.

Vancomycin (generic)
Injection (powder for reconstitution) 500mg, 1g vial = $33 and $63 respectively.

Vancomycin injection can be used to prepare an oral solution; add 10mL WFI to a 500mg vial of powder and give 2.5mL (125mg) q.i.d. diluted with water or fruit juice (other than grapefruit), 10-day course = $333.

1 Pepin J et al. (2004) Clostridium difficile-associated diarrhea in a region of Quebec from 1991 to 2003: a changing pattern of disease severity. *Canadian Medical Association Journal*. **171**: 466–472.
2 Monaghan T et al. (2008) Recent advances in Clostridium difficile-associated disease. *Gut*. **57**: 850–860.
3 Fekety R (1997) Guidelines for the diagnosis and management of Clostridium difficile-associated diarrhea and colitis. American College of Gastroenterology, Practice Parameters Committee. *American Journal of Gastroenterology*. **92**: 739–750.
4 Johnson S et al. (1990) Nosocomial Clostridium difficile colonisation and disease. *Lancet*. **336**: 97–100.
5 Starr J (2005) Clostridium difficile associated diarrhoea: diagnosis and treatment. *British Medical Journal*. **331**: 498–501.
6 Gerding DN et al. (1995) Clostridium difficile associated diarrhoea and colitis. Clinical Practice Guidelines by the Society for Healthcare Epidemiology (SHEA) and the Infectious Diseases Society of America (ISDA). *Infection Control and Hospital Epidemiology*. **16**: 459–477. Available from: www.shea-online.org/Assets/files/position_papers/Cldiff95.PDF
7 Donaldson L and Beasley C (2005) Infection caused by Clostridium difficile. Letter from the Chief Medical Officer and Chief Nursing Officer. Department of Health. Available from: www.dh.gov.uk/en/Publicationsandstatistics/Lettersandcirculars/Professionalletters/Chiefmedicalofficerletters/DH_4125069
8 Cherry R et al. (1982) Metronidazole: an alternate therapy for antibiotic-associated colitis. *Gastroenterology*. **82**: 849–851.
9 Teasley D et al. (1983) Prospective randomized trial of metronidazole versus vancomycin for Clostridium difficile-associated diarrhoea and colitis. *Lancet*. **2**: 1043–1046.
10 Gilbert DN et al. (eds) (2008) *The Sanford guide to antimicrobial therapy 2008*. Antimicrobial Therapy Inc, Sperryville.
11 Durai R (2007) Epidemiology, pathogenesis, and management of Clostridium difficile infection. *Digestive Diseases and Sciences*. **52**: 2958–2962.
12 Blondel-Hill E and Fryters S (eds) (2006) *Bugs & Drugs* (online edition) Capital Health. Edmonton. Available from: www.bugsanddrugs.ca/bugs_drugs_website/web-content/COMBINED_BandD2006_certified.pdf
13 Malnick SD and Zimhony O (2002) Treatment of Clostridium difficile-associated diarrhea. *Annals of Pharmacotherapy*. **36**: 1767–1775.
14 Tabaqchali S and Jumaa P (1995) Diagnosis and management of Clostridium difficile infections. *British Medical Journal*. **310**: 1375–1380.
15 Bricker E et al. (2005) Antibiotic treatment for Clostridium difficile-associated diarrhea in adults. *Cochrane Database Systematic Reviews*. CD004610.
16 Surawicz CM et al. (2000) The search for a better treatment for recurrent Clostridium difficile disease: use of high-dose vancomycin combined with Saccharomyces boulardii. *Clinical Infectious Diseases*. **31**: 1012–1017.
17 Dendukuri N et al. (2005) Probiotic therapy for the prevention and treatment of Clostridium difficile-associated diarrhea: a systematic review. *Canadian Medical Association Journal*. **173**: 167–170.

HELICOBACTER PYLORI GASTRITIS

Helicobacter pylori infection of the stomach is ubiquitous, with a global prevalence of about 50% of the adult population. However, infection rates are uneven; it is more prevalent among low socio-economic groups and in developing countries. The prevalence in the Canadian general public is 20–40%, increasing with age.[1,2] Infection is generally acquired in childhood, and long-term infection predisposes to chronic gastritis, GI ulceration and subsequent gastric cancer.[3,4] Eradication of *H. pylori* with antibacterials and gastric acid suppressants (PPIs or H_2-receptor antagonists) is more cost-effective than acid suppression alone in relation to:
- relieving non-ulcer dyspepsia[5]
- healing peptic ulcers[6]
- preventing recurrent ulceration and bleeding.[7]

It is uncertain whether *H. pylori* eradication lowers the risk of gastric cancer.[2,8–14]

H. pylori-associated type B chronic atrophic gastritis facilitates the development of gastropathy during treatment with NSAIDs (see p.249), and eradication probably improves the GI safety of NSAIDs.[9,15] Thus testing for and eradicating *H. pylori* is important in patients starting regular NSAID treatment, particularly if they have dyspepsia, a history of ulceration or a high risk of ulceration (see Box 5.C, p.250).[2,14-16]

The benefit of eradication is debatable in patients with established ulcers who need to continue taking an NSAID or low-dose aspirin.[17] However, Canadian guidelines advise eradication in all *H. pylori*-positive patients with proven GI ulcers, even if NSAIDs are the likely cause.[2,13,14] In relation to ulcer healing, when given after discontinuing an NSAID in patients with NSAID-related bleeding peptic ulcer, eradication is no more effective than **omeprazole** alone.[17]

Management strategy

If possible, stop the NSAID

Patients on an NSAID who develop symptoms suggesting a GI ulcer should ideally stop taking the NSAID (or minimize the dose if this is not possible), be tested for *H. pylori* and receive eradication treatment if the test is positive.[2]

Test for H. pylori

For patients starting on regular NSAID treatment or those with symptoms suggestive of an *uncomplicated* ulcer (e.g. gnawing or burning epigastric pain, worse at night or when the stomach is empty, and relieved by food or antacids), non-invasive tests are appropriate. However, local availability of these tests varies across Canada:

- urea breath tests, the preferred option,[13,14] involve ingesting [13]C- or ^{14}C-labelled urea, which is broken down by *H. pylori* to produce ammonia and labelled CO_2. This is then detected in expired air. These tests have excellent specificity, sensitivity and reliability, and detect *active* infection.[2,14,18] They cost about $60, and are funded under some provincial medical plans. However, to avoid false-positive results, PPIs or H_2-receptor antagonists must be stopped 1–2 weeks before the test, and patients must fast for 6h immediately before[2,18]
- the serological antibody test is now regarded as less useful than urea breath tests, but is still widely used in Canada.[14] This test has specificity and sensitivity rates of 75–85% and cannot distinguish between present and past infection with *H. pylori*. It can give false-positive results, particularly when the prevalence of *H. pylori* in the population is low, e.g. in adults <45 years old[13,14]
- stool (fecal) antigen tests detect *H. pylori*-associated antigens in feces using specific antibodies. Although these tests detect *active* infection and have a specificity and sensitivity of >90% when performed accurately,[19] Canadian guidelines do not yet recommend them for diagnosing *H. pylori* in the community because of lack of data regarding their reliability when performed in non-specialist laboratories.[14] However, some provinces allow their use where available.[20]

An endoscopic examination and biopsy is recommended for patients with symptoms suggesting a *complicated* ulcer or gastric cancer (i.e. otherwise unexplained GI bleeding, iron-deficiency anemia, GI obstruction or mass, dysphagia, persistent vomiting, anorexia or weight loss, severe abdominal pain suggesting perforation, or suspicious barium meal, particularly if the patient is ≥50 years old).[2] Endoscopy is also recommended for patients >50 years old who have unexplained persistent dyspepsia alone.[13]

Eradicate the organism

Many *H. pylori* eradication regimens exist. With triple therapy (two antibacterials and a gastroprotective drug, generally a PPI) for 10–14 days, eradication is successful in 80–90% of patients if there is good adherence.[21] On the other hand, simpler regimens (one antibacterial and a PPI) have a success rate of <50% and an increased likelihood of antibacterial resistance.[22] Pharmaco-economic studies confirm that triple therapy is more cost-effective.[22] In patients with ulcer symptoms, resolution generally occurs in ≤1 week. In Canada, as in the UK, 1-week triple therapy regimens are recommended; eradication is achieved in about 85% of patients with fewer undesirable effects and greater adherence than 2-week regimens.[23]

The Canadian Helicobacter Study Group considers regimens which achieve an eradication rate of >80% suitable for first-line treatment, and currently recommends three main options (Box 6.D).[13,14] Other regimens are endorsed for use in specific circumstances, e.g. when a patient is allergic to a particular antibacterial, or when local resistance patterns govern choice.[13]

If first-line therapy is unsuccessful, susceptibility testing should be considered before selecting a second-line regimen.[14]

The quadruple therapy regimen was promoted to first-line status in Canada in 2004, after RCTs showed that it was as effective and well tolerated as triple therapy, and that adherence rates were similar despite the complexity of the quadruple regimen. Potential advantages are a lower susceptibility to emerging resistance and an improved cure rate because of the longer treatment duration.[14] However, in practice, there are reservations regarding adherence to this regimen, and hence the potential for eradication failure.[14] For palliative care patients, it also imposes a higher medication burden than triple therapy; it involves taking 14 tablets/capsules plus 120mL of liquid each day for up to 2 weeks. Thus, from a practical perspective, the 1-week triple therapy regimens are a more acceptable choice in the palliative care setting.

Box 6.D Canadian Helicobacter Study Group recommended eradication regimens for *Helicobacter pylori*[13,14]

Triple therapy regimens
Regimen 1
Three drugs are taken b.i.d. for 1 week:
- a standard-dose PPI (e.g. lansoprazole 30mg, omeprazole 20mg or pantoprazole 40mg)
- amoxicillin 1g
- clarithromycin 500mg.

Regimen 2 (suitable for patients allergic to penicillins)
Three drugs are taken b.i.d. for 1 week:
- a standard-dose PPI, as above
- clarithromycin 250mg or 500mg
- metronidazole 500mg.

Quadruple therapy regimen
Four drugs are taken for 10–14 days:
- a standard-dose PPI b.i.d., as above
- bismuth subsalicylate (Pepto-Bismol® oral liquid) 30mL q.i.d.; the chewable tablets are unsuitable because they contain calcium carbonate, which interferes with the absorption of tetracycline from the GI tract[24]
- metronidazole 500mg q.i.d.
- tetracycline 500mg q.i.d.

If necessary, confirm eradication

Patients with, or at high risk of, ulcer complications (e.g. perforation or bleeding) should be retested to confirm eradication, even if asymptomatic. Urea breath tests can be used, but are affected by antibacterials and PPIs. It is necessary to delay urea breath retesting for 4 weeks after finishing antibacterial-containing eradication regimens and 1 week after completing a course of PPIs. Stool antigen tests are used successfully for this purpose in other countries, e.g. the UK, but are awaiting validation in Canada. Serological testing does not help because antibodies persist long after *H. pylori* has been eradicated.[2,14,15]

Supply

For **lansoprazole** and **omeprazole**, see Proton pump inhibitors, p.21.
For **amoxicillin** and **clarithromycin**, see Acute inflammatory episodes, p.359.
For **metronidazole**, see p.356.

Tetracycline (generic)
Capsules 250mg, 10 or 14 days @ 500mg q.i.d. = $5 and $7 respectively.

Bismuth subsalicylate
Pepto-Bismol® (Procter and Gamble)
Oral liquid 17.6mg/mL, 10 or 14 days @ 30mL q.i.d. = $30 and $42 respectively.

Combination packs
HP-Pac® (TAP Pharmaceuticals)
Suitable for triple therapy regimen 1 (Box 6.D). Each pack contains *two doses* (i.e. 1 day's treatment). Each dose comprises one **lansoprazole** 30mg capsule, two **amoxicillin** 500mg capsules, and one **clarithromycin** 500mg tablet.
7 days @ 1 dose b.i.d. = $88.

1 Veldhuyzen van Zanten SJ et al. (1994) Increasing prevalence of Helicobacter pylori infection with age: continuous risk of infection in adults rather than cohort effect. *Journal of Infectious Diseases*. **169**: 434–437.

2 Hunt R and Thomson AB (1998) Canadian Helicobacter pylori consensus conference. Canadian Association of Gastroenterology. *Canadian Journal of Gastroenterology*. **12**: 31–41.

3 Czinn SJ (2005) Helicobacter pylori infection: detection, investigation, and management. *Journal of Pediatrics*. **146 (suppl)**: s21–26.

4 Guarner J (2004) The spectrum of gastric disease associated with Helicobacter pylori and other infectious gastritides. *Current Gastroenterology Reports*. **6**: 441–446.

5 Moayyedi P et al. (2005) Eradication of Helicobacter pylori for non-ulcer dyspepsia. *Cochrane Database Systematic Review*. **1**.

6 Ford A et al. (2003) Eradication therapy for peptic ulcer disease in Helicobacter pylori positive patients. *Cochrane Database Syst Rev*. **4**: CD003840.

7 Gisbert JP et al. (2004) H. pylori eradication therapy vs. antisecretory non-eradication therapy (with or without long-term maintenance antisecretory therapy) for the prevention of recurrent bleeding from peptic ulcer. *Cochrane Database Syst Rev*. **2**: CD004062.

8 McCormack K (1989) Mathematical model for assessing risk of gastrointestinal reactions to NSAIDs. In: K Rainsford (ed) *Azapropazone – over two decades of clinical use*. Kluwer Academic Publishers, Boston, pp. 81–93.

9 Becker JC et al. (2004) Current approaches to prevent NSAID-induced gastropathy – COX selectivity and beyond. *British Journal of Clinical Pharmacology*. **58**: 587–600.

10 Sung JJ (2004) Should we eradicate Helicobacter pylori in non-steroidal anti-inflammatory drug users? *Alimentary Pharmacology and Therapeutics*. **20 (suppl 2)**: 65–70.

11 Chang CC et al. (2005) Eradication of Helicobacter pylori significantly reduced gastric damage in nonsteroidal anti-inflammatory drug-treated Mongolian gerbils. *World Journal of Gastroenterology*. **11**: 104–108.

12 Di Leo V et al. (2005) Effect of Helicobacter pylori and eradication therapy on gastrointestinal permeability. Implications for patients with seronegative spondyloarthritis. *Journal of Rheumatology*. **32**: 295–300.

13 Hunt R et al. (1999) Canadian Helicobacter pylori Consensus Conference update: infections in adults. *Canadian Journal of Gastroenterology*. **13**: 213–217.

14 Hunt R et al. (2004) Canadian Helicobacter Study Group Consensus Conference: Update on the management of Helicobacter pylori–an evidence-based evaluation of six topics relevant to clinical outcomes in patients evaluated for H pylori infection. *Canadian Journal of Gastroenterology*. **18**: 547–554.

15 DTB (2005) H. pylori eradication in NSAID-associated ulcers. *Drug and Therapeutics Bulletin*. **43**: 37–40.

16 Hunt RH and Bazzoli F (2004) Review article: should NSAID/low-dose aspirin takers be tested routinely for H. pylori infection and treated if positive? Implications for primary risk of ulcer and ulcer relapse after initial healing. *Alimentary Pharmacology & Therapeutics*. **19 (suppl 1)**: 9–16.

17 Chan FK et al. (1998) Does eradication of Helicobacter pylori impair healing of nonsteroidal anti-inflammatory drug associated bleeding peptic ulcers? A prospective randomized study. *Alimentary Pharmacology and Therapeutics*. **12**: 1201–1205.

18 Fallone CA et al. (2000) The urea breath test for Helicobacter pylori infection: taking the wind out of the sails of endoscopy.[see comment]. *CMAJ Canadian Medical Association Journal*. **162**: 371–372.

19 Schenk BE et al. (2000) Effect of Helicobacter pylori eradication on chronic gastritis during omeprazole therapy. *Gut*. **46**: 615–621.

20 Guidelines and Protocols Advisory Committee (2003) Helicobacter pylori infection-detection and treatment in adult patients. British Columbia Medical Association and British Columbia Ministry of Health. Available from: www.bcguidelines.ca/gpac/pdf/hpylori.pdf

21 University of Michigan Health System (2005) Guidelines for Clinical Care. Peptic Ulcer Disease. Available from: cme.med.umich.edu/pdf/guideline/PUD05.pdf

22 ASHP (2001) Therapeutic position statement on the identification and treatment of Helicobacter pylori-associated peptic ulcer disease in adults. *American Journal of Health System Pharmacy*. **58**: 331–337.

23 BNF (2008) Section 1.3 Ulcer-healing drugs: Test for Helicobacter pylori. In: *British National Formulary* (No. 55). British Medical Association and Royal Pharmaceutical Society of Great Britain, London. Current BNF available from: www.bnf.org/bnf/bnf/current/.

24 Regier L (1999) H. pylori eradication regimens 1-2-3 cured. Available from: www.rxfiles.ca/rxfiles/uploads/documents/hpylori.pdf

7: ENDOCRINE SYSTEM AND IMMUNOMODULATION

BISPHOSPHONATES

Indications: Licensed indications vary between products; consult the manufacturers' Product Monographs for details; they include tumour-induced hypercalcemia, prophylactic use to reduce skeletal events associated with osteolytic lesions (multiple myeloma, metastatic cancer), prevention/treatment of osteoporosis, Paget's disease. Also used as an adjunct for †metastatic bone pain.[1]

Contra-indications: Creatinine clearance <30mL/min.

Pharmacology

The bisphosphonates are stable analogues of pyrophosphate, a naturally occurring regulator of bone metabolism. They have a high affinity for calcium ions, and bind rapidly to hydroxyapatite crystals in mineralized bone. Bisphosphonates are subsequently released and taken up by osteoclasts, interfering with their function and/or inducing their apoptosis (programmed cell death). Nitrogen-containing bisphosphonates (e.g. **pamidronate disodium, zoledronic acid**) inhibit the mevalonate pathway vital for normal cellular function (e.g. vesicular trafficking, cell signalling, cytoskeleton function) and non-nitrogen-containing bisphosphonates (**clodronate disodium, etidronate disodium**) form cytotoxic adenosine triphosphate (ATP) analogues.[2,3] These cellular effects also extend to macrophages, reducing the production of cytokines, and this anti-inflammatory effect may contribute to the analgesic effect of bisphosphonates.[4,5] Bisphosphonates interfere with the cancer-related increase in the number and activity of osteoclasts which cause bone pain by:

- producing an increasingly acidic environment (stimulating acid-sensing receptors on sensory nerves)
- destroying sensory nerves (producing neuropathic pain)
- causing mechanical instability as a result of the loss of bone mineral (stimulating mechanoreceptors on sensory nerves in the periosteum).[6]

In vitro and in animals, bisphosphonates also have a direct anticancer effect via inhibition of matrix metalloproteinase, altered cell adhesion, anti-angiogenic activity, reduction in release of local growth factors from bone and induction of apoptosis.[7,8] However, a cancer-promoting effect has been seen in some animal studies.[9] Bisphosphonates have no impact on the effect of parathyroid-related protein (PTHrP) or on renal tubular resorption of calcium.

Bisphosphonates are poorly absorbed PO and this is reduced further by food. They are rapidly taken up by the skeleton, particularly at sites of bone resorption and where the mineral is more exposed, and they remain there for weeks to months.[10] Most of the remainder is bound to plasma proteins. Bisphosphonates are not metabolized and are excreted unchanged via the kidneys. The plasma proportion of the drug is eliminated generally within 24h. Thereafter, elimination is much slower as the remainder gradually seeps out of bone.[11] Comparison of the halflives of different bisphosphonates is complicated by this multiphasic elimination. Other pharmacokinetic details are shown in Table 7.1.

Table 7.1 Bisphosphonates and the initial treatment of hypercalcemia[12,13]

	Zoledronic acid	Pamidronate disodium
IV dose	4mg	30–90mg
Onset of effect	<4 days	<3 days
Time to maximum effect	4–7 days	5–7 days
Duration of effect	4 weeks	2.5 weeks
Restores normocalcemia	90%	70–75%

Tumour-induced hypercalcemia

Bisphosphonates given IV are the treatment of choice for hypercalcemia of malignancy.[14] The initial response is higher with **zoledronic acid** (~90%) than with **pamidronate disodium** (~75%). A longer duration of response can be obtained with **zoledronic acid** compared with **pamidronate disodium**.[13] The Product Monograph for **pamidronate disodium** recommends a scale of doses depending on the initial *corrected* calcium concentration (see p.375), with higher doses for higher initial calcium concentrations. However, one systematic review suggests that 90mg (the maximum recommended dose) should always be given to increase the likelihood of a response, and prolong its duration.[14]

Prophylactic use in patients with myeloma or bone metastases

Pamidronate disodium and **zoledronic acid** IV given *long-term* decrease the incidence of new skeletal events in patients with bone metastases. Benefit is most evident for patients with breast cancer or myeloma and is less clear for other types of cancers.[15–20] Only studies ≥6 months in duration have shown a reduction in vertebral and non-vertebral fractures, hypercalcemia and the need for radiation therapy. Studies ≥2 years in duration have also shown a reduced need for orthopedic surgery. The incidence and severity of pain is reduced with an NNT of 11 at 4 weeks and 7 at 12 weeks. There is no impact on survival or the occurrence of spinal cord compression.

Various national guidelines recommend, with caveats, the routine use of bisphosphonates for the treatment and prevention of skeletal complications in patients with:
- breast cancer with symptomatic bone metastases[21,22]
- myeloma whether or not bone lesions are evident[23,24]
- hormone-resistant prostate cancer with bone metastases (± symptoms); also for the relief of bone pain.[25,26]

The optimal duration of treatment is unclear, but bisphosphonates are generally continued for as long as they are tolerated, or there is a substantial decline in the patient's performance status. There is no consensus on the use of bisphosphonates in other cancers, although it has been suggested that in any patient with a prognosis of ≥4–6 months and multiple bone metastases, it is reasonable to consider their use.[1]

The ability of bisphosphonates to prevent the development of bone metastases is being investigated.[27]

Bisphosphonates as adjuvant analgesics

Bisphosphonates have been used for metastatic bone pain and several regimens have been recommended for use when more conventional methods have been exhausted.[4,28–31] An effect is generally seen within 2 weeks. The evidence suggests that benefit is more likely in patients with breast cancer or myeloma, and with an IV bisphosphonate.[31]

Prophylactic use in patients treated for breast or prostate cancer

Estrogen deficiency is induced in women treated for breast cancer by chemotherapy ± aromatase inhibitors. This increases the rate of bone loss and risk of fracture.[32] Oral bisphosphonates, e.g. **risedronate** 35mg once a week, can prevent the loss following chemotherapy and ongoing studies are examining their use with aromatase inhibitors.[32,33]

The increased bone loss associated with androgen deprivation treatment in men with prostate cancer is also prevented by bisphosphonate therapy, e.g. **zoledronic acid** 4mg every 3 months.[34]

Systemic inflammatory reactions following IV bisphosphonates

Acute systemic inflammatory reactions causing symptoms such as fever, myalgia, arthralgia, nausea and vomiting, occur in 25–50% of patients following IV bisphosphonates. They are possibly related to the release of cytokines from inflammatory cells. Generally, the onset is within 2 days of the infusion, the fever is mild, although rigors occasionally occur. There may be bone pain, generally within 12h of the infusion. These effects can be treated with **acetaminophen** or NSAIDs and resolve completely within 1–2 days; they generally lessen with repeat doses, or with prophylactic **acetaminophen** or NSAID given before the infusion.[35]

Renal toxicity

Bisphosphonates can affect renal function. High-dose (200–1,500mg/day for 2–5 days), short-duration (<2h) IV infusions of **clodronate disodium** and **etidronate disodium** can cause oliguria, tubulo-interstitial damage and acute renal failure, possibly via the formation of an insoluble calcium-bisphosphonate complex in the blood.[36,37] **Pamidronate disodium** can also rarely cause collapsing focal segmental glomerulosclerosis, particularly in high doses, e.g. 180mg every 2–4 weeks. The probable mechanism is a direct toxic effect on glomerular capillary podocytes and renal tubules.[38] The more potent third-generation bisphosphonates are given in much smaller doses and reach lower concentrations in the renal tubules. Nevertheless, renal impairment has occurred with **zoledronic acid** (see p.378).[39–42] The risk of renal toxicity is reduced by adhering to the recommended dose and infusion rate, ensuring adequate hydration, monitoring renal function and adjusting the dose of bisphosphonate as appropriate or discontinuing treatment if there is deterioration, and avoiding the concurrent use of other nephrotoxic drugs.

Jaw osteonecrosis

All bisphosphonates have been implicated as a risk factor for jaw osteonecrosis.[43–45] Most reports involve the long-term use of **zoledronic acid** or **pamidronate disodium** for metastatic bone disease.[46] Although osteonecrosis has been reported after as little as 4 months of bisphosphonate use, generally, patients have been receiving bisphosphonates for years (mean and median duration of use vary around 1 and 2–3 years respectively). The true incidence of osteonecrosis is difficult to identify, but some studies put it as high as 10% of patients receiving long-term **zoledronic acid** and 4% of those receiving **pamidronate disodium**.[46] Other risk factors for jaw osteonecrosis include dental procedures (reported in about 60% of patients), poor dental health, blood clotting disorders, anemia, and possibly chemotherapy and corticosteroids.

The jaw bones may be particularly susceptible to osteonecrosis because of the combination of repeated low-level local trauma (e.g. from chewing, dentures) and ease of infection from microbes. Trauma and infection increase the demand for bone repair which the bisphosphonate-inhibited bone cannot meet, resulting in localized bone necrosis; the anti-angiogenic effect of bisphosphonates may also contribute.[46]

Osteonecrosis can present as an asymptomatic bony exposure in one or more sites in the mandible or maxilla, or with orofacial pain, trismus, offensive discharge from a cutaneous fistula, chronic sinusitis because of an oro-antral fistula and numbness in the mandible or maxilla.[35] If probed, the necrotic bone is usually non-tender and may not bleed. There may be osteomyelitis with oral-cavity flora or *Actinomyces* species. Osteonecrosis may show as mottled bone on a plain radiograph and be confused with bone metastases on a bone scan. Pathological fracture can occur.

Management is based on clinical experience. Long-term outcomes are generally poor with relatively few patients experiencing improvement or resolution. Thus, prevention is an important part of the recommended approach:[35]

- *preventive dental treatment* before commencing long-term bisphosphonates, e.g. treat infection, teeth extractions
- *encourage good dental hygiene* including regular dental cleaning by a dentist or dental hygienist
- avoid invasive dental procedures during treatment
- *minimize trauma*, e.g. patients with dentures should wear soft liners.

If osteonecrosis occurs:

- *discontinue the bisphosphonate* but new lesions may continue to appear
- *treat infection*, e.g. antimicrobials, **chlorhexidine** mouthwash, periodic minor debridement and wound irrigation (major debridement is avoided as it may worsen the situation)
- *avoid major surgery* unless there is no alternative, e.g. due to sequestered bone, pathological fracture, or oro-antral fistula.

If urgent treatment precludes a prior dental examination, a dental referral and any treatment should be undertaken within 1–2 months for those patients anticipated to continue to receive regular bisphosphonates in the long-term.[46]

Ocular toxicity

A rare undesirable effect is ocular inflammation, causing eye pain, redness, swelling, abnormal vision or impaired eye movement (due to rectus muscle edema).[47,48] Typically, the onset is within 2 days of the first or second infusion and affects both eyes. There may be other symptoms of an acute systemic inflammatory reaction (see above). An urgent ophthalmology assessment is required, followed by appropriate treatment. Patients with mild reactions, e.g. those which settle quickly without treatment, can generally continue to receive the same bisphosphonate. Those with more severe reactions, e.g. uveitis, scleritis, should not receive the same bisphosphonate again; some tolerate a switch to a non-nitrogen-containing bisphosphonate, but specialist advice should be sought from the ophthalmologist ± endocrinologist.[35]

Other emerging toxicities

Severe (sometimes incapacitating) musculoskeletal pain has been reported after days, months or years of bisphosphonate treatment. It has generally occurred with PO bisphosphonates used for osteoporosis and Paget's disease, but the US FDA is also investigating a possible link with IV bisphosphonates. The pain is distinct from the arthralgia/myalgia associated with an acute systemic inflammatory reaction (see above), and may respond to temporary or permanent discontinuation of the bisphosphonate.[49]

The US FDA is investigating a possible association between the use of bisphosphonates and the development of atrial fibrillation.[50]

Cautions

Serious drug interactions: concurrent use with aminoglycoside antibacterials may produce symptomatic hypocalcemia if given with long-term oral **disodium clodronate** therapy;[51] prolonged hypocalcemia and hypomagnesemia may occur with aminoglycosides and **zoledronic acid**. Risk of renal impairment increased by concurrent use with other nephrotoxic drugs.

Renal impairment (correct hypovolemia before treatment and monitor renal function), hypocalcemia, hypophosphatemia or hypomagnesemia. Vitamin D deficiency (increased risk of hypocalcemia);[52] unless being treated for tumour-related hypercalcemia, patients should receive oral **calcium** and **vitamin D** supplements. Invasive dental procedures (risk of osteonecrosis of the jaw).

Undesirable effects

For full list, see manufacturer's Product Monograph.

Very common (>10%): transient pyrexia and influenza-like symptoms (more common with IV nitrogen-containing bisphosphonates), fatigue, headache, anxiety, hypertension, anemia, thrombocytopenia, cough, arthralgia, myalgia, bone pain, asymptomatic hypocalcemia, hypomagnesemia, hypophosphatemia. Oral products in particular may cause anorexia, dyspepsia, nausea, vomiting, abdominal pain, diarrhea or constipation.

Common (<10%, >1%): sleep disturbance, psychosis, tachycardia, atrial fibrillation or flutter, syncope, dyspnea, leucopenia, infusion site reactions, deterioration in renal function, increased serum creatinine, hypokalemia, jaw osteonecrosis.

Rare (<0.1%, >0.01%): ocular inflammation, angioedema, collapsing focal segmental glomerulosclerosis (**pamidronate disodium**), nephrotic syndrome (**pamidronate disodium**), symptomatic hypocalcemia (e.g. tetany).

Very rare (<0.01%): anaphylaxis, bronchospasm.

Also see Other emerging toxicities (above).

Dose and use

On the grounds of cost, **pamidronate disodium** is still widely used as the bisphosphonate of first choice, and **zoledronic acid** tends to be reserved for patients who fail to respond to **pamidronate**. The guidance below relates to **pamidronate**; for **zoledronic acid**, see p.378.

Tumour-induced hypercalcemia

Stop and think! Are you justified in correcting a potentially fatal complication in a moribund patient?

The Canadian Product Monograph for **pamidronate disodium** recommends a dose dependent on the initial albumin-corrected plasma calcium concentration (Box 7.A. and Table 7.2). However, it has been suggested that the higher dose should be given irrespective of the initial calcium level to increase the probability of a response and prolong its duration:[14]

- patients should be well hydrated, using 0.9% saline if necessary
- standard and maximum recommended dose is 90mg IV/treatment
- dilute the dose in 1L of 0.45% saline, 0.9% saline or 5% dextrose (glucose); the Product Monograph advises that the concentration should not exceed 90mg/250mL
- infuse over at least 2h; the Product Monograph advises that the infusion rate should not exceed 60mg/h in patients with normal renal function, but 22.5mg/h (90mg in 500mL over 4h) in patients with tumour-induced hypercalcemia or multiple myeloma. Patients with mild–moderate renal impairment (creatinine clearance 30–90mL/min) do not require dose reduction but the infusion rate should not exceed 90mg/4h
- do not give to patients with a creatinine clearance <30mL/min
- repeat after 1 week if initial response inadequate
- repeat every 3–4 weeks according to plasma calcium concentration
- measure serum creatinine before each dose, no dose adjustment is required in mild–moderate renal impairment.

In palliative care, treatment with a bisphosphonate is unlikely to be started in patients with hypercalcemia and severe renal impairment (creatinine clearance <30mL/min). However, if considered appropriate, note the information given below on the prophylactic use of **pamidronate disodium** in bone metastases caused by multiple myeloma or breast cancer and obtain specialist renal/endocrinologist advice; treatment can be justified only if the potential benefits clearly outweigh the potential undesirable effects.

If the IV route is inaccessible, **pamidronate disodium** can be administered by CSCI, 90mg in 1L 0.9% saline over 12–24h.[53,54]

Box 7.A   Correcting plasma calcium concentrations

If the mean normal plasma albumin for the local laboratory is 40g/L:
Corrected calcium (mmol/L) = measured calcium + (0.022 × (40 − albumin g/L))
  e.g. measured calcium = 2.45; albumin = 30
    corrected calcium = 2.45 + (0.022 × 10) = 2.67mmol/L
    (normal range 2.12–2.65mmol/L)

Table 7.2   IV disodium pamidronate for hypercalcemia[a]

Corrected plasma calcium concentration (mmol/L)	Dose (mg)
<3	30
3–3.5	30 or 60
3.5–4	60 or 90
>4	90

a. manufacturer's recommendations.

Prophylactic use to reduce the incidence of skeletal-related events in patients with multiple myeloma or breast cancer with bone metastases

For **pamidronate disodium**:

- patients should be well hydrated, using 0.9% saline if necessary
- with breast cancer with bone metastases give 90mg in 250mL of 0.45% saline, 0.9% saline or 5% dextrose (glucose) IVI over 2h every 3–4 weeks
- with multiple myeloma a greater dilution and slower infusion rate is recommended because of the greater risk of renal toxicity; give 90mg in 500mL of 0.45% saline, 0.9% saline or 5% dextrose (glucose) IVI over 4h every 4 weeks

- for both breast cancer and multiple myeloma patients, serum creatinine should be measured before each dose. Treatment should be withheld if creatinine increases by:
  - ▷ ≥44micromol/L in patients with a normal baseline creatinine concentration (i.e. <124micromol/L), or
  - ▷ ≥88micromol/L in patients with a raised baseline creatinine concentration (i.e. >124micromol/L)
- treatment may be resumed at the same dose as before when the serum creatinine returns to within 10% of the baseline value
- discontinue treatment permanently if the serum creatinine does not return to within 10% of the baseline value after 4–8 weeks
- because of limited pharmacokinetic and safety data, patients with bone lesions and severe renal impairment (creatinine clearance <30mL/min) should not be treated.

Metastatic bone pain

Several regimens have been recommended for when more conventional methods have been exhausted:

- **pamidronate disodium** 90mg IV (50% of patients respond, generally within 1–2 weeks); if helpful repeat 60–90mg every 3–4 weeks for as long as benefit is maintained[4]
- **pamidronate disodium** 120mg IV, repeated p.r.n. every 2–4 months[30]
- **pamidronate disodium** 90–120mg IV repeated p.r.n. In patients not responding to a first treatment, a second can be tried but, if still no response, discontinue.[31]

Supply

For **zoledronic acid**, see p.380.
Pamidronate disodium (generic)
Injection 3mg/mL, 10mL (30mg) vial = $89; 6mg/mL, 10mL (60mg) vial = $177; 9mg/mL, 10mL (90mg) vial = $266.

Aredia® (Novartis Pharmaceuticals Canada)
Injection (powder for reconstitution) 30mg vial = $176; 90mg vial = $521.

1 Body JJ (2006) Bisphosphonates for malignancy-related bone disease: current status, future developments. *Supportive Care in Cancer.* **14**: 408–418.
2 Fleisch H (1998) Bisphosphonates: mechanisms of action. *Endocrine Reviews.* **19**: 80–100.
3 Russell R *et al.* (1999) Bisphosphonates: pharmacology, mechanisms of action and clinical uses. *Osteoporosis International.* **9 (suppl 2)**: s66–s80.
4 Crosby V *et al.* (1998) A randomized controlled trial of intravenous clodronate. *Journal of Pain and Symptom Management.* **15**: 266–268.
5 Harada H *et al.* (2004) Effects of bisphosphonates on joint damage and bone loss in rat adjuvant-induced arthritis. *Inflammation Research.* **53**: 45–52.
6 Mantyh PW (2006) Cancer pain and its impact on diagnosis, survival and quality of life. *Nature Reviews Neuroscience.* **7**: 797–809.
7 Neville-Webbe H *et al.* (2002) The anti-tumour activity of bisphosphonates. *Cancer Treatment Reviews.* **28**: 305–319.
8 Green JR (2004) Bisphosphonates: preclinical review. *Oncologist.* **9 (suppl 4)**: 3–13.
9 Sevcik MA *et al.* (2004) Bone cancer pain: the effects of the bisphosphonate alendronate on pain, skeletal remodeling, tumor growth and tumor necrosis. *Pain.* **111**: 169–180.
10 Rogers MJ *et al.* (2000) Cellular and molecular mechanisms of action of bisphosphonates. *Cancer.* **88 (suppl 12)**: 2961–2978.
11 Barrett J *et al.* (2004) Ibandronate: a clinical pharmacological and pharmacokinetic update. *Journal of Clinical Pharmacology.* **44**: 951–965.
12 Purohit O *et al.* (1995) A randomised, double-blind comparison of intravenous pamidronate and clodronate in hypercalcaemia of malignancy. *British Journal of Cancer.* **72**: 1289–1293.
13 Major P *et al.* (2001) Zoledronic acid is superior to pamidronate in the treatment of hypercalcaemia of malignancy: a pooled analysis of two randomized, controlled clinical trials. *Journal of Clinical Oncology.* **19**: 558–567.
14 Saunders Y *et al.* (2004) Systematic review of bisphosphonates for hypercalcaemia of malignancy. *Palliative Medicine.* **18**: 418–431.
15 Wong R and Wiffen PJ (2002) Bisphosphonates for the relief of pain secondary to bone metastases. *Cochrane Database Systematic Reviews.* **2**: CD002068.
16 Ross JR *et al.* (2003) Systematic review of role of bisphosphonates on skeletal morbidity in metastatic cancer. *British Medical Journal.* **327**: 469.
17 Body JJ *et al.* (2004) Oral ibandronate reduces the risk of skeletal complications in breast cancer patients with metastatic bone disease: results from two randomised, placebo-controlled phase III studies. *British Journal of Cancer.* **90**: 1133–1137.
18 Body JJ *et al.* (2004) Oral ibandronate improves bone pain and preserves quality of life in patients with skeletal metastases due to breast cancer. *Pain.* **111**: 306–312.
19 Yuen KK *et al.* (2006) Bisphosphonates for advanced prostate cancer. *Cochrane Database Systematic Reviews.* CD006250.
20 Pavlakis N *et al.* (2005) Bisphosphonates for breast cancer. *Cochrane Database Systematic Reviews.* CD003474.
21 Warr D *et al.* (2004) Use of biphosphonates in women with breast cancer. Practice guideline report #1-11. In: *Cancer Care Ontario program in evidence-based care.* Available from: www.cancercare.on.ca/common/pages/UserFile.aspx?fileId = 34182

22 SIGN (Scottish Intercollegiate Guidelines Network) (2005) *Management of breast cancer in women. A national clinical guideline.* (No. 84). SIGN publication, Edinburgh (Scotland).

23 Imrie K *et al.* (2007) The role of biphosphonates in the management of skeletal complications for patients with multiple myeloma: a clinical practice guideline. In: *Cancer Care Ontario program in evidence-based care.* Available from: www.cancercare.on.ca/common/pages/UserFile.aspx?fileId=14146

24 Smith A *et al.* (2006) Guidelines on the diagnosis and management of multiple myeloma 2005. *British Journal of Haematology.* **132**: 410–451.

25 British Association of Urological Surgeons (2005) Systemic management of metastatic bone disease. In: *Guidelines on the Management and Treatment of Metastatic Prostate Cancer,* UK.

26 Berry S *et al.* (2005) The use of biphosphonates in men with hormone-refractory prostate cancer. Practice guideline report #3-14. In: *Cancer Care Ontario Program in Evidence-based Care.* Available from: www.cancercare.on.ca/common/pages/userFile.aspx?fileId=14032

27 Clemons M and Verma S (2005) Should oral bisphosphonates be standard of care in women with early breast cancer? *Breast Cancer Research and Treatment.* **90**: 315–318.

28 Vorreuther R (1993) Biphosphonates as an adjunct to palliative therapy of bone metastases from prostatic carcinoma. A pilot study on clodronate. *British Journal of Urology.* **72**: 792–795.

29 O'Rourke N *et al.* (1995) Double-blind, placebo-controlled, dose response trial of oral clodronate in patients with bone metastases. *Journal of Clinical Oncology.* **13**: 929–934.

30 Vinholes J *et al.* (1996) Metabolic effects of pamidronate in patients with metastatic bone disease. *British Journal of Cancer.* **73**: 1089–1095.

31 Mannix K *et al.* (2000) Using bisphosphonates to control the pain of bone metastases: evidence-based guidelines for palliative care. *Palliative Medicine.* **14**: 455–461.

32 Eastell R (2007) Breast cancer and the risk of osteoporotic fracture: a paradox. *Journal of Clinical Endocrinology and Metaboloism.* **92**: 42–43.

33 Greenspan SL *et al.* (2007) Prevention of bone loss in survivors of breast cancer: a randomized, double-blind, placebo-controlled clinical trial. *Journal of Clinical Endocrinology and Metabolism.* **92**: 131–136.

34 Smith MR (2003) Bisphosphonates to prevent osteoporosis in men receiving androgen deprivation therapy for prostate cancer. *Drugs Aging.* **20**: 175–183.

35 Tanvetyanon T and Stiff PJ (2006) Management of the adverse effects associated with intravenous bisphosphonates. *Annals of Oncology.* **17**: 897–907.

36 Bounameaux HM *et al.* (1983) Renal failure associated with intravenous diphosphonates. *Lancet.* **1**: 471.

37 Kanis JA *et al.* (1983) Effects of intravenous diphosphonates on renal function. *Lancet.* **1**: 1328.

38 Markowitz GS *et al.* (2001) Collapsing focal segmental glomerulosclerosis following treatment with high-dose pamidronate. *Journal of the American Society of Nephrology.* **12**: 1164–1172.

39 Rosen LS *et al.* (2001) Zoledronic acid versus pamidronate in the treatment of skeletal metastases in patients with breast cancer or osteolytic lesions of multiple myeloma: a phase III, double-blind, comparative trial. *Cancer Journal* **7**: 377–387.

40 Rosen LS *et al.* (2004) Zoledronic acid is superior to pamidronate for the treatment of bone metastases in breast carcinoma patients with at least one osteolytic lesion. *Cancer.* **100**: 36–43.

41 Markowitz GS *et al.* (2003) Toxic acute tubular necrosis following treatment with zoledronate (Zometa). *Kidney International.* **64**: 281–289.

42 Chang JT *et al.* (2003) Renal failure with the use of zoledronic acid. *New England Journal of Medicine.* **349**: 1676–1679.

43 FDA (2004) Drug Safety Revisions: Food and Drugs Administration Update. *P&T.* **29**: 733.

44 CHM (2006) Osteonecrosis of the jaw with bisphosphonates. In: *Current Problems in Pharmacovigilance.* Commission on Human Medicines. Available from: www.mhra.gov.uk/Publications/Safetyguidance/CurrentProblemsinPharmacovigilance/CON2023859

45 Ruggiero SL *et al.* (2004) Osteonecrosis of the jaws associated with the use of bisphosphonates: a review of 63 cases. *Journal of Oral and Maxillofacial Surgery.* **62**: 527–534.

46 Woo SB *et al.* (2006) Narrative [corrected] review: bisphosphonates and osteonecrosis of the jaws. *Annals of Internal Medicine.* **144**: 753–761.

47 Fraunfelder FW and Fraunfelder FT (2003) Bisphosphonates and ocular inflammation. *New England Journal of Medicine.* **348**: 1187–1188.

48 Australian Adverse Drug Reactions Bulletin (2004) Bisphosphonates and ocular inflammation. Available from: www.tga.gov.au/adr/aadrb/aadr0404.htm#3

49 FDA (2008) Information for healthcare professionals. Bisphosphonates (marketed as Actonel, Actonel+Ca, Aredia, Boniva, Didronel, Fosamax, Fosamax+D, Reclast, Skelid, and Zometa). Food and Drugs Administration. Available from: www.fda.gov/Drugs/DrugSafety/PostmarketDrugSafetyInformationforPatientsandProviders/ucm101551.htm

50 FDA (2008) Early communication of an ongoing safety review. Bisphosphonates: alendronate (Fosamax, Fosamax Plus D), etidronate (Didronel), ibandronate (Boniva), pamidronate (Aredia), risedronate (Actonel, Actonel W/Calcium), tiludronate (Skelid), and zoledronic acid (Reclast, Zometa). Food and Drug Administration. Available from: www.fda.gov/Drugs/DrugSafety/PostmarketDrugSafetyInformationforPatientsandProviders/DrugSafetyInformationforHealthcareProfessionals/ucm070303.htm

51 Johnson M and Fallon M (1998) Symptomatic hypocalcaemia with oral clodronate. *Journal of Pain and Symptom Management.* **15**: 140–142.

52 Broadbent A *et al.* (2005) Bisphosphonate-induced hypocalcemia associated with vitamin D deficiency in a patient with advanced cancer. *American Journal of Hospice and Palliative Care.* **22**: 382–384.

53 Roemer-Becuwe C *et al.* (2003) Safety of subcutaneous clodronate and efficacy in hypercalcemia of malignancy: a novel route of administration. *Journal of Pain and Symptom Management.* **26**: 843–848.

54 Duncan AR (2003) The use of subcutaneous pamidronate. *Journal of Pain and Symptom Management.* **26**: 592–593.

ZOLEDRONIC ACID

Class: Bisphosphonate.

Indications: Tumor-induced hypercalcemia; prophylactic use to reduce the incidence of skeletal-related events in patients with multiple myeloma or bone metastases from solid tumors; †bone pain.

Pharmacology

Zoledronic acid is a third-generation bisphosphonate and the most potent currently available.[1,2] In patients with hypercalcemia, zoledronic acid 4mg compared with **pamidronate disodium** 90mg is more effective in achieving normocalcemia (90% vs. 70%) and provides a longer median time to relapse, approximately 4 weeks vs. 2.5 weeks (see Table 7.1, p.372).[3] Normocalcemia is achieved in 50% but the median duration of response is only 2 weeks.[3] Because of concerns about renal impairment with an 8mg dose, doses higher than 4mg are not recommended, and are off-label.[4]

When used prophylactically to prevent skeletal-related events (pain, pathological fracture), 4mg every 2 weeks is no better than every 4 weeks.[5] In patients with breast cancer, compared with placebo, zoledronic acid 4mg IV given every 4 weeks for 1 year reduces the risk of skeletal complications (e.g. vertebral and non-vertebral fractures, hypercalcemia, need for radiation therapy) by about 40%.[6] Zoledronic acid is at least as effective as **pamidronate disodium** in reducing skeletal complications and pain scores in patients with multiple myeloma or breast cancer.[7–9] In one study, patients receiving zoledronic acid required less radiation therapy and less surgery than those receiving **pamidronate disodium**. NNTs were 4 and 20 respectively.[8] Zoledronic acid has reduced pain and markers of bone turnover in patients with breast cancer who have developed a skeletal-related event or progressive bone disease despite receiving **pamidronate disodium** or **clodronate disodium**.[10]

In patients with prostate cancer, compared with placebo, zoledronic acid 4mg IV given every 3 weeks for up to 2 years reduces the risk of skeletal complications by about 36%.[11,12] Baseline bone pain levels were low (mean composite Brief Pain Inventory score of 2/10) and over the course of the study, pain increased slightly in both groups; this was to a lesser degree with zoledronic acid which was significant at some but not all time points. However, about 1/3 of patients had what is considered a clinically relevant improvement in bone pain (⩾2 point change in their pain score).[13]

Although approved for all solid tumours, the evidence of benefit is generally weaker for other tumour types.[9] The combination of zoledronic acid with radionucleotides, e.g. Strontium-89 and Samarium-153, is being explored to reduce skeletal complications. The ability of zoledronic acid to prevent the development of bone metastases is also being explored.[14] *In vitro*, zoledronic acid is a more potent inhibitor of prostate cancer cell growth than **pamidronate disodium**.[15]

Zoledronic acid is tolerated as well as **pamidronate disodium**.[8,9,11,12,16] It has a long terminal elimination halflife because of its slow release from bone back into the systemic circulation and is excreted unchanged by the kidney. Dose reduction is required in patients with mild–moderate renal impairment (see Table 7.3, p.380). In direct comparisons, the incidence of decreased renal function with zoledronic acid 4mg is similar to **pamidronate disodium** 90mg over 2h (about 10%).[4,9] Decreased renal function was defined as an increase in serum creatinine ⩾44micromol/L for patients with a normal baseline serum creatinine (i.e. <124micromol/L) and ⩾88micromol/L for patients with an abnormal baseline serum creatinine of (i.e. ⩾124micromol/L), or a doubling or more of the baseline value.

With zoledronic acid 4mg, increases in serum creatinine lead to treatment delay or discontinuation in about 1% and 3% of patients respectively and increases in creatinine levels >3 times the upper limit of normal were seen in 0.4% of patients.[8,17] There have been rare case reports of life-threatening renal failure because of toxic acute tubular necrosis in patients treated with zoledronic acid, e.g. 72 cases among >430,000 patients (i.e. <0.02%).[18–20] Other risk factors were often present, including dehydration, pre-existing renal impairment, and concurrent use of other nephrotoxic drugs. Onset of decreased renal function can be after any number of treatments, but is generally apparent within 6–8 weeks of starting treatment. Mild impairment generally recovers within several months of discontinuing zoledronic acid, sometimes within a few days. However, in those with renal failure, the damage is generally permanent.[21] Thus, the risk of renal toxicity is reduced by:

- adhering to the recommended dose and infusion rate
- ensuring adequate hydration
- avoiding the concurrent use of other nephrotoxic drugs
- monitoring renal function.

The dose of zoledronic acid should be adjusted as appropriate or discontinued if there is deterioration in renal function (see Dose and use).

Onset of action normocalcemia achieved by a median of 4 days (ranging up to 10); pain relief up to 14 days.

Plasma halflife 1.75h; terminal elimination halflife 1 week.

Duration of action 4 weeks.

Cautions

Serious drug interactions: concurrent use with other nephrotoxic drugs, aminoglycosides (risk of prolonged hypocalcemia and hypomagnesemia), loop diuretics (risk of hypocalcemia and dehydration), or **thalidomide** (increased risk of renal impairment in multiple myeloma patients).

Not recommended in severe renal impairment, i.e. creatinine clearance < 30mL/min (see Table 7.3, p.380), hypocalcemia, hypophosphatemia or hypomagnesemia. Correct hypovolemia before treatment and monitor renal function.

To minimize the risk of jaw osteonecrosis, patients should undergo a dental examination before starting zoledronic acid and avoid invasive dental procedures during treatment (see p.373).

Undesirable effects

For full list, see manufacturer's Product Monograph.

Very common (>10%): fever, influenza-like syndrome (fatigue, rigors, malaise, and flushing), headache, insomnia, dizziness, anxiety, depression, confusion, agitation, fatigue, weakness, paresthesia, anemia, neutropenia, cough, dyspnea, weight loss, abdominal pain, nausea, vomiting, constipation or diarrhea, bone pain, myalgia, hypophosphatemia, hypomagnesemia, hypokalemia.

Common (<10%, >1%): asthenia, drowsiness, chest pain, leg edema, hypotension, granulocytopenia, thrombocytopenia, pancytopenia, pleural effusion, stomatitis, mucositis, anorexia, renal impairment, jaw osteonecrosis, arthralgia, hypocalcemia.

Rare (<0.1%): uveitis, episcleritis.

There have been reports of severe (sometimes incapacitating) musculoskeletal pain, arising days, months or years after starting bisphosphonate treatment (generally with PO use for osteoporosis and Paget's disease), which may respond to temporary or permanent discontinuation. The US FDA is investigating a possible link with all bisphosphonates, including zoledronic acid.[22]

The US FDA is investigating a possible association between the use of bisphosphonates and the development of atrial fibrillation.[23]

Dose and use

Tumour-induced hypercalcemia (corrected serum calcium > 3mmol/L)

Stop and think! Are you justified in correcting a potentially fatal complication in a moribund patient?

- patients should be well hydrated
- give 4mg IVI in 100mL 0.9% saline or 5% dextrose (glucose) over 15min
- if serum calcium does not normalize, repeat after 1 week[16]
- 8mg has been used in refractory hypercalcemia[3] but is off-label because of concerns relating to renal impairment (see Pharmacology)
- measure serum creatinine before each dose; no dose adjustment is needed in mild–moderate renal impairment for patients being treated for hypercalcemia

In palliative care, treatment with bisphosphonates will probably not be initiated in patients with hypercalcemia and severe renal impairment. If it is considered appropriate, seek specialist renal/endocrinologist advice.

Prophylactic use to reduce the incidence of skeletal-related events in patients with cancer involving the bones and for metastatic bone pain when more conventional methods have been exhausted

- patients should be well hydrated
- for dose in patients with renal impairment, see Table 7.3

- otherwise, give 4mg IVI in 100mL 0.9% saline or 5% dextrose (glucose) over 15min every 3–4 weeks; with appropriate support, these have been given in the home setting[24,25]
- daily supplements of elemental **calcium** 500mg and **vitamin D** 400 international units are recommended[26]
- measure serum creatinine before each dose; withhold treatment if creatinine increases by:
  ▷ ≥44micromol/L in patients with a normal baseline creatinine concentration (i.e. <124micromol/L)
  or
  ▷ ≥88micromol/L in patients with a raised baseline creatinine concentration (i.e. >124micromol/L)
- treatment may be resumed at the same dose as before when serum creatinine returns to within 10% of the baseline value
- discontinue treatment permanently if serum creatinine fails to improve after 4–8 weeks.

Table 7.3 Dose reduction for zoledronic acid in patients with cancer involving the bones and mild–moderate renal impairment[a,b,c]

Baseline creatinine clearance (mL/min)	Recommended dose (mg)	Amount of concentrate (mL)
>60	4.0 (i.e. no reduction)	5
50–60	3.5	4.4
40–49	3.3	4.1
30–39	3.0	3.8

a. manufacturer's recommendations for patients with multiple myeloma or bone metastases
b. no data exist for severe renal impairment (creatinine clearance <30mL/min) because these patients were excluded from the studies
c. reduced doses are diluted in 100mL 0.9% saline or 5% dextrose (glucose) and given IVI over 15min.

Supply

Zometa® (Novartis Pharmaceuticals Canada)
Injection (concentrate for dilution and use as an infusion) 4mg/5mL, 5mL vial = $593.

The manufacturer operates a sponsored programme called the Access Zometa programme. This includes drug cost assistance and infusion at home. For more information, contact 1-866-4765.

1 Green J et al. (1994) Preclinical pharmacology of CGP 42'446 a new, potent, heterocyclic bisphosphonate compound. *Journal of Bone and Mineral Research.* **9**: 745–751.
2 Neville-Webbe H and Coleman RE (2003) The use of zoledronic acid in the management of metastatic bone disease and hypercalcaemia. *Palliative Medicine.* **17**: 539–553.
3 Major P et al. (2001) Zoledronic acid is superior to pamidronate in the treatment of hypercalcaemia of malignancy: a pooled analysis of two randomized, controlled clinical trials. *Journal of Clinical Oncology.* **19**: 558–567.
4 Rosen LS et al. (2001) Zoledronic acid versus pamidronate in the treatment of skeletal metastases in patients with breast cancer or osteolytic lesions of multiple myeloma: a phase III, double-blind, comparative trial. *Cancer Journal.* **7**: 377–387.
5 Mystakidou K et al. (2006) A prospective randomized controlled clinical trial of zoledronic acid for bone metastases. *American Journal of Hospice & Palliative Medicine.* **23**: 41–50.
6 Kohno N et al. (2005) Zoledronic acid significantly reduces skeletal complications compared with placebo in Japanese women with bone metastases from breast cancer: a randomized, placebo-controlled trial. *Journal of Clinical Oncology.* **23**: 3314–3321.
7 Berenson J et al. (2001) Zoledronic acid reduces skeletal-related events in patients with osteolytic metastases. *Cancer.* **91**: 1191–1200.
8 Rosen LS et al. (2003) Long-term efficacy and safety of zoledronic acid compared with pamidronate disodium in the treatment of skeletal complications in patients with advanced multiple myeloma or breast carcinoma: a randomized, double-blind, multicenter, comparative trial. *Cancer.* **98**: 1735–1744.
9 Rosen LS et al. (2004) Zoledronic acid is superior to pamidronate for the treatment of bone metastases in breast carcinoma patients with at least one osteolytic lesion. *Cancer.* **100**: 36–43.
10 Clemons MJ et al. (2006) Phase II trial evaluating the palliative benefit of second-line zoledronic acid in breast cancer patients with either a skeletal-related event or progressive bone metastases despite first-line bisphosphonate therapy. *Journal of Clinical Oncology.* **24**: 4895–4900.
11 Rosen LS et al. (2004) Long-term efficacy and safety of zoledronic acid in the treatment of skeletal metastases in patients with nonsmall cell lung carcinoma and other solid tumors: a randomized, Phase III, double-blind, placebo-controlled trial. *Cancer.* **100**: 2613–2621.
12 Saad F et al. (2004) Long-term efficacy of zoledronic acid for the prevention of skeletal complications in patients with metastatic hormone-refractory prostate cancer. *Journal of the National Cancer Institute.* **96**: 879–882.

13 Weinfurt KP et al. (2006) Effect of zoledronic acid on pain associated with bone metastasis in patients with prostate cancer. Annals of Oncology. **17**: 986–989.

14 Clemons M and Verma S (2005) Should oral bisphosphonates be standard of care in women with early breast cancer? Breast Cancer Research and Treatment. **90**: 315–318.

15 Lee M et al. (2001) Bisphosphonate treatment inhibits the growth of prostate cancer cells. Cancer Research. **61**: 2602–2608.

16 Perry CM and Figgitt DP (2004) Zoledronic acid: a review of its use in patients with advanced cancer. Drugs. **64**: 1197–1211.

17 Vogel CL et al. (2004) Safety and pain palliation of zoledronic acid in patients with breast cancer, prostate cancer, or multiple myeloma who previously received bisphosphonate therapy. Oncologist. **9**: 687–695.

18 Chang JT et al. (2003) Renal failure with the use of zoledronic acid. New England Journal of Medicine. **349**: 1676–1679.

19 Markowitz GS et al. (2003) Toxic acute tubular necrosis following treatment with zoledronate (Zometa). Kidney International. **64**: 281–289.

20 Munier A et al. (2005) Zoledronic Acid and renal toxicity: data from French adverse effect reporting database. Annals of Pharmacotherapy. **39**: 1194–1197.

21 Tanvetyanon T and Stiff PJ (2006) Management of the adverse effects associated with intravenous bisphosphonates. Annals of Oncology. **17**: 897–907.

22 FDA (2008) Information for healthcare professionals. Bisphosphonates (marketed as Actonel, Actonel+Ca, Aredia, Boniva, Didronel, Fosamax, Fosamax+D, Reclast, Skelid, and Zometa). Food and Drugs Administration. Available from: www.fda.gov/Drugs/DrugSafety/PostmarketDrugSafetyInformationforPatientsandProviders/ucm101551.htm

23 FDA (2008) Early communication of an ongoing safety review. Bisphosphonates: alendronate (Fosamax, Fosamax Plus D), etidronate (Didronel), ibandronate (Boniva), pamidronate (Aredia), risedronate (Actonel, Actonel W/Calcium), tiludronate (Skelid), and zoledronic acid (Reclast, Zometa). Food and Drug Administration. Available from: www.fda.gov/Drugs/DrugSafety/PostmarketDrugSafetyInformationforPatientsandProviders/DrugSafetyInformationforHeathcareProfessionals/ucm070303.htm

24 Italiano A et al. (2006) Home infusions of biphosphonate in cancer patients: a prospective study. Journal of Chemotherapy. **18**: 217–220.

25 Wardley A et al. (2005) Zoledronic acid significantly improves pain scores and quality of life in breast cancer patients with bone metastases: a randomised, crossover study of community vs hospital bisphosphonate administration. British Journal of Cancer. **92**: 1869–1876.

26 Dhillon S et al. (2008) Zoledronic acid: a review of its use in the management of bone metastases of malignancy. Drugs. **68**: 507–534.

SYSTEMIC CORTICOSTEROIDS

Indications: Suppression of inflammatory and allergic disorders, cerebral edema, nausea and vomiting with chemotherapy, hypercalcemia associated with cancer; †see Box 7.B.

Box 7.B Off-label indications for systemic corticosteroids in advanced cancer[1,2]

This list of off-label uses does not claim to be totally comprehensive. Further, inclusion does not mean that a systemic corticosteroid is necessarily the treatment of choice.

Specific
Spinal cord compression[3]
Nerve compression
Breathlessness
  pneumonitis (after radiation therapy)
  lymphangitis carcinomatosa
  tracheal compression/stridor
Superior vena caval obstruction
Obstruction of hollow viscus
  bronchus
  ureter
  bowel[4,5]
Radiation-induced inflammation
Discharge from rectal tumour
(can give either PO or PR)
Paraneoplastic fever

Pain relief
Nerve compression
Spinal cord compression[3]
Pain caused by a tumour in a confined organ or body cavity, e.g. raised intracranial pressure, bone pain

Anticancer hormone therapy
Breast cancer[6]
Prostate cancer[7]
Hematological malignancies
Lymphoproliferative disorders

General ('tonic')
To improve appetite
To enhance sense of wellbeing

Pharmacology

The adrenal cortex secretes **hydrocortisone** (cortisol) which has glucocorticoid activity and weak mineralocorticoid activity.[8] It also secretes aldosterone which has mineralocorticoid activity. Thus, in deficiency states, physiological replacement is best achieved with a combination of **hydrocortisone** and **fludrocortisone**, a mineralocorticoid.

In many disease states, corticosteroids are used primarily as potent anti-inflammatory agents. The anti-inflammatory action is mediated via several interacting mechanisms,[8] in contrast to the more specific impact of NSAIDs on prostaglandin synthesis (see p.244). Thus, as anti-inflammatory agents, corticosteroids are potentially more effective than NSAIDs. However, certainly when used long-term, corticosteroids are likely to cause more numerous and more serious undesirable effects (see below).

When comparing the relative anti-inflammatory (glucocorticoid) potencies of corticosteroids, their water-retaining properties (mineralocorticoid effect) should also be borne in mind (Table 7.4). Thus, **hydrocortisone** is not used for long-term disease suppression because large doses would be required and these would cause troublesome fluid retention. On the other hand, the moderate anti-inflammatory effect of **hydrocortisone** makes it a useful corticosteroid for topical use in inflammatory skin conditions; undesirable effects are minimal, both topical and systemic.

Prednisone is the most frequently used corticosteroid for disease suppression. **Dexamethasone**, with high glucocorticoid activity but insignificant mineralocorticoid effect, is particularly suitable for high-dose anti-inflammatory therapy. It is 6–12 times more potent than **prednisone**, i.e. 2mg of **dexamethasone** is approximately equivalent to 15–25mg of **prednisone** (Box 7.C) and it has a long duration of action (Table 7.4). Some corticosteroid esters, e.g. of **betamethasone** and of **beclomethasone**, exert a marked topical effect; use is made of this property with skin applications and bronchial inhalations (see p.94 and p.458).

The non-specific 'tonic' use of corticosteroids is based on the known general effects of this group of drugs. RCTs of corticosteroids as appetite stimulants have used daily doses of **prednisone** 15–40mg (or equivalent).[9–12] All showed significant benefit compared with placebo. In one, benefit was comparable for daily doses of **dexamethasone** of either 3mg or 6mg (equivalent to **prednisone** 20mg or 40mg). Overall, some 50–75% of the patients reported benefit, and the increase in appetite was still significant after 4 weeks.[9,11] However, both corticosteroids and progestins (see p.399) should *not* be regarded as 'anticachexia' agents. Any weight gain, rather than representing increased skeletal muscle and fat, is a less helpful retention of fluid ± increased fat. This could make mobilizing more difficult in an already debilitated patient. In addition, the catabolic effect of corticosteroids on skeletal muscle, exacerbated by reduced levels of physical activity, may well further weaken the patient.

Dexamethasone is an integral part of standard management of severe chemotherapeutic vomiting.[13–15] Its anti-emetic effect is possibly mediated by a corticosteroid-induced reduction in the permeability of the chemoreceptor trigger zone and of the blood-brain barrier to emetogenic substances, and a reduction in the neuronal content of gamma-aminobutyric acid (GABA) in the brain stem.

In palliative care, **dexamethasone** is often used when all else fails as an 'add-on' anti-emetic (see p.183). On the other hand, in an RCT in patients with advanced cancer receiving **metoclopramide**, **dexamethasone** 20mg/24h failed to further reduce chronic nausea.[16] In obstructive syndromes (see Box 7.B, p.381), **dexamethasone** may help by reducing inflammation at the site of the block, thereby increasing the lumen of the obstructed hollow viscus.[4,5,16]

For pharmacokinetic details, see Table 7.4

Cautions

Diabetes mellitus, psychotic illness. Although there is only a small increased risk of peptic ulceration with corticosteroids alone,[19] when given concurrently with NSAIDs, the risk is increased *15 times*.[20]

Corticosteroids antagonize oral hypoglycemics and insulin (glucocorticoid effect), anti-hypertensives and diuretics (mineralocorticoid effect). Increased risk of hypokalemia if high doses of corticosteroids are prescribed with β_2-agonists (e.g. **salbutamol**, **terbutaline**).

The metabolism of corticosteroids is accelerated by anti-epileptics (**carbamazepine**, **phenobarbital**, **phenytoin**, **primidone**) and **rifampin**. This effect is more pronounced with long-acting glucocorticoids; thus **phenytoin** may reduce the bio-availability of **dexamethasone** to 25–50%, and larger doses (double or more) will be needed when prescribed concurrently.[21] **Dexamethasone** itself can affect plasma **phenytoin** concentrations (may either rise or fall).

Undesirable effects

For full list, see manufacturer's Product Monograph.
See Box 7.D–Box 7.F

Table 7.4 Selected pharmacokinetic details of commonly used corticosteroids[17,18]

Drug	Anti-inflammatory potency	Approximate equivalent dose (mg)	Sodium-retaining potency	Oral bio-availability (%)	Onset of action	Peak plasma concentration	Plasma halflife (h)	Duration of action (h)	Relative affinity for lung tissue	Daily dose (mg) above which adrenal suppression possible	
										Male	Female
Hydrocortisone	1	20	1	96	No data	No data	1.5	8–12	1	20–30	15–25
Prednisone[a] and prednisolone	4	5	0.25	75–85	No data	1h PO	3.5	12–36	1.6	7.5–10	7.5
Dexamethasone	25–50[b]	0.5–1	<0.01	78	8–24h IM[c]	1–2h PO	4.5	36–54	1	1–1.15	1
Betamethasone				98	No data	10–36min IV	6.5	24–48			

a. biologically inert prednisone is converted by the liver to prednisolone
b. thymic involution assay
c. acute allergic reactions.

Box 7.C   Approximate equivalent anti-inflammatory doses of corticosteroids[a]

Hydrocortisone	20mg
Prednisone	5mg
Prednisolone	5mg
Methylprednisolone	4mg
Triamcinolone	4mg
Betamethasone	750microgram
Dexamethasone	750microgram

a. this list takes no account of either mineralocorticoid effects or variations in duration of action.

Box 7.D   Undesirable effects of corticosteroids

Glucocorticoid effects
Diabetes mellitus
Osteoporosis
Avascular bone necrosis
Mental disturbances
  insomnia
  paranoid psychosis
  depression
  euphoria
Muscle wasting and weakness (Box 7.E)
Peptic ulceration (if given with an NSAID)[21,22]
Infection (increased susceptibility)
  candidosis (debatable, see p.351)
  septicemia (may delay recognition)
  tuberculosis (may delay recognition)
  chickenpox,[a] measles (increased severity)
Suppression of growth (in child)

Mineralocorticoid effects
Sodium and water retention
  → edema
Potassium loss
Hypertension

Cushing's syndrome
Moonface
Striae
Acne

Steroid cataract
Prednisone 15mg/daily for several years
or equivalent = 75% risk; also
associated with long-term inhaled
steroids[21]

a. if exposed to infection, should be given immunoglobulin (either varicella-zoster or normal).

Box 7.E   Systemic corticosteroid myopathy[24,25]

Onset generally in the third month of treatment with dexamethasone >4mg daily or prednisone >40mg daily. Can occur earlier and with lower doses.

If the chronological sequence fits with corticosteroid myopathy, a presumptive diagnosis should be made and the following steps taken:
• explanation to patient and family
• discuss need to compromise between maximizing therapeutic benefit and minimizing undesirable effects
• halve corticosteroid dose (generally possible as a single step)
• consider changing from dexamethasone to prednisone (non-fluorinated corticosteroids cause less myopathy)
• attempt further reductions in dose at intervals of 1–2 weeks
• arrange for physiotherapy (disuse exacerbates myopathy)
• emphasize that weakness should improve after 3–4 weeks (provided cancer-induced weakness does not supervene).

Box 7.F   Steroid pseudorheumatism

Patients receiving corticosteroids for rheumatoid arthritis occasionally develop diffuse pains, malaise and pyrexia, so-called steroid pseudorheumatism.[26]

It is sometimes also seen in cancer patients receiving large doses of corticosteroids or when a very high dose is reduced rapidly to a lower dose. Most likely to be affected are those:
- receiving 100mg of prednisone daily for several days in association with chemotherapy
- with spinal cord compression given dexamethasone 96mg IV daily for 3 days[27] (followed by a rapidly reducing oral dose)[a]
- on high doses of dexamethasone to reduce raised intracranial pressure associated with brain metastases
- reducing to an ordinary maintenance dose after a prolonged course.

---

a. such a high dose is unnecessary; 10mg IV is as effective as 96mg.[28,29]

Dose and use
For inhaled corticosteroids, see p.94.
For depot corticosteroid injections, see p.433.
For topical corticosteroids, see p.458.

If expected to take corticosteroids for ≥3 weeks, patients should be given a *Steroid Treatment* card (Box 7.G).

Box 7.G   Example of a *Steroid Treatment* card

I am a patient on STEROID treatment which must not be stopped suddenly.

- If you have been taking this medicine for more than 3 weeks, the dose should be reduced gradually when you stop taking steroids unless your doctor says otherwise.
- Read the patient information leaflet given with the medicine.
- Always carry this card with you and show it to anyone who treats you (for example a doctor, nurse, pharmacist, or dentist).
- For 1 year after you stop the treatment, you must mention that you have taken steroids.
- If you become ill, or if you come into contact with anyone who has an infectious disease, consult your doctor promptly.
- If you have never had chickenpox, you should avoid close contact with people who have chickenpox or shingles. If you do come into contact with chickenpox, see your doctor urgently.
- Make sure that the information on the card about your current dose is kept up to date.

Except for **hydrocortisone**, corticosteroids can be given in a single daily dose each morning; this eases compliance and reduces the likelihood of corticosteroid-induced insomnia. Even so, **temazepam** or **diazepam** at bedtime is sometimes needed to counter insomnia or agitation. The initial daily dose varies according to indication and fashion.

Replacement therapy: hydrocortisone 20mg each morning, 10mg each evening with **fludrocortisone** 100–300microgram.
Anti-emetic: e.g. **dexamethasone** 8–20mg each morning (see Pharmacology section above; also p.183).[13–15]
Anorexia: **dexamethasone** 2–6mg or **prednisone** 15–40mg.[9–12]
Raised intracranial pressure: **dexamethasone** 8–16mg each morning.[30,31]
Obstruction of hollow viscus: **dexamethasone** 6–16mg each morning.[4]
Spinal cord compression: **dexamethasone** 16mg each morning.[29]
Discharge from rectal tumour or acute post-radiation proctitis: **hydrocortisone** retention enema 100mg every 1–2 days. If topical application is not feasible or not tolerated, PO corticosteroids can be used.

Stopping corticosteroids

If after 7–10 days the corticosteroid fails to achieve the desired effect, it should be stopped. It is often possible to stop corticosteroids abruptly (Box 7.H).[32] However, if there is uncertainty about disease or symptom resolution, withdrawal should be guided by monitoring disease activity or the symptom.

After whole-brain radiation, **dexamethasone** 4mg should be maintained for at least 1 week and the dose then reduced at the rate of 1mg/week.[33] In dying patients who are no longer able to swallow medication, it is generally acceptable to discontinue corticosteroids abruptly.

Occasionally, a patient with a brain tumour or multiple brain metastases requests that **dexamethasone** is stopped because, despite its continued use, there is progressive physical deterioration and/or cognitive impairment. In this circumstance, it is often best to reduce the **dexamethasone** step by step on a daily basis. This gives the patient time to reconsider. Extra analgesics should be prescribed in case headache develops as the intracranial pressure increases:

- if already taking **acetaminophen**, prescribe a weak opioid or a weak opioid-**acetaminophen** combination p.r.n.
- if already taking a weak opioid, prescribe **morphine** 10–20mg PO or **morphine** 5–10mg SC p.r.n.
- if >2 p.r.n. doses have been given in the last 24h, increase the regular analgesic dose
- if the patient becomes drowsy or swallowing becomes difficult, switch PO anti-epileptics to a non-oral route, e.g. SC **midazolam** or **phenobarbital** and possibly give both **morphine** and the anti-epileptic by CSCI.

If the patient becomes semicomatose and cannot communicate clearly, the presence of headache may manifest as grimacing or general restlessness. However, as in all moribund patients, it is important to exclude other common reasons for agitation, e.g. a full bladder or rectum, and discomfort and stiffness secondary to immobility.

Box 7.H   Recommendations for withdrawing systemic corticosteroids[32]

Abrupt withdrawal
Systemic corticosteroids may be stopped abruptly in those whose disease is unlikely to relapse *and* have received treatment for <3 weeks *and* are not in the groups below.

Gradual withdrawal
Gradual withdrawal of systemic corticosteroids is advisable in patients who:
- have received more than 3 weeks treatment
- have received prednisone >40mg daily or equivalent, e.g. dexamethasone 4–6mg
- have had a second dose in the evening
- are taking a short course within 1 year of stopping long-term treatment
- have other possible causes of adrenal suppression.

During corticosteroid withdrawal the dose may initially be reduced rapidly (e.g. halving the dose daily) to physiological doses (prednisone 7.5mg daily or equivalent) and then more slowly (e.g. 1–2mg per week) to allow the adrenals to recover and to prevent a hypo-adrenal crisis (malaise, profound weakness, hypotension, etc.). The patient should be monitored during withdrawal in case of deterioration.

Supply

Prednisone (generic)
Tablets 1mg, 5mg, 50mg, 28 days @ 15mg once daily = $2.

Prednisolone (generic)
Oral liquid 5mg/5mL, 28 days @ 15mg once daily = $31.

Pediapred® (Sanofi-Aventis Canada)
Oral liquid 5mg/5mL, 28 days @ 15mg once daily = $55.

Dexamethasone (generic)
Note: **dexamethasone** 1mg = **dexamethasone** *phosphate* 1.2mg = **dexamethasone** *sodium phosphate* 1.3mg.

Tablets dexamethasone 500microgram, 750microgram, 2mg, 4mg, 28 days @ 2mg once daily = $11.
Oral solution (elixir) 500microgram/5mL, 28 days @ 2mg once daily = $168.
Injection dexamethasone *sodium phosphate* 4mg/mL, 5mL vial = $9; 10mg/mL, 1mL, 10mL vials = $1.50, and $15 respectively.

Dexasone® (Valeant)
Tablets dexamethasone 500microgram, 750microgram, 4mg, 28 days @ 2mg once daily = $12.

Rectal products
Hydrocortisone
Cortenema® (Axcan)
Retention enema hydrocortisone 100mg/60mL, 60mL single-dose disposable unit = $7.

Hycort® (Valeant)
Retention enema hydrocortisone 100mg/60mL, 60mL single-dose disposable unit = $6.

1 Hanks GW et al. (1983) Corticosteroids in terminal cancer – a prospective analysis of current practice. *Postgraduate Medical Journal.* **59**: 702–706.
2 Hardy J et al. (2001) A prospective survey of the use of dexamethasone on a palliative care unit. *Palliative Medicine.* **15**: 3–8.
3 Greenberg HS et al. (1980) Epidural spinal cord compression from metastatic tumor: results with a new treatment protocol. *Annals of Neurology.* **8**: 361–366.
4 Feuer D and Broadley K (1999) Systematic review and meta-analysis of corticosteroids for the resolution of malignant bowel obstruction in advanced gynaecological and gastrointestinal cancers. *Annals of Oncology.* **10**: 1035–1041.
5 Laval G et al. (2000) The use of steroids in the management of inoperable intestinal obstruction in terminal cancer patients: do they remove the obstruction? *Palliative Medicine.* **14**: 3–10.
6 Minton MJ et al. (1981) Corticosteroids for elderly patients with breast cancer. *Cancer.* **48**: 883–887.
7 Tannock I et al. (1989) Treatment of metastatic prostatic cancer with low–dose prednisolone: evaluation of pain and quality of life as pragmatic indices of response. *Journal of Clinical Oncology.* **7**: 590–597.
8 Rhen T and Cidlowski JA (2005) Antiinflammatory action of glucocorticoids-new mechanisms for old drugs. *New England Journal of Medicine.* **353**: 1711–1723.
9 Moertel C et al. (1974) Corticosteroid therapy for preterminal gastrointestinal cancer. *Cancer.* **33**: 1607–1609.
10 Willox JC et al. (1984) Prednisolone as an appetite stimulant in patients with cancer. *British Medical Journal.* **288**: 27.
11 Bruera E et al. (1985) Action of oral methylprednisolone in terminal cancer patients: a prospective randomized double-blind study. *Cancer Treatment Reports.* **69**: 751–754.
12 Twycross RG and Guppy D (1985) Prednisolone in terminal breast and bronchogenic cancer. *Practitioner.* **229**: 57–59.
13 Gralla R et al. (1999) Recommendations for the use of antiemetics: evidence-based, clinical practice guidelines. *Journal of Clinical Oncology.* **17**: 2971–2994.
14 Editorial (1991) Ondansetron versus dexamethasone for chemotherapy-induced emesis. *Lancet.* **338**: 478.
15 Sridhar K et al. (1992) Five-drug antiemetic combination for cisplatin chemotherapy. *Cancer Investigation.* **10**: 191–199.
16 Bruera E et al. (2004) Dexamethasone in addition to metoclopramide for chronic nausea in patients with advanced cancer: a randomized controlled trial. *Journal of Pain and Symptom Management.* **28**: 381–388.
17 Swartz S and Dluhy R (1978) Corticosteroids: clinical pharmacology and therapeutic use. *Drugs.* **16**: 238–255.
18 Demoly P and Chung K (1998) Pharmacology of corticosteroids. *Respiratory Medicine.* **92**: 385–394.
19 Ellershaw J and Kelly M (1994) Corticosteroids and peptic ulceration. *Palliative Medicine.* **8**: 313–319.
20 Naesdal J and Brown K (2006) NSAID-associated adverse effects and acid control aids to prevent them: a review of current treatment options. *Drug Safety.* **29**: 119–132.
21 Chalk J et al. (1984) Phenytoin impairs the bioavailability of dexamethasone in neurological and neurosurgical patients. *Journal of Neurology, Neurosurgery, and Psychiatry.* **47**: 1087–1090.
22 Piper JM et al. (1991) Corticosteroid use and peptic ulcer disease: role of nonsteroidal anti-inflammatory drugs. *Annals of Internal Medicine.* **114**: 735–740.
23 Jick S et al. (2001) The risk of cataract among users of inhaled steroids. *Epidemiology.* **12**: 229–234.
24 Dropcho EJ and Soong S-J (1991) Steroid induced weakness in patients with primary brain tumours. *Neurology.* **41**: 1235–1239.
25 Eidelberg D (1991) Steroid myopathy. In: DA Rottenberg (ed) *Neurological Complications of Cancer Treatment.* Butterworth-Heineman, Boston, pp. 185–191.
26 Rotstein J and Good R (1957) Steroid pseudorheumatism. *AMA Archives of Internal Medicine.* **99**: 545–555.
27 Greenberg H et al. (1979) Epidural spinal cord compression from metastatic tumour: results with a new treatment protocol. *Annals of Neurology.* **8**: 361–366.
28 Delattre J-Y et al. (1988) High dose versus low dose dexamethasone in experimental epidural spinal cord compression. *Neurosurgery.* **22**: 1005–1007.
29 Vecht C et al. (1989) Initial bolus of conventional versus high-dose dexamethasone in metastatic spinal cord compression. *Neurology.* **39**: 1255–1257.
30 Galicich JH and French LA (1961) The use of dexamethasone in the treatment of cerebral oedema resulting from brain tumours and brain surgery. *American Practitioner.* **12**: 169.
31 Kirkham S (1988) The palliation of cerebral tumours with high-dose dexamethasone: a review. *Palliative Medicine.* **2**: 27–33.
32 CSM (Committee on Safety of Medicines and Medicines Control Agency) (1998) Withdrawal of systemic corticosteroids. *Current Problems in Pharmacovigilance.* **24 (May)**: 5–7.
33 Vecht C et al. (1994) Dose-effect relationship of dexamethasone on Karnofsky performance in metastatic brain tumors. A randomized study of doses of 4, 8 and 16 mg per day. *Neurology.* **44**: 675–680.

DESMOPRESSIN

Class: Vasopressin analogue.

Indications: Pituitary diabetes insipidus, post–hypophysectomy polydipsia and polyuria, post head-trauma polydipsia and polyuria, nocturnal enuresis (tablets only).

Contra-indications: Moderate-severe renal impairment (creatinine clearance < 50mL/min), current or previous hyponatremia. Coronary insufficiency, psychogenic polydipsia, polydipsia associated with alcohol abuse, concurrent use with diuretics. Type IIB or platelet-type (pseudo) von Willebrand's disease.

Pharmacology

Desmopressin is an analogue of the pituitary antidiuretic hormone, **vasopressin**. It increases water resorption by the renal tubules, thereby reducing urine volume. Desmopressin is ineffective in nephrogenic diabetes insipidus. Desmopressin has a longer duration of action than **vasopressin**.

Bio-availability 3–4% intranasal; 0.1–5% PO.
Onset of action 1h intranasal; 2h PO.
Plasma halflife 0.4–4h intranasal; 1.5–2.5h PO.
Duration of action 5–24h intranasal; 6–8h PO.

Cautions

Serious drug interactions: the concurrent use of drugs which increase the endogenous secretion of vasopressin increases the risk of symptomatic hyponatremia, notably TCAs, SSRIs, **chlorpromazine**, opioid analgesics, NSAIDs, **lamotrigine** and **carbamazepine**. **Loperamide** triples the desmopressin plasma concentration after PO administration.[1]

Hypertension, CHF, raised intracranial pressure. Take care to avoid fluid overload; with excessive water intake there is a higher risk of hyponatremia.

The effect of desmopressin is likely to be potentiated by drugs which cause fluid retention, e.g. NSAIDs and corticosteroids.

Undesirable effects

For full list, see manufacturer's Product Monograph.

Common (<10%, >1%): tablets and high doses of nasal spray (≥40microgram/24h): headache, abdominal pain, nausea. Nasal spray: nosebleeds, nasal congestion or rhinitis, sore throat.

Rare or very rare (<0.1%): water retention and hyponatremia; in extreme cases this may result in hyponatremic seizures.

Dose and use

Note: worldwide post-marketing data indicate a higher incidence of hyponatremia in patients being treated with intranasal formulations compared with oral formulations.

Keep to the recommended starting doses to minimize the risk of hyponatremic seizures. Advise patients to restrict fluids in the evenings, particularly if they are at risk of developing raised intracranial pressure, or if using desmopressin for nocturia. They should stop taking desmopressin if they develop persistent nausea and vomiting, or diarrhea, and seek medical advice.

Pituitary diabetes insipidus

- start with 100microgram PO t.i.d., 60microgram SL t.i.d. or 10–20microgram intranasally at bedtime
- if ineffective, increase dose progressively every few days
- effective dose is generally 100–400microgram PO t.i.d., 60–240microgram SL t.i.d. or 10–20microgram at bedtime–b.i.d.

Refractory nocturia
Treat only with PO tablets:
- start with 200microgram PO at bedtime
- if ineffective, increase dose progressively every few days to a maximum of 600microgram PO at bedtime.

Supply
Desmopressin (generic)
Tablets 100microgram, 200microgram, 28 days @ 200microgram t.i.d. = $167.
Nasal spray (pump) 10microgram/metered spray, 50 dose bottle = $71.

DDAVP® (Ferring)
Tablets 100microgram, 200microgram, 28 days @ 200microgram t.i.d. = $238.
Tablets SL (DDAVP® Melt) 60microgram, 120microgram, 28 days @ 120microgram t.i.d. = $179.
Intranasal solution (DDAVP® Rhinyle®) 100microgram/mL, 50 dose bottle = $101. *Store in refrigerator at 2–8°C.*
Nasal spray (aerosol) (DDAVP® Spray) 10microgram/metered spray, 25 and 50 dose bottle = $51 and $101 respectively. *Store upright at room temperature 15–30°C.*

---

1 Callreus T et al. (1999) Changes in gastrointestinal motility influence the absorption of desmopressin. *European Journal of Clinical Pharmacology.* **55**: 305–309.

DRUGS FOR DIABETES MELLITUS

Indications: Diabetes mellitus not controlled by diet.

Contra-indications: Because of their long plasma halflives (and increased risk of hypoglycemia), **chlorpropamide** and **glyburide** should not be used in the elderly, those with renal (creatinine clearance < 60mL/min) or hepatic impairment, during severe infection, after major trauma, or peri-operatively.
  Because of the risk of lactic acidosis, **metformin** should not be used in patients receiving medication for CHF, hypoxemic states, or with renal impairment. Avoid in patients with excessive alcohol intake, severe hepatic impairment, patients undergoing radiologic studies involving intravascular administration of iodinated contrast materials, during severe infection, after major trauma, or peri-operatively.
  Thiazolidinediones, e.g. **pioglitazone**, **rosiglitazone**, should not be used in patients with NYHA class 3 and class 4 CHF, severe hepatic impairment or concurrently with nitrates or insulin.[1]

Clinical background
There are two main types of diabetes mellitus (Box 7.1).
In patients with symptoms suggestive of diabetes mellitus (e.g. polyuria and/or thirst, polydipsia), a diagnosis can be made on the basis of the following criteria:
- fasting plasma glucose concentrations of ≥7.0mmol/L (normal < 5.6mmol/L) *or*
- casual (random) plasma glucose concentrations of ≥11.1mmol/L *or*
- 2h post-load plasma glucose ≥11.1mmol/L (normal < 7.8mmol/L) during oral 75g glucose tolerance test.

In patients who do not have symptoms suggestive of diabetes mellitus, these criteria should be confirmed by repeat testing on another day.[2,3] However, the renal threshold increases with age, and older patients may not develop typical symptoms until their fasting blood glucose concentration exceeds 18mmol/L.
  Glucose intolerance is one of the first metabolic consequences of cancer and is found in nearly 40% of non-diabetic cancer patients given an oral or IV glucose tolerance test.[4] Corticosteroids are the most common precipitant of diabetes in advanced cancer.[5] Thiazide diuretics, **furosemide**, **octreotide**, and atypical antipsychotic medications such as **risperidone** and **olanzapine** may also produce hyperglycemia.

Box 7.1 Classification of diabetes mellitus

Type 1 (the minority, 5–10% in North America)
Typically develops in children, young people, and adults <30 years old. There is a lack of insulin because of immune-mediated destruction of the β-cells in the pancreas. Symptoms develop rapidly and the diagnosis is based on the presence of characteristic symptoms plus a high blood glucose concentration.

Injections of insulin are an essential life-long treatment, including the last days of life. However, in order to avoid hypoglycemia, the dose will need to be reduced as dietary intake declines.

Type 2 (the majority)
Typically develops in adults >40 years old, although it is increasingly manifesting in younger people because of obesity. The pancreas does not produce sufficient insulin for the body's needs and generally there is also marked insulin resistance, i.e. cells are not able to respond to the insulin that is produced. Symptoms tend to develop gradually, with a long delay (possibly years) before diagnosis. Treatment is based on modification of diet and weight loss, together with various glucose-lowering drugs.

Note: *some Type 2 diabetics need insulin.* However, when an illness such as cancer leads to a reduced dietary intake and weight loss, it is often possible to reduce or discontinue insulin, and sometimes oral hypoglycemic drugs as well.

The main goal of diabetic management in palliative care is to preserve quality of life. Thus, the aim of treatment is the prevention of symptoms from hyper-or hypoglycemia, keto-acidosis and hyperosmolar non-ketotic states; concern about long-term complications is no longer relevant.[6] Although glycated hemoglobin (HbA$_{1c}$) is measured to determine the overall level of glycemic control over 6–8 weeks, this will be irrelevant in most palliative care patients (normal = 6%; aim in diabetes = <9–10%, preferably <7%).[7]

Pharmacology
There are several different classes of antidiabetic drugs, with differing modes of action (Table 7.5) In newly diagnosed symptomatic patients, the Canadian Diabetes Association (www.diabetes.ca) recommends **metformin** as the first-line oral hypoglycemic.[8] However, **metformin** is associated with weight loss, making it unattractive for most patients with end-stage cancer. It is also contra-indicated in patients with CHF or renal impairment because of the increased risk of lactic acidosis. **Metformin** is also best not used in all elderly debilitated patients, particularly those with hepatic impairment or COPD.

Thus, in debilitated or elderly patients, a sulfonylurea may be a more appropriate choice. A relatively short-acting sulfonylurea such as **gliclazide** or **tolbutamide** should be prescribed with a realistic safe target, e.g. fasting blood glucose 8–12mmol/L. The dose should be reduced if the fasting blood glucose is consistently <8mmol/L.

Alternatively, a meglitinide can be used, e.g. **repaglinide**. This new class of drugs acts in a similar way to the sulfonylureas but more rapidly and for a shorter time. This permits 'pulse dosing' before meals. For pharmacokinetic details, see Table 7.6.

Thiazolidinediones are contra-indicated in patients with end-stage CHF because they cause fluid retention.[1,7] All patients taking a thiazolidinedione should be monitored for symptoms and signs of CHF, e.g. excessive/rapid weight gain, cough, increasing breathlessness, and/or edema.

Insulin is sometimes needed in patients with advanced cancer and newly diagnosed diabetes mellitus. The dose is monitored to achieve a fasting blood glucose of 8–12mmol/L. Doses of 0.5units/kg/day of a *long-acting* **insulin analogue**, e.g. **insulin glargine**, **insulin detemir** (both given once daily) or **isophane (NPH) insulin** (given b.i.d., or just at bedtime) will provide only a basal insulin supply, and thus it does not matter if a patient on this amount is not eating

Table 7.5 Selected oral antidiabetic drugs

Class	Examples	Mechanism of action	Risk of hypoglycemia	Comment
Biguanides	Metformin	Decrease hepatic gluconeogenesis, and increase the uptake of glucose by muscle	−	Tend to cause weight loss; may cause nausea and diarrhea; low risk of lactic acidosis
DPP-4 (dipeptidyl peptidase-4) inhibitors	Sitagliptin	Increase insulin secretion and lower glucagon secretion	±	Newly introduced; little experience
Meglitinides	Repaglinide	Increase insulin secretion	−	Relatively fast onset and short duration of action permits a more flexible regimen
Sulfonylureas	Gliclazide	Increase insulin secretion	++ with longer-acting drugs, e.g. glyburide, chlorpropamide	Original class of oral antidiabetic drugs; relatively inexpensive
Thiazolidinediones	Pioglitazone, rosiglitazone	Enhance the effect of insulin	−	Cause fluid retention, and exacerbate CHF[9,10]

Table 7.6 Pharmacokinetics of selected oral hypoglycemic drugs

	Repaglinide	Tolbutamide	Gliclazide
Bio-availability	56%	>95%	78%
Onset of action	15–60min	1–3h	3–4h
Time to peak plasma concentration	1h	3–5h	2–4h
Plasma halflife	1h	4.5–6.5h	10–12h
Duration of action	4–6h	≤12h	12–24h

(see below for timing). However, in patients who are still eating, requiring larger doses than this, **insulin glargine** or **insulin detemir** are a better choice than **isophane (NPH) insulin** because there is less likelihood of interprandial hypoglycemia. A SC sliding scale of a *rapid-acting* **insulin analogue** (e.g. **insulin aspart**, **insulin lispro**, available as pen devices) is occasionally necessary. An IV sliding scale of rapid-acting **regular (soluble) insulin** is generally reserved for patients with diabetic keto-acidosis or used peri-operatively.

Further, if prescribed a corticosteroid, patients with pre-existing non-insulin-dependent diabetes on maximal doses of **gliclazide** or **tolbutamide** may require **insulin** *in addition*. Although 10 units of **insulin glargine**, **insulin detemir** or **isophane (NPH) insulin** may suffice, a much higher total daily dose of **insulin** is sometimes necessary, occasionally as much as 100 units.[6] Note:

• it is unnecessary to maintain theoretically ideal blood glucose levels to avoid long-term complications[6]
• rigid dietary control is not indicated when life expectancy is short
• when stable, monitoring is generally adequate with a fasting blood glucose fingerstick test twice a week.

Cautions

Patients starting treatment with **insulin** should not drive a motor vehicle until their physician confirms that it is safe for them to do so. If concerned about the ongoing safety of a patient to drive, physicians are required to inform the Motor Registration/Vehicle department in the province or territory in which that patient is licensed.

Patients with impaired awareness of the onset of hypoglycemia or frequent hypoglycemic episodes should be informed that they are at high risk of experiencing symptomatic hypoglycemia when driving. They should make efforts to minimize the risk, including measuring blood glucose levels periodically before and during driving.[11] For more information, see www.diabetes.ca/Section_About/aboutdriveguide.asp.

After discontinuation, **chlorpropamide** and **glyburide** can produce hypoglycemia for 2–3 days, and up to 4 days if there is renal or hepatic impairment.

In patients with long-standing diabetes, autonomic neuropathy may remove both the warning symptoms (sweating, tremor, pounding heart beat) and the counter-regulatory mechanism of an epinephrine-induced increase in blood glucose. Such patients tend to present with pallor, mental detachment ± drowsiness ± clumsiness. Some become irritable and aggressive, and others slip rapidly into hypoglycemic coma. Malnourished patients with reduced hepatic glycogen stores also have a reduced capacity to counteract hypoglycemia (Box 7.J).[12]

Box 7.J   Treatment of hypoglycemia

If conscious, give glucose 10–20g PO. Approximately 15g of glucose is contained in:
- 4 Dex4® glucose tablets (total 16g glucose) or 3 BD® glucose tablets (total 15g glucose)
- 2/3 Insta-Glucose® gel tube (1 tube = 24g glucose)
- 3 teaspoons or 15mL of sugar dissolved in water
- 15mL (tablespoon) of honey
- 90mL of Coca-Cola® (not diet version)
- 120–180mL of fruit juice (squeezed or concentrate).

If drowsy and swallowing unsafe, or unconscious, give glucagon 1mg IM or IV; can be given SC, but will act more slowly.

If no response in 10min, give glucose 20% 50mL IV.

Undesirable effects
See manufacturer's Product Monograph.
GI symptoms, e.g. nausea and diarrhea, are common with **metformin**, particularly initially.

Dose and use

Any patient admitted to a palliative care service or a hospice with a diagnosis of end-stage CHF and type 2 diabetes mellitus, and who is still taking a thiazolidinedione, should stop this medication immediately. This sometimes leads to significant improvement in the patient's condition and quality of life. Thiazolidinediones should also be stopped in patients with severe hepatic impairment.

Hypoglycemic drugs may need to be reduced or stopped if the patient loses weight and/or becomes anorexic, or if nausea and vomiting results in a much reduced food intake.[6]

Gliclazide
- start with 40–80mg each morning (with breakfast)
- if necessary, increase every 3 days to a maximum of 160mg b.i.d.

Tolbutamide
- start with 500mg b.i.d.
- if necessary, increase every 3 days to a maximum of 1g b.i.d.

Metformin
- start with 500mg each morning (with breakfast), or b.i.d. (e.g. with breakfast and evening meal)
- if necessary, increase by 500mg at weekly intervals
- maximum dose 2,550mg/24h, i.e. 850mg t.i.d. with meals.

Repaglinide
- take before main meals; frequency changes if eating pattern changes
- start with 500microgram if no previous treatment with oral hypoglycemic drugs
- start with 1mg if previously treated with an alternative oral hypoglycemic drug
- if necessary, increase the dose at 1–2 week intervals, to a maximum of 4mg q.i.d.

Insulin
- if the patient is already taking the maximum dose of an oral hypoglycemic, and the fasting blood glucose is >12mmol/L, prescribe a long-acting **insulin analogue**, e.g. **insulin glargine** 10 units once daily at bedtime[13]
- adjust the dose according to the response
- a preprandial sliding scale of a SC rapid-acting **insulin analogue**, e.g. **insulin aspart** or **insulin lispro** is occasionally necessary (Table 7.7).

Table 7.7 Preprandial sliding scale of SC *rapid-acting* insulin analogue[a]

Preprandial blood glucose (mmol/L)	Rapid-acting insulin analogue dose (units)
10–15	6
15–18	8
18–22	10
>22[b]	12

a. responses to insulin vary widely and sliding scales need to be individualized
b. patients with marked hyperglycemia should have monitoring 2h after meals as well until the blood glucose is better controlled.

Supply
Gliclazide (generic)
Tablets 80mg (scored), 28 days @ 80mg each morning = $8.

Diamicron® (Servier Canada)
Tablets 80mg (scored), 28 days @ 80mg each morning = $12.

Tolbutamide (generic)
Tablets 500mg, 28 days @ 500mg b.i.d. = $3.

Metformin (generic)
Tablets 500mg, 850mg, 28 days @ 500mg b.i.d. = $7.

Glucophage® (Sanofi-Aventis Canada)
Tablets 500mg, 850mg, 28 days @ 500mg b.i.d. = $29.

Repaglinide
Gluconorm® (Novo Nordisk Canada)
Tablets 500microgram, 1mg, 2mg, 28 days @ 500microgram t.i.d. = $26.

Sitagliptin
Januvia® (Merck Frosst Canada)
Tablets 100mg, 28 days @ 100mg daily = $85.

Insulin analogues
Rapid-acting insulin analogues
Insulin lispro
Humalog® (Eli Lilly Canada)
Injection 100 units/mL, 10mL multidose vial = $29.

Injection (cartridge for use with re-usable pen injector device), 100 units/mL, 5×3mL cartridge = $60.
Injection (disposable prefilled pen injector), 100 units/mL, 5×3mL pen = $75.

Insulin lispro is also available with **insulin lispro protamine** as an intermediate-acting combination.

Insulin aspart
Novorapid® (Novo Nordisk Canada)
Injection 100 units/mL, 10mL multidose vial = $30.
Injection (cartridge for use with re-usable PenFill® injector device), 100 units/mL, 5×3mL cartridge = $58.

Long-acting insulin analogues
Insulin detemir
Levemir® (Novo Nordisk Canada)
Injection (cartridge for use with re-usable PenFill® injector device), 100 units/mL, 3mL cartridge = $24.

Insulin glargine
Lantus® (Sanofi-Aventis Canada)
Injection 100 units/mL, 10mL multidose vial = $61.
Injection (cartridge for use with re-usable injector device), 100 units/mL, 5×3mL cartridge = $95.
Injection (disposable prefilled pen injector), SoloStar®, 100 units/ml, 5×3mL pen = $95.

1   Nesto RW *et al.* (2004) Thiazolidinedione use, fluid retention, and congestive heart failure: a consensus statement from the American Heart Association and American Diabetes Association. *Diabetes Care.* **27**: 256–263.
2   World Health Organization (1999) *Definition, diagnosis and classification of diabetes mellitus and its complications; Part 1: Diagnosis and classification of diabetes mellitus.* WHO, Geneva.
3   ADA (American Diabetes Association) (2008) Diagnosis and classification of diabetes mellitus. *Diabetes Care.* **31 (suppl 1)**: S55–60.
4   Glicksman A and Rawson R (1956) Diabetes and altered carbohydrate metabolism in patients with cancer. *Cancer.* **9**: 1127–1134.
5   Poulson J (1997) The management of diabetes in patients with advanced cancer. *Journal of Pain and Symptom Management.* **13**: 339–346.
6   Usborne C and Wilding J (2003) Treating diabetes mellitus in palliative care patients. *European Journal of Palliative Care.* **10**: 186–188.
7   Diabetes Care (2008) Executive Summary: Standards of Medical Care in Diabetes—31 (**1**): S5. Available from: *http://care.diabetesjournals.org/cgi/reprint/31/Supplement_1/S5?eaf*
8   Canadian Diabetes Association (2008) Clinical practice guidelines for the prevention and management of diabetes in Canada. Available from: www.diabetes.ca/files/cpg2008/cpg-2008.pdf
9   Page RL, 2nd *et al.* (2003) Possible heart failure exacerbation associated with rosiglitazone: case report and literature review. *Pharmacotherapy.* **23**: 945–954.
10 Cheng AY and Fantus IG (2004) Thiazolidinedione-induced congestive heart failure. *Annals of Pharmacotherpy.* **38**: 817–820.
11 Begg IS *et al.* (2003) Canadian Diabetes Association's clinical practice guidelines for diabetes and private and commerical driving. *Canadian Journal of Diabetes.* **27**: 128–140.
12 Holroyde C *et al.* (1975) Altered glucose metabolism in metastatic carcinoma. *Cancer Research.* **35**: 3710–3714.
13 Yki-Jarvinen H *et al.* (1992) Comparison of insulin regimens in patients with non-insulin-dependent diabetes mellitus. *New England Journal of Medicine.* **327**: 1426–1433.

*OCTREOTIDE

Class: Synthetic hormone.

Indications: Acromegaly; †unresectable hormone-secreting tumours, e.g. carcinoid, VIPomas, glucagonomas; †prevention of complications after elective pancreatic surgery;[1] †bleeding esophageal varices;[2] †salivary, pancreatic and enterocutaneous fistulas;[3,4] †intractable diarrhea related to high output ileostomies,[5,6] †AIDS, radiation therapy, chemotherapy or bone marrow transplant;[3,7] †inoperable bowel obstruction in patients with cancer;[8,9] †hypertrophic pulmonary osteo-arthopathy;[10] †ascites in cirrhosis and cancer;[11,12,13] †buccal fistula,[14] †death rattle, †bronchorrhea,[15] †reduction of tumour-related secretions.[11]

Pharmacology

Octreotide is a synthetic analogue of somatostatin with a longer duration of action.[16] Somatostatin is an inhibitory hormone found throughout the body. In the hypothalamus it inhibits the release of growth hormone, thyroid-stimulating hormone (TSH), prolactin and adrenocorticotrophic hormone (ACTH). It inhibits the secretion of insulin, glucagon, gastrin and other peptides of the gastro-enteropancreatic system (i.e. peptide YY, neurotensin, VIP and substance P), reducing splanchnic blood flow, portal blood flow, GI motility, gastric, pancreatic and small bowel secretion, and increasing water and electrolyte absorption.[17] In Type I diabetes mellitus, octreotide decreases insulin requirements. However, in Type 2 diabetes, octreotide suppresses both insulin and glucagon release, leaving plasma glucose concentrations either unchanged or slightly elevated.[18,19] Octreotide has a direct anticancer effect on solid tumours of the GI tract and prolongs survival.[20–23] In hormone-secreting tumours, octreotide improves symptoms by inhibiting hormone secretion, e.g.

- 5HT in carcinoid (improving flushing and diarrhea)
- VIP in VIPomas (improving diarrhea)
- glucagon in glucagonomas (improving rash and diarrhea).

In patients with cancer and inoperable bowel obstruction, octreotide rapidly improves symptoms in ≥75% of patients.[8,9,24] Doses of ≤1,200microgram/24h were used but a beneficial effect is generally apparent with ≤600microgram/24h. Octreotide 300microgram/24h appears to reduce NG (nasogastric) tube output more effectively and rapidly than **hyoscine (scopolamine) butylbromide** 60mg/24h, although both allowed NG tube removal after about 5 days.[24] (Although no head-to-head comparison has been published to date, it is likely that the same is true for **glycopyrrolate**.)

Octreotide 300microgram SC b.i.d. can suppress diuretic-induced activation of the renin-aldosterone-angiotensin system and its addition has improved renal function and Na+ and water excretion in patients with cirrhosis and ascites receiving **furosemide** and **spironolactone**.[13] Octreotide is also reported to reduce the rate of formation of malignant ascites.[11,12] It may interfere with ascitic fluid formation through a reduction in splanchnic blood flow or as a result of a direct tumour antisecretory effect. Octreotide may also help improve the efficacy of diuretics as in cirrhosis.[25] Octreotide could be considered in patients with rapidly accumulating ascites requiring frequent paracentesis despite diuretic therapy (see **Spironolactone**, p.42). Octreotide may also help resolve chylous ascites[26,27] and pleural effusion secondary to cirrhosis.[28,29] Octreotide is reported to improve mucous discharge from rectal cancers,[11] and to provide rapid pain relief in a patient with hypertrophic pulmonary osteo-arthopathy that had not improved with more traditional analgesia.[10] Octreotide reduces salivary production and may be of use in buccal fistulas[14] (see **scopolamine (hyoscine) hydrobromide** p.195, **hyoscine (scopolamine) butylbromide** p.11, **glycopyrrolate** p.465). Octreotide led to rapid and complete control of bronchorrhea (>1L/day) in a patient with adenocarcinoma of the lung.[15]

At doses far below those necessary for an antisecretory effect (e.g. 1microgram SC t.i.d.), octreotide protects the stomach from NSAID-related injury, probably via its ability to reduce NSAID-induced neutrophil adhesion to the microvasculature.[30] Somatostatin receptors have been identified on leucocytes and, in rats, octreotide has been shown to suppress inflammation.[31] Octreotide is also of value in chronic non-malignant pancreatic pain caused by hypertension in the scarred pancreatic ducts.[32,33] Suppressing exocrine function by administering **pancreatin** supplements also reduces pain in 50-75% of patients with chronic pancreatitis.[34] The benefit reported with octreotide could therefore be secondary to its antisecretory action.[35] Octreotide is generally given as a bolus SC or by CSCI.[36] It can be given IV when a rapid effect is required.

Octreotide has also been administered IT.[37] Long-acting depot formulations are also available for octreotide.[38] Their use has been evaluated only in hormone-secreting tumours.

Lanreotide is an alternative sandostatin analogue. It is available as a depot injection via the Special Access Programme. It is approved in the UK and USA for the long-term treatment of acromegaly which has not responded to, or cannot be treated with, surgery or radiation therapy, and for symptoms associated with neuro-endocrine tumours, particularly carcinoid.

Onset of action 30min.
Time to peak plasma concentration 30min SC.
Plasma halflife 1.5h SC (may be increased in cirrhosis).
Duration of action 8h.

Cautions

Serious drug interactions: octreotide markedly reduces plasma **cyclosporine** concentrations and inadequate immunosuppression may result. Increase the **cyclosporine** dose by 50% before starting octreotide, and monitor the plasma concentration daily to guide further adjustments.[39]

May cause gallstones (manufacturer advises ultrasound examination of the gallbladder before treatment and then every 6–12 months for patients on long-term treatment). Avoid abrupt withdrawal of short-acting octreotide after long-term treatment (may precipitate biliary colic caused by gallstones/biliary sludge).

Insulinoma: may potentiate hypoglycemia. In Type I diabetes mellitus, **insulin** requirements may be reduced by up to 50%; monitor plasma glucose concentrations to guide any dose reduction needed with **insulin** or oral hypoglycemic agents.[39]

May cause bradycardia, conduction defects or other arrhythmias; use with caution in at-risk patients. Monitor thyroid function during long-term treatment; may cause hypothyroidism.

Undesirable effects

For full list, see manufacturer's Product Monograph.
Bolus injection SC is painful (but less if the vial is warmed to room temperature), fatigue, headache, dizziness, bradycardia, conduction defects, arrhythmia, ECG changes including QT interval prolongation, dry mouth, flatulence (lowers esophageal sphincter tone), anorexia, nausea, vomiting, abdominal pain, diarrhea, steatorrhea, impaired glucose tolerance, hypoglycemia (shortly after starting treatment), persistent hyperglycemia (during long-term treatment), gallstones (10–20% of patients on long-term treatment), pancreatitis (associated with gallstones), back pain.

Dose and use

Dose varies according to indication (Table 7.8). Some of the recommendations are based on experience with only a small number of patients, so the dose should always be titrated according to effect. Once improvement in the symptom is achieved, reduction to the lowest dose that maintains symptom control can be tried.

Extrapolation from t.i.d. dosing may explain why 300–600microgram/24h CSCI is a common recommendation. However, because of ampoule size, rounding down to 250–500microgram is more convenient and more cost-effective.

Octreotide can be painful if given as an SC bolus. This can be reduced if the ampoule is warmed in the hand to body temperature before injection. To reduce the likelihood of inflammatory reactions at the skin injection site with CSCI, dilute to the largest volume possible and consider the use of 0.9% saline (see Diluent section in Chapter 18, p.515).

There are 2-drug compatibility data for octreotide in 0.9% saline with **haloperidol, hyoscine (scopolamine) butylbromide, scopolamine (hyoscine) hydrobromide, midazolam, morphine sulfate, ondansetron**. Incompatibility may occur with **dexamethasone**.
For more details and 3-drug compatibility data see Charts A4.1–A4.4 (p.591). Compatibility data in WFI can be found on www.palliativedrugs.com *Syringe Driver Survey Database.*

Table 7.8 Typical dose recommendations for SC octreotide

Indication	Starting dose	Usual maximum
Hormone-secreting tumours		
acromegaly	100–200microgram t.i.d.	600microgram/24h[17]
carcinoid, glucagonomas	50microgram once daily or b.i.d.; increased to 200microgram t.i.d.	1,500microgram/24h; rarely 6,000microgram/24h[40]
VIPomas	100microgram b.i.d.–t.i.d.	As for carcinoid (above)
Intractable diarrhea	50–500microgram/24h	1,500microgram/24h,[41] occasionally higher[42]
Bowel obstruction	250–500microgram/24h	750microgram/24h, occasionally higher
Tumour-antisecretory effect	50–100microgram b.i.d.	600microgram/24h[11]
Ascites	200–600microgram/24h	600microgram/24h[12]
Bronchorrhea	300–500microgram/24h[15]	
Hypertrophic pulmonary osteo-arthopathy	100microgram b.i.d.[10]	

Depot formulation

A depot formulation of octreotide 10–30mg, given every 4 weeks is available. There is limited experience of its use for the long-term management of malignant bowel obstruction, although benefit in a small number of patients with ovarian cancer for up to 15 months has been reported.[43] Thus, in palliative care, the long-acting formulation is most likely to be used in patients with a chronic intestinal fistula or intractable diarrhea. Generally, it will be used only when symptoms have first been controlled with SC octreotide, and when cost is not prohibitive. The Canadian manufacturer advises that patients who have not previously received octreotide should be treated with SC octreotide for 2 weeks to exclude any undesirable effects before switching to the depot injection and, in acromegaly, this must have been brought under control. The depot octreotide product requires deep IM injection into the gluteal muscle.

In acromegaly, stop the SC dose of octreotide when the first depot injection is given; for other neuro-endocrine tumours continue the SC dose for a further 2 weeks.

Lanreotide

See Product Monograph. Give depot formulation by deep SC injection into the gluteal region.

Supply

Octreotide (generic)
Injection 50microgram/mL, 1mL vial = $6; 100microgram/mL, 1mL vial = $9; 500microgram/mL, 1mL vial = $39; 200microgram/mL, 5mL vial = $78. *Unopened vials can be kept for up to 2 weeks at room temperature. For prolonged storage, unopened vials should be kept in a refrigerator. Once opened, multidose vials must be refrigerated and used within 2 weeks.*

Sandostatin® (Novartis Pharmaceuticals Canada)
Injection 50microgram/mL, 1mL amp = $6; 100microgram/mL, 1mL amp = $11; 500microgram/mL, 1mL amp = $48; *for prolonged storage, keep unopened ampules in a refrigerator; unopened ampules can be kept for up to 2 weeks at room temperature.*

Sandostatin LAR® (Novartis Pharmaceuticals Canada)
Depot injection (microsphere powder for aqueous suspension) 10mg vial = $1,350; 20mg vial = $1,744; 30mg vial = $2,238 (all supplied with diluent and syringe), for IM injection every 28 days. *Keep in a refrigerator and protect from light; vial should be brought up to room temperature 30–60min before administration but must only be reconstituted immediately before injection.*

Lanreotide

Somatuline Autogel® (Ipsen)
Available via Special Access: McKesson Logistics Solutions (1-888-288-8143).

Depot injection (prefilled syringe) 60mg = $1,102; 90mg = $1,470; 120mg = $1,840. *Keep in a refrigerator and protect from light; the syringe should be brought up to room temperature 30min before administration but should only be removed from its sealed pouch immediately before injection.*

1 Bassi C et al. (1994) Prophylaxis of complications after pancreatic surgery: results of a multicenter trial in Italy. Italian Study Group. Digestion. **55 (suppl 1)**: 41–47.

2 Sung J (1993) Octreotide infusion or emergency sclerotherapy for variceal haemorrhage. Lancet. **342**: 637–641.

3 Harris A (1992) Octreotide in the treatment of disorders of the gastrointestinal tract. Drug Investigation. **4**: 1–54.

4 Spinell C et al. (1995) Postoperative salivary fistula: therapeutic action of octreotide. Surgery. **117**: 117–118.

5 Farthing MJ (1994) Octreotide in the treatment of refractory diarrhoea and intestinal fistulae. Gut. **35 (suppl 3)**: s5–10.

3 Dorta G (1999) Role of octreotide and somatostatin in the treatment of intestinal fistulae. Digestion. **60 (suppl 2)**: 53–56.

7 Crouch M et al. (1996) Octreotide acetate in refractory bone marrow transplant-associated diarrhea. Annals of Pharmacotherapy. **30**: 331–336.

8 Mercadante S et al. (1993) Octreotide in relieving gastrointestinal symptoms due to bowel obstruction. Palliative Medicine. **7**: 295–299.

9 Riley J and Fallon M (1994) Octreotide in terminal malignant obstruction of the gastrointestinal tract. European Journal of Palliative Care. **1**: 23–25.

10 Johnson S et al. (1997) Treatment of resistant pain in hypertrophic pulmonary arthropathy with subcutaneous octreotide. Thorax. **52**: 298–299.

11 Harvey M and Dunlop R (1996) Octreotide and the secretory effects of advanced cancer. Palliative Medicine. **10**: 346–347.

12 Caims W and Malone R (1999) Octreotide as an agent for the relief of malignant ascites in palliative care patients. Palliative Medicine. **13**: 429–430.

13 Kalambokis G et al. (2005) Renal effects of treatment with diuretics, octreotide or both, in non-azotemic cirrhotic patients with ascites. Nephrology, Dialysis, Transplantation. **20**: 1623–1629.

14 Lam C and Wong S (1996) Use of somatostatin analog in the management of traumatic parotid fistula. Surgery. **119**: 481–482.

15 Hudson E et al. (2006) Successful treatment of bronchorrhea with octreotide in a patient with adenocarcinoma of the lung. Journal of Pain and Symptom Management. **32**: 200–202.

16 Lamberts SWJ et al. (1996) Octreotide. New England Journal of Medicine. **334**: 246–254.

17 Gyr K and Meier R (1993) Pharmacodynamic effects of sandostatin in the gastrointestinal tract. Digestion. **54**: 14–19.

18 Davies R et al. (1989) Somatostatin analogues in diabetes mellitus. Diabetic Medicine. **6**: 103–111.

19 Lunetta M et al. (1997) Effects of octreotide on glycaemic control, glucose disposal, hepatic glucose production and counterregulatory hormone secretion in type 1 and type 2 insulin treated diabetic patients. Diabetes Research and Clinical Practice. **38**: 81–89.

20 Cascinu S et al. (1995) A randomised trial of octreotide vs best supportive care only in advanced gastrointestinal cancer patients refractory to chemotherapy. British Journal of Cancer. **71**: 97–101.

21 Pandha H and Waxman J (1996) Octreotide in malignant intestinal obstruction. Anti-cancer Drugs. **7**: 5–10.

22 Kouroumalis E et al. (1998) Treatment of hepatocellular carcinoma with octreotide: a randomised controlled study. Gut. **42**: 442–447.

23 Deming DA et al. (2005) A dramatic response to long-acting octreotide in metastatic hepatocellular carcinoma. Clinical Advances in Hematology & Oncology. **3**: 468–472; discussion 472–464.

24 Ripamonti C et al. (2000) Role of octreotide, scopolamine butylbromide, and hydration in symptom control of patients with inoperable bowel obstruction and nasogastric tubes: a prospective randomized trial. Journal of Pain and Symptom Management. **19**: 23–34.

25 Kalambokis G et al. (2006) The effects of treatment with octreotide, diuretics, or both on portal hemodynamics in nonazotemic cirrhotic patients with ascites. Journal of Clinical Gastroenterology. **40**: 342–346.

26 Widjaja A et al. (1999) Octreotide for therapy of chylous ascites in yellow nail syndrome. Gastroenterology. **116**: 1017–1018.

27 Ferrandiere M et al. (2000) Chylous ascites following radical nephrectomy: efficacy of octreotide as treatment of ruptured thoracic duct. Intensive Care and Medicine. **26**: 484–485.

28 Dumortier J et al. (2000) Successful treatment of hepatic hydrothorax with octreotide. European Journal of Gastroenterology and Hepatology. **12**: 817–820.

29 Pfammatter R et al. (2001) Treatment of hepatic hydrothorax and reduction of chest tube output with octreotide. European Journal of Gastroenterology and Hepatology. **13**: 977–980.

30 Scheiman J et al. (1997) Reduction of NSAID induced gastric injury and leucocyte endothelial adhesion by octreotide. Gut. **40**: 720–725.

31 Karalis K et al. (1994) Somatostatin analogues suppress the inflammatory reaction in vivo. Journal of Clinical Investigations. **93**: 2000–2006.

32 Okazaki K et al. (1988) Pressure of papillary zone and pancreatic main duct in patients with chronic pancreatitis in the early state. Scandinavian Journal of Gastroenterology. **23**: 501–506.

33 Donnelly PK et al. (1991) Somatostatin for chronic pancreatic pain. Journal of Pain and Symptom Management. **6**: 349–350.

34 Mossner J et al. (1989) Influence of treatment with pancreatic extracts on pancreatic enzyme secretion. Gut. **3**: 1143–1149.

35 Lembcke B et al. (1987) Effect of the somatostatin analogue sandostatin on gastrointestinal, pancreatic and biliary function and hormone release in man. Digestion. **36**: 108–124.

36 Mercadante S (1995) Tolerability of continuous subcutaneous octreotide used in combination with other drugs. Journal of Palliative Care. **11 (4)**: 14–16.

37 Chrubasik J (1985) Spinal infusion of opiates and somatostatin. Hygieneplan, Germany.

38 Scherubl H et al. (1994) Treatment of the carcinoid syndrome with a depot formulation of the somatostatin analogue lanreotide. European Journal of Cancer. **30A**: 1591–1591.

39 Baxter K (ed) (2008) Stockley's Drug Interactions (8e). Pharmaceutical Press, London.

40 Harris A and Redfern J (1995) Octreotide treatment of carcinoid syndrome: analysis of published dose-titration data. Alimentary Pharmacology and Therapeutics. **9**: 387–394.

41 Cello J et al. (1991) Effect of octreotide on refractory AIDS-associated diarrhea. A prospective, multicenter clinical trial. Annals of internal medicine. **115**: 705–710.

42 Cherny N (2008) Evaluation and management of treatment-related diarrhea in patients with advanced cancer: a review. Journal of Pain and Symptom Management. **36**: 413–423.

43 Matulonis UA et al. (2005) Long-acting octreotide for the treatment and symptomatic relief of bowel obstruction in advanced ovarian cancer. Journal of Pain and Symptom Management. **30**: 563–569.

PROGESTINS

Class: Sex hormones.

Indications: Licensed indications vary between products; consult the manufacturers' Product Monographs for details. Uses include hormone therapy in breast and endometrial cancers, renal advanced prostate cancer (stage D_2); anorexia and cachexia in cancer, AIDS or †other conditions, †post-castration hot flashes in both women and men.

Contra-indications: Medroxyprogesterone acetate (**MPA**): Hepatic impairment, history of (or high risk of developing) thrombo-embolism, partial or complete loss of vision because of ophthalmic vascular disease, migraine, active thrombophlebitis, estrogen-progestin-dependent neoplasia, undiagnosed abnormal vaginal bleeding, pregnancy (known or suspected).

Pharmacology

In addition to natural **progesterone**, there are several classes of synthetic progestins, e.g. derivatives of retroprogesterone, progesterone, and 17α-hydroxyprogesterone (**cyproterone**, **MPA**, **megestrol acetate**).[1] Whereas all derivatives have a progestogenic effect on the uterus, there are differences in other biological effects (Table 7.9).

Table 7.9 Comparison of the biological effects of natural progesterone and selected synthetic progestins[1]

Progestin	Effect[a]		
	Androgenic	Anti-androgenic	Anti-mineralocorticoid
Progesterone	−	+	+
Cyproterone acetate	−	++	−
Megestrol acetate	+	+	−
MPA	+	−	−

Key: ++ = effect present; + = weak effect; − = no effect.
a. all the above possess similar progestogenic, anti-gonadotrophic, anti-estrogenic and glucocorticoid effects.

Hormonal manipulation with a progestin is used in the treatment of several cancers, notably of the breast, prostate and endometrium.[2–5] Treatment is not curative but may induce remission in 15–30% of patients, occasionally for years. Tumour response and treatment toxicity need to be monitored, and treatment changed if progression occurs or undesirable effects exceed benefit.

Progestins are also used in cachexia-anorexia, although their efficacy in cachexia is debatable (see next section). Progestins may improve appetite by increasing levels of orexigenic neurotransmitters in the hypothalamus (e.g. neuropeptide Y), counteracting the anorexic effects of cytokines on the hypothalamus, or by interfering with the production of cytokines via their glucocorticoid anti-inflammatory effect.[6,7] In vitro, cytokine release from peripheral blood mononucleocytes are inhibited by both **megestrol acetate** and **MPA** in concentrations that would be achieved by daily doses of 320–960mg and 1,500–2,000mg respectively.[6] The release of serotonin was also inhibited and was considered one possible mechanism by which progestins have an anti-emetic effect.[6]

Megestrol acetate is not very water-soluble and thus its bio-availability is low. Bio-availability is improved if taken with food. Both **MPA** and **megestrol acetate** are highly protein-bound, mainly to albumin. The majority of **megestrol acetate** is excreted unchanged in the urine. **MPA** is metabolized extensively in the liver, and excreted mostly as glucuronide conjugates. For pharmacokinetic details, see Table 7.10.

Cachexia and anorexia

Cachexia is common in cancer and other chronic diseases, impairing quality of life and increasing morbidity and mortality.[9] It is characterized by the loss of skeletal muscle and body fat. Loss of skeletal muscle is associated with impaired physical function and quality of life, whereas loss of fat (the body's main energy store) is associated with reduced survival.

Table 7.10 Selected pharmacokinetic data[8]

	Megestrol acetate	MPA
Bio-availability	No data	1–10%
Time to peak plasma concentration	1–3h	2–7h
Plasma halflife	13–105h (mean 30h)	38–46h

In cancer, the two main mechanisms are a reduced food intake (anorexia) and abnormal host metabolism resulting from factors produced by the cancer, e.g. proteolysis-inducing factor, or by the host in response to the cancer, e.g. cytokines.[10] One outcome of this is a chronic inflammatory state, the level of which relates to the degree and rate of weight loss.[11] Cytokines such as interleukin-1 and tumour necrosis factor-α act on the hypothalamus and skeletal muscle leading to anorexia, inefficient energy expenditure, loss of body fat and wasting of skeletal muscle. The management of cachexia requires both of these main mechanisms to be addressed, and explains why increasing nutritional intake alone is generally ineffective.[10,12–14]

Megestrol acetate is used to stimulate appetite and weight gain in patients with cancer or AIDS. Several systematic reviews of the literature (about 30 trials, >4,000 patients) have concluded that appetite (NNT 3) and weight (NNT 8) is improved in patients with cancer, but have been unable to comment for other groups, because of insufficient numbers. For appetite stimulation, 160mg/day is as effective as a higher dose. For weight gain there appears to be more of a dose-response, although one review found no difference in outcomes between ≤800mg and >800mg daily.[15–17] However, the studies in the reviews used body weight as a primary outcome measure, and none accurately evaluated changes in body composition.

In those studies that have evaluated body composition, both **megestrol acetate** and **MPA** appear to increase fat mass, but not fat-free mass, the part which includes skeletal muscle.[7,18–20] Thus it is likely that the gain in weight with progestins (and corticosteroids), rather than representing the ideal increase in skeletal muscle *and* fat, is a less helpful retention of fluid or increase in fat only. This could make mobilizing more difficult in an already debilitated patient. In addition, the catabolic effect of progestins on skeletal muscle could further weaken the patient. Catabolism may result from the glucocorticoid effect of progestins but they also suppress the amount and function of testosterone, which is anabolic.

Others have noted that progestins lead to a substantial improvement in appetite in <30% of patients, or have questioned the clinical relevance of the magnitude of weight gain seen (≈1kg), or have highlighted the occurrence of undesirable effects of deep vein thrombosis (5%) and male impotence (10–25%).[7,18,20–25] Further, in the USA, where **megestrol acetate** is increasingly used in frail, elderly nursing home residents with weight loss from any cause, a recent study suggests its use is associated with a significant increase in all-cause mortality but not weight. The reasons for this are unclear but venous thrombo-embolism may play a role as the incidence of DVT was 6-fold higher with **megestrol acetate**.[26]

Progestins are much more expensive than **dexamethasone, prednisone, or prednisolone**. **Megestrol acetate** 800mg/day and **dexamethasone** 3mg/day are comparable with regard to appetite stimulation and non-fluid weight gain, although the latter was not accurately evaluated.[27] In this study, a high proportion of patients discontinued **dexamethasone** (36%) or **megestrol acetate** (25%) because of undesirable effects. **Dexamethasone** was more likely to cause cushingoid changes, myopathy, heartburn and peptic ulcers; **megestrol acetate** was associated with increased thrombo-embolism.[27] **Dexamethasone** is a fluorinated corticosteroid, a class which is more prone to cause muscle catabolism.[28] Thus, ideally, the use of **dexamethasone** should be limited to short-term use only.

If long-term use of a corticosteroid is contemplated, a switch to the non-fluorinated **prednisone** or **prednisolone** 10–20mg/day should be considered.[7] However, for patients expected to live months rather than weeks, progestins may be more appropriate. Caution is still required as long-term progestins can also cause cushingoid changes (25% of patients after 3 months in one study),[29] muscle catabolism and suppression of the hypothalamic-pituitary-adrenal axis. The latter may present with non-specific symptoms and a high level of clinical suspicion is required.[30] Additional corticosteroid replacement therapy would be a reasonable precaution in patients with serious infections or undergoing surgery.[7,31,32] Adrenal suppression is secondary to a central glucocorticoid effect on the hypothalamus and is dose-related; maximal suppression is seen with daily doses of **megestrol acetate** 200mg and **MPA** 1,000mg.[29]

The combination of a progestin and an NSAID has been investigated.[33,34] **Megestrol acetate** 160mg t.i.d. together with **ibuprofen** 400mg t.i.d. resulted in improved quality of life and weight gain. However, this was probably caused by fluid retention, because total body water increased *even though there was no clinical edema.*[33] The combination of **MPA** 500mg b.i.d. and **celecoxib** 200mg b.i.d. also stabilized weight and improved systemic symptoms.[34] Because the NSAID probably provided benefit by reducing the chronic inflammatory response (CRP levels were reduced), others have used **indomethacin** alone.[35]

In conclusion, progestins and systemic corticosteroids (see p.381) are useful *appetite stimulants* which can increase calorie intake and as such may be indicated in selected patients for anorexia. Progestins may be a more appropriate choice for long-term use than corticosteroids, but significant undesirable effects can occur. Starting doses should be low and titrated to the lowest effective dose. Both progestins and corticosteroids are best *not* regarded as *'anticachexia' agents*; any weight gain is likely to be because of an increase in fat and fluid retention, and the catabolism of skeletal muscle *increased*, particularly in inactive people.

Cautions

Possibility of glucocorticoid effects. May cause or worsen diabetes mellitus. May suppress the hypothalamic-pituitary-adrenal axis.

MPA: discontinue if any of the following develop: jaundice, hepatic impairment, significant increase in blood pressure, thrombo-embolic event (e.g. stroke, myocardial infarction, DVT, pulmonary embolism), new onset migraine, severe visual disturbances. May exacerbate existing migraine, epilepsy, asthma, cardiac or renal impairment.

Megestrol acetate: history of thrombophlebitis, severe hepatic impairment.

Undesirable effects

For full list, see manufacturer's Product Monograph.
Thrombo-embolism (5%).
Frequency not stated: hyperglycemia, depression, insomnia, fatigue, hypertension, edema/fluid retention, nausea, vomiting, constipation, cushingoid changes, bone mineral density loss, reduced libido, impotence, altered menstruation, breast tenderness, urticaria, acne.
Rare (<0.1%): jaundice, alopecia, hirsutism.

Dose and use

Advanced breast cancer
- **megestrol acetate** 40mg q.i.d.

Endometrial cancer
- **megestrol acetate** 40–320mg/24h in divided doses.

Prostate cancer (stage D2)
- **megestrol acetate** 120mg PO once daily together with **diethylstilbestrol** 100microgram.

Appetite stimulation
- start with **megestrol acetate** 80–160mg PO each morning
- if initial response poor, consider doubling the dose after 2 weeks[36,37]
- maximum dose generally 800mg PO daily.

MPA 400mg PO each morning–b.i.d. is an alternative countries where higher strength tablets are available (e.g. 100mg, 200mg and 400mg).

Hot flashes after surgical or chemical castration
MPA 5–20mg b.i.d.–q.i.d. or **megestrol acetate** 40mg each morning.[38] The effect manifests after 2–4 weeks.

Supply

Megestrol acetate (generic)
Tablets 40mg, 160mg, 28 days @ 160mg each morning = $120.

Megace® OS (Bristol-Myers Squibb Canada)
Oral suspension 40mg/mL, 28 days @ 160mg each morning = $188.

Medroxyprogesterone acetate (generic)
Tablets 2.5mg, 5mg, 10mg, 100mg, 28 days @ 5mg b.i.d. = $9.

Provera® (Pfizer Canada)
Tablets 2.5mg, 5mg, 10mg, 100mg, 28 days @ 5mg b.i.d. = $19.

---

1 Schindler AE et al. (2003) Classification and pharmacology of progestins. Maturitas. **46 (suppl 1)**: s7–s16.
2 Early Breast Cancer Trialists' Collaborative Group (1992) Systemic treatment of early breast cancer by hormonal, cytotoxic, or immune therapy: 133 randomised trials involving 31,000 recurrences and 24,000 deaths among 75,000 women. Lancet. **339**: 1–15 & 71–85.
3 Stuart NS et al. (1996) A randomised phase III cross-over study of tamoxifen versus megestrol acetate in advanced and recurrent breast cancer. European Journal of Cancer. **32A**: 1888–1892.
4 Martin-Hirsch P et al. (1999) Progestagens for endometrial cancer. Cochrane Database Systematic Review. **4**: CD001040.
5 Harris KA and Reese DM (2001) Treatment options in hormone-refractory prostate cancer: current and future approaches. Drugs. **61**: 2177–2192.
6 Mantovani G et al. (1998) Cytokine involvement in cancer anorexia/cachexia: role of megestrol acetate and medroxyprogesterone acetate on cytokine downregulation and improvement of clinical symptoms. Critical Reviews in Oncogenesis. **9**: 99–106.
7 MacDonald N (2005) Anorexia-cachexia syndrome. European Journal of Palliative Care. **12 (suppl)**: 8s–14s.
8 Par Pharmaceuticals Data on file.
9 Laviano A et al. (2003) Cancer anorexia: clinical implications, pathogenesis, and therapeutic strategies. Lancet Oncol. **4**: 686–694.
10 Gordon JN et al. (2005) Cancer cachexia. Quarterly Journal of Medicine. **98**: 779–788.
11 Scott HR et al. (2002) The systemic inflammatory response, weight loss, performance status and survival in patients with inoperable non-small cell lung cancer. British Journal of Cancer. **87**: 264–267.
12 Davis MP et al. (2004) Appetite and cancer-associated anorexia: a review. Journal of Clinical Oncology. **22**: 1510–1517.
13 Ramos EJ et al. (2004) Cancer anorexia-cachexia syndrome: cytokines and neuropeptides. Current Opinion in Clinical Nutrition & Metabolic Care. **7**: 427–434.
14 Laviano A et al. (2005) Therapy insight: Cancer anorexia-cachexia syndrome—when all you can eat is yourself. Nature Clinical Practice Oncology. **2**: 158–165.
15 Pascual Lopez A et al. (2004) Systematic review of megestrol acetate in the treatment of anorexia-cachexia syndrome. Journal of Pain and Symptom Management. **27**: 360–369.
16 Berenstein EG and Ortiz Z (2005) Megestrol acetate for the treatment of anorexia-cachexia syndrome. Cochrane Database of Systematic Reviews. **2**: CD004310.
17 Lesniak W et al. (2008) Effects of megestrol acetate in patients with cancer anorexia-cachexia syndrome-a systematic review and meta-analysis. Polskie Archiwum Medycyny Wewnetrznej. **118**: 636–644.
18 Loprinzi CL et al. (1993) Phase III evaluation of four doses of megestrol acetate as therapy for patients with cancer anorexia and/or cachexia. Journal of Clinical Oncology. **11**: 762–767.
19 Loprinzi C et al. (1993) Body-composition changes in patients who gain weight while receiving megestrol acetate. Journal of Clinical Oncology. **11**: 152–154.
20 Simons JP et al. (1998) Effects of medroxyprogesterone acetate on food intake, body composition, and resting energy expenditure in patients with advanced, nonhormone-sensitive cancer: a randomized, placebo-controlled trial. Cancer. **82**: 553–560.
21 Jatoi A et al. (2002) Dronabinol versus megestrol acetate versus combination therapy for cancer-associated anorexia: a North Central Cancer Treatment Group study. Journal of Clinical Oncology. **20**: 567–573.
22 Jatoi A et al. (2003) On appetite and its loss. Journal of Clinical Oncology. **21 (suppl 9)**: 79–81.
23 Jatoi A et al. (2004) An eicosapentaenoic acid supplement versus megestrol acetate versus both for patients with cancer-associated wasting: a North Central Cancer Treatment Group and National Cancer Institute of Canada collaborative effort. Journal of Clinical Oncology. **22**: 2469–2476.
24 Kropsky B et al. (2003) Incidence of deep-venous thrombosis in nursing home residents using megestrol acetate. Journal of the American Medical Directors Association. **4**: 255–256.
25 Garcia VR and Juan O (2005) Megestrol acetate-probably less effective than has been reported! Journal of Pain and Symptom Management.. **30**: 4; author reply 5–6.
26 Bodenner D et al. (2007) A retrospective study of the association between megestrol acetate administration and mortality among nursing home residents with clinically significant weight loss. American Journal Geriatric Pharmacotherapy. **5**: 137–146.
27 Loprinzi CL et al. (1999) Randomized comparison of megestrol acetate versus dexamethasone versus fluoxymesterone for the treatment of cancer anorexia/cachexia. Journal of Clinical Oncology. **17**: 3299–3306.
28 Faludi G et al. (1966) Factors influencing the development of steroid-induced myopathies. Annals of the New York Academy of Sciences. **138**: 62–72.
29 Willemse PH et al. (1990) A randomized comparison of megestrol acetate (MA) and medroxyprogesterone acetate (MPA) in patients with advanced breast cancer. European Journal of Cancer. **26**: 337–343.
30 Dev R et al. (2007) Association between megestrol acetate treatment and symptomatic adrenal insufficiency with hypogonadism in male patients with cancer. Cancer. **110**: 1173–1177.
31 Naing KK et al. (1999) Megestrol acetate therapy and secondary adrenal suppression. Cancer. **86**: 1044–1049.
32 Lambert C et al. (2002) Effects of testosterone replacement and/or resistance exercise on the composition of megestrol acetate stimulated weight gain in elderly men: a randomized controlled trial. Journal of Clinical Endocrinology and Metabolism. **87**: 2100–2106.
33 McMillan DC et al. (1999) A prospective randomized study of megestrol acetate and ibuprofen in gastrointestinal cancer patients with weight loss. British Journal of Cancer. **79**: 495–500.
34 Cerchietti LC et al. (2004) Effects of celecoxib, medroxyprogesterone, and dietary intervention on systemic syndromes in patients with advanced lung adenocarcinoma: a pilot study. Journal of Pain and Symptom Management. **27**: 85–95.
35 Bosaeus I et al. (2002) Dietary intake, resting energy expenditure, weight loss and survival in cancer patients. Journal of Nutrition. **132 (suppl)**: 3465s–3466s.

---

36 Donnelly S and Walsh TD (1995) Low-dose megestrol acetate for appetite stimulation in advanced cancer. *Journal of Pain and Symptom Management.* **10**: 182–183.
37 Vadell C *et al.* (1998) Anticachectic efficacy of megestrol acetate at different doses and versus placebo in patients with neoplastic cachexia. *American Journal of Clinical Oncology.* **21**: 347–351.
38 Loprinzi CL *et al.* (1996) Megestrol acetate for the prevention of hot flashes. *New England Journal of Medicine.* **331**: 347–352.

DANAZOL

Class: Anabolic steroid (17α-alkyl androgen).

Indications: Endometriosis, benign fibrocystic breast disease, †hereditary angioedema,[1,2] †pruritus associated with obstructive jaundice, †idiopathic immune thrombocytopenia †gynecomastia.

Contra-indications: Thrombo-embolic disorders; severe cardiac, hepatic or renal impairment (*except when indicated for cholestatic pruritus*, see Box 5.O, p.339); androgen-dependent tumour; undiagnosed genital bleeding; porphyria; pregnancy; breast-feeding.

Pharmacology

Danazol is a chemically modified testosterone. It suppresses the pituitary-ovarian axis by inhibiting the pituitary output of gonadotrophins. The beneficial effect of 17α-alkyl androgens in hepatic (cholestatic) pruritus was discovered serendipitously some 60 years ago when the co-incidental use of **methyltestosterone** (not Canada) in a patient with primary biliary cirrhosis resulted in relief from the associated pruritus.[3] Hepatic pruritus is central in origin and is associated with enhanced opioidergic tone, secondary to the increased production of endogenous opioids.[4–6] In intrahepatic cholestasis, an opioid antagonist such as **naloxone** (see p.343) or **naltrexone** (see p.345) is the treatment of choice.[7]

It is possible that, when opioids are needed for concurrent cancer pain, a 17α-alkyl androgen is one alternative.[8] The mechanism of action is uncertain, but 17α-alkyl androgens are directly toxic to hepatocytes.[9–11] Thus, it is possible that danazol causes focal cell damage which limits the ability of the cholestatic liver to produce enkephalins. Androgens themselves can cause cholestatic jaundice[12] and have occasionally caused severe hepatic impairment.[13]

By mouth, 17α-alkyl androgens (e.g. **methyltestosterone**) are more bio-available than other androgens (e.g. **testosterone**) because of the reduction in first-pass hepatic metabolism in androgens with a 17α-alkyl radical.[14] Danazol also has additional effects on the liver which are not shared by **testosterone**.[15] The antipruritic effect is maintained even if the cholestasis is exacerbated by the androgen itself.[14]

Androgens and estrogens sometimes relieve non-specific pruritus in the elderly.[16] An anecdotal report suggests that some patients with AIDS may benefit from anabolic steroids in terms of weight gain and increased strength.[17]

Bio-availability 11% (fasting), 44% (after lipid-rich meal);[18] doubling the dose, increases the plasma concentration by only 35–40%.
Onset of action 5–10 days in hepatic pruritus.
Time to peak plasma concentration < 2h.
Plasma halflife 4.5h (single dose); > 24h (multiple doses).
Duration of action > 24h.

Cautions

Hepatic or renal disease, fluid retention, cardiovascular disease, hypertension, epilepsy, diabetes mellitus, lipoprotein disorder, polycythemia, migraine. Discontinue if female virilization occurs (may become irreversible if treatment continued), or if symptoms of raised intracranial pressure or thrombo-embolism arise.

Danazol inhibits CYP3A4 and may enhance the activity of several drugs, including **carbamazepine**, **cyclosporine**, **insulin**, **warfarin**, and possibly **tacrolimus**.

Monitor liver function and blood count every 6 months during long-term treatment. May cause false results with thyroid function tests.

Undesirable effects

For full list, see manufacturer's Product Monograph.

Related to inhibition of the pituitary-ovarian axis: amenorrhea, hot flashes, sweating, reduction in breast size, reduced libido, vaginitis, emotional lability.

Related to androgenic activity: acne, oily skin or hair, mild hirsutism, deepening of the voice, androgenic alopecia, and rarely clitoral hypertrophy. Paradoxically, testicular atrophy may occur.

Other effects: include cramps, nausea, photosensitivity, severe hepatotoxicity (occasional), benign intracranial hypertension (rare).

Dose and use

Pruritus

Moisturizing the skin with an emollient is always the first step. In patients with an extrahepatic obstruction (e.g. because of pancreatic cancer, lymphadenopathy), the treatment of choice is generally stenting of the bile duct.

When this is not feasible or when associated with intrahepatic cholestasis, one of several drugs can be used, and the choice depends on both individual circumstances and local fashion:

- **naltrexone** 12.5–250mg once daily[5–7]
- **rifampin** 75–300mg once daily[19]
- **paroxetine** 5–20mg once daily [20]
- danazol 200mg once daily–t.i.d.[21]

Benefit from danazol is generally seen after about 5–10 days.[22,23] Androgenic changes may be ameliorated by reducing the dose from once daily to 3 times weekly or even less.[14]

Supply

Cyclomen® (Sanofi-Aventis Canada)
Capsules 50mg, 100mg, 200mg, 28 days @ 200mg daily = $62.

1 Hosea SW and Frank MM (1980) Danazole in the treatment of hereditary angioedema. *Drugs.* **19**: 370–372.
2 MacFarlane JT and Davies D (1981) Management of hereditary angio-oedema with low-dose danazol. *British Medical Journal (Clinical Research Ed).* **282**: 1275.
3 Ahrens E et al. (1950) Primary biliary cirrhosis. *Medicine.* **29**: 299–364.
4 Jones E and Bergasa N (1990) The pruritus of cholestasis. From bile acids to opiate agonists. *Hepatology.* **11**: 884–887.
5 Jones E and Dekker L (2000) Florid opioid withdrawal-like reaction precipitated by naltrexone in a patient with chronic cholestasis. *Gastroenterology.* **118**: 431–432.
6 Jones E and Bergasa N (2004) The pruritus of cholestasis and the opioid neurotransmitter system. In: Z Zylicz et al. (eds) *Pruritus in advanced desease.* Oxford University Press, Oxford, pp. 56–68.
7 Jones E and Bergasa N (1999) The pruritus of cholestasis. *Hepatology.* **29**: 1003–1006.
8 Twycross RG et al. (2003) Itch: scratching more than the surface. *Quarterly Journal of Medicine.* **96**: 7–26.
9 Welder A et al. (1995) Toxic effects of anabolic-androgen steroids in primary rat hepatic cell cultures. *Journal of Pharmacological and Toxicological Methods.* **33**: 187–195.
10 Ohsawa T and Iwashita S (1986) Hepatitis associated with danazol. *Drug Intelligence and Clinical Pharmacy.* **20**: 889.
11 Fermand JP et al. (1990) Danazol-induced hepatocellular adenoma. *American Journal of Medicine.* **88**: 529–530.
12 Boue F et al. (1986) Danazol and cholestatic hepatitis. *Annals of Internal Medicine.* **105**: 139–140.
13 Gurakar A et al. (1994) Androgenic/anabolic steroid-induced intrahepatic cholestasis: a review with four additional case reports. *Journal of Oklahoma State Medical Association.* **87**: 399–404.
14 Lloyd-Thomas H and Sherlock S (1952) Testosterone therapy for the pruritus of obstructive jaundice. *British Medical Journal.* **ii**: 1289–1291.
15 Fernandez L et al. (1994) Stanozolol and danazol, unlike natural androgens, interact with the low affinity glucocorticoid-binding sites from male rat liver microsomes. *Endocrinology.* **134**: 1401–1408.
16 Feldman S et al. (1942) Treatment of senile pruritus with androgens and estrogens. *Archives of Dermatology and Syphilology Chicago.* **46**: 112–127.
17 Berger J et al. (1993) Effect of anabolic steroids on HIV-related wasting myopathy. *Southern Medical Journal.* **86**: 865–866.
18 Sunesen VH et al. (2005) Effect of liquid volume and food intake on the absolute bioavailability of danazol, a poorly soluble drug. *European Journal of Pharmaceutical Sciences.* **24**: 297–303.
19 Ghent C and Carruthers S (1988) Treatment of pruritus in primary biliary cirrhosis with rifampin. Results of a double-blind crossover randomized trial. *Gastroenterology.* **94**: 488–493.
20 Zylicz Z et al. (2003) Paroxetine in the treatment of severe non-dermatological pruritus: a randomized, controlled trial. *Journal of Pain and Symptom Management.* **26**: 1105–1112.
21 Twycross RG and Zylicz Z (2004) Systemic therapy: making rational choices. In: Z Zylicz et al. (eds) *Pruritus in advanced disease.* Oxford University Press, London, pp. 161–178.
22 Sherlock S (1981) *Diseases of the Liver and Biliary System* (6e). Blackwell Scientific, Oxford.
23 Sherlock S and Dooley J (1993) *Diseases of the Liver and Biliary System* (9e). Blackwell Scientific, Oxford.

*THALIDOMIDE

Class: Immunomodulator.

Indications: There are no licensed indications for thalidomide. Unlicensed uses include: †cutaneous manifestations of lepromatous leprosy (erythema nodosum leprosum), †multiple myeloma (with concurrent **dexamethasone**), †graft versus host disease (GVHD), †recurrent aphthous stomatitis in HIV infection and connective tissue disease (Behcet's syndrome), †paraneoplastic sweating, †paraneoplastic and uremic pruritus, †cachexia in HIV and cancer, †intractable GI bleeding, †intractable **irinotecan**-induced diarrhea, †discoid lupus erythematosus, †rheumatoid arthritis, †prevention of graft rejection.[1,2]

Contra-indications: Thalidomide should never be used in women who are pregnant or may become so.

Pharmacology

Thalidomide is an immunomodulator with anticytokine, anti-integrin, and anti-angiogenic properties.[3] It was withdrawn from use as a non-barbiturate hypnotic with anti-emetic properties in the early 1960s after it became apparent that it caused severe congenital abnormalities (absent or shortened limbs) when given to women in the first trimester of pregnancy.[4] Subsequently, it has been found to have immunomodulatory properties with potential for the treatment of various conditions.[5] Thalidomide inhibits the synthesis of the pro-inflammatory cytokine tumour necrosis factor α (TNF-α) by monocytes.[6] It also inhibits chemotaxis of neutrophils and monocytes. Thalidomide antagonizes PGE_2, PGF_2, histamine, serotonin, and acetylcholine.[7] It also affects several other mechanisms associated with inflammation and immunomodulation.[8] These properties probably account for the prevention of **irinotecan**-induced diarrhea,[9] and for the amelioration of paraneoplastic sweating[10] and paraneoplastic pruritus.[11]

Thalidomide also inhibits angiogenesis, a property which is the basis for investigational studies in oncology.[12,13] This effect is mediated by suppression of vascular endothelial growth factor (VEGF), a potent angiogenic factor secreted by cancer cells in response to hypoxia. This property provides the rationale underlying the use of thalidomide in refractory GI bleeding.[14-17]

Except for teratogenicity in pregnant women, the most serious undesirable effect is peripheral neuropathy.[8] This is caused by axonal degeneration without demyelination, with sensory nerves affected predominantly.[18] Neuropathy occurs in up to 30% of cases. The likelihood of developing neuropathy increases with cumulative dosing but has been reported after only 2.8g.[19] It is not related to age. Symptoms include numbness, paresthesia, hyperesthesia for pain and temperature of the hands and feet, and leg cramps. The lower limbs are more commonly involved than the upper limbs. Findings include diminished ankle jerks and decreased sensation to vibration and position.[20] Although thalidomide is sometimes continued despite electrophysiological abnormalities, if a patient develops symptomatic neuropathy thalidomide should be stopped to decrease the likelihood of chronic painful neuropathy.[19,20] Thalidomide appears to undergo non-enzymatic hydrolysis in plasma; hepatic metabolism is minor. Studies in patients with hepatic and renal impairment have not been performed. Thalidomide causes an increase in plasma **acetaminophen** concentration but this is not clinically important.[9]

Analogues of thalidomide with similar anti-angiogenic, immunomodulatory and anti-inflammatory properties are being developed for use in hematological malignancies.[21,22] For example, **lenalidomide** is approved in the USA and Europe for myelodysplastic syndromes (associated with a deletion 5q cytogenetic abnormality) causing transfusion-dependent anemia.[23-25] Although effective in reducing the need for red blood cell transfusions in 2/3 of patients, undesirable effects are common, particularly thrombocytopenia and neutropenia. It is also approved for use with concurrent **dexamethasone** in the treatment of multiple myeloma in patients who have received at least one previous therapy.

Lenalidomide is also associated with an increased risk of DVT and pulmonary embolism. Further, like thalidomide, **lenalidomide** is presumed to carry serious teratogenic risk. Thus, it has no obvious advantages over thalidomide, at least in relation to its use in palliative care. Both thalidomide and **lenalidomide** are restricted in their availability.

Bio-availability 67–93% PO in animals, no data in humans.
Onset of action varies from 2 days for lepromatous leprosy and paraneoplastic sweating to 1–2 months for GVHD and 2–3 months for rheumatoid arthritis.

Time to peak plasma concentration 2–6h, delayed by food.
Plasma halflife 6h (200mg/24h)–18h (800mg/24h).[8]
Duration of action 24h.

Cautions

Treat as a 'cytotoxic' when handling. Pregnant women or women planning to become pregnant should not handle thalidomide. Thalidomide is present in semen, and men taking thalidomide should use latex condoms when having sexual intercourse.

Thalidomide potentiates the sedative properties of barbiturates and alcohol, and increases the likelihood of extrapyramidal effects with **chlorpromazine** and **reserpine**.[7] Thalidomide should be used cautiously with drugs that cause drowsiness, neuropathy or reduce the effectiveness of oral contraception (e.g. HIV protease inhibitors, **rifampin**, **rifabutin**, **phenytoin** and **carbamazepine**).[7,26]

Undesirable effects

Teratogenicity if given to pregnant women in the first trimester and peripheral neuropathy in up to 30% of patients. In clinical trials, 10–20% of patients stopped taking thalidomide, mostly because of drowsiness, skin rashes and peripheral neuropathy.[27–30] Rash may occur even when thalidomide is given with **dexamethasone**. Drowsiness and sedation are dose-dependent. Myelosuppression is rare. Thalidomide can increase HIV viral load.[31]

A dose-dependent decrease in supine systolic and diastolic pressures is seen up to 2h after dosing.[32] Headache, dizziness, and delirium occur more often at higher doses.[26,32] Other undesirable effects include seizures,[33] dry mouth, constipation, bradycardia, altered temperature sensitivity, irregular menstrual cycles, hypothyroidism, edema, and Stevens-Johnson syndrome.[26,33–35] Cancer patients may have an increased susceptibility to thalidomide-associated undesirable effects, including thrombo-embolism.[33]

Dose and use

In palliative care, thalidomide will always be a treatment of 'last resort'. In other words, to be used only when conventional treatments have failed, specialist colleague advice sought, and a full review of the potential pros and cons undertaken.

Recommendations include:
Aphthous ulcers in HIV+ disease: 100–200mg at bedtime for 10 days.[36]
Paraneoplastic sweating: 100–200mg at bedtime.[37,38]
Paraneoplastic and uremic pruritus: 100mg at bedtime.[11,39]
Cachexia in HIV+ disease and cancer: 100–200mg at bedtime.[40,41]
GI bleeding: 300mg at bedtime.[17]
Intractable irinotecan-induced diarrhea: 400mg at bedtime.[9,42]

Female patients prescribed thalidomide must be counseled about the need for contraception and male patients must use a condom. Written consent should be obtained.[43]

Supply

Thalidomide is available through a distribution programme called the Canadian Thalomid Access Program (CANTAP). Clinicians wishing to use thalidomide must be registered with the programme. Authorization to distribute may be obtained by contacting the program at 1-888-611-6817.

Lenalidomide is available through a similar controlled distribution programme, RevAid. Details can be obtained from www.RevAid.ca or by calling 1-888-738-2431.

Thalomid® (Celgene)
Capsules 50mg, 28 days @ 200mg at bedtime = $13,420.

1 Calabrese L and Fleischer A (2000) Thalidomide: current and potential clinical applications. *American Journal of Medicine.* **108**: 487–495.

2 Jacobson J (2000) Thalidomide: a remarkable comeback. *Expert Opinion in Pharmacotherapy.* **1**: 849–863.

3 Davis M and Dickerson E (2001) Thalidomide: dual benefits in palliative medicine and oncology. *American Journal of Hospice and Palliative Care.* **18**: 347–351.

4 Marriott J *et al.* (1999) Thalidomide as an emerging immunotherapeutic agent. *Trends in Immunology Today.* **20**: 538–540.

5 Peuckmann V *et al.* (2000) Potential novel uses of thalidomide: focus on palliative care. *Drugs.* **60**: 273–292.

6 Sampaio E *et al.* (1991) Thalidomide selectively inhibits tumour necrosis factor alpha production by stimulated human monocytes. *Journal of Experimental Medicine.* **173**: 699–703.

7 Radomsky C and Levine N (2001) Thalidomide. *Dermatologic Clinics.* **19**: 87–103.

8 Bousvaros A and Mueller B (2001) Thalidomide in gastrointestinal disorders. *Drugs.* **61**: 777–787.

9 Govindarajan R *et al.* (2000) Effect of thalidomide on gastrointestinal toxic effects of irinotecan. *Lancet.* **356**: 566–567.

10 Deaner P (2000) The use of thalidomide in the management of severe sweating in patients with advanced malignancy: trial report. *Palliative Medicine.* **14**: 429–431.

11 Smith J *et al.* (2002) Use of thalidomide in the treatment of intractable itch. In: International Journal of Palliative Nursing (ed) *Palliative Care Congress*; Sheffield. Mark Allen.

12 Eisen T (2000) Thalidomide in solid tumors: the London experience. *Oncology (Williston Park).* **14(12) (suppl 13)**: 17–20.

13 Eleutherakis-Papaiakovou V *et al.* (2004) Thalidomide in cancer medicine. *Annals of Oncology.* **15**: 1151–1160.

14 Bauditz J *et al.* (2004) Thalidomide for treatment of severe intestinal bleeding. *Gut.* **53**: 609–612.

15 Craanen ME *et al.* (2006) Thalidomide in refractory haemorrhagic radiation induced proctitis. *Gut.* **55**: 1371–1372.

16 Karajeh MA *et al.* (2006) Refractory bleeding from portal hypertensive gastropathy: a further novel role for thalidomide therapy? *European Journal of Gastroenterology and Hepatology.* **18**: 545–548.

17 Lambert K and Ward J (2009) The use of thalidomide in the management of bleeding from a gastric cancer. *Palliative Medicine.* **23**: 473–475.

18 Fullerton P and O'Sullivan D (1968) Thalidomide neuropathy: a clinical, electrophysiological, and histological follow up study. *Journal of Neurology, Neurosurgery and Psychiatry.* **31**: 543–551.

19 Gardner-Medwin J *et al.* (1994) Clinical experience with thalidomide in the management of severe oral and genital ulceration in conditions such as Behcet's disease. *Annals of Rheumatic Diseases.* **128**: 443–450.

20 Ochonisky S *et al.* (1994) Thalidomide neuropathy incidence and clinico-electrophysiologic findings in 42 patients. *Archives of Dermatology.* **130**: 66–69.

21 Anderson KC (2005) Lenalidomide and thalidomide: mechanisms of action-similarities and differences. *Seminars in Hematology.* **42**: S3–8.

22 Dredge K *et al.* (2005) Orally administered lenalidomide (CC-5013) is anti-angiogenic in vivo and inhibits endothelial cell migration and Akt phosphorylation in vitro. *Microvascular Research.* **69**: 56–63.

23 List A *et al.* (2005) Efficacy of lenalidomide in myelodysplastic syndromes. *New England Journal of Medicine.* **352**: 549–557.

24 Giagounidis AA *et al.* (2006) Biological and prognostic significance of chromosome 5q deletions in myeloid malignancies. *Clinical Cancer Research.* **12**: 5–10.

25 Naing A *et al.* (2006) Developmental therapeutics for myelodysplastic syndromes. *Journal of the National Comprehensive Cancer Network.* **4**: 78–82.

26 Thomas D and Kantarjian H (2000) Current role of thalidomide in cancer treatment. *Current Opinion in Oncology.* **12**: 564–573.

27 Vogelsang G *et al.* (1992) Thalidomide for the treatment of chronic graft-versus-host disease. *New England Journal of Medicine.* **326**: 1055–1058.

28 Hamuryudan V *et al.* (1998) Thalidomide in the treatment of the mucocutaneous lesions of the Behcet syndrome. A randomized, double-blind, placebo-controlled trial. *Annals of Internal Medicine.* **128**: 443–450.

29 Ehrenpreis E *et al.* (1999) Thalidomide therapy for patients with refractory Crohn's disease: an open label trial. *Gastroenterology.* **117**: 1271–1277.

30 Vasilauskas E *et al.* (1999) An open label study of low-dose thalidomide in chronically active, steroid-dependent Crohn's disease. *Gastroenterology.* **117**: 1278–1287.

31 Marriott J *et al.* (1997) A double-blind placebo-controlled phase II trial of thalidomide in asymptomatic HIV-positive patients: clinical tolerance and effect on activation markers and cytokines. *AIDS Research and Human Retroviruses.* **13**: 1625–1631.

32 Noormohamed F *et al.* (1999) Pharmacokinetics and hemodynamic effects of single oral doses of thalidomide in asymptomatic human immunodeficiency virus-infected subjects. *AIDS Research and Human Retroviruses.* **15**: 1047–1052.

33 Clark T *et al.* (2001) Thalidomid (Thalidomide) capsules: A review of the first 18 months of spontaneous postmarketing adverse event surveillance, including off-label prescribing. *Drug Safety.* **24**: 87–117.

34 Adlard J (2000) Thalidomide in the treatment of cancer. *Anticancer Drugs.* **11**: 787–791.

35 Galani E *et al.* (2000) Thalidomide and dexamethasone combination for refractory multiple myeloma. *Annals of Oncology.* **4**: 97.

36 Jacobson J *et al.* (1997) Thalidomide for the treatment of oral aphthous ulcers in patients with human immunodeficiency virus infection. *New England Journal of Medicine.* **336**: 1487–1493.

37 Deaner P (1998) Thalidomide for distressing night sweats in advanced malignant disease. *Palliative Medicine.* **12**: 208–209.

38 Calder K and Bruera E (2000) Thalidomide for night sweats in patients with advanced cancer. *Palliative Medicine.* **14**: 77–78.

39 Silva S *et al.* (1994) Thalidomide for the treatment of uremic pruritus: a crossover randomized double-blind trial. *Nephron.* **67**: 270–273.

40 Boasberg P *et al.* (2000) Thalidomide induced cessation of weight loss and improved sleep in advanced cancer patients with cachexia. ASCO Online. **Abstract 2396**.

41 Mantovani G *et al.* (2001) Managing cancer-related anorexia/cachexia. *Drugs.* **61**: 499–514.

42 Govindarajan R (2000) Irinotecan and thalidomide in metastatic colorectal cancer. *Oncology (Williston Park).* **14(12) (suppl 13)**: 29–32.

43 Powell R and Gardner-Medwin J (1994) Guideline for the clinical use and dispensing of thalidomide. *Postgraduate Medical Journal.* **70**: 901–904.

8: URINARY TRACT DISORDERS

TAMSULOSIN

Class: Uroselective α_1-adrenergic receptor antagonist.[1]

Indications: Symptoms associated with benign prostatic hypertrophy (particularly hesitancy of micturition), †radiation-induced urethritis, †medical management of urinary stones.[2]

Contra-indications: Symptomatic postural hypotension.

Pharmacology

Tamsulosin is a selective and competitive antagonist at post-synaptic α_1-adrenergic receptors, particularly subtype α_{1A}, in the prostate. It relaxes the smooth muscle of the prostate gland and bladder neck,[3-6] thereby reducing functional prostatic obstruction and increasing maximum urinary flow rate. RCT data indicate that tamsulosin improves lower urinary tract symptoms by at least 25% in up to 80% of patients.[7-9] Tamsulosin may also antagonize α_{1A}- and α_{1D}-adrenergic receptors in the bladder, inhibiting detrusor contractions and improving detrusor instability and urinary storage symptoms such as frequency, urgency and incontinence. Inhibition of α-adrenergic receptors in the sympathetic nervous system and spinal cord may also contribute to its effects.[6] Tamsulosin 400–800microgram/24h also relieves external beam radiation-induced urethritis in patients with prostate cancer.[10] When started 2–3 weeks before prostate radiation brachytherapy, tamsulosin also reduces short-term urinary irritation and obstruction, the need for a urinary catheter and for transurethral resection of the prostate.[11] Symptom improvement is dose-related up to a ceiling dose of 400microgram/24h.[12,13] Tamsulosin is metabolized in the liver, primarily by CYP2D6 and CYP3A4; <10% is excreted unchanged in the urine.

Other less specific α_1-adrenergic receptor antagonists are available, e.g. **prazosin**. Symptomatic and urodynamic efficacy is similar but, unlike **prazosin**, tamsulosin generally does *not* cause postural hypotension either when given alone or with commonly used antihypertensive drugs, e.g. **atenolol, enalapril** and **nifedipine**.[14-16] **Prazosin** also needs to be taken b.i.d. rather than daily; lower cost is its only advantage.

Muscarinic drugs and anticholinesterases provide an alternative approach to the management of urinary hesitancy, e.g. **bethanechol** 10–25mg t.i.d. Also, because they have a different mechanism of action, they can be used concurrently with tamsulosin.

Bio-availability SR ~100% PO fasting, reduced by 30% p.c.;[6] Flomax CR® 55–59%, not affected by food.

Onset of action SR 4–8h; maximum benefit 4–8 weeks.

Time to peak plasma concentration 1h; SR 4h fasting, 6h p.c.;[6] Flomax CR® 4–6h, not affected by food.

Plasma halflife 5–7h; SR 9–13h (healthy volunteers), 14–15h (elderly);[6] Flomax CR® 12–15h.

Duration of action <24h.

Cautions

Severe hepatic or renal impairment. Concurrent use with epidural **morphine**, **sildenafil** or other α_1-adrenergic receptor antagonists increases the risk of postural hypotension. Tamsulosin may increase the anticoagulant effect of **warfarin**. *In vitro* studies suggest that **diclofenac** and **warfarin** may increase the elimination of tamsulosin. **Cimetidine** decreases the elimination of tamsulosin.[6]

Undesirable effects

For full list, see manufacturer's Product Monograph.

Very common (>10%): dizziness, headache and rhinitis.

Common (<10%, >1%): asthenia, drowsiness or insomnia, amblyopia, chest pain, sinusitis, pharyngitis, cough, bitter taste, nausea, abdominal discomfort, diarrhea, back pain, reduced libido, ejaculatory impairment.

Uncommon (<1%, >0.1%): syncope, vertigo, palpitations, postural hypotension, vomiting, constipation, rash, pruritus.

Very rare (<0.01%, >0.001%): priapism.

Dose and use
Hesitancy of micturition
- tamsulosin 400microgram SR once daily (take at the same time each day, preferably 30min p.c.)
- if necessary, increase to 800microgram once daily after 2–4 weeks[6]
- to avoid damaging their SR properties, do not open, crush or chew the capsules.

Supply

Tamsulosin (generic)
Capsules SR 400microgram, 28 days @ 400microgram once daily = $17.

Flomax CR® (Boehringer Ingelheim Canada)
Tablets SR 400microgram, 28 days @ 400microgram once daily = $18.

1 Hieble JP *et al.* (1995) International Union of Pharmacology. X. Recommendation for nomenclature of alpha 1-adrenoceptors: consensus update. *Pharmacological Reviews.* **47**: 267–270.
2 Dellabella M *et al.* (2005) Randomized trial of the efficacy of tamsulosin, nifedipine and phloroglucinol in medical expulsive therapy for distal ureteral calculi. *Journal of Urology.* **174**: 167–172.
3 Hieble J and Ruffolo R (1996) The use of alpha-adrenoceptor antagonists in the pharmacological management of benign prostatic hypertrophy: an overview. *Pharmacological Research.* **33**: 145–160.
4 Kenny B *et al.* (1996) Evaluation of the pharmacological selectivity profile of alpha 1 adrenoceptor antagonists at prostatic alpha 1 adrenoceptors: binding, functional and *in vivo* studies. *British Journal of Pharmacology.* **118**: 871–878.
5 Pupo A *et al.* (1999) Effects of indoramin in rat vas deferens and aorta: concomitant alpha 1-adrenoceptor and neuronal uptake blockade. *British Journal of Pharmacology.* **127**: 1832–1836.
6 Lyseng-Williamson KA *et al.* (2002) Tamsulosin: an update of its role in the management of lower urinary tract symptoms. *Drugs.* **62**: 135–167.
7 Abrams P *et al.* (1995) Tamsulosin, a selective alpha 1c-adrenoceptor antagonist: a randomized, controlled trial in patients with benign prostatic 'obstruction' (symptomatic BPH). The European Tamsulosin Study Group. *British Journal of Urology.* **76**: 325–336.
8 Chapple CR *et al.* (1996) Tamsulosin, the first prostate-selective alpha 1A-adrenoceptor antagonist. A meta-analysis of two randomized, placebo-controlled, multicentre studies in patients with benign prostatic obstruction (symptomatic BPH). European Tamsulosin Study Group. *European Urology.* **29**: 155–167.
9 Lee M (2000) Tamsulosin for the treatment of benign prostatic hypertrophy. *Annals of Pharmacotherapy.* **34**: 188–199.
10 Prosnitz RG *et al.* (1999) Tamsulosin palliates radiation-induced urethritis in patients with prostate cancer: results of a pilot study. *International Journal of Radiation Oncology, Biology, Phyisics.* **45**: 563–566.
11 Merrick GS *et al.* (2000) Temporal resolution of urinary morbidity following prostate brachytherapy. *International Journal of Radiation Oncology, Biology, Physics.* **47**: 121–128.
12 Lepor H (1998) Phase III multicenter placebo-controlled study of tamsulosin in benign prostatic hyperplasia. Tamsulosin Investigator Group. *Urology.* **51**: 892–900.
13 Narayan P and Tewari A (1998) A second phase III multicenter placebo controlled study of 2 dosages of modified release tamsulosin in patients with symptoms of benign prostatic hyperplasia. United States 93–01 Study Group. *Journal of Urology.* **160**: 1701–1706.
14 Lowe FC (1997) Coadministration of tamsulosin and three antihypertensive agents in patients with benign prostatic hyperplasia: pharmacodynamic effect. *Clinical Therapeutics.* **19**: 730–742.
15 Michel MC *et al.* (1998) Tamsulosin: real life clinical experience in 19,365 patients. *European Urology.* **34 (suppl 2)**: 37–45.
16 Clifford G and Farmer R (2000) Medical therapy for benign prostatic hyperplasia: a review of the literature. *European Urology.* **38**: 2–19.

OXYBUTYNIN

Class: Antimuscarinic (anticholinergic).

Indications: Symptoms of an overactive bladder, including urge incontinence, urinary frequency, urgency, caused by either idiopathic detrusor instability or a neurogenic bladder (detrusor hyperreflexia).

Contra-indications: Bladder outflow obstruction, GI obstruction including paralytic ileus, glaucoma and myasthenia gravis.

Pharmacology

Oxybutynin hydrochloride has an antimuscarinic effect on bladder innervation and a direct papaverine-like antispasmodic effect on the smooth muscle (detrusor) of the bladder.[1] It inhibits bladder contraction, relieves spasm induced by various stimuli, increases bladder capacity, and delays the desire to void in patients with a neurogenic bladder. Oxybutynin also has a topical anesthetic effect on the bladder mucosa.[2] The plasma halflife of oxybutynin increases in the elderly, generally allowing smaller doses to be given less frequently. It has an active metabolite. An alternative drug may be more appropriate for some patients (Box 8.A).
Bio-availability 6% PO.
Onset of action 30–60min.
Time to peak plasma concentration 30–60min.
Plasma halflife 2–3h (4–5h in the elderly).
Duration of action 6–10h.

Box 8.A   Alternative drugs for urinary frequency and bladder spasms

Antimuscarinics are the drugs of choice even though treatment may be limited by other antimuscarinic effects:
- tolterodine 2mg b.i.d. is as effective as oxybutynin 5mg t.i.d. but has fewer antimuscarinic effects;[3] it is more expensive
- amitriptyline or imipramine 25–50mg at bedtime.

Musculotropic drugs, flavoxate 200–400mg t.i.d.

NSAIDs, e.g. naproxen 250–500mg b.i.d.

Vasopressin analogues, e.g. desmopressin, are of value in refractory nocturia; hyponatremia is a possible complication.

Cautions

See Antimuscarinics, p.5.

Undesirable effects

For full list, see manufacturer's Product Monograph.
Dry mouth, other antimuscarinic effects (see p.5), cognitive impairment and delirium in the elderly,[4] nausea, abdominal discomfort.
   SR and TD formulations produce fewer undesirable effects but are more expensive.

Dose and use
Normal-release
- start with 2.5–5mg b.i.d.
- if necessary, increase to 5mg q.i.d.

Sustained-release
- start with 5mg once daily
- if necessary, increase in 5mg/day steps at weekly intervals
- maximum recommended dose 30mg once daily.

TD patches
- apply 1 patch (3.9mg/24h) twice weekly to clean, dry skin on abdomen, hip or buttock; avoid application to same site within 1 week.

Supply
Oxybutynin (generic)
Tablets 2.5mg, 5mg, 28 days @ 5mg b.i.d. = $14.
Oral solution 1mg/mL, 28 days @ 5mg b.i.d. = $21.

Sustained-release
Ditropan® XL (Janssen-Ortho)
Tablets SR 5mg, 10mg, 28 days @ 10mg once daily = $64.

Uromax® (Purdue)
Tablets SR 10mg, 15mg, 28 days @ 10mg once daily = $39.

Transdermal
Oxytrol® (Watson)
TD patches 36mg (releasing 3.9mg/24h), 28 days @ 1 patch twice weekly = $55.

---

1 Andersson K (1988) Current concepts in the treatment of disorders of micturition. *Drugs.* **35**: 477–494.
2 Robinson T and Castleden C (1994) Drugs in focus: 11. Oxybutynin hydrochloride. *Prescribers' Journal.* **34**: 27–30.
3 Hills C *et al.* (1998) Tolterodine. *Drugs.* **55**: 813–820.
4 Donnellan C *et al.* (1997) Oxybutynin and cognitive dysfunction. *British Medical Journal.* **315**: 1363–1364.

METHENAMINE MANDELATE AND NITROFURANTOIN

The use of urinary antiseptics is no longer widespread. Except for recurrent cystitis in otherwise healthy women, clinicians generally prefer to treat acute (symptomatic) cystitis with an appropriate antibiotic. However, as one way of reducing the frequency of catheter blockage, a urinary antiseptic is of potential benefit in some patients with a long-term indwelling urinary catheter.

Class: Urinary antiseptics.

Indications: †Prophylaxis against blockage of indwelling urinary catheters.

Contra-indications: Methenamine *mandelate* should not be used in severe renal impairment (creatinine clearance <10mL/min), metabolic acidosis, hepatic impairment, severe dehydration, or gout. Nitrofurantoin should not be given with a creatinine clearance of <60mL/min or elevated plasma creatinine.

Pharmacology
In an acid environment (pH <5.5), methenamine *mandelate* dissociates into methenamine and mandelic acid. Methenamine is then converted to formaldehyde which is responsible for the bactericidal effect.[1,2] Urea-splitting bacteria, e.g. *Pseudomonas aeruginosa*, by producing ammonia tend to raise the pH of urine and could thereby inhibit the formation of formaldehyde; however, mandelic acid maintains an acidic environment. Nearly all bacteria are sensitive to formaldehyde at concentrations of ≥20microgram/mL.

Nitrofurantoin is an alternative urinary antiseptic which also works best in an acid environment. Because of its rapid excretion from the blood, nitrofurantoin reaches significant concentrations only in the bladder.[3] With renal impairment, antibacterial concentrations in the bladder are less likely to be achieved, and toxic plasma levels are correspondingly more likely. Nitrofurantoin is reduced by flavoproteins to reactive intermediates which inactivate or alter bacterial ribosomal proteins and other macromolecules. As a result, protein synthesis, aerobic metabolism, DNA synthesis, RNA synthesis and cell wall synthesis are inhibited. This broad mode of action is probably the reason why acquired bacterial resistance to nitrofurantoin is rare.

The need for antibacterials for treatment of symptomatic urinary tract infections in patients with an indwelling urinary catheter was significantly less in those receiving prophylactic regimens of methenamine *hippurate* and nitrofurantoin compared with controls.[4] Methenamine *hippurate* (not available in Canada) reduces sediment and catheter blockage, and doubles the interval between catheter changes.[5] Because their mechanisms of action are identical, methenamine *mandelate* can be expected to have a comparable impact.

In terms of symptom-free days, in an RCT in otherwise healthy women with urinary tract infection treated for up to 1 year, methenamine *hippurate* was less effective than nitrofurantoin.[6]

For pharmacokinetic details, see Table 8.1. When taken after food, the amount of nitrofurantoin absorbed and the duration of therapeutic urine concentrations is substantially increased,[7] GI tolerance may improve, and bio-availability increases by about 40% (see Product Monograph for Macrobid®).

Table 8.1 Pharmacokinetics of urinary antiseptics PO

	Methenamine mandelate	Nitrofurantoin
Bio-availability	Readily absorbed	Up to 90% (higher after food)[7]
Onset of action	>2h	2.5–4.5h
Plasma halflife	4h	60min
Duration of action	No data	5h fasting, 8h after food

Cautions

With chronic use, the formaldehyde produced from methenamine may irritate and inflame the bladder mucosa, and lead to painful and frequent voiding, hematuria and proteinuria.

Methenamine *mandelate* should not be administered concurrently with sulfonamides because of the possibility of crystalluria. Concurrent administration with **magnesium salts** reduces the absorption of nitrofurantoin. Neither methenamine *mandelate* nor nitrofurantoin should be given concurrently with alkalinizing agents, e.g. **potassium citrate**, because of the need for an acid urinary environment. Uricosuric drugs, e.g. **probenecid** and **sulfinpyrazone**, may inhibit renal tubular secretion of nitrofurantoin which could lead to increased systemic toxicity and decreased efficacy.

Rarely, nitrofurantoin is associated with an acute allergic pulmonary reaction.[8,9] This occurs within 3 weeks of first exposure to nitrofurantoin, and is characterized by fever, cough, dyspnea, abnormal chest radiograph, and leukocytosis, with rapid resolution after nitrofurantoin is discontinued. Chronic use of nitrofurantoin over many months is occasionally associated with pulmonary fibrosis (<1/1,000 chronic users). Although CT shows changes typical of chronic irreversible fibrosis, discontinuation leads to resolution.[10] Diagnosis is based on clinical suspicion (pattern recognition) and exclusion of other causes. If drug-induced pulmonary fibrosis is suspected, nitrofurantoin should be stopped immediately.

Rarely, the chronic use of nitrofurantoin causes hepatitis, which tends to be insidious in onset. It is thus advisable for patients receiving nitrofurantoin long-term to have their LFTs checked every 3–6 months.

Undesirable effects

For full list, see manufacturer's Product Monograph.
Both methenamine *mandelate* and nitrofurantoin may cause dyspepsia, nausea and vomiting. Nitrofurantoin may cause headache and discolouration of the urine (dark yellow or brown); it also enhances predisposition to peripheral neuropathy, e.g. in diabetes mellitus.

Dose and use

Methenamine *mandelate* and nitrofurantoin should *not* be used to treat infection of the *upper* urinary tract, i.e. pyelonephritis.

The optimum dose for a urinary antiseptic in patients with an indwelling catheter is unknown, but is likely to be lower than that recommended for acute cystitis. Further, in relation to catheterized patients, the substitution of nitrofurantoin for mandelamine is justified only by extrapolation. However, on the grounds of cost and convenience, nitrofurantoin (as normal-release tablets) would seem to be the urinary antiseptic of first choice. The following reflects the practice at some centres:

- methenamine *mandelate* 1g b.i.d.–q8h[2,11]
- nitrofurantoin 50–100mg once daily, preferably p.c.[6]

Supply

Methenamine *mandelate*
Mandelamine® (Erfa Canada)
Tablets 500mg, 28 days @ 1g b.i.d. = $11.

Nitrofurantoin (generic)
Capsules 50mg, 100mg, 28 days @ 100mg at bedtime = $18.
Tablets 50mg, 100mg, 28 days @ 100mg at bedtime = $7.

Sustained-release
Macrobid® (Procter and Gamble Canada)
Capsules SR 100mg, 28 days @ 100mg at bedtime = $21.

1 Strom JJ and Jun H (1993) Effect of urine pH and ascorbic acid on the rate of conversion of methenamine to formaldehyde. *Biopharmaceutics and Drug Disposition.* **14**: 61–69.
2 Sweetman SC (ed) (2007) *Martindale: The Complete Drug Reference.* (35e). Pharmaceutical Press, London, pp. 266–267.
3 Hooper D (1995) Urinary tract agents: nitrofurantoin and methenamine. In: G Mandell *et al.* (eds) *Mandell, Douglas and Bennett's Principles and Practice of Infectious Diseases* Vol 1 (4e). Churchill Livingstone, New York, pp. 376–381.
4 Nyren P *et al.* (1981) Prophylactic methenamine hippurate or nitrofurantoin in patients with an indwelling urinary catheter. *Annals of Clinical Research.* **13**: 16–21.
5 Norberg A *et al.* (1980) Randomized double-blind study of prophylactic methenamine hippurate treatment of patients with indwelling catheters. *European Journal of Clinical Pharmacology.* **18**: 497–500.
6 Brumfitt W *et al.* (1981) Prevention of recurrent urinary infections in women: a comparative trial between nitrofurantoin and methenamine hippurate. *Journal of Urology.* **126**: 71–74.
7 Gleckman R *et al.* (1979) Drug therapy reviews: nitrofurantoin. *American Journal of Hospital Pharmacy.* **36**: 342–351.
8 Jick SS *et al.* (1989) Hospitalizations for pulmonary reactions following nitrofurantoin use. *Chest.* **96**: 512–515.
9 Boggess KA *et al.* (1996) Nitrofurantoin-induced pulmonary toxicity during pregnancy: a report of a case and review of the literature. *Obstetrical and Gynecological Survey.* **51**: 367–370.
10 Sheehan RE *et al.* (2000) Nitrofurantoin-induced lung disease: two cases demonstrating resolution of apparently irreversible CT abnormalities. *Journal of Computer Assisted Tomography.* **24**: 259–261.
11 Cronberg S *et al.* (1987) Prevention of recurrent acute cystitis by methenamine hippurate: double blind controlled crossover longterm study. *British Medical Journal.* **294**: 1507–1508.

CRANBERRY JUICE

Class: Herbal remedy.

Indications: †Prophylaxis against urinary tract infections (UTIs).

Pharmacology

Cranberry juice inhibits bacterial adherence to the urinary tract mucosa by disrupting the binding of bacterial macromolecules to receptors on mucosal epithelial cells.[1,2] This effect, which has been demonstrated *in vitro* in *Escherichia coli*, is produced by the pro-anthrocyanidins (tannins) and fructose present in cranberries.[3,4] Cranberry juice has also shown *in vitro* activity against *Staphylococcus aureus, Klebsiella pneumoniae, Pseudomonas aeruginosa* and *Proteus mirabilis*.[5] Blueberry juice also contains pro-anthrocyanidins, and may possess anti-adhesive activity, but clinical trials are lacking.[3] These natural juices could be a useful alternative to antibacterials for preventing UTIs, and could thus reduce the development of resistant organisms.[3]

The benefit of cranberry juice is limited to the prevention of UTIs; it does not cure established infection.[5,6] It reduces the frequency of symptomatic UTIs caused by *Escherichia coli*,[7] and the frequency of infections over 1 year in women with recurrent UTIs.[4] The addition of **ascorbic acid** (vitamin C) is not necessary. Evidence for effectiveness in the elderly (both men and women) is less clear, and there is no evidence of effectiveness in people with an indwelling urinary catheter.[3,4,8]

The optimum dose form is not clear, but most research has been done with the fruit juice.[4] Juices with a fruit content of 25–33% have been used in most studies;[2,3] and Health Canada recommends ⩾30%.[9] The optimum daily dose is also unknown;[2] Health Canada suggests up to 750mL/24h,[9] but volumes larger than 300mL/24h did not increase efficacy in clinical studies, and are associated with more undesirable effects.[5,7] Further, the relatively high drop-out rate in the clinical studies suggests that long-term consumption of cranberry juice may be unacceptable to some patients.[4] There is little research regarding the efficacy of cranberry capsules.[5]

Pharmacokinetic data not available.

Cautions

Like many other fruits and berries, cranberry juice contains significant amounts of salicylic acid (7mg/L). Theoretically, large amounts of cranberry juice could trigger an allergic reaction in people with **aspirin** allergy or asthma.[5] In very large doses, e.g. 3–4L/24h of juice, cranberry can cause GI upset and diarrhea. Consuming more than 1L/24h over a prolonged period may increase the risk of uric acid kidney stone formation (300mL of cranberry juice contains approximately 19mg of oxalate).[5]

Cranberry juice contains various anti-oxidants, including flavonoids, which are known to inhibit cytochrome P450 activity.[10] This was originally thought to explain several case reports, including one fatality,[11–14] in which the regular use of cranberry juice was linked to an increase in or fluctuation of INR values in patients taking **warfarin**, a drug predominantly metabolized by CYP2C9 (see p.551).[15] These cases led the UK authorities to recommend avoiding the concurrent use of cranberry products and **warfarin**, unless the benefit (prevention of UTI) outweighed the risks.[12] However, Health Canada does not consider the risk sufficiently proven to issue a regulatory warning.[16] Further, more recent research suggests that this interaction is unlikely to occur with the amounts of cranberry juice now recommended for the treatment of UTI. Patients on stable **warfarin** doses who drank cranberry juice 250mL once daily for 1 week showed no significant increase in anticoagulant activity.[17] Further, in volunteers, drinking cranberry juice 200mL t.i.d. did not significantly affect the pharmacokinetic profiles of **warfarin**, **tizanidine** or **midazolam**, which are probes for CYP2C9, CYP1A2 and CYP3A4 respectively.[18] Nonetheless, because the quantities of flavonoids in different commercial brands of cranberry juice may differ, and it is not clear whether other mechanisms are also involved, an interaction with **warfarin** cannot be ruled out, particularly if large volumes of cranberry juice are drunk regularly or when cranberry products other than juice are taken.[19–21] Thus, the INR should be monitored more closely in patients on **warfarin** if they consume large amounts of cranberry juice or take other cranberry supplements.[21]

Dose and use

Drink as fruit juice, preferably ≥30%, 150mL b.i.d. or 300mL once daily, or take as capsules containing dried juice 400–1,200mg once daily. Benefit is seen only after 4 weeks or more.[9]

Supply

Available OTC.

1 Liu Y (2006) Role of cranberry juice on molecular-scale surface characteristics and adhesion behaviour of Escherichia coli. *Biotechnology and Bioengineering.* **93**: 297–305.

2 Liu Y et al. (2008) Cranberry changes the physiochemical surface properties of E.coli and adhesion with uroepithelial cells. *Colloids and Surfaces B: Biointerfaces.* **65**: 35–42.

3 Jepson R (2007) A systematic review of the evidence for cranberries and blueberries in UTI prevention. *Molecular Nutrition & Food Research.* **51**: 738–745.

4 Jepson RG and Craig JC (2008) Cranberries for preventing urinary tract infections. In: *Cochrane Database of Systematic Reviews 1: CD001321.* Available from: www.mrw.interscience.wiley.com/cochrane/clsysrev/articles/CD001321/frame.html

5 Natural Medicines Comprehensive Database (2008) Cranberry. In: *Natural Medicines Comprehensive Database.* Available from: www.naturaldatabase.com

6 Tong H et al. (2006) Effect of ingesting cranberry juice on bacterial growth in urine. *American Journal of Health-System Pharmacy.* **63**: 1417–1419.

7 Avorn J et al. (1994) Reduction of bacteriuria and pyuria after ingestion of cranberry juice. *Journal of the American Medical Association.* **271**: 751–754.

8 McMurdo ME et al. (2005) Does ingestion of cranberry juice reduce symptomatic urinary tract infections in older people in hospital? A double-blind, placebo-controlled trial. *Age & Ageing.* **34**: 256–261.

9 Health Canada (2007) Cranberry. Available from: www.hc-sc.gc.ca/dhp-mps/prodnatur/applications/licen-prod/monograph/mono_cranberry-canneberge-eng.php

10 Hodek P et al. (2002) Flavonoids-potent and versatile biologically active compounds interacting with cytochromes P450. *Chemico-Biological Interactions.* **139**: 1–21.

11 Suvarna R et al. (2003) Possible interaction between warfarin and cranberry juice. *British Medical Journal.* **327**: 1454.

12 CSM (Committee on Safety of Medicines) (2004) Interaction between warfarin and cranberry juice: new advice. *Current Problems in Pharmacovigilance.* **30 (October)**: 10.

13 MHRA (2003) Possible interaction between warfarin and cranberry juice. *Current problems in Pharmacovigilance.* **29 (Sept)**: 8.

14 Grant P (2004) Warfarin and cranberry juice: an interaction? *Journal of Heart Valve Disease.* **13**: 25–26.

15 Rettie AE et al. (1992) Hydroxylation of warfarin by human cDNA-expressed cytochrome P-450: a role for P-4502C9 in the etiology of (S)-warfarin-drug interactions. *Chemical Research in Toxicology.* **5**: 54–59.

16 Health Canada (2004) Suspected warfarin-cranberry juice interaction. *Canadian Adverse Reaction Newsletter.* **14 (July)**: 2.

17 Li Z et al. (2006) Cranberry does not affect prothrombin time in male subjects on warfarin. *Journal of the American Dietetic Society.* **106**: 2057–2061.

18 Lilja JJ et al. (2007) Effects of daily ingestion of cranberry juice on the pharmacokinetics of warfarin, tizanidine, and midazolam–probes of CYP2C9, CYP1A2, and CYP3A4. *Clinical Pharmacology & Therapeutics.* **81**: 833–839.

19 Aston JL et al. (2006) Interaction between warfarin and cranberry juice. *Pharmacotherapy.* **26**: 1314–1319.

20 Welch J and Forster K (2007) Probable elevation in international normalized ratio from cranberry juice. *Journal of Pharmacy Technology.* **23**: 104–107.

21 O'Mara N (2007) Does a cranberry juice-warfarin interaction really exist? Detail document. *Pharmacist's Letter/Prescriber's Letter.* **23**: 1–3.

CATHETER PATENCY SOLUTIONS (URINARY BLADDER IRRIGANTS)

Indications: Catheter blockage.

General considerations

Catheters can block because of blood clots, bladder mucosal debris, small calculi and/or phosphate encrustations on the surface of an indwelling catheter. Encrustations are associated with infection of the urine by urease-producing bacteria, e.g. *Proteus mirabilis*, *Pseudomonas aeruginosa* and *Klebsiella*. Urease breaks down urea to form ammonia, increasing the alkalinity of the urine and leading to the deposition of mainly phosphate crystals on the surface of the catheter.

The main purpose of a catheter patency solution is to reduce the frequency of catheter blockage; irrigation does *not* cure infection.[1,2] Consideration should be given to the long-term use of a urinary antiseptic to acidify the urine and to reduce the frequency of infection (see **Methenamine mandelate** and **nitrofurantoin**, p.412). Repeated blockage several times per day generally means that the catheter needs to be changed.[3]

Dose and use

To reduce the likelihood of encrustations causing a blockage, latex catheters should be changed at least every 6 weeks. If the catheter is to be left for longer periods, a silicone catheter should be used.

Unless the blockage is definitely caused by encrustations, rather than mucosal debris etc.:
* start with **sodium chloride** once daily–b.i.d. (occasionally more often)
* if this is inadequate, change to **Urologic G irrigation** (or a comparable solution)
* switch back to **sodium chloride** after 4–5 days if the number of blockages reduces to 1–2 per 24h.

Supply

Sodium chloride for irrigation USP for flushing out debris and small blood clots (but not for dissolution of encrustations).
Irrigating solution 0.9% e.g. 1L = $5.

Urologic G irrigation (generic)
Irrigating solution citric acid solution containing magnesium oxide and sodium carbonate, for dissolution of phosphate calculi or encrustations. 1.62%, 1L = $24; 3.24%, 1L = $22.

Other irrigating solutions are available but are not featured here.

---

1 Getliffe K (1996) Bladder instillations and bladder washouts in the management of catheterized patients. *Journal of Advanced Nursing.* **23**: 548–554.
2 Pomfret I et al. (2004) Using bladder instillations to manage indwelling catheters. *British Journal of Nursing.* **13**: 261–267.
3 Williams C and Tonkin S (2003) Blocked urinary catheters: solutions are not the only solution. *British Journal of Community Nursing.* **8**: 321–326.

DISCOLOURED URINE

Patients need to be warned about drugs and other substances which can discolour urine (Box 8.B). If the urine is red, it may be assumed to be blood, and cause alarm.

The colour-banding in Box 8.B is approximate, i.e. a drug listed under 'brown/orange/yellow' will most likely cause discolouration at some point in that range. Sometimes the colour is pH dependent. Further information on causes of discoloured urine is available from: www.wrongdiagnosis.com/symptoms/urine_color_changes/causes.htm.

Note: urine colour will vary according to the concentration or dilution of the urine. Colouring agents in processed food can also affect urine colour.

Purple urine bag syndrome is caused by the breakdown of dietary tryptophan metabolites by bacteria in urine, ultimately producing indigo (blue) and indirubin (red) in alkaline urine.[2–4] Chronic urinary tract infection, long-term catheterization, constipation and immobility are the main risk factors. Although harmless, purple urine bag syndrome causes the urine to develop a strong, unpleasant odour, which becomes more noticeable over time and in warm conditions. This distresses patients more than the discolouration. Changing the drainage bag more frequently, e.g. every 3 days rather than every 5–7 days, helps to avoid the build-up of the odour. Indwelling long-term catheters may also need changing more often than normal.[4]

Box 8.B Selected causes of discoloured urine[a]

Black/dark brown
Iron (ferrous salts)
Methocarbamol

Brown/orange/yellow
Aloe
Carrots
Cascara
Chloroquine
Chlorzoxazone
Dantrolene
Fluorescein
Heparin
Nitrofurantoin
Paprika
Phenazopyridine
Primaquine
Quinine
Retinol (vitamin A)
Riboflavin (vitamin B2)
Rifampin
Senna (pH dependent)
Sulfasalazine
Sulfonamides
Warfarin

Brown/red/pink
Anthraquinone laxatives
Beetroot (alkaline urine)
Blackberries (acid urine)
Daunorubicin
Doxorubicin
Entacapone
Ibuprofen
Levodopa
Metronidazole (acid urine)
Napthalene-based dyes in foods and medicines, e.g. Ponceau 4R
Phenolphthalein (alkaline urine)
Phenothiazines
Phenytoin
Rhubarb (in several proprietary laxatives; pH dependent)
Senna (alkaline urine)

Purple
Degradation of tryptophan by urinary bacteria (see text)

Blue/green
Amitriptyline[1]
Chlorophyll breath mints
FD & C Dye No. 1 (used in foods and medicines)
Hydroquinone
Indomethacin
Magnesium salicylate
Phenols
Promethazine (injection)
Propofol

continued

Box 8.B   Continued

Pseudomonas aeruginosa (pyocyanin; alkaline urine)
Resorcinol
Thymol
Triamterene

Milky colour
Diffuse glomerular nephritis
Lipids
Neutrophils
Phosphates
Radiographic dyes
Urates

---

a. discolouration which occurs only when urine is left 'on standing' has not been included.

---

1 Beeley L (1986) What drugs turn urine green? *British Medical Journal.* **293**: 750.
2 Al-Jubouri MA and Vardhan MS (2001) A case of purple urine bag syndrome associated with Providencia rettgeri. *Journal of Clinical Pathology.* **54**: 412.
3 Ribeiro JP *et al.* (2004) Case report: purple urine bag syndrome. *Critical Care (London, England).* **8**: R137.
4 Robinson J (2003) Purple urinary bag syndrome: a harmless but alarming problem. *British Journal of Community Nursing.* **8**: 263–266.

9: NUTRITION AND BLOOD

ANEMIA

Anemia is common in cancer and other forms of chronic disease. The main causes are:
- anemia of chronic disease
- iron deficiency
- folate deficiency
- malignant infiltration of the marrow
- hemolytic anemia
- renal failure.

It is important to distinguish between the various types of anemia because treatment differs. The commonest form in cancer is anemia of chronic disease (ACD). This is a paraneoplastic phenomenon and relates partly to suppression of endogenous erythropoietin production (Figure 9.1).[1]

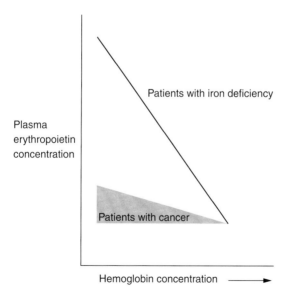

Figure 9.1 Relationship between hemoglobin and erythropoietin concentration in patients with iron deficiency and cancer-associated anemia.[1]

Diagnostic features are:
- normochromic-normocytic anemia (hypochromic-microcytic in iron deficiency)
- low/low-normal plasma transferrin concentration (TIBC) (vs. high/high-normal in iron deficiency)
- low plasma iron

- high/high-normal plasma ferritin concentration, although the ferritin rises during acute phase response, e.g. to trauma, infection and some cancers (vs. low in iron deficiency)
- bone marrow appearance generally unremarkable; may show abnormal iron distribution
- increased marrow iron stores
- reduced iron within maturing erythroblasts.

There are two potential treatment options:
- intermittent blood transfusions or
- SC **epoetin**.[2]

About 75% of patients with ACD respond to **epoetin** treatment. In patients already transfusion-dependent, about 1/2 will become transfusion-independent.[3,4] However, because of increased tumour progression and reduced survival time in cancer patients treated with **epoetin**, regulatory agencies in Canada, the USA and Europe now recommend that **epoetin** is restricted in cancer to patients receiving chemotherapy (Box 9.A). The UK MHRA advises that blood transfusion may be preferable for patients with advanced or metastatic cancer who have a good survival prognosis.[5]

Box 9.A   Epoetin

Epoetin is recombinant human erythropoietin, the hormone responsible for the maintenance of erythropoiesis.[6] The drug binds to and activates receptors on erythroid progenitor cells which then develop into mature erythrocytes.[7] Epoetin increases the reticulocyte count, hemoglobin concentration (Hgb) and hematocrit in a dose-proportional manner.

Response to epoetin in patients receiving chemotherapy has been shown in RCTs and confirmed by meta-analysis.[3] RCTs also show a higher rate of tumour progression and reduced survival in cancer patients receiving epoetin, with or without chemotherapy.[8,9]

In a study in renal patients with a target Hgb of 135g/L (13.5g/dL), epoetin was associated with an increase in cardiovascular complications (myocardial infarction, hospitalization for CHF, stroke and death).[8]

As a result, regulatory authorities in Canada, the UK and the USA have issued new guidelines for use:
- epoetin products should be used *only* for their approved indications (i.e. for renal patients, cancer patients with chemotherapy-related anemia or HIV patients with zidovudine-related anemia)
- the risks should be weighed against the potential need for and risks of blood transfusion
- they should *not* be used in cancer patients not on chemotherapy
- the dose recommendations in each manufacturer's product information should be strictly adhered to
- cancer patients on chemotherapy should:
  ▷ have the potential risks of progression and shortened survival explained to them before starting or continuing on epoetin
  ▷ receive the lowest possible dose to relieve the symptoms of anemia
  ▷ stop epoetin once the course of chemotherapy is completed
- the target Hgb should be no more than 120g/L (12g/dL) and, if the Hgb rises above this or if there is an increase of $\geqslant$10g/L ($\geqslant$1g/dL) in any 2-week period, the next dose should be withheld.[10–14]

---

1 Miller C et al. (1990) Decreased erythropoietin response in patients with the anemia of cancer. *New England Journal of Medicine*. **322**: 1689–1692.

2 Ludwig H (2002) Anemia of hematologic malignancies: what are the treatment options? *Seminars in Oncology*. **29 (3 suppl 8)**: 45–54.

3 Seidenfeld J et al. (2001) Epoetin treatment of anemia associated with cancer therapy: a systematic review and meta-analysis of controlled clinical trials. *Journal of the National Cancer Institute*. **93**: 1204–1214.

4 Turner R et al. (2001) Epoetin alfa in cancer patients: evidence-based guidelines. *Journal of Pain and Symptom Management*. **22**: 954–965.

5 MHRA (2008) Drug safety update. **2 (1, August)**: 3–4. Available from: www.mhra.gov.uk/Publications/Safetyguidance/index.htm

6 Engert A (2000) Recombinant human erythropoietin as an alternative to blood transfusion in cancer-related anaemia. *Disease Management and Health Outcomes.* **8**: 259–272.
7 Dunn C and Markham A (1996) Epoetin beta. A review of its pharmacological properties and clinical use in the management of anaemia associated with chronic renal failure. *Drugs.* **51**: 299–318.
8 Steensma DP (2007) Erythropoiesis stimulating agents. *British Medical Journal.* **334**: 648–649.
9 Bohlius J (2009) Recombinant human erythropoiesis-stimulating agents and mortality in patients with cancer: a meta-analysis of randomized trials. *Lancet.* **373**: 1532–1542.
10 Health Canada (2007) Important safety information and prescribing information for the erythropoiesis-stimulating agents (ESAs) Aranesp (darbepoetin alfa) and Eprex (epoetin alfa) for health professionals. Available from: http://www.hc-sc.gc.ca/dhp-mps/medeff/advisories-avis/prof/_2007/aranesp_eprex_hpc-cps-eng.php
11 EMEA (2007) Public statement. European Medicines Agency starts review of the safety of epoetins. European Agency for the Evaluation of Medicinal Products. Available from: www.emea.europa.eu/pdfs/human/press/pus/18806807en.pdf
12 FDA (2007) Information for healthcare professionals. Erythropoiesis stimulating agents. Food and Drugs Administration. Available from: www.fda.gov/Drugs/DrugSafety/PublicHealthAdvisories/ucm054721.htm
13 FDA (2007) Medwatch 2007 safety alert: Aranesp (darbepoetin alfa). Food and Drugs Administration. Available from: www.fda.gov/Safety/MedWatch/SafetyInformation/SafetyAlertsforHumanMedicalProducts/ucm150816.htm and www.fda.gov/Safety/MedWatch/SafetyInformation/SafetyAlertsforHumanMedicalProducts/ucm150817.htm
14 FDA (2008) Communication about an Ongoing Safety Review: Erythropoiesis-Stimulating Agents (ESAs) Epoetin alfa (marketed as Procrit, Epogen) Darbepoetin alfa (marketed as Aranesp). Available from: www.fda.gov/Drugs/DrugSafety/PostmarketDrugSafetyInformationforPatientsandProviders/DrugSafetyInformationforHeathcareProfessionals/ucm072280.htm

FERROUS SULFATE

Class: Elemental salt.

Indications: Prevention and treatment of iron deficiency anemia.

Contra-indications: Anemia not caused by iron deficiency. Hemosiderosis, hemochromatosis.

Pharmacology

Ferrous salts are better absorbed than ferric salts. Because there are only marginal differences in terms of efficiency of iron absorption, the choice of ferrous salt is based mainly on the incidence of undesirable effects and cost. Undesirable effects relate directly to the amount of elemental iron, and improved tolerance after switching to another salt may be because the elemental iron content is less (Table 9.1). SR formulations are designed to reduce undesirable effects by releasing iron gradually as the tablet or capsule passes down the GI tract. However, these products are likely to carry most of the iron past the first part of the duodenum into parts of the intestine where iron absorption is poor. Such products have no therapeutic advantage and should not be used.[1]

Table 9.1 Elemental ferrous iron content of different iron salts

Iron salt	Amount (mg)	Ferrous content (mg)
Ferrous fumarate	200	65
Ferrous sulfate, dried (anhydrous)	200	65
Ferrous sulfate	300	60
Ferrous gluconate	300	35

Some oral formulations contain **ascorbic acid** to aid absorption, or the iron is in the form of a chelate. These modifications have been shown experimentally to produce a modest increase in the absorption of iron. However, the therapeutic advantage is minimal, and the cost may be increased. Further, **ascorbic acid** may increase GI irritation.[1] There is no clinical justification for the inclusion of other therapeutically active ingredients such as the B group of vitamins (except **folic acid** for pregnant women).

In the treatment of iron deficiency, Hgb should rise by about 1g/dL/week. After the Hgb has risen to normal, treatment should be continued for a further 3 months to replenish the iron stores. Epithelial tissue changes such as atrophic glossitis and koilonychia also improve but generally more slowly.

Cautions

Because of decreased absorption of either iron or the other drug, or both, ferrous sulfate should not be administered concurrently with antacids, bisphosphonates, **calcium salts**, **cholestyramine**, **levodopa**, **penicillamine**, quinolone antibacterials, tetracyclines, **thyroxine**, **vitamin E** and **zinc.**[1]

Undesirable effects

For full list, see manufacturer's Product Monograph.

Dyspepsia, nausea, epigastric pain, constipation and diarrhea. Elderly patients are more likely to develop constipation, occasionally leading to fecal impaction; SR products are more likely to cause diarrhea.

Note: liquid formulations may stain teeth. Urine and stools are discolored (black), and this may result in a false positive fecal occult blood test.

Dose and use

The diagnosis of iron deficiency should be confirmed before iron supplements are prescribed (see Anemia, p.421):

- prescribe ferrous sulfate 300mg b.i.d.–t.i.d. (elemental iron 120–180mg/24h); doses >900mg/24h exceed the maximal absorption capacity and increase undesirable effects
- if undesirable GI effects occur:
  ▷ reduce the dose
  ▷ take with food (but may reduce absorption by ⩽50%)
  ▷ switch to an alternative iron salt with a lower elemental iron content
  ▷ switch to a liquid formulation (may be less damaging to GI mucosa)[2]
- dilute liquid formulations and swallow through a straw to prevent discoloration of the teeth.

Consider prophylaxis in patients at high risk of iron deficiency, e.g. those with a poor diet, malabsorption, and after total or sub-total gastrectomy:

- prescribe ferrous sulfate 300mg once daily (elemental iron 60mg).

Supply

Ferrous sulfate (generic)
Tablets 300mg (60mg iron), 28 days @ 300mg b.i.d. = $2.50 available OTC.
Oral syrup 150mg (30mg iron)/5mL, 28 days @ 300mg (10mL) b.i.d. = $32 available OTC.

Ferrous gluconate (generic)
Tablets 300mg (35mg iron), 28 days @ 300mg b.i.d. = $3.

Ferrous fumarate
Palafer (Glaxosmithkline Consumer Healthcare Inc.)
Capsules 300mg (100mg iron) 28 days @ 300mg daily = $12.
Suspension 300mg (100mg iron)/5mL 28 days @ 300mg (5mL) daily = $22.

---

1 Rutledge Harding S (2007) Chapter 87. Common Anemias. In: J Gray (ed) *Therapeutic Choices 5th Edition*. Canadian Pharmacists Association, Ottawa, pp. 1114–1130.
2 Ji H and Yardley JH (2004) Iron medication-associated gastric mucosal injury. *Archives of Pathology & Laboratory Medicine*. **128**: 821–822.

ASCORBIC ACID (VITAMIN C)

Class: Vitamin.

Indications: Scurvy, †decubitus ulcers, †furred tongue (topical), †urinary infection.

Pharmacology

Ascorbic acid (vitamin C) is a powerful reducing agent. It is obtained from dietary sources of fresh fruit and vegetables, particularly blackcurrants and kiwifruit, broccoli, red pepper and oranges; it cannot be synthesized by the body. It is involved in the hydroxylation of proline to hydroxyproline, which is necessary for the formation of collagen. The failure of this accounts for most of the clinical effects found in deficiency (scurvy), e.g. keratosis of hair follicles with 'corkscrew hair', perifollicular hemorrhages, swollen spongy infected and bleeding gums, loose teeth, spontaneous bruising and hemorrhage, anemia and failure of wound healing. Repeated infections are also common. In healthy adults, a dietary intake of 30–60mg/24h is necessary; in scurvy, a rapid clinical response is seen with 100–200mg/24h. Absorption occurs mainly from the proximal small intestine by a saturable process. In health, body stores of ascorbic acid are about 1.5g, although larger stores may occur with intakes higher than 200mg/24h. It is excreted as oxalic acid, unchanged ascorbic acid and small amounts of dehydro-ascorbic acid. Ascorbic acid is used to acidify urine in patients with alkaline urine and recurrent urinary infections.

A beneficial effect of megadose ascorbic acid therapy has been claimed for many conditions,[1] including the common cold, asthma, atherosclerosis, cancer, psychiatric disorders, increased susceptibility to infections related to abnormal leucocyte function, infertility and osteogenesis imperfecta. Ascorbic acid has also been tried in the treatment of wound healing, pain in Paget's disease and opioid withdrawal. There are few controlled studies to substantiate these claims. High-dose vitamin C is not effective against advanced cancer.[2] Vitamin C alone or with β-carotene and vitamin E does not prevent the development of colorectal adenoma.[3] However, ascorbic acid does reduce the severity of a cold but not its incidence.[4] On the other hand, enthusiasm for high-dose ascorbic acid for HIV+ people waned after many died from disease progression.[5] Although it has been postulated that ascorbic acid might help prevent ischemic heart disease, in contrast to other anti-oxidant vitamins, little benefit is seen in controlled studies.[6,7] Of more concern are data which indicate that a total daily dose as small as 500mg has a pro-oxidant effect which could result in genetic mutation.[8]

Vitamin C deficiency is common in cancer patients and patients with low plasma concentrations have been shown to have a shorter survival.[9]

Undesirable effects
For full list, see manufacturer's Product Monograph.
GI symptoms may occur at doses of >1g/24h.[10] Doses of >3g/24h may result in acidosis, diarrhea, glycosuria, oxaluria and renal stones. Tolerance may occur with prolonged use of large doses, resulting in symptoms of deficiency when intake is returned to normal. If allowed to dissolve in the mouth, the acidity of effervescent tablets can break down tooth enamel and may cause localized esophagitis if patients lie down immediately after taking them.

Dose and use
The doses below take into account the fact that only 500mg and 1g tablets are available in Canada.

Furred tongue
- place 1/4 of a 1g effervescent tablet on the tongue and allow it to dissolve; repeat up to q.i.d. for <1 week
- do not use if the patient has a sore mouth.
Pineapple is also used for removing coating from the tongue and oral mucosa (see p.443).

Acidification of urine
- 250mg b.i.d. or 500mg once daily; test urine with litmus paper until constant acid result is obtained (note: may alter the excretion of some drugs).

Scurvy
- 250mg b.i.d. or 500mg once daily for 4 weeks.

Supply
Ascorbic acid (generic)
Tablets 500mg, 28 days @ 500mg once daily = $2.50.
Tablets chewable 500mg, 28 days @ 500mg once daily = $3.

Redoxon® (Bayer Consumer)
Tablets effervescent 1g, 28 days @ 1/4 of a tablet q.i.d. = $3.

1 Ovesen L (1984) Vitamin therapy in the absence of obvious deficiency. What is the evidence? *Drugs.* **27**: 148–170.
2 Moertel C *et al.* (1985) High-dose vitamin C versus placebo in the treatment of patients with advanced cancer who have had no prior chemotherapy. A randomized double-blind comparison. *New England Journal of Medicine.* **312**: 137–141.
3 Greenberg E *et al.* (1994) A clinical trial of antioxidant vitamins to prevent colorectal adenoma. Polyp Prevention Study Group. *New England Journal of Medicine.* **331**: 141–147.
4 Hemila H (1994) Does vitamin C alleviate the symptoms of the common cold? a review of current evidence. *Scandinavian Journal of Infectious Diseases.* **26**: 1–6.
5 Abrams D (1990) Alternative therapies in HIV infection. *AIDS.* **4**: 1179–1187.
6 Rimm E (1993) Vitamin E consumption and the risk of coronary heart disease in men. *New England Journal of Medicine.* **328**: 1450–1456.
7 Stampfer M (1993) Vitamin E consumption and the risk of coronary disease in women. *New England Journal of Medicine.* **328**: 1444–1449.
8 Podmore I *et al.* (1998) Vitamin C exhibits pro-oxidant properties. *Nature.* **392**: 559.
9 Mayland CR *et al.* (2005) Vitamin C deficiency in cancer patients. *Palliative Medicine.* **19**: 17–20.
10 Beveridge C (2002) Basic Nutrition. In: C Repchinsky and C LeBlanc (eds) *Patient Self Care* (1e). Canadian Pharmacists Association, Ottawa, pp. 339–358.

PHYTONADIONE (VITAMIN K₁)

Class: Vitamin.

Indications: Vitamin K deficiency, reversal of anticoagulant effects of **warfarin**, †bleeding tendency in patients with hepatic impairment in advanced cancer. Vitamin K may have a role in hypoprothrombinemia induced by salicylates, sulfonamides, **quinidine**, **quinine** and broad-spectrum antibacterials if interference with vitamin K activity is clearly the cause.

Pharmacology

Phytonadione (vitamin K₁) is the active form of vitamin K. It is necessary for the production of blood clotting factors and proteins involved in bone calcification. Because vitamin K is fat-soluble, patients with fat malabsorption may become deficient, e.g. in biliary obstruction or liver disease. Oral coumarin anticoagulants (e.g. **warfarin**) act by interfering with vitamin K metabolism in the liver and their effects are antagonized by giving exogenous vitamin K.

Vitamin K hepatic stores are depleted in less than 3 days of dietary restriction. Based on low plasma vitamin K, 22% of patients with advanced cancer have been shown to be vitamin K deficient.[1]

Vitamin K is not indicated routinely in hepatic failure, nor even in moribund patients with manifestations of a bleeding diathesis (e.g. petechiae, purpura, multiple bruising, nose and gum bleeds), and it should not be used merely to prevent an imminent inevitable death. Its use is limited to conscious patients with a reasonable performance status for whom other supportive measures are deemed appropriate (e.g. blood transfusion). Failure to respond to vitamin K may indicate that a coagulation defect exists or that the condition is unresponsive to vitamin K.

Plasma halflife 1.5–3h.

Cautions

Oral absorption is reduced by co-administration with **cholestyramine** or **mineral oil (liquid paraffin)**.

Undesirable effects

For full list, see manufacturer's Product Monograph.

Hypersensitivity/anaphylactic reactions after IV use. Injection site reactions after IM use.

Dose and use

Partial reversal of warfarin anticoagulation

• The American College of Chest Physicians evidence-based clinical practice guidelines should be followed[2]

Correction of a bleeding tendency in hepatic failure

• give phytonadione injection 10mg IVI in 50–100mL of 5% dextrose, infused over 30–60min, repeat p.r.n.

Prevention of vitamin K deficiency in malabsorption
- give phytonadione 10mg PO once daily (injection is used orally, tablets only available via Special Access Programme)
- in patients with decreased bile secretion, bile salts should be given with each dose of phytonadione to ensure absorption.

Supply
Phytonadione (generic)
Injection 1mg/0.5mL (hospital only), 0.5mL amp = $2.50; 10mg/mL, 1mL amp = $2.50 (injection may be given orally).

Mephyton (Merk)
Tablets 5mg (via Special Access Programme).

1 Harrington DJ et al. (2008) A study of the prevalence of vitamin K deficiency in patients with cancer referred to a hospital palliative care team and its association with abnormal haemostasis. *Journal of Clinical Pathology.* **61**: 537–540.
2 Hirsh J et al. (2008) Executive summary: American College of Chest Physicians Evidence-Based Clinical Practice Guidelines (8th Edition). *Chest.* **133 (6 suppl)**: 71S–109S. [Erratum appears in Chest. 2008 Oct;134(4):892.]

POTASSIUM

Class: Elemental salt.

Indications: Hypokalemia (<3.5mmol/L).

Pharmacology
In palliative care, hypokalemia is most common in patients receiving non-potassium-sparing diuretics, particularly if also taking a corticosteroid. Hypokalemia is also associated with chronic diarrhea and persistent vomiting. Correction of hypokalemia is important in patients taking **digoxin** or other anti-arrhythmic drugs because of the risk of an arrhythmia. Potassium supplements are seldom required with small doses of diuretics given to treat hypertension.

When larger doses of thiazide or loop diuretics are given to eliminate edema, potassium-sparing diuretics (e.g. **amiloride, spironolactone**) rather than potassium supplements are preferable for the prevention of hypokalemia. Dietary supplements also help to maintain plasma potassium; 10mmol of potassium is contained in a large banana and in 250mL of orange juice.

When treating hypokalemia, potassium chloride is generally the salt of choice because of associated hypochloremia. However, occasionally, hypokalemia is associated with metabolic acidosis, and an alkalinizing salt will be preferable, e.g. potassium citrate. Co-existing hypomagnesemia should always be corrected (see p.429).

Cautions
For full list, see manufacturer's Product Monograph.
Hyperkalemia may result if used concurrently with drugs which increase the plasma potassium concentration, e.g. ACE inhibitors, potassium-sparing diuretics, **cyclosporine**. Use smaller doses of potassium if there is renal insufficiency (common in the elderly).

Undesirable effects
For full list, see manufacturer's Product Monograph.
Esophageal or GI ulceration, nausea and vomiting. Liquid formulations are distasteful.

Dose and use
The dose of potassium supplements depends on the requirements of the individual patient. The usual adult dietary intake of potassium is 40–80mmol/day. Whenever possible, orange juice and bananas should be used as a palatable source of potassium (see above). To minimize nausea

and vomiting, potassium supplements are best taken during or after a meal. SR products are large, and some patients are unable to swallow them.

Prevention of hypokalemia
Typical oral total daily doses are 20–40mmol/day:
- potassium chloride 600mg SR 1–2 tablets t.i.d. (24–48mmol/day) *or*
- prescribe a potassium-sparing diuretic, e.g. **amiloride** 5–20mg once daily, **spironolactone** 25–200mg/day.

Treatment of hypokalemia
Typical oral total daily doses are 40–80mmol (max 100mmol/day):
- potassium chloride 600mg SR 2 tablets t.i.d. (48mmol/day)
- potassium chloride 1.5g SR 2 tablets b.i.d. (80mmol/day)
- potassium chloride oral solution 15mL b.i.d. (40mmol/day).

If hypokalemia persists, investigate for possible magnesium deficiency (see p.429).

Emergency treatment of hyperkalemia
Stop and think! Are you justified in correcting a potentially fatal complication in a moribund patient? The use of β_2-agonists (e.g. **salbutamol**) for this indication is included here to allow practitioners to institute treatment without undue delay. However, this is only part of the management of hyperkalemia and specialist advice should be obtained as necessary:
- when ECG abnormalities are present, first give **calcium gluconate** 10mL of 10% solution IV to protect against arrhythmia; this is important because initially β_2-agonists may transiently increase the plasma potassium concentration[1,2]
- **salbutamol** 1,200microgram (12 puffs) inhaled over 2min via a spacer device *or*
- **salbutamol** 10–20mg nebulized (use 5mg/mL formulation) over 10–30min
- effective within 5–30min; duration of effect 1–2h or more
- if necessary, repeat dose[3]
- others use smaller doses, **salbutamol** 2.5mg nebulized every 20min as tolerated
- if the above is ineffective or hyperkalemia is severe (i.e. ⩾6mmol/L), combine the above with **insulin** and **dextrose** (glucose).[2]

Supply
Potassium chloride (generic)
Tablets SR 600mg (8mmol K$^+$), 28 days @ 2 t.i.d. = $7.

Slow K$^{\circledR}$ (Novartis Pharmaceuticals Canada Inc.)
Tablets SR 600mg (8mmol K$^+$), 28 days @ 2 t.i.d. = $11.

K-Dur$^{\circledR}$ (Schering-Plough Canada Inc.)
Tablets SR 1.5g (20mmol K$^+$), 28 days @ 2 b.i.d. = $18.

Micro-K Extencaps$^{\circledR}$ (Paladin Labs)
Capsules SR 600mg (8mmol K$^+$), 28 days @ 2 t.i.d. = $17.

K10$^{\circledR}$ (Glaxosmithkline)
Oral solution 1.5g (20mmol K$^+$)/15mL, 28 days @ 15mL b.i.d. = $14.

Potassium citrate
K-Lyte $^{\circledR}$ (Wellspring)
Tablets effervescent (orange flavoured and coloured when dissolved in water) potassium citrate 2.5g (25mmol K$^+$), 28 days @ 1 b.i.d. = $35.

1 Mandelberg A *et al.* (1999) Salbutamol metered-dose inhaler with spacer for hyperkalemia: how fast? How safe? *Chest.* **115**: 617–622.
2 Evans KJ and Greenberg A (2005) Hyperkalemia: a review. *Journal of Intensive Care Medicine.* **20**: 272–290.
3 Mahoney BA *et al.* (2005) Emergency interventions for hyperkalaemia. *Cochrane Database of Systematic Reviews.* **2**: CD003235.

MAGNESIUM

Class: Metal element.

Indications: Hypomagnesemia, constipation (see p.34), †arrhythmia, †eclampsia, †asthma, †myocardial infarction.

Pharmacology

Magnesium is the second most abundant intracellular ion after potassium, and is an essential component of numerous biochemical and physiological functions, particularly in muscle and nerve tissue.[1] This includes all functions involving adenosine triphosphate. It also acts as an NMDA-receptor-channel blocker (see **ketamine**, p.468) which probably accounts for its analgesic effect.[2–5]

The recommended total daily intake is generally considered to be 300–400mg/24h, but recent work suggests that 120–240mg/24h may be sufficient.[6] Magnesium competes with calcium for absorption in the small intestine, probably by active transport. Magnesium salts are generally poorly absorbed PO and have a laxative effect. The normal serum magnesium is 0.7–1.1mmol/L. Intracellular magnesium is mostly bound to ribosomes, phospholipids and nucleotides.[1] Magnesium is excreted by the kidneys, 3–12mmol/24h. Magnesium and calcium share the same transport system in the renal tubules and there is a reciprocal relationship between the amounts excreted. The minimum total daily dietary requirement of magnesium is 10–20mmol.

Magnesium deficiency can result from an inadequate dietary intake, alcoholism, reduced absorption (e.g. small bowel resection, cholestasis, pancreatic insufficiency), excessive loss from the GI tract (e.g. diarrhea, stoma, fistula) or kidney (e.g. due to interstitial nephritis, acute tubular necrosis, aminoglycosides, **amphotericin**, **cisplatin**, **cyclosporine** or loop diuretic). The risk of hypomagnesemia with **cisplatin** is dose-dependent and increases with cumulative doses (40% cycle 1 → 100% cycle 6).[7] It can also persist for 4–5 months and sometimes years after cessation.[8,9] Although generally mild and asymptomatic, it can be severe and symptomatic.

When magnesium deficiency develops acutely, the symptoms may be obvious and severe, particularly muscle cramps, which aids diagnosis (Box 9.B). In chronic deficiency, symptoms may be insidious in onset, less severe and non-specific.

Box 9.B Symptoms and signs of magnesium deficiency and excess

Magnesium deficiency	Magnesium excess
Muscle	Muscle
weakness	weakness
tremor	hypotonia
twitching	loss of reflexes
cramps	Sensation of warmth (IV)
tetany (positive Chvostek's sign)	Flushing (IV)
Paresthesia	Drowsiness
Apathy	Slurred speech
Depression	Double vision
Delirium	Delirium
Choreiform movements	Hypotension
Seizures	Cardiac arrhythmia
Prolonged QT interval	Respiratory depression
Cardiac arrhythmia	Nausea and vomiting
Increased pain (?)	Thirst
Hypomagnesemia[a]	Hypermagnesemia
Hypokalemia	
Hypocalcemia	
Hypophosphatemia	

a. not always present.

Magnesium deficiency in animals rapidly leads to a release of substance P and other mediators from nerve endings. These cause immune cells to release histamine and cytokines, which trigger a pro-inflammatory state with resultant production of oxy-radicals and nitric oxide. This leads to, for example, cutaneous erythema, hyperemia and edema, hyperalgesia, leucocytosis, an enhanced response to immune and oxidative stress, atherogenesis and inflammatory lesions within cardiac muscle.[10,11] In humans, deficiency is associated with several chronic diseases, e.g. diabetes, cardiac failure, hypertension.[11] Less is known about the benefit of replacement, but plasma magnesium is an independent predictor of muscle performance and improved exercise capacity has been reported in patients with coronary artery disease.[12,13]

Hypermagnesemia is rare and is seen most often in patients with renal impairment who take OTC medicines containing magnesium. Serum concentrations >4mmol/L produce drowsiness, vasodilation, slowing of atrioventricular conduction and hypotension. Over 6mmol/L there is profound CNS depression and muscle weakness (Box 9.B). **Calcium gluconate** IV is used to help reverse the effects of hypermagnesemia.

When drugs such as **cisplatin** cause severe renal wasting of magnesium, hypomagnesemia is generally present and aids diagnosis. If necessary, this can be confirmed by the high urinary excretion of magnesium. In deficiency states which develop more insidiously, the serum magnesium is an insensitive guide to total body stores and hypomagnesemia is not always present.[14] In this situation, the finding of a low urinary excretion of magnesium helps diagnosis. *Hypokalemia not responding to supplementation (± hypocalcemia) should also raise the possibility of magnesium deficiency.* The best method for detecting magnesium deficiency is the magnesium loading test (Box 9.C).[14–16]

Box 9.C   The magnesium loading test[15]

Collect pre-infusion urine sample for urinary magnesium (Mg)/creatinine (Cr) ratio. Measure Mg and Cr in mmol/L; divide the Mg value by the Cr value to calculate the Mg/Cr ratio.

By IVI over 4h, give 0.1mmol/kg of elemental magnesium, using magnesium sulfate 500mg (2mmol)/mL diluted to 50mL with 5% glucose.

Simultaneously, start a 24h urine collection for magnesium and creatinine. Measure the total amounts of magnesium and creatinine excreted in mmol (*not* the concentrations in mmol/L).

Calculate % magnesium retention:

$$1 - \left[\frac{\text{24h urinary Mg (mmol)} - (\text{pre-infusion urinary Mg/Cr ratio (mmol/L)} \times \text{24h urinary Cr (mmol)})}{\text{dose of elemental magnesium infused (mmol)}} \right] \times 100$$

>50% retention implies definite deficiency.

Cautions
Risk of hypermagnesemia in patients with renal impairment.

Undesirable effects
For full list, see manufacturer's Product Monograph.
Flushing, sweating and sensation of warmth IV; diarrhea PO. Also see Box 9.B, p.429.

Dose and use
Magnesium supplements can be given IV or PO. Because correcting a chronic deficiency generally involves the need to replace >1mmol/kg of magnesium, the route of choice is IV, generally given in divided doses over 3–5 days.[17,18] If the cause of the magnesium deficiency persists, PO maintenance therapy will be required.

Prevention
• magnesium-rich foods, e.g. meat, seafood, green leafy vegetables, cereals and nuts
• potassium-sparing diuretics also preserve magnesium, e.g. **amiloride**.

IV correction of chronic deficiency

Because the degree of deficiency is difficult to determine from the serum magnesium, replacement is empirical, guided by symptoms, serum magnesium and renal function:

- typically 50mmol is given on the first day, followed by 25mmol/day until the deficiency is corrected; give as 12.5–25mL of magnesium sulfate 500mg (2mmol)/mL added to 250mL 0.9% saline or 5% glucose (equivalent to a concentration of 0.1–0.2mmol/mL); infuse over 1.5–4h
- to avoid venous irritation the maximum recommended concentration for IVI is 200mg (0.8mmol)/mL
- to avoid saturating renal tubular resorption of magnesium, with resultant urinary loss, the rate of IVI should not exceed 150mg (0.6mmol)/min
- in renal impairment, reduce doses by 50% and monitor serum magnesium daily
- when there is need to replace >1mmol/kg of magnesium, the route of choice is IV, generally given in divided doses over 3–5 days.[17,18]

Patients receiving cisplatin chemotherapy

Routine monitoring of magnesium levels and the provision of magnesium supplementation in the IV hydration fluid is recommended (Table 9.2).[7]

Table 9.2 Magnesium supplementation in patients receiving cisplatin

Cisplatin dose (mg/m^2)	Amount of magnesium/cycle (mmol)
≤60	40
61–100	60
>100	80

PO maintenance

PO is used unless poorly tolerated or ineffective, e.g. malabsorption. The main limiting factor is diarrhea, generally seen at doses ≥40mmol/24h. It may be reduced by taking magnesium with food. The following regimens provide 30–40mmol of elemental magnesium/24h:

- magnesium glucoheptonate oral solution 100mg (0.21mmol elemental magnesium)/mL, e.g. 5g (50mL) t.i.d.–q.i.d.
- magnesium complex tablets 50mg, 100mg and 250mg (2.1mmol, 4.2mmol and 10.5mmol elemental magnesium respectively), e.g. 250mg (1 tablet) t.i.d.–q.i.d.
- magnesium oxide tablets 420mg (10.5mmol elemental magnesium), e.g. 420mg (1 tablet) t.i.d.–q.i.d.

Supply

Magnesium *glucoheptonate* (Rougier)
Oral solution 100mg (0.21mmol elemental magnesium)/mL, 500mL and 2L = $19 and $75 respectively.

Magnesium *complex* (Jamieson)
Includes magnesium oxide, citrate, fumarate, malate, succinate and glutamate.
Tablets 50mg, 100mg, 250mg (2.1mmol, 4.2mmol, 10.5mmol elemental magnesium respectively), 100 = $10, $12, $14 *OTC retail pricing*.

Magnesium *oxide*
Tablets 420mg (10.5mmol), 90 = $6 *OTC retail pricing*.

Magnesium *sulfate* (4mmol elemental magnesium/1g magnesium sulphate)
Injection 500mg (2mmol elemental magnesium)/mL, 2mL, 10mL and 50mL amp = $2, $4, and $6 respectively.

1 Romani A (2006) Regulation of magnesium homeostasis and transport in mammalian cells. *Archives of Biochemistry and Biophysics.* **458**: 90–102.

2 Mauskop A *et al.* (1995) Intravenous magnesium sulphate relieves migraine attacks in patients with low serum ionised magnesium levels: a pilot study. *Clinical Science.* **89**: 633–636.

3 Tramer M *et al.* (1996) Role of magnesium sulphate in postoperative analgesia. *Anesthesiology.* **84**: 340–347.

4 Crosby V et al. (2000) The safety and efficacy of a single dose (500mg or 1g) of intravenous magnesium sulfate in neuropathic pain poorly responsive to strong opioid analgesics in patients with cancer. *Journal of Pain and Symptom Management.* **19**: 35–39.

5 Bondok RS and Abd El-Hady AM (2006) Intra-articular magnesium is effective for postoperative analgesia in arthroscopic knee surgery. *British Journal of Anaesthesia.* **97**: 389–392.

6 Hunt CD and Johnson LK (2006) Magnesium requirements: new estimations for men and women by cross-sectional statistical analyses of metabolic magnesium balance data. *American Journal of Clinical Nutrition.* **84**: 843–852.

7 Hodgkinson E et al. (2006) Magnesium depletion in patients receiving cisplatin-based chemotherapy. *Clinical Oncology (Royal College of Radiologists).* **18**: 710–718.

8 Schilsky RL et al. (1982) Persistent hypomagnesemia following cisplatin chemotherapy for testicular cancer. *Cancer Treatment Reports.* **66**: 1767–1769.

9 Buckley JE et al. (1984) Hypomagnesemia after cisplatin combination chemotherapy. *Archives of Internal Medicine.* **144**: 2347–2348.

10 Mazur A et al. (2006) Magnesium and the inflammatory response: Potential physiopathological implications. *Archives of Biochemistry and Biophysics.* **458**: 48–56.

11 Tejero-Taldo MI et al. (2006) The nerve-heart connection in the pro-oxidant response to Mg-deficiency. *Heart Failure Reviews.* **11**: 35–44.

12 Dominguez LJ et al. (2006) Magnesium and muscle performance in older persons: the InCHIANTI study. *American Journal of Clinical Nutrition.* **84**: 419–426.

13 Pokan R et al. (2006) Oral magnesium therapy, exercise heart rate, exercise tolerance, and myocardial function in coronary artery disease patients. *British Journal of Sports Medicine.* **40**: 773–778.

14 Dyckner T and Wester P (1982) Magnesium deficiency – guidelines for diagnosis and substitution therapy. *Acta Medica Scandinavica.* **661**: 37–41.

15 Ryzen E et al. (1985) Parenteral magnesium testing in the evaluation of magnesium deficiency. *Magnesium.* **4**: 137–147.

16 Crosby V et al. (2000) The importance of low magnesium in palliative care. *Palliative Medicine.* **14**: 544.

17 Flink E (1969) Therapy of magnesium deficiency. *Annals of the New York Academy of Science.* **162**: 901–905.

18 Miller S (1995) Drug-induced hypomagnesaemia. *Hospital Pharmacy.* **30**: 248–250.

10: MUSCULOSKELETAL AND JOINT DISEASES

DEPOT CORTICOSTEROID INJECTIONS

Indications: Inflammation of joints and soft tissues, †pain in superficial bones (e.g. rib, scapula, iliac crest), †pain caused by spinal metastases, †malignant (peritoneal) ascites.

Contra-indications: Untreated local or systemic infection.

Pharmacology
Corticosteroids have an anti-inflammatory effect, i.e. they reduce the concentration of algesic substances present in inflammation and which thereby sensitize nerve endings.[1] When injected locally, they also have a direct inhibitory effect on spontaneous activity in excitable damaged nerves.[2] For many years, they have been given epidurally in selected patients with sciatica.[3–5] By extrapolation, they have also been used in some patients with intractable pain associated with spinal metastases. A recent Cochrane review found no strong evidence for or against the effectiveness of ED corticosteroids in subacute and chronic low back pain.[6] However, patients with radiculopathy (spinal nerve root damage) were excluded, pending a specific review of this subject. Although definitive conclusions must await the outcome, accumulated clinical experience indicates that ED corticosteroids can be helpful in palliative care patients with otherwise difficult-to-treat pain when spinal involvement may be a factor.

Cautions
May mask or alter presentation of infection in immunocompromised patients; such patients should not receive live vaccines and should receive *Varicella zoster* immunoglobulin if exposed to chickenpox. Depot formulations may result in symptomatic hyperglycemia for several days in patients with diabetes mellitus, and suppression of the hypothalamic-pituitary-adrenal axis for up to 4 weeks. Injection under a rib may be complicated by a pneumothorax.

Undesirable effects
For full list, see manufacturer's Product Monograph.
Antagonism of antihypertensive, antidiabetic and diuretic drugs. Enhanced effect of potassium-wasting drugs (see Systemic corticosteroids, p.381). Occasionally, a patient develops lipodystrophy (local fat necrosis) which results in an indentation of the overlying skin.

Dose and use
Injection into and/or over painful bone secondary[7]
- infiltrate the skin and SC tissues overlying the point of maximal bone tenderness with local anesthetic
- with the tip of the needle pressing against the tender bone, inject depot **methylprednisolone acetate** 80mg in 2mL
- if there are 2 painful bones, inject 40mg at each spot; generally limit the total amount given at any one time to 80mg.

In addition, for rib lesions, reposition the needle under the rib and inject 5mL of **bupivacaine** 0.5% to anesthetize the intercostal nerve. Complete or good relief occurs in about 70% of patients. If of benefit, injections can be repeated if the pain returns but not more than every 2 weeks.

Epidural injection[3]

Depot **methylprednisolone** *acetate* 80mg in 2mL. A single ED injection is given, or once daily for 3 days, via an indwelling catheter. The effect of ED corticosteroids is unpredictable and may not peak until 1 week after injection; some patients obtain weeks of benefit from one injection. Further injections can be given at monthly or longer intervals. Depot corticosteroids cannot be injected through an epidural bacterial filter.

Some centres use depot **triamcinolone** or a *non-depot* formulation of **dexamethasone sodium phosphate** for ED injection; check with your local anesthetist for details.

Malignant (peritoneal) ascites

After a preliminary paracentesis, inject intra-abdominally:
- **triamcinolone** *hexacetonide* 10mg/kg, up to a maximum of 640mg *or*
- **triamcinolone** *acetonide* 8mg/kg, up to a maximum of 520mg *or*
- **methylprednisolone** *acetate* 10mg/kg, up to a maximum of 640mg.

In an open study, mean interval between paracenteses increased from 9 to 18 days.[8]

Supply

Methylprednisolone *acetate*
Depo-Medrol® (Pfizer)
Depot injection (aqueous suspension) 20mg/mL, 5mL vial = $13; 40mg/mL, 2mL vial = $11, 5mL vial = $20; 80mg/mL, 1mL vial = $11, 5mL vial = $43.

Triamcinolone *acetonide*
Kenalog-10® (Westwood-Squibb)
Depot injection (aqueous suspension) 10mg/mL, 5mL vial = $17.

Kenalog-40® (Westwood-Squibb)
Depot injection (aqueous suspension) 40mg/mL, 1mL vial = $8, 5mL vial = $27.

Triamcinolone *hexacetonide*
Aristospan® (Valeo Pharma)
Depot injection 20mg/mL, 1mL vial = $7.

---

1 Pybus P (1984) Osteoarthritis: a new neurological method of pain control. *Medical Hypothesis.* **14:** 413–422.
2 Devor M *et al.* (1985) Corticosteroids reduce neuroma hyperexcitability. In: HL Fields *et al.* (eds) *Advances in Pain Research and Therapy* Vol 9. Raven Press, New York, pp. 451–455.
3 McQuay HJ and Moore A (1996) Epidural steroids for sciatica. *Anaesthesia and Intensive Care.* **24:** 284–285.
4 Watts RW and Silagy CA (1995) A meta-analysis on the efficacy of epidural corticosteroids in the treatment of sciatica. *Anaesthesia and Intensive Care.* **23:** 564–569.
5 Koes BW *et al.* (1995) Efficacy of epidural steroid injections for low-back pain and sciatica: a systematic review of randomized clinical trials. *Pain.* **63:** 279–288.
6 Staal JB *et al.* (2009) Injection therapy for subacute and chronic low back pain: an updated Cochrane review. *Spine.* **34:** 49–59.
7 Rowell NP (1988) Intralesional methylprednisolone for rib metastases: an alternative to radiotherapy? *Palliative Medicine.* **2:** 153–155.
8 Mackey J *et al.* (2000) A phase II trial of triamcinolone hexacetonide for symptomatic recurrent malignant ascites. *Journal of Pain and Symptom Management.* **19:** 193–199.

RUBEFACIENTS AND OTHER TOPICAL PRODUCTS

Indications: Soft tissue pains (rubefacients, topical NSAIDs), †notalgia paresthetica.

Contra-indications: Inflamed or broken skin.

Pharmacology

Rubefacients act by counter-stimulation of the skin, thereby closing the pain 'gate' in the dorsal horn of the spinal cord.[1,2] **Menthol** is a component of various traditional OTC products. On application to the skin, the **menthol** causes local vasodilation, and this produces a sensation of either warmth or cooling which may last for several hours.[3] **Menthol**-containing rubefacients have been used as 'home remedies' for tension headache, muscle spasm and joint pain. (**Menthol** is also an ingredient in several topical antipruritic products, see p.460.)

Capsaicin is a naturally occurring alkaloid found in the fruits of various species of *Solanaceae* (the nightshade family) and in pepper plants of the genus *Capsicum* (chilli peppers).[4] It affects the synthesis, storage, transport and release of substance P (SP) in nociceptive fibres. In animals, **capsaicin** has also been shown to be neurotoxic, principally affecting nociceptive C fibres.[5] Application of **capsaicin** causes an initial release of SP from C fibres with subsequent depletion on continued use. Axonal transport of SP to synaptic terminals is reduced and synthesis is inhibited.[6] **Capsaicin** may also elevate the thresholds for the release of SP and other neurotransmitters. Reduced availability of SP diminishes pain transmission. Following cessation of **capsaicin** application, SP stores revert to pretreatment levels and neuronal sensitivity returns to normal.[7-9]

In an open study of topical **capsaicin** 0.025% in post-axillary dissection pain, 14/18 women continued treatment.[10] Twelve reported benefit after 4 weeks, 8 of whom had good or excellent responses; after 6 months most still had good relief. A placebo-controlled RCT of **capsaicin** cream 0.075% for 6 weeks gave comparable results.[11] Thus, 8/13 patients had ≥50% improvement, 5 of whom had a good or excellent result. Benefit was seen mainly in relation to stabbing pain.

Topical **capsaicin** also relieves localized pruritus in uremia, and pruritus caused by notalgia paresthetica (nerve damage, often caused by entrapment, of the dorsal ramus of the T2–T6 thoracic nerves which causes pruritus and/or altered sensation in the areas of skin between or below the shoulder blade on either side of the back).[12,13]

Topically applied salicylates and certain other NSAIDs can achieve high local SC concentrations and therapeutically effective concentrations within synovial fluid and peri-articular tissues similar to those seen after oral administration.[14-16] The benefit of topical **ibuprofen** has been demonstrated in an RCT; a trial with **piroxicam** failed to show benefit.[17,18]

Onset of action generally immediate, although the effects of **capsaicin** may take 2–4 weeks to become apparent in neuralgia.

Duration of action 3–6h.

Undesirable effects

For full list, see manufacturer's Product Monograph.
The most frequently reported undesirable effect of **capsaicin** cream is tingling, stinging or burning at the site of application. This effect is thought to be related to the initial release of SP from C fibres. The stinging and burning usually decreases with continued applications, often clearing in a few days. In others, dysesthesia may persist for 4 weeks or more.

Large quantities of topical NSAIDs have been associated with systemic effects, e.g. hypersensitivity, rash, asthma and renal impairment.[19]

Dose and use

Capsaicin cream 0.025–0.075%:
• apply t.i.d.–q.i.d.
Application less frequently than t.i.d. is associated with a prolongation of the burning sensation. If the burning is severe, topical **lidocaine** can be applied before **capsaicin** in the first few weeks of treatment. Because heat and humidity influence the dysesthesia, patients should avoid excessive sweating, and not take a hot bath immediately before application. Occlusion and tight bandaging should also be avoided.

Patients should apply the cream using gentle massage, avoiding contact with eyes, mucous membranes and broken/inflamed skin. *Patients must wash their hands after applying the cream to avoid subsequent unintentional contact with the eyes.*

Topical NSAIDs:
• generally apply b.i.d.–q.i.d.
• **diclofenac diethylamine** gel is a new product marketed for acute muscle and joint injuries. The manufacturer advises applying 2–4g t.i.d.–q.i.d. for a maximum of 1 week; treatment duration can be extended if recommended by a physician, and depends on the clinical response, the natural course of healing, and the effect of rest.

Supply

Capsaicin (generic)
Cream 0.025%, 60g = $18.
Forte Cream 0.075%, 60g = $23.

Zostrix® (Medicis)
Cream 0.025%, 60g = $25.

Antiphlogistine Rub A-535® (Church & Dwight)
Cream 0.05%, 65mL = $20.

Zostrix HP® (Medicis)
Cream 0.075%, 60g = $32.

Diclofenac
Pennsaid® (Paladin Pharmaceuticals)
Topical solution 1.5%, 60mL = $42.

Diclofenac diethylamine
Voltaren® Emulgel (Novartis)
Gel 1.16%, 50g = $11, 100g = $15. Available OTC.

*Topical preparations containing **diclofenac** 2–5% or **ketoprofen** 5–20% can be compounded for individual patients; contact your local compounding pharmacy for details.*

1 Melzack R and Wall P (1965) Pain mechanisms: a new theory. *Science*. **150**: 971–979.
2 Melzack R (1991) The gate control theory 25 years later: new perspectives on phantom limb pain. In: M Bond *et al.* (eds) *Proceedings of the VIth World Congress on Pain*. Elsevier Science, Amsterdam, pp. 9–21.
3 Anonymous (1993) How does menthol work? *Pharmaceutical Journal*. **251**: 480.
4 Towlerton GR and Rice AS (2003) Topical analgesics for chronic pain. In: AS Rice *et al.* (eds) *Clinical Pain Management: Chronic Pain*, pp. 213–226.
5 Chung JM *et al.* (1993) Chronic effects of topical application of capsaicin to the sciatic nerve on responses of primate spinothalamic neurons. *Pain*. **53**: 311–321.
6 Gamse R *et al.* (1982) Capsaicin applied to peripheral nerve inhibits axoplasmic transport of substance P and somatostatin. *Brain Research*. **239**: 447–462.
7 Gamse R *et al.* (1981) Differential effects of capsaicin on the content of somatostatin, substance P, and neurotensin in the nervous system of the rat. *Naunyn Schmiedebergs Archives of Pharmacology*. **317**: 140–148.
8 Fitzgerald M (1983) Capsaicin and sensory neurones: a review. *Pain*. **15**: 109–130.
9 LaMotte RH *et al.* (1988) Hypothesis for novel classes of chemoreceptors mediating chemogenic pain and itch. In: R Dubner *et al.* (eds) *Proceedings of the Vth World Congress on Pain*. Elsevier, New York, pp. 529–535.
10 Watson C *et al.* (1989) The postmastectomy pain syndrome and the effect of topical capsaicin. *Pain*. **38**: 177–186.
11 Watson CPN and Evans RJ (1992) Post-mastectomy pain syndrome and topical capsaicin: a randomized trial. *Pain*. **51**: 375–379.
12 Bernstein JE (1988) Capsaicin in dermatologic disease. *Seminars in Dermatology*. **7**: 304–309.
13 Breneman D *et al.* (1992) Topical capsaicin for treatment of hemodialysis-related pruritus. *Journal of the American Academy of Dermatology*. **26**: 91–94.
14 Mondino A *et al.* (1983) Kinetic studies of ibuprofen on humans. Comparative study for the determination of blood concentrations and metabolites following local and oral administration. *Medizinische Welt*. **34**: 1052–1054.
15 Chlud K and Wagener H (1987) Percutaneous nonsteroidal anti-inflammatory drug (NSAID) therapy with particular reference to pharmacokinetic factors. *EULAR Bulletin*. **2**: 40–43.
16 Peters H *et al.* (1987) Percutaneous kinetics of ibuprofen (German). *Aktuelle Rheumatologie*. **12**: 208–211.
17 Kageyama T (1987) A double blind placebo controlled multicenter study of piroxicam 0.5% gel in osteoarthritis of the knee. *European Journal of Rheumatology and Inflammation*. **8**: 114–115.
18 DTB (1990) More topical NSAIDs: worth the rub? *Drugs and Therapeutics Bulletin*. **28**: 27–28.
19 O'Callaghan C *et al.* (1994) Renal disease and use of topical NSAIDs. *British Medical Journal*. **308**: 110–111.

SKELETAL MUSCLE RELAXANTS

Skeletal muscle relaxants are used to relieve painful chronic muscle spasm and spasticity associated with neural injury, e.g. paraplegia, post-stroke, multiple sclerosis and (sometimes) motor neurone disease (amyotrophic lateral sclerosis).[1] †**Baclofen** is also used to relieve hiccup. **Baclofen, diazepam** and **tizanidine** act principally on spinal and supraspinal sites within the CNS; **dantrolene** and **quinine** act on muscle (Table 10.1). The use of **diazepam** as a muscle

Table 10.1 Oral drugs used to treat spasticity

Drug	Starting dose	Maximum dose	Undesirable effects	Monitoring	Precautions
Diazepam	5mg at bedtime	60mg/24h	Weakness, sedation, cognitive impairment, depression	Accumulation; prolongation of plasma halflife with cimetidine	Abrupt cessation may result in rebound anxiety and insomnia
Baclofen	5mg once daily–t.i.d.	20mg q.i.d.	Weakness, sedation, fatigue, dizziness, nausea, hepatotoxicity	Periodic LFTs	Abrupt cessation may result in agitation and psychosis; seizures may also occur
Tizanidine	2–4mg at bedtime	12mg t.i.d.	Drowsiness, dry mouth, dizziness, hepatotoxicity	Periodic LFTs	Do not use with antihypertensives or clonidine
Dantrolene	25mg once daily	100mg q.i.d.	Weakness, sedation, diarrhea, hepatotoxicity	Periodic LFTs	

relaxant is discussed elsewhere (see p.108 and p.113). There is no clear evidence that any one drug is superior to any other.[2] **Baclofen** and **diazepam** are preferred at some centres because they are the cheapest options.

1 Zafonte R et al. (2004) Acute care management of post-TBI spasticity. *Journal of Head Trauma Rehabilitation.* **19:** 89–100.
2 Chou R et al. (2004) Comparative efficacy and safety of skeletal muscle relaxants for spasticity and musculoskeletal conditions: a systematic review. *Journal of Pain and Symptom Management.* **28:** 140–175.

BACLOFEN

Class: Skeletal muscle relaxant.

Indications: Painful muscle spasm, spasticity, †hiccup.

Contra-indications: Peptic ulcer.

Pharmacology

Baclofen is a chemical congener of the naturally occurring neurotransmitter, GABA.[1] It acts upon the GABA-receptor, inhibiting the release of the excitatory amino acids glutamate and aspartate, principally at the spinal level, and thereby decreases spasm in skeletal muscle. Baclofen relieves hiccup, possibly by a direct effect on the diaphragm.[2,3] It is preferable to **diazepam** when the likely duration of use introduces the risk of **diazepam** dependence (e.g. patients with chronic neurological disease such as multiple sclerosis).

Bio-availability >90% PO.
Onset of action 3–4 days.
Time to peak plasma concentration 0.5–3h.
Plasma halflife 3.5h; 4.5h in the elderly.
Duration of action 6–8h.[4]

Cautions

Withdrawal: abrupt withdrawal of PO baclofen may produce increased spasticity, hyperactivity, hyperthermia, pruritus, anxiety, disorientation, hallucinations and occasionally seizures. The manufacturer advises discontinuing by gradual dose reduction over 1–2 weeks, or longer if withdrawal symptoms occur. Similarly, sudden withdrawal of IT baclofen or failure of the IT pump may lead to a potentially fatal withdrawal syndrome (hyperthermia, altered mental status, exaggerated rebound spasticity and muscle rigidity, occasionally progressing to rhabdomyolysis and multiple organ-system failure). Seizures, DIC, cardiac depression and coma have also been reported. Regular checking and maintenance of IT pumps is thus of paramount importance.[5]

History of peptic ulceration, severe psychiatric disorders, epilepsy, liver disease (monitor LFTs), renal impairment (reduce dose), respiratory impairment, diabetes mellitus, hesitancy of micturition (may precipitate urinary retention), patients who use spasticity to maintain posture or to aid function. Drowsiness may affect skilled tasks and driving; effects of alcohol enhanced.

Undesirable effects

For full list, see manufacturer's Product Monograph.

Very common (>10%): sedation, drowsiness, muscular hypotonia, nausea, urinary frequency or incontinence, dysuria.

Common (<10%, >1%): dizziness, fatigue, muscle weakness, ataxia, tremor, insomnia, headache, visual disturbances, psychiatric disturbances, hypotension, respiratory depression, dry mouth, vomiting, constipation or diarrhea, hyperhidrosis, rash.

Uncommon, rare or very rare (<1%, >0.001%): seizures (particularly in known epileptics), muscle pain, paresthesia, taste disturbance, abdominal pain, hepatic impairment, urinary retention, impotence. Occasional patients have developed increased spasticity as a paradoxical reaction.

Dose and use

Starting doses are the same for muscle spasm, spasticity and hiccup:
- start with 5mg b.i.d.–t.i.d., preferably p.c.
- increase if necessary by 5mg b.i.d.–t.i.d. every 3 days but more slowly if troublesome undesirable effects, particularly in the elderly
- effective doses for hiccup are often relatively low, e.g. 5–10mg t.i.d., although it may be necessary to increase the dose to 20mg t.i.d.
- for spasticity, the effective dose is generally ≤20mg t.i.d. (maximum total daily dose 100mg)
- effective doses for muscle spasm fall somewhere in the middle.

With spasticity, if no improvement with maximum tolerated dose after 6 weeks, withdraw gradually over 1–2 weeks.

An undesirable degree of hypotonia may occur, but can generally be relieved by reducing the daytime dose and increasing the evening dose.

Supply

Baclofen (generic)
Tablets 10mg, 20mg, 28 days @ 5mg and 20mg t.i.d. = $13 and $48 respectively.

Lioresal® (Novartis Pharmaceuticals)
Tablets (scored) 10mg, 20mg, 28 days @ 5mg and 20mg t.i.d. = $29 and $112 respectively.
*Intrathecal injection 50microgram/mL, 1mL amp (for test dose) = $15; 500microgram/mL, 20mL amp (for use in implantable pump) = $212; 2mg/mL, 5mL amp (for use in implantable pump) = $214.

1 Zafonte R et al. (2004) Acute care management of post-TBI spasticity. *Journal of Head Trauma Rehabilitation.* **19**: 89–100.
2 Ramirez FC and Graham DY (1992) Treatment of intractable hiccup with baclofen: results of a double-blind randomized, controlled, crossover study. *American Journal of Gastroenterology.* **87**: 1789–1791.
3 Guelaud C et al. (1995) Baclofen therapy for chronic hiccup. *European Respiratory Journal.* **8**: 235–237.
4 Kochak GM et al. (1985) The pharmacokinetics of baclofen derived from intestinal infusion. *Clinical Pharmacology and Therapeutics.* **38**: 251–257.
5 Mohammed I and Hussain A (2004) Intrathecal baclofen withdrawal syndrome- a life-threatening complication of baclofen pump: a case report. *BMC Clinical Pharmacology.* **4**: 6.

DANTROLENE SODIUM

Class: Skeletal muscle relaxant.

Indications: Chronic severe spasticity of skeletal muscle.

Contra-indications: Hepatic impairment, particularly active liver disease, e.g. hepatitis or cirrhosis (may cause severe liver damage); compromised pulmonary function, particularly COPD; acute muscle spasm or where spasm is useful in maintaining posture, balance or walking.

Pharmacology

Dantrolene acts directly on skeletal muscle, reducing the amount of intracellular calcium available for contraction.[1] It produces fewer central undesirable effects than **baclofen** and **diazepam** and, if necessary, it can be used concurrently with them.
Bio-availability 35% PO.
Onset of action up to 1 week.
Time to peak plasma concentration up to 3h.
Plasma halflife 5–9h.
Duration of action no data.

Cautions

The dose of dantrolene must be built up slowly, by not more than 25mg per week. Because of the risk of hepatotoxicity with long-term use, discontinue if no benefit is observed after 6 weeks of treatment. Perform LFTs before starting treatment and then at regular intervals, e.g. monthly, throughout treatment; if possible, avoid concurrent use of other hepatotoxic drugs.

Undesirable effects

For full list, see manufacturer's Product Monograph.
Transient drowsiness, dizziness, muscle weakness, diarrhea. Rarely severe hepatotoxicity develops after 1–6 months in people over 30 years of age; fatalities have occurred only with doses over 200mg/24h.[2,3]

Dose and use

- starting dose 25mg once daily
- increase by 25mg weekly
- usual effective dose 75mg t.i.d.; maximum dose 100mg q.i.d.

Some centres increase the dose more rapidly because of the patient's limited prognosis.

Supply

Dantrium® *(Procter & Gamble Pharmaceuticals)*
Capsules 25mg, 100mg, 28 days @ 75mg t.i.d. = $34.

---

1 Zafonte R *et al.* (2004) Acute care management of post-TBI spasticity. *Journal of Head Trauma Rehabilitation.* **19**: 89–100.
2 Utili R *et al.* (1977) Dantrolene-associated hepatic injury. Incidence and character. *Gastroenterology.* **72**: 610–616.
3 Wilkinson S *et al.* (1979) Hepatitis from dantrolene sodium. *Gut.* **20**: 33–36.

TIZANIDINE

Class: Skeletal muscle relaxant.

Indications: Spasticity in multiple sclerosis, spinal cord injury or disease.

Contra-indications: Severe hepatic impairment, patients for whom spasm is useful in maintaining posture, balance or walking, concurrent use with potent CYP1A2 inhibitors, e.g. **ciprofloxacin** and **fluvoxamine**.

Pharmacology

Tizanidine, like **clonidine**, is a central α_2-agonist within the CNS at supraspinal and spinal levels.[1] This results in inhibition of spinal polysynaptic reflex activity. This reduces the sympathetic outflow which in turn reduces muscle tone. Tizanidine has no direct effect on skeletal muscle, the neuromuscular junction or on monosynaptic spinal reflexes. Tizanidine reduces pathologically increased muscle tone, including resistance to passive movements, and alleviates painful spasms and clonus.[2] In spasticity, tizanidine is comparable in efficacy to **diazepam** and **baclofen**.[3] Tizanidine is well absorbed but undergoes extensive first-pass metabolism in the liver to inactive metabolites which are mostly excreted by the kidneys. Wide interindividual variability in the effective plasma concentrations means that the optimal dose must be titrated over 2–4 weeks for each patient. Maximum effects occur within 2h of administration.[4]
Bio-availability 40% PO.
Onset of action 1–2h; peak response 8 weeks.
Time to peak plasma concentration 1.5h.
Plasma halflife 2.5h; up to 14h ± 10h in renal failure.[5]
Duration of action no data.

---

www.palliativedrugs.com

Cautions

Renal impairment; elderly; concurrent administration with drugs which prolong the QT interval; concurrent administration with hypotensive drugs or **digoxin** which may potentiate hypotension or bradycardia. LFTs should be monitored monthly for the first 4 months.

Undesirable effects

For full list, see manufacturer's Product Monograph.
Drowsiness, weakness and dry mouth in over 2/3 of those taking it,[6] although drowsiness and weakness may be less than with **diazepam** and **baclofen**.[7] Also reduction in blood pressure and dizziness. Less frequently insomnia, bradycardia, hallucinations and hepatotoxicity.

Dose and use

- starting dose 2mg once daily
- increase by 2mg every 3–4 days according to response
- doses above 2mg should be divided and given b.i.d.–q.i.d.
- usual dose up to 24mg/24h in 3–4 divided doses
- maximum total daily dose 36mg.

A slow titration helps minimize undesirable effects. Elderly patients and those with renal impairment (creatinine clearance <25mL/min) should undergo an even slower titration. Because of the prolonged plasma halflife, slow titration with a *single* daily dose is recommended by the manufacturers.

Supply

Tizanidine (generic)
Tablets 4mg, 28 days @ 8mg t.i.d. = $86.

Zanaflex® (Paladin)
Tablets 4mg, 28 days @ 8mg t.i.d. = $100.

1 Zafonte R *et al.* (2004) Acute care management of post-TBI spasticity. *Journal of Head Trauma Rehabilitation.* **19**: 89–100.
2 Wallace J (1994) Summary of combined clinical analysis of controlled clinical trials with tizanidine. *Neurology.* **44 (suppl 9)**: s60–s69.
3 Lataste X *et al.* (1994) Comparative profile of tizanidine in the management of spasticity. *Neurology.* **44 (suppl 9)**: s53–s59.
4 Wagstaff A and Bryson H (1997) Tizanidine. A review of its pharmacology, clinical efficacy and tolerability in the management of spasticity associated with cerebral and spinal disorders. *Drugs.* **53**: 435–452.
5 Keyser E and Ohnhaus E (1986) *Data on file.* Pharmacokinetic study with Sirdalud (tizanidine, DS 103–282) in patients with renal insufficiency.
6 Nance P *et al.* (1997) Relationship of the antispasticity effect of tizanidine to plasma concentration in patients with multiple sclerosis. *Archives of Neurology.* **54**: 731–736.
7 Smith H and Barton A (2000) Tizanidine in the management of spasticity and musculoskeletal complaints in the palliative care population. *American Journal of Hospice and Palliative Care.* **17 (1)**: 50–58.

QUININE

Class: Antimalarial.

Indications: †Nocturnal leg cramps.

Contra-indications: Myasthenia gravis, optic neuritis, hypoglycemia, history of blackwater fever. Discontinue if signs of toxicity occur, e.g. tinnitus or thrombocytopenic purpura.

Pharmacology

Quinine reduces the amount of intracellular calcium available for muscle contraction. Controlled trials show that quinine reduces the frequency of cramps by about 25% in ambulatory patients and improves sleep,[1] but does not always reduce cramp severity.[2] However, benefit was generally less in three unpublished trials than in four published ones.[3] Maximum benefit takes up to 4 weeks. Smoking can block the effect of quinine.[4]

Bio-availability 76–88% PO.
Onset of action <1h.
Time to peak plasma concentration 1–3h PO.
Plasma halflife 8–12h.
Duration of action 4–8h.

Cautions

Quinine is very toxic in overdose and fatalities have occurred. It can cause ventricular arrhythmias, hypersensitivity reactions (including anaphylaxis), and serious skin reactions (e.g. Stevens-Johnson syndrome). The FDA considers the risk associated with the use of quinine is justified in relation to malaria, but not for preventing or treating leg cramps. Although Health Canada and the National Association of Pharmacy Regulatory Authorities (NAPRA) do not consider a similar safety warning necessary at present, the situation is being kept under review, and the prescribing of quinine for leg cramps remains off-label.[5]

Undesirable effects

For full list, see manufacturer's Product Monograph.
Tinnitus, other symptoms of cinchonism (i.e. headache, hot flushed skin, nausea, abdominal pain, rashes, visual disturbances/temporary blindness, confusion), thrombocytopenia, DIC, acute renal failure, hypoglycemia (unlikely with oral administration).

Dose and use

- quinine *sulfate* 200–300mg at bedtime[6–8] or 200mg with evening meal and 100mg at bedtime.[6] Stop if no benefit after 4 weeks; interrupt treatment every few months to see if quinine is still needed.

Supply

Quinine sulfate (generic)
Capsules 200mg, 300mg, 28 days @ 200mg and 300mg at bedtime = $7 and $11 respectively.
Tablets 200mg, 300mg, 28 days @ 200mg and 300mg at bedtime = $7 and $11 respectively.

---

1 Man Son Hing M and Wells G (1998) Quinine for nocturnal leg cramps. A meta-analysis including unpublished data. *Journal of General Internal Medicine*. **13**: 600–606.
2 Connolly PS *et al.* (1992) The treatment of nocturnal leg cramps: a crossover trial of quinine versus vitamin E. *Archives of Internal Medicine*. **152**: 1877–1880.
3 Anonymous (2001) Quinine for nocturnal leg cramps. *Bandolier*. **8 (6)**: 4–5.
4 Kasdon D (1986) Controversies in the surgical management of spasticity. *Clinical Neurosurgery*. **35**: 523–529.
5 Health Canada and NAPRA (2007) Health Canada health products and food branch bilateral meeting program, April 23 2007. Record of decisions. Available from: www.hc-sc.gc.ca/dhp-mps/prodpharma/activit/assoc/2007-04-23-eng.php
6 Jansen P *et al.* (1997) Randomised controlled trial of hydroquinine in muscle cramps. *Lancet*. **349**: 528–532.
7 Warburton A *et al.* (1987) A quinine a day keeps the leg cramps away? *British Journal of Clinical Pharmacology*. **23**: 459–465.
8 Man Son Hing M and Wells G (1995) Meta-analysis of efficacy of quinine for treatment of nocturnal leg cramps in elderly people. *British Medical Journal*. **310**: 13–17.

11: EAR, NOSE AND OROPHARYNX

MOUTHWASHES

Mouthwashes cleanse and freshen the mouth. Unless the tongue or oral mucosa is coated, warm tap water, saline solution or **compound sodium chloride mouthwash BP** is probably as beneficial as any. Mouth *swabs* containing **glycerin** should *not* be used because **glycerin** tends to have a rebound drying effect. However, it is difficult to avoid **glycerin**-containing *mouthwashes* because many of the commercial mouthwashes available in Canada contain **glycerin**. This includes all brands of **chlorhexidine** mouthwash, Betadine® (**povidone-iodine**), and Scope® (OTC).

Mouthwashes containing an oxidizing agent, such as **hydrogen peroxide**, froth when in contact with oral debris and help to debride a heavily furred tongue. A **sodium bicarbonate**-containing mouthwash, e.g. **compound sodium chloride mouthwash BP**, is probably equally effective, as is gentle brushing with a child's soft toothbrush. **Ascorbic acid** (vitamin C) effervescent tablets can also be used for debriding the tongue (see p.424) but should not be used in patients with a sore mouth. Pineapple contains a proteolytic enzyme, ananase, and can also be used to clean a coated mouth.[1,2] Any form of pineapple can be used except pineapple tinned in *syrup* because the syrup destroys the ananase. Pineapple is unsuitable for patients with an inflamed or ulcerated mouth because the juice is acidic.

Chlorhexidine inhibits the formation of plaque on teeth and may be a useful adjunct to other measures for oral infection or when toothbrushing is not possible. It does not remove established plaque, which should be removed by professional cleaning, ideally by a dental hygienist or dentist. Particularly in tea and coffee drinkers, **chlorhexidine** can stain the teeth (and tongue); this can be removed by cleaning. All the commercial **chlorhexidine** mouthwashes currently available in Canada contain alcohol. This may cause mucosal discomfort and irritate inflamed tissue. Diluting the mouthwash with an equal amount of water may help reduce both teeth-staining and discomfort.[3]

Chlorhexidine mouthwash should *not* be used at the same time as **nystatin** oral suspension because **chlorhexidine** binds to **nystatin**, and both drugs are inactivated. This problem is avoided if **chlorhexidine** is used ⩾30min before **nystatin**.[4–7]

Povidone-iodine is useful for mucosal infections but does not inhibit plaque. It should not be used for more than 2 weeks because a significant amount of iodine is absorbed.

Supply and use

For liquid mouthwashes, rinse the mouth with the recommended volume for about 30sec–1min, and then spit out.

Pineapple juice can be applied to the oral mucosa using an oral swab (sponge-tipped stick). Alternatively, a piece of fresh pineapple, or pineapple tinned in water or its own juice, can be sucked or held in the side of the mouth for 5–10min.

Saline solution

Add 1 heaped teaspoonful of table salt to a glass of warm water (about 250mL) and stir well to dissolve. Use p.r.n.

Sodium chloride mouthwash BP

Mouthwash containing **sodium chloride** 1.5g, **sodium bicarbonate** 1g, concentrated peppermint emulsion 2.5mL, double-strength chloroform water 50mL, water to 100mL. Dilute 15mL with an equal volume of warm water and use p.r.n.

Chlorhexidine gluconate
Oro-Clense® oral rinse (Germiphene)
Mouthwash 0.12%, 480mL = $22; *contains alcohol 10%, glycerin 3–7%, pH 5–7.* Use 15mL (1 capful) undiluted or diluted with an equal volume of water b.i.d.

Perichlor® (Pharmascience)
Mouthwash 0.12%, 475mL = $8; *contains alcohol 14.7%, glycerin 12%, pH 5–7.* Use 15mL (1 capful) undiluted or diluted with an equal volume of water b.i.d.

Peridex® (3M Canada)
Mouthwash 0.12%, 475mL = $11; *contains alcohol 11.6%, glycerin 1–10%, pH 5–7.* Use 15mL (1 capful) undiluted or diluted with an equal volume of water b.i.d.

Periogard® (Colgate Oral Pharmaceuticals)
Mouthwash 0.12%, 470mL = $9; *mint flavour; contains alcohol 11.6%, glycerin (amount not stated), pH 5–7.* Use 15mL (1 capful) undiluted or diluted with an equal volume of water b.i.d.

Hydrogen peroxide
Peroxyl® (Colgate Oral Pharmaceuticals)
Mouthwash 1.5%, 237mL = $9; *mint flavour; contains alcohol 6%, pH 3–6.* Use 10mL undiluted after meals and at bedtime.

Povidone-iodine
Betadine® (Purdue Pharma)
Mouthwash 1%, 250mL = $8; *contains alcohol 8%, glycerin (*amount not stated*), pH 4–6.* Use 10mL undiluted or diluted with an equal volume of warm water up to q.i.d. for up to 14 days.

---

1 Regnard C et al. (1997) Mouth care, skin care, and lymphoedema. *British Medical Journal.* **315**: 1002–1005.
2 Twycross RG et al. (2009) *Symptom Management in Advanced Cancer.* (4e). palliativedrugs.com Ltd., Nottingham, pp. 64–65.
3 Sweeney P (2005) Oral hygiene. In: A Davies and I Finlay (eds) *Oral Care in Advanced Disease.* Oxford University Press, Oxford, pp. 21–35.
4 Feber T (1995) Mouth care for patients receiving oral irradiation. *Professional Nurse.* **10**: 666–670.
5 Ellepola AN and Samaranayake LP (2001) Adjunctive use of chlorhexidine in oral candidoses: a review. *Oral Diseases.* **7**: 11–17.
6 Hancock PJ et al. (2003) Oral and dental management related to radiation therapy for head and neck cancer. *Journal of the Canadian Dental Association.* **69**: 585–590.
7 NHS Institute for Innovation and Improvement (2007) Clinical knowledge summary. Candida-oral. Management: what drug interactions can occur with nystatin? Available from: http://cks.library.nhs.uk/candida_oral/management/medicines_management/topical_antifungals/nystatin/what_drug_interactions_can_occur_with_nystatin#

ARTIFICIAL SALIVA

Severe dry mouth (xerostomia) is managed by saliva substitutes or stimulants. Although 99% of saliva is water, the remaining 1% consists of a wide range of electrolytes and molecules important for saliva's many roles, e.g. lubricant, antimicrobial, cleansing, buffering, digestion, taste and mineralization of teeth.[1] This may explain why sipping water, iced drinks or sucking ice chips gives only short-lived relief. Artificial saliva is also a poor substitute for natural saliva, and the use of saliva stimulants is preferable.[2] For example, chewing gum acts as a saliva stimulant.[3] The gum should be sugar-free and, in patients with dentures, low-tack, e.g. Orbit® sugar-free gum or Biotene® dry mouth gum. Topical acids stimulate the flow of saliva, e.g. ascorbic acid (see p.424), citric acid (e.g. lemon juice) and malic acid (in some artificial saliva products), although long-term use will cause dental demineralization. If dry mouth remains a major problem, the use of **pilocarpine** or **bethanechol** should be considered (see p.446).

If using artificial saliva, a gel-based product is more effective than a spray,[4] although patient preference is evenly divided.[5] Ideally, artificial saliva should reflect the composition of natural saliva, particularly in dentate patients, i.e. should have a neutral pH (to prevent demineralization) and contain electrolytes (including fluoride, to enhance remineralization). Some products contain **lactoperoxidase** which in natural saliva enhances the production of hypothiocyanite, an antibacterial ion. Thus, theoretically, **lactoperoxidase** could enhance the benefit of artificial saliva. However, there is no evidence that this is the case.

Undesirable effects
For full list, see manufacturers' Product Monograph.
Unpleasant taste, irritation of the mouth, nausea and/or diarrhea in ⩽30% of patients.[3,6]

Dose and use

Artificial salivas with a neutral pH are preferred by *PCF* for long-term use. Acidic artificial salivas or acidic topical saliva stimulants should be avoided in dentate patients with a prognosis of >2–3 months (demineralization of teeth) or in those with mucositis (increased pain).

The duration of effect of artificial saliva is relatively short because it will inevitably be swallowed.[7,8] In a post-irradiation study of Oralbalance® synthetic polymer gel, the mean duration of effect was about 1h during the daytime and >4h during the night.[9] A herbal product, Mouth-Kote®, is said to have a mean duration of effect of almost 2h (www.parnellpharm.com). Even so, for maximum effect, most varieties of artificial saliva will need to be taken every 30–60min, and before and during meals.

Supply
Biotene® (GSK)
Saliva replacement gel (sugar-free) Oralbalance® dry mouth moisturizing gel, containing **lactoperoxidase**, glucose oxidase, lactoferrin, lysozyme and xylitol in a synthetic polymer gel (polyglycerylmethacrylate) base, 42g = $13, available OTC; *pH 4.9–5.5.*
Mouth moisturizing liquid (sugar-free) Oralbalance® dry mouth moisturizing liquid, containing **lactoperoxidase**, glucose oxidase, milk-derived proteins and minerals in a **cellulose** and **xanthan gum** base, 45mL spray bottle = $13, available OTC.
Mouthwash containing **lactoperoxidase**, glucose oxidase, lactoferrin, lysozyme, calcium lactate and xylitol, 473mL = $11, available OTC; *mint flavour, alcohol free; pH 5.0–5.5.*
Toothpaste containing **lactoperoxidase**, glucose oxidase, lactoferrin, lysozyme, sodium monofluorophosphate and calcium lactate, 125g (4.5oz) = $12, available OTC; *gentle mint or fresh mint flavour, also available in a formulation for sensitive teeth.*
Chewing gum (sugar-free) Dry mouth gum, containing **lactoperoxidase** and glucose oxidase, 16-piece pack = $5, available OTC; *mint flavour.*

Moi-Stir® Dry mouth solution spray (Pendopharm)
Saliva replacement solution (sugar-free) containing electrolytes normally present in saliva (**calcium chloride** 150microgram/mL, **magnesium chloride** 50microgram/mL, **potassium chloride** 1.2mg/mL, **sodium chloride** 50microgram/mL, **dibasic sodium phosphate** 280microgram/mL) and **glycerin** 1% in a **sodium carboxymethylcellulose** and **sorbitol** base, 120mL spray = $14, available OTC; *mint flavour, pH 6.5–7.5.*

Mouth-Kote® Oral Spray (Oryx)
Saliva replacement solution (sugar-free) containing *Yerba santa* mucilage, xylitol, sorbitol and citric acid, 60mL = $12, 240mL = $19, available OTC; *lemon-lime flavour, alcohol-free, glycerin-free, pH 4.*

1 Davies A (2005) Salivary gland dysfunction. In: A Davies and I Finlay (eds) *Oral Care in Advanced Disease.* Oxford University Press, Oxford, pp. 97–114.
2 Twycross R et al. (2009) *Symptom Management in Advanced Cancer.* (4e). palliativedrugs.com Ltd., Nottingham, pp. 64–65.
3 Davies AN (2000) A comparison of artificial saliva and chewing gum in the management of xerostomia in patients with advanced cancer. *Palliative Medicine.* **14**: 197–203.
4 Furumoto EK et al. (1998) Subjective and clinical evaluation of oral lubricants in xerostomic patients. *Special Care in Dentistry.* **18**: 113–118.
5 Davies A (2006) Personal communication.
6 Davies A et al. (1998) A comparison of artificial saliva and pilocarpine in the management of xerostomia in patients with advanced cancer. *Palliative Medicine.* **12**: 105–111.

7 Daniels TE and Wu AJ (2000) Xerostomia – clinical evaluation and treatment in general practice. *Journal of the California Dental Association.* **28**: 933–941.
8 Wynn RL and Meiller TF (2000) Artificial saliva products and drugs to treat xerostomia. *General Dentistry.* **48**: 630–636.
9 Regelink G *et al.* (1998) Efficacy of a synthetic polymer saliva substitute in reducing oral complaints of patients suffering from irradiation-induced xerostomia. *Quintessence International.* **29**: 383–388.

PILOCARPINE

Class: Parasympathomimetic.

Indications: Xerostomia (dry mouth) after radiation therapy for head and neck cancer, dry mouth (and dry eyes) in Sjögren's syndrome and †drug-induced dry mouth.

Contra-indications: Intestinal or urinary obstruction, or where increased intestinal or urinary tract motility could be harmful (e.g. after recent surgery); asthma; when miosis could be harmful (e.g. narrow-angle glaucoma, acute iritis).

Pharmacology

Pilocarpine is a parasympathomimetic (predominantly muscarinic) drug with mild β-adrenergic activity which stimulates secretion from exocrine glands, including salivary glands.[1] The *prophylactic* use of pilocarpine 5mg q.i.d. in patients receiving head and neck radiation (starting simultaneously and continuing for 4–6 weeks after the radiation is completed) has been shown to reduce the decrease in unstimulated salivary flow,[2,3] and to actually increase it in about 1/4 of patients.[2,3] Despite this objective improvement, a large placebo-controlled trial (n = 245) failed to show symptomatic benefit.[2] On the other hand, about 50% of patients with dry mouth several weeks or months *after* radiation therapy will respond to pilocarpine although benefit may take 3 months to become apparent.[4,5] Thus, failure to show symptomatic benefit from *prophylactic* use may relate to too short a treatment period or the presence of concurrent problems, e.g. mucositis.

About 90% of patients with drug-induced dry mouth respond to pilocarpine with benefit seen immediately.[5] In a controlled study, 1/2 of the patients preferred pilocarpine because it was more effective, and 1/2 preferred **mucin**-based artificial saliva (not Canada) mainly because it was a spray and not a tablet.[5] Undesirable effects were much more common in patients receiving pilocarpine (84% vs. 22%), which resulted in 1/4 of the patients withdrawing from the study.

Cheaper alternatives to pilocarpine, e.g. **bethanechol** are used at some centres.[6–9] Chewing gum also acts as a saliva stimulant. It is as effective as, and preferred to, **mucin**-based artificial saliva,[10] and thus provides a useful alternative in Canada, where **mucin**-based artificial saliva is unavailable. The gum should be sugar-free and, in patients with dentures, low-tack, e.g. Freedent® sugar-free gum or Biotene® dry mouth gum (see p.445).
Bio-availability 96% PO.
Onset of action 20min (drug-induced dry mouth); up to 3 months (after radiation).
Time to peak plasma concentration 1h.
Plasma halflife 1h.
Duration of action 3–5h (single dose).

Cautions

Pilocarpine may antagonize the effects of antimuscarinics, e.g. inhaled **ipratropium bromide**. Concurrent use with β-adrenergic receptor antagonists (β-blockers) may cause cardiac conduction disturbances.

Cognitive or psychiatric disorder, epilepsy, parkinsonism. Miosis may affect vision and driving ability, particularly at night. Cardiovascular disease (changes in hemodynamics or heart rhythm), hyperthyroidism, COPD (increased bronchial smooth muscle tone, airway resistance and bronchial secretions). Peptic ulcer (increased acid secretion), gallstones or biliary tract disease (increased biliary smooth muscle contraction). Mild–moderate hepatic impairment (reduce dose); avoid in severe hepatic impairment (no human data on metabolism and excretion). Renal impairment (no reliable human data on metabolism and excretion), kidney stones (potential for renal colic). Increased sweating may exacerbate dehydration in patients unable to drink sufficient fluids.

Undesirable effects
For full list, see manufacturer's Product Monograph.
Very common (>10%): headache, flu-like syndrome, nausea, urinary frequency, sweating.
Common (<10%, >1%): dizziness, asthenia, chills, blurred vision, eye pain, conjunctivitis, flushing, palpitations, hypertension (after initial hypotension), rhinitis, abdominal pain, dyspepsia, nausea, vomiting, diarrhea or constipation, rash, pruritus.

Dose and use
In drug-induced dry mouth the effective dose is generally 5mg t.i.d. or less, whereas after radiation therapy the effective dose is generally 5–10mg t.i.d.:
- start with 5mg t.i.d. with meals; the last dose of the day should be taken with the evening meal
- if necessary and if tolerated, increase the dose after 2 days if the dry mouth is drug-induced, and after 4 weeks if radiation-induced
- maximum dose 10mg t.i.d.
- if no improvement, stop after 2 days if the dry mouth is drug-induced, and after 12 weeks if radiation-induced.

In patients with mild–moderate hepatic impairment start on a lower dose, e.g. 5mg once daily, and work up to 5mg t.i.d. if well tolerated.

It is cheaper to give pilocarpine *eyedrops* PO than to prescribe tablets, e.g. pilocarpine 4% 2–3 drops t.i.d. = 4–6mg. Maximum cost/month about $5, whereas tablets would cost $99.

If **bethanechol** is used instead for drug-induced dry mouth:
- start with 25mg t.i.d. 30min a.c.
- reduce dose to 10mg t.i.d. if patients experience excessive salivation.
Undesirable effects are similar to pilocarpine but generally less severe, either because the equivalent dose is less or the muscarinic receptor binding pattern of **bethanechol** is different.

Supply
Pilocarpine
Isopto Carpine® liquid 4% (Alcon)
Eyedrops 4% (40mg/1mL), 15mL lasts 33–50 days @ 2–3 drops PO t.i.d. = $5.

Salagen® (Pfizer Canada)
Tablets 5mg, 28 days @ 5mg t.i.d. = $99.

Bethanechol
Duvoid® (Paladin)
Tablets 10mg, 25mg, 50mg, 28 days @ 25mg t.i.d. = $39.

1 Anonymous (1994) Oral pilocarpine for xerostomia. *Medical Letter on Drugs and Therapeutics.* **36**: 76.
2 Scarantino C et al. (2006) Effect of pilocarpine during radiation therapy: results of RTOG 97-09, a phase III randomized study in head and neck cancer patients. *Journal of Supportive Oncology.* **4**: 252–258.
3 Nyarady Z et al. (2006) A randomized study to assess the effectiveness of orally administered pilocarpine during and after radiotherapy of head and neck cancer. *Anticancer Research.* **26**: 1557–1562.
4 Rieke JW et al. (1995) Oral pilocarpine for radiation-induced xerostomia: integrated efficacy and safety results from two prospective randomized clinical trials. *International Journal of Radiation Oncology, Biology, Physics.* **31**: 661–669.
5 Davies A et al. (1998) A comparison of artificial saliva and pilocarpine in the management of xerostomia in patients with advanced cancer. *Palliative Medicine.* **12**: 105–111.
6 Everett H (1975) The use of bethanechol chloride with tricyclic antidepressants. *American Journal of Psychiatry.* **132**: 1202–1204.
7 Epstein J et al. (1994) A clinical trial of bethanechol in patients with xerostomia after radiation therapy. A pilot study. *Oral Surgery, Oral Medicine and Oral Pathology.* **77**: 610–614.
8 Taylor SE (2003) Efficacy and economic evaluation of pilocarpine in treating radiation-induced xerostomia. *Expert Opinion on Pharmacotherapy.* **4**: 1489–1497.

9 Davies A (2005) Salivary gland dysfunction. In: A Davies and I Finlay (eds) *Oral Care in Advanced Disease*. Oxford University Press, Oxford, pp. 97–114.

10 Davies AN (2000) A comparison of artificial saliva and chewing gum in the management of xerostomia in patients with advanced cancer. *Palliative Medicine*. **14**: 197–203.

DRUGS FOR ORAL INFLAMMATION AND ULCERATION

'Stomatitis' is a general term applied to diffuse inflammatory, erosive and ulcerative conditions affecting the mucous membranes of the mouth, whereas 'mucositis' tends to be restricted to stomatitis caused by chemotherapy or local radiation therapy. The causes of ulceration of the oral mucosa include trauma, recurrent aphthous ulcers, infection, cancer and nutritional deficiencies. It is important to determine the cause so that, if appropriate, specific as well as symptomatic treatment is given. For example, teeth and dentures should be checked, and ill-fitting dentures replaced or relined. Oral mucositis associated with radiation therapy or chemotherapy is the commonest cause of severe oral inflammation and ulceration in patients with cancer.[1] Mouth care before, during and after treatment reduces the severity of mucositis.[2–6]

When treating established mucositis, some centres use a locally compounded oral rinse (e.g. Magic mouthwash, Pink Lady). The composition of such mixtures varies. However, the inclusion of a corticosteroid may increase the likelihood of candidosis, and **diphenhydramine** (a topical analgesic/antihistamine, see opposite) may result in contact sensitization.

Management strategy

For aphthous ulcers, treatment generally comprises local corticosteroids ± antibacterial mouthwashes (Box 11.A).[7]

Box 11.A   Treatment of aphthous ulcers

Corticosteroids
Corticosteroids are useful for recurrent attacks. Use as soon as symptoms/ulcers appear; avoid in oral infections:
- triamcinolone acetonide 0.1% oral paste (Oracort® dental paste) b.i.d.–q.i.d. (preferably p.c. and at night) for up to 1 week; press a small amount onto the ulcers without rubbing until the paste forms a film, can be difficult to apply
- nasal aerosols sprayed into the mouth, when a more potent corticosteroid is needed for sites such as the soft palate and oropharynx, e.g. budesonide (generic or Rhinocort Aqua®, 64microgram/metered spray), triamcinolone acetonide (Nasacort AQ®, 55microgram/metered spray)
- hydrocortisone and lidocaine mouthwash when ulcers are widespread.

Antibacterial mouthwashes
Useful when there are multiple ulcers and when not accessible to covering pastes, e.g.:
- tetracycline suspension 250mg in 10mL t.i.d.–q.i.d. for 3 days (prepared by mixing the contents of a capsule with a small quantity of water); hold in the mouth for 2–3min and then spit out[8]
- minocycline suspension 10mg in 5mL of water q.i.d.; rinse around the mouth for 1min and then spit out.[9]

For stomatitis and mucositis generally, in addition to prophylactic measures and disease-specific treatment, a range of symptomatic options is available (see below).[10] A step by step approach is preferable, for example:
- *Step 1* topical non-opioid analgesic
- *Step 2* topical local anesthetic ± topical non-opioid analgesic

- *Step 3* topical **morphine** ± systemic **morphine**
- *Step 4* concurrent use of 'burst' **ketamine** (see p.468)
- *Step 5* concurrent use of **thalidomide** (see p.450 and p.405).

Topical non-opioid analgesics

Topical non-opioid analgesics have a definite but limited role in the management of painful oral ulceration, including chemotherapy and radiation-induced mucositis. When applied topically their action is of relatively short duration; pain relief cannot be maintained continuously throughout the day. **Diphenhydramine**, an antihistamine with a topical analgesic effect, is often used in compounded mouthwashes (Box 11.B).

Box 11.B   The use of diphenhydramine hydrochloride for oral mucositis[11]

The adult solutions of diphenhydramine commercially available in Canada contain alcohol 10–13.3%; *use solutions with a low alcohol content* to avoid causing additional discomfort. (Note: Benadryl® children's liquid 6.25mg/5mL contains no alcohol.)

Formulations include:
- diphenhydramine hydrochloride (12.5mg/5mL) and magnesium hydroxide in equal parts
- diphenhydramine in Kaopectate® (equal parts of diphenhydramine elixir 12.5mg/5mL and Kaopectate®); the pectin in the Kaopectate® helps the diphenhydramine adhere to inflamed/ulcerated mucosa
- stomatitis cocktail ('magic mouthwash'), National Cancer Institute, USA (equal parts of lidocaine viscous 2%, diphenhydramine elixir 12.5mg/5mL and Maalox®, a proprietary antacid similar to Almagel®)

Use up to 30mL q2h. Spread around the mouth with the tongue and then swallow or spit out after 2–3min.

A recent study suggests that there may be a place for topical **doxepin** as an oral rinse in the management of painful oral mucositis.[12] In some countries, NSAID products for topical oral use are used, e.g. **benzydamine** oral rinse, **choline salicylate** oral gel.

Topical local anesthetics

The efficacy of topical local anesthetics relates to the formulation, duration of application (at least 5min is required) and site of application; they are less effective in more keratinized areas of the mouth, e.g. the palate.[13] Some systemic absorption of the local anesthetic occurs, which is increased by mucosal inflammation. However, plasma levels are generally low, and toxicity has been reported only in exceptional circumstances (see Systemic local anesthetics, p.44).

With all topical local anesthetics care must be taken not to produce anesthesia of the pharynx before meals because this might lead to aspiration and choking:
- **benzocaine** buccal liquid 20%
- **benzocaine** oral (dental) paste 20%, applied up to q.i.d. p.r.n.
- **benzocaine** oral swabs 20% q.i.d. p.r.n.
- **lidocaine** 2% viscous solution, use 15mL q3h p.r.n.; swish around the mouth for 1–2min and then spit out; maximum 120mL/24h
- 'Pink Lady' 1/3 lidocaine viscous 2% with 2/3 antacid (e.g. Almagel®), use 5–10mL q4h p.r.n.; swish around the mouth then spit out.[14]

Duration of effect varies, but may be only 20–45min.

Topical opioids

Opioids have a topical analgesic effect on inflamed tissue and can be used as a mouthwash or oral spray. Some recommend that the mouthwash is subsequently swallowed in order to combine a systemic analgesic effect with the topical one:
- **morphine sulfate** 0.2% (2mg/mL) solution (compounded) or an alcohol-free proprietary product, take 10mg in 5mL q4h–q3h, hold in the mouth for 2min *and then spit out or swallow*; some patients need higher doses, occasionally 30mg q4h–q3h[15,16]

- **morphine sulfate** gel 1–5mg/mL (compounded, see p.306), initially 3mL q8h-q4h, hold in mouth for 10min *and then spit out or swallow*
- **hydromorphone** oral spray 0.05–0.1% (compounded); particularly useful for patients unable to tolerate the application of a paste to the back of the mouth.

Systemic analgesics

Non-opioids and opioids should be given as for other pains, balancing benefit against undesirable effects. For severe mucositis (patient unable to eat ± unable to drink) inadequately relieved by topical measures, a parenteral opioid should be administered, e.g. **morphine**. Chemotherapy patients often have a permanent IV access, e.g. Hickman line, and this can be used for patient-controlled analgesia (PCA).[17] In other patients, and in palliative care generally, CSCI is likely to be more convenient.

Some patients have benefited from short-term ('burst') treatment with **ketamine** (see Box 13.C, p.470).

Immunomodulators

*†**Thalidomide** 100mg at bedtime or b.i.d. for 10 days is sometimes used in resistant cases of mouth ulceration in patients with AIDS. Its use is restricted because it causes severe congenital abnormalities (absent or shortened limbs) and irreversible peripheral neuropathy. *The use of* **thalidomide** *is best limited to centres with the necessary expertise* (see p.405).

Other management options

Coating agents

Coating agents are of limited value. They can be difficult to apply, and they do not relieve persistent pain caused by oral inflammation, but by adhering to and coating the raw surface they help reduce contact pain, e.g. from eating or drinking. Available agents include:

- **hydroxypropylcellulose** gel (Zilactin®) or **sodium carboxymethylcellulose** (**carmellose sodium**) paste (Orabase® paste) apply to the sore area p.c.[18]
- **sucralfate** is *not* of benefit in chemotherapy or radiation-induced mucositis,[19,20] but may help in less severe stomatitis; it can be given in a suspension 1g/5mL q.i.d.

Growth factors

Palifermin is a recombinant human keratinocyte growth factor which stimulates the proliferation and differentiation of epithelial cells, reducing the incidence and severity of mucositis. It is expensive, and is unlikely to be used in palliative care.

Supply

The following list is selective.

Corticosteroids
Triamcinolone acetonide
Oracort® dental paste (Taro)
Oral paste 0.1% in adhesive base, 7.5g = $9.

Nasacort AQ® (Sanofi-Aventis Canada)
Nasal spray (aqueous) 55microgram/metered spray, 120-dose spray = $25.

Budesonide (generic)
Nasal spray (aqueous) 64microgram/metered spray, 120-dose (10mL) spray = $11.

Rhinocort Aqua® (AstraZeneca Canada)
Nasal spray (aqueous) 64microgram/metered spray, 120-dose spray = $11.

Antibiotic mouthwashes
Tetracycline (generic)
Capsules 250mg, 3 days @ 250mg t.i.d. = $0.50.

Minocycline (generic)
Mouthwash 10mg/5mL, compounded from capsules 50mg, 3 days @ 10mg q.i.d. = $2.50.

Topical non-opioid analgesics
Diphenhydramine
Mouthwash compounded from diphenhydramine oral solution (elixir) 12.5mg/5mL.

Topical local anesthetics
Benzocaine
Orajel® (Church & Dwight)
Buccal liquid containing **benzocaine** 20%, 13mL = $7.
Oral gel containing **benzocaine** 10%, 9.5g = $6; 20%, 9.5g = $7.
Oral paste containing **benzocaine** 20%, 5.3g = $9.
Oral swabs containing **benzocaine** 20%, pack of 8 = $9.

Zilactin B® (ANB)
Oral gel containing **benzocaine** 10% in a **hydroxypropylcellulose** gel base, 6g = $9.

Kank-a-Liq® (Blistex)
Buccal liquid containing **benzocaine** 20%, **cetylpyridinium chloride** 0.1%, 10mL = $8.

Oragard-B® (Colgate Oral Pharmaceuticals)
Oral paste containing **benzocaine** 20%, 6g = $9, available OTC.

Lidocaine viscous (generic)
Oral topical solution 2%, 50mL = $8, 100mL = $12, available OTC; *alcohol-free, glycerin-free* (Odan). Note: PMS *product contains glycerin.*

Xylocaine Viscous® (AstraZeneca Canada)
Oral topical solution 2%, 100mL = $16, available OTC; *alcohol-free, glycerin-free.*

Topical opioids
Morphine
Mouthwash 0.2% (2mg/mL in water), can be compounded for individual patients.
Oral gel 0.1–0.5% (1–5mg/mL), can be compounded for individual patients.

Hydromorphone
Oral spray 0.05–0.1% (0.5–1mg/mL), can be compounded for individual patients.

Coating agents
Orabase® (ConvaTec Canada)
Oral paste containing **carboxymethylcellulose sodium** 13.3%, **gelatin** 13.3% and **pectin** 13.3%, 7.5g = $12, available OTC.

Zilactin® (Associated National Brokerage)
Oral gel containing **benzyl alcohol** 10% in a **hydroxypropylcellulose** gel base, 6g = $9, available OTC.

Sucralfate
Sucralfate Suspension Plus® (Axcan)
Oral suspension 1g/5mL, 500mL = $51; *alcohol-free, contains approximately 20% glycerin.*

---

1 Wilkes J (1998) Prevention and treatment of oral mucositis following cancer chemotherapy. *Seminars in Oncology.* **25**: 535–551.
2 Larson P et al. (1998) The PRO-SELF mouth aware program: an effective approach for reducing chemotherapy-induced mucositis. *Cancer Nursing.* **21**: 263–268.
3 Brennan MT et al. (2006) Alimentary mucositis: putting the guidelines into practice. *Supportive Care in Cancer.* **14**: 573–579.
4 Lalla RV et al. (2006) Anti-inflammatory agents in the management of alimentary mucositis. *Supportive Care in Cancer.* **14**: 558–565.
5 Ngeow WC et al. (2008) Management of radiation therapy-induced mucositis in head and neck cancer patients. Part I: clinical significance, pathophysiology and prevention. *Oncology Reviews.* **2**: 102–113.
6 Ngeow WC et al. (2008) Management of radiation therapy-induced mucositis in head and neck cancer patients. Part II: supportive treatments. *Oncology Reviews.* **2**: 164–182.
7 Davies A and Finlay I (eds) (2005) *Oral Care in Advanced Disease.* Oxford University Press, Oxford.
8 Barrons RW (2001) Treatment strategies for recurrent oral aphthous ulcers. *American Journal of Health-System Pharmacy.* **58**: 41–50; quiz 51–43.
9 Gorsky M et al. (2007) Topical minocycline and tetracycline rinses in treatment of recurrent aphthous stomatitis: a randomized cross-over study. *Dermatology Online Journal.* **13**: 1.
10 Turhal N et al. (2000) Efficacy of treatment to relieve mucositis-induced discomfort. *Support Care Cancer.* **8**: 55–58.
11 NIH Consensus Development Conference Statement (1989) Oral complications of cancer therapies, prevention and treatment. *NIH Consensus Statement.* **7**: 1–11.

---

12 Epstein JB et al. (2007) Management of pain in cancer patients with oral mucositis: follow-up of multiple doses of doxepin oral rinse. *J Pain Symptom Manage.* **33**: 111–114.

13 Meecham J (2005) Oral pain. In: A Davies and I Finlay (eds) *Oral Care in Advanced Disease.* Oxford University Press, Oxford, pp. 134–143.

14 Latimer EJ (2002) Mouth care – treating the often overlooked symptoms. *Canadian Journal of Diagnosis.* **March**: 43–52.

15 Cerchietti LC et al. (2002) Effect of topical morphine for mucositis-associated pain following concomitant chemoradiotherapy for head and neck carcinoma.[erratum appears in Cancer. 2003; 97:1137.]. *Cancer.* **95**: 2230–2236.

16 Cerchietti L and Cerchietti L (2007) Morphine mouthwashes for painful mucositis.[comment]. *Supportive Care in Cancer.* **15**: 115–116; author reply 117.

17 Coda B et al. (1997) Comparative efficacy of patient-controlled administration of morphine, hydromorphone, or sufentanil for the treatment of oral mucositis pain following marrow transplantation. *Pain.* **72**: 333–346.

18 Ship JA et al. (2000) Recurrent aphthous stomatitis. *Quintessence International.* **31**: 95–112.

19 Loprinzi C et al. (1997) Phase III controlled evaluation of sucralfate to alleviate stomatitis in patients receiving fluorouracil-based chemotherapy. *Journal of Clinical Oncology.* **15**: 1235–1238.

20 Meredith R et al. (1997) Sucralfate for radiation mucositis: results of a double-blind randomized trial. *International Journal of Radiation, Oncology, Biology and Physics.* **37**: 275–279.

CERUMENOLYTICS

Indications: Impacted ear wax (cerumen).

Contra-indications: perforated ear drum, presence of myringotomy tubes (grommets), recent ear surgery.

Pharmacology

Ear wax is secreted to provide a protective film on the skin of the external auditory meatus. It is generally expelled naturally, but if it accumulates and becomes impacted, it can cause hearing loss, pain, dizziness, tinnitus or chronic cough.[1] The risk of impaction is increased in children, the elderly and patients with learning disabilities, and if natural expulsion is obstructed, e.g. by anatomical abnormalities of the external auditory meatus, hearing aids, or using cotton-tipped applicators (Q-tips®) to clean the ears.[1,2]

Keratin is a major constituent of ear wax. Disintegration is facilitated by keratin cell hydration and lysis.[3] Keratolysis, and thus liquefying of ear wax, is optimal in aqueous solutions, e.g. water, 0.9% saline or 5% **sodium bicarbonate**.[4,5] In contrast, even after 1 week, organic-based products have little or no disintegrating effect, and should thus *not* be used for this purpose.[5,6] Oils, e.g. **olive oil**, act by lubricating the impacted wax plug, facilitating its natural expulsion or removal by syringing. Cerumol® (**chlorobutanol** 5%, **dichlorobenzene** 2%, **turpentine oil** 10%, **arachis** (peanut) **oil** 57%) causes meatal irritation,[7] and is not recommended.

Systematic reviews and a later RCT concluded that tap or sterile water or 0.9% saline was as effective as more expensive commercial products or **sodium bicarbonate** ear drops.[8–10] However, the evidence is weak, and practice varies widely.

Dose and use

PCF regards tap water as the cerumenolytic of choice.

Ear wax should be removed only if it causes symptoms, e.g. deafness, or prevents examination of the ear drum.[1,2] Although the use of a cerumenolytic over several days may obviate the need,[9] syringing is likely to be necessary to remove a firmly impacted plug of ear wax. The patient should lie down with the affected ear uppermost; then to soften the wax before syringing:

- fill the ear with warm tap water and wait for 15–30min[11] or
- instil **olive oil** and wait for 5min.

If syringing is unsuccessful, instil warm water b.i.d. for 3 days, and then repeat syringing.[1]

Supply

Although several OTC products exist, their relative effectiveness is unproven and appears to be no better than that of water or 0.9% saline. Thus, none is recommended.

0.9% Saline (generic)
Injection (use as ear drops) 5mL in plastic amp, 3 days @ 1amp b.i.d. = $2.
Ear drops compounded.

Rhinaris® saline solution (PharmaScience Inc.)
Nose drops (use as ear drops), 45mL = $6; available OTC.

1 McCarter DF *et al.* (2007) Cerumen impaction. *American Family Physician.* **75**: 1523–1528.
2 Browning G (2008) Ear Wax. In: *BMJ Clinical Evidence.* Available from: http://clinicalevidence.bmj.com/ceweb/conditions/ent/0504/0504-get.pdf
3 Robinson A *et al.* (1989) The mechanism of ceruminolysis. *Journal of Otolaryngology.* **18**: 268–273.
4 Robinson AC and Hawke M (1989) The efficacy of ceruminolytics: everything old is new again. *Journal of Otolaryngology.* **18**: 263–267.
5 Chalishazar U and Williams H (2007) Back to basics: finding an optimal cerumenolytic (earwax solvent). *British Journal of Nursing.* **16**: 806–808.
6 Horowitz H (1968) Solvent for ear wax. *British Medical Journal.* **4**: 583.
7 Bellini M *et al.* (1989) An evaluation of common cerumenolytic agents: an in-vitro study. *Clinical Otolaryngology.* **14**: 23–25.
8 Burton MJ and Doree CJ (2003) Ear drops for the removal of ear wax. *Cochrane Database Systematic Reviews.* CD004400.
9 Hand C and Harvey I (2004) The effectiveness of topical preparations for the treatment of earwax: a systematic review. *British Journal of General Practice.* **54**: 862–867.
10 Roland PS *et al.* (2004) Randomized, placebo-controlled evaluation of Cerumenex and Murine earwax removal products. *Archives of Otolaryngology – Head & Neck Surgery.* **130**: 1175–1177.
11 Pavlidis C and Pickering JA (2005) Water as a fast acting wax softening agent before ear syringing.[see comment]. *Australian Family Physician.* **34**: 303–304.

12: SKIN

EMOLLIENTS

Indications: Dry or rough skin.

Pharmacology

Emollients are indicated for all causes of dry flaky skin that has lost epidermal lubrication. In palliative care, common causes include:

- age (asteotic dermatitis)
- drying environments
- overwashing
- diuretics
- drug reactions
- radiation-induced dermatitis.

Asteotic dermatitis typically affects the legs (particularly the shins) and less commonly the trunk and arms. The skin assumes a 'crazy paving' appearance with large scales demarcated by fine red superficial fissures; purpura and capillary bleeding can occur.

By adding oil and water to the skin, emollients (moisturizers) soothe and smooth the skin, and restore some of the skin's function as a barrier.[1] Less water is lost from skin in a good condition, and the risk of infection is reduced. In the past, it was possible to classify topical products into distinct categories. However, methods of manufacture have become so sophisticated that the distinction between, for example, creams and oily lotions is no longer meaningful (Table 12.1).

Table 12.1 Topical applications

Ointments	Creams	Lotions
Grease-based	Emulsions of water and oil; vary from more greasy products (water-in-oil, 'rich creams') to more aqueous ones (oil-in-water, 'light creams')	Solutions, suspensions or emulsions from which water evaporates leaving a thin coating of powder or oil
Application once daily; generally sufficient	Require more frequent application	Only emulsions containing oil have an emollient effect; other lotions are drying
Messy to apply; difficult if skin is very hairy; may occlude hair follicles	Massage well into skin; cosmetically more acceptable	Shake suspensions well before use; apply lotions to the skin without friction

The properties of oily lotions are comparable to light creams but, because they are more liquid, oily lotions can be applied more easily to large areas. Both light creams and oily lotions have a cooling effect on the skin (heat lost by evaporation of the water content).

Ointments are greasy because of their structure, even when their water content is high. Anhydrous ointments shield the skin; this results in a build-up of heat and moisture. Subsequent swelling of the horny layer of the epidermis allows added agents to reach the deeper layers of the skin more easily.

Some creams contain propylene glycol. This gives them a smoother texture, and facilitates application. Propylene glycol is also a humectant (see below). However, on broken skin, it is irritating. Thus, with broken skin, a propylene glycol-free cream or an ointment is generally preferable.

Some products contain humectants, e.g. alpha-hydroxy acids, propylene glycol and urea. These help to attract moisture to, and retain it in, the stratum corneum.[2] However, humectants may be irritating. Adequate hydration is generally obtained with 5–10% urea,[3,4] whereas concentrations of 20–30% are antipruritic, break down keratin, decrease the thickness of the stratum corneum, and are used in scaling conditions such as ichthyosis.[3]

Proprietary emollients often contain additives and fragrances (perfumes) which are potentially allergenic (Table 12.2). However, concern about lanolin is largely misplaced; many emollients contain highly purified ('hypo-allergic') lanolin which is rarely responsible for contact dermatitis.[5]

Table 12.2 Some potential skin allergens to which patients may be exposed

Allergen	Comment
Fragrances (perfumes)[3,6]	
Preservatives (particularly parabens and cresols)[3,6]	In many creams
Emulsifying agents and ointment bases (particularly sodium lauryl sulfate and cetostearyl alcohols)[3,6]	In many creams and ointments
Wool fat derivatives (including lanolin)[3,6]	In many creams and ointments
Topical local anesthetics	
Neomycin	
Ethyl alcohol	In some products and skin wipes
Rubber additives (plasticizers, preservatives)	Undersheets, elastic stockings, etc.
Paraphenylenediamine, chromates	In leather
Tea tree oil[7]	

Dose and use

Emollients should be applied liberally, generally once daily (ointments) or b.i.d. (creams). It is helpful to show the use of the recommended emollient (or one of comparable consistency) to the patient and the family/informal carers. This is particularly useful in patients with unsightly skin who may feel ostracized, and for whom physical contact (touch) generally provides real psychological benefit.

Further, for patients with persistent dry skin despite the conscientious use of an emollient, greater benefit can be obtained by applying the emollient at the time when the skin is most hydrated, i.e. immediately after a bath. The patient can be advised to shake off excess water (like a dog) or lightly dab dry with a soft towel, and then to apply the emollient to the still damp skin.

Average quantities required for b.i.d. application for 1 week are shown in Table 12.3. Choice of emollient involves consideration of:
- patient preference
- area to be treated, e.g. ointment acceptable for legs and trunk but not face and hands
- ingredients (does it contain known or potential allergens?)
- the consistency required
- packaging, e.g. risk of in-use contamination with pots; patients with weak hands may find removing screw-top lids or squeezing tubes difficult. Compounded creams are often packed in disposable syringes; this avoids contamination, allows the application of measured amounts, and the contents are generally easy to push out
- patient's lifestyle
- availability; some products may not be widely available in all provinces. Check with your pharmacy regarding any locally-used products
- cost-effectiveness, e.g. **aqueous cream BP** and Atlas Base® are similar to, but cheaper than, Glaxal Base®.

Table 12.3 Quantities required for b.i.d. application for 1 week

	Creams and ointments (g)	Lotions (mL)
Face	15–30	100
Groins and genitalia	15–25	100
Both hands	25–50	200
Scalp	50–100	200
Both arms or both legs	100–200	200
Trunk	400	500

There is a dearth of RCT data about emollients.[8,9] However, in practice, *the best emollient is the one which a patient is happy to use long-term*. This implies that it is both cosmetically acceptable and effective, and preferably should not be expensive. For example, many patients like the silky feel of Aveeno® (**colloidal oatmeal**), particularly on their hands and face.

Emollients containing **arachis** (peanut) **oil** should not be used by patients with peanut or soya allergy.[10] However, few such emollients are now available.

An aqueous (light) cream or emollient lotion b.i.d. (e.g. **aqueous cream BP**, Atlas Base®, Glaxal Base® or Moisturel® lotion) generally suffices with mild–moderate degrees of dryness (Table 12.4). Some patients may need to apply a **petrolatum** (**white soft paraffin**)-based ointment b.i.d. initially. Thick emollients, e.g. ointments, should be used with caution on hairy

Table 12.4 Emollient and additive content of selected topical products[a]

	Wool fat derivatives, e.g. lanolin	Petrolatum (white soft paraffin) or mineral oil (liquid paraffin)	Sensitizing preservative	Fragrance
Oils				
Coconut oil	–	–	–	–
Mineral oil (liquid paraffin)	–	+	–	–
Ointments				
Petroleum jelly (petrolatum, white soft paraffin)	–	+	–	–
Creams				
Aqueous cream BP	–	+	–	–
Atlas Base®	–	+	+	–
Atrac-Tain®	–	–	–	–
Aveeno®	–	+	+	–
Complex-15® Face cream	–	–	–	–
Complex-15® Hand cream	–	+	–	–
Eucerin Original®	+	+	–	–
Glaxal Base®	–	+	+	–
Lubriderm Advanced Moisture Therapy®	–	+	+	–
Lubriderm Intense Dry Skin Repair®	–	+	+	–
Moisturel®	–	+	+	–
Uremol 10®	–	+	–	–
Lotions				
Aveeno®	–	+	+	–
Complex-15® Body lotion	–	–	–	–
Eucerin Original®	+	+	–	–
Glaxal Base®	–	+	+	–
Lac-hydrin®	–	+	+	–
Lubriderm®	+	+	+	+
Lubriderm Intense Dry Skin Repair®	–	+	+	–
Moisturel®	–	+	+	–
Uremol 10®	–	–	–	–

a. products which do not contain wool fat derivatives or petrolatum/mineral oil generally contain plant-based oils or fatty acid derivatives.

parts of the body because they can block the hair follicles and cause folliculitis. The likelihood of this happening is reduced by massaging in the direction of hair growth.

Soap should *not* be used because of its drying effect on the skin. Cleansers such as **aqueous cream BP**, Cetaphil Gentle Skin Cleanser® or Cetaphil Gentle Cleansing Bar® can be used instead. An emollient bath additive, such as Keri Moisturizing Shower and Bath Oil®, can also be used when bathing. It is advisable to use a mat to prevent slipping when using such products in the bath or shower.

When the skin is cracked, emollients can cause stinging. In this circumstance, particularly if the skin is inflamed, apply a low-potency topical corticosteroid instead for 1 week, e.g. **desonide** 0.05%, and then recommence the emollient. To minimize undesirable effects from topical corticosteroids, they should be applied thinly once daily or b.i.d. to the affected area only. If the skin is broken, use a combination product containing a topical corticosteroid and an antibacterial and/or antifungal.

If emollient-related contact dermatitis is suspected, patch testing with the standard set of potential allergens may identify an allergen. If allergy is confirmed, a product which does not contain the allergen and, ideally, any other added preservatives or fragrances, should be prescribed. However, not all contact dermatitis is allergic; sometimes it is caused by direct chemical irritation.

Lymphedema

Skin care is just one component of multimodal lymphedema management.[11,12] The following advice must be applied within the broader management context.

Although the following all contain **petrolatum** (**white soft paraffin**), the choice will depend on the state of the skin:[13]
- if not obviously dry and flaky, a bland cream such as **aqueous cream BP**, Atlas Base® or Glaxal Base® can be applied once daily–b.i.d. as a prophylactic measure
- if the skin is dry ± cracked, apply **mineral oil** (**liquid paraffin**) in **petrolatum** 50/50 b.i.d.
- If there is a build-up of scales, apply **petrolatum**, e.g. **petroleum jelly**.

The application of **petroleum jelly** is done best after soaking the limb in a bucket of warm water for 15–20min. Cover the **petroleum jelly** with a hydrocolloid dressing and bandage for 2 days. Repeat the process until the skin condition is good. Note: if there are toe web fissures, take scrapings to look for fungus and, if present, treat appropriately.

Note:
- ointments are generally not necessary for more than 1 week
- some people prefer coconut oil because it has a skin-cooling effect
- after 2 days of soaking/softening, the **petroleum jelly** can be applied with a circular motion; this helps to lift off the softened hyperkeratotic plaques.

Antipruritic emollients

If pruritus is caused by dry skin, rehydration of the skin will correct it. Thus, all emollients are antipruritic in this sense. However, some products have a specific antipruritic agent added, and can provide added benefit in some patients (see p.460).

Supply

The following list is highly selective.

Pharmaco-economics

Before prescribing a relatively expensive proprietary product, check to see whether, content for content, there is a cheaper essentially equivalent product.

Non-soap cleansers
Cetaphil Gentle Cleansing Bar® (Galderma)
127g = $7.

Cetaphil Gentle Skin Cleanser® (Galderma)
250mL = $11, 500mL = $20.

Bath oil
Keri Moisturizing Bath Oil® (Bristol-Myers Squibb)
450mL = $12.

Emollients
Aqueous cream BP
Cream containing **emulsifying ointment BP** 30%, phenoxyethanol 1%, water to 100%, 450g = $12. (**Emulsifying ointment BP** contains **emulsifying wax** 30%, **petrolatum (white soft paraffin)** 50%, **mineral oil (liquid paraffin)** 20%.)

Atlas Base® (Atlas)
Cream containing **petrolatum, mineral oil**, 450g = $16.

Colloidal oatmeal
Aveeno® (Johnson & Johnson)
Cream Skin relief moisturizing cream®, 312g = $20.
Lotion Skin relief moisturizing lotion®, 354mL = $14.

Eucerin Original® (Beiersdorf)
Cream containing **petrolatum, mineral oil, lanolin**, 473mL = $17.
Lotion containing **petrolatum, mineral oil, lanolin**, 473mL = $16.

Glaxal Base® (Wellspring)
Cream containing **petrolatum, mineral oil**, 100g = $12, 450g = $29.
Lotion 227g = $12.

Lubriderm® (Pfizer)
Lotion containing **lanolin, mineral oil, petrolatum**, 580mL = $12.

Lubriderm Intense Dry Skin Repair® (Pfizer)
Cream 140g = $12.
Lotion 480mL = $12.

Lubriderm Advanced Moisture Therapy® (Pfizer)
Cream containing **glycerin, mineral oil**, 100g = $9.

Moisturel® (Novartis Consumer Health Canada)
Cream containing **dimethicone** 1%, **petrolatum** 30%, 120g = $13.
Lotion containing **dimethicone** 3%, **petrolatum** 6%, 225mL = $9, 400mL = $14.

Petroleum jelly (generic)
White petrolatum, 100g = $3, 454g = $7.

Vaseline® petroleum jelly (Lever Pond's)
White petrolatum, 100g = $3, 375g = $6.

With humectants
Atrac-Tain® (Sween)
Cream containing **urea** 10%, **alpha-hydroxyl acid (lactic acid)** 4%, 140g = $17.

Complex 15® (Schering)
Face cream containing **dimethicone, lecithin**, 100mL = $11.
Hand cream containing **dimethicone, lecithin**, 100mL = $11.
Body lotion containing **dimethicone, lecithin**, 300 mL = $11.

Lac-Hydrin® (Novartis)
Lotion containing **lactic acid** (as ammonium lactate) 12%, 225mL = $13.

Uremol 10® (Stiefel)
Cream containing **urea** 10%, 75g = $11, 120g = $14.
Lotion containing **urea** 10%, 250mL = $16.

Low-potency topical corticosteroid
Desonide (generic)
Cream 0.05%, 15g = $5, 60g = $18.
Ointment 0.05%, 60g = $18.

1 Ryan TJ (2004) The first commandment: Oil it! *Community Dermatology.* 1: 1–16.
2 Kraft JN and Lynde CW (2005) Moisturizers: what thye are and a practical approach to product selection. *Skin Therapy Letter.* **10** (5): 1–8.
3 Sibbald D (2002) Dermatitis. In: C Repchinsky (ed) *Patient Self-care* (2e). Canadian Pharmacists Association, Ottawa, pp. 479–505.
4 Fluhr JW et al. (2008) Emollients, moisturizers, and keratolytic agents in psoriasis. *Clinics in Dermatology.* **26**: 380–386.
5 Hoppe U (ed) (1999) *The Lanolin Book.* Beierdorf AG, Hamburg.
6 Voegeli D (2008) Care or harm: exploring essential components in skin care regimens. *British Journal of Nursing.* **17**: 24–30.
7 Rubel DM et al. (1998) Tea tree oil allergy: what is the offending agent? Report of three cases of tea tree oil allergy and review of the literature. *Australasian Journal of Dermatology.* **39**: 244–247.
8 Hoare C et al. (2000) Systematic review of treatments for atopic eczema. *Health Technology Assessment.* **4**: 1–191.
9 Peters J (2005) Exploring the use of emollient therapy in dermatological nursing. *British Journal of Nursing.* **14**: 494–502.
10 MHRA (2003) Medicines containing peanut (arachis) oil. *Current Problems in Pharmacovigilance.* **29 (September)**: 5.
11 Twycross R et al. (2009) *Symptom Management in Advanced Cancer* (4e). palliativedrugs.com, Nottingham, pp. 298–311.
12 Twycross RG et al. (2000) *Lymphoedema.* Radcliffe Medical Press, Oxford.
13 Linnitt N (2000) Skin management in lymphoedema. In: RG Twycross et al. (eds) *Lymphoedema.* Radcliffe Medical Press, Oxford, pp. 118–129.

TOPICAL ANTIPRURITICS

Indications: Pruritus.

Cautions

Because of the risk of contact sensitization (causing contact dermatitis), *discourage* the use of topical products containing:
• local anesthetics
• H_1-antihistamines.
Because of their drying effect, *discourage* the use of products containing **calamine**.

Pharmacology

Traditional topical antipruritics include **phenol, menthol** (see p.434) and **camphor**. **Phenol** 0.5–3% acts by anesthetizing cutaneous nerve endings, whereas **menthol** 0.5–2% and **camphor** 0.5–3% act as counter-irritants. Topical products containing these agents may be available OTC, or they can be prepared by a compounding pharmacist if a plain emollient is inadequate.[1]

Capsaicin products (see p.434) are sometimes used for pruritus associated with psoriasis and prurigo nodularis. A **coal tar**-based shampoo, e.g. Polytar®, has a long tradition of use with scalp pruritus.

Some products contain a local anesthetic instead, e.g. **benzocaine, lidocaine, pramoxine** (**pramocaine**), **tetracaine** (**amethocaine**). Products containing **pramoxine** may sting when initially applied; thus avoid contact with eyes and nasal mucosa, and wash hands after use.[2] All 'caines' can cause contact dermatitis to a variable extent. Thus, their use is best restricted to a few days. Local anesthetic products are available OTC.

Crotamiton 10% lotion (Eurax®) has a mild antiscabetic effect which is probably the reason for its reputation as an antipruritic. However, in a controlled trial, **crotamiton** was no more effective than plain aqueous cream,[3] and thus it is not recommended generally as a antipruritic agent.

Topical H_1-antihistamines such as **diphenhydramine** are of benefit only when the pruritus is cutaneous in origin, and related to histamine release.[4] **Diphenhydramine** can cause contact dermatitis and photosensitivity, and so avoid use, or limit use to a few days.

Topical doxepin

Doxepin, marketed primarily as a TCA, is a potent H_1- and H_2-receptor antagonist. Its affinity for H_2-receptors is 6 times that of **cimetidine**.[5] It also blocks muscarinic receptors.[6] **Amitriptyline** is similar in potency to **doxepin** as an H_1-antihistamine, but other TCAs are much less so.[7] Patients with chronic urticaria who do not respond to conventional H_1-antihistamines may well benefit from **doxepin** 10–75mg at bedtime.[6]

Doxepin as a 5% cream (commercially unavailable in Canada) is reported to be of benefit in some patients with atopic dermatitis[5,8,9] but long-term independent studies are lacking.[10] It is not generally suitable for use in children. About 15% of patients complain initially of localized stinging or burning, and, because there can be significant absorption, a similar proportion complain of drowsiness. Thus, it is possible that the benefit is systemic rather than topical. **Doxepin** cream is less effective than systemic treatment.[11]

As with TCAs generally, MAOIs should be discontinued at least 2 weeks before starting treatment with **doxepin**. Patients prescribed **doxepin**, either systemically or topically, should also avoid the concurrent use of drugs which inhibit cytochrome P450, e.g. **cimetidine**, imidazole antifungals and macrolide antibacterials (see Cytochrome P450, p.551).

Use

Whenever possible, the treatment of pruritus should be cause-specific.[4,12] For example:
- scabies → treat patient and the whole family with **permethrin**
- atopic dermatitis → topical corticosteroid (+ emollient)
- contact dermatitis → topical corticosteroid, identify causal substance and avoid further contact
- systemic opioid (rare) → switch opioid ± H$_1$-antihistamine (also see p.290).

A topical antipruritic should be considered when more specific options have been exhausted, e.g. in the treatment of pruritus of unknown cause. Although topical products are not convenient to apply regularly to the whole body, many patients with generalized pruritus have patches of more intense discomfort, and may benefit from more limited application.

Because pruritus is often associated with dry skin, an emollient (moisturizer) should be tried first (see p.455). A light cream, e.g. **aqueous cream BP**, Atlas Base® or Glaxal Base® often suffices with mild–moderate degrees of dryness. Products containing **colloidal oatmeal** (Aveeno®) are popular because of their silky feel.

Keeping creams and lotions cool in a refrigerator may increase benefit.

Supply

Menthol and **phenol** are time-honoured antipruritic agents. Either can be added to **aqueous cream BP** (or alternative emollient) to make a 0.5–2% compounded cream, and applied topically 3–4 times/24h.

Calamine can be helpful but, because it is unsightly, it is unlikely to be acceptable except on a short-term basis, e.g. in acute contact dermatitis. **Calamine lotion BP** contains **phenol** 0.5%, and can be strengthened by adding a further 0.5%. Although the vehicle is drying, it can be compounded into an oily lotion. **Phenolated calamine lotion USP** contains **phenol** 1%.

Many topical antipruritics are available OTC; a sample is listed below.

Lotions
Sarna P® lotion (Stiefel)
Camphor 0.5%, **menthol** 0.5%, **pramoxine hydrochloride** 1% in an emollient base, 150mL = $16.

Aveeno anti-itch® lotion (Johnson & Johnson)
Pramoxine hydrochloride 1%, **calamine** 3%, 118mL = $13.

Solarcaine® Medicated First Aid lotion (Schering-Plough Canada)
Lidocaine hydrochloride 0.5%, 170mL = $9.

Cream
Aveeno anti-itch® cream (Johnson & Johnson)
Pramoxine hydrochloride 1%, **calamine** 3%, 28g = $8.

Ointments
Petro Carbo Salve® (Watkins)
Phenol 1.2%, 124g = $11. Obtainable from www.watkinsonline.com.

Vicks VapoRub® (Procter & Gamble)
Camphor 4.73%, **menthol** 2.6%, **eucalyptus oil** 1.2%, 57mL = $8, 115mL = $13, 190mL = $19; *pruritus is an off-label use, the product is marketed for relief of cold symptoms.*

Gels
Deep Cold Gel® (The Mentholatum Company of Canada)
Regular strength gel menthol 2%, 100g = $7, 225g = $11, 500g = $18.
Extra strength gel menthol 3%, 230mL = $11.

Solarcaine® Medicated Lidocaine gel (Schering-Plough Canada)
Lidocaine hydrochloride 0.5%, 220mL = $11.

Topical patch
Deep Cold Pain Patch® (The Mentholatum Company of Canada)
Menthol 5%, pack of 6 = $11.

Shampoos
Polytar® (Stiefel)
Regular strength shampoo coal tar 1%, 150mL = $11, 350mL = $20.
Mild shampoo coal tar 0.5%, 150mL = $11, 350mL = $20.

Doxepin products
Doxepin hydrochloride (generic)
Capsules 25mg, 75mg, 28 days @ 25mg or 75mg at bedtime = $6 and $16 respectively.

Sinequan® (Erfa Canada)
Capsules 10mg, 75mg, 28 days @ 10mg or 75mg at bedtime = $8 and $25 respectively.

1 Anonymous (2005) Pharmacy information pointers. The preparation of menthol (1 per cent w/w) in aqueous cream BP. *Pharmaceutical Journal.* **274**: 469.
2 Sweetman SC (ed) (2007) *Martindale: The complete drug reference* (35e). Pharmaceutical Press, London, pp. 266–267.
3 Smith E et al. (1984) Crotamiton lotion in pruritus. *International Journal of Dermatology.* **23**: 684–685.
4 Zylicz Z et al. (eds) (2004) *Pruritus in Advanced Disease.* Oxford University Press, Oxford.
5 Drake L et al. (1994) Relief of pruritus in patients with atopic dermatitis after treatment with topical doxepin cream. The Doxepin Study Group. *Journal of the American Academy of Dermatology.* **31**: 613–616.
6 Figueiredo A et al. (1990) Mechanism of action of doxepin in the treatment of chronic urticaria. *Fundamental and Clinical Pharmacology.* **4**: 147–158.
7 Figge J et al. (1979) Tricyclic antidepressants: potent blockade of histamine H₁ receptors of guinea pig ileum. *European Journal of Pharmacology.* **58**: 479–483.
8 Breneman D et al. (1997) Doxepin cream relieves eczema-associated pruritus within 15 minutes and is not accompanied by a risk of rebound upon discontinuation. *Journal of Dermatological Treatment.* **8**: 161–168.
9 DTB (2000) Doxepin cream for eczema? *Drug and Therapeutics Bulletin.* **38**: 31.
10 Hoare C et al. (2000) Systematic review of treatments for atopic eczema. *Health Technology Assessment.* **4**: 1–191.
11 Smith P and Corelli R (1997) Doxepin in the management of pruritus associated with allergic cutaneous reactions. *Annals of Pharmacotherapy.* **31**: 633–635.
12 Twycross R et al. (2009) *Symptom Management in Advanced Cancer* (4e). palliativedrugs.com, Nottingham, pp. 321–329.

BARRIER PRODUCTS

Indications: Skin protection, diaper rash.

Pharmacology

Barrier products contain water-repellent substances which help to protect the skin. They can be used around stomas, and in the perineal and peri-anal areas in patients with urinary or fecal incontinence. Traditional formulations include **zinc oxide** ointments. Desitin® (**zinc oxide** and cod-liver oil) and Zincofax® (**zinc oxide**) are commonly available barrier products. Some products include **dimethicone**, e.g. Critic-Aid Clear®, or other water-repellant silicone.

A cream is less sticky and is sometimes advantageous because it is easier to apply and wash off, e.g. **zinc oxide** cream, Baza Protect® (**zinc oxide** and **dimethicone**) or Sween 24® (**dimethicone**).

Cautions

It is important to ensure any signs of infection are treated promptly with antibacterials and/or antifungals, as appropriate. Most topical skin products are intended to be applied to intact skin.

Dose and use
Intertrigo
Microbes (fungi and bacteria) thrive in the warm, wet, dark environment of macerated skin between two apposed skin surfaces. Of these, it is the wet component which is most easily modified. Before moving to maintenance treatment with a barrier product alone, it may be necessary to treat any local infection (most likely fungal).

Thus, for some patients, initial treatment will include the *topical* use of a broad-spectrum antifungal, e.g. **clotrimazole**, **miconazole** (both available OTC), **ketoconazole**. Sometimes, if the area is inflamed, the use of a topical low-potency corticosteroid for 3–7 days accelerates improvement, e.g. **desonide** 0.05% (see p.458). Thus, initial treatment (after topical cleansing and blow-drying with a hand-held hairdryer) may comprise:
- topical antimicrobial or topical corticosteroid
- barrier product
- corn starch powder (absorbent; better than talc which can be an irritant) is sometimes used, but opinion is divided on whether it may act as a culture medium for bacteria and *Candida albicans*.[1,2]

Protection around the stoma
Many specialist products designed to protect the skin around a stoma from liquid effluent are available; a stoma nurse can advise on product selection. Sprays or wipes which dry to form a protective film are commonly used. An alcohol-free formulation is preferable because it is less likely to sting or irritate the skin, e.g. Cavilon No-Sting Barrier Film®.

Incontinence
After cleansing and gently drying, apply a barrier product to the affected area whenever the dressing or padding is changed.

Supply
The following is only a selection of the available products. All the products listed are available OTC except **ketoconazole**.

Ointments
Desitin® diaper rash ointment (Johnson & Johnson)
Zinc oxide 37%, cod-liver oil 14%, 60g = $7, 130g = $10.

Zincofax® (Squire)
Zinc oxide 15%, 50g = $7, 130g = $11; available in original and fragrance-free formulations.

Zincofax® Extra Strength (Squire)
Zinc oxide 40%, 100g = $11.

Critic-Aid Clear® (Coloplast)
Dimethicone, white petrolatum 71.5%, 4g single-use pack = $1, 71g = $13.

Proshield Plus® treatment film ointment (Healthpoint)
Dimethicone 1%, 115g = $16.

Creams
Barrier cream 20%® (Wellspring)
Silicone 20%, 50g = $6, 100g = $10, 450g = $35.

Cavilon Durable® barrier cream (3M)
Dimethicone, coconut oil, mineral oil, petrolatum (paraffin), 92g = $9.

Zinc oxide 15% (generic), 50g = $6, 130g = $6, 450g = $20.

Baza Protect® (Coloplast)
Zinc oxide 12%, **dimethicone** 1%, 60g = $6, 140g = $12.

Sween 24® (Coloplast)
Dimethicone 6%, glycerin, 4g single-use pack = $1, 90g = $9.

Stoma products
Cavilon® no-sting barrier film (3M)
Wipes 25 × 1mL = $36.
Pump spray 28mL = $24.

Antifungal products
Clotrimazole 1% (generic)
Cream 20g = $8, 30g = $12, 50g = $17.

Canesten® topical cream (Bayer)
Cream 15g = $10, 30g = $16.

Ketoconazole 2%
Ketoderm® (Taro)
Cream 30g = $10.

Miconazole 2%
Micatin® (Wellspring Pharmaceutical Canada)
Cream 30g = $17.
Spray 85g = $11.

Monistat-Derm® (Johnson & Johnson)
Cream 15g = $11, 30g = $20.

Topical corticosteroid
For **desonide** 0.05%, see p.459.

---

1 Sibbald D (2002) Dermatitis. In: C Repchinsky (ed) *Patient Self-care* (2e). Canadian Pharmacists Association, Ottawa, pp. 479–505.
2 Mitchell W and Lynh P (1996) *Principles and Practice of Dermatology (2e)*. Churchill Livingstone, New York, pp. 419–426.

13: ANESTHESIA

GLYCOPYRROLATE (GLYCOPYRRONIUM)

Class: Antimuscarinic (anticholinergic).

Indications: Smooth muscle spasm (e.g. intestine, †bladder), drying secretions (including surgical premedication, control of upper airway secretions, †sialorrhea, †drooling, †noisy respiratory secretions (death rattle) and †inoperable intestinal obstruction), †paraneoplastic pyrexia and sweating, †hyperhidrosis.

Pharmacology

Glycopyrrolate (rINN glycopyrronium) is a synthetic ionized quaternary ammonium antimuscarinic that penetrates biological membranes slowly and erratically.[1] In consequence it rarely causes sedation or delirium.[2,3] Absorption PO is poor and the IV to PO potency ratio is about 35:1.[4] Even so, glycopyrrolate 200–400microgram PO t.i.d. produces plasma concentrations associated with an antisialogogic effect lasting up to 8h.[5–7] By injection, glycopyrrolate is 2–5 times more potent than **scopolamine (hyoscine) hydrobromide** as an antisecretory drug,[4] and may be effective in some patients who fail to respond to **scopolamine**. However, the efficacy of **scopolamine hydrobromide**, hyoscine (**scopolamine**) **butylbromide** and glycopyrrolate as antisialogogues is generally similar, with noisy respiratory secretions (death rattle) reduced in 1/2–2/3 of patients.[8] The optimal parenteral single dose is 200microgram.[9] Compared with **scopolamine hydrobromide**, the onset of action of glycopyrrolate is slower.[10] It has fewer cardiac effects because of a reduced affinity for muscarinic-type 2 receptors.[11–13] Although at standard doses glycopyrrolate does not change ocular pressures or pupil size, it can precipitate narrow-angle glaucoma. It is excreted by the kidneys and lower doses are effective in patients with renal impairment.[1,14] Glycopyrrolate has also been used for paraneoplastic pyrexia and sweating, localized hyperhidrosis[15,16] and (inhaled or nebulized) as a bronchodilator.[17]
Bio-availability <5% PO.
Onset of action 1min IV; 30–40min SC, PO.
Time to peak plasma concentration immediate IV; no data SC, PO.
Plasma halflife 1.7h.
Duration of action 7–8h.

Cautions

Competitively blocks the prokinetic effect of **metoclopramide** and **domperidone**.[18] Increases the peripheral antimuscarinic toxicity of antihistamines, phenothiazines and TCAs (see Antimuscarinics, p.5). Use with caution in conditions predisposing to tachycardia (e.g. thyrotoxicosis, heart failure, concurrent β_2-agonists), and bladder outflow obstruction (prostatism). Likely to exacerbate acid reflux. Narrow-angle glaucoma may be precipitated in those at risk, particularly the elderly. Use in hot weather or pyrexia may lead to heatstroke.

Undesirable effects

For full list, see manufacturer's Product Monograph.
Peripheral antimuscarinic effects (see p.5).
Very common (>10%): inflammation at the injection site.
Common (<10%, >1%): dysphagia, photosensitivity.

Dose and use

Glycopyrrolate is an alternative to **scopolamine** *hydrobromide*, **hyoscine** *butylbromide* and **atropine**.[19–21]

Glycopyrrolate is compatible with fentanyl, lorazepam, morphine sulfate, meperidine and promethazine. It is incompatible with dexamethasone, diazepam, dimenhydrinate, methylprednisolone and phenobarbital (also see Charts A4.1–A4.4, p.591).

Drooling

Administer as a compounded solution PO:
- start with 200microgram PO stat and q8h
- if necessary, increase dose progressively every 2–3 days to 500–600microgram q8h
- occasionally doses of up to 2mg q8h are needed.

A subsequent reduction in dose may be possible, particularly when initial dose escalation has been rapid. Can be given by gastrostomy tube.[7]

Several formulae are available for compounded oral solutions with examples shown in Box 13.A.[22,23] It is much cheaper to use the powder than the injection for compounding; 10mg of glycopyrrolate costs $93 using 50mL of injection from 20mL vials, but only $1 using powder.

Box 13.A   Examples of compounded oral solutions of glycopyrrolate

Based on glycopyrrolate injection
Glycopyrrolate 100microgram/mL (1mg/10mL)[23]
Combine 25mL of Ora-Plus® and 25mL of Ora-Sweet®; add to 50mL of preservative-free glycopyrrolate injection USP 200microgram/mL to make up to 100mL, and mix well.
Stable for 35 days at room temperature or in a refrigerator (refrigeration minimizes risk of microbial contamination).
In a taste test, this formulation masked the bitter taste of glycopyrrolate better than water or syrup-based vehicles, and was preferred by 4/5 patients.

Based on glycopyrrolate powder
Glycopyrrolate 500microgram/mL (5mg/10mL)[22]
Add 5mL of glycerin to 50mg of glycopyrrolate powder and mix to form a smooth paste. Add 50mL of Ora-Plus® in portions and mix well. Add sufficient Ora-Sweet® or Ora-Sweet SF® to make a total volume of 100mL.
This solution is stable for 90 days at room temperature or in a refrigerator.

Noisy respiratory secretions (death rattle)
- 200microgram SC stat and p.r.n.[24] *or*
- 200microgram SC stat and 600–1,200microgram/24h CSCI.

Antispasmodic and inoperable intestinal obstruction
- 200microgram SC stat and p.r.n. *or*
- 200microgram SC stat and 600–1,200microgram/24h CSCI.

Paraneoplastic pyrexia and sweating
- for long-term use and higher doses, use a compounded aqueous solution (Box 13.A)
- start with 200microgram PO t.i.d.
- if necessary, increase progressively to 2mg PO t.i.d.

Localized hyperhidrosis
- apply topically as a 0.5–4% cream (Box 13.B) or aqueous solution once daily–b.i.d., avoiding the nose, mouth and particularly the eyes; do not wash treated skin for 3–4h[16,25]
- if severe, or if alternative treatments fail, 1–2mg PO as a compounded solution b.i.d.–t.i.d., titrated to response.[15]

Box 13.B Compounded glycopyrrolate cream 1%[26]

Mix 1g of glycopyrrolate powder with propylene glycol to make a paste. Incorporate into a water-washable cream base until smooth, making a total of 100g. Refrigerate after compounding. Expiry date: 60 days.

Supply
Glycopyrrolate (generic)
Injection 200microgram/mL, 1mL amp = $4, 2mL amp = $7, 20mL vial = $37.

Glycopyrrolate (Galenova)
Compounding powder for oral solutions and topical formulations (See Box 13.A and Box 13.B), obtainable from www.galenova.com, 1g = $99, 5g = $458.

---

1 Mirakhur R and Dundee J (1983) Glycopyrrolate pharmacology and clinical use. *Anaesthesia.* **38**: 1195–1204.
2 Gram D *et al.* (1991) Central anticholinergic syndrome following glycopyrrolate. *Anesthesiology.* **74**: 191–193.
3 Wigard D (1991) Glycopyrrolate and the central anticholinergic syndrome (letter). *Anesthesiology.* **75**: 1125.
4 Mirakhur R and Dundee J (1980) A comparison of the effects of atropine and glycopyrrollate on various end organs. *Journal of the Royal Society of Medicine.* **73**: 727–730.
5 Ali-Melkkila T *et al.* (1989) Glycopyrrolate; pharmacokinetics and some pharmacodynamics findings. *Acta Anaesthesiologica Scandinavica.* **33**: 513–517.
6 Blasco P (1996) Glycopyrrolate treatment of chronic drooling. *Archives of Paediatric and Adolescent Medicine.* **150**: 932–935.
7 Olsen A and Sjogren P (1999) Oral glycopyrrolate alleviates drooling in a patient with tongue cancer. *Journal of Pain and Symptom Management.* **18**: 300–302.
8 Hughes A *et al.* (2000) Audit of three antimuscarinic drugs for managing retained secretions. *Palliative Medicine.* **14**: 221–222.
9 Mirakhur R *et al.* (1978) Evaluation of the anticholinergic actions of glycopyrronium bromide. *British Journal of Clinical Pharmacology.* **5**: 77–84.
10 Back I *et al.* (2001) A study comparing hyoscine hydrobromide and glycopyrrolate in the treatment of death rattle. *Palliative Medicine.* **15**: 329–336.
11 Mirakhur R *et al.* (1978) Atropine and glycopyrronium premedication. A comparison of the effects on cardiac rate and rhythm during induction of anaesthesia. *Anaesthesia.* **33**: 906–912.
12 Warren J *et al.* (1997) Effect of autonomic blockade on power spectrum of heart rate variability during exercise. *American Journal of Physiology.* **273**: 495–502.
13 Scheinin H *et al.* (1999) Spectral analysis of heart rate variability as a quantitative measure of parasympatholytic effect-integrated pharmacokinetics and pharmacodynamics of three anticholinergic drugs. *Therapeutic Drug Monitoring.* **21**: 141–151.
14 Ali-Melkkila T *et al.* (1993) Pharmacokinetics and related pharmacodynamics of anticholinergic drugs. *Acta Anaesthesiologica Scandinavica.* **37**: 633–642.
15 Solish N *et al.* (2007) A comprehensive approach to the recognition, diagnosis, and severity-based treatment of focal hyperhidrosis: recommendations of the Canadian Hyperhidrosis Advisory Committee. *Dermatologic Surgery.* **33**: 908–923.
16 Kim WO *et al.* (2008) Topical glycopyrrolate for patients with facial hyperhidrosis. *British Journal of Dermatology.* **158**: 1094–1097.
17 Hansel TT *et al.* (2005) Glycopyrrolate causes prolonged bronchoprotection and bronchodilatation in patients with asthma. *Chest.* **128**: 1974–1979.
18 Schuurkes JAJ *et al.* (1986) Stimulation of gastroduodenal motor activity: dopaminergic and cholinergic modulation. *Drug Development Research.* **8**: 233–241.
19 Rashid H *et al.* (1997) Management of secretions in esophageal cancer patients with glycopyrrolate. *Annals of Oncology.* **8**: 198–199.
20 Lucas V and Amass C (1998) Use of enteral glycopyrrolate in the management of drooling. *Palliative Medicine.* **12**: 207.
21 Davis M and Furste A (1999) Glycopyrrolate: a useful drug in the palliation of mechanical bowel obstruction. *Journal of Pain and Symptom Management.* **18**: 153–154.
22 Anonymous (2004) Glycopyrrolate 0.5mg/mL oral liquid. *International Journal of Pharmaceutical Compounding.* **8**: 218.
23 Landry C *et al.* (2005) Stability and subjective taste acceptability of four glycopyrrolate solutions for oral administration. *International Journal of Pharmaceutical Compounding.* **9**: 396–398.
24 Bennett M *et al.* (2002) Using anti-muscarinic drugs in the management of death rattle: evidence based guidelines for palliative care. *Palliative Medicine.* **16**: 369–374.
25 Kavanagh GM *et al.* (2006) Topical glycopyrrolate should not be overlooked in treatment of focal hyperhidrosis. *British Journal of Dermatology.* **155**: 477–500.
26 Glasnapp A and BJ S (2001) Topical therapy for localized hyperhidrosis. *International Journal of Pharmaceutical Compounding.* **5**: 28–29.

---

*KETAMINE

Class: General anesthetic.

Indications: †pain unresponsive to standard treatments (postoperative, neuropathic, inflammatory, ischemic limb, myofascial and procedure-related).[1-3]

Contra-indications: Any situation in which an increase in blood pressure or intracranial pressure would constitute a hazard. Acute intermittent porphyria.

Pharmacology

The NMDA-glutamate receptor is a calcium channel closely involved in the development of central (dorsal horn) sensitization (Figure 13.1).[4] At normal resting membrane potentials, the channel is blocked by magnesium and inactive.[5] When the resting membrane potential is changed as a result of prolonged excitation, the channel unblocks with a reduction in opioid-responsiveness and the development of allodynia and hyperalgesia. These effects are probably mediated by the intracellular formation of nitric oxide.[6]

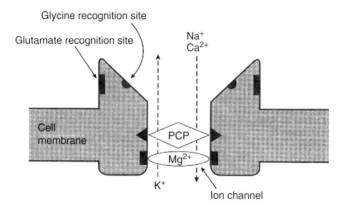

Figure 13.1 Diagram of NMDA (excitatory) receptor-channel complex. The channel is blocked by Mg^{2+} when the membrane potential is at its resting level (voltage-dependent block) and by drugs which act at the phencyclidine (PCP) binding site in the glutamate-activated channel, e.g. dextromethorphan, ketamine, methadone (use-dependent block).[4]

Ketamine is a dissociative anesthetic which has analgesic properties in sub-anesthetic doses.[3,7] Ketamine is the most potent NMDA-receptor-channel blocker available for clinical use, binding to the phencyclidine site when the channels are in the open activated state.[8] It also binds to a second membrane-associated site which does not require the channel to be open and thereby decreases the frequency of channel opening.[9] In some countries, both the racemic mixture and the S-enantiomer are commercially available for clinical use; only the racemic mixture is available in Canada. Because of its greater affinity and selectivity for the NMDA-receptor, the S-enantiomer (parenterally) is about 4 times more potent as an analgesic than the R-enantiomer and twice as potent as the racemic mixture.[10-12] When equi-analgesic doses are compared, the S-enantiomer is also associated with lower levels of undesirable effects, e.g. anxiety, tiredness, cognitive impairment.[11,13] However, no significant differences in efficacy or tolerability were found between the PO racemic mixture (median dose 320mg/24h), the S-enantiomer or placebo in patients with cancer-related neuropathic pain.[14] Ketamine has other actions which may also contribute to its analgesic effect, including interactions with other calcium and sodium channels, dopamine receptors, cholinergic transmission, noradrenergic and serotoninergic re-uptake inhibition (intact descending inhibitory pathways are necessary for analgesia) μ, δ and κ opioid-like effects and an anti-inflammatory effect.[15,16] Ketamine also appears to have an antidepressant effect in patients with major depression.[17,18]

A systematic review of sub-anesthetic doses of ketamine as an adjunct to opioid-based postoperative analgesia identified 37 double-blind RCTs, and concluded that IV or ED ketamine was effective and did not increase undesirable effects. CIVI (generally 0.12–0.6mg/kg/h) was best for surgery associated with high opioid requirements, although a single IV dose (generally 0.15–1mg/kg) may suffice for minor surgery. Adding ketamine to IV patient-controlled analgesia (PCA) was *not* effective. Ketamine reduced the incidence of chronic post-surgical pain, e.g. post-thoracotomy pain.[19] Conversely, a systematic review of ketamine as an adjuvant to opioids for cancer pain found only two studies and concluded that there was insufficient robust evidence to reach a conclusion.[20] Thus, in patients with cancer, evidence of ketamine's efficacy as an analgesic is mainly from case reports, retrospective surveys or uncontrolled studies in patients with neuropathic pain.[21–30] A few prospective studies or RCTs have been published in refractory pain in cancer, including neuropathic, bone and mucositis-related.[31–36] In chronic non-cancer pain, evidence of benefit is mixed and undesirable effects occur in about 1/2 of patients.[3,37] Ketamine may be less effective in neuropathic pain of long duration ($\geqslant$3 years).[12,38] Generally, ketamine is used in addition to **morphine** or alternative strong opioid when further opioid increments have been ineffective or precluded by unacceptable undesirable effects. When used in this way, ketamine is generally administered PO or SC.[23,29] It can also be administered IM, IV, SL, intranasally, PR and spinally (preservative-free formulation; not Canada).[34,38–43]

There is some evidence that short-term 'burst' treatment with ketamine may have relatively long-term benefit. For example, in patients taking regular strong opioids for ischemic limb pain, a single 4h IV infusion of ketamine 0.6mg/kg reduced opioid requirements during a week of observation.[44] Ketamine 100mg/24h by CIVI for 2 days in a cancer patient, repeated a month later, reduced opioid requirements by 70%.[45] In several case series of cancer patients with severe intractable pain from various causes, 'burst' ketamine 100–500mg/24h by CSCI for 3–5 days relieved pain in about 50% of patients.[31,35,46] Relief lasted from several days to 4 weeks, and occasionally for 2 months. In one study using this regimen, although there were no withdrawals, 1/4 of patients experienced severe undesirable effects, such as sedation and confusion.[31]

PO ketamine undergoes extensive first-pass hepatic metabolism mainly to norketamine (via CYP3A4).[47] As an *anesthetic*, norketamine is about 1/3 as potent as parenteral ketamine. However, as an *analgesic* it is equipotent. The maximum blood concentration of norketamine is greater after PO administration than after injection,[48] and in chronic use norketamine may be the main analgesic agent. This possibly explains why, when switching from CSCI to PO after weeks-months, an equi-analgesic PO dose is *smaller* than the parenteral dose. It can be as little as 25–50% of the previous parenteral dose.[26] Less than 10% of ketamine is excreted unchanged, 1/2 in the feces and 1/2 renally. Long-term use of ketamine leads to hepatic enzyme induction and enhanced ketamine metabolism.

Ketamine causes tachycardia and intracranial hypertension. Most patients experience vivid dreams, misperceptions, hallucinations and alterations in body image and mood as emergent (psychotomimetic) phenomena after anesthetic use, i.e. as the effects of a bolus dose wear off. These occur to a lesser extent with the sub-anesthetic analgesic doses given PO or CSCI, and generally can be controlled by a benzodiazepine or **haloperidol**.[34,49,50] Sub-anesthetic doses of ketamine are associated with impaired attention, memory and judgement and it is used as a pharmacological model for acute schizophrenia.[3]

Bio-availability 93% IM; 30% SL; 20% PO.[51]
Onset of action 5min IM; 15–30min SC; 30min PO.
Time to peak plasma concentration no data SC; 30min PO; 1h norketamine.[52]
Plasma halflife 1–3h IM; 3h PO; 12h norketamine.[53]
Duration of action 30min–2h IM; generally given by CSCI; 4–6h, sometimes longer PO.[54]

Cautions

Epilepsy, hypertension, heart failure, ischemic heart disease and a history of cerebrovascular accidents.[55] Plasma concentration increased by **diazepam**.

Undesirable effects

For full list, see manufacturer's Product Monograph.
Occur in about 40% of patients when given CSCI; less PO: psychotomimetic phenomena (euphoria, dysphasia, blunted affect, psychomotor retardation, vivid dreams, nightmares, poor concentration, illusions, hallucinations, altered body image), delirium, dizziness, diplopia, blurred vision, nystagmus, altered hearing, hypertension, tachycardia, erythema and pain at injection site.

When used at higher doses in anesthesia, tonic-clonic movements are very common (>10%); however, these have not been reported after oral use or with the lower parenteral doses used for analgesia.

Dose and use

Dose recommendations vary considerably but ketamine is often started in a low dose PO (Box 13.C). An oral solution can be compounded by the pharmacy (Box 13.D). Alternatively, patients can be supplied with vials of ketamine and 1mL graduated syringes. Two needles (one as an air vent) should be inserted in the stopper of the vial to facilitate withdrawing the ketamine; sterility is not necessary for PO administration. Long-term success, i.e. both pain relief and tolerable undesirable effects, varies from <20% to about 50%.[27,38,40,56]

Box 13.C   Dose recommendations for ketamine

PO[23,29,57–59]

Use direct from vial or dilute for convenience to 50mg/5mL (patient adds flavouring of choice, e.g. fruit juice, to mask the bitter taste):
- start with 10–25mg t.i.d.–q.i.d. and p.r.n.
- if necessary, increase dose in steps of 10–25mg up to 50mg q.i.d.
- maximum reported dose 200mg q.i.d.[57,59]
- give a smaller dose more frequently if psychotomimetic phenomena or drowsiness occurs which does not respond to a reduction in opioid.

SL[43]
- start with 10–25mg
- place SL and ask patient not to swallow for 2min
- use a high concentration to minimize dose volume; retaining >2mL is difficult.

SC[29]
- typically 10–25mg p.r.n., some use 2.5–5mg
- if necessary, increase dose in steps of 25–33%.

CSCI[21–23,25,49,60]

Because ketamine is irritant, dilute to the largest practical volume, preferably using 0.9% saline (see CSCI, Diluent section, p.515):
- start with 1–2.5mg/kg/24h
- if necessary, increase by 50–100mg/24h
- maximum reported dose 3.6g/24h.
Alternatively, give as short-term 'burst' therapy:[31,35,46]
- start with 100mg/24h
- if 100mg not effective, increase after 24h to 300mg/24h
- if 300mg not effective, increase after further 24h to 500mg/24h
- stop 3 days after last dose increment.
Fifty percent of patients respond and the regimen can be repeated p.r.n.; the duration of benefit varies and undesirable effects are common. The use of prophylactic diazepam, lorazepam, midazolam or haloperidol is recommended (see text).

IV[29,61]

For cancer pain:
- 2.5–5mg.
To cover procedures which may cause severe pain:
- 0.5–1mg/kg (typically 25–50mg; some start with 5–10mg), given over 1–2min preceded by lorazepam 1mg or midazolam 0.1mg/kg (typically 5–10mg; some start with 1–2mg) to reduce emergent phenomena (also see p.313).
The right dose should provide analgesia within 1–5min lasting for 10–20min. Procedures of longer duration may require ketamine CIVI; obtain advice from an anesthetist.

Box 13.D   Preparation of ketamine oral solution: pharmacy guidelines

Use ketamine 50mg/mL 10mL vials because this is the cheapest concentration. Simple syrup USP can be used for dilution but this is too sweet for some patients. Alternatively, use purified water as the diluent and ask patients to add their own flavouring, e.g. fruit juice, just before use to disguise the bitter taste.

To prepare 100mL of 50mg/5mL oral solution:
• 2 × 10mL vials of ketamine 50mg/mL for injection
• 80mL purified water.
Store in a refrigerator with an expiry date of 1 week from manufacture.

When given by CSCI, ketamine is often mixed with **morphine** ± other drugs. Most likely mixtures are known to be compatibile in 0.9% saline (see Charts A4.1–A4.4, p.591). Compatibility data in WFI can be found on www.palliativedrugs.com *Syringe Driver Survey Database* (SDSD). Note: UK manufacturer's data on file states that ketamine forms precipitates with barbiturates and **diazepam**, and thus should not be mixed. Mixing **lorazepam** with ketamine is also not recommended; there is a lack of compatibility data and a risk of adsorption to the tubing.

Some centres routinely reduce the opioid dose by 25–50% when commencing parenteral ketamine. The dose of opioid should be reduced if the patient becomes drowsy. If a patient experiences dysphoria or hallucinations, the dose of ketamine should be reduced and a benzodiazepine prescribed, e.g. **diazepam** 5mg PO stat & at bedtime, **lorazepam** 1mg PO/SL stat & b.i.d., **midazolam** 5mg SC stat and 5–10mg CSCI, or **haloperidol**, e.g. 2–5mg PO stat & at bedtime, 2–5mg SC stat and 2–5mg CSCI.[50] In patients at greatest risk of dysphoria, i.e. those with high anxiety levels, these measures may be more effective if given before starting ketamine.[8]

After weeks–months of use, when switching from CSCI to PO ketamine, a *smaller* total daily dose (25–50% of the parenteral dose) maintains a similar level of analgesia, e.g. CSCI 400mg/24h → PO 150mg/24h (see Pharmacology).[26] However, when switching from CSCI to PO after just a few days, a conversion ratio of 1:1 should be used.[28]

After long-term use it may be preferable to discontinue ketamine gradually; whole body hyperalgesia and allodynia have been reported after the sudden cessation of ketamine after 3 weeks of use.[62]

Ketamine is sometimes used with **fentanyl** and **midazolam** to control intractable pain and agitation.[63,64]

Supply

Unless stated otherwise, all products are **Schedule 1 controlled drugs** under the Controlled Drugs and Substances Act, and listed in the Schedule to the Narcotic Control Regulations.

Ketamine (generic)
Injection 10mg/mL, 2mL vial = $3, 20mL vial = $23; 50mg/mL, 2mL vial = $9, 10mL vial = $38.

Ketalar® (Erfa Canada)
Injection 10mg/mL, 20mL vial = $30; 50mg/mL, 10mL vial = $49.
Although its use as an analgesic is off-label, ketamine injection can be prescribed both in hospitals and in the community.

---

1 Persson J et al. (1998) The analgesic effect of racemic ketamine in patients with chronic ischemic pain due to lower extremity arteriosclerosis obliterans. *Acta Anaesthesiologica Scandinavica.* **42**: 750–758.

2 Graven-Nielsen T et al. (2000) Ketamine reduces muscle pain, temporal summation, and referred pain in fibromyalgia patients. *Pain.* **85**: 483–491.

3 Visser E and Schug SA (2006) The role of ketamine in pain management. *Biomedicine and Pharmacotherapy.* **60**: 341–348.

4 Richens A (1991) The basis of the treatment of epilepsy: neuropharmacology. In: M Dam (ed) *A Practical Approach to Epilepsy.* Pergamon Press, Oxford, pp. 75–85.

5 Mayer M et al. (1984) Voltage-dependent block for Mg^{2+} of NMDA responses in spinal cord neurones. *Nature.* **309**: 261–263.

6 Elliott K et al. (1994) The NMDA receptor antagonists, LY274614 and MK-801, and the nitric oxide synthase inhibitor, NG-nitro-L-arginine, attenuate analgesic tolerance to the mu-opioid morphine but not to kappa opioids. *Pain.* **56**: 69–75.

7 Fallon MT and Welsh J (1996) The role of ketamine in pain control. *European Journal of Palliative Care.* **3**: 143–146.

8 Oye I (1998) Ketamine analgesia, NMDA receptors and the gates perception. *Acta Anaesthesiologica Scandinavica.* **42**: 747–749.

9 Orser B et al. (1997) Multiple mechanisms of ketamine blockade of N-methyl-D-aspartate receptors. *Anesthesiology.* **86**: 903–917.

---

10 Oye I et al. (1991) The chiral forms of ketamine as probes for NMDA receptor function in humans. In: T Kameyama (ed) NMDA Receptor Related Agents: Biochemistry, Pharmacology and Behavior. NPP, Ann Arbor, Michigan, pp. 381–389.
11 White PF et al. (1980) Pharmacology of ketamine isomers in surgical patients. Anesthesiology. 52: 231–239.
12 Mathisen L et al. (1995) Effect of ketamine, an NMDA receptor inhibitor, in acute and chronic orofacial pain. Pain. 61: 215–220.
13 Pfenninger EG et al. (2002) Cognitive impairment after small-dose ketamine isomers in comparison to equianalgesic racemic ketamine in human volunteers. Anesthesiology. 96: 357–366.
14 Fallon M Personal communication.
15 Meller S (1996) Ketamine: relief from chronic pain through actions at the NMDA receptor? Pain. 68: 435–436.
16 Kawasaki C et al. (2001) Ketamine isomers suppress superantigen-induced proinflammatory cytokine production in human whole blood. Canadian Journal of Anaesthetics. 48: 819–823.
17 Berman R et al. (2000) Antidepressant effects of ketamine in depressed patients. Biological Psychiatry. 47: 351–354.
18 Zarate CA, Jr. et al. (2006) A randomized trial of an N-methyl-D-aspartate antagonist in treatment-resistant major depression. Archives of General Psychiatry. 63: 856–864.
19 Subramaniam K et al. (2004) Ketamine as adjuvant analgesic to opioids: a quantitative and qualitative systematic review. Anesthesia and Analgesia. 99: 482–495, table of contents.
20 Bell RF et al. (2003) Ketamine as adjuvant to opioids for cancer pain. A qualitative systematic review. Journal of Pain and Symptom Management. 26: 867–875.
21 Oshima E et al. (1990) Continuous subcutaneous injection of ketamine for cancer pain. Canadian Journal of Anaesthetics. 37: 385–392.
22 Cherry DA et al. (1995) Ketamine as an adjunct to morphine in the treatment of pain. Pain. 62: 119–121.
23 Luczak J et al. (1995) The role of ketamine, an NMDA receptor antagonist, in the management of pain. Progress in Palliative Care. 3: 127–134.
24 Mercadante S (1996) Ketamine in cancer pain: an update. Palliative Medicine. 10: 225–230.
25 Bell R (1999) Low-dose subcutaneous ketamine infusion and morphine tolerance. Pain. 83: 101–103.
26 Fitzgibbon EJ et al. (2002) Low dose ketamine as an analgesic adjuvant in difficult pain syndromes: a strategy for conversion from parenteral to oral ketamine. Journal of Pain and Symptom Management. 23: 165–170.
27 Kannan TR et al. (2002) Oral ketamine as an adjuvant to oral morphine for neuropathic pain in cancer patients. Journal of Pain and Symptom Management. 23: 60–65.
28 Benitez-Rosario M et al. (2003) A retrospective comparison of the dose ratio between subcutaneous and oral ketamine. Journal of Pain and Symptom Management. 25: 400–402.
29 Kotlinska-Lemieszek A and Luczak J (2004) Subanesthetic ketamine: an essential adjuvant for intractable cancer pain. Journal of Pain and Symptom Management. 28: 100–102.
30 Fitzgibbon EJ and Viola R (2005) Parenteral ketamine as an analgesic adjuvant for severe pain: development and retrospective audit of a protocol for a palliative care unit. Journal of Palliative Medicine. 8: 49–57.
31 Jackson K and Howell D Personal communication.
32 Yang CY et al. (1996) Intrathecal ketamine reduces morphine requirements in patients with terminal cancer pain. Canadian Journal of Anaesthesia. 43: 379–383.
33 Lauretti G et al. (1999) Oral ketamine and transdermal nitroglycerin as analgesic adjuvants to oral morphine therapy and amitriptyline for cancer pain management. Anesthesiology. 90: 1528–1533.
34 Mercadante S et al. (2000) Analgesic effect of intravenous ketamine in cancer patients on morphine therapy: a randomized, controlled, double-blind, crossover, double-dose study. Journal of Pain and Symptom Management. 20: 246–252.
35 Jackson K et al. (2001) 'Burst' ketamine for refractory cancer pain: an open-label audit of 39 patients. Journal of Pain and Symptom Management. 22: 834–842.
36 Lossignol DA et al. (2005) Successful use of ketamine for intractable cancer pain. Supportive Care in Cancer. 13: 188–193.
37 Hocking G and Cousins MJ (2003) Ketamine in chronic pain management: an evidence-based review. Anesthesia and Analgesia. 97: 1730–1739.
38 Haines D and Gaines S (1999) N of 1 randomised controlled trials of oral ketamine in patients with chronic pain. Pain. 83: 283–287.
39 Lin T et al. (1998) Long-term epidural ketamine, morphine and bupivacaine attenuate reflex sympathetic dystrophy neuralgia. Canadian Journal of Anaesthesia. 45: 175–177.
40 Batchelor G (1999) Ketamine in neuropathic pain. The Pain Society Newsletter. 1: 19.
41 Beltrutti D et al. (1999) The epidural and intrathecal administration of ketamine. Current Review of Pain. 3: 458–472.
42 Carr DB et al. (2004) Safety and efficacy of intranasal ketamine for the treatment of breakthrough pain in patients with chronic pain: a randomized, double-blind, placebo-controlled, crossover study. Pain. 108: 17–27.
43 Mercadante S et al. (2005) Alternative treatments of breakthrough pain in patients receiving spinal analgesics for cancer pain. Journal of Pain and Symptom Management. 30: 485–491.
44 Mitchell AC and Fallon MT (2002) A single infusion of intravenous ketamine improves pain relief in patients with critical limb ischaemia: results of a double blind randomised controlled trial. Pain. 97: 275–281.
45 Mercadante S et al. (2003) Burst ketamine to reverse opioid tolerance in cancer pain. Journal of Pain and Symptom Management. 25: 302–305.
46 Wilcock A (2005) Data on file. Burst ketamine in cancer patients.
47 Hijazi Y et al. (2002) Contribution of CYP3A4, CYP2B6, and CYP2C9 isoforms to N-demethylation of ketamine in human liver microsomes. Drug Metabolism & Disposition. 30: 853–858.
48 Clements JA et al. (1982) Bio-availability, pharmacokinetics and analgesic activity of ketamine in humans. Journal of Pharmaceutical Sciences. 71: 539–542.
49 Hughes A et al. (1999) Ketamine. CME Bulletin Palliative Medicine. 1: 53.
50 Giannini A et al. (2000) Acute ketamine intoxication treated by haloperidol: a preliminary study. American Journal of Therapeutics. 7: 389–391.
51 Chong CC et al. (2006) Bioavailability of Ketamine After Oral or Sublingual Administration. Pain Medicine. 7: 469–469.
52 Grant IS et al. (1981) Pharmacokinetics and analgesic effects of IM and oral ketamine. British Journal of Anaesthesia. 53: 805–810.
53 Domino E et al. (1984) Ketamine kinetics in unmedicated and diazepam premedicated subjects. Clinical Pharmacology and Therapeutics. 36: 645–653.
54 Rabben T et al. (1999) Prolonged analgesic effect of ketamine, an N-methyl-D-aspartate receptor inhibitor, in patients with chronic pain. Journal of Pharmacology and Experimental Therapeutics. 289: 1060–1066.
55 Ward J and Standage C (2003) Angina pain precipitated by a continuous subcutaneous infusion of ketamine. Journal of Pain and Symptom Management. 25: 6–7.

56 Enarson M et al. (1999) Clinical experience with oral ketamine. *Journal of Pain and Symptom Management*. **17**: 384–386.
57 Clark JL and Kalan GE (1995) Effective treatment of severe cancer pain of the head using low–dose ketamine in an opioid-tolerant patient. *Journal of Pain and Symptom Management*. **10**: 310–314.
58 Broadley K et al. (1996) Ketamine injection used orally. *Palliative Medicine*. **10**: 247–250.
59 Vielvoye-Kerkmeer A (2000) Clinical experience with ketamine. *Journal of Pain and Symptom Management*. **19**: 3.
60 Lloyd-Williams M (2000) Ketamine for cancer pain. *Journal of Pain and Symptom Management*. **19**: 79–80.
61 Mason KP et al. (2002) Evolution of a protocol for ketamine-induced sedation as an alternative to general anesthesia for interventional radiologic procedures in pediatric patients. *Radiology*. **225**: 457–465.
62 Mitchell AC (1999) Generalized hyperalgesia and allodynia following abrupt cessation of subcutaneous ketamine infusion. *Palliative Medicine*. **13**: 427–428.
63 Berger J et al. (2000) Ketamine-fentanyl-midazolam infusion for the control of symptoms in terminal life care. *American Journal of Hospice and Palliative Care*. **17 (2)**: 127–132.
64 Enck R (2000) A ketamine, fentanyl, and midazolam infusion for uncontrolled terminal pain and agitation. *American Journal of Hospice and Palliative Care*. **17 (2)**: 76–77.

*PROPOFOL

Class: General anesthetic.

Indications: Induction and maintenance of general anesthesia, continuous conscious sedation (surgical or diagnostic procedures, intubated and mechanically ventilated patients on intensive therapy units). †Refractory agitated delirium or intolerable distress in the imminently dying, †intractable nausea and vomiting.[1]

Contra-indications: Continuous conscious sedation in children ≤18 years. When used for sedation in children in intensive care, the death rate was increased 2–3 times.[2] Allergy to eggs or soya (the available products contain purified egg phosphatide as an emulsifying agent and soya bean oil).[3]

Pharmacology

Propofol is an ultrafast-acting IV anesthetic drug. It is rapidly metabolized, mainly in the liver, to inactive compounds which are excreted in the urine. The incidence of untoward hemodynamic changes is low. Propofol reduces cerebral blood flow, cerebral metabolism and, less consistently, intracranial pressure.[4] The reduction in intracranial pressure is greater if the baseline pressure is raised. On discontinuation, patients rapidly regain consciousness (10–30min) without a hangover effect.

Propofol is used to relieve refractory agitated delirium or intolerable distress in the imminently dying. Careful titration generally permits 'conscious sedation', i.e. patients open their eyes on verbal command, possess intact autonomic reflexes and tolerate mild noxious stimuli.[1]

Propofol also has an anti-emetic effect resulting in less postoperative vomiting compared with other anesthetic agents.[5–7] Specific postoperative anti-emetic regimens have been designed.[8–10] Chemotherapy-related nausea and vomiting is also helped by adjunctive propofol.[11] In patients receiving non-platinum regimens who were refractory to a combination of **dexamethasone** and a 5HT$_3$-receptor antagonist, propofol was of benefit in ≥80%.[12] Propofol has also been used to relieve refractory nausea and vomiting in dying patients.[1] It was more effective in relieving nausea than vomiting, although most of the patients probably had bowel obstruction.

Animal studies suggest that the mechanism of action of propofol as an anti-emetic is by inhibition of serotonin release by enhancing GABA activity, possibly by direct GABA-mediated action on 5HT$_3$-receptors in the area postrema/chemoreceptor trigger zone.[13]

Propofol also has antipruritic, anxiolytic, bronchodilatory, muscle relaxant and anti-epileptic properties. A possible role in refractory status epilepticus requires further clarification.[14,15] Transient excitatory phenomena are seen occasionally (e.g. myoclonus, opisthotonus, tonic-clonic activity), during induction or recovery when blood levels are low, and presumably at a time when inhibitory centres but not excitatory centres have been depressed.[4,16]

Onset of action 0.5min.

Time to peak effect 5min.

Plasma halflife 2–4min initial distribution phase; 30–60min slow distribution and initial elimination phase; 3–12h terminal elimination phase. The terminal elimination halflife may increase with prolonged use.

Duration of action 3–10min after single IV bolus.[17,18]

Cautions

Risk of cardiorespiratory depression. Involuntary movements and seizures have been reported, particularly in epileptics, during induction or recovery.[16,19] With prolonged use in acute intensive care, metabolic acidosis, hyperlipidemia and hepatomegaly have been reported.[2] Although in this setting it is good practice to check plasma lipid levels in patients receiving propofol for ⩾3 days, it is unnecessary in patients whose expected prognosis is only days.

Disodium edetate (EDTA), the preservative in Diprivan®, is a chelating agent which can reduce circulating concentrations and increase urinary losses of trace metals, e.g. zinc. Supplements should be considered for patients who are likely to receive prolonged propofol treatment, particularly those at particular risk of deficiency, e.g. from fluid loss, catabolic states or infection.

Undesirable effects

For full list, see manufacturer's Product Monograph.
Very common (>10%): local pain at the injection site.
Common (<10%, >1%): headache, hypotension, bradycardia, transient apnea.
Uncommon (<1%, >0.1%): thrombosis, phlebitis.

Dose and use

Propofol is an emulsion of oil-in-water. This gives it a white appearance and makes it a potential growth medium. Diprivan® contains the preservative EDTA, but in a concentration (0.005%) sufficient only to *retard* microbial growth. The generic propofol products available in Canada contain no preservatives. Thus, strict aseptic technique must be employed to prevent microbial contamination *and the container and IV line renewed every 6–12h, in accordance with the individual manufacturer's instructions.*

The use of propofol requires specialist palliative care units to have access to the necessary expertise and equipment. It is generally given by CIVI as an undiluted 1% (10mg/mL) solution through a computer-controlled volumetric infusion pump or IV syringe pump. Pain at the injection site can be minimized by using a large vein in the fore-arm and:
- by co-administering the first dose with **lidocaine**:
  ▷ give 1mL of **lidocaine** 1% IV before starting propofol *or*
  ▷ mix **lidocaine** with propofol immediately before starting the infusion; do not exceed a concentration of 20mg lidocaine/200mg propofol because this can cause the emulsion to separate.

If necessary, the injection can be diluted with 5% dextrose (glucose) immediately before administration. In some countries, dilution is advised if propofol is given through a less sensitive infusion control device, e.g. a drop counter or in-line burette, because the weaker concentration reduces the risk of a severe overdose if the infusion runs fast. Diluted propofol should be used within 6h.

Compatibility: propofol injection 1% is compatible with **alfentanil** and **lidocaine**, and can be diluted with 5% dextrose (glucose) before use (see manufacturer's Product Monograph for details). Propofol can be added through a Y-connector to a running infusion of 5% dextrose, 5% dextrose +0.45% saline, 5% dextrose +0.2% saline, lactated Ringer's solution or lactated Ringer's solution +5% dextrose; the Y-connector should be placed as close to the injection site as possible.

Refractory agitated delirium or intolerable distress in the imminently dying
Consider propofol only if standard treatments have failed (Figure 13.2).[1,20–22] Generally, **phenobarbital** should be used in preference to propofol because it is less complicated for clinical staff to titrate and monitor. At some Canadian centres, **phenobarbital** is given by SC bolus as an adjunct to **midazolam** CSCI (see p.226).

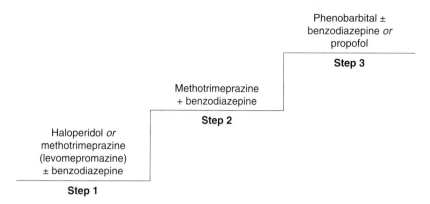

Figure 13.2 Drug treatment for irreversible agitated delirium in the last days of life.

Aim to titrate the dose until conscious sedation is achieved, i.e. patients open their eyes on verbal command but are not distressed by nursing interventions (e.g. mouth care, turning):
- generally start with propofol 1mg/kg/h IV
- if necessary, increase by 0.5mg/kg/h every 5–10min until a satisfactory level of sedation is achieved; smaller dose steps can be used to fine-tune the treatment; most patients respond well to 1–2mg/kg/h
- to increase the level of sedation quickly, a bolus dose can be given by increasing the rate to 1mg/kg/min for 2–5min
- monitor the patient closely during the first hour of treatment with respect to symptom relief and/or level of sedation, and then after 2, 6, and 12h
- continue to monitor the effect of propofol and the level of sedation at least twice daily
- if the patient is too sedated (i.e. does not respond to a verbal command to open their eyes, shows no response to noxious stimuli) and/or there is evidence of drug-induced respiratory depression, the infusion should be turned off for 2–3min and restarted at a lower rate; occasionally this leads to a progressive reduction in dose because the patient has become unconscious as a result of their disease
- tolerance can develop, necessitating a dose increase, but generally not within 1 week
- long-term use of doses >4mg/kg/h is not recommended because of increasing risk of undesirable effects
- if the patient does not respond to propofol 4mg/kg/h alone, supplement with **midazolam** by CSCI
- it is important to replenish the infusion quickly when a container empties, because the effect of propofol wears off after 10–30min
- because propofol has no analgesic properties, analgesics should be continued.

Intractable nausea and vomiting
The use of propofol as an anti-emetic should be considered only if all other treatments have failed (see p.183).[1] Dose titration is generally slower for intractable nausea and vomiting than for terminal agitation:
- generally start with propofol 0.5mg/kg/h
- if necessary, increase by 0.25–0.5mg/kg/h every 30–60min until a satisfactory response is obtained; smaller dose steps can be used to fine-tune the treatment
- most patients respond well to 0.5–1mg/kg/h; doses >1mg/kg/h may result in sedation
- monitor the patient closely during the first hour of treatment with respect to symptom relief and/or level of sedation and then after 2, 6, and 12h
- continue to monitor the effect of propofol and level of sedation at least twice daily
- if the patient is too sedated, the infusion should be turned off for 2–3min and then restarted at a lower rate
- if the patient responds well, reduce the infusion rate on a trial basis after 18–24h

- tolerance can develop, necessitating a dose increase, but generally not within 1 week
- it is important to replenish the infusion quickly when a container empties, because the effect of propofol wears off after 10–30min
- when used solely for its anti-emetic effect in the last days of life, some centres reduce the dose of, or even discontinue, propofol when the patient becomes unconscious.

Supply

Propofol (generic)
Injection (emulsion) 10mg/mL (1%), 20mL amp = $8, 50mL vial = $19, 100mL vial = $38.

Diprivan® (AstraZeneca, Canada)
Injection (emulsion) 10mg/mL (1%), 20mL amp = $10, 50mL vial = $25, 100mL vial = $49.

1 Lundstrom S et al. (2005) When nothing helps: propofol as sedative and antiemetic in palliative cancer care. *Journal of Pain and Symptom Management*. **30**: 570–577.
2 Anonymous (2001) Propofol (Diprivan) infusion: sedation in children aged 16 years or younger contraindicated. *Current Problems in Pharmacovigilance*. **27**: 10.
3 Hofer KN et al. (2003) Possible anaphylaxis after propofol in a child with food allergy. *Annals of Pharmacotherapy*. **37**: 398–401.
4 Mirenda J and Broyles G (1995) Propofol as used for sedation in the ICU. *Chest*. **108**: 539–548.
5 Tramer M et al. (1997) Meta-analytic comparison of prophylactic antiemetic efficacy for postoperative nausea and vomiting: propofol anaesthesia vs omitting nitrous oxide vs total i.v. anaesthesia with propofol. *British Journal of Anaesthesia*. **78**: 256–259.
6 Sneyd JR et al. (1998) A meta-analysis of nausea and vomiting following maintenance of anaesthesia with propofol or inhalational agents. *European Journal of Anaesthesiology*. **15**: 433–445.
7 DeBalli P (2003) The use of propofol as an antiemetic. *International Anesthesiology Clinics*. **41**: 67–77.
8 Gan TJ et al. (1997) Determination of plasma concentrations of propofol associated with 50% reduction in postoperative nausea. *Anesthesiology*. **87**: 779–784.
9 Gan TJ et al. (1999) Patient-controlled antiemesis: a randomized, double-blind comparison of two doses of propofol versus placebo. *Anesthesiology*. **90**: 1564–1570.
10 Fujii Y et al. (2001) Small doses of propofol, droperidol, and metoclopramide for the prevention of postoperative nausea and vomiting after thyroidectomy. *Otolaryngology and Head and Neck Surgery*. **124**: 266–269.
11 Scher C et al. (1992) Use of propofol for the prevention of chemotherapy-induced nausea and emesis in oncology patients. *Canadian Journal of Anaesthesia*. **39**: 170–172.
12 Borgeat A et al. (1994) Adjuvant propofol enables better control of nausea and emesis secondary to chemotherapy for breast cancer. *Canadian Journal of Anaesthesia*. **41**: 1117–1119.
13 Cechetto DF et al. (2001) The effects of propofol in the area postrema of rats. *Anesthesia and Analgesia*. **92**: 934–942.
14 Garcia Penas JJ et al. (2007) Status epilepticus: evidence and controversy. *Neurologist*. **13 (6 suppl 1)**: S62–73.
15 Rossetti AO (2007) Which anesthetic should be used in the treatment of refractory status epilepticus? *Epilepsia*. **48 (suppl 8)**: 52–55.
16 Sneyd JR (1999) Propofol and epilepsy. *British Journal of Anaesthesia*. **82**: 168–169.
17 Jungheinrich C et al. (2002) Pharmacokinetics of the generic formulation propofol 1 fresenius in comparison with the original formulation (Disoprivan 1). *Clinical Drug Investigation*. **22**: 417–427.
18 Fechner J et al. (2004) Comparative pharmacokinetics and pharmacodynamics of the new propofol prodrug GPI 15715 and propofol emulsion. *Anesthesiology*. **101**: 626–639.
19 AstraZeneca (2006) *Data on file*.
20 Mercadante S et al. (1995) Propofol in terminal care. *Journal of Pain and Symptom Management*. **10**: 639–642.
21 Moyle J (1995) The use of propofol in palliative medicine. *Journal of Pain and Symptom Management*. **10**: 643–646.
22 Cheng C et al. (2002) When midazolam fails. *Journal of Pain and Symptom Management*. **23**: 256–265.

14: GUIDANCE ABOUT PRESCRIBING IN PALLIATIVE CARE

In recent years, both national drug regulatory authorities and the general public have become increasingly concerned about the possibility of dangerous/life-threatening adverse drug events. Official documents and drug manufacturers' information increasingly include a warning along the lines of:

'Use the lowest effective dose for the shortest possible time in order to reduce the risk of serious adverse events.'

This advice is, of course, one of the general foundational principles of therapeutic drug use; the advice is simply underlining 'good practice'. Official documents and drug manufacturers' information also highlight when caution is necessary in relation to, for example, hepatic and renal impairment.

In palliative care, many patients are elderly and debilitated, and many have impaired organ function. Accordingly, in *PCF*, it is assumed that prescribers will adopt an appropriately cautious approach in relation to both dose and duration of treatment (also see Getting the most out of PCF, p.xiii).

This chapter, in addition to offering general advice about 'safe prescribing', emphasizes the special needs of children and the elderly, and examines the impact of hepatic and renal impairment.

GENERAL PRINCIPLES

Always remember: drugs are not the total answer for the relief of pain and other symptoms. For many symptoms, the concurrent use of non-drug measures is equally important, and sometimes more important. An holistic approach to patient care is outlined in various national service provision guidelines.[1–3]

The use of drugs should always be within the context of a systematic approach, which is encapsulated in the acronym *EEMMA*:

- *Evaluation* of the impact of the illness on the patient and family, and of the causes of the patient's symptoms (often multifactorial)
- *Explanation* to the patient before starting treatment about what is going on, and what is the most appropriate course of action
- *Management*: correct the correctable, non-drug treatment, drug treatment
- *Monitoring*: frequent review of the impact of treatment; optimizing the doses of symptom relief drugs to maximize benefit and minimize undesirable effects
- *Attention to detail:* do not make unwarranted assumptions; listen actively to the patient, respond to non-verbal and verbal cues.

In palliative care, the axiom *diagnosis before treatment* still holds true. Even when cancer is responsible, a symptom may be caused by different mechanisms. For example, in lung cancer, vomiting may be caused by hypercalcemia or by raised intracranial pressure (to name just two possible causes). Treatment often varies with the cause.

Attention to detail

Attention to detail includes *precision in taking a drug history*. Thus, if a patient says, 'I take **morphine** every 4 hours', the doctor should ask, 'Tell me, when do you take your first dose?' 'And your second dose?', etc. When this is done, it often turns out that the patient is taking **morphine** q.i.d. rather than q4h, and possibly p.r.n. rather than prophylactically. One 90-year-old woman interpreted '**acetaminophen** four times a day' as meaning 0800h, 1200h, 1600h, and 2000h. Regrettably, she regularly woke between 0200h and 0300h in excruciating pain – so much so that she dreaded going to bed at night.

Attention to detail also means giving *clear instructions for drug regimens*. 'Take as much as you like, as often as you like', is a recipe for anxiety and poor symptom relief. The drug regimen should be written out for the patient and their family to work from. Times to be taken, name of drugs, reason for use ('for pain', 'for bowels', etc.) and dose (x mL, y tablets) should all be stated (Figure 14.1 and Figure 14.2). (This will need to be modified if both the patient and the immediate family cannot read.) The patient should also be advised how to obtain further supplies, e.g. from the family physician.

When prescribing an additional drug, it is important to ask:
'What is the treatment goal?'
'How can it be monitored?'
'What is the risk of undesirable effects?'
'What is the risk of drug interactions?'
'Is it possible to stop any of the current medications?'

Safe prescribing

Safe prescribing is a skill, and is crucial to success in symptom management. It extends to considering size, shape and taste of tablets and solutions, and avoiding doses which force patients to take more tablets, and/or open more containers, than would be the case if doses were 'rounded up' to a more convenient tablet size. For example, SR **morphine** 100mg (one tablet, one container) is easier for the patient than 90mg (two tablets and two containers: 60mg + 30mg).

Safe prescribing requires good communication with patients, carers, and other professionals. Poor communication contributes to 1/2 of preventable drug errors.[4] A lack of information and involvement may leave patients dissatisfied.[5] Good communication includes clear documentation (e.g. allergies, co-morbidities, prescription writing).[6–8] The use of a patient's 'logbook' is to be encouraged; this would include important contact names and telephone numbers.

Safe prescribing practice is particularly important in palliative care where polypharmacy, debility, co-morbidities (e.g. renal impairment), involvement of multiple health professionals, and the use of higher risk medications are among the many factors which make such patients particularly vulnerable to problems with adherence (compliance), undesirable effects, medication errors, drug interactions and other potentially preventable burdens.

Monitoring medication

It is often difficult to predict the optimum dose of a symptom relief drug, particularly opioids, laxatives and psychotropics. Further, undesirable effects put drug adherence in jeopardy. Thus, arrangements must be made for monitoring the effects of medication. The responsibility for such monitoring must be clearly stated. Shared decision-making is a definite risk factor for medication errors.[5,9]

Compromise is sometimes necessary

It may be necessary to compromise on complete relief in order to avoid unacceptable undesirable effects. Antimuscarinic effects, e.g. dry mouth or visual disturbance, may limit dose escalation. Also, with inoperable bowel obstruction, it may be better to aim to reduce the incidence of vomiting to once or twice a day rather than to seek to abolish it altogether.

Hospice Home Care

Name Linda Berton   **Age** 58   **Date** 15 December 2009

Tablets/medicines	2 am	On waking	10 am	2 pm	6 pm	Bed time	Purpose
Morphine Solution (2 mg in 1 mL)		10 mL	10 mL	10 mL	10 mL	20 mL	pain relief
Metoclopramide (10 mg tablet)		1	1	1	1	1	anti-sickness
Ibuprofen (400 mg tablet)		2		2		2	pain relief
Sennosides (8.6 mg tablet)			2			2	for bowels
Trazodone (50 mg tablet)						1	for sleep

If troublesome pain: take an extra 10 mL of MORPHINE SOLUTION between regular doses.
If bowels remain constipated: increase SENNOSIDES to 3 tablets twice a day.

- Keep this chart with you so you can show your doctor or nurse this list of what you are taking.
- Ask for a fresh supply of your medication 2–3 days before you need it.
- Sometimes your medication may be supplied in different strengths or presentations. If you have any concerns about this, check with your pharmacist.
- In an emergency, phone _____ and ask to speak to _____

Figure 14.1   Example of a patient's home medication chart (q4h).

Hospice Home Care

Name *Nicolas Crowther*   **Age** *65*   **Date** *15 December 2009*

Tablets/medicines	Breakfast	Midday meal	Evening meal	Bedtime	Purpose
Almagel (suspension)	10 mL	10 mL	10 mL	10 mL	for hiccups
Morphine SR (100 mg tablet)	1			1	pain relief
Naproxen (500 mg tablet)	1			1	pain relief
Sennosides (8.6 mg tablet)	2	2	2	2	for bowels
Haloperidol (1 mg tablet)				1	anti-sickness
Diazepam (5 mg tablet)				1	for sleeping and relaxation

If troublesome pain: take MORPHINE SOLUTION (2 mg in 1 mL) 10 mL, up to every hour.
If troublesome hiccup: take extra 10 mL of ALMAGEL, up to every 2 hours.

- Keep this chart with you so you can show your doctor or nurse this list of what you are taking.
- Ask for a fresh supply of your medication 2–3 days before you need it.
- Sometimes your medication may be supplied in different strengths or presentations. If you have any concerns about this, check with your pharmacist.
- In an emergency, phone _____ and ask to speak to
_____ .

Figure 14.2 Example of a patient's home medication chart (q.i.d.).

Rescue ('as needed') medication

Patients need advice about what to do for episodic symptoms, particularly break-through (episodic) pain. Generally with drugs, it is good practice to err on the side of generosity in relation to the recommended frequency of p.r.n. medication. However, it does depend on the class and formulation of the drug in question, and whether the patient is an inpatient or at home.

In all circumstances, it is important that the permitted frequency is stated clearly on the patient's medication chart (Figure 14.1 and Figure 14.2), and verbally explained to the patient and the family.

Regular SR strong opioid medication at home

The *corresponding* normal-release opioid analgesic formulation should also be prescribed q1h p.r.n. in an appropriate dose (see p.233).

Regular normal-release strong opioid medication at home

The *same* normal-release opioid analgesic formulation should also be prescribed routinely q1h p.r.n.

With regular normal-release strong opioid medication, if a patient needs an *occasional* rescue dose, say, 40min or less before the next regular dose is due, it may suffice to give the next regular dose early. However, opinion is divided. Some specialists say that a p.r.n. dose should be given, followed in due course by the regular dose.

Regular analgesic medication other than a strong opioid

Acetaminophen and NSAIDs are often prescribed at the maximum recommended dose. In this case, a normal-release opioid analgesic should be prescribed *q1h p.r.n.*, either a weak opioid product or a low dose of a strong opioid.

Recommendations for anti-emetics, laxatives, and psychotropics have been given in their respective sections.

Inpatients

Recommendations can be more generous because there are trained personnel to monitor the effect of any additional medication, and thus prevent serious toxicity. For example, prescribing a range of permitted doses allows nurses to increase the amount given on their own initiative.

Example: Patient taking SR **morphine** 100mg b.i.d.
Expected p.r.n. dose = 1/10–1/6 of total 24h dose, i.e. 20–30mg
Chart **morphine** tablets/suspension 20–30mg q1h p.r.n.

In practice, nurses tend to start with the lower dose, but increase to the top of the range if necessary. If two consecutive top-of-the-range doses at the maximum permitted frequency are insufficient, medical advice should be obtained, and alternative measures considered, e.g. rapid titration with IV **morphine** (see p.301 and Boxes 5.J and 5.K, p.304 and Box 5.L, p.305).

Dying patients

When a patient is likely to have difficulty with swallowing, non-oral as well as PO p.r.n. medication should be prescribed to cover common distressing situations. Some services provide the necessary medication in emergency kits. In the USA, SL, PR and TD products are generally preferred; whereas in the UK and Canada, the tendency is to use injections:
- analgesics: e.g. **morphine** SC *q1h* (p.r.n. dose depends on regular dose)
- anti-emetics: e.g. **metoclopramide** 10–20mg SC *q1h* or **methotrimeprazine** 6–25mg SC *q1h*
- sedative, anti-epileptic: e.g. **midazolam** 2.5–10mg SC *q1h*
- antisecretory drug: e.g. **hyoscine (scopolamine) butylbromide** 20mg q1h or **glycopyrrolate** 200microgram SC *q1h*
- delirium: **haloperidol** 2.5–5mg SC *q1h*.

The routine prescribing of emergency medication can form part of a Care Pathway, e.g. the Liverpool Care Pathway for the Dying Patient.[1,10–12] Pathways are particularly helpful in non-palliative care and non-hospice settings. They facilitate a review of the direction and purpose of treatment, and increase the likelihood that interventions which are becoming futile will be stopped.

COMPOUNDING PHARMACY

A compounded preparation is a prescription drug prepared locally, often for one particular patient.[13] Although all licensed pharmacists should have the skills necessary to compound drugs, the term 'compounding pharmacist' is generally restricted to pharmacists who have undertaken further training and invested in compounding equipment. Formulations include troches (dispersible tablets), capsules, powders, solutions, elixirs, syrups, emulsions, suspensions, ointments, creams, suppositories, and gels (Table 14.1). In the USA, compounded drugs are widely used in hospices and palliative care units when the oral route becomes difficult or impossible. In contrast, in the UK and Canada, proprietary parenteral formulations are generally used instead.

Table 14.1   Examples of compounded preparations in the USA

Drug	Strength	Formulation	Typical cost (US $)
ABHR[a]	1/25/1/10mg	Gel[b]	75c/mL
ABHR[a]	0.5/12.5/0.5/10mg	Suppositories	75c each
BDR[a]	12.5/4/10mg	Suppositories	$1 each
Chlorpromazine	50mg/mL	Solution	50c/mL
Chlorpromazine	25mg	Suppositories	$1.25 each
Chlorpromazine	50mg	Suppositories	$1.50 each
Dexamethasone	4mg/mL	Gel[b]	$1/mL
Dexamethasone	4mg/mL	Solution	$1.25/mL
Dexamethasone	4mg	Suppositories	$1.25 each
Diazepam	5mg	Suppositories	$1 each
Hydromorphone	4mg/mL	Oral solution	$1/mL
Ibuprofen	400mg	Suppositories	$1 each
Ketamine	100mg/mL	Gel[b]	$1/mL
Ketoprofen	50mg/mL	Gel[b]	$1/mL
Lorazepam	2mg/mL	Concentrated solution	$1.60/mL
Lorazepam	1mg/mL	Gel[b]	$1/mL
Lorazepam	2mg	Suppositories	$1.15 each
Magic mouthwash[c]	1/1/1	Solution	3c/mL
Magic mouthwash with nystatin[d]	1/1/1/1	Solution	6c/mL
Methadone	All strengths	Suppositories	$1 each
Metronidazole	10mg/mL	Paste	25c/g
Morphine	20mg/mL	Gel[b,e]	$1/mL
Prochlorperazine	25mg/mL	Gel[b]	$1/mL

a. see text for further details
b. pluronic lecithin organogel is a commonly used base for compounded topical preparations when a systemic effect is desired[14]
c. equal parts of Maalox®, diphenhydramine elixir and viscous lidocaine 2% solution; used in the management of stomatitis/mucositis
d. equal parts of Maalox®, diphenhydramine elixir, viscous lidocaine 2% solution and nystatin suspension 100,000 units/1mL; used in the management of stomatitis/mucositis caused or complicated by oropharyngeal candidosis
e. in the UK and Canada, morphine is sometimes compounded with Intrasite® gel 1mg/1mL.

The italicized preparations in Table 14.1 each contain several drugs, and are popular among hospice clinicians in the USA. However, the popularity of a multi-drug combination does not necessarily justify its use. The acronyms ABHR and BDR reflect the common USA proprietary names for **lorazepam** (Ativan®), **diphenhydramine** (Benadryl®), **haloperidol** (Haldol®) and **metoclopramide** (Reglan®) on the one hand, and **diphenhydramine** (Benadryl®), **dexamethasone** (Decadron®) and **metoclopramide** (Reglan®) on the other. However, it is difficult to justify fixed-dose polypharmacy of this nature, even when single or dual anti-emetic treatment has proved inadequate (see p.183). Accordingly, the use of such preparations is strongly discouraged by *PCF.*

When compounded drugs are used, it is important to inspect them periodically for physical changes which could imply instability. For example, capsules may become brittle, powders may cake, and liquid drug preparations may precipitate or become contaminated with microbes.

Compounded ointments, gels and creams may change in consistency or develop an unusual odour, and suppositories and troches may become abnormally hard or soft. Unfortunately, different batches of compounded drugs may differ in bio-availability, absorption, sterility, efficacy, stability, and thus safety.

PRESCRIBING FOR CHILDREN

In a survey in Canada, about 50% of those referred for pediatric palliative care were under 5 years, and 1/2 of these were under 1 year. The three main diagnostic groups were:
- disorders of the nervous system (39%)
- congenital anomalies, e.g. cardiac abnormalities, and conditions manifesting in the perinatal period (22%)
- cancer (22%).[15]

Palliative care is often needed in parallel with disease-directed treatment of the underlying condition and of any intercurrent illness. However, evaluation is inherently more difficult than in most adults (Box 14.A). Further, in children with life-limiting conditions, it is often difficult to identify the end-stage, particularly with disorders other than cancer. Ongoing care should be under the direction of a multiprofessional team, including specialist pediatric input, ideally with advice from a pediatric pharmacist.

Box 14.A Evaluation of symptoms in dying children

Common problems include cerebral irritability, intractable seizures, skeletal muscle spasm, pain, swallowing and feeding difficulties, gastro-esophageal reflux, breathlessness and troublesome secretions.

Symptom evaluation can be particularly difficult in children with cognitive impairment.[16,17] When possible, facilitate self-reporting by using tools appropriate to the child's age and cognitive ability.[18–21] A parent's report and staff observation are also important.

Symptom scales and diaries aid continuity between different carers, and across different settings, e.g. home, school, hospital, hospice, and respite centre.

There are several respected sources which provide guidance about prescribing for children.[22–26] However, there is still a dearth of pediatric data for pharmacokinetics, pharmacodynamics, and drug safety.[27] In order to increase the body of knowledge, significant undesirable effects in children should be reported to:
- in Canada:
  - ▷ Medeffect (adverse drug reporting programme) www.hc-sc.gc.ca/dhp-mps/medeff/index-eng.php,
  - ▷ Canadian Network of Palliative Care for Children http://cnpcc.ca/,
  - ▷ pediatric pain mailing list http://pediatric-pain.ca/ppml/ppmlist.html
- in the UK: PaedPalCare www.act.org.uk
- in the USA: FDA Medwatch http://www.fda.gov/Safety/MedWatch/default.htm.

And, ideally, also to www.palliativedrugs.com.

Extra care is required when prescribing for children:
- *avoid drugs as far as possible:* first consider non-drug options, and prescribe only if there is a clear indication
- *simplify regimens:* try to avoid the need to administer drugs during school time
- *limit the range of medications:* become familiar with the use of a limited range of drugs and their effects in children
- *check dose calculations.*

Children should be involved (at a level appropriate to their age and understanding) in decisions about taking drugs.

Children are at increased risk of medication errors because of:
- lack of evidence-based data
- the diversity and rarity of their conditions
- the need to calculate and adjust the dose for the age and/or weight of the child
- the lack of suitable dose formulations
- variations in recommended doses and administration regimens
- inconsistent presentation of recommended dose information (e.g. microgram/kg per dose, microgram/kg per hour, mg per dose, total 24h dose).

Particular care is required when prescribing in the neonatal period (prematurity and first 28 days of life) because of immature renal function and liver enzyme pathways, immature reticular activating systems, and differing volumes of distribution.

As far as possible, drugs should be prescribed within the terms of their licence.[28] However, as in adult palliative care, it will be necessary to prescribe some drugs 'off-label', beyond their approved indications and/or routes of administration (see p.xvii).

Deciding the dose

Pediatric dosing needs to be based on the physiological characteristics of the child, and the pharmacokinetics of the drug.[29] Dosing by age may be misleading, particularly in palliative care where, because of underlying disease, children are unlikely to be close to the mean weight for their age. Thus, for most drugs, the dose is determined by *body weight*. However, using body surface area is more accurate because it tends to mirror physiological processes more closely, and this should be used particularly when calculating doses of cytotoxic drugs. Generally, doses in children should not exceed the maximum adult dose.

There is little evidence-based data for drug doses in children, and practice has often evolved from personal experience and case series. Flexible personalized schedules are acceptable for many drugs so as to make it as straightforward as possible for the child, and thus increase adherence to the regimen and minimize disruption to schooling and sleep. However, regular timing is important for some drugs, e.g. antibiotics.

Drug formulation and administration

A liquid may be easier to administer than tablets or capsules, particularly for children who are younger, very unwell, or have dysphagia. On the other hand, some children may prefer the taste of tablets to nauseating syrups. Crushing tablets may not be appropriate because it can affect drug delivery and absorption, particularly for SR formulations (see Administering drugs via enteral feeding tubes, p.531).

Although unpleasant taste may affect adherence, the taste of a medication can often be masked with small quantities of food or fruit juice. However, medication should not be added to a feeding bottle.

An oral syringe should be used for accurate measurement and administration of liquid medicines. The use of alternative routes of administration (buccal, intranasal, PR, SC, IV) is relatively common in children. Some already have a central venous line which can be accessed by carers. This route, if available, is most appropriate for continuous infusions. Carers need to be advised and trained for this role.

Many children with life-limiting illnesses or life-threatening conditions are fed by nasogastric or gastrostomy tubes, although some may still be able to take medication orally (see p.531).[30] The presence of a feeding tube may mean that, during the last few hours or days, a CSCI/CIVI is not needed. However, vigilance is required because, close to death, enteral absorption can become impaired. There is also the risk that medicines may continue to be administered via a feeding tube, even when no longer necessary or appropriate. Regular medication review is essential.

The IM route is particularly distressing for children, and should generally be avoided. The SC route may be appropriate and acceptable for children, and is the route of choice for continuous infusions if there is no permanent central venous access.

Pharmacological considerations
Polypharmacy

Children with life-limiting or life-threatening illnesses are often on complicated regimens with multiple medications. This increases the possibility of undesirable drug effects and interactions (particularly with anti-epileptic drugs). Further, large volumes of liquid may be needed when administering multiple medications. Regimens should be reviewed regularly and simplified whenever possible. In this, the help of a pediatric pharmacist is invaluable.

Pharmacokinetics and pharmacodynamics

Compared with adults, children under 12 years tend to absorb and metabolize drugs differently:
- *neonates (<1 month)* have relatively low renal and hepatic clearances, and higher volumes of distribution, resulting in a prolonged halflife for many drugs; this may necessitate relatively lower doses at longer intervals (compared with infants and children, on a weight for weight basis). Drugs primarily metabolized by the liver should be administered with extreme care until the age of 2 months[29]
- *infants and children (1 month–12 years)* have relatively high drug clearances, and normal volumes of distribution, resulting in a shorter halflife for many drugs; this may necessitate relatively higher doses at shorter intervals (compared with adults)
- *hepatic impairment* may not necessitate dose reduction, because children have a large reserve of hepatic metabolic capacity compared with adults. Liver volumes increase with age and are more closely correlated to surface area rather than weight.[29]

Thus, special consideration is required with:
- *neonates (particularly if premature) and infants:* because liver enzyme systems may not be fully developed, metabolic pathways can differ from those in older children (e.g. **alfentanil, midazolam, morphine** all have longer elimination halflives in neonates and infants)[29]
- *hypoproteinemia:* the effect of highly protein-bound drugs (e.g. benzodiazepines, **phenytoin, prednisone, warfarin**) may be increased
- *coagulation impairment:* gives rise to an increased response to oral anticoagulants
- *hepatotoxic drugs:* more likely to cause toxicity in children with liver disease.

In addition, immaturity of renal function in children can result in lower renal drug clearance, particularly in neonates.

Monitoring drug concentrations

Monitoring plasma drug concentrations is generally of limited value, and additional venipunctures are distressing for children. Monitor the plasma concentration only when dose adjustment on a clinical basis is known to be inadequate, e.g. **gentamicin, phenobarbital, phenytoin, teicoplanin** (not Canada).

Specific cautions when prescribing for children
Anti-epileptics

Many children with life-limiting or life-threatening conditions are on complicated anti-epileptic regimens. Interactions are common between anti-epileptics, and are mostly caused by liver enzyme induction or inhibition. They are variable and unpredictable and may increase toxicity without a corresponding increase in anti-epileptic effect. Anti-epileptics also have significant interactions with other drugs (see p.202). Specialist pediatric neurology advice is recommended when titrating or reducing anti-epileptics in children.

Generally, anti-epileptic medication should *not* be stopped in the terminal phase, although absorption and administration may prove unpredictable. An alternative route of administration, and the addition or substitution of SC **midazolam** or **phenobarbital** may be necessary. Some anti-epileptics (**carbamazepine, clonazepam, diazepam, lorazepam, phenobarbital** and **valproic acid**) can be given PR, but may require dose adjustment.[31] For example, the dose of **carbamazepine** should be increased by 25% when converting from PO to PR.[32]

Rectal administration may also be possible for **lamotrigine**[33] and **vigabatrin**, but strong evidence is lacking.

Corticosteroids

Corticosteroids are most often used to relieve headache and vomiting caused by raised intracranial pressure associated with progressive intracranial tumours.

However, compared with adults, children seem to experience a more rapid onset of relatively severe undesirable effects (particularly cushingoid facies, proximal myopathy, weight gain, and changes in mood and behaviour). Thus, corticosteroids are generally used at the lowest effective dose and for the shortest possible time. Some centres use short courses of corticosteroids (e.g. **dexamethasone** ≤0.5mg/kg/day for 3–5 days) repeated as dictated by symptoms.

However, good symptom management may necessitate daily administration, despite the increased undesirable effects and increased difficulty when attempting to wean a child off corticosteroids.[34] A gastroprotective drug may need to be prescribed concurrently.

Opioids

Opioids can generally be used safely in children, just as in adults, although this may require careful explanation to parents and carers to allay fears. Alternative non-invasive routes (e.g. buccal) are often used for p.r.n. doses for break-through (episodic) pain, particularly if a rapid response is required.

The use of some drugs is limited in children by the lack of an appropriate formulation. However, **fentanyl** patches are being increasingly used as a convenient long-acting opioid formulation for children.

There is concern about the risk of respiratory depression in children, but little evidence of this except in neonates. In this group, there is a documented incidence of late respiratory depression (>4h after administration of normal-release **morphine**).[35] Compared with doses in children aged 2–12 years, the recommended doses per kg are lower in those under 2 years, and much lower in neonates (<1 month).

Of the undesirable effects of opioids, pruritus and urinary retention are probably more common, and nausea probably less common than in adults (although this may be under-diagnosed).[36]

Phenothiazines

Although evidence is sparse, children may have an age-related increased risk of dystonic reactions with D_2-receptor antagonists, e.g. phenothiazines and **metoclopramide** (also see Drug-induced movement disorders, p.561). Such drugs should be used with caution particularly in those <20 years old.[37,38]

PRESCRIBING FOR THE ELDERLY

Particular care is required when prescribing for the elderly.[39,40] The following should be kept in mind:

- *Avoid drugs whenever possible:* always consider non-drug options first; prescribe drugs only when clearly indicated
- *Simplify regimens:* avoid complicated or frequent dose regimens; whenever possible give medication once daily or b.i.d.
- *Limit the range of drugs:* become familiar with the use of a limited range of drugs and their effects in the elderly
- *Long-acting antidiabetic drugs:* **chlorpropamide** and **glyburide** are best avoided
- *Dose reduction:* doses should generally be lower than for younger patients, e.g. start with about 50% of the normal adult dose.

Beers' list of potentially inappropriate medication

In 1991, a group of geriatricians, pharmacists and geriatric psychiatrists in the USA, under the leadership of Mark Beers, compiled a list of drugs and drug classes which they considered carried a significantly greater risk of undesirable effects in the elderly (>65 years).[41] Those listed were termed 'potentially inappropriate medication'. Since then, the list has been revised twice, most recently in 2003 (Box 14.B).[40] The list is not 'evidence-based' in the narrow sense of the word (i.e. based on the results of RCTs), but reflects the consensus view of the group in the light of what is known generally about the pharmacokinetics and pharmacodynamics of drugs in the elderly.

In 1999, in the USA, the Centers for Medicare and Medicaid Services (CMS) incorporated the contents of the Beers' list in the regulatory guidelines for nursing homes. By so doing, they sent out a powerful message which is often interpreted to mean 'Do *not* prescribe these drugs for elderly patients'. However, the intention of the original consensus group was not to prohibit the use of the listed drugs but rather to remind doctors of the need to reflect more carefully before prescribing: 'Think before you ink'. Similarly, concerns about the inappropriate use of antipsychotics in patients with behavioural problems associated with advanced dementia[42–45] could hinder the appropriate use of **haloperidol** in hospice patients in some nursing homes.

Box 14.B Potentially inappropriate medication in the elderly[40]

Amiodarone	Ergot mesyloids (L)	Nifedipine, short-acting
Amitriptyline (H)	Estrogens	Nitrofurantoin
Amphetamines (excluding methylphenidate and anorexics)	Ethacrynic acid	NSAIDs, long-term use of full-dose, longer halflife, non-COX-selective (e.g. naproxen, oxaprozin, piroxicam)
	Ferrous sulfate >325mg/day	
	Fluoxetine	
Barbiturates (H)	GI antispasmodics (belladonna alkaloids, clidinium-chlordiazepoxide, dicyclomine, hyoscyamine, propantheline = all (H))	
Benzodiazepines, long-acting (chlordiazepoxide (H), diazepam (H), flurazepam (H), oxazepam (H), temazepam)		Oxybutynin, short-acting
		Pentazocine (H)
	Guanadrel	Perphenazine-amitriptyline
	Guanethidine	Promethazine
Chlorpheniramine	Hydroxyzine	Propantheline
Chlorpropamide (H)	Indomethacin (L)	Propoxyphene
Cimetidine	Isoxsuprine	Reserpine (L)
Clonidine	Ketorolac	Stimulant laxatives, long-term use except with opioid analgesics (e.g. bisacodyl, cascara sagrada, castor oil/Neoloid®)
Clorazepate	Meperidine (H)	
Cyproheptadine	Meprobamate	
Desiccated thyroid	Mesoridazine	
Digoxin >125microgram/day (H)	Methyldopa and methyldopa/hydrochlorothiazide (H)	Thioridazine
		Ticlopidine (H)
Diphenhydramine (H)	Methyltestosterone	Trimethobenzamide (H)
Dipyridamole, short-acting (L)	Mineral oil	Tripelennamine
Disopyramide (H)	Muscle relaxants (carisoprodol, chlorzoxazone, cyclobenzaprine, dantrolene, methocarbamol, orphenadrine = all (L))	
Doxazosin		
Doxepin (H)		

Key: H = high-severity-impact medication; L = low-severity-impact medication.

Antipsychotics and several drugs on the Beers' list are important drugs in specific situations in palliative care.[46] Because of the relatively short prognosis and the greater need to ensure comfort, a higher risk is generally acceptable in palliative and hospice care. Thus, for example, in an elderly patient:

- if there is a clear indication for the use of **haloperidol** (or an alternative antipsychotic), it is important that local regulations do not prevent its administration
- with cholestatic pruritus in whom stenting of the common bile duct is inappropriate or has proved technically impossible, the use of an androgen (e.g. **danazol** (UK and Canada), **methyltestosterone** (USA)) may well be the most convenient drug treatment (see Table 5.21, p.340)
- the prolonged use of an NSAID, such as **naproxen**, together with a strong opioid is generally good practice for a patient with severe cancer-related pain (see p.231).

Form of medicine

Frail elderly patients may have difficulty swallowing tablets. They should be instructed to take tablets or capsules with fluid in an upright position to minimize the possibility of them remaining in the mouth or esophagus, and causing ulceration (e.g. NSAIDs, **temazepam**). Alternative formulations (e.g. liquid) or routes of administration (e.g. SC) may be preferable.

Polypharmacy

Elderly patients are more likely to be receiving multiple drugs for existing diseases and the addition of more drugs for the relief of symptoms will increase the risk of drug interactions (see Cytochrome P450, p.551), undesirable effects, and may affect adherence (compliance). Thus, medicines should be reviewed regularly and any of doubtful benefit should be stopped. These include prophylactic drugs which become irrelevant for a patient with a poor prognosis, e.g. statins.

Pharmacokinetics

One of the most important changes to occur with increasing age, which influences the pharmacokinetics of many drugs, is the progressive decline in renal function. Drugs are excreted more slowly and a lower dose may suffice, particularly those with a narrow therapeutic ratio, e.g. **digoxin** (see Renal impairment, p.491). Acute illness, particularly accompanied by dehydration, can lead to a rapid further reduction in renal clearance.

Drug monitoring

With highly protein-bound drugs, if the plasma drug concentration is used to monitor treatment, changes in plasma protein concentrations can lead to difficulty in interpreting the results:

- *albumin* binds acidic drugs, e.g. **phenytoin**, and when reduced by malnutrition, cirrhosis, nephrotic syndrome, end-stage renal disease, etc., the proportion of unbound (active) drug is likely to increase, even though the total plasma drug concentration may decrease or remain normal
- α_1-*acid glycoprotein* (an acute phase protein) binds basic drugs, e.g. **lidocaine**, and when increased by infection, inflammatory disease, cancer, etc., the total plasma drug concentration will increase, but the proportion of unbound (active drug) may decrease or remain normal.

Thus, a patient with hypo-albuminemia may have a low total **phenytoin** plasma concentration but a therapeutic unbound concentration, and increasing the dose to achieve a 'therapeutic' total concentration may result in toxicity.

Conversely, a patient with an acute illness may have a high total **lidocaine** plasma concentration but a therapeutic unbound concentration, and reducing the dose to achieve a 'therapeutic' total concentration may result in loss of effect.

Thus, measuring free (unbound) levels of highly protein-bound drugs is preferable. If this is not possible, formulas to 'correct' for low plasma protein concentrations are available for some drugs. For example, the following formula can be used to correct the total **phenytoin** concentration in someone with hypo-albuminemia:[47]

$$\text{Corrected total phenytoin concentration} = \frac{\text{observed concentration}}{(0.02 \times \text{albumin}) + 0.1}$$

Pharmacodynamics

The aging body shows increased sensitivity to drugs, e.g. centrally-acting drugs such as opioids, benzodiazepines and antipsychotics. This increases the risk of delirium, postural hypotension and falls (Box 14.C).

Box 14.C Specific cautions when prescribing for the elderly

Antihypertensives, antiparkinsonian drugs, digoxin, psychotropics
Undesirable effects are more common. Use smaller doses and monitor closely.

Sulfamethoxazole-trimethoprim, mianserin (not Canada)
Avoid if possible because of increased risk of drug-induced bone marrow depression.

Diuretics
Do not use long-term to treat simple gravitational or hypoproteinemic edema.

Night sedatives (hypnotics)
Use a short course of a drug with a short halflife. Benzodiazepines impair balance and their use may result in falls. There is no evidence that zopiclone or zolpidem are better tolerated.

NSAIDs
Serious or fatal bleeding is more common. A special hazard in patients with heart disease (fluid retention) or renal impairment (may exacerbate). Use non-drug methods and acetaminophen before prescribing an NSAID in low dose, e.g. naproxen 250mg b.i.d. or ibuprofen 200–400mg t.i.d.

Warfarin
A lower maintenance dose is generally required, and the outcome of bleeding is often more serious.

HEPATIC IMPAIRMENT

The liver is the major site of metabolism for most drugs. Moderate–severe hepatic impairment may have a major impact on the pharmacokinetics of a drug.[48,49] The following features of liver disease can alter a patient's response to a drug.

Impaired drug metabolism

Hepatic metabolism involves:[50]
- *phase I:* cytochrome P450 enzymes in the endoplasmic reticulum (see Cytochrome P450, p.551)
- *phase II:* various enzymes, e.g. glucuronyl transferases, in the endoplasmic reticulum and cytosol
- *phase III:* active drug transport across cell membranes, e.g. P-glycoprotein.

The effect of liver disease on drug metabolism depends on:
- *drug:* generally the liver converts active lipophilic drugs into inactive hydrophilic metabolites for excretion by the kidneys; sometimes pro-drugs are metabolized into active forms, e.g. **codeine → morphine**
- *disease severity:* because of the large hepatic reserve, impaired hepatic elimination only occurs in severe disease
- *enzymes:* generally phase II enzymes are affected less than phase I enzymes, which are also affected to different degrees, e.g. CYP1A2, 2C19 > 2A6, 3A4 > 2C9, 2E1
- *disease process:* e.g. acute hepatitis impairs phase I > phase III, whereas the opposite occurs in cholestasis; drugs excreted unchanged in the bile, e.g. **rifampin, fusidic acid**, may accumulate in cholestasis.

Thus, in liver disease, the metabolism of different drugs is not uniformly affected, and it is not possible to predict from routine LFTs how the metabolism of a particular drug will be impaired.

Impaired hepatic blood flow

Cirrhosis may result in a decreased hepatic blood flow. This can increase the bio-availability of some drugs which are generally highly extracted by the liver, e.g. **chlormethiazole** (not Canada or USA), **pentazocine**, **meperidine (pethidine)**, **propranolol**, **verapamil**. However, **morphine** metabolism is generally unaffected by changes in hepatic blood flow until hepatic impairment is severe.

Impaired renal function

Severe and rapidly deteriorating liver disease is known to impair renal function (hepatorenal syndrome). However, even moderate hepatic impairment reduces renal clearance and will necessitate a reduction in dose of renally excreted drugs.[51] Serum creatinine is an insensitive guide to glomerular filtration rate (GFR) in patients with cirrhosis (reduced muscle mass; reduced conversion of creatine → creatinine). Ideally, creatinine clearance should be used, but it can overestimate GFR in cirrhosis.[50]

Hypo-albuminemia

With highly protein-bound drugs, if the plasma drug concentration is used to monitor treatment, hypo-albuminemia can lead to difficulty in interpreting the results, e.g. **phenytoin** (see p.488).

Reduced clotting

Reduced hepatic synthesis of blood-clotting factors, indicated by a prolonged prothrombin time, increases sensitivity to **warfarin** and other oral anticoagulants.

Altered pharmacodynamics

In hepatic impairment there may be increased sensitivity to drugs, e.g. centrally-acting drugs such as opioids, benzodiazepines and psychotropics (increased risk of sedation), antihypertensives (increased risk of hypotension), oral hypoglycemics (increased risk of hypoglycemia), NSAIDs (increased risk of GI bleeding).

Hepatic encephalopathy

Many drugs can precipitate hepatic encephalopathy by causing sedation (e.g. opioids, benzodiazepines and psychotropics), hypokalemia (e.g. diuretics, corticosteroids), or constipation (e.g. opioids).

Fluid overload

Edema and ascites in chronic liver disease may be exacerbated by drugs that cause fluid retention, e.g. NSAIDs, corticosteroids.

Hepatotoxic drugs

Hepatotoxicity is either dose-related (predictable) or idiosyncratic (unpredictable). Drugs causing dose-related toxicity do so at lower doses in patients with hepatic impairment, and drugs producing idiosyncratic reactions do so more frequently. These drugs should be avoided or used with extra care.

Recommendations for practice

In severe liver disease, avoid drugs whenever possible, particularly those with a narrow therapeutic index. In moderate liver disease, use renally-excreted drugs with appropriate caution (see below). Generally, use lower starting doses, slower rates of titration, consider reducing the dosing frequency, e.g. **morphine** q4h→q6h, and monitor the patient carefully.

RENAL IMPAIRMENT

Renal impairment can alter the pharmacokinetic and pharmacodynamic properties of a drug. For example:

- reduced renal excretion of a drug will cause accumulation, a prolonged halflife and a longer time to reach steady-state
- reduced renal excretion of an active drug or metabolite may cause toxicity, e.g. **digoxin, gabapentin, pregabalin, insulin, lithium, LMWH,** morphine-6-glucuronide, morphine-3-glucuronide, hydromorphone-3-glucuronide
- with highly protein-bound drugs, if the plasma drug concentration is used to monitor treatment, hypo-albuminemia can lead to difficulty in interpreting the results, e.g. **phenytoin** (see p.488)
- reduced efficacy of some drugs acting on the kidneys, e.g. diuretics
- increased sensitivity to the therapeutic and undesirable effects of some drugs, even if elimination is unimpaired, e.g. psycho-active drugs
- increased nephrotoxic effect of a drug, e.g. **allopurinol,** aminoglycosides, **cyclosporine, lithium,** NSAIDs.

Some of these problems can be overcome by:

- avoiding drugs which are nephrotoxic
- using alternative drugs which are not renally excreted
- reducing the total daily maintenance dose of a renally excreted drug, either by reducing the size of the individual doses or by increasing the interval between doses.

Advice about opioid choice in patients with renal impairment is given in the generic monograph on strong opioids (see p.295).

Principles of dose adjustment in renal impairment

The degree of renal impairment which necessitates a dose reduction depends on the extent to which the drug and any active metabolite is dependent on renal excretion and how serious any undesirable effects of the drug may be:

- for drugs with minimal undesirable effects, a simple scheme for dose reduction is sufficient, i.e. start low and monitor for efficacy and toxicity
- for drugs with a small safety margin, dose adjustments should be based on a measure of renal function, e.g. creatinine clearance, often estimated using the Cockcroft-Gault formula (see p.492)
- for drugs where both efficacy and toxicity are closely related to plasma concentration, ongoing treatment must be adjusted according to clinical response and plasma concentration, e.g. **gentamicin.**

Measuring renal function

The glomerular filtration rate (GFR) is the best overall measure of renal function, but the most accurate measures of GFR are impractical for routine use. Serum creatinine concentration has traditionally been used as a proxy but is only a rough guide because a significant proportion of renal function may be lost before creatinine levels rise above the upper limit of normal, particularly in patients with a low body muscle mass or low protein intake. One approach is to use a formula-based *estimation* of GFR (eGFR), which takes into account some of the factors that complicate serum creatinine interpretation, e.g. Modification of Diet in Renal Disease (MDRD) study formula.[52] This takes into account 4 variables, namely serum creatinine, age, sex, and ethnic origin. It is the nationally adopted standard in England[39] and is widely used in Canada. Alternatives include the Chronic Kidney Disease Epidemiology Collaboration (CKD-EPI) formula.[53] This MDRD formula is more accurate than the Cockcroft-Gault formula with 90% of estimates $<60mL/min/1.73m^2$ within 30% of the true value. Changes in MDRD eGFR are more reliable than single estimates, with a decrease of $\geq15\%$ likely to represent a true change in renal function.[52] Five stages of renal disease are categorized according to MDRD eGFR (Table 14.2).[54]

The MDRD eGFR is expressed as a normalized value, i.e. what that individual's GFR would be if they had a body surface area of $1.73m^2$. The MDRD eGFR is *not* appropriate for considering drug clearance and dose adjustment as this should be based on an individual's absolute GFR. For example, for individuals with a body surface area $<1.73m^2$, the MDRD eGFR could overestimate renal function and potentially lead to drug overdosing, with the converse being true for individuals with a body surface area $>1.73m^2$.

Table 14.2 Diagnostic stages of renal disease

Stage	eGFR (mL/min/1.73m²)	Description[a]
1	>90	Normal renal function but renal disease based on urine findings, or presence of structural abnormalities or genetic trait
2	60–89	Mildly reduced renal function in the presence of renal disease (as above); in the absence of renal disease, an eGFR ⩾60mL/min/1.73m² is considered normal
3	30–59	Moderately reduced renal function
4	15–29	Severely reduced renal function
5	<15	Very severe, established (end-stage) renal failure

a. evidence of damage or a reduced eGFR must be present for >3 months.

The MDRD formula may also be misleading in situations where creatinine production, volume of distribution or excretion rate are altered, and in patients with a clearance of <50mL/min.[55] Further, it has not been validated for use in:
- children <18 years old
- pregnancy
- acute renal impairment
- edematous states
- malnourished patients
- muscle wasting disease states
- amputees.

Thus, in palliative care patients who are elderly, malnourished, cachectic and/or edematous, renal impairment may exist even when the serum creatinine or the MDRD eGFR are within normal limits, and it may be prudent to assume that there is at least mild renal impairment in such patients. Even when abnormal, the serum creatinine or the MDRD eGFR may both underestimate the actual degree of renal impairment.

Modifying drug dose based on renal function

In patients known to have chronic renal impairment or those at high risk of renal impairment, e.g. the elderly, those with hypertension or diabetes, renal function should be checked before prescribing a drug that may need dose modification. A baseline serum creatinine and MDRD eGFR (bearing in mind the above limitations) can help to indicate the need for dose modification and serial measurements used to monitor the effect of the drug on renal function.

However, *when considering dose adjustment guidelines, an absolute eGFR or creatinine clearance should be calculated*. Because most dose adjustment guidelines are currently based on an estimated creatinine clearance using the Cockcroft-Gault formula, this should be used in preference. Alternatively, the MDRD eGFR can be converted to an absolute value:

Cockcroft-Gault formula

$$\text{Creatinine clearance} = \frac{F \times [140 - \text{age}] \times [\text{weight (kg)}]}{\text{serum creatinine (micromol/L)}}$$

F = 1.23 (male) or 1.04 (female)

Converting the MDRD eGFR to an absolute value:
Absolute eGFR (mL/min) = MDRD eGFR (mL/min/1.73m²) × (body surface area/1.73) (m²)

Body surface area (m²) = $\sqrt{((\text{height (cm)} \times \text{weight (kg)})/3{,}600)}$

The Cockcroft-Gault formula, by taking weight rather than body surface area into account, tends to overestimate or underestimate creatinine clearance in obese and underweight patients respectively. As with the MDRD eGFR, it can be misleading in situations where creatinine production, volume of distribution or excretion rate are altered and similar precautions regarding the interpretation of results in palliative care patients will apply. It is not appropriate to use when renal function is changing rapidly.

Dose adjustment can then be made following the advice given here in *PCF* and in the manufacturer's literature. Other resources include *The Renal Drug Handbook*[47] and *Drug Prescribing in Renal Failure*.[56] For *prescribing purposes*, renal impairment is generally arbitrarily divided into mild, moderate and severe, corresponding to creatinine clearances of 60–90mL/min, 30–60mL/min and < 30mL/min respectively, although these values vary slightly between sources/drugs.

When a drug dose modification has been necessary, or for drugs known to cause renal impairment, a clinical review and evaluation of renal function should be carried out within 2 weeks, or at anytime if drug-induced nephrotoxicity is suspected, e.g. symptoms such as rash, arthralgia, edema.[52]

Patients requiring dialysis

For guidance on drug use in dialysis, generally consult specialist renal pharmacists and/or the literature. For example, dialysis can remove **gabapentin** and additional doses will be required with each dialysis session.

TRANSDERMAL PATCHES AND MRI

Broadly speaking, TD patches contain the drug either in a reservoir or embedded within a matrix. This is protected by a backing on the outside, and a removable liner covering the surface to be applied to the skin. Some TD patches contain metal in their backing (Box 14.D). This is potentially dangerous because, if such a patch is worn during MRI, the patient may develop a burn under the patch.[57,58]

Box 14.D   TD patches (USA) and MRI:[59] *correct as of December 2008*

Need to remove before MRI	*No need to remove before MRI*
Androderm® (testosterone)	Alora® (estradiol)
Catapres-TTS® (clonidine)	Climara® (estradiol)
CombiPatch® (estradiol/norethindrone)	ClimaraPro® (estradiol plus levonorgestrel)
Deponit®, Transderm-nitro® (nitroglycerin)	Esclim® (estradiol)
Habitrol®, Nicoderm®, Nicotrol® (nicotine)	Estraderm® (estradiol)
Daytrana® (methylphenidate)*	Lidoderm® (lidocaine)
Duragesic® (fentanyl)ᵃ	Menostar® (estradiol)
Emsam® (selegiline)	Minitran® (nitroglycerin)
LidoSite® (lidocaine/epinephrine)	Nitro-Dur® (nitroglycerin)
PediaPatch® (salicylic acid)	OrthoEvra® (estradiol plus norelgestromin)
Synera® (lidocaine/tetracaine)	Oxytrol® (oxybutynin)
Transderm-scop® (scopolamine hydrobromide)	
Trans-Ver-Sal® (salicylic acid)	
Vivelle-Dot® (estradiol)	

---

a. in the USA, Duragesic® is a reservoir patch with metal in the backing; in contrast, in the UK, the backing of Durogesic DTrans® matrix patch is metal-free. For the generic fentanyl patches (reservoir or matrix) available in the USA, contact the manufacturer for clarification of the metal content.

TD patches with metal in the backing must be removed immediately before MRI, and replaced with a new patch immediately afterwards (Box 14.D). Although some patches have metal in the liner, this is irrelevant because the liner is removed before application.

If in doubt, double-check

Box 14.D is correct as of December 2008 for products distributed *in the USA*. For Canadian products, check the Product Monograph, and/or contact the manufacturer directly.

1 Liverpool Care Pathway and Marie Curie Cancer Care (2006) The Liverpool care pathway for the dying patient. Available from: http://www.mcpcil.org.uk/liverpool-care-pathway/

2 NICE (2004) Guidance on cancer services: improving supportive and palliative care for adults with cancer: the manual. National Institute for Clinical Excellence, London. Available from: www.nice.org.uk/page.aspx?o = csgspfullguideline

3 Thomas K (2003) The gold standards framework in community palliative care. *European Journal of Palliative Care.* **10**: 113–115.

4 Rothschild JM *et al.* (2002) Analysis of medication-related malpractice claims: causes, preventability, and costs. *Archives of Internal Medicine.* **162**: 2414–2420.

5 Spinewine A *et al.* (2005) Appropriateness of use of medicines in elderly inpatients: qualitative study. *British Medical Journal.* **331**: 935.

6 Jones TA and Como JA (2003) Assessment of medication errors that involved drug allergies at a university hospital. *Pharmacotherapy.* **23**: 855–860.

7 Kanjanarat P *et al.* (2003) Nature of preventable adverse drug events in hospitals: a literature review. *American Journal of Health-System Pharmacy.* **60**: 1750–1759.

8 Neale G *et al.* (2001) Exploring the causes of adverse events in NHS hospital practice. *Journal of the Royal Society of Medicine.* **94**: 322–330.

9 Dean B *et al.* (2002) Causes of prescribing errors in hospital inpatients: a prospective study. *Lancet.* **359**: 1373–1378.

10 Ellershaw J (2002) Clinical pathways for care of the dying: an innovation to disseminate clinical excellence. *Journal of Palliative Medicine.* **5**: 617–621.

11 Bookbinder M *et al.* (2005) Improving end-of-life care: development and pilot-test of a clinical pathway. *Journal of Pain and Symptom Management.* **29**: 529–543.

12 Luhrs CA *et al.* (2005) Pilot of a pathway to improve the care of imminently dying oncology inpatients in a Veterans Affairs Medical Center. *Journal of Pain and Symptom Management.* **29**: 544–551.

13 Coyne PJ *et al.* (2006) Compounded Drugs. *Journal of Hospice and Palliative Nursing.* **8**: 222–226.

14 Willimann H *et al.* (1992) Lecithin organogel as matrix for transdermal transport of drugs. *Journal of Pharmaceutical Sciences.* **81**: 871–874.

15 Widger K *et al.* (2007) Pediatric patients receiving palliative care in Canada: results of a multicenter review. *Archives of Pediatrics & Adolescent Medicine.* **161**: 597–602.

16 Regnard C *et al.* (2007) Understanding distress in people with severe communication difficulties: developing and assessing the disability distress assessment tool (DisDAT). *Journal of Intellectual Disability Research.* **51**: 277–292.

17 Regnard C *et al.* (2003) Difficulties in identifying distress and its causes in people with severe communication problems. *International Journal of Palliative Nursing.* **9**: 173–176.

18 Hain RD (1997) Pain scales in children: a review. *Palliative Medicine.* **11**: 341–350.

19 Gauvain-Piquard A *et al.* (1999) The development of the DEGR(R): A scale to assess pain in young children with cancer. *European Journal of Pain.* **3**: 165–176.

20 Wong D and Baker C (1988) Pain in children: comparison of assessment scales. *Pediatric Nursing.* **14(1)**: 9017.

21 Herr K *et al.* (2006) Pain Assessment in the Nonverbal Patient: Position Statement with Clinical Practice Recommendations. Available from: http://www.aspmn.org/Organization/documents/NonverbalJournalFINAL.pdf

22 International Children's Palliative Care Network (2008). Available from: www.icpcn.org.uk

23 BNFC (2007) British National Formulary for Children. In: *British National Formulary.* BMJ Publishing Group Ltd, RPS Publishing, RCPCH Publications Ltd, London. Current BNFC available from: http://bnfc.org/bnfc/bnfc/current/.

24 General Medical Council (GMC) (2007) 0–18. *Guidance for all doctors.*

25 Ballantine N and Fitzmaurice N (2006) Using Medications. In: A Goldman *et al.* (eds) *Ch 18: Oxford Textbook of Palliative Care for Children.* Oxford University Press, Oxford.

26 Royal College of Paediatrics and Child Health (RCPCH) (2007) *Medicines for Children* (3e), London.

27 Stephenson T (2005) How children's responses to drugs differ from adults. *British Journal of Clinical Pharmacology.* **59**: 670–673.

28 AAP (American Academy of Pediatrics) (2006) Uses of Drugs Not Described in the Package Insert (Off-Label Uses) Available from: http://aappolicy.aappublications.org/cgi/content/full/pediatrics/10/1/181

29 Bartelink IH *et al.* (2006) Guidelines on paediatric dosing on the basis of developmental physiology and pharmacokinetic considerations. *Clinical Pharmacokinetics.* **45**: 1077–1097.

30 White R and Bradnam V (2007) *Handbook of Drug Administration via Enteral Feeding Tubes.* Pharmaceutical Press, London.

31 Smith S *et al.* (2001) Guidelines for rectal administration of anticonvulsant medication in children. *Paediatric and Perinatal Drug Therapy.* **4**: 140–147.

32 Arvidsson J *et al.* (1995) Replacing carbamazepine slow-release tablets with carbamazepine suppositories: a pharmacokinetic and clinical study in children with epilepsy. *Journal of Child Neurology.* **10**: 114–117.

33 Birnbaum AK *et al.* (2000) Rectal absorption of lamotrigine compressed tablets. *Epilepsia.* **41**: 850–853.

34 Glaser AW *et al.* (1997) Corticosteroids in the management of central nervous system tumours. Kids Neuro-Oncology Workshop (KNOWS). *Archives of Disease in Childhood.* **76**: 76–78.

35 Zernikow B *et al.* (2006) Paediatric cancer pain management using the WHO analgesic ladder-results of a prospective analysis from 2265 treatment days during a quality improvement study. *European Journal of Pain.* **10**: 587–595.

36 Hain RDW Pharmacodynamics of morphine and M6G in children with cancer: analgesia and adverse effects. International Conference in Paediatric Palliative Care. Cardiff; 2006.

37 van Harten PN *et al.* (1999) Acute dystonia induced by drug treatment. *British Medical Journal.* **319**: 623–626.

38 Grosset KA and Grosset DG (2004) Prescribed drugs and neurological complications. *Journal of Neurology, Neurosurgery & Psychiatry.* **75 Suppl 3**: iii2–8.

39 DoH (2001) *National Service Framework for Older People.* HMSO, London.

40 Fick DM *et al.* (2003) Updating the Beers criteria for potentially inappropriate medication use in older adults: results of a US consensus panel of experts. *Archives of Internal Medicine.* **163**: 2716–2724.

41 Beers MH *et al.* (1991) Explicit criteria for determining inappropriate medication use in nursing home residents. UCLA Division of Geriatric Medicine. *Archives of Internal Medicine.* **151**: 1825–1832.

42 Howard R *et al.* (2001) Guidelines for the management of agitation in dementia. *International Journal of Geriatric Psychiatry.* **16**: 714–717.

43 Lee PE *et al.* (2004) Atypical antipsychotic drugs in the treatment of behavioural and psychological symptoms of dementia: systematic review. *British Medical Journal.* **329**: 75.

44 Sink KM *et al.* (2005) Pharmacological treatment of neuropsychiatric symptoms of dementia: a review of the evidence. *Journal of the American Medical Association.* **293**: 596–608.

45 Fossey J *et al.* (2006) Effect of enhanced psychosocial care on antipsychotic use in nursing home residents with severe dementia: cluster randomised trial. *British Medical Journal.* **332**: 756–761.

46 Bain KT and Weschules DJ (2007) Medication inappropriateness for older adults receiving hospice care: a pilot survey. *Consultant Pharmacist.* **22**: 923–934.

47 Ashley C and Currie A (2004) *The Renal Drug Handbook* (2e). Radcliffe Medical Press Ltd, Oxford.

48 Ford-Dunn S (2005) Managing patients with cancer and advanced liver disease. *Palliative Medicine.* **19**: 563–565.

49 Tegeder I *et al.* (1999) Pharmacokinetics of opioids in liver disease. *Clinical Pharmacokinetics.* **37**: 17–40.

50 Pirmohamed M (2006) Prescribing in liver disease. *Medicine.* **35**: 31–33.

51 Morgan TR (1995) Protein consumption and hepatic encephalopathy in alcoholic hepatitis. VA Cooperative Study Group #275. *Journal of the American College of Nutrition.* **14**: 152–158.

52 Anonymous (2006) The patient, the drug and the kidney. *Drug and Therapeutics Bulletin.* **44**: 89–95.

53 Levey AS *et al.* (2009) A new equation to estimate glomerular filtration rate. *Annals of internal medicine.* **150**: 604–612.

54 Royal College of Physicians of London and Renal Association (2006) Chronic Kidney disease in adults: UK guidelines for identification, management and referral. Available from: www.renal.org/CKDguide/full/CKDprintedfullguide.pdf

55 Holweger K *et al.* (2008) Novel algorithm for more accurate calculation of renal function in adults with cancer. *Annals of Pharmacotherapy.* **42**: 1749–1757.

56 Brier M and Aronoff G (2007) *Drug Prescribing in Renal Failure 5e.* ACP Press, Philadelphia.

57 Institute for Safe Medication Practices (2004) Medication Safety Alert. Burns in MRI patients wearing transdermal patches. Available from: www.ismp.org/Newsletters/acutecare/articles/20040408.asp?ptr = y

58 Health Canada (2005) Association of transdermal drug patches with thermal burns during magnetic resonance imaging procedures. Available from: www.hc-sc.gc.ca/dhp-mps/medeff/advisories-avis/prof/_2005/mri-irm_patch-timbre_nth-ah-eng.php

59 Hulisz DT (2008) Are topical patches safe during MRI or CT Scans? Medscape Pharmacists. Available from: http://www.medscape.com/viewarticle/572561

15: OPIOID DOSE CONVERSION RATIOS

General approach

This chapter provides a summary of selected opioid dose conversion ratios. These can be used to calculate equivalent doses of opioids when switching from a weak opioid to **morphine**, or from one strong opioid to another. Caution is always necessary. It is crucial to appreciate that conversion ratios are *never* more than an approximate guide because of:

- wide interindividual variation in opioid pharmacokinetics
- other variables such as nutritional status and concurrent medications
- data derived from single dose rather than chronic dose studies.

Thus, careful monitoring during conversion is necessary to avoid both underdosing and excessive dosing. This is particularly the case if:

- switching at high doses
- there has been a recent rapid escalation of the first opioid
- switching to **methadone**.

When switching at high doses (e.g. **morphine** or equivalent doses of $\geq 1\,g/24h$), it is generally good practice to prescribe a lower than calculated dose (e.g. 1/4–1/2 lower), and rely on p.r.n. doses to make up any deficit while re-titrating to a satisfactory dose of the new opioid. In a comparably cautious way, when there has been a recent rapid dose escalation of the first opioid, use the pre-escalation dose to calculate the initial dose of the second opioid.

Determining the dose of the second opioid

Select the appropriate Table based on the routes of administration:

Route	Table	Page
PO to PO	15.1	498
PO to TD	15.2	499
PO to SC/IV	15.3	500
SC/IV to SC/IV	15.4	501

The Tables relate mainly to switching to or from **morphine**. If switching from an opioid other than **morphine** to another opioid, it will be necessary to convert the dose of the first opioid to **morphine** equivalents, and then use that quantity to determine the dose of the second opioid (Tables 15.1–15.4). With any switch:

- round the calculated dose up or down to the nearest convenient dose of the formulation concerned, e.g. tablet, TD patch, ampoule
- decide on an appropriate p.r.n. dose.

The conversion ratios in this chapter are based on referenced sources given in the various individual opioid monographs. Where these differ significantly from the manufacturers' recommended ratios, the latter are included for comparison.

Table 15.1 *PCF* recommended dose conversion ratios: PO to PO

Conversion	Ratio	Calculation	Example	Monograph
Codeine to morphine	10:1	Divide 24h codeine dose by 10	Codeine 240mg/24h PO → morphine 24mg/24h PO	Codeine, p.278
Tramadol to morphine	10:1	Divide 24h tramadol dose by 10	Tramadol 400mg/24h PO → morphine 40mg/24h PO	Tramadol, p.283
Morphine to hydromorphone	5:1[a]	Divide 24h morphine dose by 5	Morphine 60mg/24h PO → hydromorphone 12mg/24h PO	Hydromorphone, p.324
	5–7.5:1[b]	*Divide 24h morphine dose by 5–7.5*	*Morphine 60mg/24h PO → hydromorphone 8–12mg/24h PO*	Hydromorphone, p.324
Morphine to methadone	Variable	See methadone, p.327		
Morphine to oxycodone	1.5:1	Divide 24h morphine dose by 1.5 (decrease dose by 1/3)	Morphine 30mg/24h PO → oxycodone 20mg/24h PO	Oxycodone, p.335
	2:1[b]	*Divide 24h morphine dose by 2*	*Morphine 30mg/24h PO → oxycodone 15mg/24h PO*	Oxycodone, p.335

a. for converse, some use 1:4, e.g. hydromorphone 8mg/24h PO → morphine 32mg/24h PO
b. italicized entries = manufacturers' recommendations.

Table 15.2 *PCF recommended dose conversion ratios: PO to TD*

Conversion	Ratio	Calculation	Example	Monograph
Morphine to fentanyl	100:1	Multiply 24h morphine dose in mg by 10 to obtain 24h fentanyl dose in microgram; divide answer by 24 to obtain microgram/h patch strength	Morphine 300mg/24h PO→ fentanyl 3,000microgram/24h→ 125microgram/h; give as 100 + 25microgram/h patches	Fentanyl, p.315
	150:1[a]	*Use the manufacturer's guidelines in the Product Monograph*	*The doses will be smaller than those obtained with the PCF preferred dose conversion ratio*	Fentanyl, p.315

a. italicized entries = manufacturers' recommendations.

For determining the appropriate p.r.n. morphine dose for patients receiving TD fentanyl, see p.322.

Table 15.3 *PCF recommended dose conversion ratios; PO to SC/IV*

Conversion	Ratio	Calculation	Example	Monograph
Hydromorphone to hydromorphone	2:1	Divide 24h hydromorphone dose by 2	Hydromorphone 32mg/24h PO → hydromorphone 16mg/24h SC/IV	Hydromorphone, p.324
Morphine to alfentanil	30–40:1	Divide 24h morphine dose by 30–40	Morphine 40mg/24h PO → alfentanil 1mg/24h SC/IV	Alfentanil, p.310
Morphine to hydromorphone	10–15:1	Divide 24h morphine dose by 10–15	Morphine 30mg/24h PO → hydromorphone 2mg/24h SC/IV	Hydromorphone, p.324
Morphine to morphine	2:1	Divide 24h morphine dose by 2	Morphine 30mg/24h PO → morphine 15mg/24h SC/IV	Morphine, p.300

Table 15.4 *PCF* recommended dose conversion ratios; SC/IV to SC/IV

Conversion	Ratio	Calculation	Example	Monograph
Morphine to alfentanil	15–20:1	Divide 24h morphine dose by 15–20	Morphine 40mg/24h SC/IV → alfentanil 2mg/24h SC/IV	Alfentanil, p.310
Morphine to hydromorphone	5:1	Divide 24h morphine dose by 5	Morphine 30mg/24h SC/IV → hydromorphone 6mg/24h SC/IV	Hydromorphone, p.324

16: MANAGEMENT OF POSTOPERATIVE PAIN IN OPIOID-DEPENDENT PATIENTS

Opioid-dependent patients include those using long-term opioids for:
- pain relief (mainly cancer but increasingly non-cancer pain)
- long-term opioid maintenance for opioid dependence
- current substance misuse.

All such patients will require *additional* opioids to relieve any superadded pain. It is thus crucially important that pre-operative, peri-operative and postoperative doses take this into account, and that *extra amounts* of a strong opioid are prescribed. Almost certainly, these will be larger than the typical doses used by non-opioid-dependent patients in these circumstances.[1]

Because tolerance to undesirable effects, e.g. respiratory depression, develops more rapidly than to analgesia (often within days or 1–2 weeks at most), opioids can be safely titrated to the higher doses required. In contrast, if only typical postoperative doses are prescribed (e.g. **morphine** 2.5mg IV q2h or 5–10mg SC/IM q4h p.r.n.), patients will at best experience no pain relief. However, because such patients are likely to be physically dependent on opioids, they may well develop an opioid withdrawal syndrome, possibly associated with *hyperalgesia*. This will magnify the postoperative pain and any other underlying pain. In short, under-prescribing could lead to devastating overwhelming pain.

As far as possible, a multidisciplinary approach should be adopted, e.g. pre-operative consultation with the patient's substance misuse team, the anesthetist and the acute pain team, to develop a pain management plan which should include intra-operative and postoperative monitoring, with dose adjustments made by an experienced anesthetist. There are no uniform recommendations, but Box 16.A outlines the general approach.[2–11]

Pain management in conjunction with long-term naltrexone therapy

The opioid antagonist **naltrexone** is approved in Canada to promote abstinence in addicts by blocking the opioid 'high'. It is also used in alcoholics. It blocks all types of opioid receptor, and is long-acting. It thus prevents/blocks opioid analgesia. Analgesia for these patients requires careful consideration and planning (see Box 5.R, p.347).[12]

1　Rapp SE et al. (1995) Acute pain management in patients with prior opioid consumption: a case-controlled retrospective review. *Pain*. **61**: 195–201.
2　Macintyre PE (2001) Safety and efficacy of patient-controlled analgesia. *British Journal of Anaesthesia*. **87**: 36–46.
3　Mitra S and Sinatra RS (2004) Perioperative management of acute pain in the opioid-dependent patient. *Anesthesiology*. **101**: 212–227.
4　Lewis NL and Williams JE (2005) Acute pain management in patients receiving opioids for chronic and cancer pain. *Continuing Education in Anaesthesia; Critical Care and Pain*. **5**: 127–129.
5　Roberts DM and Meyer-Witting M (2005) High-dose buprenorphine: perioperative precautions and management strategies. *Anaesthesia and Intensive Care*. **33**: 17–25.
6　Alford DP et al. (2006) Acute pain management for patients receiving maintenance methadone or buprenorphine therapy. *Annals of Internal Medicine*. **144**: 127–134.
7　British Pain Society (2006) *Pain and Substance Misuse: Improving the Patient Experience. A Consensus Document for Consultation*. British Pain Society, London. Available from: www.britishpainsociety.org
8　James C and Williams JE (2006) How should postoperative pain in patients on long-term opioids be managed? *British Journal of Hospital Medicine (London)*. **67**: 500.
9　Mackenzie JW (2006) Acute pain management for opioid dependent patients. *Anaesthesia*. **61**: 907–908.
10　Macintyre PE and Ready LB (2006) *Acute Pain Management – A Practical Guide* (2e). Saunders Ltd., Philadelphia, PA, p. 272.
11　Mehta V and Langford RM (2006) Acute pain management for opioid dependent patients. *Anaesthesia*. **61**: 269–276.
12　Vickers AP and Jolly A (2006) Naltrexone and problems in pain management. *British Medical Journal*. **332**: 132–133.
13　Grond S et al. (2000) Clinical pharmacokinetics of transdermal opioids: focus on transdermal fentanyl. *Clinical Pharmacokinetics*. **38**: 59–89.

Box 16.A Management of postoperative pain in opioid-dependent patients

1 Consider local anesthetic or multimodal approaches to analgesia, e.g. regional blocks, acetaminophen, NSAIDs, clonidine, etc.

2 Identify the baseline opioid dose; in patients misusing opioids this may mean a 'best guess' estimate.

3 Generally, the baseline opioid dose should be continued as a regular prescription.

4 Reduce the baseline dose if:
   • the surgery is likely to improve the pre-operative pain
   • the baseline opioid needs to be replaced by an alternative opioid; reduce the dose calculated from equipotency tables by 1/3–1/2, particularly when dealing with large doses, e.g. ≥ morphine 1g/24h PO or equivalent (see p.295).

5 If PO is not possible immediately postoperatively, an alternative route, e.g. CSCI or CIVI should be used to deliver the baseline dose. This can also be done via IV patient-controlled analgesia (PCA) (see point 11).

6 Before restarting PO SR opioids, ensure that GI function has returned to normal. Gastric stasis can lead to delayed dissolution and drug absorption, followed by 'dose-dumping' when motility improves, with consequential overdose.

7 It is sometimes recommended that fentanyl TD patches are removed before surgery. However, if the surgery is unlikely to lead to major changes in skin perfusion and the ongoing opioid requirements are unlikely to change, it is reasonable to leave TD patches in place, and give additional p.r.n. opioid.

8 Should TD patches be removed, pain relief will persist for several hours because fentanyl is sequestrated widely throughout the body, particularly in adipose tissue (see p.315). Note: in postoperative patients, after a patch has been removed, the mean time for the plasma fentanyl concentration to drop below the minimum effective level is 16h, with a range of 2–23h.[13]

9 Continue long-term ED or IT pumps unchanged unless pain is expected to be less severe as a result of the operation.

10 Prescribe an appropriate dose of a strong opioid for p.r.n. use; typically equivalent to 1/6–1/10th of the total daily dose.

11 With IV PCA, a larger bolus dose is generally necessary compared with the typical bolus dose of morphine 1mg. PCA can also be used to continuously deliver the baseline opioid dose.

Example
Patient on long-term morphine 300mg/day PO = 100mg/day IV = 4mg/h IV.
PCA background infusion = 4mg/h IV.
PCA bolus dose = 4mg IV with a 5–10min lockout period between doses.
If the patient is needing ≥3 doses/h, consider increasing the bolus dose.

With addicts, if there is considerable uncertainty about their opioid intake, it may be safer to adopt a more cautious approach, e.g. underestimate the background infusion dose and overestimate the corresponding bolus dose.

12 Close monitoring is required to:
   • identify inadequate dosing (unrelieved pain, withdrawal phenomena)
   • ensure rapid dose titration
   • prevent excessive dosing (sedation, respiratory depression).

17: ANALGESIC DRUGS AND FITNESS TO DRIVE

Several classes of centrally-acting drugs used as analgesics have the potential to influence driving performance. Doctors have a duty of care to inform patients of this risk and advise them appropriately (see www.drivesafe.com). As a minimum, patients should be reminded that it is their legal responsibility to ensure that they drive only if they feel 100% safe to do so.[1] However, the impact of ceasing to drive can be considerable and impairment from stable doses of centrally-acting analgesics is not inevitable.

This chapter summarizes the evidence regarding the effect of opioids, anti-epileptics, antidepressants, benzodiazepines and cannabinoids on driving performance and the risk of a motor vehicle accident. Although the evidence is sometimes conflicting, the information provided here will assist health professionals when advising patients. However, it must always be tailored to the individual's circumstances, e.g. the influence of the disease itself, age, visual disturbances, the presence of pain and use of other sedative drugs (e.g. antimuscarinics).

Driving performance and drugs

Evaluating the impact of drugs on driving can be difficult. Driving performance is affected by multiple mechanisms from altered attention and reaction time to impaired judgment and risk taking. Studying actual or simulated driving, or surrogate laboratory markers of such skills, may not capture all influences on driving performance.[2] Although studying analgesic use among people involved in road traffic accidents avoids this problem, confounding factors include multiple drug use and impairment caused by pain and the illness itself.[3] Further, driving performance is impaired in some patients with chronic non-cancer pain not receiving centrally-acting medication.[4] Indeed, cognitive performance may improve with effective long-term opioid analgesia.[5,6] In a comparison of cancer patients with or without **morphine** analgesia and healthy volunteers, cognitive impairment was associated with the cancer rather than **morphine** use.[7]

Guidance for patients receiving a potentially sedating analgesic

The *Criminal Code* is the relevant piece of Canadian Federal legislation concerning drugs and driving. The focus within the *Criminal Code* is on the operation or the care and control of motor vehicles and vessels (and on assisting in the operation of aircraft and railway equipment) while 'impaired' by drugs, a combination of drugs and alcohol, or alcohol alone.[1] The *Criminal Code* does not define drugs in this context, nor does it distinguish between illegal/illicit, prescription or OTC drugs. It is not the drug but the state of impairment that matters. Although not defined in the legislation, it is necessary to evaluate impairment to determine if a person has committed an offence.

The evidence, summarized in Table 17.1, suggests that patients should be warned not to drive after starting and when titrating potentially sedating medication, or after taking a dose for break-through (episodic) pain. They should be warned that sedation will be increased by the concurrent use of alcohol, even within normal alcohol driving limits, or other sedating medication, whether obtained by prescription, OTC or illicitly. They should also be advised that some OTC drugs contain potentially sedating drugs, e.g.:
- Tylenol No.1®: each caplet = acetaminophen 300mg and codeine 8mg but also caffeine 15mg
- Nytol Regular Strength® and Nytol Extra Strength®: each tablet/caplet = diphenhydramine 25mg and 50mg respectively (cf. Nytol Natural Source® which contains valerian instead).

Table 17.1 Drugs and driving: a summary of the evidence

Class of drug	Impact on risk of a motor vehicle accident	Comments
Opioids	No increased risk with chronic use of a stable dose[2,3,8–14]	Cognition and driving performance impaired for about 1 week after the start of treatment or after dose increments[15,16] Additional transient impairment with doses for break-through (episodic) pain
Anti-epileptics	No increased risk with chronic use of a stable dose[17]	Cognition impaired by multiple, high-dose anti-epileptics; marginally less with newer drugs (e.g. gabapentin) compared with older drugs (e.g. carbamazepine)[18,19]
Antidepressants	Sedative antidepressants double the risk in the elderly (>65 years) but not other age groups[17,20–23]	Sedative antidepressants impair performance for about 1 week after the start of treatment (mianserin ≥2 weeks). SSRIs appear to cause less impairment, but caution is still required[24,25]
Benzodiazepines	Double the risk[26]	Risk only partially decreases with time and is related to dose, halflife and concurrent alcohol. Risk from nocturnal use of shorter halflife hypnotic benzodiazepines is unclear[22,27]
Cannabinoids	Risk likely to be increased initially. The degree of tolerance to chronic use of stable doses of prescribed cannabinoids is uncertain	Most studies deal with illicit use, frequently confounded by alcohol consumption and risk-taking behaviours[28,29]

Patients receiving opioids, anti-epileptics and antidepressants can consider driving once a stable dose is achieved if they are not affected by drowsiness, nor impaired by the disease itself. When possible, use less sedating drugs, e.g. consider the use of an SSRI rather than a TCA when treating depression. For benzodiazepines, particularly if taken in the daytime and/or those with a long halflife, the risk is more persistent, and consideration should be given to using a less sedating alternative, e.g. **tizanidine** for muscle spasm, or not driving. Providing the patient with written information is also helpful. Examples of information leaflets used elsewhere are available at www.palliativedrugs.com; select *Document library* and search under prescribing issues, driving on medication.

Requirements for physicians to report patients who should not drive is determined at the provincial or territorial level, and readers should be familiar with their provincial/territorial legislation in this regard. Regulations vary from province to province. To be able to advise patients appropriately, it is important to be familiar with the conditions and circumstances which necessitate informing the provincial Department of Motor Vehicles. Contact details can be obtained through the following websites:

- http://www.ccmta.ca/english/alookat/faqs.cfm
- http://www.gov.ns.ca/snsmr/rmv/related.asp

Risk from specific analgesic drug classes
Opioids
Driving performance does not appear to be affected by stable doses of appropriately titrated strong opioids:[2,8–14]
- cognition returns to normal after about 1 week after the start of treatment or after dose increments[15]
- long-term opioid analgesia for cancer pain[8] and non-cancer pain[9,11] has little or no impact on surrogate laboratory measures of driving performance compared with:
  ▷ healthy volunteers[11]
  ▷ cancer patients not taking opioids[8]
  ▷ patients with various causes of cerebral impairment who had passed a standardized fitness-to-drive test[9]
- patients with non-cancer pain receiving opioids at stable doses for ≥1 week do not differ from those without opioids or from healthy volunteers in tests of actual driving performance[16]
- epidemiological studies do not show an increased risk of road traffic accidents among drivers using opioid analgesics.[3]

The optimal interval between dose initiation or increase and returning to driving is unclear and may vary between individuals and formulation used, e.g. steady-state plasma concentrations of TD **fentanyl** are generally achieved after 36–48h but, according to the manufacturers, this is sometimes achieved only after 6–12 days (see p.315).

Anti-epileptics
Several studies have examined the cognitive effects of anti-epileptic drugs in patients with epilepsy or healthy volunteers. Marked cognitive impairment is associated with the use of multiple or high-dose anti-epileptic drugs, particularly **phenobarbital**. Newer drugs, e.g. **gabapentin**, may cause marginally less impairment than older drugs, e.g. **carbamazepine** and **valproic acid**.[18,19] In a case-control study, anti-epileptic drugs did not increase the risk of a motor vehicle accident.[17]

Antidepressants
Using a standard on-the-road test, sedating antidepressants, e.g. **amitriptyline**, **doxepin**, **imipramine**, **mirtazapine**, **mianserin** (not Canada), were found initially to impair driving performance. Performance returned to baseline within 1 week, except for **mianserin** which still caused impairment when the study ended after 2 weeks.[24] Less sedating drugs, e.g. SSRIs, appear to cause less impairment, but studies of airline pilots suggest this can still be to a degree which necessitates caution.[24,25]

Even though lower doses of antidepressants are generally used for analgesia, performance in driving tests was impaired in patients with neuropathic pain after the first dose of **amitriptyline** 25mg but had returned to baseline when evaluated 2 weeks later.[4] The possibility of pharmacokinetic interactions and additive sedation with other analgesics should also be borne in mind.

In three case-control studies across all age groups, antidepressants did not increase the risk of a motor vehicle accident.[17,22,23] However, when older people were considered separately, a doubling of risk was found.[20,21]

Benzodiazepines

In case-control studies, benzodiazepines approximately double the risk of motor vehicle accidents.[26] The risk is highest in those taking higher doses, drugs with a longer halflife, or concurrent alcohol.[17,22,26] The risk only partially decreases with time.[27]

Simulated driving tests show impaired reaction times, tracking and co-ordination with the acute use of benzodiazepines. In multiple-dose studies the degree of attenuation of impairment over time was variable.[30]

The risk from a bedtime dose of a hypnotic benzodiazepine with a short halflife is unclear; studies of airline pilots suggest shorter-acting benzodiazepines do not cause a detectable sedating effect the following morning.[25] However, this may not be true in an elderly or frail population receiving multiple medications. **Zopiclone** is *not* a safer alternative.[22,26,27,30]

Cannabinoids

Most studies consider the risk from the illicit use of whole cannabis plant. Interpretation is hampered by associated alcohol consumption, risk-taking behaviour (potentially a cause and/or effect of cannabis use), and methodological limitations. However, taken together these studies suggest cannabis causes dose-dependent impairment of driving ability.[25,28,29] The risk of motor vehicle accidents is approximately doubled, and is further increased by concurrent alcohol consumption.[29] Some studies suggest a degree of insight into the impairment, and an ability to compensate partially for it (e.g. by driving more cautiously).

These studies are unlikely to reflect the risk associated with the use of stable doses of prescribed cannabinoids (see p.169). Those which controlled for alcohol use or risk-taking behaviour generally found a reduced or even absent risk.[29] Further, stable doses may allow tolerance to impairment to develop, as with many psychotropics. For example, 6 patients with multiple sclerosis and painful spasticity showed no impairment of laboratory markers of driving ability after receiving **nabilone** 2mg/day for 4 weeks.[31] However, caution is necessary particularly in physically debilitated patients, and they should be advised *not* to drive during initial dose titration. Once on a stable dose of cannabinoids, restarting driving can be discussed.

1 Department of Justice Canada (1985) Criminal Code of Canada (R.S., 1985, c.C-46). Part VIII Offences against the person and reputation. Motor vehicles, vessels and aircraft. Sections 253-258. Available from: http://laws.justice.gc.ca/en/showdoc/cs/C-46/bo-ga:l_VIII-gb:s_249/20090721/en

2 Fishbain D et al. (2003) Are opioid-dependent/tolerant patients impaired in driving-related skills? A structured evidence-based review. Journal of Pain and Symptom Management. 25: 559–577.

3 Fishbain D et al. (2002) Can patients taking opioids drive safely? A structured evidence-based review? Journal of Pain and Palliative Care Pharmacotherapy. 16 (1): 9–28.

4 Veldhuijzen DS et al. (2006) Effect of chronic nonmalignant pain on highway driving performance. Pain. 122: 28–35.

5 Tassain V et al. (2003) Long term effects of oral sustained release morphine on neuropsychological performance in patients with chronic non-cancer pain. Pain. 104: 389–400.

6 Jamison RN et al. (2003) Neuropsychological effects of long-term opioid use in chronic pain patients. Journal of Pain and Symptom Management. 26: 913–921.

7 Clemons M et al. (1996) Alertness, cognition and morphine in patients with advanced cancer. Cancer Treatment Reviews. 22: 451–468.

8 Vainio A et al. (1995) Driving ability in cancer patients receiving longterm morphine analgesia. Lancet. 346: 667–670.

9 Galski T et al. (2000) Effects of opioids on driving ability. Journal of Pain and Symptom Management. 19: 200–208.

10 Chapman S (2001) The effects of opioids on driving ability in patients with chronic pain. American Pain Society Bulletin. 11.

11 Sabatowski R et al. (2003) Driving ability under long-term treatment with transdermal fentanyl. Journal of Pain and Symptom Management. 25: 38–47.

12 Pease N et al. (2004) Driving advice for palliative care patients taking strong opioid medication. Palliative Medicine. 18: 663–665.

13 Brandman JF (2005) Cancer patients, opioids, and driving. Journal of Supportive Oncology. 3: 317–320.

14 Kress HG and Kraft B (2005) Opioid medication and driving ability. European Journal of Pain. 9: 141–144.

15 Bruera E et al. (1989) The cognitive effects of the administration of narcotic analgesics in patients with cancer pain. Pain. 39: 13–16.

16 Byas-Smith MG et al. (2005) The effect of opioids on driving and psychomotor performance in patients with chronic pain. Clinical Journal of Pain. 21: 345–352.

17 Neutel I (1998) Benzodiazepine-related traffic accidents in young and elderly drivers. Human Psychopharmacology. 13 (suppl): s115–s123.

18 Brunbech L and Sabers A (2002) Effect of antiepileptic drugs on cognitive function in individuals with epilepsy: a comparative review of newer versus older agents. Drugs. 62: 593–604.

19 Aldenkamp AP et al. (2003) Newer antiepileptic drugs and cognitive issues. Epilepsia. 44 (suppl 4): 21–29.

20 Ray WA et al. (1992) Psychoactive drugs and the risk of injurious motor vehicle crashes in elderly drivers. American Journal of Epidemiology. 136: 873–883.

21 Leveille SG et al. (1994) Psychoactive medications and injurious motor vehicle collisions involving older drivers. *Epidemiology.* **5**: 591–598.

22 Barbone F et al. (1998) Association of road-traffic accidents with benzodiazepine use. *Lancet.* **352**: 1331–1336.

23 McGwin G, Jr. et al. (2000) Relations among chronic medical conditions, medications, and automobile crashes in the elderly: a population-based case-control study. *American Journal of Epidemiology.* **152**: 424–431.

24 Ramaekers JG (2003) Antidepressants and driver impairment: empirical evidence from a standard on-the-road test. *Journal of Clinical Psychiatry.* **64**: 20–29.

25 Carter T (2006) *Fitness to drive: A guide for health professionals.* Royal Society of Medicine Press, London.

26 Thomas RE (1998) Benzodiazepine use and motor vehicle accidents. Systematic review of reported association. *Canadian Family Physician.* **44**: 799–808.

27 Hemmelgarn B et al. (1997) Benzodiazepine use and the risk of motor vehicle crash in the elderly. *Journal of the American Medical Association.* **278**: 27–31.

28 UK Department for Transport (2000) Cannabis and driving: a review of the literature and commentary (No.12). Available from: http://www.dft.gov.uk/pgr/roadsafety/research/rsrr/theme3/cannabisanddrivingareviewoft4764

29 Ramaekers JG et al. (2004) Dose related risk of motor vehicle crashes after cannabis use. *Drug and Alcohol Dependence.* **73**: 109–119.

30 Rapoport MJ and Banina MC (2007) Impact of psychotropic medications on simulated driving: a critical review. *CNS Drugs.* **21**: 503–519.

31 Kurzthaler I et al. (2005) The effect of nabilone on neuropsychological functions related to driving ability: an extended case series. *Human Psychopharmacology.* **20**: 291–293.

18: CONTINUOUS SUBCUTANEOUS INFUSIONS

CSCI in clinical practice

Continuous subcutaneous infusion (CSCI) is used extensively in palliative care in the UK, particularly in patients who can no longer swallow medication or who can do so only with increasing difficulty. Use is increasing in the USA (Table 18.1),[1,2] but as yet is not widespread in Canada.

Table 18.1 Drugs given by CSCI in 659 palliative care units in the USA[2]

≥8% of palliative care units	4–3% of palliative care units	2–1% of palliative care units
Morphine (97%)	Heparin (4%)	Dexamethasone (2%)
Hydromorphone (60%)	Meperidine (pethidine) (4%)	Hydroxyzine (2%)
Haloperidol (15%)	Octreotide (4%)	Calcitonin (1%)
Midazolam (9%)	Scopolamine (hyoscine)	Fentanyl (1%)
Metoclopramide (8%)	hydrobromide (4%)	
	Atropine (3%)	
	Lorazepam (3%)	
	Phenobarbital (3%)	

CSCI is as effective as continuous IV infusion (CIVI),[3] and at least as good as intermittent bolus injections.[4] In settings where it is difficult to be certain that intermittent regular injections will be administered on time, CSCI is likely to provide better round-the-clock comfort (Box 18.A).

Indications for CSCI

CSCI should not just be thought of as the last resort but as a useful alternative route of administration in certain circumstances.[5] CSCI is *not* 'Step 4' on the analgesic ladder, but merely an alternative method of administration. For most drugs, this method is off-label.[6] Indications for using CSCI include:

• persistent nausea and vomiting
• dysphagia
• intestinal obstruction
• coma
• poor absorption of oral drugs (rare)
• patient preference.

Before setting up a CSCI, it is important to explain to the patient and family:

• the reason(s) for using this route and method
• how the infusion device works
• the advantages and possible disadvantages of CSCI (see Box 18.A).

Box 18.A Advantages and disadvantages of CSCI

Advantages
Saving of nursing time.
Round-the-clock comfort because plasma drug concentrations are maintained without peaks and troughs.
Generally needs to be loaded once daily or less, depending on sterility guidelines.
Control of multiple symptoms with a combination of drugs.
Independence and mobility maintained because the device is lightweight and can be worn in a holster under or over clothes.

Disadvantages
Initial cost of infusion devices.
Training necessary for staff, together with need to maintain competency.
Lack of flexibility if more than one drug is being administered.
Lack of reliable compatibility data for some mixtures.
Possible inflammation and pain at the infusion site.
Although uncommon, problems with the infusion device can lead to break-through (episodic) pain (or other symptom) if the problem cannot be resolved quickly.
The fact that it is no longer necessary to give injections q4h could lead to an undesirable 'high tech-low touch' approach to care.

Although often administered by CSCI in the UK, several drugs with a long duration of action, e.g. **dexamethasone**, **methotrimeprazine** (**levomepromazine**) can be given equally well as a bolus SC or IV injection once daily or b.i.d. (Table 18.2).[7]

Table 18.2 Drugs which can be given once daily or b.i.d. instead of by CSCI

Drug	Plasma halflife (h)	Duration of action (h)
Dexamethasone	3–4.5	36–54
Furosemide	0.5–2	6–8
Granisetron	10–11	≤24
Haloperidol	13–35	≤24
Methadone	8–75	≤12
Methotrimeprazine	15–30	≤24
Promethazine	12	≥12

Phenobarbital also has a long duration of action but generally should not be given SC because of the risk of tissue necrosis. SC use in Canada in the past was with a special access preparation which is no longer available.

Drug doses

If symptoms are controlled, start the CSCI 1–2h before the effect of the medication is due to wear off. If symptoms are uncontrolled, set up the CSCI immediately with stat doses of the same drugs.

Drugs are generally *more* bio-available by injection than PO. This means that the dose of a drug given by CSCI will be *less* than the dose previously given PO, generally between 1/3 and 2/3 of the PO dose. The bio-availability data given at the end of the pharmacology section in the individual drug monographs serve as a guide to the appropriate reduction. For example, the dose of a drug with oral bio-availability of 75% should be reduced by 1/4 when given SC and, if 50% bio-available, the dose should be halved when given SC, and so on. The SC and IV routes are generally considered equipotent, and the respective doses are thus the same.[3,8]

Rescue medication

Appropriate doses of p.r.n. medication should always be prescribed, and given as separate SC injections, or via a small butterfly needle/cannula. These should be flushed with diluent according to local policy.

TD patches

As a general rule, TD opioid patches, e.g. **fentanyl** should be continued when the need for supplemental opioid via CSCI is short-term, e.g. in the last days of life (see Guidelines: Use of transdermal fentanyl patches, p.322). It is more straightforward to supplement the patch with a CSCI of **morphine** or other opioid than to convert completely to a single alternative opioid.

Drug compatibility

There is a dearth of data on CSCI practices in Canada. In the UK, it is common practice to administer 2–3 different drugs in the same syringe.[7,9,10] It is clearly important to consider drug compatibility (Box 18.B), and compatibility data from other countries may be relevant if the formulation and brand of drugs are the same. Some centres mix 4 drugs. This is generally because of a decision to add **dexamethasone** or an antisecretory drug, e.g. **hyoscine (scopolamine) butylbromide**, **scopolamine (hyoscine) hydrobromide** or **glycopyrrolate**.

Box 18.B   Drug compatibility data

Physical compatibility
If mixing two or more drugs does not result in a physical change, e.g. discolouration, clouding or crystallization, they are said to be physically compatible.

Observational data
Data from many palliative care services about the visual appearance of various drug mixtures over the infusion period (generally 24h) have been collated for use in Appendix 4. However, observational data are subjective and imprecise; generally, only major incompatibilities can be identified in this way.

Laboratory data
These are generally derived from microscopic examination of a drug mixture under polarized light at specified concentrations and several time points when kept under controlled conditions. Although more robust, these are not definitive; a solution may remain physically clear even when there is chemical incompatibility.[11]

Chemical compatibility
If mixing two or more drugs does not result in a chemical change leading to loss or degradation of one or more of the drugs, the mixture is said to be chemically compatible. Chemical compatibility data are generally obtained by analyzing the drug mixture by high-performance liquid chromatography (HPLC) at specified concentrations and several time points when kept under controlled conditions.

Occasionally, a drug combination has been shown to be chemically compatible but physically incompatible. Thus, physical compatibility should be checked before proceeding to chemical analysis.

Generally, drugs with a similar pH are more likely to be compatible than those with widely differing ones. Most drugs are acidic in solution, however, **dexamethasone, ketorolac** and **phenobarbital** are alkaline in solution and often cause compatibility problems (Table 18.3). The risk of precipitation with **dexamethasone** is reduced if it is added last to an already dilute drug mixture. On the other hand, as already noted, **dexamethasone** has a long duration of action. Thus, except when it is being given to reduce the risk of skin reactions (see p.518), there is no real need to give it by CSCI (see Table 18.2, opposite).

Table 18.3 pH values of drugs delivered by infusion devices (manufacturers' information)

Drug	pH	Drug	pH
Bupivacaine	4–6.5	Lidocaine	5–7
Clonidine	4–4.5	Methadone	3–6.5
Dexamethasone	7–8.5	Methotrimeprazine	4.5
Glycopyrrolate	2–3	Metoclopramide	4.5–6.5
Granisetron	4.7–7.3	Midazolam	3
Haloperidol	3–3.8	Morphine	2.5–6
Hydromorphone	4–5.5	Octreotide	3.9–4.5
Hyoscine (scopolamine)	3.7–5.5	Ondansetron	3.3–4
butylbromide		Phenobarbital	9.2–10.2
Ketamine	3.5–5.5	Scopolamine (hyoscine)	5–7
Ketorolac	6.9–7.9	hydrobromide[a]	

a. in the compatibility charts, listed as hyoscine hydrobromide.

Charts A4.1–A.4.4 (see p.591) summarize the compatibility data available for the more commonly used 2- and 3-drug combinations given by CSCI *in 0.9% saline*. Charts summarizing 2- and 3-drug combinations given by CSCI *in water* can be found on the www.palliativedrugs.com along with the *Syringe Driver Survey Database* (SDSD). The SDSD is a continually updated resource and contains observational compatibility data on mixing combinations of up to 4 drugs. We would ask health professionals to submit to www.palliativedrugs.com *Syringe Driver Survey Database* details of successful or unsuccessful combinations for which there are no published data. There is a particular need for information about **alfentanil** and **hydromorphone**.

Information on compatibility can also be obtained from other sources, including:
• *The Syringe Driver: Continuous Subcutaneous Infusions in Palliative Care.*[10]
• www.pallcare.info[12]
• Handbook on Injectable Drugs.[13]

It is important to ascertain if the compatibility data are relevant to the situation of intended use. Drug combinations may be compatible only at certain concentrations, thus the *concentration* of each drug in the solution (the dose of each drug divided by the total final volume used) should be compared, not the dose. The diluent used and the time period for which the infusion ran should also be checked because different diluents and longer infusion periods may also cause compatibility problems.

Other factors also affect drug stability and compatibility (Box 18.C), and these may be the reason for conflicting anecdotal reports. If there is doubt about the relevance of the compatibility data to the situation in which a given drug combination is to be used, advice should be obtained from a clinical pharmacist.

Box 18.C Factors which may affect drug stability and compatibility[13–15]

Drug concentrations.
Brand/formulation of the drug, e.g. differing or incompatible excipients.
Diluent.
Time interval.
Temperature of the surroundings:
• ambient
• whether the delivery device is worn under or over clothes.
Exposure to light.
Order of mixing, e.g. dexamethasone added first or last.
Delivery system material.[a,b]

---

a. some drugs adsorb onto the material of the container, e.g. clonazepam onto PVC infusion sets[16]
b. cloudiness can be caused by chemicals in the material of the container leaching into the solution.

Diluent

To avoid confusion, consistency of practice within individual units is important.[17] For drugs approved for this route of administration, the Product Monograph will advise about which diluent to use, but not if CSCI use is off-label. Further, the information given may not be helpful when giving more than one drug. In Canada, 0.9% saline is generally used as the first-line diluent (see Charts A4.1–A4.4, p.591), whereas water for injection (WFI) is more widely used in the UK. They both have advantages and disadvantages (Table 18.4).

Some centres in the USA use 5% dextrose in water instead, but this is acidic and unsuitable for very alkaline drugs, e.g. **furosemide** and **phenobarbital**.

Table 18.4 Comparison of diluents

Advantages	Disadvantages
Saline 0.9%[18]	
Isotonic	Generally less compatibility data available for
Less infusion site pain and skin reaction	commonly used drugs
	Incompatible with some drugs, e.g. haloperidol at high concentrations approaching 2mg/mL; cyclizine (not Canada); diamorphine > 40mg/mL (not Canada)
WFI	
Less chance of incompatibility	Large volumes are hypotonic, and may cause
Generally more compatibility data available for commonly used drugs	infusion site pain and skin reaction

Volume

The volume of the CSCI will generally depend on the infusion device being used, the total volume of the drugs, the maximum rate of delivery and the intended infusion time (see p.516, Setting up the infusion device).

If a syringe driver is used, many centres in the UK use a 10mL luerlock syringe. However, it has been suggested that a 20mL luerlock syringe should be used as the minimum final volume of the CSCI to allow greater dilution.[10] Greater dilution reduces:
- the risk of incompatibility
- the impact of priming a line (less drug in the 'dead space')
- injection site skin reactions from the drug.

When a syringe driver is used, the total volume of drugs required may exceed the maximum volume that the syringe driver can deliver in 24h. This is most likely with combinations which include higher doses of **bupivacaine**, **metoclopramide**, **midazolam** or **morphine**. This problem can generally be circumvented by using a different infusion device, prescribing drugs for a shorter infusion time, e.g. 12h, or in the case of **morphine**, by switching to **hydromorphone**,[19] **fentanyl** or **sufentanil**.

When a cartridge/cassette/bag infusion system is used, a larger final volume is possible. Even so, some centres standardize to 50mL volume with a maximum rate of 2mL/h.

Siting the CSCI

- avoid areas listed in Box 18.D
- choose a preferred site, commonly; anterior chest wall, anterolateral aspects of upper arms, sometimes; anterior abdominal wall, anterior surface of the thighs
- insert an 18-gauge butterfly needle at an angle of 30–45° into SC tissue
- use a plastic cannula in patients with a known sensitivity to metal
- where possible use fine bore tubing with a small priming volume (preferably less than 0.3mL)
- secure the tubing with a transparent semipermeable adhesive dressing (e.g. Tegaderm®), with a loop to reduce the likelihood of needle displacement.

Box 18.D   Skin areas to avoid when siting a CSCI
Edematous areas
Skin folds
Breast
Broken, inflamed or infected skin
Recently irradiated skin sites
Cutaneous tumour sites
Bony prominences
Near a joint
Anterior chest wall in cachectic patients
Upper arm in bedbound patients who need turning
Scarring

Portable infusion devices

There is currently no published information on the use of portable infusion devices in Canada. Several portable delivery systems are available (Table 18.5). The use of delivery systems with cartridges/cassettes prepared by pharmacists adds significantly to the cost, but in areas where drug diversion is a concern, these systems are more secure.

Setting up the infusion device

Full instructions can be found in the manufacturer's instruction manual. Additional good practice points are outlined below.[10,20–23]

1 Unless prepared by a pharmacy, cartridges/syringes/bags should be made up immediately before use using strict aseptic technique.

2 When prepared in a clinical area, some sources recommend discarding the solution after 24h.[24,25] However, it is unclear if this recommendation is an extrapolation from data relating to IV use. There are anecdotal Canadian reports of longer durations being safely used; local guidelines should be consulted.

3 Ensure adequate mixing has occurred; the solution should be clear and free from crystals or precipitate.

4 If using dexamethasone, it should be the last drug added to an already dilute combination of drugs in order to reduce the risk of incompatibility.

5 The cartridge/syringe/bag should be labeled with a list of its contents, taking care not to obscure the solution or any measuring scale.

6 Priming uses about 0.5mL. This is of significance when using small volumes, e.g. syringe drivers; the contents of the delivery device will thus be delivered in less than the planned time. Subsequent infusions which do not involve priming will not be affected.

7 Protect the infusion from excessive sunlight and heat, e.g. electric blankets.

8 Do not add drugs to an infusion already in place.

9 Do not increase the rate of an infusion already in place if there are multiple drugs in the infusion.

10 If changes to the infusion other than the rate are required, discard the infusion in place and make up a new infusion. Use a new line and consider giving stat doses of appropriate medication if an immediate effect is needed.

Table 18.5 Examples of portable battery-driven infusion delivery systems available in Canada

Delivery system	Type	Manufacturer	Size (HxWxD) (inches)	Weight (excluding power source) (ounces)	Power source	Website
CADD Prizm	Cartridge/cassette	Smiths Medical	$5.6 \times 4.1 \times 1.7$	17	Battery (1, 9 volt)	www.smiths-medical.com/ca-en/
Gemstar infusion systems	Cartridge/cassette	Hospira	$5.5 \times 3.8 \times 2$	17	Batteries (2, AA size) or power pack	www.hospira.ca
Graseby MS16A and MS26	Syringe driver	Graseby Medical	$6.5 \times 2.1 \times 0.9$	6.5	Battery (1, 9 volt)	http://marcalmedical.com
Baxter Ipump	Bag	Baxter				www.baxter.ca/en

Checks in use

Specific record charts should be used for checking a CSCI; examples are available in the document library on www.palliativedrugs.com. Checks should be documented within 1h of setting up the CSCI, and then q4h:

- is the device still working
- rate
- amount of time and/or solution left, and whether the infusion is running to time (based on the preceding 4h)
- appearance of the solution in the tubing and cartridge/syringe/bag
- condition of the skin site
- break-through (PCA) doses (and number of attempts).

Do not remove the cartridge/syringe/bag from the infusion device to perform these checks. If checking indicates a problem, action should be taken and then documented. For example, if the infusion needs to be resited and hence reprimed, the time, the new site and the new infusion volume/syringe length should be recorded. Other comments might include details of incompatibility and mention of any mishaps, such as the delivery device being found disconnected.

Infusion site problems

Infusion site problems may be due to various causes (Box 18.E).[10,26,27]

Box 18.E Causes of infusion site problems

Irritant drugs
Tonicity of the solution
pH of the solution
Incompatible drug/diluent mixture
Glass particles from ampoules
Infection
Sterile abscess
Allergy to nickel needle
Infrequent resiting
Anatomical site

With non-irritant drugs an infusion site may be satisfactory for ⩾1 week (and occasionally 2–3 weeks).[28] Site reactions can be reduced by:[27]

- use of a less irritant drug, e.g. **haloperidol** instead of **prochlorperazine** (Box 18.F)
- diluting the solution as much as possible, and perhaps using a shorter syringe infusion time, e.g. 12h instead of 24h, thereby halving drug concentration
- using a plastic cannula instead of a butterfly needle[29,30] (always in patients with a known metal allergy)
- changing the site prophylactically every 2–3 days
- applying **hydrocortisone** 1% cream to the skin around the needle entry site, and covering it with an occlusive dressing
- adding **dexamethasone** 1mg to the solution if compatibility data permits.[28]

Although the routine addition of **dexamethasone** has been recommended on the grounds that it extends the life of an infusion site by about 50%, the fact that some sites have lasted 2–3 weeks without **dexamethasone** suggests that routine use cannot be recommended.[28]

Converting from CSCI to PO

Some patients are able to revert from CSCI to PO medication, e.g. those being treated for nausea and vomiting. When this seems possible, convert the drugs sequentially rather than all at once. For example, convert the anti-emetic medication first and, if the nausea and vomiting do not recur, change the other medication 1–2 days later.

Remember: just as drug doses were reduced when starting CSCI, doses will generally need to be increased when reverting to PO. This is particularly the case with strong opioid analgesics, e.g. **morphine** 15mg/24h CSCI will need to be increased to **morphine** 30mg/24h PO (see p.497).

The CSCI is generally discontinued when the first dose of the PO medication is administered. It is important at this time to review p.r.n. medication, and to adjust it appropriately.

Box 18.F   Drugs which are irritant SC

Strongly irritant
Chlorpromazine: can cause local tissue necrosis } do *not* give by SC bolus
Diazepam } injection or by CSCI
Prochlorperazine: sometimes given by SC bolus; do not give by CSCI

Relatively irritant, precautions may be necessary[a]
Ketamine
Ketorolac
Methadone
Methotrimeprazine (levomepromazine)
Octreotide[b]
Ondansetron
Phenobarbital
Promethazine

---

a. see text and respective monographs
b. painful if given as SC bolus; this is reduced if warmed to body temperature before injection.

---

1 Letizia M et al. (2000) Intermittent subcutaneous injections for symptom control in hospice care: a retrospective investigation. The Hospice Journal. 15: 1–11.
2 Herndon CM and Fike DS (2001) Continuous subcutaneous infusion practices of United States hospices. Journal of Pain and Symptom Management. 22: 1027–1034.
3 Nelson KA et al. (1997) A prospective within-patient crossover study of continuous intravenous and subcutaneous morphine for chronic cancer pain. Journal of Pain and Symptom Management. 13: 262–267.
4 Watanabe S et al. (2008) A randomized double-blind crossover comparison of continuous and intermittent subcutaneous administration of opioid for cancer pain. Journal of Palliative Medicine. 11: 570–574.
5 Anderson SL and Shreve ST (2004) Continuous subcutaneous infusion of opiates at end-of-life. Annals of Pharmacotherapy. 38: 1015–1023.
6 Fonzo-Christe C et al. (2005) Subcutaneous administration of drugs in the elderly: survey of practice and systematic literature review. Palliative Medicine. 19: 208–219.
7 Wilcock A et al. (2006) Drugs given by a syringe driver: a prospective multicentre survey of palliative care services in the UK. Palliative Medicine. 20: 661–664.
8 Moulin D et al. (1991) Comparisons of continuous subcutaneous and intravenous hydromorphone infusion for management of cancer pain. Lancet. 337: 465–468.
9 O'Doherty CA et al. (2001) Drugs and syringe drivers: a survey of adult specialist palliative care practice in the United Kingdom and Eire. Palliative Medicine. 15: 149–154.
10 Dickman A et al. (2005) The Syringe Driver: Continuous Subcutaneous Infusions in Palliative Care (2e). Oxford University Press, Oxford.
11 Good PD et al. (2004) The compatibility and stability of midazolam and dexamethasone in infusion solutions. Journal of Pain and Symptom Management. 27: 471–475.
12 Back I (2001) Syringe driver drug compatibility database and patient information leaflets on the Internet. Palliative Medicine. 15: 77.
13 Trissel LA (2005) Handbook on Injectable Drugs (13e). American Society of Health System Pharmacists, Maryland, USA.
14 Kohut J, 3rd et al. (1996) Don't ignore details of drug-compatibility reports. American Journal of Health-System Pharmacy. 53: 2339.
15 Vermeire A and Remon JP (1999) Stability and compatibility of morphine. International Journal of Pharmaceutics. 187: 17–51.
16 Schneider JJ et al. (2006) Effect of tubing on loss of clonazepam administered by continuous subcutaneous infusion. Journal of Pain and Symptom Management. 31: 563–567.
17 Flowers C and McLeod F (2005) Diluent choice for subcutaneous infusion: a survey of the literature and Australian practice. International Journal of Palliative Nursing. 11: 54–60.
18 Schneider J et al. (1997) A study of the osmolality and pH of subcutaneous drug infusion solutions. Australian Journal of Hospital Pharmacy. 27: 29–31.
19 Fudin J et al. (2000) Use of continuous ambulatory infusions of concentrated subcutaneous (s.q.) hydromorphone versus intravenous (i.v.) morphine: cost implications for palliative care. American Journal of Hospice and Palliative Care. 17: 347–353.
20 NHS West Lothian Healthcare NHS Trust (2006) Subcutaneous Infusion by Graseby MS26 Daily Rate Syringe Driver. In: RAG panel. Available from: www.palliativedrugs.com

---

21 Camden Primary Care NHS Trust (2001) Syringe driver policy for Graseby MS16A. In: *RAG panel*. Available from: www.palliativedrugs.com

22 NHS Argyll and Clyde (2005) Syringe driver guidelines for Graseby MS26 (mm/24h) Available from: www.palliativedrugs.com

23 Queensland Government (2006) Centre for Palliative Care Research and Education Guidelines for syringe driver management in palliative care. In: *RAG panel*. Available from: www.palliativedrugs.com

24 National Patient Safety Agency (NPSA) (2007) Patient safety alert 20: Promoting safer use of injectable medicines. Available from: www.npsa.nhs.uk/nrls/alerts-and-directives/alerts/injectable-medicines/

25 BNF (2009) Appendix 6: Intravenous additives. In: *British National Formulary 57*. British Medical Association and Royal Pharmaceutical Society of Great Britain, London. Available from: www.bnf.org/bnf/bnf/current/

26 Oliver D (1991) The tonicity of solutions used in continuous subcutaneous infusions. The cause of skin reactions? *Hospital Pharmacy Practice*. **Sept**: 158–164.

27 Graham F (2006) Syringe drivers and subcutaneous sites: a review. *European Journal of Palliative Care*. **13**: 138–141.

28 Reymond L *et al.* (2003) The effect of dexamethasone on the longevity of syringe driver subcutaneous sites in palliative care patients. *Medical Journal of Australia*. **178**: 486–489.

29 Dawkins L *et al.* (2000) A randomized trial of winged Vialon cannulae and metal butterfly needles. *International Journal of Palliative Nursing*. **6**: 110–116.

30 Ross JR *et al.* (2002) A prospective, within-patient comparison between metal butterfly needles and Teflon cannulae in subcutaneous infusion of drugs to terminally ill hospice patients. *Palliative Medicine*. **16**: 13–16.

19: SPINAL ANALGESIA

Indications

Spinal analgesia is commonly used for obstetric or peri-operative pain relief. In the case of cancer patients receiving specialist palliative care, about 2–4% proceed to spinal analgesia because of unsatisfactory pain relief with more standard systemic analgesia.[1–7] Typical indications include:

- systemic opioid intolerance
- pathological fracture in a patient close to death
- refractory neuropathic pain (e.g. visceral neuropathic pain, lumbosacral plexopathy).

Spinal analgesia is effective in ≥50% of patients.[3,4,8–13] Good communication between palliative, pain and primary care teams is essential.

Contra-indications: Uncorrected coagulopathy, systemic or local infection, raised intracranial pressure.

Circumstances in which extra caution should be used include:

- spinal deformity
- incipient spinal cord compression
- myelosuppressive chemotherapy.

Route, placement and delivery device considerations

Analgesics are delivered to the intrathecal (IT) or epidural (ED) space via a small indwelling catheter placed by an anesthetist. The tube is generally tunnelled subcutaneously to emerge at a distant site, e.g. the supraclavicular fossa or flank, to reduce the risk of displacement and infection. This can be done using local anesthesia ± sedation, but general anesthesia is more comfortable for the patient.[4] The preferred route and delivery device are influenced by local experience and the likely duration of use (Table 19.1). Devices vary in allowing fixed vs. variable delivery rates, patient-controlled boluses, and cost.

Table 19.1 Preferred route and delivery device

Likely duration of use	Route and device	Comments
≤3 weeks	External ED device (re-usable)	Fewer initial complications than IT (8% vs. 25%); less headache from CSF leakage[14]
3 weeks–3 months	External IT device (re-usable)	Fewer later complications than ED (5% vs. 55%); less catheter occlusion[14]
≥3 months	Implantable IT device	More expensive initially, lower running costs; more cost–effective long-term[15]

Drugs delivered to the ED space diffuse through the meninges to reach the spinal cord and adjacent nerve roots. The level of the spinal cord at which the catheter is sited influences the area over which maximal analgesia is obtained. Migration or misplacement of ED catheters into the IT space (a rare event) will deliver an excessive dose resulting in significant toxicity, and may cause death secondary to respiratory arrest, unless recognized and treated urgently.

The IT route delivers drugs directly to the cerebrospinal fluid (CSF). Compared with the ED route, lower doses are required, thereby permitting the use of smaller devices and/or reducing the frequency of refilling (see below). IT administration generally provides better pain relief than the ED route.[3,14,16,17] IT is also the preferred route for long-term spinal analgesia, i.e. > 3 weeks.[3] The area of analgesia is less dependent on the site of the catheter because drugs in the CSF automatically diffuse rostrally.

Although the same delivery devices can theoretically be used for SC, IV and spinal infusion, for maximum safety it is best to use a device specifically designed for spinal delivery.[5] Distinct pumps and connectors will reduce the potential for confusion in a patient receiving concurrent spinal and SC/IV infusions.[3] However, such recommendations must be weighed against the considerable advantage of staff using a delivery device with which they are familiar from frequent SC/IV use.

Clinical services caring for patients receiving spinal analgesia require clear procedures to be in place to minimize risk at all stages of treatment. An added problem is maintaining staff competence where such approaches are required infrequently: clear clinical guidelines and 'refresher' training can be helpful.

Choice of drugs

Morphine, bupivacaine and **clonidine** are the most commonly used (see below). In cancer pain, particularly neuropathic pain, opioids are generally combined with **bupivacaine** (or alternative local anesthetic) from the outset, and **clonidine** added subsequently. **Hydromorphone** is an alternative where morphine is poorly tolerated.[3,5,6,18,19]

Opioids

Spinally administered opioids act locally and/or in the brain stem. The latter occurs through CSF diffusion and/or systemic redistribution. The advantages of spinal administration are greatest with hydrophilic opioids, e.g. **morphine** and **hydromorphone** which penetrate the spine effectively and are slowly redistributed. **Fentanyl** and other hydrophobic opioids are rapidly redistributed: their spinal administration thus has fewer advantages over their systemic use,[20] although the lower risk of catheter tip granuloma is an advantage in specific patients (see p.525).

There is considerable uncertainty about dose equivalences between routes.[3,21,22] However, the following conversion factors for **morphine** can be used when deciding the initial spinal dose and an appropriate p.r.n. dose:

- SC → ED, divide SC 24h dose by 10
- SC → IT, divide SC 24h dose by 100.

Thus, **morphine** 300mg/24h SC is replaced by 3mg/24h IT. The appropriate p.r.n. dose of SC **morphine** for this will be (as usual) 1/10–1/6 of the SC equivalent of the IT dose, i.e. 30–50mg SC.[3,19,22]

Maximum opioid concentrations and daily doses have been proposed to minimize the risk of catheter tip granuloma formation (Table 19.2).[6] These are less applicable if short-term use is anticipated, although granulomas have been reported after just 27 days.[23]

Table 19.2 Recommended maximum long-term IT drug concentrations and doses[6]

Drug	Maximum concentration (mg/mL)	Maximum dose/24h (mg)
Morphine	20	15
Hydromorphone	10	4
Bupivacaine	40	30
Clonidine	2	1

Local anesthetic

Bupivacaine is the most widely used local anesthetic for spinal analgesia.[3,5,6,19] Inherent antimicrobial properties may decrease the probability of infection.[19] Undesirable effects include dose-dependent motor and sensory impairment, affecting 4–13% and ≤7% of patients respectively, generally at doses >15mg/day.[3,5,8–10,12]

Ropivacaine is used at some centres.[24] This has similar efficacy and tolerability to **bupivacaine**.[25,26]

Clonidine

Clonidine 15–30microgram/24h (IT) or 150–300microgram/24h (ED) is generally given with an opioid and a local anesthetic. Benefit is seen particularly in neuropathic pain. Undesirable effects include dose-dependent hypotension and bradycardia (see p.50).[3,5,19] Abrupt cessation (e.g. because of pump failure) may cause severe rebound hypertension. Administer oral **clonidine** while seeking specialist advice.[6]

Other drugs

Baclofen is used for pain related to spasticity. A life-threatening withdrawal syndrome can occur if IT **baclofen** is abruptly discontinued (Box 19.A).

Ketamine's spinal use is associated with histological changes of uncertain significance within the cord.[6,27–30]

The spinal use of various other drugs is described or under investigation, including **adenosine, gabapentin, midazolam, ketorolac, ziconotide** (not available in Canada) and **octreotide**.[6,31]

Box 19.A   IT baclofen withdrawal syndrome[32]

Cause
Sudden cessation of IT baclofen (e.g. delivery device failure).
Reported with a wide range of doses (50–1500microgram/24h).

Clinical features
Symptoms evolve over 1–3 days:
- tachycardia, hypotension or labile blood pressure
- fever
- dysphoria and malaise → unconsciousness → seizures
- spasticity and rigidity → rhabdomyolysis → acute renal failure
- pruritus, paresthesia
- priapism.

Differential diagnosis
Other drug-related cardiovascular-neuromuscular syndromes:
- Neuroleptic (antipsychotic) malignant syndrome (see p.123)
- Malignant hyperpyrexia
- Serotonin toxicity (see p.140).
Autonomic dysreflexia.
Sepsis.
Undesirable effects of spinal medication (e.g. hypotension caused by clonidine or bupivacaine).

Management
Restart the IT baclofen infusion as soon as possible.
Cardiopulmonary support as indicated.
High-dose baclofen PO or by enteral feeding tube (up to 120mg/24h).
If necessary, give a benzodiazepine by CSCI/CIVI (e.g. midazolam) titrated to achieve muscle relaxation, normothermia, stabilization of blood pressure and cessation of seizures.

Drug compatibility

Unlike acute pain, with chronic intractable pain, single drug spinal analgesia is often inadequate. Combinations of **morphine** with **bupivacaine** ± **clonidine** are widely used, particularly with external devices.[8–10,16] Long-term compatibility data for drug combinations in both external devices (at room temperature) and implanted pump reservoirs (at body temperature) are limited.[5] Several factors can affect drug stability and compatibility (see Box 18.C, p.514). It is important to ascertain if the compatibility data are relevant to the situation of intended use, and confirm what is the appropriate diluent, i.e. discuss with a pharmacist.

Compatibility data at room temperature

There are compatibility data on the following combinations at room temperature:
- **morphine sulfate** with **bupivacaine** or **clonidine** 2 months[33,34]
- **morphine sulfate** with **ropivacaine** 1 month[26]
- **hydromorphone** with **bupivacaine** 3 days[35]
- **fentanyl** with **ropivacaine**[26]
- **sufentanil** with **ropivacaine**[26]
- **clonidine** with **bupivacaine** 2 weeks[36]
- **clonidine** with **ropivacaine** 1 month.[26]

Compatibility data at body temperature

There are compatibility data on the following combinations at body temperature:
- **morphine sulfate** with **clonidine** $\pm$ **bupivacaine** $\leqslant$3 months in a SynchroMed pump[37,38]
- **hydromorphone** 4 months in a SynchroMed pump[39]
- **clonidine** with **hydromorphone** 1.5 months (only stability of **clonidine** evaluated).[40]

Ideally, delivery devices with mixtures to be administered over >24h should be prepared in a sterile environment, e.g. a licensed pharmacy unit, and not on the ward/by the bedside. Drugs should be preservative-free.[5]

Undesirable effects and complications of spinal analgesia

MRI can cause implantable pumps to malfunction. Inactivation or reservoir and catheter drainage may be required: seek manufacturer's advice.

These can relate to:[41]
- the drug(s) (Table 19.3)
- medical complications, e.g. bleeding, infection (Table 19.4)
- the delivery system (Table 19.4).

All health professionals caring for patients with spinal analgesia should, as a minimum, be aware of the most serious undesirable effects and complications, and their management (Box 19.B). Respiratory failure can result from central depression of respiratory drive (opioids) or impaired motor output to the respiratory muscles at the spinal level (**bupivacaine**). Rate of onset varies: systemic redistribution of the spinally administered opioid causes respiratory depression within minutes or hours, whereas diffusion through the CSF causes a delayed onset, occurring after 6–48h. Both **bupivacaine** and **clonidine** cause hypotension, the latter also causing bradycardia.

The transient undesirable effects seen when commencing systemic opioids are also seen with spinal opioids (Box 19.C).[19,41] Clinical areas should have access to resuscitation equipment including IV fluids, **naloxone** and **ephedrine**. Before insertion of a spinal catheter, baseline blood tests will help to evaluate fitness and exclude, for example, a coagulopathy. A neurological and cardiopulmonary examination provides an essential baseline for future reference if a problem arises.

Suspected infection

In addition to the usual infective and neoplastic causes of fever in palliative care, spinal catheter-related infections can occur (often with coagulase-positive or -negative *Staphylococci*).

Exit site infection: transparent dressings allow the early identification of exit site erythema. Systemic and topical antibacterials should be started promptly; this reduces the incidence of deeper infection/meningitis.[3] However, prophylactic antibacterials should not be routinely used.

ED abscesses: present with fever, escalating pain (this is invariable; either the original pain and/or back pain at the ED site), and new neurological impairment (80%).[12] Evaluation includes blood cultures, aspiration of fluid from the spinal catheter for microscopy and culture, neurological examination, identification of other potential sources of fever and MRI (see warning about MRI above). Seek early advice from a microbiologist and spinal or neurosurgeon. The risk increases with time. Distant non-healing wounds may be a risk factor.[4]

Meningitis: presents with fever and/or meningeal irritation (neck stiffness, stretch signs). Evaluation includes blood and line microscopy and cultures, white cell count, neurological examination, and identification of other potential sources of fever. Consider also MRI, particularly if new neurological impairment is present (see warning about MRI above). Spinal catheters need

Table 19.3 Drug-related undesirable effects

Drug	Undesirable effect	Frequency (%)	Comment
Early onset and/or after titration			
Withdrawal of systemic opioids	Diarrhea and intestinal colic		Partly avoidable if laxatives stopped and then retitrated after change to spinal route
Opioids	Nausea and vomiting	33[3,12,42,43]	
Opioids	Pruritus	15	Less likely if already taking opioids[13,42,43]
Bupivacaine	Motor or sensory disturbance; dose-dependent	4–13	Persistent motor impairment, overall frequency in palliative care series[3,9,12]
Opioids, bupivacaine	Urinary retention	8–43[3,8,43]	
Opioids, bupivacaine	Respiratory depression	0.1–2[3,44]	
Bupivacaine, clonidine	Cardiovascular compromise	5–20	Symptomatic hypotension; clonidine also causes bradycardia[3]
Late onset (also see p.000)			
Opioids[a]	Catheter tip granulomas	0.1[23]	MRI screening revealed granulomas in 3% of patients with long-term IT infusions. Eighty percent were asymptomatic. Twenty percent had mild symptoms of unrecognized significance[45]
Opioids	Decreased libido, ±disturbed menstruation	70–95[46]	Endocrine effect seen with IT opioids if given >1 year but may occur sooner. In patients with a long prognosis, measure testosterone and LH at baseline and annually in men, and estradiol, progesterone, LH and FSH in women[5]
Opioids	Hypocorticalism or growth hormone deficiency	15[46]	
Opioids	Edema	6–18[5,11,47]	
Opioids	Immuno-modulation	Frequency uncertain[48]	Significance uncertain. May be more pronounced with systemic opioids

a. Less commonly described with non-opioids.

not be automatically removed and allow a means of obtaining CSF for culture.[3] Mild meningeal irritation can be a normal phenomenon post-procedure, and patients can be safely observed while awaiting CSF cultures if they are systemically well and the above reveal no evidence of infection.[64] A prolonged operation time when placing the catheter is a risk factor for serious catheter-related infection.[65]

New neurological impairment

It can be difficult to distinguish between new neurological signs and symptoms caused by complications of spinal analgesia vs. those caused by the disease itself (Box 19.D). Estimates of complication rates vary greatly, and often predominantly relate to peri-operative/obstetric spinal anaesthesia.[66] Disease-related neurological impairment is common: spinal cord compression occurs in ≤6% of patients receiving spinal analgesia.[3] ED metastases are present in ≤70% of patients with refractory cancer pain. They are associated with motor impairment, and higher **morphine** and **bupivacaine** dose requirements (although not higher pain scores). Those with spinal canal stenosis (58%) also have higher IT insertion complication rates.[67]

Table 19.4 Non-drug complications of spinal analgesia

Undesirable effect	Frequency	Comment
Traumatic catheter placement		
CSF leakage headache	25% of IT[17]	Less common in recent palliative series (0–7%), perhaps because of concurrent systemic analgesia[3,49] or more modern spinal needles[50]
ED hematoma	Rare	
Neurological tissue damage	Rare[51,52]	
Infection		
Exit site infection	≤6%	In palliative care patients cared for at home or in palliative care units[3,9,49,53]
ED abscess	≤8%[3,4,12,53]	
Meningitis	≤3%[3,4,9,12]	
Delivery system		
Device-related complications	8–27%	E.g. catheter-related (fracture, kinking, displacement or withdrawal); pump failure (battery failure, mechanical failure, programming or refilling error).
		Rates, and propensity to human error, vary between pumps[3,41,42,47,54]

Box 19.B Emergency management of life-threatening complications

Stop spinal infusion.
Administer oxygen.
Obtain IV access.
If patient arrests, follow local resuscitation procedures.

Respiratory depression (sedation often precedes bradypnea)
Sit the patient up.
If respiratory rate ≤8 breaths/min, the patient is barely rousable, and/or cyanosed, administer 20microgram boluses of naloxone every 2min until respiratory status is satisfactory (see p.344).
Further boluses may be necessary because naloxone is shorter acting than morphine and other spinal opioids.

Hypotension[a] (systolic <80mmHg)
Lay patient flat (not head down).
Check heart rate: if <40 beats/min, treat bradycardia (below) or
If no evidence of fluid overload, give an IV fluid challenge, e.g. 500mL of a colloidal plasma expander over 30min.
Examine for alternative causes such as bleeding.
If no response to fluids, give ephedrine 6mg IV.

Bradycardia[a]
ECG monitoring, if available.
Administer atropine (0.6mg boluses IV, up to total 3mg).
If atropine ineffective, give ephedrine 6mg IV.

---

a. cardiovascular disturbance also occurs with IT baclofen withdrawal syndrome (see Box 19.A).

Box 19.C Management of common undesirable effects of spinal analgesia

Opioid discontinuation (diarrhea, colic, sweating, restlessness)
Spinal delivery results in a massive reduction in the patient's total opioid dose.
Laxatives should be discontinued and retitrated. If peripheral withdrawal symptoms occur, the pre-spinal opioid should be given p.r.n. in a dose approximately 25% of the former pain-related p.r.n. dose.

Opioid-induced pruritus
In palliative care, patients receiving spinal analgesia are generally not opioid-naïve (thus reducing the probability of pruritus) and most receive bupivacaine concurrently (this tends to restrict pruritus to the face).[55]

The concurrent use of NSAIDs may reduce the incidence of pruritus.[56,57] Treat with ondansetron (see p.340).[58] Consider switching to an alternative opioid if the pruritus persists.[59]

Opioid antagonists (naloxone, naltrexone) also abolish pruritus but will reverse analgesia.[60–63]

H_1-antihistamines are ineffective because opioid-induced pruritus is initiated centrally, and is not the result of mast cell degranulation.

Urinary retention
Drug-related urinary retention may be transient; removal of the urinary catheter after 3–4 days is successful in 3/4 of patients.[8] If persistent, may be because of the underlying disease.

Box 19.D Evaluation of new neurological impairment in patients receiving spinal analgesia

Differential diagnosis
Neurological damage caused by insertion of the catheter.

Bupivacaine-induced; dose-dependent, generally seen only when IT doses exceed 15mg/day,[5] but unmasking of incipient spinal cord compression can occur with lower doses.[5,68]

Disease process, e.g. cauda equina or spinal cord compression.

Spinal catheter complications, e.g. ED abscess or hematoma, catheter tip granuloma.

Withdrawal syndrome in patients receiving IT baclofen (see Box 19.A); neuromuscular features include spasticity, rigidity and priapism.

Initial evaluation
Neurological examination (location of problem).

Timing and rate of onset:
• immediate (spinal medication, 'unmasking' of pre-clinical impairment, neurological damage at insertion)
• days or weeks (ED abscess, disease itself)
• insidious over months (catheter tip granuloma).

Features of infection (ED abscess).

Pain at the catheter site and/or recurrence of the original pain (ED abscess or hematoma, disease itself, catheter tip granuloma; pain may precede neurological impairment).

Investigation
MRI may show both disease-related causes and spinal catheter-related space-occupying lesions (see warning about MRI, p.524).

Catheter tip granulomas present with occlusion (worsening of the original pain) or local mass effects (vertebral pain, spinal cord or cauda equina compression). The risk increases with time. Pain precedes neurological features, which develop gradually over days or weeks.[69] Although more commonly a complication of ED catheters, catheter tip granulomas are also described with IT catheters, particularly where **morphine** or **hydromorphone** are used in higher concentration. The risk with **fentanyl** is thought to be lower.[6] A granuloma caused by IT **baclofen** has also been reported.[23] Masses often resolve over 2–5 months with cessation of **morphine**. In the absence of neurological impairment, consider catheter tip relocation, opioid dose reduction and/or switching opioid to **fentanyl** or a non-opioid. However, surgical excision may be required, where symptoms persist or there is neurological impairment.[23]

Exacerbation of pain

Increased pain may reflect:
- worsening of the original pain
- development of a new pain because of:
  ▷ disease progression or co-morbidity
  ▷ spinal catheter-related abscess, hematoma or granuloma
- reduced effect of the spinal infusion (delivery device malfunction).

Evaluation may reveal evidence of progression or new sites of disease, neurological impairment associated with spinal catheter-related mass, or infection. If external, the delivery system can be examined for disconnection, rate of delivery and contents.

A sudden increase in pain (e.g. as a result of catheter dislodgement) should be initially treated with p.r.n. opioid medication PO/SC while the cause is investigated. Alternatively, give **ketamine** 10–25mg PO/SC p.r.n. (see p.468), particularly if the pain is opioid poorly-responsive.

If the spinal infusion includes **baclofen**, and sudden failure of drug delivery is suspected, be alert to the presence of a severe life-threatening withdrawal syndrome (see Box 19.A). The sudden cessation of **clonidine** can cause severe rebound hypertension. Treat with oral **clonidine** while seeking specialist advice.[6]

Delivery device malfunction may involve:
- a problem with the pump itself (battery failure, mechanical failure)
- a problem with the catheter (kinking, fracture, displacement, occlusion)
- human error (wrong drug, dose or rate setting; overfilling or filling of the wrong port).

Plain radiographs may show a kinked, dislodged or disconnected catheter. Catheter position and patency can be confirmed by injection of a radiological contrast agent *after first aspirating the catheter dead-space to avoid delivery of the dead-space contents as a bolus*. The contrast agent must be appropriate for CSF use: *IT delivery of inappropriate radiological contrast agents can cause arachnoiditis or death.*

1 Zech D et al. (1995) Validation of World Health Organization guidelines for cancer pain relief: a 10-year prospective study. Pain. **63**: 65–76.
2 Hanks G et al. (2001) Morphine and alternative opioids in cancer pain: the EAPC recommendations. British Journal of Cancer. **84**: 587–593.
3 Baker L et al. (2004) Evolving spinal analgesia practice in palliative care. Palliative Medicine. **18**: 507–515.
4 Burton AW et al. (2004) Epidural and intrathecal analgesia is effective in treating refractory cancer pain. Pain Medicine. **5**: 239–247.
5 British Pain Society (2007) Intrathecal drug delivery for the management of pain and spasticity in adults; recommendations for best clinical practice. The British Pain Society. Available from: www.britishpainsociety.org
6 Deer T et al. (2007) Polyanalgesic consensus conference 2007: Recommendations for the management of pain by intrathecal (intraspinal) drug delivery; report of an interdisciplinary expert panel. Neuromodulation. **10**: 300–328.
7 Tei Y et al. (2008) Treatment efficacy of neural blockade in specialized palliative care services in Japan: a multicenter audit survey. Journal of Pain and Symptom Management. **36**: 461–467.
8 Sjoberg M et al. (1991) Long-term intrathecal morphine and bupivacaine in 'refractory' cancer pain. Results from the first series of 52 patients. Acta Anaesthesiologica Scandinavica. **35**: 30–43.
9 Mercadante S et al. (1994) Intrathecal morphine and bupivacaine in advanced cancer pain patients implanted at home. Journal of Pain and Symptom Management. **9**: 201–207.
10 Sjoberg M et al. (1994) Long term intrathecal morphine and bupivacaine in patients with refractory cancer pain. Results from a morphine:bupivacaine dose regimen of 0.5:4.75mg/ml. Anesthesiology. **80**: 284–297.
11 Hassenbusch S et al. (1995) Long-term intraspinal infusions of opioids in the treatment of neuropathic pain. Journal of Pain and Symptom Management. **10**: 527–543.
12 Smitt PS et al. (1998) Outcome and complications of epidural analgesia in patients with chronic cancer pain. Cancer. **83**: 2015–2022.
13 Smith TJ et al. (2002) Randomized clinical trial of an implantable drug delivery system compared with comprehensive medical management for refractory cancer pain: impact on pain, drug-related toxicity, and survival. Journal of Clinical Oncology. **20**: 4040–4049.

14 Crul BJP and Delhaas EM (1991) Technical complications during long term subarachnoid or epidural administration of morphine in terminally ill cancer patients: A review of 140 cases. *Regional Anesthesia.* **16**: 209–213.
15 Hassenbusch SJ et al. (1997) Clinical realities and economic considerations: economics of intrathecal therapy. *Journal of Pain and Symptom Management.* **14**: S36–48.
16 Nitescu P et al. (1990) Epidural versus intrathecal morphine–bupivacaine: assessment of consecutive treatments in advanced cancer pain. *Journal of Pain and Symptom Management.* **5**: 18–26.
17 Dahm P et al. (1998) Efficacy and technical complications of long-term continuous intraspinal infusions of opioid and/or bupivacaine in refractory nonmalignant pain: a comparison between the epidural and the intrathecal approach with externalized or implanted catheters and infusion pumps. *Clinical Journal of Pain.* **14**: 4–16.
18 Dougherty PM and Staats PS (1999) Intrathecal drug therapy for chronic pain: from basic science to clinical practice. *Anesthesiology.* **91**: 1891–1918.
19 Bennett G et al. (2000) Evidence-based review of the literature on intrathecal delivery of pain medication. *Journal of Pain and Symptom Management.* **20**: S12–36.
20 Bernards CM (2002) Understanding the physiology and pharmacology of epidural and intrathecal opioids. *Best Practice and Research Clinical Anaesthesiology.* **16**: 489—505.
21 Sylvester R et al. (2004) The conversion challenge: from intrathecal to oral morphine. *American Journal of Hospice and Palliative Medicine.* **21 (2)**: 143–147.
22 Mercadante S (1999) Problems of long-term spinal opioid treatment in advanced cancer patients. *Pain.* **79**: 1–13.
23 Deer T et al. (2008) Management of intrathecal catheter-tip inflammatory masses: an updated 2007 consensus statement from an expert panel. *Neuromodulation.* **11**: 77–91.
24 Svedberg K et al. (2002) Compatibility of ropivacaine with morphine, sufentanil, fentanyl, or clonidine. *Journal of Clinical Pharmacy and Therapeutics.* **27**: 39–45.
25 Dahm P et al. (2000) Comparison of 0.5% intrathecal bupivacaine with 0.5% intrathecal ropivacaine in the treatment of refractory cancer and noncancer pain conditions: results from a prospective, crossover, double-blind, randomized study. *Regional Anesthesia and Pain Medicine.* **25**: 480–487.
26 Simpson D et al. (2005) Ropivacaine: a review of its use in regional anaesthesia and acute pain management. *Drugs.* **65**: 2675–2717.
27 Karpinski N et al. (1997) Subpial vacuolar myelopathy after intrathecal ketamine: report of a case. *Pain.* **73**: 103–105.
28 Benrath J et al. (2005) Long-term intrathecal S(+)-ketamine in a patient with cancer-related neuropathic pain. *British Journal Anaesthesia.* **95**: 247–249.
29 Vranken JH et al. (2005) Neuropathological findings after continuous intrathecal administration of S(+)-ketamine for the management of neuropathic cancer pain. *Pain.* **117**: 231–235.
30 Vranken JH et al. (2006) Severe toxic damage to the rabbit spinal cord after intrathecal administration of preservative-free S(+)-ketamine. *Anesthesiology.* **105**: 813–818.
31 Deer T (2008) Future directions for intrathecal pain management: a review and update from the interdisciplinary polyanalgesic consensus conference 2007. *Neuromodulation.* **11**: 92–97.
32 Coffey RJ et al. (2002) Abrupt withdrawal from intrathecal baclofen: recognition and management of a potentially life-threatening syndrome. *Archives of Physical Medicine and Rehabilitation.* **83**: 735–741.
33 Trissel Lawrence A et al. (2002) Physical and chemical stability of low and high concentrations of morphine sulfate with bupivacaine hydrochloride packaged in plastic syringes. In: *International Journal of Pharmaceutical Compounding.* Available from: www.ijpc.com/editorial/SearchByIssue.cfm?PID = 100
34 Xu Quanyun A et al. (2002) Physical and chemical stability of low and high concentrations of morphine sulfate with clonidine hydrochloride packaged in plastic syringes. In: *International Journal of Pharmaceutical Compounding.* Available from: www.ijpc.com/editorial/SearchByIssue.cfm?PID = 100
35 Christen C et al. (1996) Stability of bupivacaine hydrochloride and hydromorphone hydrochloride during simulated epidural coadministration. *American Journal of Health System Pharmacy.* **53**: 170–173.
36 Trissel LA (2005) *Handbook on Injectable Drugs* (13e). American Society of Health System Pharmacists, Maryland, USA.
37 Hildebrand KR et al. (2003) Stability and Compatibility of Morphine–Clonidine Admixtures in an Implantable Infusion System. *Journal of Pain and Symptom Management.* **25**: 464–471.
38 Classen AM et al. (2004) Stability of admixture containing morphine sulfate, bupivacaine hydrochloride, and clonidine hydrochloride in an implantable infusion system. *Journal of Pain and Symptom Management.* **28**: 603–611.
39 Hildebrand KR et al. (2001) Stability and Compatibility of Hydromorphone Hydrochloride in an Implantable Infusion System. *Journal of Pain and Symptom Management.* **22**: 1042–1047.
40 Rudich Z et al. (2004) Stability of clonidine in clonidine-hydromorphone mixture from implanted intrathecal infusion pumps in chronic pain patients. *Journal of Pain and Symptom Management.* **28**: 599–602.
41 Naumann C (1999) Drug adverse events and system complications of intrathecal opioid delivery for pain: Origins, detection, manifestations and management. *Neuromodulation.* **2**: 92–107.
42 Paice JA et al. (1996) Intraspinal morphine for chronic pain: a retrospective, multicenter study. *Journal of Pain and Symptom Management.* **11**: 71–80.
43 Winkelmuller W et al. (1999) Intrathecal opioid therapy for pain: Efficacy and outcomes. *Neuromodulation.* **2**: 67–76.
44 Rawal N et al. (1987) Present state of extradural and intrathecal opioid analgesia in Sweden. A nationwide follow-up survey. *British Journal of Anaesthesia.* **59**: 791–799.
45 Deer TR (2004) A prospective analysis of intrathecal granulomas in chronic pain patients: a review of the literature and report of a surveillance study. *Pain Physician.* **7**: 225–228.
46 Abs R et al. (2000) Endocrine consequences of long-term intrathecal administration of opioids. *Journal of Clinical Endocrinology and Metabolism.* **85**: 2215–2222.
47 Winkelmuller M and Winkelmuller W (1996) Long-term effects of continuous intrathecal opioid treatment in chronic pain of nonmalignant etiology. *Journal of Neurosurgery.* **85**: 458–467.
48 Budd K and Shipton E (2004) Acute pain and the immune system and opioimmunosuppression. *Acute Pain.* **6**: 123–135.
49 Mercadante S et al. (2007) Intrathecal treatment in cancer patients unresponsive to multiple trials of systemic opioids. *Clinical Journal of Pain.* **23**: 793–798.
50 Moen V et al. (2004) Severe neurological complications after central neuraxial blockades in Sweden 1990–1999. *Anesthesiology.* **101**: 950–959.
51 Aromaa U et al. (1997) Severe complications associated with epidural and spinal anaesthesias in Finland 1987–1993. A study based on patient insurance claims. *Acta Anaesthesiologica Scandinavica.* **41**: 445–452.

52 Cook TM et al. (2009) Major complications of central neuraxial block: report on the Third National Audit Project of the Royal College of Anaesthetists. British Journal of Anaesthesia. **102**: 179–190.

53 Holmfred A et al. (2006) Intrathecal catheters with subcutaneous port systems in patients with severe cancer-related pain managed out of hospital: the risk of infection. Journal of Pain and Symptom Management. **31**: 568–572.

54 Nitescu P et al. (1995) Complications of intrathecal opioids and bupivacaine in the treatment of "refractory" cancer pain. Clinical Journal of Pain. **11**: 45–62.

55 Asokumar B et al. (1998) Intrathecal bupivacaine reduces pruritus and prolongs duration of fentanyl analgesia during labor: a prospective, randomized, controlled trial. Anaesthesia and Analgesia. **87**: 1309–1315.

56 Colbert S et al. (1999) The effect of rectal diclofenac on pruritus in patients receiving intrathecal morphine. Anaesthesia. **54**: 948–952.

57 Colbert S et al. (1999) The effect of intravenous tenoxicam on pruritus in patients receiving epidural fentanyl. Anaesthesia. **54**: 76–80.

58 Borgeat A and Stimemann H-R (1999) Ondansetron is effective to treat spinal or epidural morphine-induced pruritus. Anesthesiology. **90**: 432–436.

59 Hassenbusch SJ et al. (2004) Polyanalgesic Consensus Conference 2003: an update on the management of pain by intraspinal drug delivery–report of an expert panel. Journal of Pain and Symptom Management. **27**: 540–563.

60 Korbon G et al. (1985) Intramuscular naloxone reverses the side effects of epidural morphine while preserving analgesia. Regional Anaesthesia. **10**: 16–20.

61 Ueyama H et al. (1992) Naloxone reversal of nystagmus associated with intrathecal morphine administration (letter). Anesthesiology. **76**: 153.

62 Pierard G et al. (2000) Pharma-clinics. How I treat pruritus by an antihistamine. Revue Médicale de Liege. **55**: 763–766.

63 Kjellberg F and Tramer M (2001) Pharmacological control of opioid-induced pruritus: a quantitative systematic review of randomized trials. European Journal of Anaesthesiology. **18**: 346–357.

64 Paice JA et al. (1997) Clinical realities and economic considerations: efficacy of intrathecal pain therapy. Journal of Pain and Symptom Management. **14 (suppl)**: S14–26

65 Byers K et al. (1995) Infections complicating tunneled intraspinal catheter systems used to treat chronic pain. Clinical Infectious Diseases. **21**: 403–408.

66 Bromage PR (1997) Neurological complications of subarachnoid and epidural anesthesia. Acta Anaesthesiologica Scandinavica. **41**: 439–444.

67 Appelgren L et al. (1997) Spinal epidural metastasis: implications for spinal analgesia to treat "refractory" cancer pain. Journal of Pain and Symptom Management. **13**: 25–42.

68 van Dongen RTM et al. (1997) Neurological impairment during long-term intrathecal infusion of bupivacaine in cancer patients: a sign of spinal cord compression. Pain. **69**: 205–209.

69 Miele VJ et al. (2006) A review of intrathecal morphine therapy related granulomas. European Journal of Pain. **10**: 251–261.

20: ADMINISTERING DRUGS VIA ENTERAL FEEDING TUBES

Administering drugs via an enteral feeding tube (EFT) is generally off-label. Thus, when PO administration is not possible and continuation of drug therapy is deemed necessary, consideration should be given to using an alternative approved route, e.g. PR, SC, IV or changing to a comparable drug which is approved for tube administration.[1,2] However, administration by EFT is often preferable from a practical or personal point of view.

General guidelines for the administration of drugs via an EFT are given in Box 20.A. Similar guidelines, used at some centres in Canada, are produced by the American Society for Parenteral and Enteral Nutrition (ASPEN); these can be obtained from www.nutritioncare.org (subscription required).

Types and implications of different enteral feeding tubes

There are several types of feeding tubes (Box 20.B), which can be further classified according to:
- outer diameter of the lumen (French gauge; 1 French unit = 0.33mm)[2]
- number of lumens (single or multiple)
- duration of use (short-term, long-term/fixed).

In addition to the general guidance (Box 20.A), the following should be considered when administering drugs via EFT:
- *site of drug delivery*, with jejunal tubes, absorption may be unpredictable because of the effects of pH or because the tube may extend beyond the main site of absorption of the drug, e.g. **cephalexin, ketoconazole, metronidazole benzoate**;[1,8] care should also be taken with drugs that have a narrow therapeutic range, e.g. **digoxin, warfarin, phenytoin** and other anti-epileptics;[8] drugs which undergo extensive first-pass hepatic metabolism may have greater systemic effects because of increased absorption from the jejunum, e.g. opioids, TCAs;[2] undesirable effects may also be increased because of rapid delivery into the jejunum
- *binding to the plastic tubing*, e.g. **carbamazepine**,[9] **clonazepam, diazepam, phenytoin**; minimize by diluting with 30–50mL water and monitor the clinical response
- *diameter and length of lumen*, narrow lumen, e.g. 5–12 French, or long tubes, e.g. NJ, are more likely to block, particularly with thick oral syrups; dilute with 30–50mL water before administration; the internal diameter of equivalent French gauge tubes varies between manufacturers; wide bore tubes require larger flush volumes
- *number of lumens*, ensure the correct lumen is used with multilumen tubes; *do not use an aspiration gastric decompression port for drug administration;* some tubes have one lumen terminating in the stomach and another in the jejunum
- *function of the tube*, drugs should not be administered if the tube is on free-drainage or suction[7]
- *sterility*, with jejunal tubes use sterile water because the acid barrier in the stomach is bypassed;[1] some centres use an aseptic technique to reduce the risk of infective diarrhea
- *feeding regimen*, with continuous feeding and multiple drug administration periods, it may be necessary to adjust the feeding rate to compensate for the breaks in feed administration; if possible, the drug dosing schedule should also be rationalized, aiming for once daily drug administration.[2]

Box 20.A Guidelines for the administration of drugs via enteral feeding tubes[1]

Before using this route, check that there is documented confirmation by a doctor that the EFT is correctly positioned. Testing aspirate from nasogastric tubes with pH indicator paper will also show whether or not a tube is still in the stomach and should be performed regularly according to local guidelines.[3]

The patient should be in a sitting position to prevent regurgitation and pulmonary aspiration.

To prevent accidental parenteral administration, or the rupture of the feeding tube, use a 50mL enteral syringe, i.e. a syringe which cannot be connected to IV catheters, ports or other parenteral devices.[4]

Do not use 3-way taps and syringe tip adaptors because these can inadvertently result in connection safeguards being bypassed.[4]

Drug charts should state the route of administration, e.g. nasogastric (NG), nasojejunal (NJ), and specify the lumen to be used.

Do not add drugs to enteral feeds because this increases the risk of incompatibility, microbial contamination, tube blockage, and underdosing or overdosing if the feed rate is altered.[5]

Stop the feed and ensure any other ports are closed and airtight.

Flush the tube using a pulsating action with 15–30mL of water (*sterile if jejunal tube*). This helps to clear the tube and prevent physical interactions with the feed which could result in coagulation in the tube, e.g. acidic solutions (chlorpheniramine) or antacids.[5,6]

Check if a specific time interval is needed before and after administration to ensure maximal absorption, e.g. penicillins, and/or to reduce the risk of chemical interactions with the feed, e.g. ciprofloxacin, itraconazole, ketoconazole, phenytoin, theophylline, warfarin.[6]

Administer each drug separately in the most suitable formulation (see Choosing a suitable formulation, opposite) in a 50mL enteral syringe; flush between each drug with 10mL of water, and after the last drug with 15–30mL of water (*sterile if jejunal tube*) using a pulsating action.

Document the total volume of fluid given (including flushes) on a fluid balance chart; this is important in patients who are on restricted fluids.

Resume feeding after any necessary interval (see above).

Monitor the clinical response particularly if:
• changing from SR to normal-release formulations
• a drug has a narrow therapeutic range the
• bio-availability of the drug differs between tablet and liquid.

Do not administer bulk-forming laxatives because they may block the tube; use an enteral feed with a high fibre content instead.[7]

Box 20.B Main types of feeding tubes

Nasogastric (NG), inserted into the stomach via the nose.
Nasoduodenal (ND), inserted into the duodenum via the nose.
Nasojejunal (NJ), inserted into the jejunum via the nose.
Percutaneous endoscopic gastrostomy (PEG) or 'G-tube', inserted into the stomach via the abdominal wall.
Percutaneous endoscopic jejunostomy (PEJ) or 'J-tube', inserted into the jejunum via the abdominal wall.
Percutaneous endoscopic gastro-jejunostomy (PEGJ), inserted into the jejunum via the abdominal wall and through the stomach.

Choosing a suitable formulation

When planning drug administration by EFT, guidance should be obtained from a pharmacist. In a descending order of preference, the choice of formulation comprises:

- commercial oral liquid or soluble tablet
- compounded oral liquid
- fully dispersed tablet or capsule contents
- injection (given via EFT).

Option 1: Commercial oral liquid or soluble tablet

If available, this is generally the preferred option. Soluble tablets dissolve completely when placed in 10mL water to give a solution of the drug in contrast to dispersible or orodispersible tablets which disperse in water to give particles (see Option 3 below). Liquid formulations are not always suitable because of:

- *excipients,* osmotic diarrhea can occur because of high osmolality or sorbitol content, particularly with jejunal administration; the normal osmolality of GI secretions is 100–400mosm/kg, whereas many liquid formulations are >1,000mosm/kg;[7,8] reduce osmolality by diluting with as much water as is practical. Sorbitol in doses of ≥15g/day generally causes diarrhea
- *altered bio-availability and/or pharmacokinetics,* when converting from tablets to oral solution, e.g. **phenytoin**, **sodium fusidate**, or from SR formulations to oral solution; the dose and/or frequency may need to be changed according to the clinical response
- *tube blockage,* caused by high viscosity formulations, e.g. **amoxicillin-clavulanate**, mineral oil, syrups or by particles from suspensions; minimize by diluting with 30–50mL water and flushing well[7]
- *coagulation of the feed,* particularly if the drug formulation is acidic, i.e. pH < 4;[7] this applies to many syrups[2]
- *bezoar (insoluble concretion) formation in the tube or in the stomach,* as a result of an interaction between the drug and the feed, e.g. **sucralfate**;[10] avoid by not prescribing for patients on enteral feeds
- *large volumes,* from high doses or multiple drugs which are impractical.

Option 2: Compounded oral liquid preparations

Locally compounded preparations may be an alternative if a commercial product is not available or not suitable. They may cause the same problems as commercial products, but it may be possible for an experienced pharmacist to alter the formulation with careful consideration for quality, storage and shelf life etc., and thus make it more suitable for EFT administration. Continuity of supply upon discharge and shorter dated shelf-life may make this option impractical.

Option 3: Fully dispersed tablet or capsule contents

Commercial dispersible tablets disintegrate in water to form particles/granules, but some may be too large for administration via fine bore EFT.

Orodispersible tablets are designed to disperse on the tongue and are generally swallowed with the saliva without water. The formulations, dose equivalences and administration of orodispersible tablets vary depending on the medicine concerned and individual product details should be consulted before using via EFT.

Many tablets and capsule contents will disperse completely when mixed with 10mL water, even though they are not marketed as dispersible. Crushing the tablet/capsule contents first can sometimes facilitate this. However, crushing should be considered a last resort (Box 20.C), and great care must be taken to ensure that this is safe for both the patient and health professional.

Do not administer dispersed or crushed tablet/capsule contents which have not completely dispersed into non-visible particles in the water or which have an oily residue; sediment and oily films increase the risk of blocking the tube[7,11] (Box 20.C).

A few capsules contain liquid contents, e.g. **nifedipine**. Because of the small volume of the contents (which varies between brands) it is *not* recommended that these are used as a source of a drug for EFT administration.

Box 20.C   Guidelines for administration of dispersed tablets and capsule contents[1,12]

Administer each drug separately.[8]

Crush tablet(s) or capsule contents using a mortar and pestle or tablet crusher, and put into a clean medicine pot.

Add 10mL of tap water, allow to disperse, then mix well; *use sterile water throughout for jejunal tubes.*

Ensure the drug is completely dispersed into non-visible particles without residue, then draw up using a 50mL enteral syringe and administer via the feeding tube, according to general guidelines (Box 20.A).

Rinse the medicine pot or container with water and administer the rinsings through the tube to ensure the patient receives the whole dose.

Thoroughly clean the equipment with hot soapy water to avoid cross-contamination.

Do not crush

EC formulations (including EC capsule contents) because this will destroy the properties of the formulation, may alter bio-availability and/or block the tube.[7,11,13,14]

SR formulations (including SR capsule contents) because this may cause dangerous dose peaks and troughs.[7,11,14,15]

Cytotoxics, prostaglandin analogues, hormone antagonists or antibiotics because there are risks to the staff through inhalation and/or topical absorption.[7,11,14]

Buccal or sublingual formulations because their bio-availability may be dramatically reduced if absorbed via the GI tract.[7,11,14]

Nitrates because crushing nitrate-containing tablets could cause an explosion.[16]

Option 4: Injection (given via EFT)

Formulations for injection are often unsuitable for enteral administration. This may be for one or more of several reasons:
- high osmolality or hypertonicity; the high solute concentration can cause osmotic diarrhea
- unsuitable pH
- formulation with a different salt of unknown bio-availability
- an additive which is irritant to the GI tract, e.g. polysorbate 80 (Tween® 80) in **amiodarone**[1,17]
- risk of IV administration by mistake (but see Box 20.A)
- cost.

Generally, all injections suitable for administration via EFT should be diluted with 30–50mL water before administration.

Administration of EC and SR coated formulations

Generally, these products should *not* be administered via EFT. However, some capsules/granules/compressed tablets contain EC or SR granules for which specific procedures have been developed to allow administration of the coated granules via EFT, e.g. **esomeprazole** EC capsules, EC tablets and EC granules for oral suspension (Nexium®), **lansoprazole** EC capsules (Prevacid®) and EC orally disintegrating tablets (Prevacid FasTab®; suitable only for NG tubes ⩾8 French). See the relevant Product Monograph or consult the manufacturer for details. It is essential that the recommended procedure is strictly adhered to, and is used only for that specific formulation and the correct tube size, to avoid dangerous dose peaks and troughs or tube blockage. Care should be taken to avoid crushing the EC or SR granules. **Lansoprazole** EC orally disintegrating tablets have been cited as preferable to other oral formulations of some PPIs, based on completeness of dispersion and ease of administration for nurses, patients and carers.[18]

Drug interactions and complications

Drugs can interact with food in many ways.[6,19] Enteral feeds can cause different problems associated with bio-availability, compatibility and interactions. Because they are in liquid form, the content, consistency and pH can be very different. Generally, complications can arise from:
- binding of drugs to the EFT
- physical interaction with the feed causing coagulation
- chemical interaction between the drug and feed causing a non-absorbable drug-feed complex
- indirect drug or nutrient interactions, e.g. the **vitamin K** content of a feed affecting the action of **warfarin**[6]
- the effects of malnutrition on drug pharmacokinetics.

Drug–drug interactions can also occur. Following the guidance in Box 20.A will reduce the risk of dangerous interactions. Clinically, the most important interactions are those between drugs with a narrow therapeutic range, e.g. **digoxin, theophylline, warfarin, phenytoin** and other anti-epileptics; these may warrant plasma monitoring. Clinical response should also be monitored. Appropriate precautionary measures may need to be taken if the feed is discontinued, particularly if dose adjustments were made because of an interaction.

Unblocking enteral feeding tubes

Tube blockage may be caused by the feed, e.g. stagnant or contaminated feed, or by incorrect drug administration, e.g. particle blockage or interaction between the feed and drug. It is more likely with narrow lumens; a 35% incidence of blockage in patients with 8 French tubes has been cited.[20] Many tubes can be unblocked using 15–30mL water in a 50mL syringe and a push/pull action, although this may take 20–30min.

Various other agents have been used to unblock tubes (Box 20.D).[7] Their use is based on anecdote. Acidic solutions, e.g. **cranberry juice** and carbonated drinks, could make the situation worse by causing feed coagulation.[7]

Pancreatic enzymes help only if the blockage is caused by the feed. Sodium bicarbonate needs to be added to activate the enzymes, which may not be practical. A guide-wire or excessive force must not be used to unblock a tube because of the danger of perforation.[17] If in doubt, consult a specialist nutrition nurse if available.

Box 20.D   Agents used to unblock feeding tubes[7]

Cold or warm water
Soda water
Sodium bicarbonate
Cola
Pineapple juice
Cranberry juice
Meat tenderizer, contains papain, a mixture of proteolytic enzymes
Pancreatic enzymes

---

1   White R and Bradnam V (2007) *Handbook of Drug Administration via Enteral Feeding Tubes.* Pharmaceutical Press, London.
2   Williams NT (2008) Medication administration through enteral feeding tubes. *American Journal of Health-System Pharmacy.* **65**: 2347–2357.
3   NPSA (National Patient Safety Agency) (2005) Reducing harm caused by misplaced nasogastric feeding tubes. Interim advice for healthcare staff-February 2005. How to confirm the correct position of nasogastric feeding tubes in infants children and adults. Available from: www.npsa.nhs.uk/advice
4   NPSA (National Patient Safety Agency) (2007) Promoting safter measurement and administration of liquid medicines via oral and other enteral routes. In: *Patient Safety Alert 19.* Available from: www.npsa.nhs.uk/public/alerts
5   Engle KK and Hannawa TE (1999) Techniques for administering oral medications to critical care patients receiving continuous enteral nutrition. *American Journal of Health-System Pharmacy.* **56**: 1441–1444.
6   Baxter K (ed) (2008) *Stockley's Drug Interactions* (8e). Pharmaceutical Press, London.
7   Thomson F et al. (2000) Enteral and parenteral nutrition. *Hospital Pharmacist.* **7**: 155–164.
8   Adams D (1994) Administration of drugs through a jejunostomy tube. *British Journal of Intensive Care.* **4**: 10–17.

---

9 Clark-Schmidt AL *et al.* (1990) Loss of carbamazepine suspension through nasogastric feeding tubes. *American Journal of Hospital Pharmacy.* **47**: 2034–2037.
10 Garcia-Luna PP *et al.* (1997) Esophageal obstruction by solidification of the enteral feed: a complication to be prevented. *Intensive Care Medicine.* **23**: 790–792.
11 Gilbar P (1999) A guide to drug administration in palliative care (review). *Journal of Pain and Symptom Management.* **17**: 197–207.
12 BAPEN (British Association of Parenteral and Enteral Nutrition) (2004) Administering drugs via enteral feeding tubes. A practical guide. BAPEN. Available from: www.bapen.org.uk/res_drugs.html
13 Beckwith MC *et al.* (1997) Guide to drug therapy in patients with enteral feeding tubes: dosage form selection and administration methods. *Hospital Pharmacist.* **32**: 57–64.
14 Mitchell J (1998) Oral dosage forms that should not be crushed: 1998 update. *Hospital Pharmacist.* **33**: 399–415.
15 Schier JG *et al.* (2003) Fatality from administration of labetalol and crushed extended-release nifedipine. *Annals of Pharmacotherapy.* **37**: 1420–1423.
16 Wright D (2002) Swallowing difficulties protocol: medication administration. *Nursing Standard.* **17**: 43–45.
17 Shaw J (1994) A worrying gap in knowledge: nurses' knowledge of enteral feeding practice. *Enteral Feeding.* **July**: 656–666.
18 Johnson JL *et al.* (2008) Enteral administration of three proton-pump-inhibitor formulations. *American Journal of Health-System Pharmacy.* **65**: 2324–2325.
19 Schmidt LE and Dalhoff K (2002) Food–drug interactions. *Drugs.* **62**: 1481–1502.
20 Marcuard SP and Stegall KS (1990) Unclogging feeding tubes with pancreatic enzyme. *Journal of Parenteral Enteral Nutrition.* **14**: 198–200.

21: NEBULIZED DRUGS

Nebulizers are used in asthma and COPD for both acute exacerbations and long-term prophylaxis.[1,2] Other uses include the pulmonary delivery of antimicrobial drugs for cystic fibrosis, bronchiectasis and AIDS-related pneumonia. Nebulizers are also used in palliative care. The aim is to deliver a therapeutic dose of a drug as an aerosol in particles small enough to be inspired within 5–10min. A nebulizer is preferable to a hand-held metered dose inhaler (MDI) when:

- a large drug dose is needed
- co-ordinated breathing is difficult
- MDIs + a spacer are ineffective
- a drug is unavailable in an inhaler.

On the other hand, nebulizers are noisy, and are less efficient than MDIs at delivering drugs to the airway. They are also ineffective in patients with shallow breathing, and in those unable to sit up to at least 45°, i.e. semi-upright or more.

Commonly used nebulizers are:

Jet: the aerosol is generated by a flow of gas from, for example, an electrical compressor or an oxygen cylinder. At least 50% of the aerosol produced at the recommended driving gas flow should be particles small enough to inhale.

Ultrasonic: the aerosol is generated by ultrasonic vibrations of a piezo-electric crystal.

Aerosol output (the mass of particles in aerosol form produced/min) is not necessarily the same as drug output (the mass of drug produced/min as an aerosol). Ideally, the drug output of a nebulizer should be known for each of the different drugs given. Various factors affect the drug output and deposition:

- gas flow rate (generally air at 6–8L/min but oxygen if treating acute asthma)
- chamber design
- volume (commonly 2–5mL)
- residual volume (commonly 0.5mL)
- physical properties of the drug in solution
- breathing pattern of the patient.

The choice of nebulizer can be crucial, particularly when trying to produce an aerosol small enough to deliver a drug to the alveoli. Services which provide nebulizers will generally offer information, education and support for patients and their families (Box 21.A). Information should include:

- a description of the equipment and its use
- drugs used, doses and frequencies
- equipment maintenance/cleaning
- action to take if treatment becomes less effective
- action to take and emergency telephone number to use if equipment breaks down.

Patients should be instructed to take steady normal breaths (interspersed with occasional deep ones) and nebulization time should be less than 10min or 'to dryness'. Because there is always a residual volume, 'dryness' should be taken as 1min after spluttering starts. In general, whereas a mask can be used for bronchodilators, a mouthpiece should be used for other drugs to limit environmental contamination and/or contact with the patient's eyes. However, a mask may be preferable in patients who are acutely ill, fatigued or very young, regardless of the nature of the drug.

Nebulizers in palliative care

Nebulizers are used to ease cough and breathlessness in advanced cancer (Table 21.1 and Table 21.2); they should be reviewed after 2 days to check effectiveness. When using **lidocaine** or

Box 21.A   Advice about using a nebulizer at home

To help your breathing, your doctor has prescribed a drug to be used with a nebulizer. The nebulizer converts the drug into a fine mist which you inhale.

The apparatus
Your nebulizer system consists of the following parts:

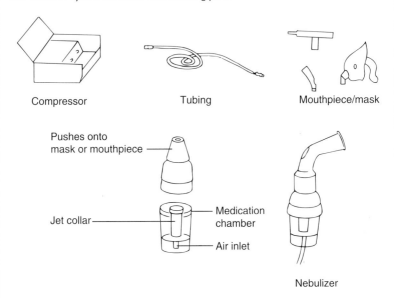

Compressor   Tubing   Mouthpiece/mask

Pushes onto
mask or mouthpiece

Jet collar

Medication
chamber

Air inlet

Nebulizer

The compressor is the portable pump which pumps air along the tubing into the nebulizer. The nebulizer is a small chamber for the liquid medicine, through which air is blown to make a mist. The nebulizer has a screw-on top onto which the mask or mouthpiece is attached.

How to use your nebulizer
Place the medication in the nebulizer, replace the screw-on top and turn the compressor on. Inhale by mouthpiece or mask while breathing at a normal rate. The mask should sit comfortably but tightly against the face to prevent mist getting into the eyes. Stop 1 minute after the nebulizer contents start spluttering or after a maximum of 10 minutes.

General advice
The nebulizer may help you cough stuff up, so have some tissues nearby. You may wish to use the nebulizer before attempting an activity which makes you feel out of breath.

If the effects of the nebulizer wear off or you have any questions or concerns about it, please speak to your doctor or nurse.

Cleaning
Wash the mouthpiece/mask and nebulizer in warm water and detergent, then rinse and dry well. Ideally this should be done after every use, but *once a day as a minimum*. Attach the tube and run the nebulizer empty for a few moments after cleaning it to make sure the equipment is dry. Once a week, unplug and wipe the compressor and tubing with a damp cloth.

Table 21.1 Nebulized drugs and cancer-related cough or breathlessness[2,5]

Class of drug	Indications	Scientific evidence	Comments
Saline 0.9%	Loosening of tenacious secretions	None	Probably underused in this setting; may also help breathlessness
Mucolytic agents, e.g. hypertonic saline, acetylcysteine	To thin viscous sputum	Conflicting evidence	May result in copious liquid sputum which the patient may still not be able to cough up
Corticosteroids, e.g. budesonide	Stridor, lymphangitis, radiation pneumonitis, cough after the insertion of a stent	None	Very limited clinical experience only; may not be more beneficial than use of inhaler or oral routes. Possible increased risk of oral candidosis[6]
Local anesthetics, e.g. lidocaine, bupivacaine	Cough, particularly if caused by lymphangitic carcinomatosis	Conflicting evidence for both breathlessness[7,8] and cough[9]	Risk of bronchospasm; reduces gag reflex, increasing risk of aspiration[3,10]
Opioids, e.g. morphine, fentanyl	Breathlessness associated with diffuse lung disease	Despite supportive anecdotal evidence,[11] a systematic review indicates no advantage compared with 0.9% saline[12,13]	Not recommended; risk of bronchospasm
Bronchodilators, e.g. salbutamol	Treatment of severe reversible airway obstruction	Extrapolated from patients with asthma and COPD	Try MDI + spacer first.[14,15] Use nebulizers only if trial of therapy shows real benefit
Furosemide	Breathlessness in cancer patients	Despite reports of benefit, RCTs do not support its use	Not recommended (see p.40)

Table 21.2 Recommended uses of nebulized drugs in palliative care

Indication	Drug	Initial regimen	Dose titration	Comments
Tenacious secretions	Saline 0.9%	5mL q6h	Up to q2h	
Reversible airway obstruction	Salbutamol	2.5mg q6h–q4h	Up to 5mg q4h	Risk of sensitivity to cardiac stimulant effects
Cough	*†Lidocaine 2%	5mL p.r.n.	Up to q6h ⎫	Risk of bronchospasm; fast for 1h after nebulization
	*†Bupivacaine 0.25%	5mL p.r.n.	Up to q8h ⎭	

bupivacaine for a dry cough (not recommended for breathlessness), in patients with asthma or COPD, pretreat with **salbutamol** because of the risk of initial bronchospasm.[3,4] After treatment with a local anesthetic, patients should be advised not to eat or drink for 1h because the reduced gag/cough reflex increases the risk of aspiration.

Because of a lack of data, e.g. physio-chemical compatibility, and aerodynamic properties, manufacturers generally do not recommend mixing nebulizer solutions. Thus, most mixtures are off-label. However:[16–21]

- some ready-mixed combinations are commercially available, e.g. **salbutamol + ipratropium bromide, fenoterol + ipratropium bromide**
- for brands available *in the UK and Germany* there are limited data indicating that certain 2-drug mixtures are physically and chemically compatible
- solutions should be mixed immediately before use, using aseptic technique; if the colour changes or cloudiness/precipitation occurs, the mixture should be discarded, and *not* used
- if dilution is necessary, sterile 0.9% saline is generally best
- if there is a lack of anticipated clinical benefit from a mixture, consider nebulizing each drug separately.

1 The Nebulizer Project Group of the British Thoracic Society Standards of Care Committee (1997) Current best practice for nebuliser treatment. *Thorax.* **52 (suppl 2)**: s1–3.
2 European Respiratory Society (2001) Guidelines on the use of nebulizers. *European Respiratory Journal.* **18**: 228–242.
3 McAlpine L and Thomson N (1989) Lidocaine-induced bronchoconstriction in asthmatic patients. Relation to histamine airway responsiveness and effect of preservative. *Chest.* **96**: 1012–1015.
4 Groeben H et al. (2000) Combined lidocaine and salbutamol inhalation for airway anesthesia markedly protects against reflex bronchoconstriction. *Chest.* **118**: 509–515.
5 Ahmedzai S and Davis C (1997) Nebulised drugs in palliative care. *Thorax.* **52 (suppl 2)**: s75–s77.
6 Davies AN et al. (2008) Oral candidosis in community-based patients with advanced cancer. *Journal of Pain and Symptom Management.* **35**: 508–514.
7 Winning A et al. (1988) Ventilation and breathlessness on maximal exercise in patients with interstitial lung disease after local anaesthetic aerosol inhalation. *Clinical Science.* **74**: 275–281.
8 Wilcock A et al. (1994) Safety and efficacy of nebulized lignocaine in patients with cancer and breathlessness. *Palliative Medicine.* **8**: 35–38.
9 Gaze M et al. (1997) Pain relief and quality of life following radiotherapy for bone metastases: a randomised trial of two fractionation schedules. *Radiotherapy and Oncology.* **45**: 109–116.
10 Barnes PJ (2007) The problem of cough and development of novel antitussives. *Pulmonary Pharmacology & Therapeutics.* **20**: 416–422.
11 Young IH et al. (1989) Effect of low dose nebulized morphine on exercise endurance in patients with chronic lung disease. *Thorax.* **44**: 387–390.
12 Jennings AL et al. (2001) Opioids for the palliation of breathlessness in terminal illness. *Cochrane Database of Systematic Reviews.* CD002066.
13 Polosa R et al. (2002) Nebulised morphine for severe interstitial lung disease. *Cochrane Database of Systematic Reviews.* CD002872.
14 Congleton J and Muers MF (1995) The incidence of airflow obstruction in bronchial carcinoma, its relation to breathlessness, and response to bronchodilator therapy. *Respiratory Medicine.* **89**: 291–296.
15 Colacone A et al. (1993) A comparison of albuterol administered by metered dose inhaler (and holding chamber) or wet nebulizer in acute asthma. *Chest.* **104**: 835–841.
16 Roberts G and Rossi S (1993) Compatibility of nebuliser solutions. *Australian Journal of Hospital Pharmacy.* **23**: 35–37.
17 McKenzie JE and Cruz-Rivera M (2004) Compatibility of budesonide inhalation suspension with four nebulizing solutions. *Annals of Pharmacotherapy.* **38**: 967–972.

18 Kamin W *et al.* (2006) Inhalation solutions: which one are allowed to be mixed? Physico-chemical compatibility of drug solutions in nebulizers. *Journal of Cystic Fibrosis.* **5**: 205–213.

19 Woodland G (2007) Which nebuliser solutions are compatible? nebuliser_compatibility100.3.doc. Welsh Medicines Information Centre and UK Medicines Information. Available from: http://www.druginfozone.nhs.uk/Record%20Viewing/ viewRecord.aspx?id=586583

20 Joseph JC (1997) Compatibility of nebulizer solution admixtures. *Annals of Pharmacotherapy.* **31**: 487–489.

21 Harriman A-M *et al.* (1996) Can we mix nebuliser solutions? Stability of drug admixtures in solutions for nebulisation. *Pharmacy in Practice.* **Oct**: 347–348.

22: PROLONGATION OF THE QT INTERVAL IN PALLIATIVE CARE

The QT interval has attained greater clinical significance because it became apparent that various factors which prolong the QT interval, particularly drugs, predispose to a potentially fatal ventricular arrhythmia, *torsade de pointes*.

An accurate diagnosis of *torsade de pointes* is important as its management differs from other forms of ventricular tachycardia. Indeed, conventional drug treatments for ventricular tachycardia can exacerbate the underlying electrochemical derangement and perpetuate *torsade de pointes*.

Palliative care clinicians caring for patients with cardiac disease, or using **methadone**, need to be particularly aware of this phenomenon.

The QT interval lies on the electrocardiograph (ECG) between the beginning of the QRS complex (which marks the start of ventricular depolarization) and the end of the T wave (which marks the end of ventricular repolarization) (Figure 22.1).

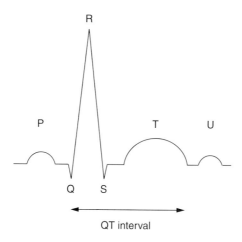

QT interval

Figure 22.1 The QT interval.

The QT interval tends to be longer with slower heart rates. For comparative purposes, it is important to adjust ('correct') the observed QT interval to take account of this. The corrected value is designated QTc. Some ECG machines automatically calculate QTc, and this is a useful guide. However, automatic calculations can be inaccurate, particularly in the presence of atrial fibrillation, frequent ventricular ectopics, or a noisy trace. Thus, manual calculation of QTc is more accurate (Box 22.A).[1] There are several ways of doing this, and local practice varies.[1,2]

Box 22.A Measuring the QT interval and calculating QTc[1]

ECG

A 12-lead ECG at 25mm/sec at 10mm/mV amplitude is generally adequate.

Measure the QT interval together with the preceding RR interval in 3–5 heart beats from leads II and V5/V6.

Calculate the mean QT and RR interval from these 3–5 measurements.

Calculate QTc using one of the following formulas:
- Bazett's (exponential square root):

$$QTc = \frac{QT\,(sec)}{\sqrt{RR\,(sec)}}$$

- Fridericia's (exponential cube root):

$$QTc = \frac{QT\,(sec)}{\sqrt[3]{RR\,(sec)}}$$

Although Bazett's formula is the most widely used, Fridericia's may be more accurate at the extremes of heart rate.

Interpretation

QTc(msec)	Male	Female
Normal	<430	<450
Borderline	430–450	450–470
Abnormal	>450	>470

Obtain advice
Obtain cardiology advice if:
- the end of the T wave is difficult to determine, e.g. because of a U wave
- there is bundle branch block
- there is atrial fibrillation.

A prolonged QT interval is a pro-arrhythmic state associated with an increased risk of ventricular arrhythmia, particularly *torsade de pointes* (Figure 22.2); this is a form of polymorphic ventricular tachycardia of varying polarity which appears to wind around the baseline and hence its name. Short runs may cause palpitation, longer ones syncope (generally without warning) or seizure-like activity; it can settle spontaneously within seconds or degenerate into fatal ventricular fibrillation.[3]

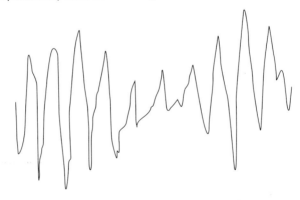

Figure 22.2 *Torsade de pointes.* Twisting complexes of ventricular tachycardia.

Treatment includes cardioversion when hemodynamically compromised and **magnesium sulfate** IV (2g bolus followed by an infusion of 2–4mg/min).[3] The risk of *torsade de pointes* grows as the QT interval increases, particularly > 500msec. A drug which leads to an increase in QTc interval of 20–60msec should also raise concern and, if by > 60msec, serious concern about the risk of arrhythmia.[4]

Drugs prolong the QT interval mainly through potassium-channel blockade (particularly I_{Kr} 'rapid' subtype) by interfering with potassium currents in (enhanced) and out (reduced) of the cardiac myocytes, modifying their repolarization and prolonging the duration of the action potential.[5] The resulting dispersion of intramural repolarization may promote triggered activity and re-entry, the electrophysiological substrate for *torsade de pointes*. Several drugs have been definitely linked with *torsade de pointes* (Box 22.B). Concerns about safety have resulted in certain drugs being withdrawn, e.g. **astemizole, terfenadine, thioridazine**, or their availability severely restricted, e.g. **cisapride, thioridazine** (available only in Canada through the Special Access Programme).

Box 22.B   Drugs associated with a prolonged QT interval and *torsade de pointes*[a,b]

Anti-arrhythmic drugs
Amiodarone
Disopyramide
Sotalol

Antimicrobial drugs
Macrolides
e.g. clarithromycin, erythromycin
Pentamidine

Antimalarial drugs
Chloroquine

Psychotropic drugs
Chlorpromazine
Droperidol[c]
Haloperidol
Pimozide
Thioridazine[c]

Miscellaneous
Arsenic trioxide[c]
Cisapride[c]
Domperidone
Methadone

a. many more drugs have been associated with *torsade de pointes*, but the evidence is inconclusive, see www.azcert.org
b. a longer list of drugs to be avoided by patients with congenital long QT syndrome is also available, see www.azcert.org
c. available through the Special Access Programme.

The incidence of *torsade de pointes* is greatest with cardiac anti-arrhythmics, particularly those with class III activity. For some drugs, the risk is present only with:[6,7]
• high doses
• IV administration
• a pharmacokinetic drug interaction, e.g. **ketoconazole** inhibits CYP3A4 and thereby impairs the metabolism of **methadone** (see Cytochrome P450, p.551)
• impaired metabolism:
  ▷ congenital, e.g. CYP2D6 poor metabolizers may be exposed to dangerously high plasma concentrations of risk-related drugs which are substrates for CYP2D6, even with normal doses
  ▷ acquired, e.g. hepatic or renal impairment.
Thus, the degree of prolongation of the QT interval is not only dose-related. The risk of drug-induced *torsade de pointes* is increased by the concurrent use of two or more drugs which prolong the QT interval, and is more likely to occur in the presence of other risk factors (Box 22.C).[6] Some patients have a subclinical congenital long QT syndrome unmasked by a QT-prolonging drug.[3]

An additional contributory factor may be central sleep apnea, which is associated with bradycardia and QT prolongation, and is reported to occur in 30% of patients on **methadone** maintenance.[8]

Box 22.C Main additional risk factors in drug-induced *torsade de pointes*

Female gender
Congenital long QT syndrome
Baseline prolonged QT interval
Electrolyte imbalance:
• hypokalemia
• hypomagnesemia

Cardiac disease, e.g.:
• bradycardia <50 beats/min
• left ventricular hypertrophy
• heart failure
• recent conversion from atrial fibrillation
• ventricular arrhythmia

Implications for practice
General recommendations to guide practice are given in Box 22.D.[2]

Box 22.D A clinical approach to drug-induced QT prolongation

When using drugs known to prolong the QT interval, a clinician needs to:
• understand the pharmacology of the drug, in particular factors which may lead to accumulation, e.g. drug–drug interaction, impaired elimination
• whenever possible, avoid the concurrent use of more than one drug which prolongs the QT interval
• use the lowest effective dose of the QT-prolonging drug
• evaluate and balance the potential benefit against the potential risk, taking into account the specific circumstances of the patient and the presence of other risk factors (see Box 22.C), e.g.:
  ▷ in patients with a known (pre-existing) prolonged QT interval, avoid the use of all QT-prolonging drugs except under specialist guidance (see Box 22.B)
  ▷ in patients with cardiac disease, drugs which prolong the QT interval should generally be avoided unless no suitable alternative exists
  ▷ in patients with cardiac disease, if a cardiac anti-arrhythmic known to prolong the QT interval is prescribed, consider undertaking an ECG before and after starting the drug, and regular monitoring of plasma potassium and magnesium concentrations to ensure these remain well within their normal ranges
  ▷ in patients without cardiac disease but with other risk factors, consider similar monitoring to above when using a QT-prolonging drug
  ▷ for advice about patients at the end of life and also methadone, see text
• explain to the patient (and family) the risk involved and the reasons for using the drug in question, to allow an informed decision to be made
• report instances of drug-related QT prolongation to Health Canada's adverse drug reporting programme
• consider *torsade de pointes* as a possible cause of palpitations, syncope or seizure-like activity.

Palliative care patients in general may be at higher risk of a prolonged QT interval given the high prevalence of multiple drug use and metabolic disturbance. Polypharmacy is the norm in palliative care,[9] and using more than one drug concurrently increases the risk of drug interactions.[10–12] However, of 300 patients referred to a specialist palliative care unit who were not imminently dying, although 48 (16%) had a prolonged QT interval, only 2 (0.7%) had a severely prolonged uncorrected QT interval of >500msec (Figure 22.3).[4,13] Both patients had ischemic heart disease and, if being considered for a QT-prolonging drug such as **methadone**, would have been identified by following the guidance to undertake an ECG in patients with one or more risk factors.

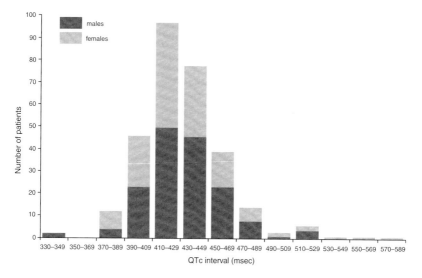

Figure 22.3   Distribution of the QT interval in 300 palliative care patients.[13]

Nonetheless, a commonsense approach should prevail and the benefit of certain drugs used in the last days of life, e.g. **haloperidol**, is likely to far outweigh any risk, and an ECG is not required.[14]

Methadone

There have been longstanding concerns relating to the occurrence of serious adverse events with **methadone**, including deaths, from apparent unintentional overdose, particularly in the first 2 weeks of administration. As the use of **methadone** has increased, for both **methadone** maintenance and chronic pain, so has the number of deaths, disproportionately more than with other opioids, resulting in the FDA issuing an alert to health professionals in 2006.[8] A major factor is considered to be a lack of knowledge among clinicians about the need to carefully monitor the use of **methadone** particularly during the first 2–4 weeks (see **methadone**, p.327). Although many of these deaths are likely to be a result of respiratory depression, *torsade de pointes* may be a contributing factor (Box 22.E).

Guidelines to minimize the risk of cardiac toxicity with **methadone** are based largely on expert opinion, and recommendations vary.[14] Although some suggest routine ECG screening, this is debatable. However, most advise an ECG in the presence of other risk factors for QT interval prolongation.[14] For example, since 2006, the UK SPC (Product Monograph) for **methadone** has recommended that it is used with caution in patients with any of the following risk factors for QT prolongation:
- a history of cardiac conduction abnormalities
- advanced heart disease or ischemic heart disease
- liver disease
- a family history of sudden death
- electrolyte abnormalities
- concurrent treatment with drugs which:
  - ▷ may cause electrolyte abnormalities
  - ▷ have a potential to prolong QT
  - ▷ inhibit CYP3A4 (see p.551).

ECG monitoring is recommended in such patients before starting **methadone** and when the dose is stabilized. ECG monitoring is also recommended in patients without recognized risk factors for QT prolongation, before dose titration above 100mg/day PO and 1 week after such up-titration (an arbitrary dose, based on expert opinion). Monitoring of serum electrolytes,

---

Box 22.E   Methadone, prolonged QT and *torsade de pointes*

The association between methadone and prolonged QT was first reported in 1973.[15] The link with *torsade de pointes* was made in 2002 when it was described in 17 patients receiving a median dose of methadone 330mg/day PO; all had QT > 500msec and most had other risk factors.[16]

Subsequently, methadone has been found to block ion channels associated with QT prolongation, and to increase the QT interval and the risk of *torsade de pointes* generally in a dose-dependent manner. However, QTc > 500msec and *torsade de pointes* have been reported with daily doses as low as 30–40mg PO.[17]

A review of 59 reports (five fatal) to the FDA confirmed that *torsade de pointes* is generally seen with higher daily doses (median 345mg, range 29–1,680mg). However, *torsade de pointes* was a confirmed cause of death in only one case, and for most reports other risk factors were present, e.g. multiple QT-prolonging drugs, drug interaction, hypokalemia, hypomagnesemia, or heart disease.[18] The frequent co-existence of other risk factors makes it difficult to quantify the risk from methadone alone and may explain the inconsistent dose-relationship seen between methadone and QT prolongation.

Although slight prolongation of the QT interval by methadone appears to be common, the clinical significance of this is unclear. A marked increase in QTc to > 500msec is seen in a small proportion of patients given methadone (generally about 2%, but 16% in one report).[17] The incidence of *torsade de pointes* and of *fatal torsade de pointes* is hard to quantify, but both are likely to be rare, e.g.:
- of the 400 adverse drug events for methadone reported to the MHRA (UK) between 1964 and 2009, 13 (3 fatal) were classified as cardiac; these included only one report each of *torsade de pointes* or ventricular fibrillation, both non-fatal; the deaths occurred after cardiopulmonary arrest or an unspecified fatal arrhythmia[19]
- the maximum mortality attributable to prolonged QT has been estimated to be 0.06 per 100 patient-years, based on the examination of deaths of patients receiving methadone maintenance therapy in Norway.[20]

IV methadone has been considered high-risk. In cancer patients receiving median IV doses of 430mg/day (range 2.4mg–2.4g):[21]
- two patients with prolonged QT died suddenly (although a definite link with *torsade de pointes* was not proven)
- QTc > 500msec occurred in a patient receiving as little as 10mg/day.

However, the formulation of methadone contained the QT-prolonging preservative chlorbutanol; this works synergistically with methadone to prolong the QT interval. Although not always readily available, chlorbutanol-free methadone can be obtained (see p.331).

---

e.g. potassium, magnesium, is generally recommended in patients taking diuretics or at risk of hypokalemia, e.g. because of vomiting or diarrhea.

Other guidelines also suggest an ECG if other risk factors develop during treatment and highlight the importance of educating patients taking **methadone** to avoid where possible the use of other drugs which can prolong QT or inhibit **methadone** metabolism, and to urgently report cardiac symptoms, e.g. palpitation, dizziness, fainting spells, seizures.[22]

Specific guidance from a palliative care perspective is limited. In the USA, an expert group has developed a guideline for the use of *parenteral* **methadone** for chronic pain and in the palliative/hospice setting. Partly because of the increased risk presented by the preservative **chlorbutanol** (Box 22.E), an ECG is recommended:
- before starting IV therapy and after 1 and 4 days of treatment
- when the dose is significantly increased
- if an additional risk factor for QT prolongation develops.[23]

Monitoring serum electrolytes in high risk patients and discussing the potential risks of prolonged QT and *torsade de pointes* with the patient and carers are also recommended. However, consideration of burden vs. benefit is paramount and, in those with life-limiting illness, the potential benefit of controlling otherwise refractory pain may far outweigh the risks, even when monitoring for arrhythmia is impractical.[23] A commonsense approach should prevail: ECG monitoring is generally irrelevant in the last days of life.[14]

On the other hand, for a patient with a reasonable prognosis, it may be appropriate to identify any risk factors for QT prolongation and consider ECG monitoring as recommended in the UK SPC (Product Monograph). Nonetheless, research is required to establish the magnitude of the risk of *torsade de pointes* with **methadone** and the overall value of adopting such an approach in the palliative care setting.

If the baseline QT is prolonged, an alternative opioid should be considered. Further, if the QT interval increases to >500msec while on **methadone**, generally it should be discontinued and an alternative used. However, there has been a report of the successful use of parenteral **methadone** for analgesia in a patient with a prolonged QT interval.[24] Implantable cardioverter-defibrillators have also been used in addicts with *torsade de pointes* who needed to remain on **methadone**.[25]

Generally, **methadone** is available only as a racemic mixture. (S)-**methadone** is a more potent blocker of the potassium channels in the cardiac myocytes than (R)-**methadone**. CYP2B6 also displays stereoselectivity for the metabolism of (S)-**methadone**, and initial findings suggest that CYP2B6 poor metabolizers (found in about 6% of Caucasians and African-Americans) have higher levels of (S)-**methadone** and may thus be at greater risk of prolonged QTc.[26] The use of (R)-**methadone** may thus be safer in this respect but, at present, it is available only in Germany.[27]

1 Goldenberg I et al. (2006) QT interval: how to measure it and what is 'normal'. *Journal of Cardiovascular Electrophysiology.* **17**: 333–336.
2 Al-Khatib SM et al. (2003) What clinicians should know about the QT interval. *Journal of the American Medical Association.* **289**: 2120–2127.
3 Gupta A et al. (2007) Current concepts in the mechanisms and management of drug-induced QT prolongation and torsade de pointes. *American Heart Journal.* **153**: 891–899.
4 Committee for Proprietary Medicinal Products (1996) Points to consider: the assessment of the potential for QT interval prolongation by non-cardiovascular medicinal products. *European Agency for the Evaluation of Medicinal Products (EMEA).* CPMP/986/96.
5 Haverkamp W et al. (2000) The potential for QT prolongation and proarrhythmia by non-antiarrhythmic drugs: clinical and regulatory implications. Report on a policy conference of the European Society of Cardiology. *European Heart Journal.* **21**: 1216–1231.
6 Zipes DP et al. (2006) ACC/AHA/ESC 2006 guidelines for management of patients with ventricular arrhythmias and the prevention of sudden cardiac death: a report of the American College of Cardiology/American Heart Association Task Force and the European Society of Cardiology Committee for Practice Guidelines (Writing Committee to Develop guidelines for management of patients with ventricular arrhythmias and the prevention of sudden cardiac death) developed in collaboration with the European Heart Rhythm Association and the Heart Rhythm Society. *Europace.* **8**: 746–837.
7 Idle JR (2000) The heart of psychotropic drug therapy. *Lancet.* **355**: 1824–1825.
8 Andrews CM et al. (2009) Methadone-induced mortality in the treatment of chronic pain: role of QT prolongation. *Cardiology Journal.* **16**: 210–217.
9 Twycross RG et al. (1994) Monitoring drug use in palliative care. *Palliative Medicine.* **8**: 137–143.
10 Wilcock A et al. (2005) Potential for drug interactions involving cytochrome P450 in patients attending palliative day care centres: a multicentre audit. *British Journal of Clinical Pharmacology.* **60**: 326–329.
11 Davies SJ et al. (2004) Potential for drug interactions involving cytochromes P450 2D6 and 3A4 on general adult psychiatric and functional elderly psychiatric wards. *British Journal of Clinical Pharmacology.* **57**: 464–472.
12 Bernard SA and Bruera E (2000) Drug interactions in palliative care. *Journal of Clinical Oncology.* **18**: 1780–1799.
13 Walker G et al. (2003) Prolongation of the QT interval in palliative care patients. *Journal of Pain and Symptom Management.* **26**: 855–859.
14 Wilcock A and Beattie JM (2009) Prolonged QT interval and methadone: implications for palliative care. *Current Opinion in Supportive and Palliative Care.* **3**: 252–257.
15 Stimmel B et al. (1973) Electrocardiographic changes in heroin, methadone and multiple drug abuse: a postulated mechanism of sudden death in narcotic addicts. *Proceedings of the National Conference on Methadone Treatment.* **1**: 706–710.
16 Krantz MJ et al. (2002) Torsade de pointes associated with very-high-dose methadone. *Annals of Internal Medicine.* **137**: 501–504.
17 Stringer J et al. (2009) Methadone-associated QT interval prolongation and torsades de pointes. *American Journal of Health System Pharmacy.* **66**: 825–833.
18 Pearson EC and Woosley RL (2005) QT prolongation and torsades de pointes among methadone users: reports to the FDA spontaneous reporting system. *Pharmacoepidemiology and Drug Safety.* **14**: 747–753.
19 MHRA (2009) Personal communication.
20 Anchersen K et al. (2009) Prevalence and clinical relevance of corrected QT interval prolongation during methadone and buprenorphine treatment: a mortality assessment study. *Addiction.* **104**: 993–999.
21 Kornick CA et al. (2003) QTc interval prolongation associated with intravenous methadone. *Pain.* **105**: 499–506.
22 Office of Alcoholism and Substance Abuse Services (2009 March) Medical advisory panel position on QTc interval screening in methadone treatment. Available from: http://www.oasas.state.ny.us/Admed/cme/QTCinterval.cfm

23 Shaiova L *et al.* (2008) Consensus guideline on parenteral methadone use in pain and palliative care. *Palliative and Supportive Care.* **6**: 165–176.

24 Sekine R *et al.* (2007) The successful use of parenteral methadone in a patient with a prolonged QTc interval. *Journal of Pain and Symptom Management.* **34**: 566–569.

25 Patel AM *et al.* (2008) Role of implantable cardioverter-defibrillators in patients with methadone-induced long QT syndrome. *American Journal of Cardiology.* **101**: 209–211.

26 Eap CB *et al.* (2007) Stereoselective block of hERG channel by (S)-methadone and QT interval prolongation in CYP2B6 slow metabolizers. *Clinical Pharmacology and Therapeutics.* **81**: 719–728.

27 Gaertner J *et al.* (2008) Methadone: a closer look at the controversy. *Journal of Pain and Symptom Management.* **36**: e4–7.

23: CYTOCHROME P450

Polypharmacy (using more than one drug concurrently) introduces the possibility of clinically important drug–drug interactions. In the past, concern about interactions focused mainly on changes in drug absorption, protein-binding in the blood and renal excretion. There was also recognition of important pharmacodynamic interactions such as serotonin toxicity observed with **meperidine** and MAOIs. However, studies over the last 25 years have shown that many of the potentially serious drug interactions involve hepatic biotransformation pathways catalyzed by the cytochrome P450 mixed-function oxidase group of enzymes. These are the major drug metabolizing enzymes catalysing mainly *oxidation* and *reduction* reactions.

The name cytochrome P450 is derived from the spectrometric characteristics of this group of enzymes; the maximum absorbance is produced at or near 450nm. The cytochromes P450 are a super-family of enzymes which exist in virtually all tissues, but their highest concentration is in the liver. In mammals, there are at least 14 families ($>40\%$ identical amino acid sequence) with some 30 active subfamilies ($>55\%$ identical amino acid sequence) (Figure 23.1). Cytochrome P450 enzymes have been assigned the root symbol CYP, followed by:

- a number designating the enzyme family
- a capital letter designating the subfamily
- a number designating the individual enzyme.

In genetic studies, the individual enzyme number is followed by an asterisk with a further number and letter to designate specific alleles (genetic variants) encoding enzymes with normal, increased or decreased activity. For example, CYP2D6*1A encodes the wild-type enzyme (i.e. the first one to be discovered), which has normal activity, whereas CYP2D6*10B contains minor mutations associated with reduced enzyme activity.[1,2]

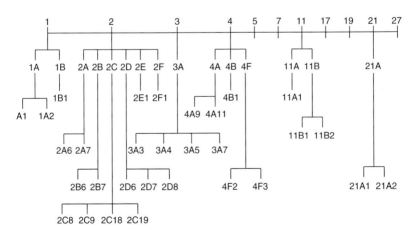

Figure 23.1 Cytochrome P450 enzyme tree.[3]

The mammalian P450 families can be divided into two major classes; those involved in the synthesis and degradation of endogenous substances, e.g. fatty acids, eicosanoids, steroids and bile acids, and those which primarily metabolize foreign substances (xenobiotics), e.g. drugs and toxins.[4] Enzymes of the CYP1, CYP2 and CYP3 families are responsible for many drug biotransformations and account for 70% of the total P450 content of the liver (Figure 23.2).

CPCF   551

Some are also present in the wall of the GI tract, e.g. CYP3A, where they can affect the bio-availability of substrate drugs and pro-drugs through first-pass metabolism.[2] Drugs responsible for interactions act either as *inhibitors* or *inducers*.

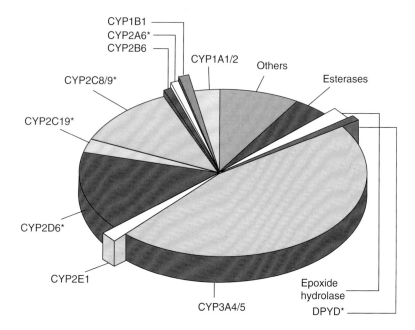

Figure 23.2 Proportion of drugs metabolized by different cytochrome P450 enzymes.[5]

Inhibition

Inhibition of drug biotransformation begins within a few hours of the administration of the inhibitor drug, leading to an increase in the plasma substrate drug concentration, drug response and toxicity, *except pro-drugs which will have a corresponding reduced effect* (see below). The mechanism of enzymatic inhibition is either reversible or irreversible. In reversible inhibition, the inhibitor drug (e.g. **cimetidine**, **ketoconazole** and macrolide antibacterials) binds to the P450 enzyme and prevents the metabolism of the substrate drug. The extent of inhibition of one drug by another depends on their relative affinities for the P450 enzyme, and the relative doses. In irreversible inhibition, the enzyme is destroyed or inactivated by the inhibitor drug or its metabolites (e.g. **chloramphenicol** and **spironolactone**).

The occurrence of serious cardiac arrhythmias seen with the concurrent administration of **ketoconazole** (an inhibitor) and **terfenadine** is an example of a non-competitive inhibitory drug interaction involving CYP3A3/4[6] (Box 23.A). Because of similar interactions, **terfenadine** and **astemizole** have been withdrawn in Canada (see Prolongation of the QT interval, p.543).

Box 23.A Ketoconazole-induced terfenadine cardiotoxicity[11]

A 39-year-old woman began a course of terfenadine and after about 1 week started ketoconazole. Two days later she developed syncopal symptoms, prolongation of her QT interval on the ECG and *torsade de pointes*. High concentrations of terfenadine and reduced concentrations of its main metabolite were found, suggesting inhibition of metabolism. It was concluded that ketoconazole-induced inhibition of terfenadine metabolism caused the cardiotoxicity.

Clopidogrel is a pro-drug activated by CYP2C19. PPIs can reduce the level of the active metabolite through inhibition of this enzyme, and thus reduce the antithrombotic effect. Individual PPIs vary in the extent to which they inhibit CYP2C19 but the general advice is to avoid concurrent use.[7–10]

Box 23.B gives examples of enhanced drug effects resulting from enzyme inhibition, and Table 23.1 gives numerous examples of cytochrome P450 enzyme inhibitors which may increase the plasma concentrations of various substrate drugs.[2,12,13]

Box 23.B   Examples of drug interactions → increased effect

Cimetidine reduces diazepam clearance → increased effect.[14]
Ciprofloxacin reduces theophylline clearance by 18–113% → increased effect.[15]
Diltiazem prolongs the halflife of propranolol and metoprolol → increased effect.[16]
Erythromycin increases cisapride concentration → possible cardiac effects.[a]
Fluvoxamine increases warfarin concentration by 65% → increased effect.[17]
Ketoconazole increases terfenadine concentration → possible life-threatening cardiac arrhythmias.[b,18]
Mexiletine reduces clearance of amitriptyline → increased effect.
SSRIs reduce clearance of TCAs → increased plasma concentrations by 50–350% → increased effect.[19–21]

---

a. cisapride is no longer marketed in Canada because of this and the same interaction with various other drugs (see Prolongation of the QT interval, p.543); it is available only through the Special Access Programme
b. terfenadine has been withdrawn because of this and the same interaction with various other drugs (see Prolongation of the QT interval, p.543).

Food-drug interactions

A food–drug interaction has been highlighted involving grapefruit juice and substrates of CYP3A enzymes such as **felodipine, nifedipine, cyclosporine, terfenadine, saquinavir, buspirone**, some benzodiazepines (**diazepam, triazolam, midazolam**) and some 'statin' lipid-lowering drugs (**atorvastatin, lovastatin, simvastatin**).[2,22–25] Grapefruit juice contains several bioflavonoids (naringenin, naringin, kaempferol and quercetin) and furanocoumarins (bergamottin) which non-competitively inhibit oxidation reactions in the CYP3A enzymes in the wall of the GI tract.[24,26,27] The effect is variable because the quantity of these components in grapefruit products varies considerably.[28,29]

The effect of grapefruit juice is maximal when ingested 30–60min before the drug. A single 250mL glass of grapefruit juice can inhibit CYP3A for 24–48h and regular intake continually suppresses GI CYP3A.[2,24] Thus, patients taking many drugs metabolized by CYP3A are warned to avoid grapefruit juice, particularly if the drug has a narrow therapeutic index, e.g. **cyclosporine**. Pomelo, Seville orange and lime juices may also inhibit CYP3A, although confirmation is required.[30,31] Apple juice has not been implicated.

Besides inhibiting CYP3A, naringin (and thus grapefruit juice) inhibits organic anion-transporting polypeptide 1A2 (OATP1A2), a carrier protein in the wall of the GI tract which is responsible for the uptake of several drugs. Orange juice (through its major flavonoid, hesperidin) has a similar effect.[32] Preliminary research suggests that apple juice also inhibits OATP1A2.[33] Drugs which may have their absorption reduced by this inhibition include **fexofenadine, etoposide**, some β-blockers (**atenolol, celiprolol, talinolol**), **cyclosporine**, quinolone antibacterials (**ciprofloxacin, levofloxacin**) and **itraconazole**.[32,33]

Cranberry juice contains various anti-oxidants, including flavonoids, which are known to inhibit cytochrome P450 activity.[34] This was originally thought to explain several case reports, including one fatality,[35–38] in which the regular use of cranberry juice was linked to an increase in or fluctuation of INR values in patients taking **warfarin**, a drug predominantly metabolized by CYP2C9.[39] However, more recent pharmacokinetic studies suggest that this interaction is unlikely to occur with the amounts of cranberry juice recommended for prophylaxis against urinary tract infections (see Cranberry juice, p.415).[40–43] Patients on stable **warfarin** doses who drank cranberry juice 250mL once daily for 1 week showed no significant increase

Table 23.1 Selected list CYP substrates, inhibitors and inducers

Enzyme	Substrates	Inhibitors	Inducers
CYP1A2	Acetaminophen Amitriptyline Caffeine Clomipramine Clozapine Ethinylestradiol Imipramine Olanzapine Propranolol Theophylline Trimipramine	Grapefruit juice Cimetidine Ciprofloxacin[a] Diltiazem Erythromycin (weak) Fluoxetine (weak)[b] Fluvoxamine[b] Mexiletine Norfloxacin (weak)[a] Paroxetine (weak)[b] Sertraline (weak)[b] Verapamil	Brassicas Charbroiled beef Smoking Omeprazole Phenobarbital Phenytoin
CYP2C8/9	Amitriptyline Diclofenac Fluvastatin Glipizide Ibuprofen Imipramine Losartan Naproxen Phenytoin Piroxicam Tolbutamide Torsemide (not Canada) Warfarin Zafirlukast	Amiodarone Cimetidine Cranberry juice (possibly; may inhibit CYP2C9 at $>600mL/24h$) Fluconazole[c] Fluvastatin (possibly) Metronidazole Miconazole Ritonavir Sulfamethoxazole Trimethoprim Zafirlukast	Barbiturates Carbamazepine Rifampin St John's wort
CYP2C19[d]	Amitriptyline Citalopram Clomipramine Clopidogrel Diazepam Fluoxetine Imipramine Lansoprazole Moclobemide Nelfinavir Omeprazole Pantoprazole Pentamidine Phenytoin Proguanil Propranolol Sertraline	Cimetidine Esomeprazole Fluoxetine[b] Fluvoxamine[b] Ketoconazole[c] Lansoprazole Moclobemide Omeprazole Rabeprazole	Phenytoin Rifampin (possibly)
CYP2D6[e]	Amitriptyline Carvedilol Clomipramine Clozapine Codeine Desipramine Dextromethorphan Flecainide Fluoxetine Haloperidol Hydrocodone Imipramine Metoprolol	Amiodarone Cimetidine Clomipramine Flecainide Fluoxetine[b] Fluvoxamine (weak)[b] Haloperidol Methotrimeprazine Paroxetine[b] Perphenazine Propafenone Quinidine[f] Sertraline (weak)[b]	

continued

Table 23.1 Continued

Enzyme	Substrates	Inhibitors	Inducers
CYP2D6[e] contd	Mexiletine Nortriptyline Ondansetron Oxycodone Paroxetine Perphenazine Propafenone Propoxyphene Propranolol Quinidine Risperidone Ritonavir Sertraline Timolol Tramadol Venlafaxine	Tramadol[g]	
CYP2E1	Acetaminophen Alcohol Caffeine Isoniazid Theophylline	Disulfiram Isoniazid	Alcohol Isoniazid
CYP3A4/5[h]	Acetaminophen Alfentanil Alprazolam Amiodarone Amitriptyline Atorvastatin Bromocriptine Carbamazepine Cisapride Clarithromycin Clomipramine Clopidogrel Clozapine Codeine Corticosteroids Cyclosporine Diazepam Diltiazem Erythromycin Ethinylestradiol Felodipine Fentanyl Imipramine Indinavir Lidocaine Losartan Lovastatin Methadone Midazolam Nelfinavir Nifedipine Omeprazole Phenytoin Pimozide Propafenone Quinidine Ritonavir	Bromocriptine Cimetidine Clarithromycin Cyclosporine Danazol Delavirdine Diltiazem Ergotamine Erythromycin Ethinylestradiol Fluconazole[c] Fluoxetine[b] Fluvoxamine[b] Grapefruit juice Indinavir Itraconazole[c] Ketoconazole[c] Miconazole Midazolam Nicardipine Nifedipine Omeprazole Paroxetine (weak)[b] Progesterone Propoxyphene Quinidine Ritonavir Saquinavir Sertraline (weak)[b] Testosterone Verapamil Zafirlukast	Carbamazepine Dexamethasone Efavirenz Nevirapine Phenobarbital Phenytoin Rifabutin Rifampin St John's wort

continued

Table 23.1 Continued

Enzyme	Substrates	Inhibitors	Inducers
CYP3A4/5[h] contd	Saquinavir		
	Sertraline		
	Sildenafil		
	Simvastatin		
	Tamoxifen		
	Theophylline		
	Triazolam		
	Venlafaxine		
	Verapamil		
	Warfarin		

a. relative inhibitory potency of fluoroquinolones: ciprofloxacin >norfloxacin >ofloxacin (almost none)
b. *in vitro* data suggest only moderate inhibition of SSRIs. CYP1A2 inhibition: fluvoxamine >all other SSRIs; CYP2D6 inhibition: paroxetine and fluoxetine >sertraline >fluvoxamine (almost none); CYP3A4 inhibition: fluvoxamine >fluoxetine >paroxetine and sertraline (almost none)
c. relative inhibitory potency of imidazoles: ketoconazole≈itraconazole >fluconazole (and possibly clotrimazole)
d. genetic polymorphism. Autosomal recessive inheritance: 2% of white Caucasians and 20% of orientals do not express this enzyme and are 'slow metabolizers'
e. genetic polymorphism. Autosomal recessive inheritance: 5–10% of white Caucasians and 1–2% of blacks and orientals do not express this enzyme and are 'slow metabolizers'
f. most potent CYP2D6 inhibitor
g. significant competitive inhibition of quinidine and propafenone metabolism has been documented with tramadol administration
h. expressed in GI mucosa resulting in substantial first-pass metabolism during absorption of some drugs.

in anticoagulant activity,[40] and, in volunteers, drinking cranberry juice 200mL t.i.d. did not significantly affect the pharmacokinetic profiles of **warfarin, tizanidine** or **midazolam** (probes for CYP2C9, CYP1A2 and CYP3A4 respectively).[41] Further, it is unclear whether the salicylate constituent of cranberry juice plays a role by producing an anti-platelet effect or displacing **warfarin** from protein-binding sites.[42]

Nonetheless, an interaction with **warfarin** cannot be ruled out, particularly when large volumes of cranberry juice are drunk regularly, or when cranberry products other than juice are taken.[42–44] Thus, the INR should be monitored more closely in patients on **warfarin** if they consume large amounts of cranberry juice or take other cranberry supplements for prophylaxis against urinary tract infections.[43]

Induction

Induction of the rate of drug biotransformation results in a decrease in the parent drug plasma concentrations and *decreased effect*, but *increased toxicity* if active metabolites are formed or if the administered drug is an inactive pro-drug. The onset and offset of enzyme induction is gradual, i.e. 2–3 weeks, because:

• onset depends on drug-induced synthesis of new enzyme
• offset depends on elimination of the enzyme-inducing drug and the decay of the increased enzyme stores.

Sequential dose adjustments, either up or down, may be necessary to maintain the desired clinical effect of the affected drug during a progressive change in CYP activity.[2]

Several molecular mechanisms for enzyme induction have been characterized, including increased DNA transcription (the most common), increased RNA processing and mRNA stabilization.

Inducer drugs like **rifampin, dexamethasone, griseofulvin** and anti-epileptics such as **carbamazepine, phenobarbital** and **phenytoin** induce members of the CYP3A subfamily. **Rifampin** is the most potent inducer of cytochrome CYP3A in clinical use. Some estrogens are metabolized by CYP3A3/4 and induction by **rifampin**, or another enzyme inducer, can cause oral contraceptive failure. Failure of protease inhibitor treatment for HIV infection has also occurred when **St John's wort** was taken concurrently.[45–47] Box 23.C gives examples of decreased drug effects as a result of enzyme induction.

Box 23.C   Examples of drug interactions → decreased effect

Carbamazepine and phenytoin increase midazolam metabolism → decreased effect.[48]
Phenytoin increases carbamazepine metabolism → possible therapeutic failure.
Quinidine inhibits biotransformation of codeine to morphine → decreased analgesic effect.[49]
Rifampin increases phenytoin clearance (halflife halved) → decreased effect.[50]

Table 23.1 gives numerous examples of CYP450 enzyme inducers which may decrease the plasma concentrations of various substrate drugs. **Carbamazepine** can potentially decrease the effect of many other drugs by decreasing their plasma concentrations (or can expedite the biotransformation of a drug to an active metabolite). For example, **carbamazepine** increases **diazepam** metabolism but, in this case, there may be no detectable clinical effect because of active metabolites.

Genetic polymorphism
Genetic differences in the amount of drug metabolized by an enzymatic pathway has resulted in the classification of individuals into slow (poor) metabolizers and rapid (extensive) meta-bolizers.[51] More recently, intermediate and ultra-rapid metabolizers have been identified for some pathways.[2] Inevitably, even within the general population of rapid metabolizers, there is a normal distribution of enzyme activity ranging from well below-average to well above-average. However, the slow metabolizers (and ultra-rapid ones) form a discontinuous genetically distinct group - they are not merely one end of a spectrum. Slow metabolizer status is generally linked to only one enzyme in any one individual, and is inherited as an autosomal recessive trait (Table 23.2). The inherited allele may encode an inactivated enzyme or one with reduced activity. Ultra-rapid metabolism may result from inheriting a more active form of the enzyme or multiple copies of an allele encoding an enzyme with normal activity.[2]

Table 23.2   Genetic polymorphism and slow (poor) metabolizer status[2,3,52]

Pathway	A selection of drugs affected	Population affected
N-acetylation	Caffeine Dapsone Hydralazine Isoniazid Procainamide	North European 60–70% American whites and blacks 50% Asians 5–10%
CYP2D6 (debrisoquine hydroxylase)	β-Blockers Codeine Debrisoquine Flecainide Oxycodone Phenothiazines SSRIs (some) TCAs (some) Tramadol	Whites 5–10% Asians 1–2%
CYP2C9	Glipizide Phenytoin Tolbutamide Warfarin	Europeans <1%
CYP2C19	Diazepam PPIs S-mephenytoin	Whites 2–5% Blacks 4% Asians 10–25%

Non-genetic circumstances in which drug metabolism may become relatively slower include liver damage (with an associated decrease in cytochrome P450 enzyme activity) and old age. In general, age-related decreases in liver mass, liver enzyme activity and hepatic blood flow result in a decrease in the overall metabolic capacity of the liver in the elderly. This is of particular importance in relation to drugs which have a high 'hepatic extraction ratio', e.g. **amitriptyline, lidocaine, propranolol, verapamil**.

Drug–drug interactions involving CYP enzymes in palliative care

Many patients attending palliative care centres are elderly and take multiple drugs for possibly several chronic conditions. This increases the likelihood of drug interactions involving CYP enzymes.

An audit of 160 patients attending UK palliative care day centres found that patients were taking a median of 7 drugs (range 1–17). About 1/5 were receiving a combination likely to produce a definitely or potentially clinically important CYP-mediated interaction (Table 23.3). Approximately 1/2 of these interactions involved corticosteroids and 1/4 analgesics. The two definitely clinically important interactions were between **omeprazole** and **diazepam** (which could result in drowsiness from increased **diazepam** levels) and between **phenytoin** and **dexamethasone** (which could result in a reduced **dexamethasone** effect).[53] Thus, it is important to be aware of drugs metabolized by CYP enzymes and to consider the possibility of interactions when adding drugs to a patient's existing medication.

Table 23.3 Drug combinations likely to produce definitely or potentially clinically important CYP-mediated interactions in 160 patients attending palliative care day centres in the UK[53]

Category	Drug combination	Frequency (number of times the combination was prescribed)	Likely outcome of the interaction (drug effect increased ($\uparrow$) or decreased ($\downarrow$))
Definitely important	Omeprazole + diazepam	3	Diazepam $\uparrow$
	Phenytoin + dexamethasone	2	Dexamethasone $\downarrow$
Potentially important	Dexamethasone + temazepam	5	Temazepam $\downarrow$
	Haloperidol + oxycodone	4	Oxycodone $\downarrow$
	Methotrimeprazine + oxycodone	3	Oxycodone $\downarrow$
	Prednisone + diazepam	3	Diazepam $\downarrow$
	Propoxyphene + tramadol	2	Tramadol $\uparrow$
	Acetaminophen-propoxyphene + codeine	1	Codeine $\downarrow$
	Carbamazepine + zopiclone	1	Zopiclone $\downarrow$
	Dexamethasone + amitriptyline	1	Amitriptyline $\downarrow$
	Dexamethasone + fentanyl	1	Fentanyl $\downarrow$
	Dexamethasone + quinine	1	Quinine $\downarrow$
	Dexamethasone + simvastatin	1	Simvastatin $\downarrow$
	Dexamethasone + tacrolimus	1	Tacrolimus $\downarrow$
	Dexamethasone + zopiclone	1	Zopiclone $\downarrow$
	Fluoxetine + codeine	1	Codeine $\downarrow$
	Haloperidol + codeine	1	Codeine $\downarrow$
	Methotrimeprazine + haloperidol	1	Methotrimeprazine $\uparrow$ Haloperidol $\uparrow$
	Methotrimeprazine + tamoxifen	1	Tamoxifen $\downarrow$
	Prednisone + amlodipine	1	Amlodipine $\downarrow$
	Prednisone + fentanyl	1	Fentanyl $\downarrow$
	Prednisone + trazodone	1	Trazodone $\downarrow$
	Prednisone + zopiclone	1	Zopiclone $\downarrow$
	Verapamil + zopiclone	1	Zopiclone $\uparrow$
Total frequency		39	
Number of patients prescribed $\geqslant$1 combination likely to produce a definitely or potentially clinically important interaction		34 (21%)	

1 Sim SC (2005) Human Cytochrome P450 (CYP). Allele Nomenclature Committee. Available from: www.imm.ki.se/CYPalleles.
2 Wilkinson GR (2005) Drug metabolism and variability among patients in drug response. *New England Journal of Medicine.* **352**: 2211–2221.
3 Riddick D (1997) Drug biotransformation. In: H Kalant and W Roschlau (eds) *Principles of Medical Pharmacology* (6e). Oxford University Press, New York.
4 Nebert DW and Russell DW (2002) Clinical importance of the cytochromes P450. *Lancet.* **360**: 1155–1162.
5 Brunton LL et al. (eds) (2005) *Goodman & Gilman's The Pharmacological Basis of Therapeutics.* (11e). McGraw-Hill, New York; London.
6 Honig P et al. (1993) Terfenadine-ketoconazole interaction. Pharmacokinetic and electrocardiographic consequences. *Journal of the American Medical Association.* **269**: 1513–1518.
7 Ho M et al. (2009) Risk of adverse outcomes associated with concomitant use of clopidogrel and proton pump inhibitors following acute coronary syndrome. *Journal of the American Medical Association.* **301**: 937–944.
8 Juurlink DN et al. (2009) A population-based study of the drug interaction between proton pump inhibitors and clopidogrel. *Canadian Medical Association Journal.* **180**: 713–718.
9 Society for Cardiovascular Angiography and Interventions (2009) A national study of the effect of individual proton pump inhibitors on cardiovascular outcomes in patients treated with clopidogrel following coronary stenting: The Clopidogrel Medco Outcomes Study. Available from: www.scai.org/drlt1.aspx?PAGE_ID = 5870.
10 MHRA (2009) Interactions between the use of clopidogrel and proton pump inhibitors. Available from: www.mhra.gov.uk/home/idcplg?IdcService = SS_GET_PAGE&ssDocName = CON051743.
11 Monahan B (1990) Torsades de Pointes occurring in association with terfenadine. *Journal of the American Medical Association.* **264**: 2788–2790.
12 Aeschlimann J and Tyler L (1996) Drug interactions associated with cytochrome P-450 enzymes. *Journal of Pharmaceutical Care in Pain and Symptom Control.* **4**: 35–54.
13 Johnson MD et al. (1999) Clinically significant drug interactions. *Postgraduate Medicine.* **105**: 193–222.
14 Klotz U and Reimann I (1980) Delayed clearance of diazepam due to cimetidine. *New England Journal of Medicine.* **302**: 1012–1014.
15 Nix D et al. (1987) Effect of multiple dose oral ciprofloxacin on the pharmacokinetics of theophylline and indocyanine green. *Journal of Antimicrobial Chemotherapy.* **19**: 263–269.
16 Tateishi T et al. (1989) Effect of diltiazem on the pharmacokinetics of propranolol, metoprolol and atenolol. *European Journal of Clinical Pharmacology.* **36**: 67–70.
17 Tatro D (1995) Fluvoxamine drug interactions. *Drug Newsletter.* **14**: 20ff.
18 Eller M (1991) Pharmacokinetic interaction between terfenadine and ketoconazole. *Clinical Pharmacology and Therapeutics.* **49**: 130.
19 Vandel S et al. (1992) Tricyclic antidepressant plasma levels after fluoxetine addition. *Neuropsychobiology.* **25**: 202–207.
20 Finley P (1994) Selective serotonin reuptake inhibitors: pharmacologic profiles and potential therapeutic distinctions. *Annals of Pharmacotherapy.* **28**: 1359–1369.
21 Pollock B (1994) Recent developments in drug metabolism of relevance to psychiatrists. *Harvard Reviews of Psychiatry.* **2**: 204–213.
22 Benton R et al. (1996) Grapefruit juice alters terfenadine pharmacokinetics, resulting in prolongation of repolarization on the electrocardiogram. *Clinical Pharmacology and Therapeutics.* **59**: 383–388.
23 Maskalyk J (2002) Grapefruit juice: potential drug interactions. *Canadian Medical Association Journal.* **167**: 279–280.
24 Dahan A and Altman H (2004) Food-drug interaction: grapefruit juice augments drug bioavailability-mechanism, extent and relevance. *European Journal of Clinical Nutrition.* **58**: 1–9.
25 MHRA (2004) Statins and cytochrome P450 interactions. *Current Problems in Pharmacovigilance.* **30 (Oct)**: 1–2.
26 Gibaldi M (1992) Drug interactions. Part II. *Annals of Pharmacotherapy.* **26**: 829–834.
27 Rouseff RL (1988) Liquid chromatographic determination of naringin and neohesperidin as a detector of grapefruit juice in orange juice. *Journal - Association of Official Analytical Chemists.* **71**: 798–802.
28 Tailor S et al. (1996) Peripheral edema due to nifedipine-itraconazole interaction: a case report. *Archives of Dermatology.* **132**: 350–352.
29 Fukuda K et al. (2000) Amounts and variation in grapefruit juice of the main components causing grapefruit-drug interaction. *Journal of Chromatography. B, Biomedical Sciences and Applications.* **741**: 195–203.
30 Savage I (2008) Forbidden fruit: interactions between medicines, foods and herbal products. *Pharmaceutical Journal.* **281**: f17.
31 Baxter K (2008) Drug interactions and fruit juices. *Pharmaceutical Journal.* **281**: 333.
32 Bailey DG et al. (2007) Naringin is a major and selective clinical inhibitor of organic anion-transporting polypeptide 1A2 (OATP1A2) in grapefruit juice. *Clinical Pharmacology & Therapeutics.* **81**: 495–502.
33 Sampson M (2008) New reasons to avoid grapefruit and other juices when taking certain drugs. Report from the 236th National Meeting of the American Chemical Society. Philadelphia, August 19th 2008. Available from: www.eurekalert.org/pub_releases/2008-08/acs-nrt072308.php.
34 Hodek P et al. (2002) Flavonoids-potent and versatile biologically active compounds interacting with cytochromes P450. *Chemico-Biological Interactions.* **139**: 1–21.
35 MHRA (2003) Possible interaction between warfarin and cranberry juice. *Current Problems in Pharmacovigilance.* **29 (Sept)**: 8.
36 Suvarna R et al. (2003) Possible interaction between warfarin and cranberry juice. *British Medical Journal.* **327**: 1454.
37 CSM (Committee on Safety of Medicines) (2004) Interaction between warfarin and cranberry juice: new advice. *Current Problems in Pharmacovigilance.* **30 (October)**: 10.
38 Grant P (2004) Warfarin and cranberry juice: an interaction? *Journal of Heart Valve Disease.* **13**: 25–26.
39 Rettie AE et al. (1992) Hydroxylation of warfarin by human cDNA-expressed cytochrome P-450: a role for P-4502C9 in the etiology of (S)-warfarin-drug interactions. *Chemical Research in Toxicology.* **5**: 54–59.
40 Li Z et al. (2006) Cranberry does not affect prothrombin time in male subjects on warfarin. *Journal of the American Dietetic Society.* **106**: 2057–2061.
41 Lilja JJ et al. (2007) Effects of daily ingestion of cranberry juice on the pharmacokinetics of warfarin, tizanidine, and midazolam-probes of CYP2C9, CYP1A2, and CYP3A4. *Clinical Pharmacology & Therapeutics.* **81**: 833–839.
42 Aston JL et al. (2006) Interaction between warfarin and cranberry juice. *Pharmacotherapy.* **26**: 1314–1319.
43 O'Mara N (2007) Does a cranberry juice-warfarin interaction really exist? Detail document. *Pharmacist's Letter/Prescriber's Letter.* **23**: 1–3.

44 Welch J and Forster K (2007) Probable elevation in international normalized ratio from cranberry juice. *Journal of Pharmacy Technology*. **23**: 104–107.

45 Flexner C (2000) Dual protease inhibitor therapy in HIV-infected patients: pharmacologic rationale and clinical benefits. *Annual Review of Pharmacology and Toxicology*. **40**: 649–674.

46 Henderson L *et al.* (2002) St John's wort (Hypericum perforatum): drug interactions and clinical outcomes. *British Journal of Clinical Pharmacology*. **54**: 349–356.

47 Piscitelli SC *et al.* (2000) Indinavir concentrations and St John's wort. *Lancet*. **355**: 547–548.

48 Backman J *et al.* (1996) Concentrations and effects of oral midazolam are greatly reduced in patients treated with carbamazepine or phenytoin. *Epilepsia*. **37**: 253–257.

49 Sindrup S *et al.* (1992) The effect of quinidine on the analgesic effect of codeine. *European Journal of Clinical Pharmacology*. **42**: 587–591.

50 Kay L *et al.* (1985) Influence of rifampicin and isoniazid on the kinetics of phenytoin. *British Journal of Clinical Pharmacology*. **20**: 323–326.

51 Meyer U (1991) Genotype or phenotype: the definition of a pharmacogenetic polymorphism. *Pharmacogenetics*. **1**: 66–67.

52 Poulsen L *et al.* (1996) The hypoalgesic effect of tramadol in relation to CYP2D6. *Clinical Pharmacology and Therapeutics*. **60**: 636–644.

53 Wilcock A *et al.* (2005) Potential for drug interactions involving cytochrome P450 in patients attending palliative day care centres: a multicentre audit. *British Journal of Clinical Pharmacology*. **60**: 326–329.

24: DRUG-INDUCED MOVEMENT DISORDERS

Drug-induced movement disorders (extrapyramidal reactions) encompass:
- parkinsonism
- acute dystonia
- acute akathisia
- tardive dyskinesia.

The features of the various syndromes are listed in Box 24.A.[1] Most extrapyramidal reactions are caused by drugs which block dopamine receptors in the CNS; these include all antipsychotics and **metoclopramide**.[2,3] Extrapyramidal reactions are dose-related. Pre-existing extrapyramidal signs increase the likelihood of a patient developing a drug-induced movement disorder; and patients with dementia are at greater risk.[4] There is probably also a genetic factor.[5]

In essence, extrapyramidal reactions are a consequence of an imbalance between two or more neurotransmitters. The imbalance varies between different causal drugs. Antipsychotic drugs and **metoclopramide** are most commonly associated with extrapyramidal reactions. With the typical antipsychotics (i.e. phenothiazines and butyrophenones), a high potency drug like **haloperidol** possesses a much greater affinity for D_2-receptors than for cholinergic receptors. The degree of imbalance between dopamine and acetylcholine increases the likelihood of extrapyramidal reactions. Compared with **haloperidol**, the atypical antipsychotics (e.g. **olanzapine** and **risperidone**) have a lower propensity for causing drug-induced movement disorders (see p.121). This is possibly because the antagonism of D_2-receptors is balanced by antagonism of serotonin (5HT).[6,7]

Numerous other drugs have been implicated,[8–10] including most classes of antidepressants, **carbamazepine, diltiazem, 5-hydroxytryptophan, levodopa, lithium, methyldopa, ondansetron** and **valproic acid**.[11–13]

A link between extrapyramidal reactions and the serotoninergic system is seen in the propensity of SSRIs to induce such disorders, including akathisia.[14] A 'four neurone model' has been proposed, embracing dopamine, muscarinic, 5HT and GABA receptors, to help explain how all these drugs cause extrapyramidal reactions.[15]

Parkinsonism

Parkinsonism develops in 30–60% of patients treated long-term with antipsychotics.[4] It is most common in those over 60 years of age. It can develop at any stage but, except in patients with dementia, generally not before the second week.[4] There may be asymmetry in the early stages. The tremor of drug-induced parkinsonism typically:
- has a frequency of <8 cycles per second
- is worse at rest
- is suppressed during voluntary movements
- is associated with rigidity and bradykinesia (Box 24.A).

This is different from drug-induced tremors of the hands, head, mouth or tongue which have a frequency of 8–12 cycles per second, and are best observed with hands held outstretched or mouth held open (Box 24.B).

Treatment
- if possible, reduce or stop causal drug
- if associated with a typical antipsychotic, consider switching to an atypical antipsychotic; they have a lower affinity for D_2-receptors and a lower risk of developing parkinsonism (see p.121)[4]

- prescribe an antimuscarinic antiparkinsonian drug, e.g.:
  - ▷ **benztropine** 1–2mg IV/IM → 2mg PO once daily–b.i.d. (occasionally more, e.g. 8–12mg/24h) *or*
  - ▷ **orphenadrine** SR 100mg once daily PO *or*
  - ▷ **procyclidine** 2.5–5mg PO t.i.d. *or*
  - ▷ **trihexyphenidyl** 2–5mg PO once daily–t.i.d.

Box 24.A Movement disorders associated with dopamine-receptor antagonists[1]

Parkinsonism
Coarse resting tremor of limbs, head, mouth and/or tongue
Muscular rigidity (cogwheel or lead pipe)
Bradykinesia, notably of face
Sialorrhea (drooling)
Shuffling gait

Acute dystonias
one or more of
Abnormal positioning of head and neck (retrocollis, torticollis)
Spasms of jaw muscles (trismus, gaping, grimacing)
Tongue dysfunction (dysarthria, protrusion)
Dysphagia
Laryngopharyngeal spasm
Dysphonia
Eyes deviated up, down or sideways (oculogyric crisis)
Abnormal positioning of limbs or trunk

Acute akathisia
one or more of
Fidgety movements or swinging of legs
Rocking from foot to foot when standing
Pacing to relieve restlessness
Inability to sit or stand still for several minutes

Tardive dyskinesia
Exposure to antipsychotic medication for >3 months (>1 month if >60 years of age)
Involuntary movement of tongue, jaw, trunk or limbs:
- choreiform (rapid, jerky, non-repetitive)
- athetoid (slow, sinuous, continual)
- rhythmic (stereotypic)

Box 24.B Drug-induced (non-parkinsonian) tremor[16]

Anti-epileptics
 valproic acid

Antidepressants
 SSRIs
 TCAs

Antipsychotics
 butyrophenones
 phenothiazines

β_2-Agonists
 salbutamol
 salmeterol

Lithium

Methylxanthines
 caffeine
 aminophylline
 theophylline

Psychostimulants
 dextroamphetamine
 methylphenidate

Acute dystonia

Acute dystonias occur in up to 10% of patients treated with antipsychotics.[4,17] They are most common in young adults. They develop abruptly within days of starting treatment, and are accompanied by anxiety (Box 24.A).

Treatment

If possible, discontinue or reduce the dose of the causal drug; if caused by **metoclopramide**, substitute **domperidone**. For immediate relief, give an injection of:

- an antimuscarinic antiparkinsonian drug, e.g. **benztropine** 1–2mg IV/IM, or
- **diazepam** 5mg IV[18] or
- an antihistaminic antimuscarinic drug, e.g. **dimenhydrinate** or **diphenhydramine** 25–50mg IV/IM.

With antimuscarinic drugs, benefit is typically seen in 10–20min. If necessary, repeat the injection after 30min. Continue treatment PO for 1 week with:

- SR **orphenadrine** 100mg once daily or
- **dimenhydrinate** or **diphenhydramine** 25–50mg b.i.d.–q.i.d.

Acute akathisia

Akathisia is a form of motor restlessness in which the subject is compelled to pace up and down or to change the body position frequently (Box 24.A).[19] It occurs in 20% or more of patients receiving typical antipsychotics.[4] The prevalence is no longer considered to be age-related, but younger patients may respond better to treatment than elderly ones.[4]

Akathisia can develop within days of starting treatment, and generally resolves within a week of stopping the causal drug. If the drug is continued, it may progress to parkinsonism. **Haloperidol** and **prochlorperazine** carry the highest risk.[20,21] It is uncommon for **metoclopramide** to cause akathisia.

Treatment

- if possible, discontinue or reduce the dose of the causal drug
- switch to an atypical antipsychotic or to a typical antipsychotic with more antimuscarinic activity
- if necessary, add **propranolol** 10mg t.i.d., increasing if necessary every few days to a maximum daily dose of 120mg (further benefit above this level is unlikely)[22]
- if the patient is very distressed, a benzodiazepine can be prescribed in addition for a few days, e.g. **diazepam** 5–10mg/24h,[18] **clonazepam** 0.5–1mg/24h, **lorazepam** 1–3mg/24h.

Although **propranolol**, a highly lipophilic non-selective β-adrenergic receptor antagonist (β-blocker), has a proven anti-akathisia effect, selective β_1-adrenergic receptor antagonists such as **atenolol** and **metoprolol** are either less or not effective.[22] This suggests that the effect is a central one, and that both β_1- and β_2-receptor antagonism is necessary to reduce akathisia.

Antimuscarinic antiparkinsonian drugs are sometimes helpful.[22] However, response in **haloperidol**-induced akathisia is less likely.[23] It has been suggested that benefit from antimuscarinic antiparkinsonian drugs occurs only if akathisia is associated with drug-induced parkinsonism.[24]

Diphenhydramine may also be of benefit.[18] Other possible treatments include **buspirone** and **clonidine**.[22,25]

Tardive dyskinesia

Tardive (late) dyskinesia is caused by the long-term administration of drugs that block dopamine receptors, particularly D_2-receptors.[26] It occurs in 20% of patients receiving a typical antipsychotic for > 3 months, particularly in the elderly and in those on high doses, e.g. **chlorpromazine** 300mg/24h or more.[4,27] It is less common in patients receiving atypical antipsychotics, e.g. **risperidone**.[27] Tardive dyskinesia is also associated with the long-term use of metoclopramide.[28]

Tardive dyskinesia typically manifests as involuntary stereotyped chewing movements of the tongue and orofacial muscles (Box 24.A). The involuntary movements are made worse by anxiety and reduced by drowsiness and during sleep.

Tardive dyskinesia is associated with akathisia in 25% of cases. In younger patients, tardive dyskinesia may present as abnormal positioning of the limbs and tonic contractions of the neck and trunk muscles causing torticollis, lordosis or scoliosis. In younger patients, tardive dyskinesia may occur if antipsychotic treatment is stopped abruptly.

Early diagnosis

'*Open your mouth and stick out your tongue.*'
The following indicate a developing tardive dyskinesia:
- worm-like movements of the tongue
- inability to protrude tongue for more than a few seconds.

Treatment

Often responds poorly to drug treatment; *antimuscarinic antiparkinsonian drugs may exacerbate*. Withdrawal of the causal drug leads to resolution in 30% in 3 months and a further 40% in 5 years; sometimes irreversible, particularly in the elderly. Drug treatment to consider:

- **tetrabenazine**, depletes presynaptic dopamine stores and blocks post-synaptic dopamine receptors; best not used in depressed patients; start with 12.5mg b.i.d. → 25mg t.i.d., increasing the dose slowly to avoid troublesome hypotension
- **levodopa**, may produce long-term benefit after causing initial deterioration
- **clonidine** 50–200microgram/24h
- **baclofen**, **clonazepam**, **diazepam** and **valproic acid**, all act by potentiating GABA inhibition, but all give inconsistent results
- **pyridoxine** up to 400mg/24h
- **branched-chain amino acids** (Tarvil®) 222mg/kg t.i.d.[29]

Paradoxically, increasing the dose of the causal drug may help, but should be considered only in desperation because it could exacerbate the dyskinesia.

1 APA (American Psychiatric Association) (1994) Neuroleptic-induced movement disorders. In: *Diagnostic and Statistical Manual of Mental Disorders* (4e). American Psychiatric Association, New York, pp. 736–751.
2 Tonda M and Guthrie S (1994) Treatment of acute neuroleptic-induced movement disorders. *Pharmacotherapy.* **14**: 543–560.
3 Jackson N *et al.* (2008) Neuropsychiatric complications of commonly used palliative care drugs. *Postgraduate Medical Journal.* **84**: 121–126.
4 Caligiuri MR *et al.* (2000) Antipsychotic-induced movement disorders in the elderly: epidemiology and treatment recommendations. *Drugs Aging.* **17**: 363–384.
5 Tang S *et al.* (2009) MDPD: an integrated genetic information resource for Parkinson's disease. In: *Nucleic Acids Research.* Available from: http://nar.oxfordjournals.org/cgi/content/full/37/suppl_1/D858
6 Hoes M (1998) Recent developments in the management of psychosis. *Pharmacy and World Science.* **20**: 101–106.
7 Geddes J *et al.* (2000) Atypical antipsychotics in the treatment of schizophrenia: systematic overview and meta-regression analysis. *British Medical Journal.* **321**: 1371–1376.
8 Zubenko G et al. (1987) Antidepressant-related akathisia. *Journal of Clinical Psychopharmacology.* **7**: 254–257.
9 Anonymous (1994) Drug-induced extrapyramidal reactions. *Current Problems in Pharmacovigilance.* **20**: 15–16.
10 Tarsy D and Simon DK (2006) Dystonia. *New England Journal of Medicine.* **355**: 818–829.
11 Arya D (1994) Extrapyramidal symptoms with selective serotonin reuptake inhibitors. *British Journal of Psychiatry.* **165**: 728–733.
12 Matthews H and Tancil C (1996) Extrapyramidal reaction caused by ondansetron. *The Annals of Pharmacotherapy.* **30**: 196.
13 Anonymous (2009) Neuroleptic-induced extrapyramidal reactions. In: *Drugdex®Consults* Micromedex, Thompson Healthcare. Available from: http://www.micromedex.com/products/drugdex/
14 Lane R (1998) SSRI-induced extrapyramidal side-effects and akathisia: implications for treatment. *Journal of Psychopharmacology.* **12**: 192–214.
15 Hamilton M and Opler L (1992) Akathisia, suicidality, and fluoxetine. *Journal of Clinical Psychiatry.* **53**: 401–406.
16 APA (American Psychiatric Association) (1994) Medication-induced postural tremor. In: *Diagnostic and Statistical Manual of Mental Disorders* (4e). American Psychiatric Association, New York, pp. 749–751.
17 Launer M (1996) Selected side-effects: 17. Dopamine-receptor antagonists and movement disorders. *Prescribers' Journal.* **36**: 37–41.
18 Gagrat D *et al.* (1978) Intravenous diazepam in the treatment of neuroleptic-induced acute dystonia and akathisia. *American Journal of Psychiatry.* **135**: 1232–1233.
19 White C and Jackson N (2005) Acute akathisia in palliative care. *European Journal of Palliative Care.* **12 (1)**: 5–7.
20 Gattera J *et al.* (1994) A retrospective study of risk factors of akathisia in terminally ill patients. *Journal of Pain and Symptom Management.* **9**: 454–461.
21 Kawanishi C *et al.* (2007) Unexpectedly high prevalence of akathisia in cancer patients. *Palliative & Supportive Care.* **5**: 351–354.
22 Miller CH and Fleischhacker WW (2000) Managing antipsychotic-induced acute and chronic akathisia. *Drug Safety.* **22**: 73–81.
23 Van Putten T *et al.* (1984) Akathisia with haloperidol and thiothixene. *Archives of General Psychiatry.* **41**: 1036–1039.
24 Braude W *et al.* (1993) Clinical characteristics of akathisia: a systematic investigation of acute psychiatric in-patient admission. *British Journal of Psychiatry.* **143**: 139–150.
25 Poyurovsky M and Weizman A (1997) Serotonergic agents in the treatment of acute neuroleptic-induced akathisia: open-label study of buspirone and mianserin. *International Clinical Psychopharmacology.* **12**: 263–268.
26 APA (American Psychiatric Association) (1992) *Tardive dyskinesia: a task force report of the American Psychiatric Association.* American Psychiatric Association, Washington, DC.
27 Jeste D (2000) Tardive dyskinesia in older patients. *Journal of Clinical Psychiatry.* **61 (suppl 4)**: 27–32.
28 Sewell DD and Jeste DV (1992) Metoclopramide-associated tardive dyskinesia: An analysis of 67 cases. *Archives of Family Medicine.* **1**: 171–278.
29 Bezchlibnyk-Butler KZ and and Jeffries JJ (eds) (2006) *Clinical Handbook of Psychotropic Drugs* (16 edn). Hogrefe, Toronto.

25: ANAPHYLAXIS

Anaphylaxis is a life-threatening systemic allergic reaction. It manifests as a constellation of features but there is disagreement about which are essential. The confusion arises partly because systemic allergic reactions can be mild, moderate or severe. In practice, the term 'anaphylaxis' is best reserved for cases where there is:
- respiratory difficulty (related to laryngeal edema or bronchoconstriction) *or*
- hypotension (presenting as fainting, collapse or loss of consciousness) *or*
- both.[1]

Urticaria, angioedema or rhinitis alone are best not described as anaphylaxis because neither respiratory difficulty nor hypotension is present.[1]

Causes

In anaphylaxis, an allergic reaction results from the interaction of an allergen with specific IgE antibodies bound to mast cells and basophils. This leads to activation of the mast cell with release of chemical mediators (including histamine) stored in granules as well as rapidly synthesized additional mediators. A rapid major systemic release of these mediators causes capillary leakage and mucosal edema, resulting in shock and respiratory difficulty.[1]

In contrast, anaphylactoid reactions are caused by activation of mast cells and release of the same mediators, but without the involvement of IgE antibodies. For example, certain drugs act directly on mast cells. In terms of management, it is not necessary to distinguish anaphylaxis from an anaphylactoid reaction. This difference is relevant only when investigations are being considered.

Anaphylaxis is rare in palliative care and is generally associated with antibacterials, **aspirin** or another NSAID. A possible case has been recorded in a woman with known peanut allergy who received an **arachis** (peanut) **oil** enema.[2] Anaphylaxis is:
- specific to a given drug or chemically-related class of drugs
- more likely after parenteral administration
- more frequent in patients with aspirin-induced asthma or systemic lupus erythematosus.

Clinical features

No single set of criteria will identify all anaphylactic reactions, but anaphylaxis is likely when all three of the following criteria are met:
- sudden onset and rapid progression of symptoms
- life-threatening respiratory or circulatory problems
- skin and/or mucosal changes.

Anaphylaxis causes a range of signs and symptoms (Box 25.A).[3] Bronchospasm occurs in only 10% of patients. Skin and mucosal changes occur in 80% of patients, but may be subtle. Angioedema may develop anywhere in the body but often involves the lips, eyes, hands or feet. Edema of the larynx may lead to stridor and acute airway obstruction.[4]

Management

National guidelines vary slightly; the advice included here is based primarily on guidance published by the UK Resuscitation Council.[3] Anaphylaxis requires urgent treatment with **epinephrine** followed by an antihistamine and **hydrocortisone** (Box 25.B). However, corticosteroids are only of secondary value because their impact is not immediate.

The best site for IM injections is the anterolateral aspect of the middle third of the thigh.[3] If there is doubt about the adequacy of the circulation, **epinephrine** can be given as a dilute IV solution, i.e. 1 in 10,000 (1mg/10mL), *using 50microgram (0.5mL) boluses, titrated to response*. However, because injecting **epinephrine** IV too rapidly can cause ventricular arrhythmias, IV administration is discouraged unless given by a specialist, and intensive care facilities are available.[3,8] Occasionally, emergency tracheotomy and assisted respiration are necessary.

Box 25.A   Clinical features of anaphylaxis

Essential
Sudden onset of life-threatening circulatory and/or respiratory problems, e.g.

Circulatory problems
Tachycardia
Hypotension
Shock
Decreased consciousness
Cardiac arrest

Respiratory problems
Airway
  pharyngeal/laryngeal edema
  hoarse voice
  stridor
Breathing
  breathlessness
  wheeze/bronchospasm
  cyanosis
  respiratory arrest

Possible

Skin/mucosal changes
Flushing or pallor
Erythema of skin
Urticaria
Angioedema[a]

Other
Agitation
Confusion
Abdominal pain
Vomiting
Diarrhea
Incontinence
Tingling of the extremities
Rhinitis
Conjunctivitis

a. angioedema is swelling in the dermis, subcutaneous and submucosal tissues.

Box 25.B   Management of anaphylaxis in adults

1 Stop causal agent, e.g. IV antibiotic.

2 Oxygen is of primary importance (>10L/min).

3 Epinephrine 1:1,000 (1mg/1mL), 500microgram (0.5mL) IM; repeat every 5min until blood pressure, pulse and breathing are satisfactory.

4 If an epinephrine auto-injector is used, 300microgram (0.3mL) is generally sufficient.

5 Diphenhydramine to counter histamine-induced vasodilation
  • 25–50mg IM or IV over 1min
  • if necessary, repeat up to a maximum of 400mg/24h
  • prescribe 25–50mg PO q.i.d. for 3–4 days to prevent relapse.[5]

6 Hydrocortisone sodium succinate 200mg IM or slow IV for patients with bronchospasm, and for all severe or recurrent reactions to prevent further deterioration. Note: may take up to 6h to act.

7 Also prescribe prednisone 40–50mg once daily for 3–4 days to prevent a relapse.[6]

8 If still shocked, give 1–2L of IV fluid; a crystalloid, e.g. 0.9% saline, may be safer than a colloid.[7]

9 If bronchospasm has not responded to the above, give a nebulized β_2-agonist, e.g. salbutamol 5mg.

Some centres also give an H_2-receptor antagonist, e.g. **ranitidine** 50mg IV stat or 150mg PO stat.[5,9] However, H_2-receptors are involved only to a limited extent in anaphylaxis, and the use of an H_2-receptor antagonist in this situation is not essential.[10]

1   Ewan P (1998) ABC of allergies: anaphylaxis. *British Medical Journal.* **316**: 1442–1445.
2   Pharmax (1998) *Data on file.*
3   Resuscitation Council (UK) (2008) Emergency treatment of anaphylactic reactions: Guidelines for healthcare providers. Available from: www.resus.org.uk/pages/reaction.pdf
4   CKS (2007) Angio-oedema and Anaphylaxis (Topic Review). In: *Clinical Knowledge Summary Service.* Available from: www.cks.library.nhs.uk/angio_oedema_and_anaphylaxis
5   Ellis AK and Day JH (2003) Diagnosis and management of anaphylaxis. *Canadian Medical Association Journal.* **169**: 307–311.
6   Poon M and Reid C (2004) Best evidence topic reports. Oral corticosteroids in acute urticaria. *Emergency Medicine Journal.* **21**: 76–77.
7   Schierhout G and Roberts I (1998) Fluid resuscitation with colloid or crystalloid solutions in critically ill patients: a systematic review of randomised trials. *British Medical Journal.* **316**: 961–964.
8   BNF (2008) Section 3.4.3 Anaphylaxis. In: *British National Formulary* (No. 55). British Medical Association and the Royal Pharmaceutical Society of Great Britain, London. Current BNF available from: www.bnf.org/bnf/bnf/current/
9   Mayumi *et al.* (1987) Intravenous cimetidine as an effective treatment for systemic anaphylaxis and acute allergic skin reaction. *Annals of Allergy.* **58**: 447–450.
10 Ellis AK and Day JH (2003) Anaphylaxis treatment: the details. *Canadian Medical Association Journal.* **169**: 1148–1149.

Appendix 1: Synopsis of pharmacokinetic data

Table A1.1 contains selected pharmacokinetic data for most of the drugs featured in *PCF*. Three reference books have been used to obtain most of the data.[1-3] However, where there is strong evidence for an alternative figure, this has been used, and the source referenced in the respective monograph. Information about **methylnaltrexone** has been taken from the manufacturer's Product Monograph.

Interindividual variation of pharmacokinetic parameters is often considerable. For example:
- bio-availability of different formulations of a drug may vary significantly
- the clearance of a drug often varies up to 5 times, and sometimes much more, e.g. **methadone** and **warfarin**.

Further, optimum plasma concentrations differ and, even when available, 'therapeutic plasma concentrations' are only an approximate guide.

Key for Table A1.1
\# connects a value in the Table with the information in the Comments column.

a. A = acid; Aa = amino acid; Amf = ampholyte; B = base; B_4 = base with quaternary ammonium group; Gly = glycoside; Pep = peptide; S = steroid; Sa = substituted amide
b. the pH at which the drug is 50% ionized
c. the fraction of the drug eliminated by non-renal pathways in normal individuals; 1 − [fraction] gives an estimate of how much of the drug is excreted unchanged in the urine
d. pharmacologically active metabolite(s)
e. metabolite(s) with possible pharmacological activity
f. apparent volume of distribution at steady-state
g. after oral administration unless stated otherwise.

BC after buccal administration
IV after intravenous administration
IM after intramuscular administration
PO after oral administration
PR after rectal administration
SC after subcutaneous administration
SL after sublingual administration
TD after transdermal administration (halflife, where stated, is calculated after a patch has been removed and not replaced).

1 Holford N (ed) (1998) *Clinical Pharmacokinetics: Drug Data Handbook* (3e). Adis International, Auckland.
2 Lacy C *et al.* (eds) (2003) *Lexi-Comp's Drug Information Handbook* (11e). Lexi-Comp and the American Pharmaceutical Association, Hudson, Ohio.
3 Sweetman SC (ed) (2007) *Martindale: The Complete Drug Reference* (35e). Pharmaceutical Press, London.

Table A1.1 Pharmacokinetic drug data

	Nature[a]	pKa[b]	Bio-availability[g] (%)	Clearance (L/h)	Plasma halflife (h)	Volume of distribution (L)	Protein binding (%)	Non-renal elimination[c]	
Acetaminophen[d]	A	9.5	60–90 (40–60[PR])	19.3	1.25–3 (2–3[IV])	65.8	Low#	1.0[d]	#At therapeutic doses
Acetylcysteine			9	58#/8###	2#/5.5###	42#/35###[f]		0.7#	#Reduced acetylcysteine ##Total acetylcysteine
Alfentanil		6.5		20	1.5	49	90		
Amantadine[e]	B	10.1		16.5[PO]	15	560#[PO]		0.1[e]	#Possibly dose-dependent
Amiloride[e]	B	8.7	50	~31[PO]	~9.6	~350[PO]		0.25[e]	
Amitriptyline[d]	B	9.4	48	51	9–25	1,085[f]	95	1.0[d]	
Aspirin[d]	A	3.5	68	39	0.25 / 2–30[d]	10.5	~70	1.0##	
Atropine	B	9.25		70	2.2	231	50	0.45	
Baclofen[e]	A	3.9/9.6	> 90		3.5		30	0.15[e]	
Beclomethasone dipropionate	S		60–90		15				
Betamethasone	S		72	11	6.5	126	6.4	0.95	
Bromocriptine[e]	Pep	4.9	6	56	3	~238	90	1.0[e]	
Budesonide	S		10#	84	2.7	308	88	0.95	
Bumetanide[e]	A		90	12	1.75	16.8	96	0.35[e]	
Bupivacaine	B	8.1		35	2.7	70[f]	96	0.95	
Buprenorphine	B	8.49/10.03	30[SL]	70	24–69[SL] / 3–16[IV] / 13–36[TD]	140	~96	1.0	#High first-pass metabolism

continued

Table A1.1 Continued

	Nature[a]	pKa[b]	Bio-availability[g] (%)	Clearance (L/h)	Plasma halflife (h)	Volume of distribution (L)	Protein binding (%)	Non-renal elimination[c]	
Bupropion[d]			5–20#		21		82–88		#In animals
Carbamazepine[d]	Sa		80	1.1/4.5[PO]	8–24	84[PO]	75	1.0[d]	
Cefuroxime	A	~2.5		8	1.3	17.5	~40	0.07	
Celecoxib	36	11		400	97		0.4		
Cetirizine	3			7–10	35	93		1.0	
Chloral hydrate[d]	A	10.04			8[d]		~35[d]	1.0[d]	
Chlordiazepoxide[d]	B	4.8	>86	1	20	28	96	0.8[d]	
Chlorpheniramine[d]	B	9.2		7.2	20	238	72	1.0[d]	
Chlorpromazine[d]	B	9.3	20	38[IM]	30	1,470[IM]	98	0.2[d]	
Chlorpropamide[d]	A	4.8	>90	0.13[PO]	40	~10.5[PO]	90	0.3	
Cimetidine	B	6.8	70[IM] >90[IM]	36	2	91	20		
Citalopram				21	33	980	50	0.9	
Clindamycin[e]	B	7.45	87	12	3	56	93	0.9[e]	#Terminal elimination phase t½ = 13h
Clobazam[d]			100	2[PO]	10–30	98[PO]	85	1.0[d]	
Clodronate disodium				6	2#			~0.1	
Clomipramine[d]	B			45	20	1,162	98	1.0[d]	
Clonazepam	Amf	1.5/10.5	98	~6[PO]	20–40	210[PO]	85	1.0	
Clonidine[e]	B	8.25	90	0.16–0.6#	6.2–12.8#	241.5	20	0.4[e]	#Dose-dependent

continued

Table A1.1 Continued

	Nature[a]	pKa[b]	Bio-availability[g] (%)	Clearance (L/h)	Plasma half life (h)	Volume of distribution (L)	Protein binding (%)	Non-renal elimination[c]	
Codeine[d]	B	7.95	40	98##[PO]	2.5–3.5	378##[PO]	~7	1.0[d]	#Corrected for bio-availability
Dalteparin					3–5[SC]				
Danazol			11#		4.5## >24####				#Fasting ##Single dose ####Multiple dose
Dantrolene[d]	A	7.5			~9			0.95[d]	
Darbepoetin alfa	Pep				49[SC]	0.06			
Desipramine[d]	B	10.2	51	130[PO]	22	1,568[PO]	80	1.0[d]	
Dexamethasone	S		80	14.7	3	52.5	77	1.0	
Diazepam[d]	B	3.3	100	1.8	24–48 48–120[d]	140	95–98	1.0	
Diclofenac[e]	A		50## 41### 50[PR]	15.6	1–2	10.5	>99	1.0[e]	#Enteric coated ##Dispersible and SR
Diflunisal	A		100	0.35–0.49#	5–20#	7.7	99	0.95	#Dose-dependent
Digoxin#	Gly		70	4.5	40	420	27	0.3	#Therapeutic plasma concentration 0.8–2microgram/L
Diltiazem		7.7	41	60	5.1	315	98	1.0	
Diphenhydramine[e]	B	8.3	42	47	5	280	98.5	0.9[e]	
Diphenoxylate	B	7.07			2.5	322			
Domperidone			12–18## 12[PR]		7–16		>90	0.7	#Fasting

continued

Table A1.1 Continued

	Nature[a]	pKa[b]	Bio-availability[g] (%)	Clearance (L/h)	Plasma halflife (h)	Volume of distribution (L)	Protein binding (%)	Non-renal elimination[c]	
Dronabinol[d]			10–20		19–24#	2.5–6.4	97–99	0.35	#49–53 for metabolites
Duloxetine			90	33–261	12		96		
Enoxaparin			91	1.24	4.2#	7			#Anti-factor Xa activity (Antithrombin activity 2.1h)
Epoetin alfa	Pep				4–13#	9			#In chronic renal failure
Erythromycin	B	8.8	35	26	1.3–2.4#	35–70#	73	0.8	#Dose-dependent
Erythropoietin	Pep		21.5	0.18#^{IV}	8#^{IV}	2.1#^{IV}		0.9	#In dialysis patients
Esomeprazole	B		40	23	1–1.5	16	97	0.2	
Ethinylestradiol	S				13	203	97		
Ethosuximide[e]	A	9.3		0.7	54	49	<10	0.8[e]	
Etidronate disodium	A		1–6		1–6#		>99		#Halflife in bone >90days
Etodolac				2.8	6	28.7	>99	1.0	
Fentanyl[e]	B	8.43		47	6#, 13–22^{TD}	~210	83	0.95[e]	#Oral transmucosal
Flecainide[d]			95	42.8#	12#/19.5###	588#	52	0.7[d]	Therapeutic plasma concentration <800microgram/L #Healthy volunteers ###Arrhythmia patients
Fluconazole			90		30	56	11	0.3	
Fludrocortisone					0.5		75		

continued

Table A1.1 Continued

	Nature[a]	pKa[b]	Bio-availability[g] (%)	Clearance (L/h)	Plasma halflife (h)	Volume of distribution (L)	Protein binding (%)	Non-renal elimination[c]	
Fluoxetine				40 10#	48 96#	1,400 2,940#	94	0.97	#Multiple doses
Flurbiprofen	A		>85	1.3[PO]	3–6	7[PO]	>99	0.9	
Fluticasone					8		91		
Fluvoxamine			77		20	1,400		0.95	
Furosemide	A	3.9	60–70	8	1	21	97	0.35	
Gabapentin			60#	7.5	5–7	49	0		#Reduced at higher doses
Glyburide[d]		5.3		5.5	1.5–10#	10.5	>99	1.0[d]	#Divergent values reported
Glycopyrrolate			~10		~0.5				
Granisetron			60	14.7	10–11	231		0.9	Wide interindividual differences
Guaifenesin					~1				
Haloperidol	B	8.3	60–70	46	13–35	1,400	90	1.0	
Heparin	A		0	2.5#	1.5#	4.9	95###	0.8	#Dose- and assay-dependent ##Lipoproteins
Hydrocortisone	S		37–62	21–30#	1.3–1.9#	21–35#	75–95#		#Dose-dependent
Hydromorphone					2.5			0.96	
Hydroxyzine[d]					20				
Ibuprofen	A	4.4/5.2	90#	3.5[PO]	2	9.8[PO]	99	1.0	#Dose-dependent
Imipramine[d]	B	9.5	27	58	18	1,470	89	1.0[d]	#Dose-dependent
Insulin	Pep			10–40#	0.25–2#		~5	0.4	#Divergent values reported

continued

Table A1.1 Continued

	Nature[a]	pKa[b]	Bio-availability[g] (%)	Clearance (L/h)	Plasma halflife (h)	Volume of distribution (L)	Protein binding (%)	Non-renal elimination[c]	
Ipratropium bromide	B				~3.5			0.3	
Isosorbide-5-mononitrate			93	7.6	4.4	49	0	0.8	
Itraconazole			40	60	30#		>99		#At steady rate
Ketamine[e]		7.5	20[IM]		3	140	12	1.0[e]	
Ketoconazole		2.9/6.5			8		99	1.0	
Ketoprofen	A		>85	5.2	1.4	7.7	<94	0.75	
Ketorolac		3.49	100	2	5	17.5	99		
Lamotrigine			95–100	1.9	23–36	80.5	56	0.9	
Lansoprazole	B				2			1.0	
Levodopa[d]	Aa	2.3/8.7			1.4			1.0[d]	
Levothyroxine sodium				0.1	150	~14	>99		
Lidocaine#	B	7.86	35	40	3.9	210	60	0.95	#Therapeutic plasma concentration 2–5mg/L
Lithium#			>85	1.6	27	56		1.02	#Therapeutic plasma concentration 0.4–1.2mmol/L
Loperamide[e]	B	8.7			10	105[PO]	97	1.0[e]	
Lorazepam	Amf	1.3/11.5	93	3[PO]	10–20	210	90	1.0	
Meclizine					6				
Medroxyprogesterone[e]	S			~76[PO, IM]	~36	~42 [PO, IM]	94	0.55[e]	
Megestrol[e]					15–20				
Meloxicam					15–20	10	>99		

continued

Table A1.1 Continued

	Nature[a]	pKa[b]	Bio-availability[g] (%)	Clearance (L/h)	Plasma halflife (h)	Volume of distribution (L)	Protein binding (%)	Non-renal elimination[c]	
Meperidine[d]	B	6.3	54	38	6.9	280	70	0.9[d]	#Terminal elimination t½ ~10h
Metformin	B	8.25	50	26–42	1.5–4.5#	70–280	<5	0.01	#Altered by urine pH (see p.000)
Methadone	B	8.4	40–100	7.5	8–75#	280	80	0.6	
Methylnaltrexone			82[SC]	28/51#	8	1.1–2.0	11–5.3	~0.5	#d-enantiomer
Methylphenidate			30 / 5#		2 / 3.7#	186/126##			
Methylprednisolone	S	4.6	82	15	3	49		1.0	
Metoclopramide	B		50–80	23–38#	2.5–5#	210	30	0.7	#Possibly dose-dependent
Metronidazole[d]	B?	2.62	100[PR] / 70[PR]	3	8	49	<20	0.85[d]	
Mexiletine[e]#		8.75	85	27	10	350	70	0.8[e]	#Therapeutic plasma concentration 0.8–2mg/L
Miconazole[e]		6.65	27	46	23	1,400	99	1.0[e]	
Midazolam	B	6.1	35–44 / 75[BC] / >90[IM]	20	2–5	84	95	1.0	#When given by CSCI
Mirtazapine[d]			50		20–40		85	0.15	#Parent drug undetectable in plasma after oral dose
Misoprostol[d]					1.5#		85		
Morphine[e]	Amf	9.85/7.87	15–64 / 25[PR]	72	2.5 / 2.5[d]#	245	35	0.9[d]	#Morphine-6-glucuronide (increases to ≤7.5h in renal failure)

continued

Table A1.1 Continued

	Nature[a]	pKa[b]	Bio-availability[g] (%)	Clearance (L/h)	Plasma halflife (h)	Volume of distribution (L)	Protein binding (%)	Non-renal elimination[c]	
Nabilone[d]			85		2 35[d]				
Nabumetone	B	7.94	38[d]#		24[d]			0.99	#Parent drug undetectable in plasma after oral dose
Naloxone[e]			6	104	1	210	20	~1.0e	
Naltrexone			5–40	94	4 13[d]	994		1.0	
Naproxen	A	4.15	99–100	0.3	12–15	7	99	0.9	
Nifedipine			50	42	1.8	98	97	1.0	
Nitrazepam	Amf	3.4/10.8	78	4	30	175	85	1.0	
Nitrofurantoin[d]	A	7.2	87	41	1	56	~40	0.7[d]	
Nitroglycerin				~1,260	0.05	~210			
Nordiazepam[d]#	Amf	11.65/3.35	50	1.5	80	175	97	1.0[d]	#Active metabolite of diazepam
Nortriptyline[d]	B	9.73	51	40	28	1,470	93	1.0[d]	
Octreotide	Pep		<5	11.4	1.5	23.8		0.9	
Olanzapine			60	18.2	34	721–1,288	93		
Omeprazole	Amf	3.97/8.8	67	35	0.5	24.5	95	1.0	
Ondansetron			56–71 60[PR]	29	3–5	161	70–76		
Orphenadrine	B	8.4			18		20		
Oxazepam	Amf	11.51/1.56	>90	8[PO]	7	70[PO]	>95	1.0	

continued

Table A1.1 Continued

	Nature[a]	pKa[b]	Bio-availability[g] (%)	Clearance (L/h)	Plasma halflife (h)	Volume of distribution (L)	Protein binding (%)	Non-renal elimination[c]	
Oxcarbazepine[d]					8[d]	52.5[d]	40[d]	1.0	
Oxybutynin[d]					2–3				
Oxycodone[d]			75		3.5				
Pamidronate disodium			1–3		27				
Pantoprazole	B		77		1	11–24	98	0.18	
Paroxetine			50		24		95	0.98	
Penicillin V	A	2.73			0.5	~35	80	0.6	
Phenobarbital#	A	7.2	>90	0.3	48–144	49	50	0.7	#Therapeutic plasma concentration 10–35mg/L
Phenytoin#	A	8.33	90–95	##	9–40	56	90	1.0	#Therapeutic plasma concentration 10–20mg/L ###Dose-dependent
Pilocarpine					~1–1.5[PO]				
Prednisone[d]#			78				65–91##		#Converted to prednisolone ###Concentration-dependent.
Pregabalin			≥90		5–9				
Prochlorperazine	B	3.73/8.1	6 14[BC]		14–17				
Promethazine	B	9.1	25	68	7–14	910[f]			
Propofol	B			104	0.05:0.5:4#	280[f]		1.0	#Tri-exponential
Propoxyphene	B	6.3		66	2.7	189	78	~1.0	

continued

Table A1.1 Continued

	Nature[a]	pKa[b]	Bio-availability[g] (%)	Clearance (L/h)	Plasma half-life[f] (h)	Volume of distribution (L)	Protein binding (%)	Non-renal elimination[c]	
Propranolol[d]	B	9.45	~30	63	4	196	93	1.0[d]	
Quetiapine			≥75		7		83	0.25	
Quinine	B	4.3/8.4	50	5.5	14	112	90	0.8	
Ranitidine[d]	B	2.7	50	35	2	105	15	0.3[d]	
Risperidone[d]			99		24#	105	90		#Active fraction (risperidone plus 9-OH risperidone)
Salbutamol	B	9.3	10.3		~5				
Salmeterol					67		95–98		
Scopolamine (hyoscine) hydrobromide	B	7.55	23 / 60–80[SL]	45	5–6	140		0.45	
Sertraline			>44		22–36	>1,400	99	1.0	
Spironolactone[d]	S		70		19[d]		98[d]	1.0[d]	
Sufentanil		8.01		44	2.6	140	93		
Sulindac[d]	A	4.5	>88		7 / 18[d]		96	1.0#	
Tamsulosin			~100		4–6 / 10–13#		94–99		#SR
Temazepam	B	1.31	>80	4[PO]	13	70[PO]	97	1.0	
Tenoxicam				0.13	72	14	99	1.0	
Terazosin			82	3.3	12	21	90	0.9	

continued

Table A1.1 Continued

	Nature[a]	pKa[b]	Bio-availability[g] (%)	Clearance (L/h)	Plasma halflife (h)	Volume of distribution (L)	Protein binding (%)	Non-renal elimination[c]	
Terbutaline	Amf	10.1/11.2/8.8		13	15	112[f]	25	0.45	
Tetracycline	Amf	7.7/3.3/9.5	77	15[PO]	6	140[PO]		0.12	
Thalidomide[e]			67–93#	10	5–7	120	50	0.993	#In animals
Theophylline[d]#	Amf	8.6/3.5	96	3	8	35		0.9[d]	#Therapeutic plasma concentration 10–20mg/L
Tinzaparin					3–4	3–5			
Tizanidine			40	120#	2.5	144#	30		#Based on a 60kg person
Tolbutamide	A	5.43		~1[PO]	7	10.5[PO]	95#		#Concentration-dependent
Tramadol[d]			65–75 77[PR]	26	6 7.4[d]	231	4	0.7[d]	
Tranexamic acid	A	4.3/10.6	34	6.7	10			0.03	
Tranylcypromine					1.5–3				
Trazodone[d]	S		65		7		93		
Triamcinolone				45–70#	1.4	98–147#		1.0	#Dose-dependent
Trimethoprim	B	7.2	100	4.5[PO]	11	91[PO]	45	0.45	
Trimipramine[e]	B		41	67	23	2,170	95	1.0[e]	
Valproic acid[d]#	A	4.95	100	0.5	7–17	10.5	90	0.03	#Therapeutic plasma concentration 50–100mg/L
Vancomycin				4.0	10	42[f]	<10–55	0.03	
Venlafaxine	B		13 45#		5 11[d]	525 400[d]	27		#SR

continued

Table A1.1 Continued

	Nature[a]	pKa[b]	Bio-availability[g] (%)	Clearance (L/h)	Plasma halflife (h)	Volume of distribution (L)	Protein binding (%)	Non-renal elimination[c]	
Vigabatrin			80–90	5.6	6	56	0	0	
Warfarin[d]	A	5.0	100	0.2/0.15#	35/50#	10.5	99	1.0[d]	#S and R enantiomers
Zoledronic acid			60[IV]	7[PO] 2–5[IM]		1.5	99	0.7	
Zopiclone			80	14.8	4.9	98	45	1.0	

\# connects a value in the Table with the information in the Comments column

a. A = acid; Aa = amino acid; Alc = alcohol; Amf = ampholyte; B = base; B$_4$ = base with quaternary ammonium group; Gly = glycoside; Pep = peptide; S = steroid; Sa = substituted amide
b. the pH at which the drug is 50% ionized
c. the fraction of the drug eliminated by non-renal pathways in normal individuals; 1 – [fraction] gives an estimate of how much of the drug is excreted unchanged in the urine
d. pharmacologically active metabolite(s)
e. metabolite(s) with possible pharmacological activity
f. apparent volume of distribution at steady-state
g. after oral administration unless stated otherwise.

BC   after buccal administration
IV   after intravenous administration
IM   after intramuscular administration
PO   after oral administration
PR   after rectal administration
SC   after subcutaneous administration
SL   after sublingual administration
TD   after transdermal administration (halflife, where stated, is calculated after a patch has been removed and not replaced).

Appendix 2: Emergency kits in palliative care

Emergency kits are used to help avoid a crisis at home, particularly in the last few days of a patient's life if new symptoms develop, or old ones recur.[1–3] The kit typically includes medication to relieve pain, nausea and vomiting, breathlessness, noisy upper airway secretions ('death rattle'), restlessness/agitation, delirium and seizures.[4] The kits are well accepted by patients, their families and health professionals; and their use reduces the incidence of emergency room visits and hospitalization.[4]

The contents of emergency kits vary considerably between palliative care services. However, the ideal is to 'keep it simple', i.e. to restrict the number of products to no more than 6–7 (Table A2.1).

Table A2.1 An example of an emergency kit

Medication	Quantity	Indication
Haloperidol injection 5mg/mL or	5 amps	Delirium/agitation,
Methotrimeprazine injection 25mg/mL	10 amps	nausea and vomiting
Atropine eyedrops 1% (for SL use) or	1 bottle	
Scopolamine TD patch	2	Noisy upper airway secretions
Lorazepam SL tablets 1mg or	10	
Midazolam injection 10mg/2mL	10 amps	Restlessness/agitation
Hydromorphone injection 10mg/mL	10 amps	Pain, breathlessness
Phenobarbital injection 120mg/mL	10 amps	Seizures

The alternatives used by different services are numerous (Table A2.2). Centres without a 24h on-call service provide a larger quantity of a wider range of drugs (typically 20–30, compared with 5 or 6 in the 'minikits' issued by centres with a 24h service). All the kits we reviewed in Canada include injections, although it was often expected that these would be administered SL rather than SC. Many kits include suppositories. At one centre, **phenytoin** capsules were included in kits for patients at risk of developing seizures.

Typically, if it is likely that emergency medication could soon be necessary, the kit is ordered and dispensed either directly from the palliative care service or through a retail pharmacy. To avoid delivery charges, the kits are generally collected by the family, but when necessary, some centres have the kit delivered to the patient's home using an approved courier.

The cost of an emergency kit depends on its source and contents. The kit provided by Fraser Health, BC, which contains sufficient supplies for approximately 3 days of comprehensive home management, costs $390 for the drugs and $15 for equipment (syringes, cannulas, alcohol swabs, etc.). More basic emergency kits will be correspondingly cheaper, e.g. $50–100. Some palliative care services purchase the initial kit contents, then bill the patient for the specific items used. This avoids any patient concern over the initial cost outlay.

There are two other issues which require consideration. The first is the appropriate storage of the kit during delivery to the patient's home and in the home. Kits should generally be stored in a cool, dry, low-access area. For practical reasons, products which require refrigeration, e.g. **lorazepam** injection, are avoided.

Table A2.2 Range of drugs used in emergency kits in Canada

Medication	Quantity (if known)
Pain, breathlessness	
Hydromorphone normal-release tablets 1mg, 2mg and 4mg	10 of each
Hydromorphone injection 2mg/mL and 10mg/mL	10 amps of each
Hydromorphone injection 50mg/mL	2 amps
Morphine oral syrup 10mg/mL (for SL use)	50mL
Morphine normal-release tablets 10mg	10
Morphine injection 10mg/mL and 50mg/mL	10 amps of each
Sufentanil injection 50microgram/mL (for SL use in break-through (episodic) pain)	10 amps
Pain, fever	
Acetaminophen suppositories 650mg	6
Diclofenac suppositories 100mg	10
Anti-emetics	
Dimenhydrinate tablets 50mg	10
Dimenhydrinate injection 50mg/mL	10 amps
Dimenhydrinate suppositories 100mg	10
Haloperidol injection 5mg/mL	5 amps
Methotrimeprazine injection 25mg/mL	10 amps
Metoclopramide tablets 10mg	10
Metoclopramide injection 10mg/2mL	10 amps
Prochlorperazine tablets 10mg	10
Prochlorperazine suppositories 10mg	10
Prochlorperazine injection 10mg/2mL	10
Scopolamine TD patches	2
Corticosteroid (e.g. for intractable vomiting, spinal cord compression, raised intracranial pressure, bowel obstruction)	
Dexamethasone tablets 4mg	10
Dexamethasone injection 10mg/mL	10 vials
Dexamethasone injection 20mg/5mL	2 vials
Delirium/restlessness/agitation	
Diazepam injection 5mg/mL	10 amps
Haloperidol tablets 500microgram and 5mg	10 of each
Haloperidol injection 5mg/mL	5 amps
Lorazepam SL tablets 1mg (for SL or oral use)	10
Methotrimeprazine tablets 5mg	20
Methotrimeprazine injection 25mg/mL	10 amps
Midazolam injection 10mg/2mL	10 amps
Noisy upper airway secretions	
Atropine eyedrops 1% (for SL use)	1 bottle
Atropine injection 600microgram/mL	10 amps
Glycopyrrolate injection 400microgram/2mL	5 vials
Scopolamine (hyoscine) hydrobromide injection 600microgram/mL	5 amps
Scopolamine TD patches	2
Seizures	
Diazepam injection 5mg/mL	10 amps
Midazolam injection 10mg/2mL	10 amps
Phenobarbital injection 120mg/mL	10 amps
Breathlessness	
Furosemide tablets 40mg	10
Furosemide injection 10mg/mL	4 amps
Salbutamol inhaler 200microgram/metered dose	1
Antispasmodic (e.g. for colic)	
Hyoscine (scopolamine) butylbromide injection 20mg/mL	5 amps

The second issue is security of the kit during the acquisition process, while stored in the patient's home, and during return to the pharmacy after use. In order to confirm that medication has not been unlawfully diverted, there must be a 'paper trail' documenting the ordering, dispensing and delivery of the medication to the patient, and return of unused medication to the pharmacy.

A medication log is also included in the kit which can act as both an administration record and a stock balance sheet. The kit should be in a suitably robust container, fastened with a combination lock or a tamper-evident security tag. Unless specifically directed otherwise, it should be opened only by the community nurse who will be preparing the drugs for use by the patient/carer, or by a physician.

It is also essential that the patient and caregiver are told about:
- the contents of the emergency kit
- the proper use of the medication in the kit, including training in the administration of SC drugs where necessary
- who to contact in the event of an emergency.

The administration of emergency medication in a patient's home at the end of life carries a high risk for error. In order to avoid confusion at the time of use, concise, well-written and illustrated patient and carer information material should be included in the kit.

1 LeGrand S et al. (2001) Dying at home: emergency medications for terminal symptoms. American Journal of Hospice and Palliative Care. 18: 421–423.
2 Amass C and Allen M (2005) How a "just in case" approach can improve out-of-hours palliative care. The Pharmaceutical Journal. 275: 22–23.
3 Bishop MF et al. (2009) Medication kits for managing symptomatic emergencies in the home: a survey of common hospice practice. Journal of Palliative Medicine. 12: 37–44.
4 Wowchuk SM et al. (2009) The palliative medication kit: an effective way of extending care in the home for patients nearing death. Journal of Palliative Medicine. 12: 797–803.

Appendix 3: Taking controlled and prescription drugs to other countries

Some patients receiving palliative care travel to other countries and need to take medication with them. Practitioners can help ensure a trouble-free journey by advising them, if relevant, about travelling with opioid analgesics and other controlled drugs (Box A3.A). Travellers must consider the laws of both Canada and the country/countries to which (and through which) they will be travelling. The laws governing the classification of narcotic and controlled drugs are not uniform throughout Canada. However, the various legal classifications, together with lists of the drugs in each category, are available from www.hc-sc.gc.ca/hc-ps/substancontrol/pol/reg-docs/int-eng.php, http://napra.ca/pages/Schedules/default.aspx and http://napra.ca/pages/Schedules/Search.aspx.

Box A3.A   The Canadian Pharmacists Association's classification of opioid analgesics and other controlled drugs[1]

Narcotic drugs
Products containing one narcotic drug, or one narcotic plus one active non-narcotic ingredient, and all parenteral narcotics. Includes all strong opioid analgesics, codeine (unless classed as a narcotic preparation below), propoxyphene (dextropropoxyphene), cocaine, ketamine. Written prescription required. Refills and transfers not permitted. Record and retain documents for all transactions. Sales reports required except for propoxyphene (dextropropoxyphene).

Narcotic preparations
Products containing one narcotic drug plus two or more active non-narcotic ingredients in a recognized therapeutic dose. Includes exempted codeine products (those containing up to 8mg/solid dose form, or 20mg/30mL in liquid form, plus two or more active non-narcotic ingredients). Prescriptions may be written or verbal. Refills and transfers not permitted. Record and retain documents for all transactions. Sales reports not required.

Controlled drugs
Part I
Amphetamines, methylphenidate, pentobarbital and preparations containing one of these drugs plus one or more active non-controlled drug. Prescriptions may be written or verbal. Refills permitted for written prescriptions under certain conditions. Transfers not permitted. Record and retain documents for all transactions. Sales reports required except for controlled drug preparations.

Part II
Other barbiturates, butorphanol, diethylpropion, nalbuphine and preparations containing one of these drugs plus one or more active non-controlled drug. Prescriptions may be written or verbal. Refills permitted for written and verbal prescriptions under certain conditions. Transfers not permitted. Record and retain documents for all transactions. Sales reports not required.

Part III
Anabolic steroids. Prescriptions may be written or verbal. Refills permitted for written and verbal prescriptions under certain conditions. Transfers not permitted. Record and retain documents for all transactions. Sales reports not required.

continued

Box A3.A Continued

Benzodiazepines and other targeted substances
Includes benzodiazepines, ethchlorvynol and meprobamate. Prescriptions may be written or verbal. Refills permitted for written and verbal prescriptions under certain conditions; fewer restrictions on the prescription details and dispensing records required for refills compared with narcotics and controlled drugs. A single transfer of a prescription is permitted. Record and retain documents for all transactions. Sales reports not required.

Note: Loss or theft of any narcotic, controlled drug or targeted substance must be reported to the Office of Controlled Substances within 10 days.

Transfer of a prescription means either that the patient takes a refill request or a part-fill prescription installment to a different pharmacy from the one they generally use, or that a prescription has been written by a practitioner in one province, but is presented for dispensing at a pharmacy in another province. A Canadian pharmacist cannot fill a prescription (i.e. receive a transfer) from a foreign country. A transfer of a Canadian prescription and the ability to fill in another country depends on the policy of the foreign country.

The following is general advice, based on current Canadian regulations, but should not be regarded as formal legal advice. Detailed advice can be obtained from the regulatory authorities, embassies or consulates for the relevant destination countries. A list of embassy contact details is available from the Foreign Affairs and International Trade section of the Canadian government website at www.international.gc.ca/protocol-protocole/foreign_reps.aspx?lang = eng.

Guidance for departure from and re-entry into Canada
Whenever possible, patients should take sufficient medication and equipment, e.g. syringes, to last their whole trip, plus a few extra days' supply in case return is delayed. However, the maximum quantities of medication for personal use which can be taken abroad (exported), or brought back into Canada (imported), are limited to:
- narcotic and controlled drugs which are *not* listed in Appendix 1 of the Section 56 class exemption document:[2]
  ▷ a single course for acute treatment, *or*
  ▷ 30 days' supply (whichever is less)
- other prescription drugs, including benzodiazepines:[3,4]
  ▷ a single course for acute treatment, *or*
  ▷ 90 days' supply (whichever is less)
- OTC medicines:[3,4]
  ▷ generally, 3 months' supply may be imported, subject to border controls and OTC status in Canada.
  Export depends on the OTC or prescription status of the medicine in the destination country.

If a patient will be away for longer than these periods, or is moving abroad permanently, they should contact a doctor in the destination country to arrange further prescriptions and supplies.

The patient or their accompanying carer should carry a copy of the prescription, stating the generic and brand names of the drugs, and a covering letter from the prescribing doctor stating the medical reason for the prescription. If syringes are needed, a medical certificate stating the reason for their use should also be carried.[2–4]

Drugs should be transported in their pharmacy- or hospital-dispensed and labelled containers, which should state the contents and dose. They should be carried in the patient's or accompanying carer's hand luggage (together with the covering letter and prescription copy) in case customs officials want to examine them.[2–4] However, because of security considerations, some items may not be allowed in airline hand luggage, e.g. syringes; *check any restrictions with the airline before travelling*.[3,5]

It is illegal for individuals to export/import controlled drugs by mail or courier, or to export/import any substance listed in Appendix 1 of the Section 56 class exemption document, e.g. cannabis products, heroin.[2,4]

On returning to Canada, patients should declare any drugs they are importing to the Canada Border Services Agency (CBSA) officer on arrival, bearing in mind that some drugs which can be legally obtained abroad may be illegal or subject to different prescription requirements in Canada. They should also inform their family practitioner and hospital physician about any medication obtained while abroad.

In some countries, other drugs may have identical or closely similar brand names to Canadian brand names. Thus, generic drug names should be used in all documents relating to travel abroad.

Travelling to or through other countries

It is important to fulfil the controlled drug import/export requirements for *all* the countries in which the patient will have to pass through customs, otherwise entry may be refused. Some drugs which are legal in Canada may be illegal elsewhere, or have different prescription requirements.

The International Narcotics Control Board has produced a list of suggested maximum quantities for personal import/export of internationally controlled substances (Table A3.1), and a model import/export certificate (Box A3.B). It is also advisable to carry a duplicate copy of the prescription, preferably stamped by the pharmacy from which the drugs were obtained. *However, patients should check exact legal details and the quantities they are allowed to import/export with the relevant embassies or consulates before travelling.*

Table A3.1 Suggested maximum quantities of controlled substances for international travellers[a,6]

Drug	Quantity
Codeine	12g
Diazepam	300mg
Dronabinol	1g
Fentanyl transdermal patches[b]	100mg
Fentanyl (other formulations)	20mg
Hydrocodone	450mg
Hydromorphone	300mg
Lorazepam	75mg
Methadone	2g
Morphine	3g
Oxycodone	1g

a. this is not a complete list; see referenced source for more details
b. approximately, this adds up to 6 fentanyl 100microgram/h patches, and 8, 12, 24, 48 of the 75, 50, 25, 12microgram/h patches respectively.

Box A3.B Model certificate for personal import/export of internationally controlled substances[6]

Country and place of issue
Country of issue
Place of issue
Date of issue
Period of validity[a]

Prescribing physician
Last name, first name
Address
Telephone (including country code)
Professional licence number

Patient
Last name, first name
Sex
Place of birth
Date of birth
Home address
Passport or identity card number
Intended country of destination

Prescribed medical preparation
Trade name of drug (or composition)
Formulation (ampoules, tablets, etc.)
Number of tablets, etc.
rINN of the active substance
Concentration of the active substance
Total quantity of the active substance
Instructions for use
Duration of prescription in days
Remarks

Issuing authority
Official name of the authority
Address
Telephone (country code, local code, number)
Official seal of the authority
Signature of the responsible officer

a. the recommended duration is 3 months.

Other useful travel information

A range of booklets, posters and other documents about travelling abroad with medicines, and travel health in general, can be downloaded from the following:

- www.voyage.gc.ca/drugs_drogues/menu-eng.asp
- www.voyage.gc.ca/publications/menu-eng.asp
- www.voyage.gc.ca/faq/medical-eng.asp
- www.pharmacists.ca/content/consumer_patient/resource_centre/working/pdf/TravellingwithRx Meds.pdf.

---

1 Canadian Pharmacists Association (ed) (2008) *Appendix 1: Narcotic and Controlled Drugs, Benzodiazepines and Other Targeted Substances.* Canadian Pharmacists Association, Ottawa, pp. A1–A2.
2 Health Canada (2005) Section 56 class exemption for travellers who are importing or exporting prescription drug products containing a narcotic or a controlled drug. Available from: www.hc-sc.gc.ca/hc-ps/substancontrol/pol/pol-docs/travellers-voyageurs-eng.php
3 Foreign Affairs and International Trade Canada (2008) Medical matters–FAQ. Available from: www.voyage.gc.ca/faq/medical-eng.asp
4 Health Canada (2009) Frequently asked questions. What you need to know about medicine for human use and international borders. Available from: www.hc-sc.gc.ca/dhp-mps/compli-conform/int/export-import/medicinebord-medicamentsext_tc-tm-eng.php
5 Canadian Air Transport Security Authority (2009) Permitted and non-permitted items. Available from: www.catsa-acsta.gc.ca/english/travel_voyage/list.shtml
6 International Narcotics Control Board (2004) Guidelines for travelers. Available from: www.incb.org/incb/guidelines_travellers.html

Appendix 4: Compatibility charts

Charts A4.1–A4.4 summarize the compatibility data available for the more commonly used 2-drug and 3-drug combinations given by CSCI in 0.9% saline, which is the usual diluent for CSCI in Canada. The charts have been compiled from clinical observations submitted to the www.palliativedrugs.com *Syringe Driver Survey Database* (SDSD) by palliative care services around the world, and from published data (see reference list). The SDSD is continually updated and contains compatibility data on mixing up to four drugs in either 0.9% saline or water for injection (WFI). Additional charts are available on www.palliativedrugs.com, alongside the SDSD (Box A4.A).

Box A4.A   Additional charts available on SDSD on www.palliativedrugs.com

Compatibility charts in 0.9% saline
Diamorphine: three drugs
Morphine tartrate: three drugs
Oxycodone: three drugs

Compatibility charts in WFI
Two drugs
Alfentanil: three drugs
Diamorphine: three drugs
Morphine sulfate: three drugs
Morphine tartrate: three drugs
Oxycodone: three drugs
Non-opioids: three drugs

The charts use a traffic light system to summarize the data available:
• *red* = do not use (available information indicates a compatibility problem)
• *amber* = proceed with caution (possible compatibility problem, depending on the order of mixing or drug concentrations)
• *green* = reported compatible (data may be observational, physical or chemical).
More information about each combination may be available on the SDSD, and the individual drug monographs may contain additional information, e.g. **hydromorphone** (see p.324). If there is doubt about the relevance of the compatibility data in any particular situation, advice should be obtained from a clinical pharmacist.

Because several factors affect drug stability and compatibility (see Box 18.C, p.514), conflicting reports can occur. Health professionals are urged to contact hq@palliativedrugs.com if their experience indicates that the code for a combination should be changed. Submissions to the SDSD of details of successful combinations for which there are no published data are also welcome.

Note: **dexamethasone** often causes compatibility problems. It should always be the last drug to be added to an already dilute combination of drugs, thus reducing the risk of precipitation. However, because **dexamethasone** has a long duration of action, it can generally be given as a bolus SC injection once daily.

In the charts, hyoscine (the recommended International Non-proprietary Nomenclature, rINN) is given priority over scopolamine. Thus:
• hyoscine butylbromide = hyoscine (scopolamine) butylbromide
• scopolamine hydrobromide = hyoscine (scopolamine) hydrobromide.

Ambados F (1995) Compatibility of morphine and ketamine for subcutaneous infusion. *Australian Journal of Hospital Pharmacy.* **25**: 352.

Anonymous (2007) Summary of product characteristics (SPC) for levomepromazine UK. Available from: http://emc.medicines.org.uk/

Back I (2006) Syringe driver database. Available from: www.pallcare.info

Barcia E et al. (2003) Compatibility of haloperidol and hyoscine-N-butyl bromide in mixtures for subcutaneous infusion to cancer patients in palliative care. *Supportive Care in Cancer.* **11**: 107–113.

Chin A et al. (1996) Stability of granisetron hydrochloride with dexamethasone sodium phosphate for 14 days. *American Journal of Health-System Pharmacy.* **53**: 1174–1176.

Dickman A et al. (2005) *The Syringe Driver: Continuous Subcutaneous Infusions in Palliative Care* (2e). Oxford University Press, Oxford.

Frimley Park Hospital NHS Trust (1998) Personal communication.

Gardiner P (2003) Compatibility of an injectable oxycodone formulation with typical diluents, syringes, tubings, infusion bags and drugs for potential co-administration. *Hospital Pharmacist.* **10**: 354–361.

Good PD et al. (2004) The compatibility and stability of midazolam and dexamethasone in infusion solutions. *Journal of Pain and Symptom Management.* **27**: 471–475.

Grassby P and Hutchings L (1997) Drug combinations in syringe drivers: the compatibility and stability of diamorphine with cyclizine and haloperidol. *Palliative Medicine.* **11**: 217–224.

Hagan R et al. (1996) Stability of ondansetron hydrochloride and dexamethasone sodium phosphate in infusion bags and syringes for 32 days. *American Journal of Health-System Pharmacy.* **53**: 1431–1435.

Hughes A et al. (1997) Ketorolac: continuous subcutaneous infusion for cancer pain. *Journal of Pain and Symptom Management.* **13**: 315–317.

Ingallinera TS et al. (1979) Compatibility of glycopyrrolate injection with commonly used infusion solutions and additives. *American Journal of Hospital Pharmacy.* **36**: 508–510.

Mehta AC and Kay EA (1997) Storage time can be extended:A stability study of alfentanil and midazolam admixture stored in plastic syringes. *Pharmacy in Practice.* **7**: 305–308.

Mendenhall A and Hoyt DB (1994) Incompatibility of ketorolac tromethamine with haloperidol lactate and thiethylperazine maleate. *American Journal of Hospital Pharmacy.* **51**: 2964.

Middleton M and Reilly CS (1994) Do morphine and ketamine keep? The stability of morphine and ketamine separately and combined for use as an infusion. *Hospital Pharmacy Practice.* **4**: 57–58.

Negro S et al. (2002) Physical compatibility and *in vivo* evaluation of drug mixtures for subcutaneous infusion to cancer patients in palliative care. *Supportive Care in Cancer.* **10**: 65–70.

NUH (Nottingham University Hospitals) NHS Trust (2002) *Data on file.* Hayward House, Nottingham.

Palliativedrugs.com (2006) *Syringe Driver Survey Results.* In: June/July 2006 newsletter. Palliativedrugs.com Ltd. Available from: www.palliativedrugs.com

Palliativedrugs.com (2007) *Syringe Driver Survey Database.* Available from: www.palliativedrugs.com

Peterson G et al. (1991) A preliminary study of the stability of midazolam in polypropylene syringes. *Australian Journal of Hospital Pharmacy.* **21**: 115–118.

Schneider JJ (2001) Personal communication.

SIGN (2000) Control of pain in patients with cancer. Scottish Intercollegiate Guidelines Network. Guideline 44. Available from: www.sign.ac.uk/guidelines/fulltext/44/index.html

Stewart JT et al. (1998) Stability of ondansetron hydrochloride and 12 medications in plastic syringes. *American Journal of Health-System Pharmacy.* **55**: 2630–2634.

Storey P et al. (1990) Subcutaneous infusions for control of cancer symptoms. *Journal of Pain and Symptom Management.* **5**: 33–41.

Trissel LA et al. (1994) Compatibility and stability of ondansetron hydrochloride with morphine sulfate and with hydromorphone hydrochloride in 0.9% sodium chloride injection at 4, 22, and 32 degrees C. *American Journal of Hospital Pharmacy.* **51**: 2138–2142.

Trissel LA (2006) *Handbook on Injectable Drugs (Interactive CD version)* (13e). American Society of Health System Pharmacists, Maryland, USA.

Virdee H et al. (1997) The chemical stability of diamorphine and ketorolac in 0.9% sodium chloride stored in plastic syringes. *Pharmacy in Practice.* **February**: 82–83.

Watson DG et al. (2005) Compatibility and stability of dexamethasone sodium phosphate and ketamine hydrochloride subcutaneous infusions in polypropylene syringes. *Journal of Pain and Symptom Management.* **30**: 80–86.

General key for charts

▮ (dark)	Do *not* use, incompatible at usual concentrations
▯ (light box)	Use with caution, compatibility may depend on order of mixing or drug concentrations
a,b,c, etc.	Some reports of incompatibility, but may be compatible at other concentrations (see footnotes)
▬ (grey)	Reported compatible (data may be observational, physical or chemical)
?	No data. Please provide information on this combination to the SDSD, www.palliativedrugs.com
▮ (grey)	Not applicable or not generally recommended, e.g. seek specialist advice when combining multiple anti-emetics
#	Use non-PVC tubing, clonazepam adsorbs onto PVC tubing
##	Dexamethasone sodium phosphate should generally be given by SC bolus injection. If given by CSCI, to minimize the risk of incompatibility, it should always be the last constituent added to a maximally diluted syringe

Alf	Alfentanil
Clzm	Clonazepam (injections not Canada)
Cyc	Cyclizine (not Canada)
Dex/Dexamethasone	Dexamethasone sodium phosphate
Dia	Diamorphine (not Canada)
Gly	Glycopyrrolate
Gra	Granisetron
Hal	Haloperidol
HBBr	Hyoscine (scopolamine) *butylbromide*
HHBr	Hyoscine (scopolamine) *hydrobromide*
Keta	Ketamine
Ketor	Ketorolac
Meth	Methotrimeprazine (levomepromazine)
Meto	Metoclopramide
Mid	Midazolam
MS	Morphine sulfate
MT	Morphine tartrate (not Canada)
Oct	Octreotide
Ond	Ondansetron
Oxy	Oxycodone (injections not Canada)

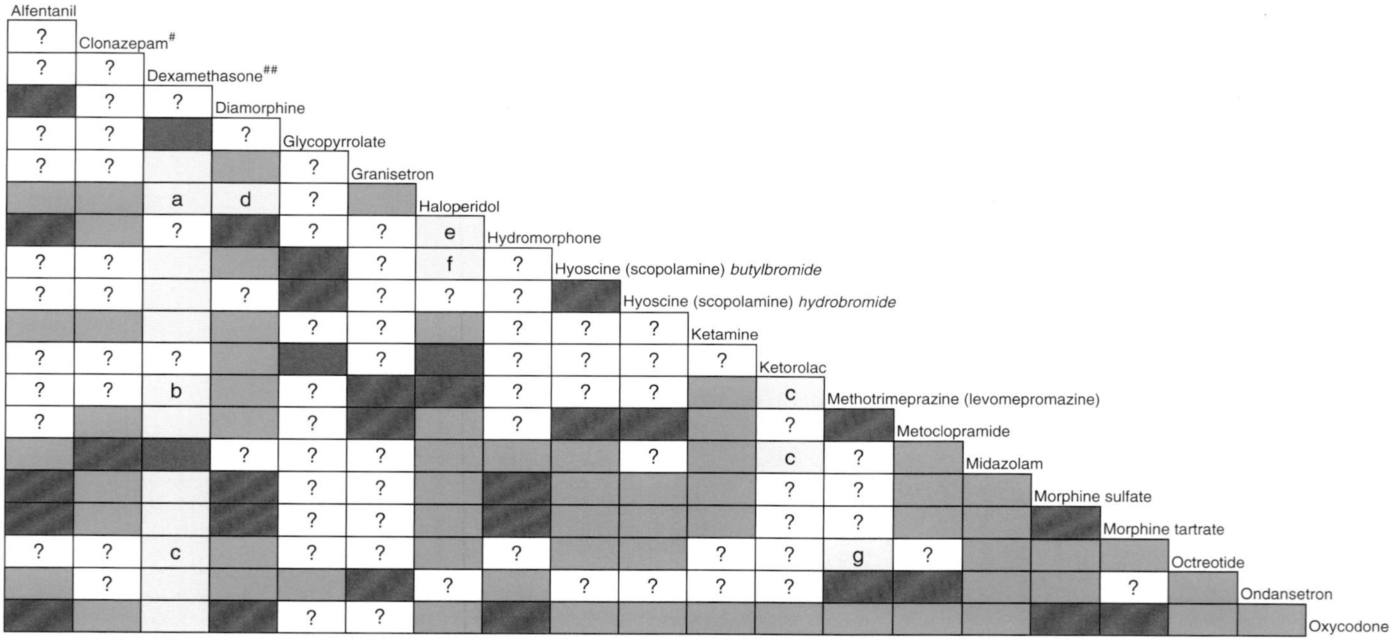

Alfentanil
Clonazepam #
Dexamethasone ##
Diamorphine
Glycopyrrolate
Granisetron
Haloperidol
Hydromorphone
Hyoscine (scopolamine) *butylbromide*
Hyoscine (scopolamine) *hydrobromide*
Ketamine
Ketorolac
Methotrimeprazine (levomepromazine)
Metoclopramide
Midazolam
Morphine sulfate
Morphine tartrate
Octreotide
Ondansetron
Oxycodone

Note: This chart summarizes the compatibility information available for drug combinations in **0.9% saline** used for CSCI over 24h in palliative care units and in the literature (see p.592). Further information about some combinations may be available at www.palliativedrugs.com on the *Syringe Driver Survey Database* (SDSD). Charts with drug combinations diluted in WFI can also be found on the SDSD.

Chart A4.I Compatibility chart for two drugs in 0.9% saline.

Chart A4.1 footnotes

All drug concentration values (mg/mL) specified below are the *final* concentrations of each drug in the syringe after mixing and dilution. For full reference details, see p.592.

a. dexamethasone sodium phosphate 0.15mg/mL + haloperidol 0.38mg/mL reported compatible (Dickman *et al.* 2005)
   dexamethasone sodium phosphate 0.63mg/mL + haloperidol 1.33mg/mL reported *incompatible* (Negro *et al.* 2001)

b. dexamethasone sodium phosphate 0.29mg/mL + methotrimeprazine (levomepromazine) 1.79mg/mL reported *incompatible* (Dickman *et al.* 2005)

c. observational reports of *incompatibility* from miscellaneous sources

d. diamorphine + haloperidol *incompatibility* at high concentrations in WFI (Grassby and Hutchings 1997) and also at haloperidol concentrations approaching 2mg/mL in 0.9% saline (Dickman *et al.* 2005)

e. haloperidol 0.06mg/mL + hydromorphone 2.78mg/mL reported compatible (Dickman *et al.* 2005)
   haloperidol 2mg/mL + hydromorphone 10mg/mL reported *incompatible* in WFI (Storey *et al.* 1990)

f. haloperidol 0.62mg/mL + hyoscine (scopolamine) *butylbromide* 5mg/mL reported compatible (Negro *et al.* 2001)
   haloperidol 1.25mg/mL + hyoscine (scopolamine) *butylbromide* 2.5mg/mL reported *incompatible* in certain long-term storage conditions (Barcia *et al.* 2003)

g. methotrimeprazine (levomepromazine) + octreotide conflicting reports of compatibility and *incompatibility* from miscellaneous sources.

	Alf + Clzm[#]	Alf+Dex[##]	Alf + Gly	Alf + Gra	Alf + Hal	Alf + HBBr	Alf + HHBr	Alf + Keta	Alf + Ketor	Alf + Meth	Alf + Meto	Alf + Mid	Alf + Oct
Dexamethasone[##]	?												
Glycopyrrolate	?	?											
Granisetron	?	?	?										
Haloperidol		?	?	?									
Hyoscine (scopolamine) *butylbromide*	?	?		?	?								
Hyoscine (scopolamine) *hydrobromide*		?		?	?								
Ketamine		?	?	?		?	?						
Ketorolac	?	?	?	?		?	?	?					
Methotrimeprazine (levomepromazine)	?	?	?				?	?	?				
Metoclopramide	?	?			?				?				
Midazolam		?		?		?	?		?				
Octreotide	?	?	?	?	?	?	?	?	?			?	
Ondansetron	?	?			?	?	?	?	?				?

Note: This chart summarizes the compatibility information available for drug combinations in 0.9% saline used for CSCI over 24h in palliative care units and in the literature (see p.592). Further information about some combinations may be available at www.palliativedrugs.com on the *Syringe Driver Survey Database* (SDSD). Charts with drug combinations diluted in WFI can also be found on the SDSD.

Chart A4.2 Compatibility chart for alfentanil: three drugs in 0.9% saline.

Chart A4.2 No footnotes

Dexamethasone##
Glycopyrrolate
Granisetron
Haloperidol
Hyoscine (scopolamine) *butylbromide*
Hyoscine (scopolamine) *hydrobromide*
Ketamine
Ketorolac
Methotrimeprazine (levomepromazine)
Metoclopramide
Midazolam
Octreotide
Ondansetron

MS + Clzm# MS+Dex## MS + Gly MS + Gra MS + Hal MS + HBBr MS + HHBr MS + Keta MS + Ketor MS + Meth MS + Meto MS + Mid MS + Oct

Note: This chart summarizes the compatibility information available for drug combinations in 0.9% saline used for CSCI over 24h in palliative care units and in the literature (see p.592). Further information about some combinations may be available at www.palliativedrugs.com on the *Syringe Driver Survey Database* (SDSD). Charts with drug combinations diluted in WFI can also be found on the SDSD.

Chart A4.3 Compatibility chart for morphine sulfate: three drugs in 0.9% saline.

Chart A4.3 footnotes

All drug concentration values (mg/mL) specified below are the *final* concentrations of each drug in the syringe after mixing and dilution. For full reference details, see p.592.

a. morphine sulfate + dexamethasone sodium phosphate + midazolam observational reports of *incompatibility* (Schneider 2001).

	Dex## + Hal	Dex## + Keta	Dex## + Mid	Hal + HBBr	Hal + Meto	HBBr + Keta	HBBr + Ketor	HHBr + Meth	Meth + Oct
Glycopyrrolate	?		?		?				
Hyoscine (scopolamine) *butylbromide*	a	?							
Methotrimeprazine (levomepromazine)	?	c	?	?			?		
Metoclopramide	b	?							
Midazolam	d		?			?	?		
Octreotide	?	?	?	?	?	?		?	?

Note: This chart summarizes the compatibility information available for drug combinations in 0.9% saline used for CSCI over 24h in palliative care units and in the literature (see p.592). Further information about some combinations may be available at www.palliativedrugs.com on the *Syringe Driver Survey Database* (SDSD). Charts with drug combinations diluted in WFI can also be found on the SDSD.

Chart A4.4 Compatibility chart for non-opioids: three drugs in 0.9% saline.

Chart A4.4 footnote

All drug concentration values (mg/mL) specified below are the *final* concentrations of each drug in the syringe after mixing and dilution. For full reference details, see p.592.

a. dexamethasone sodium phosphate 1.33mg/mL + haloperidol 0.62mg/mL + hyoscine (scopolamine) *butylbromide* 5mg/mL reported *incompatible* (Negro et al. 2001)
b. dexamethasone sodium phosphate 1.33mg/mL + haloperidol 0.62mg/mL + metoclopramide 3.33mg/mL reported *incompatible* (Negro et. al. 2001)
c. observational reports of *incompatibility* (NUH 2002)
d. *incompatibility* with 2-drug combination of dexamethasone sodium phosphate and midazolam (Good et al. 2004 and Negro et al. 2001).

Index of Generic Drug Names

Note: Main references are in **bold**

Index of Proprietary Drug Names

Topic Index

Note: A textbook on pain and symptom management should be consulted for a full discussion of these topics

1. **Words** in **bold type** indicate chapter or appendix titles.
2. **Numbers** in **bold type** indicate the main entry for that topic.